Electrocardiology

Peter W. Macfarlane · Adriaan van Oosterom · Michiel Janse · Paul Kligfield ·
John Camm · Olle Pahlm (Eds.)

Electrocardiology

Comprehensive Clinical ECG

Springer

Editors
Peter W. Macfarlane
University of Glasgow
Glasgow
UK

Adriaan van Oosterom
Radboud University Nijmegen
Nijmegen
The Netherlands

Olle Pahlm
Lund University
Lund
Sweden

Paul Kligfield
Weill Cornell Medical College
New York, NY
USA

Michiel Janse
University of Amsterdam
Amsterdam
The Netherlands

John Camm
St. George's, University of London
London
UK

ISBN 978-0-85729-873-7
DOI 10.1007/978-0-85729-874-4

Library of Congress Control Number: 2011943329

First published in 2010 as part of Comprehensive Electrocardiology, 2nd Edition (ISBN 978-1-84882-045-6)

Printed on acid-free paper

Springer is part of Springer Science+Business Media (www.springer.com)

Editors-in-Chief

Peter W. Macfarlane
University of Glasgow
Glasgow
UK

Paul Kligfield
Weill Cornell Medical College
New York, NY
USA

Adriaan van Oosterom
Radboud University Nijmegen
Nijmegen
The Netherlands

Michiel Janse
University of Amsterdam
Amsterdam
The Netherlands

Olle Pahlm
Lund University
Lund
Sweden

John Camm
St. George's, University of London
London
UK

Preface

The first edition of *Comprehensive Electrocardiology* was published in 1989, when e-mail was still in its infancy (!!), and it was never envisaged at that time that a new edition would be prepared. It is probably fair to say that the majority of physicians would have regarded electrocardiography in particular as having reached its maximum usefulness with little additional information to be obtained therefrom. The intervening 20 years have shown how untrue this was.

An update to the book is long overdue. Sadly, some of our former contributors have died since the first edition was published and it is with regret that I note the passing of Philippe Coumel, Rudolph van Dam, Karel den Dulk, Ramesh Gulrajani, Kenici Harumi, John Milliken, Jos Willems and Christoph Zywietz. Where relevant, their contributions continue to be acknowledged but in some cases, chapters have been completely rewritten by new contributors. On the other hand, eight completely new chapters have been added and the appendices restructured.

The publisher felt it would be opportune to produce separate paperback versions of each of the four volumes of the second edition of *Comprehensive Electrocardiology* – hence this book entitled. *Comprehensive Clinical Electrocardiography.*

In some ways, it is inconceivable what has taken place in the field of electrocardiology since the first edition. New ECG patterns have been recognised and linked with sudden death, new prognostic indices have been developed and evaluated, the ECG has assumed a pivotal role in the treatment of an acute coronary syndrome and among many other things, automated ECG interpretation is now commonplace. Significant advances have been made in the field of mathematical modeling and a solution to the inverse problem is now applied in routine clinical use. Electrophysiological studies have taken giant steps over the past 20 years and biventricular pacing is a relatively recent innovation. Electrocardiology has certainly not stood still in the last 20 years. Of course there have been parallel advances in imaging techniques but the ECG still retains a unique position in the armamentarium of the physician, let alone the cardiologist.

For this edition, my previous co editor, Professor T.D. Veitch Lawrie, decided to step aside and I wish to congratulate him on reaching his 91st birthday in September 2011. However, I am pleased that other very eminent individuals agreed to assist with the editing of the book, namely Adriaan van Oosterom, Olle Pahlm, Paul Kligfield, Michiel Janse and John Camm. In the nature of things, some of these co editors undertook much more work than others. For this book, I particularly have to acknowledge the support of Olle Pahlm and Paul Kligfield. Without their support, this revised version of the material in the first edition would not have been possible.

Locally, I am very much indebted to my secretary Pamela Armstrong for a huge contribution in checking and subediting every chapter which went out from my office to the publisher. This was a Herculean task carried out with great aplomb. I would also like to thank Ms. Julie Kennedy for her contribution to a variety of tasks associated with preparing selected chapters, including enhancements to the English presentation on occasions.

I also wish to thank the publishers Springer for their considerable support throughout. Grant Weston initially commissioned the book and I am grateful to him for his confidence in supporting the preparation of a new edition. Jennifer Carlson and her team in New York also assisted significantly. I am also indebted to Mr. R. Samuel Devanand and his team at SPi Global, in India, for production of the paperback edition.

I again must thank my long suffering wife Irene who has had to fight to gain access to our home PC every night over these past few years!

Comprehensive Electrocardiology aims to bring together truly comprehensive information about the field and *Basic Electrocardiology* provides a strong theoretical foundation to the principles of electrocardiography. A book can never be completely up to date given the speed of publication of research findings over the internet these days but hopefully this publication will continue to be of significant use to readers for many years to come. *Basic Electrocardiology*, together with the other three paperback versions of the other volumes of *Comprehensive Electrocardiology*, contains much information that should be of use both to the practising clinician and the experienced researcher.

Now that this huge effort has been completed and the book is available electronically, it should be much easier to produce the next edition...!!

Peter Macfarlane
Glasgow
Autumn

Table of Contents

List of Contributors

Iwona Cygankiewicz
Medical University of Lodz
Lodz
Poland

Paul Khairy
Montreal Heart Institute
Montreal, QC
Canada

T.D. Veitch Lawrie
University Of Glasgow
Glasgow
UK

Jerome Liebman
Case Western Reserve University
School of Medicine
Cleveland, OH
USA

Mário G. Lopes
Institute of Preventive Cardiology
Lisbon
Portugal

Peter W. Macfarlane
University of Glasgow
Glasgow
UK

J.E. Madias
Mount Sinai School of Medicine
New York, NY
USA

Ariane J. Marelli
McGill University Health Centre
Montreal, QC
Canada

Nuno Marques
Institute of Preventive Cardiology
Lisbon
Portugal

John A. Milliken
Queens University
Kingston, ON
Canada

Peter M. Okin
Weill Cornell Medical College
New York, NY
USA

Fernando de Pádua
Institute of Preventive Cardiology
Lisbon
Portugal

Armando Pereirinha
Institute of Preventive Cardiology
Lisbon
Portugal

Ronald H. Selvester
University of Southern Carolina
Columbia, SC
USA

David G. Strauss
Lund University
Lund
Sweden

Borys Surawicz
The Care Group at St Vincent Hospital
Indianapolis, IN
USA

Galen S. Wagner
Duke University
Durham, NC
USA

Wojciech Zareba
University of Rochester Medical Centre
Rochester, NY
USA

1 The Normal Electrocardiogram and Vectorcardiogram

Peter W. Macfarlane · T.D. Veitch Lawrie

P. W. Macfarlane et al. (eds.), *Electrocardiology*, DOI 10.1007/978-0-85729-874-4_1,

1.1 Introduction

As with all biological phenomena, there can be no clear-cut distinction between normal and abnormal, yet some attempt has to be made to define the limits of normality of the ECG. The only sound basis for the interpretation of the ECG is a thorough understanding of the way in which the ECG pattern in normal, healthy individuals varies from infancy to old age, between male and female, from one racial group to another, and so on. A knowledge of intraindividual variation is also necessary in order to avoid false-positive interpretations and to look for subtle changes in the ECG, even within the normal range of measurements.

In recent years, other noninvasive investigations, such as echocardiography and magnetic resonance imaging, have been added to the diagnostic armamentarium of the physician. Yet, electrocardiography still remains one of the most basic cardiological investigations beyond physical examination and can provide information that is not obtainable by any other means. Even now, it is unlikely that the full potential of the ECG has been realised because of the failure to establish well-defined limits of normality, which vary according to the different factors mentioned above. Furthermore, with the increasing application of computer technology to the interpretation of the ECG, the potential for setting up comprehensive cooperative studies of normal individuals to establish large databases for refining the limits of normality exists, in order to improve the diagnostic capability of the ECG. The alternative of taking ECGs from apparently healthy individuals enrolled in clinical trials, though not fully medically examined, has recently been adopted, enabling large numbers of individuals to be studied [1].

Technology has advanced rapidly, and it is perfectly conceivable that every electrocardiograph could contain facilities for some form of computer-based ECG interpretation (see ➋ Chap. 5 of *Specialized Aspects of ECG*). However, not all healthcare systems can afford such technology, and simple ECG recorders with no interpretation or measurement facility will survive for years to come. This gives added impetus to the need for a careful appraisal, if not further development, of methods for defining the normal variation of the ECG.

The classic treatise on the normal ECG is that of Simonson [2] who elegantly summarized all the material available at that time, *c.*1960. He himself contributed greatly to the understanding of the variability of the normal ECG, and much of his own thinking still influences present-day electrocardiographers. Nonetheless, technology has advanced dramatically since then, and the availability of computer techniques for the measurement of the ECG and vectorcardiogram (VCG) component amplitudes has greatly facilitated further study of normal limits.

In an assessment of the normal scalar ECG recorded from a few hundred healthy volunteers, Lundh [3] pointed out that if the order of 100 measurements are made on the ECG with each varying independently (which is unlikely to be the case), then only 1% of the ECGs could be expected to fall within normal limits on the basis of utilizing 95% confidence intervals for defining the normal range of each measurement. This, of course, is carrying matters to an extreme, but it does point to the need for a careful development of diagnostic criteria even given well-defined normal ranges. In other words, it has to be made clear from the outset that the availability of normal ranges does not mean that once a single measurement exceeds an upper limit by a small amount, the ECG has to be regarded as abnormal. This point cannot be emphasized too strongly.

1.2 The Establishment of Normal Limits

1.2.1 Sampling Methods

There are a number of different approaches to tackling the problem of establishing normal limits through large-scale population studies. One of the first questions to be resolved is whether the population should be based on apparently healthy individuals in the community or whether it should be derived from persons under investigation in hospitals for problems unrelated to cardiovascular disease. There can be no doubt that the latter offers the convenience of subjects being available close at hand to the recording center, but it is clearly open to question as to whether such individuals can be regarded as healthy. It could be argued that patients in an orthopedic ward who have been admitted for the treatment of a recent injury are no different from an apparently healthy individual in the community, always assuming that the relevant medical history is uneventful. Alternatively, such a source of volunteers is unlikely to yield an adequate distribution of subjects with respect to age and sex.

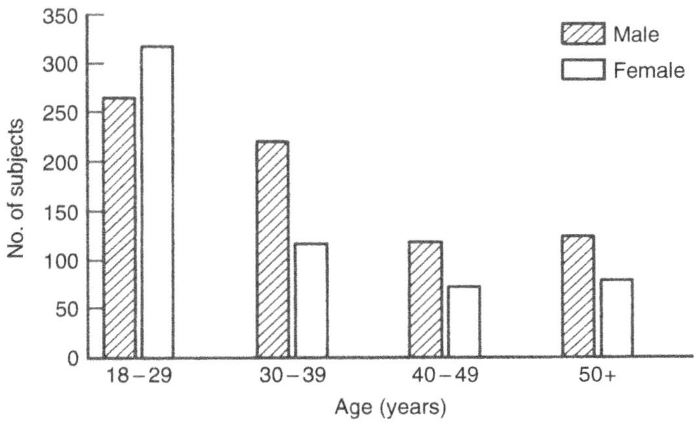

Fig. 1.1
The distribution of the 1,338 subjects in the Glasgow study of apparently healthy individuals. A very small number of individuals aged 17 years were included, but are not shown on this graph

The most satisfactory solution is to obtain apparently healthy subjects from the community at large. Different approaches to population sampling can be adopted. Some investigators favor the use of sampling a population register. For example, Lundh [3] selected every 50th man and woman born between 1915 and 1953 from the local civil registry. Although an even distribution of subjects by age and sex was not obtained, there being a predominance of younger individuals, it was claimed that this reflected the population distribution in the catchment area – a town that had expanded in recent years.

The approach of Macfarlane et al. [4] was to seek volunteers from a variety of departments in the local government within the city of Glasgow and the region of Strathclyde. In this way, a spread of occupations was covered from sedentary office work, such as in finance and library administration, to outdoor occupations, such as in parks and recreation departments. The distribution of the volunteers obtained in this study is shown in ➲ Fig. 1.1, where again it can be seen that there is a predominance of younger persons. In this case, there is a different reason for such a distribution. It is evident that younger persons who feel healthy are quite willing to volunteer for such a study, whereas older individuals appear to be more reluctant to come forward in case some hitherto unsuspected abnormality is detected that might result in further medical investigation that would be regarded as inconvenient and potentially job threatening. In addition, because many married women cease employment with the arrival of a family and then only return to work perhaps 10 or 15 years later, there is a lack of female volunteers in the 25–40 age-group. This can be compensated for by concentrating on selecting volunteers from the appropriate age and sex group when, after some time, it becomes apparent that a shortfall is present in a particular category.

A third approach that has been used in a number of studies is simply to investigate a group of employees in a particular industry or government department. Normally, such an approach is associated with screening (see ➲ Chap. 8 of *Specialized Aspects of ECG*), but it could be regarded as an alternative to the determination of normal limits, always assuming that there was a reasonable distribution of employees by age and sex.

1.2.2 Cardiovascular Screening

When the population sampling method has been chosen, it must then be decided what investigations are necessary in order to establish that an individual is healthy. In studies undertaken in the authors' laboratory and reported later in this chapter, it was decided to undertake a simple clinical examination of volunteers in order to exclude those with any evidence of an illness known to affect the cardiovascular system. In addition, blood-pressure measurements were obtained.

The list of illnesses known to have some influence on the ECG is lengthy, but of major importance are endocrine, respiratory, renal, neurological, alimentary, and hematological disorders, as well as the various cardiovascular diseases, either congenital or acquired. In the authors' study, subjects were asked to volunteer if they were apparently healthy, but, nevertheless, it was clear that a few individuals used the opportunity of participating in such a study as a means of having a checkup on earlier illnesses, which in fact precluded them from entry.

The value of a chest x-ray is questionable. In the first 500 patients in the above study in whom chest x-rays were routinely recorded, there was no single instance in which an apparently healthy volunteer had to be excluded from the study on the basis of an abnormal chest x-ray being the only positive factor. It was therefore decided that in view of the expense and inconvenience involved in arranging chest x-rays, this would not be a necessary requirement for determining that an individual was apparently healthy.

From the outset in this study, it was also decided that the need for routine blood tests was negligible. Again the expense and expected yield of abnormalities did not appear to justify the workload of such an additional test. Thus, the cohort consisted of volunteers regarded as healthy on the basis of history, blood pressure, and physical examination.

It is of interest to note that a group of electrocardiographers in North America [5] reached a similar conclusion. In other words, subjects "not actively seeking medical care" can be accepted as apparently healthy on the basis of physical examination and history, without the need for either a chest x-ray or blood tests to be available.

It can be seen that volunteers are initially regarded as healthy without recourse to ECG findings. On the other hand, it is well known that a right bundle branch block (RBBB) occurs in a small percentage of healthy persons [6] and that an ECG is sometimes the only indicator of myocardial infarction (MI) [7]. In at least two studies – one in Framingham, Massachusetts [8] and the other in Israel [9] – it was found that the ECG provided the only evidence of myocardial infarction in up to 50% of patients in whom it was agreed that a definite infarct had occurred. Notwithstanding these examples, it has to be accepted that individuals must be regarded as apparently healthy on the basis of a clinical examination, history, and other test results excluding the ECG. Thereafter, it is for the statistical techniques to deal with the question of normal ranges.

1.2.3 Statistical Considerations

1.2.3.1 Sample Size

From a statistical point of view, the larger the population studied, the more soundly based will be the results that are derived therefrom. However, consider a simple example and assume that it is desired to study the adult population in the age range of 20–70 years. (The question of variation in infancy and childhood is discussed separately below.) One approach would be to divide the population sample into decades of age so that, for the proposed sample, there would be five age-groups, namely, 20–29, 30–39, 40–49, 50–59, and 60 years and over. Likewise, the population would be split in two on the basis of sex, thereby giving ten subgroups. It is known that the ECG can be influenced by race, and hence if the population is further stratified into black and white (which is a major simplification) the number of subgroups increases to 20. From a practical point of view, if 200 entries could be obtained for each of the groups, then 4,000 individuals are required to constitute a basic population survey. Selvester and colleagues in North America, in proposing the establishment of a normal database, have indicated that up to 30,000 individuals would be required from a statistical point of view [5]. While this may be scientifically desirable, it raises many practical problems, since it entails the need for a multicenter approach. Such a method would cause difficulties in the standardization of methods, not to mention a need for the transfer of data to a central coordinating department that has the ability to analyze the massive amounts of data obtained. Nevertheless, such numbers have been obtained in a more indirect way, as already mentioned [1].

An approximate estimate of numbers required for a particular test can be obtained from the consideration of a simplified example. In a discussion of clinical trials, Schwartz et al. [10] quoted the following equation that is useful, for example, in estimating the number of people, n, required in each group when it is wished to show a significant difference, say of 0.4 mV, in the mean R amplitude between males and females of the same age-group:

$$n = (e_\alpha + e_\beta)^2 B^2 / A^2$$

where A is the difference being assessed (here, 0.4 mV), B is the standard deviation of R amplitude distribution (perhaps derived from a pilot study), e_α denotes the percentage point from the standard normal distribution corresponding to the chosen significance level α of the test, and e_β is the percentage point from the standard normal distribution corresponding to the chosen power β of the test, where β is the maximum probability of failing to detect a difference. It can be shown that 49 people would be required in each group depending on the chosen e_α, e_β, and A. If the difference being assessed is expected to be 0.2 mV, then the number increases to 195 in each group.

1.2.3.2 Normal Ranges

If a set of amplitudes, for example, the R-wave amplitude in V_5, is obtained from a group of apparently healthy individuals within a well-defined age range, there will clearly be a spread of measurements obtained with a predominance of values in the middle of the group and a smaller number at either side. In a classical situation, where there is an even spread of measurements around a central value with the distribution as shown in ➋ Fig. 1.2, there is said to be a normal distribution. A point on the bell-shaped curve simply indicates the number of people in the group who have an amplitude of a certain value. Clearly, when the distribution is symmetrical, the mean of the values will be in the middle of the range. Given the set of values, it becomes possible to calculate a mean and standard deviation for the parameter of interest. The standard deviation, SD, is calculated from the formula

$$\mathrm{SD} = \left[\frac{\sum_{i=1}^{n}(x_i - \bar{x})^2}{n-1}\right]^{1/2}$$

where $\bar{x}$ is the mean value, x_i represents the individual values, and n is the number of values in the sample. With a classical normal distribution, the mean plus or minus twice the standard deviation delineates approximately 95% of the range of values, as shown in ➋ Fig. 1.2. Hence, if it could be shown that a set of values possessed a normal distribution, then one method of defining the normal range would simply be to calculate the mean and standard deviation and proceed to derive the upper and lower limits of the normal 95 percentile range. By taking such limits, where 2.5% of the values are excluded at either end of the distribution, so-called outliers can be excluded.

With respect to ECG measurements, however, it was pointed out by Simonson [2] many years ago that the range of measurements for most ECG parameters is not normal, that is, it tends to have a skewed distribution, as shown in

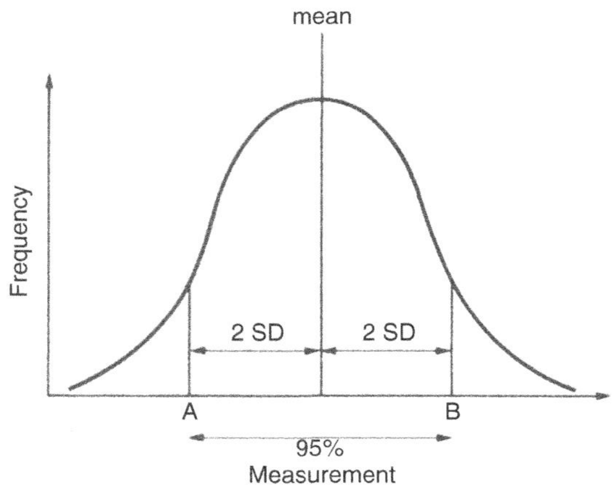

Fig. 1.2
An illustration of a normal distribution of a set of measurements. The mean value in this case is in the center of the distribution with two standard deviations, 2SD, being shown on each side of the mean; the distance AB includes approximately 95% of the measurements

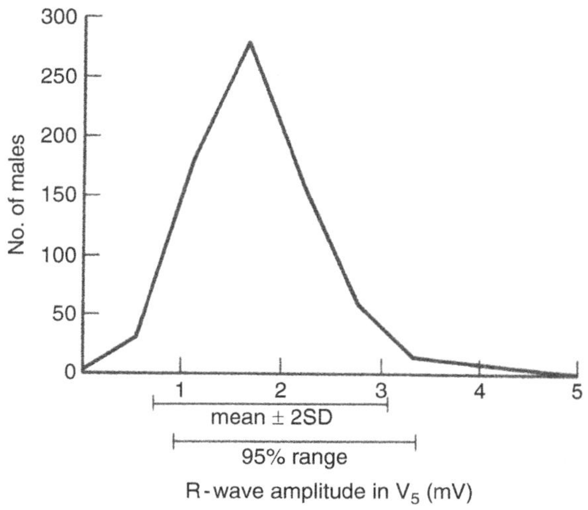

Fig. 1.3
The distribution of the R-wave amplitude in V_5 in 738 males in the Glasgow study. It can be seen that the distribution is skewed to the right, that is, toward the larger measurements. The mean ± 2SD has a different range compared to the 95 percentile range obtained by excluding 2.5% at either extreme of the distribution. Note that in many ECG studies, a 96 percentile range is used (see text)

Fig. 1.3 for the R-wave amplitude in V_5. The longer tail of the distribution is toward the higher values with the shorter tail being toward the lower values. Thus, if the 95 percentile range based on the mean ± 2SD is used, a large percentage of values at the upper end of the range are likely to be excluded.

To avoid this difficulty, an alternative approach for deriving the 95 percentile limits can be adopted; namely, 2.5% of values at the upper end of the range are excluded as are 2.5% of values at the lower end. The difference between the two ranges calculated using the alternative techniques is shown in Fig. 1.3.

In many electrocardiographic studies, the 96 percentile range has been adopted, whereby 2% of values at either extreme were removed in calculating what then became known as the "normal range." There are no scientific reasons for choosing 96% rather than 95% other than that in a study of 100 or 200 individuals, it is simpler to remove 2% as opposed to 2.5% of values, since in the latter, interpolation methods would have to be used. The different approaches to the latter were outlined by Simonson [2], but in the context of samples of adequate size, this would appear to be an unnecessary refinement.

Much of the data presented later in this chapter in respect of normal ranges and elsewhere in the Appendices is based on the above concept of the normal range. Mean values and standard deviations are also provided for completeness, wherever possible.

The use of 96% ranges means that an unusually long QRS duration as obtained from a healthy volunteer with RBBB would be excluded from the normal range, as such an abnormality occurs in less than 0.5% of a mixed community [6]. Similar conditions would apply to broad Q waves encountered in persons with silent myocardial infarction.

Another approach to defining a normal limit, particularly where there is a need to consider a continuous limit over a range of ages, is to calculate an upper 95% confidence level for the distribution. This can be done by first obtaining a set of values such as the R-wave amplitude in V_5 for a group of persons, perhaps males aged 18–65 years, as shown in Fig. 1.3. With the use of statistical methods, it is then possible to assess the effect of age and body mass, for example, with respect to their contributions to the amplitude distribution. If it can be shown that the major component contributing to the variation is age, then it is appropriate to calculate the mean amplitude values for various age ranges.Given this data and knowledge of the appropriate standard deviation, it then becomes feasible to calculate the 95% confidence interval for the mean from the following equation:

$$\text{Mean} \pm K \times \frac{\text{SD}}{(\text{group\_size})^{1/2}}$$

where K is approximately 2 for a group that is normally distributed.

Alternatively, the upper and lower 95% limits of the range of values (i.e., 2.5% of values are excluded at each extreme of an assumed normal distribution) are given by

$$\text{Mean} \pm 2 \times \text{SD}\left(1 + \frac{1}{n}\right)^{1/2}$$

where n is the number of subjects in the group.

The above applies where a single age-group, for example, is being assessed, but the process can, of course, be repeated for the different age ranges. Of interest is the possibility of deriving a continuous equation for predicting the upper limit of normal for a given age. Consider that all R-wave amplitudes in V_5 are known for a group of males aged 18–65 years. The mean and standard deviation of R in V_5 can then be calculated. If the distribution is reasonably normal and it has to be accepted that there will be some error in this assumption, these two values can be used as shown below. Similar considerations apply to age, and again the assumption of a normal distribution would be open to question. The fifth value required is the correlation coefficient. In summary, if $\bar{x}$ denotes the mean of age, S_x is the standard deviation of age, $\bar{y}$ denotes the mean of the R-wave amplitude, S_y is the standard deviation of amplitude, and r is the correlation coefficient between age and amplitude, then the expression depicting the upper 97.5% limit is

$$\left\{\bar{y} + \beta(x - \bar{x}) + 25\left[1 + \frac{1}{n} + \frac{(x - \bar{x})^2}{(n-1)S_x^2}\right]^{1/2}\right\}^2$$

where n is the number of subjects in the study, $\beta = rS_y/S_x$, x denotes age, and $S = S_y(1 - r^2)^{1/2}$. From the authors' own data for males, this equation reduces to

$$\left\{46.8 - 0.01(\text{age}) + 1.96 \times 6.702\left[1 + \frac{1}{736} + \frac{(\text{age} - 435.67)^2}{(144.52)^2 \times 735}\right]^{1/2}\right\}^2$$

where age is in months and amplitude is in microvolts. This line is plotted in Fig. 1.4 together with discrete limits of normality for different age ranges.

This expression can, without any real loss of accuracy (given the assumptions under which it was derived), be reduced to

$$[46.8 - 0.123(\text{age}) + 13.13]^2 \mu\text{V}$$

where age is in years, and clearly further to

$$\text{Upper normal limit} = (59.93 - 0.123\,\text{age})^2 \mu\text{V}$$

Thus, the upper limit of normal is 3.04 mV at age 39 and 3.026 mV at age 40. This compares with a change of 0.5 mV between these two particular ages when discrete limits are used (see Fig. 1.4).

The use of 95 percentile confidence limits where a continuous value can be derived from the equation is at first sight attractive. Clearly, the upper limit of normal for an individual should not change overnight as he changes from one age-group to another as discussed above. Jain and Rautaharju [11] have investigated the use of continuous variables with respect to diagnostic classification capabilities and have suggested that these are possibly of greater significance

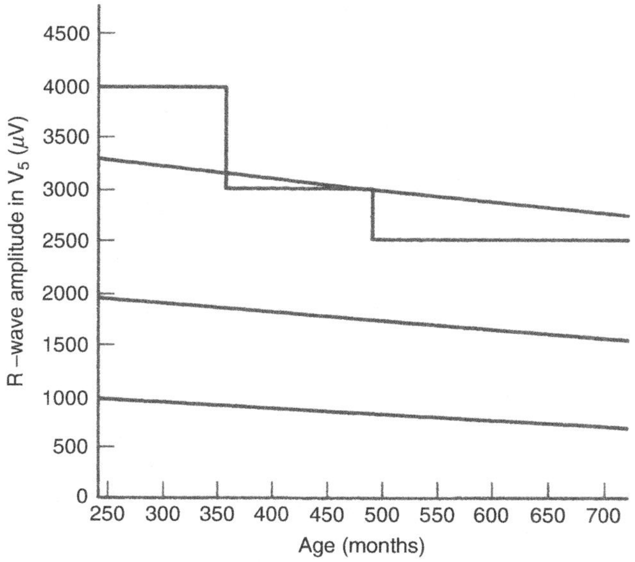

Fig. 1.4
A plot of normal limits of the R-wave amplitude in V_5 (in microvolts) against age (in months). The topmost curve or step function illustrates the upper limit of normal for this parameter for three discrete age-groups, 18–29, 30–39, and 40+. Note that within each group the level is fixed, but there is marked discontinuity at 29–30 and 39–40. The three continuous curves show, respectively, the upper 97.5 percentile distribution, the mean, and the lower 2.5 percentile limit, as derived from the equations presented in the text. In this case, the change between ages 29–30 and 39–40 is of the order of approximately 15 μV

than the use of discrete variables where limits change from one age range to another. This is an area that has not been explored intensively and is one where further study would appear to be merited if the year-to-year variation of the ECG interpretation is to be minimized. This could be important in the context of an annual company medical, for example, where a computer-based interpretation might be employed with discontinuous limits of normality being used for different age-groups. Undoubtedly, this approach would be facilitated with the availability of large databases of normal ECGs.

Indeed, in the Glasgow ECG analysis program for automated analysis of ECGs [12, 13], continuous limits of normality are extensively used. Furthermore, smoothed criteria have been introduced so that thresholds between normal and abnormal can also be blurred [14, 15]. ➋ Figure 1.5 illustrates this concept.

1.2.3.3 Angular Data

The treatment of angular data can be difficult. For example, if three vectors are oriented at 0° (360°), 120°, and 240°, what is the mean value? Fortunately, in many situations, the angular data tend to cluster around a prevalent direction and a normal range can be estimated in the manner discussed in ➋ Sect. 1.2.3.2. In more difficult situations, an alternative strategy has to be considered. Liebman (see Appendix 1) discusses the matter fully, but a summary is given here.

If a group of vectors is imagined to lie in space, a sphere of suitably small radius, R, could intercept all such vectors. The coordinates of each intercept would then be $(xR/L, yR/L, zR/L)$, where x, y, z are the components of the original vector of length L. The mean value $(\bar{x}, \bar{y}, \bar{z})$ of all such intercepts can then be found; for example,

$$\bar{x} = \sum \frac{(xR/L)}{N}$$

where N is the number of vectors. The prevalent direction can then be calculated.

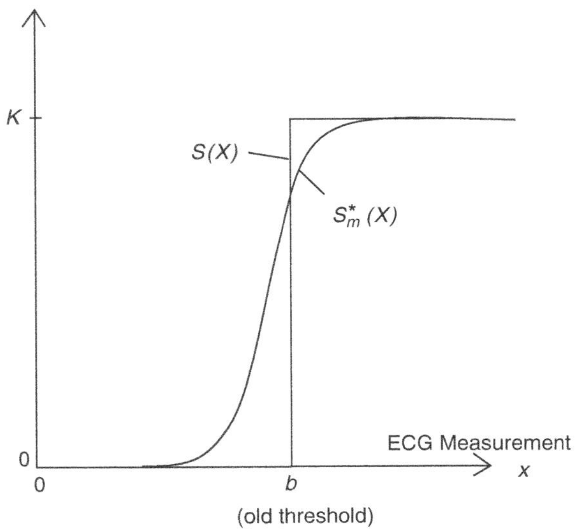

Fig. 1.5
A comparison of two scoring methods, namely, a fixed threshold and a continuous function. With the use of a fixed threshold at *b*, *K* points are scored when the threshold is exceeded. Only two values of the score are possible, namely, 0 and *K*. With the continuous function, an infinite number of values of the score between 0 and *K* are possible as the measurement increases and then exceeds *b* (Reproduced from J Electrocardiol 1993; 26(Suppl): 101–7 by kind permission of Elsevier)

1.2.3.4 Sensitivity and Specificity

The importance of normal ranges lies in the assessment of specificity of diagnostic criteria. It would therefore seem relevant to introduce the concept of sensitivity and specificity, to which reference is made in other chapters.

Consider that a group of apparently healthy individuals have ECGs recorded, while a separate group of patients with cardiac diseases known to predispose to left ventricular hypertrophy (LVH) also have an ECG recorded. It is conceivable that the distribution of S-wave amplitude in V_2 for each of the groups would appear as in ➋ Fig. 1.6. The development of criteria should be such as to obtain the optimum separation between the two groups. It can be seen from this hypothetical example that there is a considerable overlap between the two sets of measurements, which in practice is usually the case. In selecting a borderline value for a simple test to discriminate between the two groups, the investigator must first decide the level of specificity desired. This is the percentage of normal patients that will be correctly reported as normal by the test. Each of these normals is regarded as a true-negative (TN) result. The remainder of the normals wrongly reported as abnormal because their S-wave amplitude lay above the borderline value selected would be classed as false positives (FP). Thus,

$$TN + FP = \text{total number of normals}$$

With respect to the abnormal group, those patients with ventricular hypertrophy (VH) who are correctly reported as having the abnormality because their S-wave amplitude values exceed the borderline criterion, would be regarded as true positives (TP). The remainder of this group of patients would then fail to have been reported as having hypertrophy. They would thus falsely have been regarded as normal and are said to constitute the false-normal or false-negative (FN) group. Clearly,

$$TN + FN = \text{Total number of patients}$$

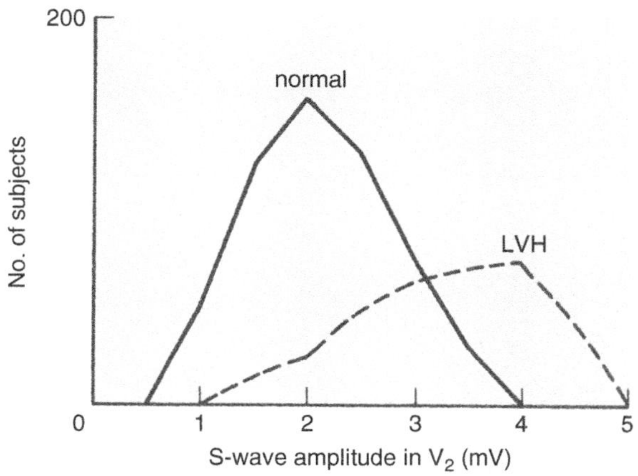

Fig. 1.6
A hypothetical example of the distribution of the S-wave amplitude in V_2 in a group of normal subjects and a group with proven left ventricular hypertrophy (LVH). If a value of 4 mV is selected to differentiate between normal and abnormal, over 50% of the cases of LVH would not be detected. The reverse would be true if 2 mV were to be selected; over 50% of the normals would be reported as having LVH

The following definitions can therefore be given.

$$\text{Specificity} = \frac{\text{Number of normals correctly reported as normal}}{\text{Total number of normals}} \times 100\%$$

$$= \frac{\text{TN}}{\text{TN} + \text{FP}} \times 100\%$$

$$\text{Sensitivity} = \frac{\text{Number of abnormals correctly reported as abnormal}}{\text{Total number of abnormals}} \times 100\%$$

$$= \frac{\text{TP}}{\text{TP} + \text{FN}} \times 100$$

When commenting on the accuracy of diagnostic criteria, in addition to sensitivity and specificity, the following measurements are also often used.

$$\text{Predictive value of an abnormal result} = \frac{\text{TP}}{\text{TP} + \text{FP}} \times 100\%$$

$$\text{Predictive value of a normal result} = \frac{\text{TN}}{\text{TN} + \text{FN}} \times 100\%$$

$$\text{Association index} = \text{sensitivity} + \text{specificity} - 100$$

In the authors' view, specificity should be selected at a high level with the desired aim of maintaining a very low rate of occurrence of false positives. The exact relationship between specificity and sensitivity can be seen more closely in ➔ Fig. 1.7. In this illustration, two situations are described [16]. In each case, the distribution of a set of normal values of a particular parameter is shown under the left-hand curve, while the distribution of the corresponding parameter from a set of patients with a particular abnormality is shown under the right-hand shaded curve. The normal group and the set of patients is the same in each case, but the parameter used in II shows a clearer separation between the two groups. If the dividing line between normal and abnormal is chosen at different points, here labelled 1–7 or 1–9

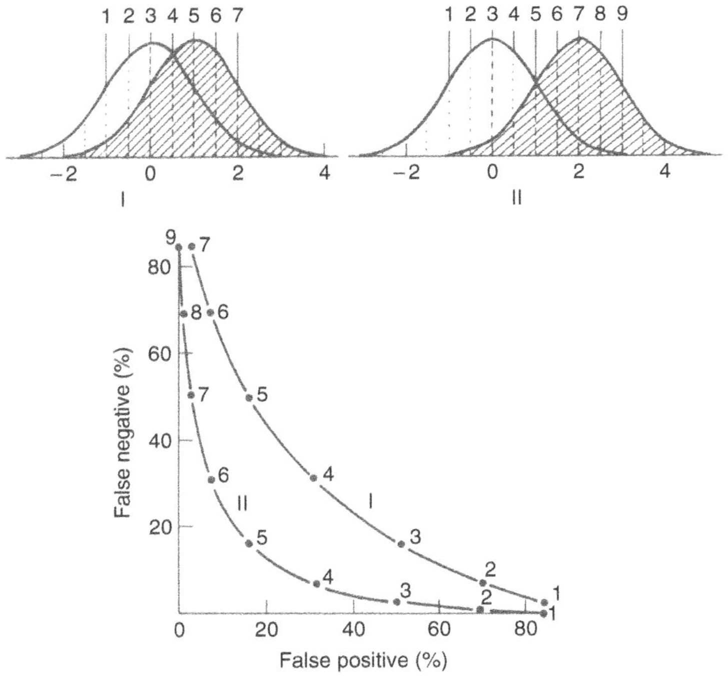

Fig. 1.7
The top curves compare the distributions of two parameters (I and II) in two groups of patients. One is a normal group and the other is an abnormal group (shaded distributions). Parameter II clearly provides a better separation between the two groups. Although this is seen visually in the top right set of curves, the findings can be presented as a set of receiver operating characteristic (ROC) curves. The numbers 1–7 represent points at which the separation between normal and abnormal can be taken so that with 1, for example, there would be a high diagnostic sensitivity and very many false-positive interpretations, whereas with 7 there would be very few false-positive interpretations but a poor diagnostic sensitivity. The curve that most closely approaches the origin is superior, and, in this case, parameter II is the better (After Dudeck and Michaelis [16]. © North-Holland, Amsterdam. Reproduced with permission)

as the case may be, then the corresponding number of false-positive and false-negative cases for each discriminating value can be plotted. The curves arising from such plots are known as "receiver operating curves" or "receiver operating characteristics" (ROC curves). For particular distributions, they allow the user to select a level of specificity (100% false positive), and from this, the corresponding sensitivity (100% false negative) can be determined from the curve. It can be argued that the value closest to the origin produces the best results, whereby false-positive and false-negative values are minimized. For example, in this case (Fig. 1.7), the lower curve denoted II indicates that this parameter is better than that of I for separating normal and abnormal. This can be a useful way of assessing the best discriminating values for use in the development of diagnostic criteria as evidenced by a recent study of different criteria [17].

The above discussion for illustrative purposes has concentrated on a two-group classification of normal and abnormal. Rautaharju et al. [18] agreed that this approach enhances sensitivity and specificity estimates, and that the relative numbers in the two groups can distort the true picture. They suggested that the comparison should not be between normal and abnormal (i.e., a particular abnormality), but between patients with such an abnormality and all others. In other words, in assessing the specificity of criteria for LVH for example, all normals and other patients known not to have LVH but who might perhaps have a myocardial infarction should be included in the "non-LVH" group, and not simply the normals alone. The alternative definitions that follow from this are summarized in Table 1.1.

Table 1.1
Definition of sensitivity (SE), specificity (SP), mean performance (MP), association index (AI), accuracy of positive test (AP), accuracy of negative test (AN), fraction of subjects with a positive test (F), and overall diagnostic accuracy (D). See text for a discussion on the meaning of negative test

Definitions	
SE = TP/(TP + FN)	AP = TP/(TP + FP)
SP = TN/(FP + TN)	AN = TN/(FN + TN)
MP = (SE + SP)/2	F = (TP + FP)/(TP + FP + FN + TN)
AI = SE + SP − 1	D = F.AP + (1 − F)AN

TP true positive, *FP* false positive, *FN* false negative, *TN* true negative

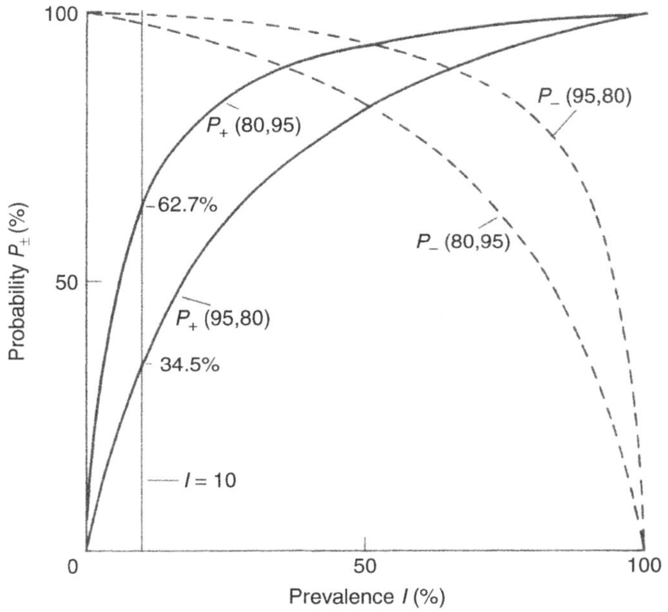

Fig. 1.8
The relationship between the probability of an ECG interpretation being correct with respect to a particular diagnosis and the prevalence of that abnormality in the population. The two curves on the left show the probability of a true-positive result, and the two curves on the right show the probability of a true-negative result. Each curve corresponds to a different set of criteria with different sensitivity and specificity. For example, with a sensitivity of 80% and a specificity of 95%, the probability that an ECG interpretation stating a particular abnormality true-positive result, given that the prevalence of the abnormality is 10%, is 62.7%. Likewise, the probability that the omission of such a diagnosis is a true negative is approximately 97% (After Bailey [19]. © Engineering Foundation, New York. Reproduced with permission)

A final point to bear in mind is that positive and negative predictive value depend on the prevalence of a particular disease in the population being studied. In other words, in assessing criteria for myocardial ischemia, it would be quite possible to produce a set of criteria that proved to have a high positive predictive value when evaluated in a population where the prevalence of ischemic heart disease is known to be high. Conversely, it is likely that the same criteria applied to a population where ischemic heart disease is known to be low would result in many false-positive diagnoses and a low positive predictive value. The two curves on the left of Fig. 1.8 show the probability of an ECG interpretation of a particular abnormality being correct (true positive) given the varying prevalence of such an abnormality in the population and a knowledge of the sensitivity and specificity of two sets of criteria [19]. In many ways, these are ROC curves for given populations where the prevalence of the abnormality is known. Conversely, the probability of a negative interpretation being correct (true negative) is also shown for the same two sets of criteria. Note that the sensitivity and specificity of the two sets of criteria are fixed, while the prevalence varies from 0% to 100%. It can be seen that, for a prevalence of disease of 10%, the criteria that are 95% specific produce a higher probability of a true-positive interpretation compared to those that are 80% specific. The equations for calculating the probabilities are as follows [19].

The probability of a correct positive result, P_+, is

$$P_+(Se, Sp) = \frac{SeI}{SeI + (1 - Sp)(1 - I)}$$

where *Se* is the sensitivity of the criteria, *Sp* is the specificity of the criteria, and *I* denotes the prevalence of that abnormality or disease in the patient population.

The probability of a correct negative result, P_-, is

$$P_-(Se, Sp) = \frac{Sp(1 - I)}{Sp(1 - I) + (1 - Se)I}$$

1.2.4 Methods of Measurement

In early studies on normal limits, the quality of the ECG-recording equipment was such that recommendations [20, 21] referred to measuring from the top of the baseline at a particular reference point. At that time, all measurements were made manually in some studies, and later, further suggestions for reference points were published [22, 23]. It was recommended by the American Heart Association [21] that the ST segment, the T wave, and the P wave should all be measured with respect to the isoelectric part of the tracing before the P wave. This recommendation was based on the avoidance of the atrial repolarization potentials, which can produce "depression" of the baseline prior to the QRS onset.

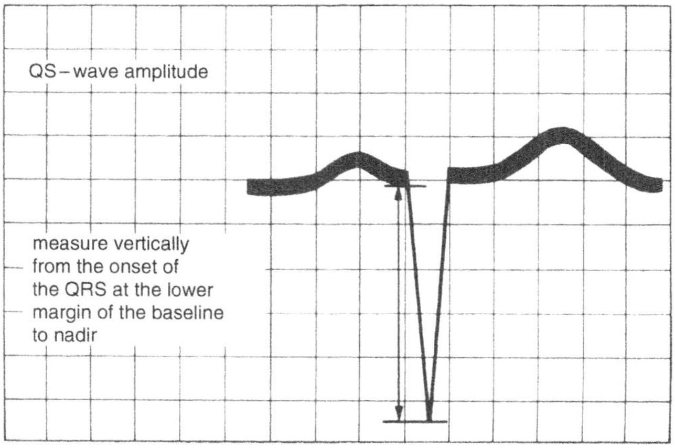

Fig. 1.9
Recommendations from the Minnesota code manual on how to measure the depth of the QS wave (After Prineas et al. [22]. © Springer, London. Reproduced with permission)

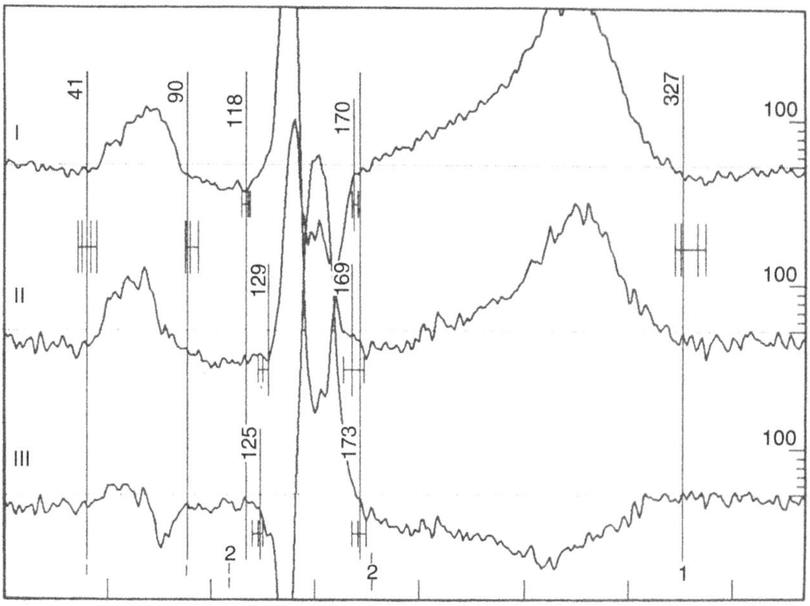

Fig. 1.10
Three simultaneously recorded leads, I, II, and III, shown expanded in time and gain. The vertical bars indicate estimates of wave onsets and offsets made by five cardiologists. The agreed onset for lead I differed from that of lead II by 11 sample points in the digitized data, that is, 22 ms (From Willems JL ed. CSE Atlas of ECGs. 1983 ACCO Leuven. Reproduced with permission)

Nowadays, with the use of computer technology, recommendations relating to the baseline "thickness" are a little less meaningful, although for manual coding, such rules [22] still apply (➋ Fig. 1.9). The general approach to a measurement involves one form of averaging or another. Normally, a set of beats of similar configuration is grouped together, and from this, an average beat is formed. Measurements are then made on this average beat. Alternative approaches do exist whereby a set of measurements (e.g., six R-wave amplitudes) is obtained and these are then averaged. A further approach is simply to select one single beat that appears to be most representative of the recording. Further details are available in ➋ Chap. 5 of *Specialized Aspects of ECG*. The use of averaging, however, theoretically leads to an improved signal-to-noise ratio and, hence, more accurate amplitude measurements. The accuracy of computer-derived durations is still under discussion (see below), but it should be noted that if a reference point is wrongly determined (the QRS onset, for example), then any amplitude measured with respect to such a point is open to error. To minimize such errors, most programs find a reference level by averaging in the vicinity of, say, the QRS onset or else fit a smooth curve from which the reference can be taken. In general terms, with respect to ECGs recorded from normal individuals, such small errors in amplitude are not of great significance and have to be set against normal day-to-day variation of measurements, which can be significantly larger [24].

While the above discussion has concentrated on amplitudes, it should also be noted that the possibility of different approaches to measuring durations of ECG components now arises from using technology, whereby all leads are recorded simultaneously. ➋ Figure 1.10 shows an actual example from three simultaneously recorded leads of a 12-lead ECG where the QRS complex in lead I appears to commence earlier than in lead II. This is perfectly feasible given an understanding of the concept of projections of electrical activity onto different cardiac axes, as discussed in ➋ Chap. 11 of *Basic Electrocardiology: Cardiac Electrophysiology, ECG Systems and Mathematical Modeling.*

However, with respect to ➋ Fig. 1.10, the question then arises as to whether the duration of the wave in lead II should be measured from the earliest QRS onset in any of the leads, or whether it should be measured from the apparent onset of the R wave in that particular lead. The difference could be over 20 ms as in this case. Again, the reader must therefore be aware of another possible source of discrepancy when considering published values for normal limits of wave-component durations.

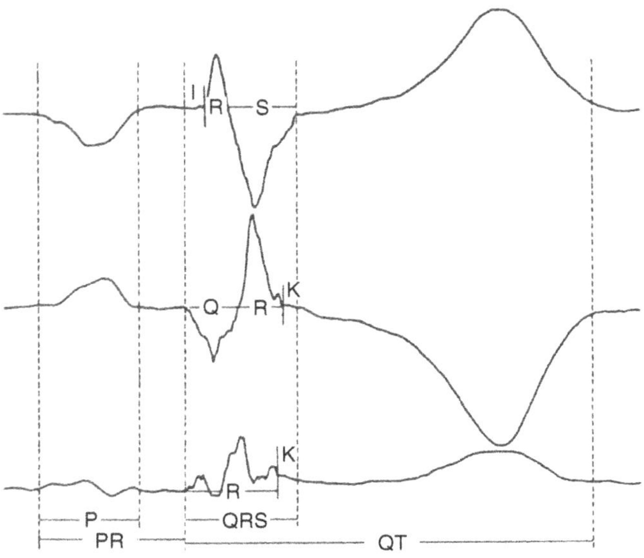

Fig. 1.11
An illustration of the definitions of isoelectric segments at the onset (I) and termination (K) of the QRS complex (After CSE Working Party [25]. © Academic Press, London. Reproduced with permission)

The availability of simultaneously recorded leads and the possibility of detecting "isoelectric" segments in some leads either at the beginning or end of waves have led the EEC working party on Common Standards in Electrocardiography (CSE) to recommend that such segments, denoted I and K for the QRS complex (see Fig. 1.11), be separately measured when detected [25].

A final point that can be made with respect to methods of measurement relates to the determination of QRS axis. Where the VCG is available and all leads have been recorded simultaneously, it is quite feasible to derive any required axis (see Chap. 11 of *Basic Electrocardiology : Cardiac Electrophysiology, ECG Systems and Mathematical Modeling*). Where the 12-lead ECG is involved, possibly with leads not recorded simultaneously, a different approach has to be utilized. There have been many suggested methods for measuring QRS axis [26–29]. However, the ad hoc Task Force of the World Health Organization (WHO) and the International Society and Federation for Cardiology (ISFC) [30] have recommended that the QRS axis should be measured on the basis of utilizing the areas under the QRS complex in leads I, II, and III. Since two pairs of leads can be selected from the three leads in three different ways, the recommendation is that the QRS axis be calculated using three different pairs of leads with an average value ultimately being derived. This recommendation has clearly been made with computer technology in mind.

An alternative approach is to utilize the sum of the signed Q (negative), R (positive) wave, and S (negative) wave amplitudes in these leads and to calculate similarly a QRS axis. In either case, a function $f(\mathrm{I})$, for example, can be used to represent the measurement (area or component sum) derived in this case from lead I. The following calculation shows how the use of the three standard limb leads I, II, and III, from which three measurements $f(\mathrm{I})$, $f(\mathrm{II})$, and $f(\mathrm{III})$ are obtained, allows an estimate of a frontal plane axis and avoids the need for repeated calculation and averaging as suggested by the WHO Task Force [30].

Consider that leads I, II, and III with lead directions as conceived in the Einthoven triangle (see Fig. 1.2) are superimposed on a Cartesian coordinate system, as shown in Fig. 1.12. Then, $OL = f(\mathrm{I})$, $OM = f(\mathrm{II})$, and $ON = f(\mathrm{III})$ represent the amplitude of the projection of the desired axis (or vector $\overrightarrow{OA}$) onto the lead axes I, II, and III, as shown in Fig. 1.12.

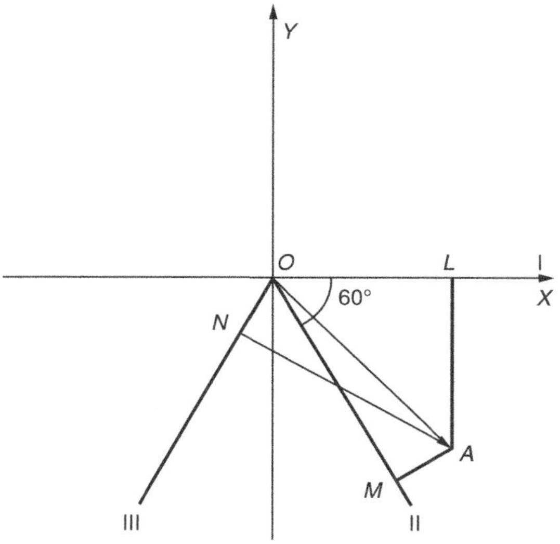

Fig. 1.12
An illustration relating to the calculation of the mean QRS vector given measurements from leads I, II, and III. The resultant vector is depicted as OA and has been calculated from a knowledge of its projection onto the three different leads I, II, and III, namely, OL, OM, and ON, respectively (See text for detailed discussion)

Thus, the Cartesian coordinates of these projections, that is, the coordinates of L, M, and N are as follows:

axis projection on lead I: $L = (f(\mathrm{I}),\ 0)$
axis projection on lead II: $M = (f(\mathrm{II})\ \cos 60°,\ f(\mathrm{II})\ \sin 60°)$
axis projection on lead III: $N = (-f(\mathrm{III})\ \cos 60°,\ f(\mathrm{III})\ \sin 60°)$

It should be noted that the functions $f(\mathrm{I})$, $f(\mathrm{II})$, and $f(\mathrm{III})$ are signed values.

It follows from the above and from the preceding section on angular data (Sect. 1.2.3.3) that the coordinates of the desired mean axis, that is, OA, on a circle of suitably small radius, R, intercepting all vectors, are given by the average component values:

$$\frac{R}{3\cdot \mathrm{OA}}\{[f(\mathrm{I})+f(\mathrm{II})\cos 60° - f(\mathrm{III})\cos 60°],[f(\mathrm{II})\sin 60° + f(\mathrm{III})\sin 60°]\}$$
$$=\frac{R}{3\cdot \mathrm{OA}}\left\{f(\mathrm{I})+\frac{1}{2}[f(\mathrm{II})-f(\mathrm{III})],\frac{\sqrt{3}}{2}[f(\mathrm{II})+f(\mathrm{III})]\right\}$$

The required angle is therefore obtained from the arc tangent of the ratio of the two components:

$$\tan^{-1}\left\{\frac{\frac{\sqrt{3}}{2}[f(\mathrm{II})+f(\mathrm{III})]}{f(\mathrm{I})+\frac{1}{2}[f(\mathrm{II})-f(\mathrm{III})}\right\}=\tan^{-1}\left\{\frac{\sqrt{3}[f(\mathrm{II})+f(\mathrm{III})]}{2f(\mathrm{I})+f(\mathrm{II})-f(\mathrm{III})}\right\}$$

This equation is based on the assumption that leads I, II, and III are related according to the equilateral Einthoven triangle (see Fig. 11.2 of *Basic Electrocardiology: Cardiac Electrophysiology, ECG Systems and Mathematical Modeling*). It can be used to calculate the P, QRS, or T axis provided the relevant measurement (e.g., P, QRS, or T area in leads I, II, and III) is substituted appropriately.

The experience of the authors' laboratory is contrary to that of the recent recommendations [30] in that the use of the area proved slightly less acceptable than the use of signed amplitudes when compared with angles derived from the VCG [31]. In a number of pathological situations (e.g., RBBB), a broad S wave can distort the measurement of the QRS axis using the area method.

1.2.5 Use of Computers

Computers first began to be utilized for analysis of the ECG in the early 1960s (see ➔ Chap. 5 of *Specialized Aspects of ECG*). Probably, the first use of the technique in the assessment of the normal limits of the ECG was that of Draper [32] from Pipberger's laboratory. In this study of 510 normal men, computer techniques were used for deriving the amplitude and duration of the P, QRS, and T components of the orthogonal leads X, Y, and Z as well as for calculating selected vector magnitudes and orientations. From this, 96 percentile ranges were derived.

It should not be assumed that because a computer is used for measurement, the ECG component amplitudes and durations are perfectly "correct." Several studies (see ➔ Chap. 5 of *Specialized Aspects of ECG*) indicate that there is variation between different programs with respect to computer measurement of amplitude, duration, and so on. It should also be noted that different authors measure wave components in different manners. While many workers have taken the QRS onset as a reference point with respect to which all other amplitudes have been measured, there are different recommendations available. For example, the American Heart Association [23] specifies that the T-wave amplitude should be measured with respect to the end of the T wave. The CSE Working Party indicated that the P-wave amplitude should be measured with respect to P-wave onset [25]. This is an approach that has not been adopted in all centers. ➔ Figure 1.13 shows three different approaches to the measurement of the P-wave amplitude, namely, with respect to the P-wave onset [23, 25], with respect to the QRS onset [33], and finally with respect to a straight line fitted between the P onset and termination [34].

Although in the vast majority of cases, and particularly when dealing with normal subjects in sinus rhythm, there will be very little difference between measurements. Nevertheless, there are obvious sources of discrepancy in the presence of a sinus tachycardia above 130 bpm and in pathological situations. The reader is therefore urged to look carefully at the different recommendations.

On the other hand, it is known that cardiologists also initially vary when defining wave onsets and terminations, as demonstrated in one of the CSE studies [35]. Furthermore, it would be extremely difficult for a physician to measure hundreds of amplitudes and durations and to calculate vector magnitudes and orientations on a multitude of ECGs. Thus, while the possibility of computer error, like human error, has to be acknowledged, automated methods provide a major step forward in defining normal ranges.

The introduction of computers and the ability to exchange data between different collaborating centers, as demonstrated by the CSE study [25, 35, 36], does support the possibility of developing more extensive databases including those from apparently healthy individuals. As already mentioned, the databases gathered from clinical trials involving one commercial company have been used to assess the limits of normality on 46,219 individuals with a very low probability of having any disease that would affect the ECG [1]. Such a task would simply be impossible without automated assistance. Although the skill of the experienced physician may still be required in reviewing a computer-based ECG interpretation, the capacity of computer systems to remember various normal limits stratified by parameters such as age, sex, and race is far beyond that of the individual. A valid second opinion is therefore provided in such cases by the automated interpretation, which supplements the experience of the physician.

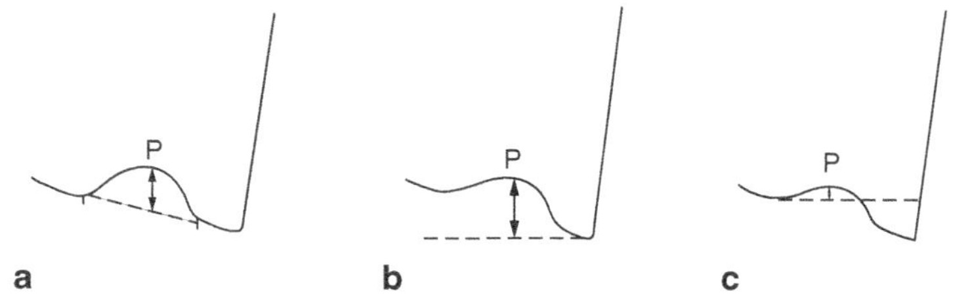

Fig. 1.13
An illustration of three methods of measuring the P-wave amplitude. They are with respect to (a) a straight line fitted between P onset and P termination, (b) QRS onset, and (c) P onset. Clearly the amplitude will differ under the various situations depicted here

1.3 Sources of Error

1.3.1 Technical Sources

Improvements in technology, as discussed in ➋ Chap. 12 of *Basic Electrocardiology: Cardiac Electrophysiology, ECG Systems and Mathematical Modeling*, mean that nowadays the accuracy of ECG recording is high. Digital recording with direct analog-to-digital conversion of the ECG within the modern computer-based electrocardiograph removes a number of sources of potential error in the recording technique.

The approach to population surveying can vary from a straightforward recording of the ECG on paper with manual measurement through to fully automated ECG recording and measurement of amplitudes, and so forth. In the former, a significant problem may arise with manual calibration of the ECG recorder. A 5% error in the setting of the 1 mV calibration signal might be difficult to avoid. Thereafter, the measurement of wave amplitudes and durations would be subject to various sources of error, not the least of which would be human error owing to fatigue. With the use of magnifying glasses for ECG measurement, the baseline written on to the chart recorder naturally appears thick, and measurement rules [37] suggest that amplitudes should be obtained by measuring from the top of the baseline to the top of the R wave, or from the bottom of the baseline to the tip of the Q wave, for example (➋ Fig. 1.9). The S-wave amplitude should be derived by measuring from the foot of the baseline to the bottom of the S wave. Such recommendations are still relevant when applying the Minnesota code, for example [22], to paper-based copies of the ECG. Likewise, the determination of the onset and offset of various components is extremely difficult using manual techniques, particularly if only a single-channel recording is available. Calibration errors can be minimized by the use of a correction factor (CF). For example, if the normal calibration of 1 mV = 10 mm is used, then the correction factor (CF) to be used would be

$$\mathrm{CF} = 10/X$$

where X = actual calibration amplitude (mm). All measured amplitudes would have to be multiplied by this correction factor.

The use of computers for the measurement of ECG parameters is also not without error. While many of the above problems, such as thickness of baseline, are avoided, the computer is still more prone to error in defining reference points, such as P onset and T termination. However, the definition of such reference points can prove troublesome even to experienced ECG reviewers, as evidenced by data from the CSE study [36, 38]. For example, given five referees' estimates of T termination, the standard deviation of the different estimates about each referee's individual mean value in a sample of 250 ECGs ranged from 12.6 to 17.8 ms. Similarly, the standard deviation of nine X, Y, and Z computer program estimates versus the mean of the computer programs ranged from 13.2 to 25.6 ms. In general terms, it is probably true to say that the measurement of amplitude by a computer will be more reliable than the measurement of durations. Some computer programs can measure small Q or R waves of the order of 8 ms duration. This is now the recommended minimum wave duration [25].

If a computer measures an extremely small primary r wave, perhaps of the order of 10 ms duration and 24 μV amplitude, care has to be taken that any larger following r′ wave is correctly utilized. ➋ Figure 1.14 illustrates this concept.

It could be argued that these difficulties are of minor significance compared with the actual repeat and day-to-day variation in the ECG itself. Each of these points will now be discussed.

1.3.2 Repeat Variation

If an ECG is recorded on the same individual twice within a short period of time and if the electrode positions are not marked on the chest, there can be marked variation in PQRST amplitudes from one recording to another. The source of this variation can be a result of a number of causes.

A principal source is undoubtedly simply that of the accuracy of placement of electrodes. In population surveys, where there is only one opportunity of recording the ECG, it is therefore of importance that an experienced technician records the ECG, paying meticulous attention to electrode placement.

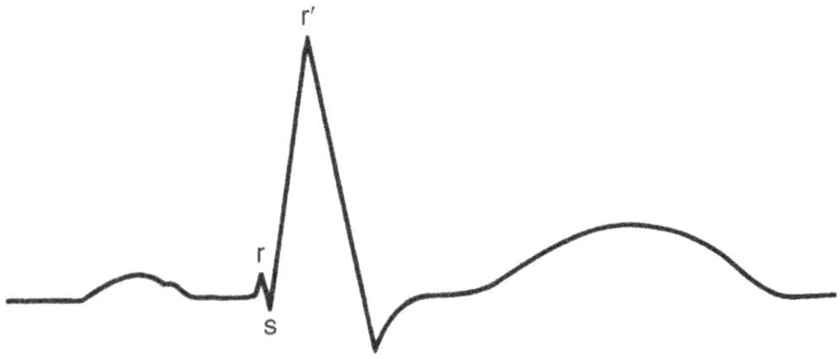

Fig. 1.14
In this ECG, a small primary r wave leads to the principal deflection being termed an r′ wave. This could lead to an error in computer diagnoses if criteria for an abnormally high amplitude R wave check only r amplitude and not r′ amplitude in addition

Table 1.2
Day-to-day, beat-to-beat, and percentage variation of QRS amplitude measurements: only upper limit of 96% variation is presented. R_X denotes the R-wave amplitude in lead *X*, and so on

	Increased amplitude (mV)				Decreased amplitude (mV)			Ranges (mV)		
Measurement	Variation (%)	Mean	SD[a]	96% day-to-day variation	Variation (%)	Mean	SD[a]	96% day-to-day variation	96% beat-to-beat variation	Maximal variation
R_X	13	0.16	0.14	0.41	17	0.22	0.17	0.52	0.377	0.52
R_Y	18	0.16	0.097	0.36	20	0.17	0.13	0.35	0.257	0.36
R_Z	17	0.099	0.082	0.24	14	0.10	0.07	0.23	0.13	0.24
Maximum spatial QRS vector	12	0.19	0.16	0.46	22	0.25	0.17	0.54	0.26	0.54

[a] Standard deviation

Where it has been possible to mark the correct electrode positions on the chest, perhaps with intracutaneous dye injection, repeat variation is minimized [39, 40] but by no means eliminated. Using the orthogonal-lead ECG, Willems et al. [39] showed that the day-to-day variation could be reduced by 25% by using marked electrode positions compared to using unmarked positions. In another study from which the data in Table 1.2 were taken [41], the electrode positions were unmarked. Table 1.2 shows the repeat variation of R-wave amplitudes in the orthogonal leads when ECGs were repeated twice, ECGs being recorded on three different days. It can be seen that the 96 percentile day-to-day variation in component amplitude ranged up to 0.52 mV, a sizable change. In a corresponding fashion, the maximum change in the spatial QRS vector was 0.54 mV.

It was pointed out by Simonson [42] that patients with coronary heart disease exhibit much more variability in repeat ECGs taken at 6-week intervals compared to a similar group of apparently healthy individuals. For example, the variation in the frontal plane T-wave axis in patients with coronary artery disease and an abnormal ECG was of the order of 64°, whereas it was only 27° for those with proven coronary artery disease and a normal ECG, while only approximately 10° for normal individuals.

Other factors influencing the repeat variation of the ECG include the phase of respiration in which the ECG is recorded, cigarette smoking [43], drinking of iced water [44], proximity to meals [45], anxiety [46], and so on. While all of these factors can influence ECG appearances in the one-off situation, by implication they must therefore affect repeat and day-to-day variation in the ECG. The experienced electrocardiographer will often have a subjective impression that suspicious appearances in an ECG may be "technical" in origin and will ask for a repeat ECG to be undertaken to make certain that an abnormality can be confirmed. The term "electrocardiographogenic disease" has been applied by

Marriott to the situation where a healthy individual may be categorized as having heart disease on account of an "abnormal" ECG [47]. A knowledge of the causes of day-to-day and repeat variation therefore assists in avoiding heart disease of electrocardiographic origin.

1.4 Factors Influencing Variability

1.4.1 Age

The factor that most influences the variation in ECG appearances is age. While other factors also have a role to play as discussed below, the effects of age are apparent from birth to death. On the other hand, influences due to the sex of an individual, for example, tend to be important in young adulthood but have a much less important role to play at either extremes of age.

As is well known, the ECG varies considerably over the first few days of life as the cardiovascular system adapts to its new role. In general, QRS voltage tends to increase toward adolescence and then begins to decrease thereafter. This can be seen in the composite illustration of ➋ Fig. 1.15 based on two different studies, one involving children and the other, adults. While this trend is demonstrated from different age-groups and different samples, the same conclusion has been demonstrated in a longitudinal study of persons in the Framingham study. ECGs recorded 40 years apart from the same individuals show a decrease in QRS amplitude in the second recording compared to the first. This is shown in ➋ Fig. 1.16. While it has always been assumed by electrocardiographers that the implication of the results of serial studies in different populations could be applied to the same individual in a longitudinal study, it is thought that this is the first time that such a finding has been demonstrated (Levy, D., personal communication, 1987).

As well as influencing ECG amplitudes, age affects intervals on the ECG. It has been shown that the PR interval increases slightly with increasing age [2], and in our study of adults, this finding has been reproduced as shown in ➋ Table 1.3. Likewise, QRS duration is shorter in older subjects compared to young persons (see ➋ Table 1.3).

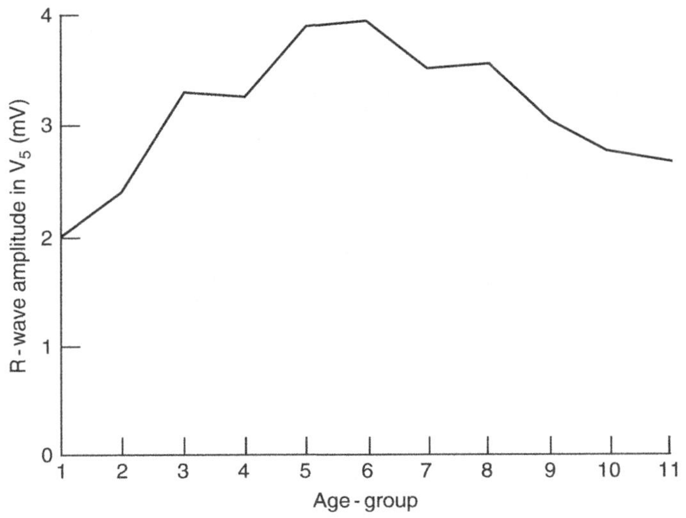

Fig. 1.15
A composite illustration of the upper limit of normal R-wave amplitude in V_5 from birth to 50 years and over in males. The peak occurs at age 8–12 years. The age-groups are as follows: (1) 0–1 day, (2) 3–7 days, (3) 1–3 months, (4) 6–12 months, (5) 3–5 years, (6) 8–12 years, (7) 12–16 years, (8) 18–29 years, (9) 30–39 years, (10) 40–49 years, and (11) over 50 years

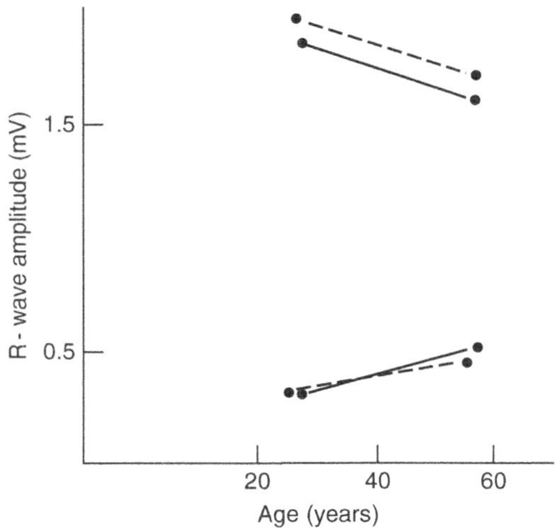

Fig. 1.16
Change in the mean R-wave amplitude in V_5 (upper two curves) and in aVL (lower two curves) over a 40-year period. Solid curves are from data kindly provided by Dr. D Levy of the Framingham heart study, while the dashed curves are from the Glasgow database. Framingham data are from the same individuals recorded 40 years ago; Glasgow data are from different individuals

Table 1.3
Means ± standard deviations and 96% ranges of PR, QRS, QT, and QT_c

Age-group	Sex	No. of subjects (*n*)	PR interval (ms)	QRS duration (ms)	QT interval (ms)	QT_c interval[a] (ms)	QT_c interval[b] (ms)
18–29	Male	265	152.5 ± 23.0	96.4 ± 8.6	385.5 ± 28.9	403.6 ± 19.0	413.9 ± 23.1
			112–208	80–114	336–442	368–444	370–463
	Female	317	145.9 ± 19.7	87.7 ± 7.8	380.0 ± 27.8	411.6 ± 18.0	429.7 ± 22.9
			114–194	72–104	332–440	378–451	386–477
30–39	Male	218	155.7 ± 21.4	95.4 ± 9.8	385.5 ± 29.5	404.8 ± 19.4	416.0 ± 22.9
			116–206	78–114	326–448	366–448	375–468
	Female	115	145.7 ± 18.6	88.6 ± 7.3	386.6 ± 27.7	415.2 ± 16.9	432.6 ± 20.9
			114–184	76–106	330–438	384–445	395–473
40–49	Male	119	157.2 ± 21.8	94.4 ± 9.9	390.8 ± 29.3	409.2 ± 17.9	420.0 ± 21.9
			116–210	78–114	340–450	377–450	377–464
	Female	72	154.9 ± 20.4	89.4 ± 7.9	386.1 ± 27.0	415.2 ± 22.5	433.7 ± 28.4
			108–200	74–108	328–434	347–457	350–483
50	Male	123	161.5 ± 18.9	92.7 ± 9.3	385.5 ± 26.0	407.4 ± 17.5	420.9 ± 22.7
			120–196	74–112	320–434	374–444	380–475
	Female	79	155.6 ± 16.9	87.1 ± 8.7	390.7 ± 31.5	419.5 ± 22.7	438.2 ± 24.8
			122–196	68–104	336–488	376–486	392–506

[a] QT_C corrected according to Hodges et al. [106]
[b] QT_C corrected according to Bazett [105]

1.4.2 Sex

The second important factor affecting appearances in the ECG is that of sex. Sex differences in the ECG are most apparent in young adulthood and tend to diminish to a certain extent thereafter. As an example, ➋ Fig. 1.17 shows the mean S-wave amplitude in V_2 for males and females in the authors' own study. Significant differences exist in the age-group 18–30 years, while by the age of 50, there tends to be little difference between S-wave amplitudes recorded from males and females.

It is possible that to some extent this difference in the younger age-group is a reflection of the level of physical activity undertaken by individuals. To investigate this effect, a subgroup of 483 persons aged 18–29 years from the population of the authors' study was subdivided into those who undertook regular exercise and those who did not. It was found that mean amplitudes of S waves in V_2 were lower in the group who did not undertake exercise, but, nevertheless, there were still significant differences between males and females who engaged in regular training activities and also between males and females who did not (➋ Table 1.4).

Another cause of lower ECG amplitudes in women is thought to be a higher fat content [2] and the influence of breast tissue. LaMonte and Freiman [48] assessed the effects of mastectomy and noted an increased QRS amplitude in women following this operation. On the other hand, Rautaharju et al. studied the effect of breast tissue on ECG amplitudes in women and concluded that there was no significant effect [49].

T-wave amplitudes in women also tend to be lower than in men, particularly in the precordial leads, where, apart from V_1, the lower limit of the normal T-wave amplitude is positive in both men and women. In the Appendices, data on T-wave amplitudes show that in V_1, T-wave inversion is much more prevalent in women than men. Indeed, T-wave inversion in V_2 and very occasionally in V_3 can be found in healthy women. On the other hand, in the limb leads, it is well known that apparently healthy young women, and sometimes men, may on occasions exhibit ST-T "changes" (slight ST depression and/or minimal T-wave inversion), particularly in the inferior leads. Since the T wave in III may often be inverted in normal persons, it is aVF that assumes more significance in this case. The exact mechanism for such T-wave changes has never been satisfactorily demonstrated. However, this applies in cases where the QRS complex is mainly upright. A leftward QRS axis shift may be accompanied by a leftward T axis shift so that an inverted T wave may appear in aVF in the presence of a dominant S wave but be of little significance. In such cases, the frontal plane QRS-T angle is small. Increasing the QRS-T angle is associated with increasing degrees of coronary artery calcification in older adults aged 66 or over [50].

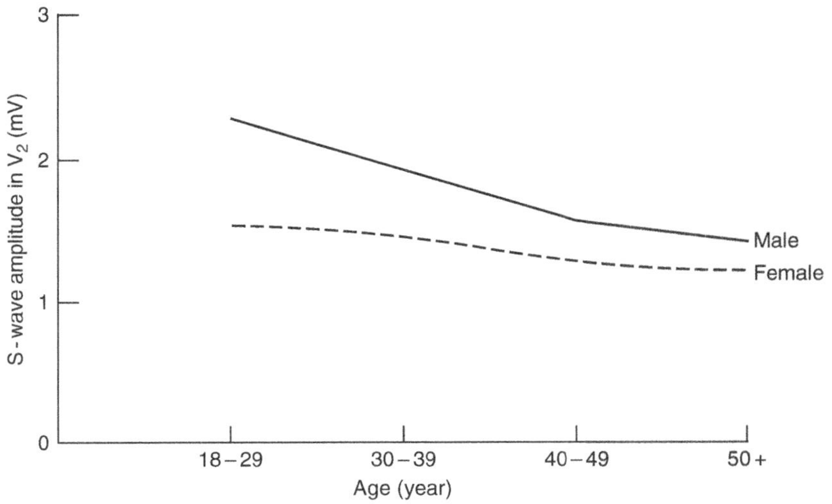

Fig. 1.17
The mean S-wave amplitude in V_2 stratified by age. Data were derived from the subjects in the Glasgow study

Table 1.4

Mean values and 96% ranges of the S-wave amplitude in V_2 for young men and women aged 18–29 years, inclusive, divided into two groups: those taking exercise and those who did not

	Sex	No. of subjects (*n*)	Mean value of wave amplitude (mV)	96% range of S-wave amplitude (mV)
Regular exercise	Male	96	2.43	0.80–4.5
	Female	95	1.53	0.59–3.04
No regular exercise	Male	128	2.18	0.77–3.76
	Female	164	1.53	0.39–2.81

Sex differences can also influence the various intervals in the ECG (➋ Table 1.3). The authors' study group showed a shorter PR interval in women (96 upper percentile = 0.196 s compared to men whose corresponding upper limit was 0.21 s). This might logically be explained on the basis of the average male heart being somewhat larger than that of the average female, necessitating a slightly longer conduction time between the sinus node and the ventricles. It was also found that women had a shorter QRS duration (88 ms, as compared to 95 ms for men) and a longer corrected QT interval (➋ Table 1.3). For some unknown reason, these basic facts are not used in ECG interpretation where most cardiologists will slavishly adhere to 120 ms as the upper limit of normal QRS for males and females and use such a value in clinical decisions on the use of cardiac resynchronization therapy, for example, irrespective of the patient's sex and of the accuracy of QRS measurement [51].

1.4.3 Race

The influence of race on the ECG has been known for some time but, despite the recent availability of computer techniques, has not been used to any significant extent in the interpretation of the ECG.

As early as 1946, Littmann [52] reported on the "persistence of the juvenile pattern in the precordial leads of healthy adult blacks." His study did not involve the use of precordial leads referred to the Wilson central terminal but utilized bipolar chest leads with the indifferent electrode being on the left leg. Since then, there has been controversy over whether or not such T-wave findings are truly representative of the black population: For example, Keller and Johnston [53], using precordial leads based on the Wilson central terminal, were unable to confirm the findings of Littman. On the other hand, Walker and Walker [54] demonstrated that T-wave inversion was found in young South African Bantu subjects. Recent work involving over 1,200 ECGs recorded from healthy adults living in Nigeria using a digital electrocardiograph, and analyzed in Glasgow, paradoxically showed more precordial T-wave inversion (➋ Fig. 1.18) in healthy black females than in healthy black males [55].

In a comparison between Japanese and North American men and women, Simonson [2] showed significant differences in most electrocardiographic parameters. In general terms, the Japanese group showed higher voltages in the precordial leads compared to the American group. The reverse appeared to be true for the limb leads.

In contrast, in a large computer-assisted study involving the authors [56], it was found that precordial voltages of young Chinese men and women were significantly lower than their Western counterparts. This difference diminished with increasing age (➋ Fig. 1.19). In general terms, there was little difference between the two populations with respect to intervals and durations. It should be stressed that the same computer program [57] was used for the analysis of all ECGs in this study. P-wave amplitudes were higher in Caucasians than Chinese, while almost 10% of Chinese women aged between 40 and 49 years had a negative T-wave component in V_3. These comparisons were derived from a study of over 500 apparently healthy Chinese undertaken in Taipei by Chen et al. [58] and from the authors' own normal data. More recently, Wu et al. found very similar normal ranges in a large Chinese cohort [59].

In the Washington code developed by Pipberger et al. [60], different limits of normal are used for white and black subjects and for males and females. The code was developed partly from a study of 518 normal men including 186 black subjects [61] and, probably, a separate study on women, which appeared much later from the same laboratory [62] although racial differences were not considered (despite a significant percentage of black women being included).

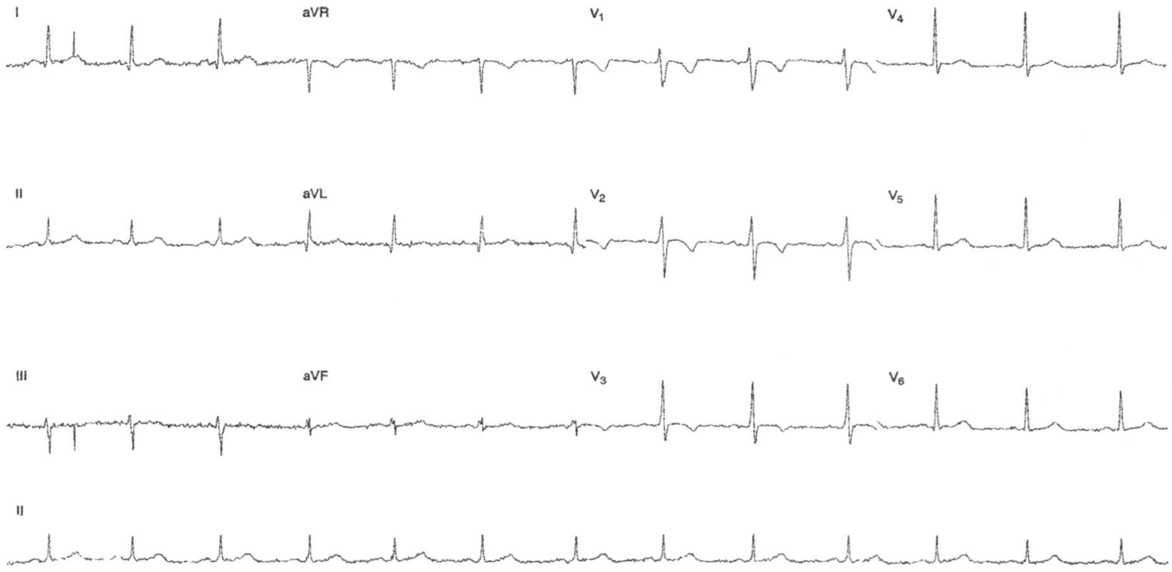

Fig. 1.18
An ECG recorded from a 31-year-old healthy Nigerian lady. Note the T-wave inversion in V_2 and V_3. This illustration is reproduced with permission of Dr. I.A. Katibi, University of Ilorin, Nigeria

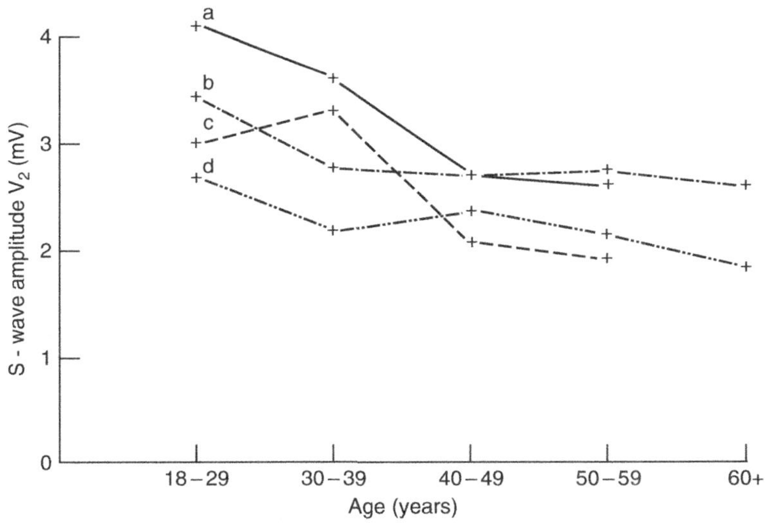

Fig. 1.19
Variation in the upper limit of normal of the S-wave amplitude in V_2 in white and Chinese populations. The white subjects were from the Glasgow study, while the Chinese data were obtained from 503 apparently healthy Chinese [56]: (a) white males, (b) Chinese males, (c) white females, and (d) Chinese females

However, a closer inspection of the published data reveals that with respect to scalar QRS amplitude data from males, the upper limit of normal voltage differed only in RZ (R amplitude in lead Z equivalent to SV_2) where the black limit was almost 30% higher than the white limit. Many other differences, while of statistical significance, were not of practical value. The exception to this is the much smaller Q/R ratio found in the lateral (X) and inferior (Y) leads in black subjects.

This is one area in particular where the continued development of large databases will lead to further enlightenment with regard to the effect of race on ECG wave amplitudes and durations.

1.4.4 Other Constitutional Variables

Other variables that might influence the ECG are those of height and weight. To a certain extent, these can be related by the use of various indices, such as weight/height^2 (Quetelet index, [63], more commonly known as body mass index) and so on. While certain variations and correlations in the ECG can be demonstrated between measurements and such indices (e.g., weight and amplitude [61]), these have never been used to any significant extent in ECG interpretation. Their use is complex in that they add an extra complication to the involvement of age and sex in diagnostic criteria. Likewise, because of the lack of availability of large databases where significant numbers in different groups can be obtained, a full study of the effect of such variables is still awaited. Matthes and coworkers [64] pointed out that some of the variation in the QRS amplitude could in fact be accounted for by an inverse relationship between body mass index and increasing age. They used

$$\frac{W \times 100}{H - 100}\%$$

as an index (where W is the weight in kilograms and H is the height in centimeters). Data from the authors' own study show the relation between the S-wave amplitude in V_2 and the Quetelet index both for males and females (➋ Fig. 1.20). The results are a little confusing. If data for males alone are considered, then there is a significant correlation between the S amplitude in V_2 and age ($r = 0.466$), which accounts for almost 22% of the variation. There was no correlation of amplitude with height as would be expected, but limited correlation with weight ($r = 0.199$), which therefore accounts for only 4% of the variation: The Quetelet index showed an intermediate relationship to the S amplitude ($r = 0.282$), and therefore accounts for 8% of the variation. Of the two (constitutional) variables, height and weight, the latter is clearly of more significance within the male group as a whole. A similar pattern was found for females although the correlation was less in each case, being 0.216 for age and 0.148 for weight with respect to the S amplitude in V_2, which was treated as a negative number.

If males and females are treated as a single group, then the correlation of the S amplitude in V_2 with age changes to 0.307 and not surprisingly height then shows a negative correlation with the S amplitude ($r = -0.227$). Conversely, the correlation of the S amplitude with weight becomes almost zero.

These results strengthen the existing generalized approach of considering only age and sex when interpreting the ECG. This is also in agreement with the view of Simonson [2] who indicated that "over-all, the effect of age on the ECG is more pronounced and consistent than the effect of relative body weight," overweight, underweight, and so on.

1.4.5 Physical Fitness

The question of fitness affecting the ECG was alluded to above when dealing with the limits of normal voltage in younger persons. With the continued interest in marathon running and the need for individuals to increase the amount of exercise taken in order to reduce cardiovascular risk factors, there have been a number of studies dealing with the effects of physical training on the heart. A review by Oakley and Oakley [65] specifically dealt with the ECG in athletes. As might be expected, an increase in precordial voltage was noted in highly trained athletes together with T-wave abnormalities. It is known from echocardiographic studies [66, 67] that there is an increase in internal left ventricular (LV) diameter together with an increase in posterior LV wall thickness and septal thickness in athletes involved in a variety of sports. It is therefore not surprising that some increase in ECG voltage is obtained. ➋ Figure 3.9 shows the ECG from a marathon runner whose echocardiogram indicated that his LV mass was at the upper limit of normal. T-wave changes can be seen in several leads.

➋ Figure 1.21 shows the ECG from a 22-year-old healthy athlete who had a normal echocardiogram and a normal cardiac magnetic resonance image scan. Marked T-wave inversion can be seen in I, aVL, V_2, and V_3. A recent publication suggested that such individuals are at increased risk of cardiomyopathy in later life [68].

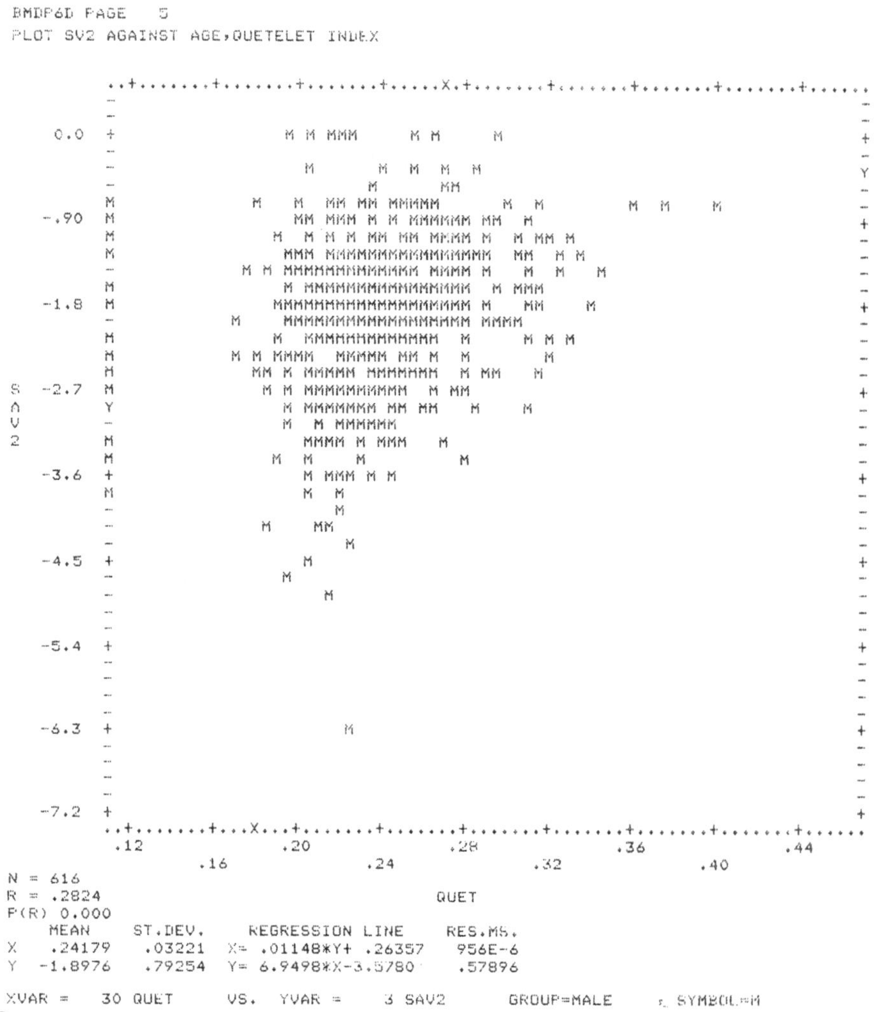

a

Fig. 1.20a
Scattergram of S amplitude in V_2 versus the Quetelet index, shown for 616 males. Note that the S amplitude is plotted as a negative number

In a balanced sample from an apparently healthy population, the occasional abnormality, such as isolated T-wave inversion as shown in Fig. 1.21, would be excluded by the use of the 96 percentile ranges of normal. Alternatively, in developing normal ranges, it might be reasonable to exclude highly trained athletes from a sample of healthy persons. On the other hand, when interpreting an ECG, it is necessary to be aware of the different ECG patterns that can be encountered in the so-called athlete's heart. In an editorial on the subject, Oakley [69] stated that "there is at present no published evidence to suggest that training-induced hypertrophy of whatever type represents anything other than cardiovascular fitness. If a positive diagnosis of cardiomyopathy cannot be made, the patient must be vigorously reassured that he has no abnormality." Indeed, Oakley's patients, many of whom had initially been advised to give up training prior to referral, were subsequently advised to restart training following a detailed investigation including cardiac catheterization.

Unusual, rather than abnormal, ECG findings in sportsmen have been well documented, for example, [68, 70]. On the other hand, some countries, particularly Italy, have been very keen to promote guidelines relating to screening of

BMDP6D PAGE 6
PLOT SV2 AGAINST AGE,QUETELET INDEX

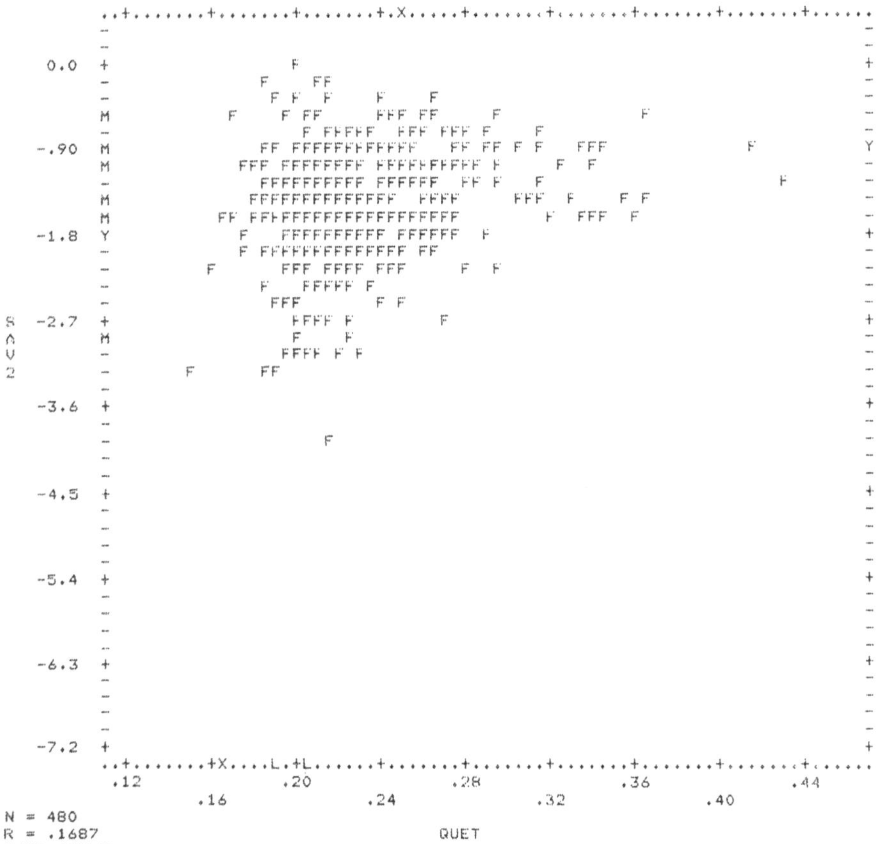


```
N = 480
R = .1687
P(R) 19E-5
     MEAN      ST.DEV.     REGRESSION LINE       RES.MS.
X    .22827    .03756   X= .01078*Y+ .24408     .00137
Y   -1.4662    .58755   Y= 2.6383*X-2.0684      .33610

XVAR =   30 QUET      VS.   YVAR =   3 SAV2       GROUP=FEMALE   ; SYMBOL=F
```

b

Fig. 1.20b
Scattergram of S amplitude in V_2 versus the Quetelet index, shown for 480 females. Note that S amplitude is plotted as a negative number

apparently healthy individuals prior to participation in sport. These have led to internationally approved guidelines [71] that involve ECG recording to exclude the presence of left ventricular hypertrophy as well as other adverse signs, such as the Brugada pattern (see ➋ Chap. 2) and long QT (see ➋ Chap. 7).

1.4.6 Heart Position

For many years, it was fashionable to describe an ECG as belonging to a particular category based on the orientation of the QRS axis which, in turn, was supposed to be related to the position of the heart. Wilson et al. in 1943 [72] described five positions of the heart on the basis of ECG appearances. These were horizontal, semihorizontal, intermediate, semivertical, and vertical. (They also mentioned a sixth indeterminate position.) An illustration of different positions is indicated in

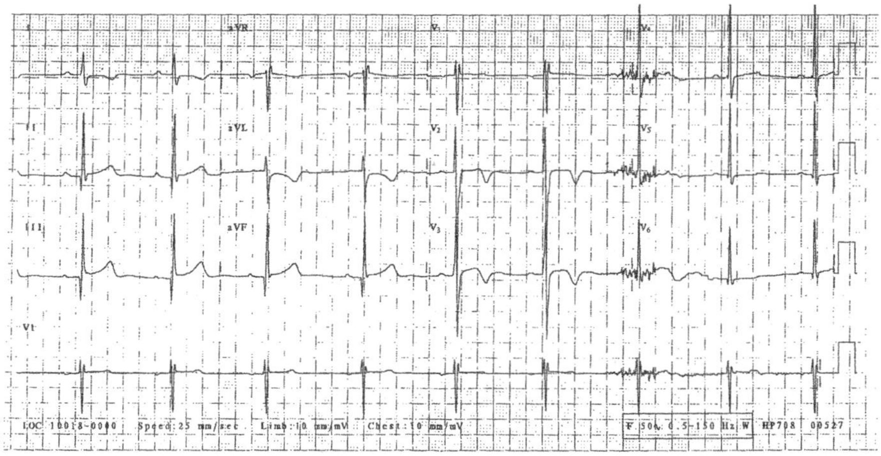

Fig. 1.21
The 12-lead ECG from a 22-year-old healthy male athlete. Note the T-wave inversion in I, aVL, V_2, and V_3. There are also deep but narrow Q waves in the inferior leads. Both the echocardiogram and cardiac MRI scan were normal in this individual

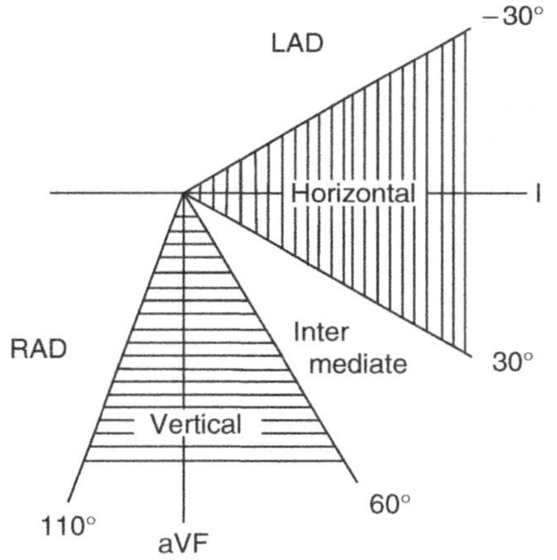

Fig. 1.22
The division of the frontal plane into different regions depending on the orientation of the mean QRS vector. *LAD* left axis deviation, *RAD* right axis deviation

Fig. 1.22. Later, Simonson [2] modified these by suggesting that the semihorizontal and semivertical positions could be omitted, hence leaving three categories. In essence, if the frontal plane QRS axis were oriented at 60° or more, the heart was said to be in the vertical position, whereas if it were superior to 30°, it was in the horizontal position. ECGs with a QRS axis between 30° and 60° were said to lie in an intermediate position. Such a definition relates to the QRS axis in the different leads although when the description was introduced at first, the definitions essentially related to QRS morphology. Thus, the horizontal heart had a dominant R wave in aVL similar to appearances in V_5 and V_6, while the QRS morphology in aVF resembled V_1 and V_2. On the other hand, in the vertical heart, there is a dominant R wave in aVF similar to V_5 and V_6, while the QRS morphology in aVL resembles that in V_1 and V_2.

A moment's reflection will show that there are bound to be statistically significant differences between R-wave amplitudes in aVF in patients with a vertical heart compared to those with a horizontal heart. However, these are of limited practical significance. What is probably of more value is the relation between the QRS and T axes in these groups.

Table 1.5
Labels of the three positional groups according to the direction of the frontal Q axis and characteristic features in the ECG

Label of positional group	Mean frontal Q axis	Number of Q waves in extremity leads	Q wave in aVL	Q wave in III
Q left	<0°	1–4	+	–
Q intermediate	0–90 °	5–6	±	±
Q right	>90°	1–4	–	+

For example, a T-wave axis around 0° is not uncommon in subjects with a horizontal heart, whereas in a patient with a vertical heart, such a T-wave axis is often regarded with much more suspicion. In other words, the QRS-T angle is larger in this latter situation. Lundh proposed a new classification system [3] for the normal ECG that included a knowledge of the heart position. His positional classification was based on the appearance of small Q waves in the limb leads, leading to the calculation of the so-called Q axis. The classification is based on the Q axes, as outlined in Table 1.5. Note that the presence of a small Q wave in aVL would correspond to a Q axis around −30° (opposite to conventional calculation).

He used this classification to determine different limits of normality for certain electrocardiographic parameters although the conclusion ultimately drawn was that further clinical work was required to prove that the system could be of diagnostic value.

1.5 The Normal Electrocardiogram

1.5.1 Evolutionary Development of the Electrocardiogram

Almost from birth onward, the ECG changes with time as the heart adapts to its new working environment. A number of significant changes occur over the first few days of life before the ECG settles for approximately the first year of life. Thereafter, as the individual continues to grow, the ECG also continues to change likewise until early adulthood when a period of regression of voltages sets in.

A number of authors (see Sect. 1.10) have been responsible for assessing normal limits of the pediatric ECG, and their results are presented in Appendix 2. In particular, Liebman [73] has contributed much to the field of pediatric electrocardiography and deals with this topic elsewhere in the book (Chap. 9). His data, particularly from orthogonal-lead ECGs in healthy children, have been incorporated into the Appendix 2 in this book and are gratefully acknowledged. Together with others, he has also published on ECGs in premature infants [74, 75].

Davignon et al. [76] have published data on the normal 12-lead ECG standards for infants and children. They have chosen to represent their data as a series of charts showing the percentile distributions of various amplitudes and durations versus age. All of these are presented in Appendix 2. With respect to the evolution of the ECG, it is helpful to study the R-wave amplitude in V_1, as shown in Fig. 1.23. Here, it can be seen that the upper 98% limit of normal is maximal during the first 3 days of life and, thereafter, steadily decreases over the first month until by the age of 1–3 months, its value is approximately 70% of that at birth. Over the next 12–16 years, this R-wave amplitude decreases to approximately 55% of its value at 1–3 months. Thus, the change in the upper limit of normal over the first month or two of life is almost as much as the change over the following 15 years.

Conversely, in keeping with a clockwise rotation of the cardiac axis in the horizontal plane over the first years of life, the R-wave amplitudes in the lateral leads increase over the first month and continue to increase more slowly thereafter.

The frontal QRS axis lies between 92° and 185° in 90% of newborn children [76], but by the age of 1–3 months, the corresponding range has altered considerably to 47–105° (see Appendix 2). Similar findings have been reported by others [77].

Another important parameter is the T-wave amplitude in V_1. In newborns, this can either be positive or negative, although, by the end of 7 days, it is always negative according to the data of Davignon et al. [76]. By the age of 5 years, a small percentage of children exhibit negative T waves in V_1. In Davignon's study, the T-wave amplitude was always positive in V_2 in the 12–16 years age-group. However, it is known from other studies [78] that some adolescents have inverted T waves in V_1 and V_2, these appearances sometimes being known as the juvenile T-wave pattern.

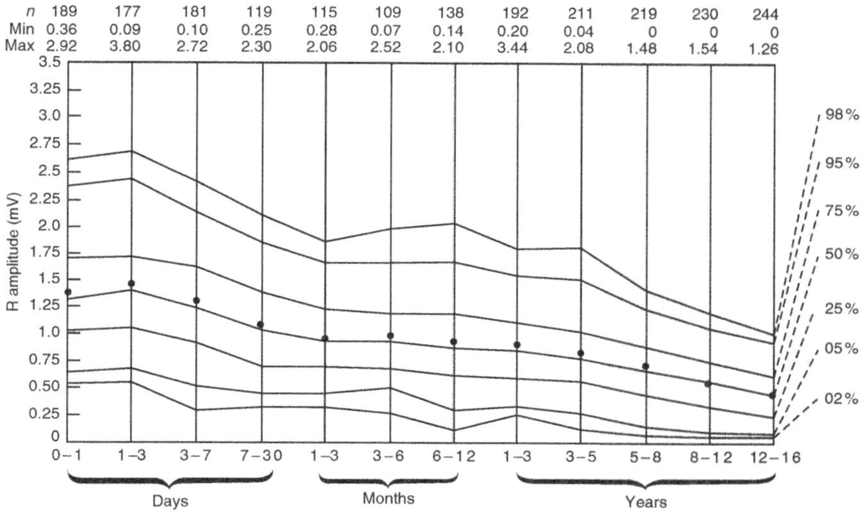

Fig. 1.23
A distribution of the R-wave amplitude in V_1 from birth to 16 years of age. The various *curves* denote the different percentiles of the distribution, while the *dots* represent the mean values (After Davignon et al. [76], © Springer, New York. Reproduced with permission)

Our own study [79] of over 1,500 neonates, infants, and children found similar data, which are presented in detail for the first time in the Appendix 2. The group included 500 neonates whose ECGs were sampled at 500 samples/s compared to the 333 samples/s of Davignon [76]. These showed some very interesting findings, e.g., the variation in the S-wave amplitude in V_2 over the first 3 months of life (➋ Fig. 1.24) and even a differing QRS duration between boys and girls from an early age (➋ Fig. 1.25).

Other significant collections of ECGs from children are those of Rijnbeek et al. [80], where 1,912 ECGs from children aged from 11 days to 15 years were studied to provide normal ranges, and of Sun et al. [81], who recorded 1,166 ECGs in Chinese children. The normal ranges from Rijnbeek et al. tended to show similar trends to those from Glasgow [79], e.g., the QRS duration was slightly longer in boys compared to girls from about 1 year of age onward. Sun et al. [81] also compared ECG appearances in healthy Chinese infants to North American counterparts [81]. R amplitude in V_5 tended to be higher in North American children compared to Chinese children, but surprisingly, R amplitude in V_2 demonstrated the reverse.

The same evolutionary changes can also be seen in the VCG. In the frontal plane, the vast majority of all newborns show a QRS axis oriented vertically or to the right [82], and over the first month or two, it shifts counterclockwise so that the frontal axis is in the range 20–120°, the prevalent direction being 80° [73]. Similarly, in the transverse plane, there is clockwise rotation of the main QRS vector over the first few months of life. The T vector in the newborn child in the transverse plane is tightly distributed between 130° and 168°, but by 3 days this range has expanded, being 90°–302° [82]. This corresponds to the development of T-wave inversion in V_1. Note, however, that the normal *XYZ*-lead ECG does not always have an upright T in *Z* (*Z* being directed positively to the back).

1.5.2 Examples of the Normal Electrocardiogram

This chapter has already stressed the variety of factors that affect the appearances of the ECG and by implication, the range of normality of ECG patterns. It should therefore be apparent that there is no one ECG or VCG that can be displayed as an example of normality. To this end, a series of ECGs recorded from apparently healthy individuals, including a newborn, is shown in ➋ Figs. 1.26–1.29. These ECGs have been selected to show the range of normality and to illustrate the influence of age and sex on ECG appearances.

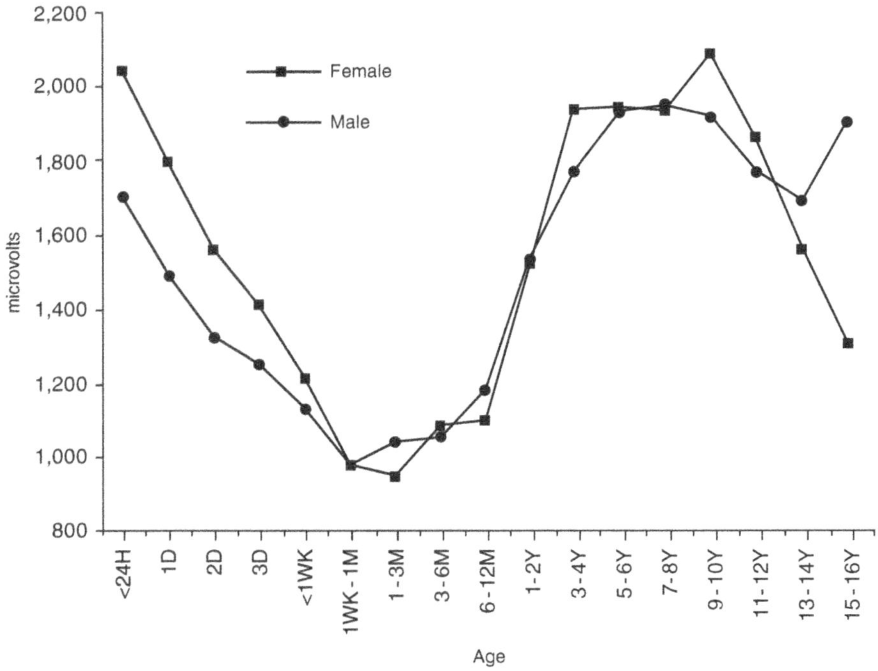

Fig. 1.24
The mean S-wave amplitude in V_2 in 1,780 healthy neonates, infants, and children. Note that the scale is nonlinear. There is a remarkable loss of amplitude over the first few days of life followed by a recovery over the first decade. The amplitude then tails off in females around puberty (Reproduced from [79] with permission)

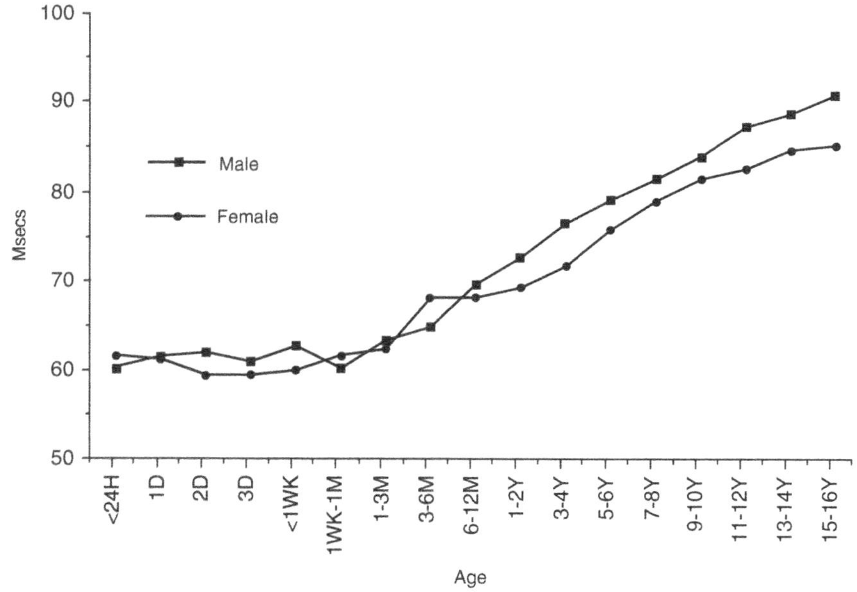

Fig. 1.25
Mean QRS duration versus age in 1,780 healthy neonates, infants, and children. Note that the scale is nonlinear. There is a clear separation between males and females from around 1 year of age (Reproduced from [79] with permission)

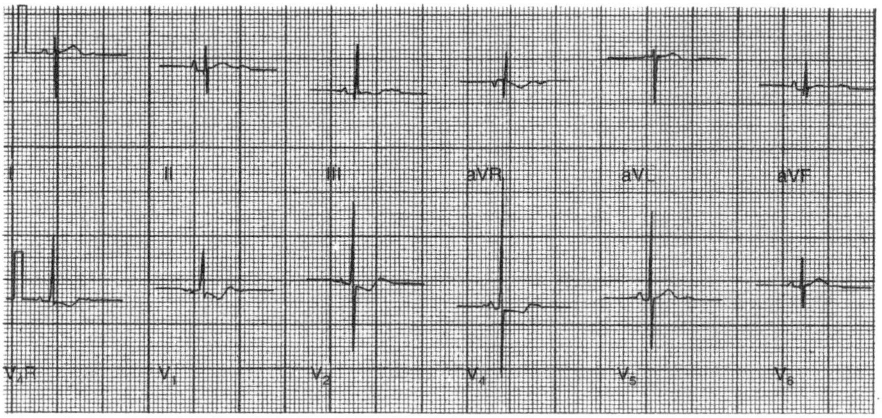

Fig. 1.26
ECG from a 4-day-old baby girl. Note the dominant R wave in V_4 R and V_1 typical of the right ventricular preponderance pattern found in the healthy newborn. Average beats are presented

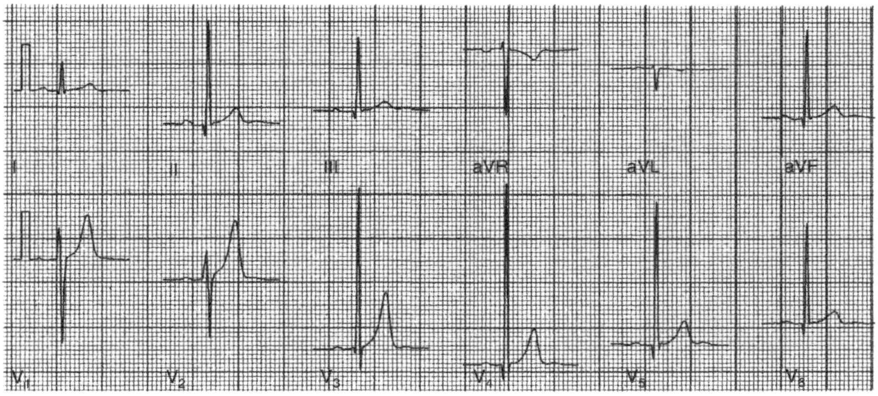

Fig. 1.27
ECG recorded from a 35-year-old apparently healthy male. Note the marked change in appearances between V_2 and V_3, which, in this case, delineates the so-called transitional zone, which is the point where the rS complex changes to the Rs configuration. The QRS axis is 74°, and there is a vertical heart. Note how aVL essentially resembles the configuration in V_1 although there are gross amplitude differences. Likewise, aVF resembles V5 typically as in a vertical heart. Average beats are displayed

For those readers who are relatively inexperienced in electrocardiography, it is sometimes of help to consider that there are only two basic QRST configurations that need to be remembered in the 12-lead ECG in order to differentiate between normal and abnormal. These two patterns and the leads in which they appear are shown in Fig. 1.30. As there is a certain amount of redundancy in the 12-lead ECG (see Chaps. 10 and 11 of *Basic Electrocardiology : Cardiac Electrophysiology, ECG Systems and Mathematical Modeling*), it is often helpful for the inexperienced electrocardiographer to consider analyzing only leads I, aVF, V_1, V_2, V_4, and V_5. Even the experienced electrocardiosgrapher will be surprised by the amount of information that can be obtained from only these six leads. With respect to this scheme, leads I, aVF, V_4, and V_5 tend to have the same pattern, whereas V_1 and V_2 have the other morphology, as shown in Fig. 1.29. The only exception to this simplified approach is in V_1 where the T wave may often be inverted.

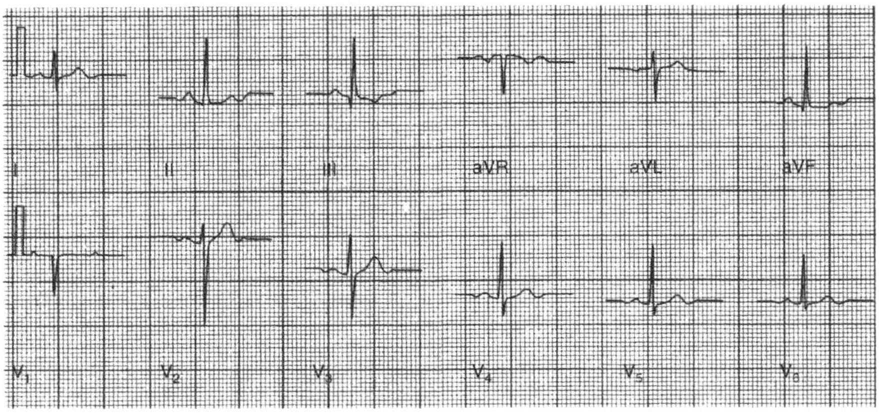

Fig. 1.28
ECG recorded from a 34-year-old healthy female. Note the slight ST depression in several leads

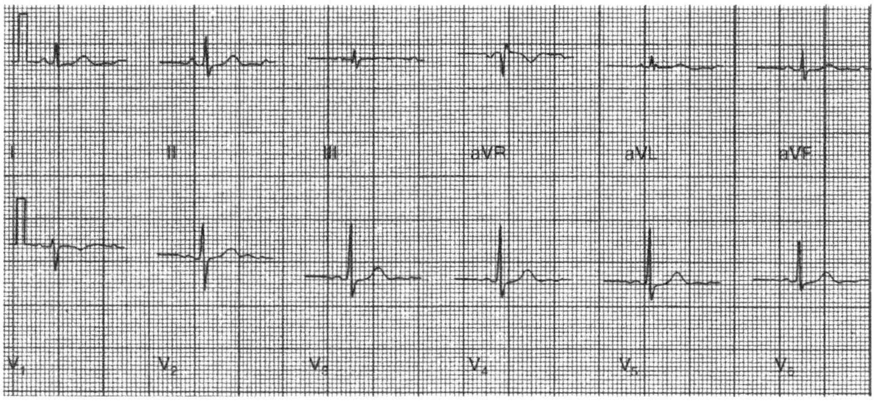

Fig. 1.29
ECG recorded from a healthy 60-year-old female. Note the normal T-wave inversion in VI. The QRS axis is 25°, which suggests a horizontal heart. aVF approximately resembles V_1, while there is a small dominant R in aVL

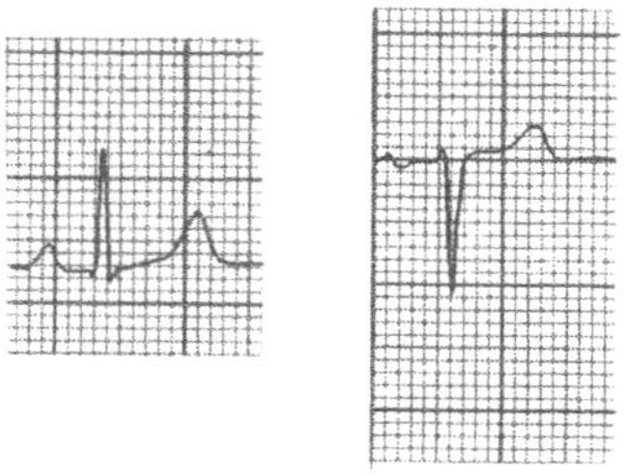

Fig. 1.30
Two complexes typifying the principal types of morphology obtained in the normal ECG. The waveform shown on the *left* is typically found in I, aVF, V_4, and V_5, and the waveform on the *right* is generally seen in V_1 and V_2. They may, of course, be found in other leads, but the use of six leads for the beginner may be helpful (See text for further discussion)

1.6 The Normal Vectorcardiogram

1.6.1 Examples of the Normal Vectorcardiogram

The normal VCG also has a wide range of appearances. Some examples are shown in ➋ Figs. 1.31–1.33. In general, however, its appearance in the three different planes (see ➋ Chap. 11 of *Basic Electrocardiology : Cardiac Electrophysiology, ECG Systems and Mathematical Modeling*) can be summarized as follows.

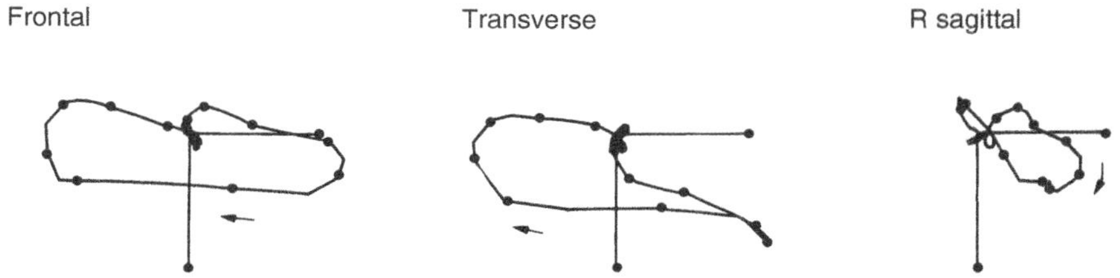

Fig. 1.31
The VCG from the newborn whose 12-lead ECG is shown in ➋ Fig. 1.26. In this case, the VCG loops have been derived from the 12-lead ECG using the inverse Dower technique (see ➋ Chap. 11 of *Basic Electrocardiology : Cardiac Electrophysiology, ECG Systems and Mathematical Modeling* for further details). All three loops show clockwise inscription of the (normal) QRS loop. The transverse loop indicates the almost total anterior displacement of the loop owing to normal right ventricular preponderance at this age. Dots are printed on the QRS loop at 4 ms intervals (R sagittal denotes right sagittal plane)

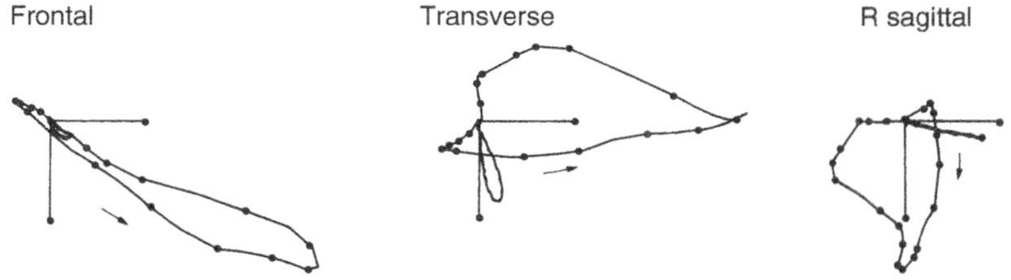

Fig. 1.32
VCG corresponding to the 12-lead ECG of ➋ Fig. 1.27. The loops were derived using the inverse Dower technique. There is counterclockwise inscription of the QRS loop in the frontal and transverse planes and clockwise inscription of the R sagittal plane. The T-wave loop is prominent in the transverse plane being at one extreme of the normal range. Dots are printed at 4 ms intervals

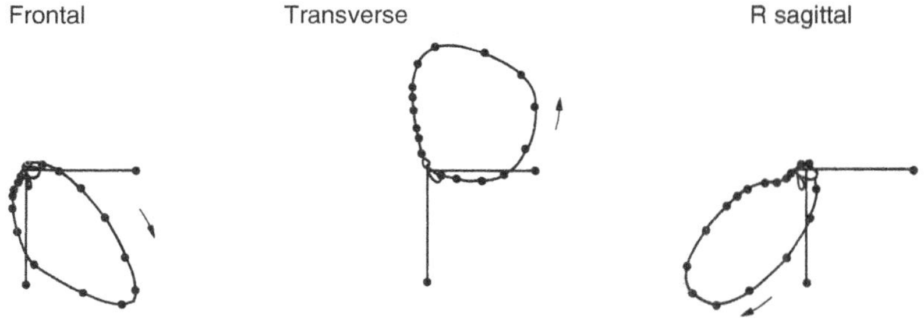

Fig. 1.33
VCG corresponding to the 12-lead ECG of ➋ Fig. 1.28. The loops were derived using the inverse Dower technique. Note the openness of this type of normal VCG loop. Dots are printed at 4 ms intervals. In the frontal and R sagittal planes, the QRS loop shows clockwise inscription, and in the transverse plane, it shows counterclockwise inscription

1.6.1.1 Frontal Plane

In the frontal plane, the P loop tends to be inscribed counterclockwise. On the other hand, the QRS loop can be inscribed either in a clockwise or counterclockwise direction. Chou and Helm [83] have suggested that about 65% of individuals have a loop that is inscribed in a clockwise direction. On average, the initial QRS vectors in the frontal plane are directed superiorly to the right, corresponding to small Q waves in X and Y. However, the absence of such small Q waves will alter the orientation of the initial vectors (the two are intimately related). For example, a Q wave in lead X *per se* means that the initial QRS vector is directed to the right, whereas a Q wave in lead Y means that the initial QRS vector is directed superiorly. There are therefore four possible combinations all of which can occur in the normal VCG.

The T loop in the frontal plane can be inscribed in either direction that need not necessarily be the same as that of the QRS loop. The maximum T vector is generally directed inferiorly to the left with a mean of around 35°.

1.6.1.2 Transverse Plane

The initial portion of the P loop in the transverse plane is always described in a counterclockwise direction. The whole loop may be similarly directed although there is often a figure-of-eight appearance. The maximum T vector can lie to either side of the X axis giving a wide range of normal values. The QRS loop is almost always inscribed in a counterclockwise direction in this plane. In a very small percentage of subjects, there may be a narrow figure-of-eight configuration where the initial part of the loop is inscribed in a counterclockwise direction with the early QRS vectors being oriented anteriorly. Likewise, the T loop is more often than not inscribed in a clockwise direction. Occasionally, however, the loop may be narrow, there being difficulty in determining an exact direction of inscription at least in one particular plane. In this case, the explanation is that the loop itself is essentially perpendicular to the transverse plane so that its projection produces a thin elongated loop.

1.6.1.3 Right Sagittal Plane

It is probably true to say that the right sagittal plane is utilized least of all by vectorcardiographers. The reason is that if appearances in the frontal and transverse planes are available, then the total information is already on display. However, the redundancy of information is often helpful in confirming impressions gained from other projections. In this plane, the P loop tends to be oriented vertically with the inscription always being clockwise. The QRS loop also has a generally inferior displacement and is usually inscribed in a clockwise direction. As with the transverse plane, the initial forces are directed anteriorly and either superiorly or inferiorly depending on the presence or absence, respectively, of a Q wave in lead Y. The T loop in this plane is also inscribed in a clockwise direction in most cases.

1.7 Normal Limits

1.7.1 Electrocardiographic Parameters

The methods of measuring ECG variables have already been discussed in ➋ Sect. 1.2.4. Before presenting and discussing the normal limits, it remains to describe in more detail the actual measurements to be tabulated. The principal measurements of the ECG waveform are outlined in ➋ Fig. 1.34. Note that these amplitudes and durations are referred to well-defined onsets and terminations of the component waves. In practice, as shown earlier in ➋ Fig. 1.10, the onset of the first wave in one lead need not necessarily coincide with the apparent onset in other leads. This leads to the concept of introducing isoelectric segments within the QRS complex, as shown in ➋ Fig. 1.11. The diagnostic significance of these segments has not yet been evaluated, but they have a relationship to vector orientations in a certain sense.

When computer analysis is available for the measurement of wave amplitudes and durations, it becomes feasible to make a number of additional measurements to assist in the characterization of a waveform. While the human eye at a glance may be able to say whether or not an ST segment is concave or convex upward, it requires several measurements

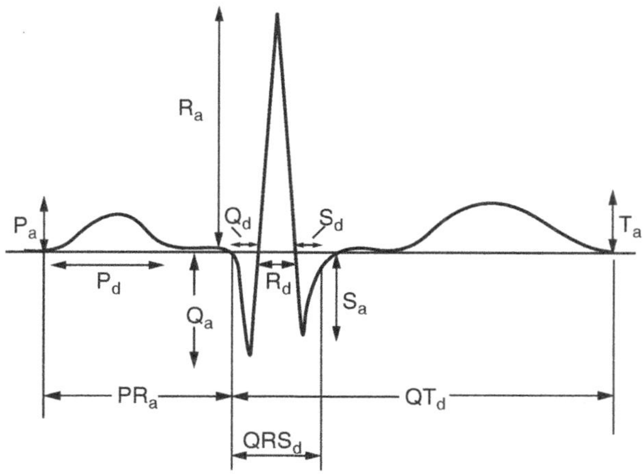

Fig. 1.34
Various component amplitudes (subscript a) and durations (subscript d) normally measured by a computer program. Note that here the reference level for all amplitude measurements is the QRS onset

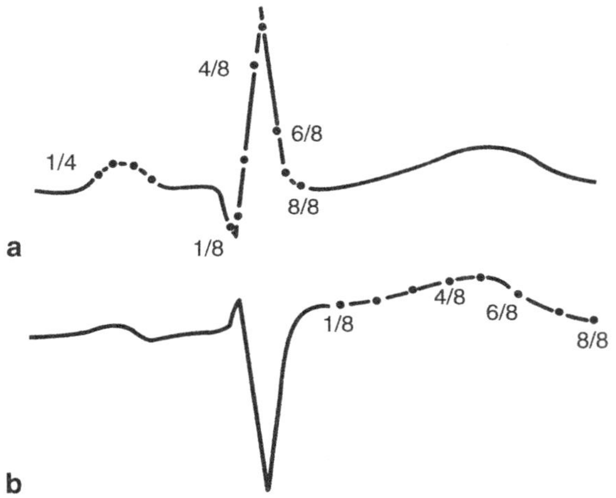

Fig. 1.35
An illustration of time normalization of (a) the P wave, which is divided into four, and the QRS complex, which is divided into eight, and (b) the ST-T segment, which is divided into eight equally spaced intervals

to establish this when using a computer program. For this reason, Pipberger and coworkers [32] introduced the concept of time normalization. With this approach, a component of the ECG such as the QRS complex can be divided into eight equal time intervals and the measurement made at the end of each of these. The ST-T segment can be dealt with in the same way. It was also subsequently suggested [84] that the P wave be divided into four equal time-normalized segments (➋ Fig. 1.35). This approach has certain advantages, but it can suffer from errors in determining the onset and termination of the components.

Another approach for categorizing the P and ST-T segments is to use a simple classification dealing with the number of components – up to two – together with a sign indicating whether the first component is positive or negative. As shown in ➋ Fig. 1.36, the P or T waves can be negative–positive or positive–negative in configuration, giving a categorization −2 or +2, respectively. An upright T wave would be classed as +1, and an inverted T wave as −1. This simple approach can also be very helpful in automated interpretation.

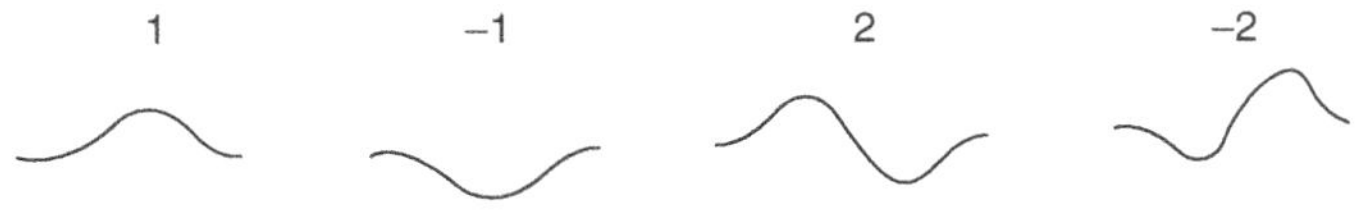

Fig. 1.36
A simplistic approach to classification of P waves or T waves depending on the number of components present and whether the first is positive or negative

Table 1.6
Expressions for estimation of the magnitude and orientation of the projection of the maximum spatial vector onto the frontal, sagittal, and transverse planes. *X, Y,* and *Z* are the amplitude values of leads *X, Y,* and *Z* at the instant the maximum spatial vector occurs

Plane	Magnitude	Orientation
Frontal	$(X^2+Y^2)^{1/2}$	$\tan^{-1}(Y/X)$
Right sagittal	$(Y^2+Z^2)^{1/2}$	$\tan^{-1}(-Y/Z)$
Left sagittal	$(Y^2+Z^2)^{1/2}$	$\tan^{-1}(Y/Z)$
Transverse	$(X^2+Z^2)^{1/2}$	$\tan^{-1}(-Z/X)$

The use of the VCG leads to many new parameters. While time normalization has been introduced for the measurement of scalar amplitudes, it can, of course, be carried over to vectorcardiography on a one-to-one basis so that vector magnitudes and orientations at 1/8, 2/8, QRS, and so on can be determined. In vectorcardiography, it has also been a custom to measure vector amplitudes and orientations at 10 ms intervals following QRS onset and prior to QRS termination. Such parameters are known as the 0.01 s QRS vector, the −0.01 s QRS vector, and so on.

The various vector amplitudes can be described in a number of ways. The amplitude of a vector is calculated simply from the following equation:

$$(X^2+Y^2+Z^2)^{1/2}$$

where *X, Y,* and *Z* represent the amplitude of each of the leads *X, Y,* and *Z* at a particular instant in time (see Chap. 2 of *Basic Electrocardiology: Cardiac Electrophysiology, ECG Systems and Mathematical Modeling*). It is clear that the leads must be recorded simultaneously to ensure perfect time alignment. While this expression can be used to calculate the maximum spatial vector, there are a number of other possibilities that arise. For example, with the use of the three planes described previously, it becomes possible to estimate the magnitude and orientation of the projection of the maximum spatial vector onto each of these three planes. This can be obtained from the expressions in Table 1.6.

Other parameters sometimes utilized are those such as the half area vector, that is, the vector that divides the spatial loop into two equal areas. The direction of inscription of the loop can be calculated mathematically from the cross product of two vectors:

$$\vec{C} = \vec{A} \times \vec{B}$$

where $\vec{C}$ is a vector pointing either upward or downward, depending on whether the rotation of the vector between *A* to *B* is clockwise or counterclockwise, respectively. One final parameter of interest in dealing with the VCG is known as spatial velocity [85].

In some ways, this term is a misnomer in that it is supposed to represent the rate of movement of the tip of the cardiac vector through space, whereas the following equation for spatial velocity, SV, demonstrates that this is not actually the case.

$$SV = \frac{1}{\Delta t}[(\Delta X)^2 + (\Delta Y)^2 + (\Delta Z)^2]^{1/2}$$

where ΔX is the change in amplitude of *X* in time Δt, etc.

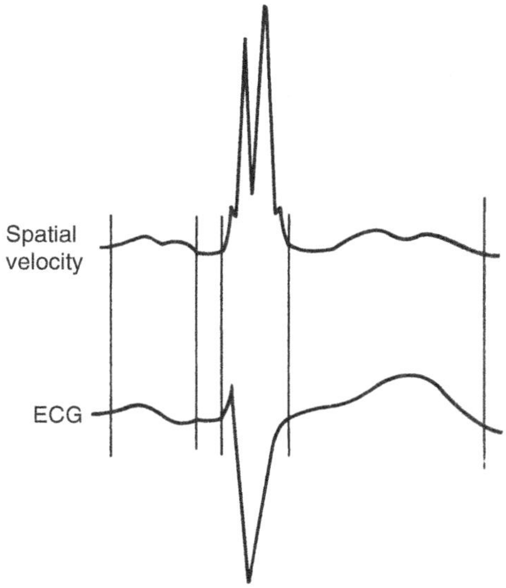

Fig. 1.37
A typical curve of spatial velocity and its time relationship to the ECG

A simplified estimate [86] of this measurement is given by the following equation, which is much more suited to rapid execution on a computer:

$$SV = \left|\frac{\Delta X}{\Delta t}\right| + \left|\frac{\Delta Y}{\Delta t}\right| + \left|\frac{\Delta Z}{\Delta t}\right|$$

Whichever equation is used, the appearance of the spatial velocity is as shown in Fig. 1.37. Through the years, there have been various publications [87, 88] that have suggested that the spatial velocity is of some help in discriminating between the different diagnostic classifications. In the main, however, it has tended to be used recently within computer programs in order to define the onset and termination of various ECG wave components. It has undoubted value in identifying parts of a vector loop where inscription slows. This would be found, for example, in the latter part of the QRS complex in an RBBB, where descriptive terms such as terminal slowing of the QRS inscription would be utilized.

1.7.2 P Wave

The normal limits of the P-wave amplitudes in various leads are as shown in Appendix 1. There are no statistically significant differences between mean P-wave amplitudes in men and women. In general, there is little tendency for the upper limits of the P-wave amplitude to decrease with increasing age in adults, as illustrated for lead II in Fig. 1.38. Of some interest may be the P terminal force in V_1, sometimes known as the Morris index [89], which is used in some diagnostic criteria such as the Romhilt-Estes criteria for LVH (see Chap. 3). Table 1.7 shows the normal limits for this estimate which does have a higher upper limit of normal in men compared to women.

It can also be seen from Appendix 2 that the P-wave amplitude in children in lead II, for example, varies very little between birth and 16 years of age and the upper limit of normal remains essentially static at 0.25 mV during this period.

The duration of the P wave is sometimes used in determining whether there is an abnormality of the left atrium. The normal P wave may often have two components, i.e. it may exhibit an M-shaped complex, and in general terms it has a duration that is less than 0.12 s (Table 1.7). A duration beyond this may possibly arise from the left atrial enlargement, causing a delay in the depolarization of the left atrium, or else from an intra-atrial conduction abnormality (see Chap. 2). Thus, in the presence of broad P waves, there is a tendency to diagnose a left atrial abnormality, that is,

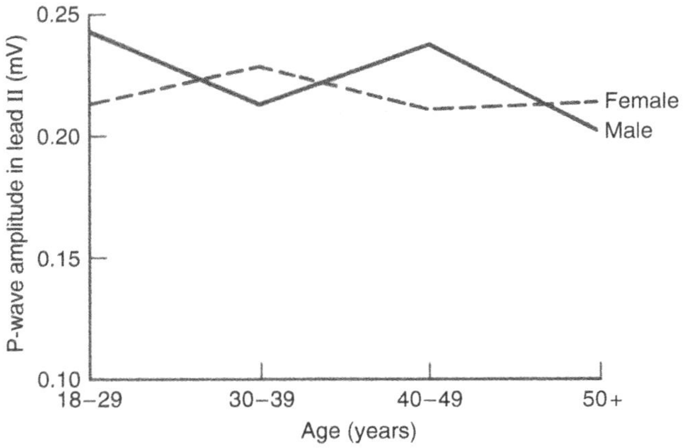

Fig. 1.38
The normal upper limit of the P-wave amplitude in lead II. Clearly, there is no age or sex dependence

Table 1.7
Mean ± standard deviations and 96% range of P terminal force in V_1 and P-wave durations

		P terminal force (mV ms)			P-wave duration (ms)		
Age-group	Sex	No of subjects (*n*)	Mean ± SD	96% range	No. of subjects (*n*)	Mean ± SD	96% range
18–29	Male	265	1.09 ± 1.33	0.00–4.62	266	103.0 ± 14.2	72 – 128
	Female	316	0.75 ± 1.03	0.00–3.54	318	99.0 ± 12.7	70 – 122
30–39	Male	219	1.61 ± 1.21	0.00–3.94	221	105.0 ± 12.3	78 – 130
	Female	118	1.02 ± 1.25	0.00–4.29	118	99.0 ± 11.6	72 – 122
40–49	Male	117	1.49 ± 1.44	0.00–4.42	119	106.0 ± 11.2	84 – 128
	Female	73	1.57 ± 1.40	0.00–5.50	73	104.0 ± 12.9	78 – 128
50+	Male	125	1.47 ± 1.44	0.00–5.45	125	110.0 ± 10.5	86 – 134
	Female	79	1.42 ± 1.37	0.00–4.05	80	106.0 ± 9.5	88 – 126

a nonspecific interpretation is made. There is a small increase in the P-wave duration with increasing age both in men and women (➋ Table 1.7), but this is of limited practical significance.

1.7.3 P Vector

The normal limits of the P-vector amplitude are shown in Appendix 1. In general terms, the P-vector loop is small and difficult to analyze, so there is not much additional benefit to be gained from the VCG in terms of the diagnostic value of the P wave.

1.7.4 QRS Complex

The means, standard deviations, and upper and lower limits of normal are set out in the various tables and illustrations in the Appendices. The scalar data relating to children have been taken from the work of Liebman [73] and Davignon et al. [76] as well as from the authors' lab. By way of explanation, a further illustration (➋ Fig. 1.39) dealing with the Q-wave amplitude in V_5 is reproduced for illustrative purposes. The graphs depict the percentile ranges of the Q-wave amplitude

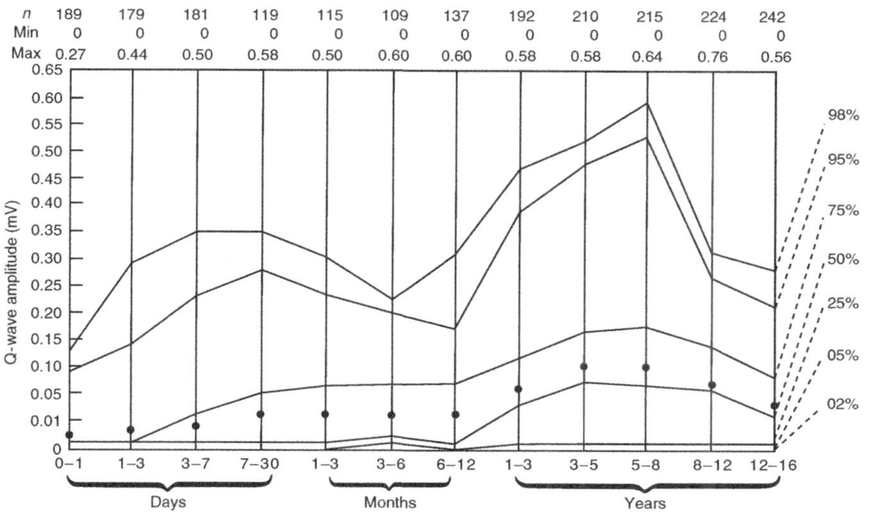

Fig. 1.39
The distribution of the Q-wave amplitude in V_5 in normal infants and children from birth to 16 years of age. In broad terms, the Q-wave amplitude increases to a maximum at 5–8 years before decreasing again. Note the scale is nonlinear (After Davignon et al. [76]. © Springer, New York. Reproduced with permission)

from birth to 16 years of age. The upper 98 percentile graph indicates the values within which 98% of the population studied had their Q-wave amplitude; for example, in the age-group 5–8 years, 98% of the 215 children studied had a Q wave in V_5 that was less than 0.60 mV. On the other hand, the lower 2 percentile curve indicates the value above which 98% of the groups studied had a Q-wave amplitude. Thus, in the same age-group of 5–8 years, there were 75% of the children who had a Q wave that was discernible. Within the meaning of 96 percentile ranges as discussed above, the 2 percentile and 98 percentile lines contain the 96% range of the amplitudes. Thus, these values can be regarded as the lower and upper normal limits of the range. The actual maximum value recorded in the study from which the graph was drawn was 0.65 mV for the age-group of 5–8 years. It should be noted that the mean value for the same group was 0.1 mV, which emphasizes the point previously made that the distribution of ECG measurements tends to be skewed, that is, it is not symmetrical about the mean. It is of importance to note that a Q wave in V_5 in excess of 0.5 mV is found in 5% of apparently healthy children in the above age range. In general terms, R-wave amplitudes tend to decrease with increasing age in children in the right precordial leads, whereas, as would be expected, they tend to increase in the left precordial leads.

➋ Table 1.8 summarizes some of the sex differences in R-wave amplitudes found by Davignon et al. in the age-group of 12–16 years. These data would tend to confirm findings of the authors' study, for example, where highly significant differences between men and women were found in the precordial leads.

From about the end of the first month of life, the R/S ratio in V_1 begins to decrease from an upper limit of approximately seven toward the adult value of approximately one. By the age of 5 years, the upper limit of normal has reduced quite considerably to a value of two. It is, of course, still very relevant to bear this in mind when interpreting ECGs from children. The data of Liebman and colleagues are also reproduced in Appendix 2. These show in numerical form the various limits of normality as determined manually from different groups of children. The same general trends can be seen both from the numerical and the graphical representation of results: scalar and vector data are presented.

The normal ranges of the adult ECG will be discussed mainly with respect to the authors' own data gathered from a study of apparently healthy individuals in Glasgow, as described in ➋ Sect. 1.2.1. The results presented mainly in Appendix 1 in numerical form have been derived from computer analysis of the ECG, where all leads were recorded simultaneously. Means, standard deviations, and 96 percentile normal ranges are presented for different age-groups that are also stratified according to sex. In order to compress some of the findings for the purposes of discussion, the upper

Table 1.8

Sex differences in R-wave amplitudes in the age-group 12–16 years. Mean values (mV), standard deviations (SD), and percentile limits are listed separately for 105 boys and 142 girls. D denotes the amplitude difference between the sexes

				Percentile limit				
Lead	Sex	Mean	Standard Deviation	02%	05%	50%	95%	98%
aVR	female	0.11	0.11	0.00	0.01	0.09	0.35	0.40
	Male	0.13	0.12	0.00	0.01	0.12	0.37	0.42
	D	0.02 NS[a]						
aVL	Female	0.23	0.18	0.01	0.03	0.18	0.62	0.70
	Male	0.23	0.20	0.01	0.02	0.19	0.60	0.86
	D	0.00 NS						
aVF	Female	0.96	0.33	0.27	0.35	0.95	1.53	1.66
	Male	1.05	0.41	0.17	0.33	1.06	1.73	2.04
	D	0.09 NS						
V_1	Female	0.37	0.23	0.01	0.04	0.35	0.85	0.96
	Male	0.44	0.25	0.02	0.05	0.42	0.94	1.03
	D	0.07[b]						
V_2	Female	0.92	0.36	0.28	0.36	0.87	1.63	1.72
	Male	1.11	0.40	0.23	0.44	1.11	1.79	1.94
	D	0.19[c]						
V_4	Female	1.76	0.57	0.61	0.76	1.74	2.79	3.32
	Male	2.58	0.72	1.11	1.36	2.55	3.81	3.94
	D	0.82[c]						
V_5	Female	1.66	0.50	0.63	0.83	1.63	2.73	2.99
	Male	2.40	0.60	1.09	1.29	2.41	3.39	3.47
	D	0.74[c]						
V_6	Female	1.23	0.30	0.59	0.72	1.22	1.78	1.91
	Male	1.58	0.40	0.80	1.01	1.59	2.23	2.41
	D	0.35[c]						

[a]Nonsignificant difference
[b]$p < 0.05$
[c]$p < 0.0001$

limits of normal for various measurements and different age-groups have been amalgamated into graphs following the style of Simonson [2]. In addition, the limb leads have been, on occasion, treated similarly, and the continuity of sequence in the limb-lead axes, namely aVL, I, −aVR, II, aVF, and III is maintained as shown in ➲ Figs. 1.40–1.42. The presentation of scalar leads in this sequence was suggested by Cabrera [90] and is favored by many Europeans, particularly in Scandinavia. This presentation was also used by Lundh in his illustrations [3].

The upper limits of normal voltage for the QRS complex in the precordial leads decrease with increasing age. This is more evident for males than it is for females. Conversely, in the limb leads, the upper limit of normal in the lateral leads I and aVL remains stable although the mean value increases with age, which is in keeping with the rotation of the mean QRS axis superiorly in the frontal plane. This corresponds to the upper limit of normal of the frontal plane QRS axis shifting from -10° to -30° as age changes from young adulthood to middle age. A corollary of this is that the R-wave amplitude in aVF decreases with increasing age.

The sum of the S-wave amplitude in V_1 plus the R-wave amplitude in V_5 (one of the Sokolow and Lyon criteria [91] for LVH) is often used by electrocardiographers. The illustration of ➲ Fig. 1.43 shows that in apparently healthy young males, the index can have an upper limit of 5.0 mV. Thus, the commonly used threshold of 3.5 mV for LVH would be somewhat nonspecific if applied to younger individuals.

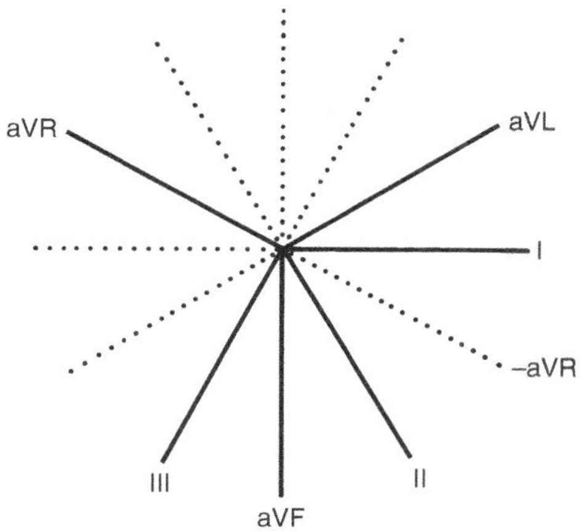

Fig. 1.40
The hexaxial lead system showing the relationship of aVR, that is, an inverted aVR to the other limb leads

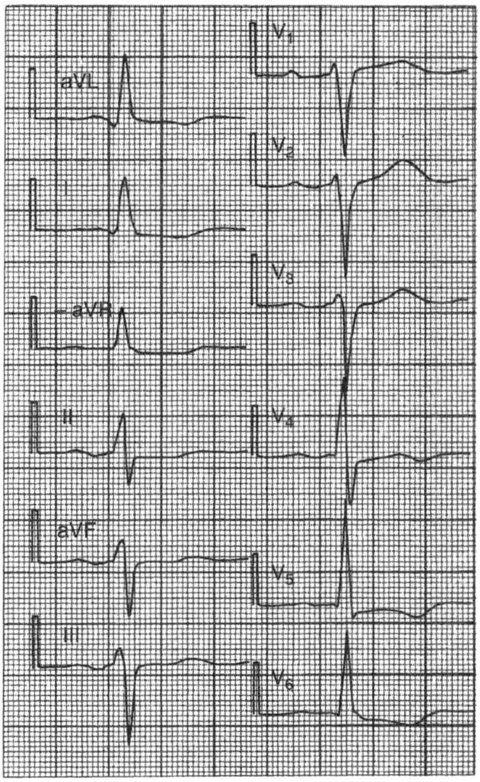

Fig. 1.41
A 12-lead ECG displayed using the format suggested by Cabrera. All 12 leads were recorded simultaneously. Note the presence of aVR and the sequence of the limb leads in keeping with the order of the lead axes, as shown in Fig. 1.40

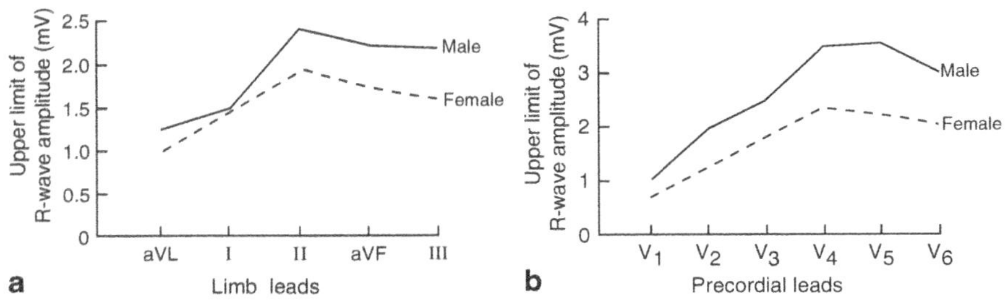

Fig. 1.42
The upper limit of the R-wave amplitude in (a) limb leads and (b) precordial leads derived from apparently healthy individuals aged 18–29 years inclusive. Note the large differences between upper limits for males and females

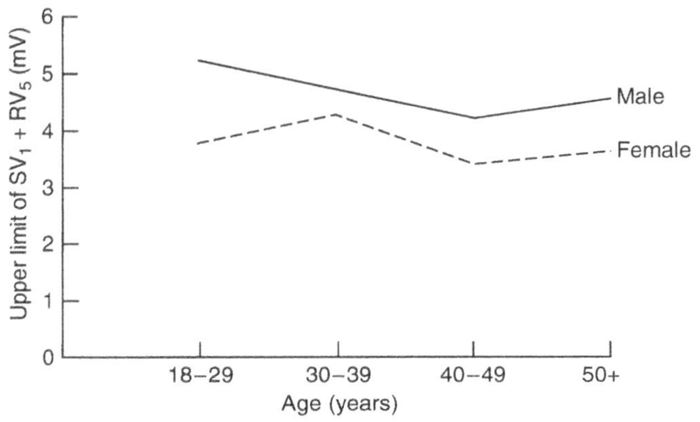

Fig. 1.43
The upper limit of normal of the Sokolow and Lyon index [91], that is, $SV_1 + RV_5$, for males and females, as derived from the Glasgow data. Note in particular how this exceeds the classically used limit of 3.5 mV, particularly in males

1.7.5 Additional Chest Leads

The use of right-sided chest leads (V_4R, for example) in adults has been confined to diagnosing right ventricular hypertrophy (RVH) and, more recently, right ventricular involvement in inferior myocardial infarction. Data on normal limits of such leads are sparse, but Andersen et al. [92] studied 109 subjects without evidence of heart disease in order to derive data on leads V_3R–V_7R. The R-wave amplitude and ST junctional deviation are presented in Table 1.9.

Additional data can be found in the Appendices. Reddy et al. also published a short note on the normal limits of V_7–V_9 [93]. More recently, in our own lab, normal limits of additional chest leads V_7–V_9 as well as V_3R–V_6R were derived from 200 adults [94]. In broad terms, an upper limit of 0.05 mV for the ST_j amplitude is applicable in all such leads except for males in V_3R and V_4R where 0.1 mV is a more specific limit to apply. This work led to such recommendations in a recent guidelines paper [95]. A typical set of waveforms from six simultaneously recorded right-sided chest leads is shown in Fig. 1.44. In children, V_4R is used widely even up to adolescence, while some centers also use V_3R.

The availability of computer methods for the estimation of durations has probably not been capitalized on to any great extent so far. Figure 1.45 shows the normal range of Q-wave durations in aVF for 1,334 adults in our series. From this, it can be seen that the 96 percentile upper limit of normal is approximately 25 ms for males and a little less for females. Conventional criteria [96] for interpreting Q-wave durations normally utilize 30 ms or even 40 ms Q waves. This, of course, is a reflection on manual methods of measurement, and our new data would suggest that, together with other signs of myocardial injury, such as ST- or T-wave change, a Q-wave duration in excess of 25 ms would provide reasonable

Table 1.9
Mean and 95% ranges of r, S, and r′ amplitudes in right precordial leads

	Median	95% fractile values	Mean $\bar{x}$	Range	Number *n*
r-wave amplitude (mm)	V_3R 1.5	0.4–3.9	1.7	0.1–4.3	107
	V_4R 1.0	0.3–3.3	1.2	0.2–4.2	101
	V_5R 1.0	0.3–2.4	1.0	0.2–5.0	79
	V_6R 0.7	0.2–2.6	0.9	0.2–5.1	59
	V_7R 0.5	0.3–3.6	1.0	0.3–5.6	37
S-wave amplitude (mm)	V_3R 5.1	1.7–11.4	5.7	0.9–13.5	108
	V_4R 3.6	1.1–8.0	3.9	0.9–9.7	104
	V_5R 3.6	1.0–7.7	3.5	0.5–8.8	89
	V_6R 2.5	0.7–6.4	2.9	0.4–7.3	70
	V_7R 2.7	0.8–5.4	2.8	0.7–6.8	45
Secondary r-wave (qr, rSr′) amplitudes (mm)	V_3R 0.8	0.5–1.5	0.9	0.4–1.5	6
	V_4R 0.7	0.2–1.8	0.8	0.2–1.8	11
	V_5R 0.8	0.3–2.5	1.0	0.2–2.5	36
	V_6R 0.9	0.3–3.6	1.3	0.2–4.2	50
	V_7R 0.9	0.3–3.6	1.2	0.1–4.8	71

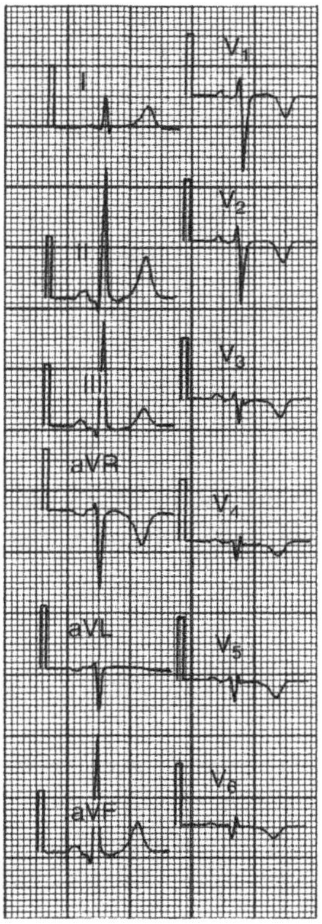

Fig. 1.44
Six simultaneously recorded right-sided chest leads are shown together with the limb leads. These were recorded from a healthy 45-year-old male. Note that the labels V_1–V_6 are equivalent to V_2, V_1, V_3R–V_6R

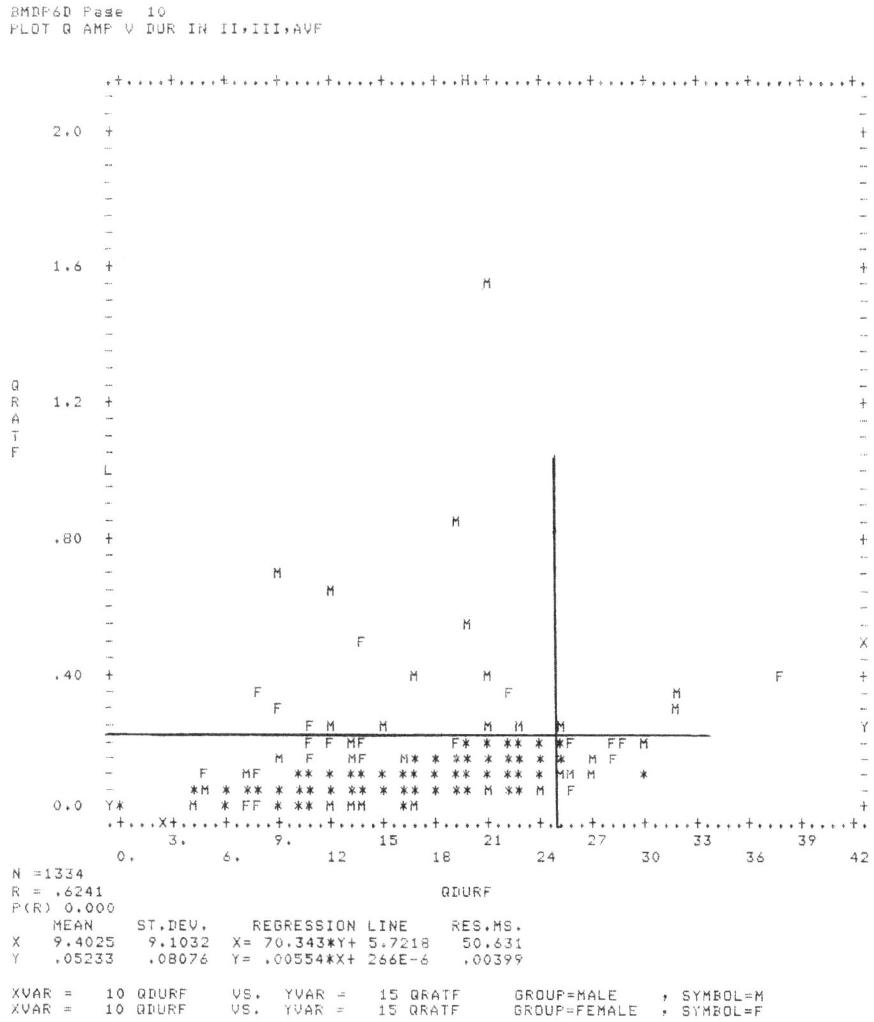

Fig. 1.45
Scattergram of Q duration in aVF against the Q/R ratio in aVF for 1,334 adults in the Glasgow study. The 96 percentile limits for each are shown, that is, the *bottom left-hand square* contains the normal values. *M* male, *F* female; *, more than one value at the same point on the plot

grounds for suggesting that myocardial infarction was present. The same figure shows that the upper limit of normal Q:R in aVF is almost exactly 1:4.

The significance of a Q wave in V_1 has been the matter of some controversy. The authors' data show that many apparently healthy individuals (1.42%) have a Q wave in V_1, while 0.67% have a Q wave in both V_1 and V_2. On the other hand, Lundh [3] raised the question of whether the Q wave in V_1 might be related to the presence or absence of a Q wave in V_6. He suggested that a Q wave in V_1 in the absence of such a wave in V_6 was abnormal. The authors' own normal data suggests that this finding has a specificity of 100%.

The effect of race on QRS amplitudes has already been mentioned in ➲ Sect. 1.4.3. In this respect, there has been a dearth of large-scale studies on which to confirm the findings. Data available from studies on 1,329 Japanese [97] are presented in Appendix 1. In this study, published in 1963, data were measured by hand and 100% ranges were quoted. A search of the literature has revealed no substantial publications dealing with studies on South Asians, while other studies on Chinese individuals [56, 59, 98, 99] have suggested that there may be a modest difference between such populations and Caucasians with respect to QRS amplitudes and some other measures. This would tend to be at variance with the larger studies on Japanese individuals.

1.7.6 QRS Loop

The various limits of normal for the QRS vectors are detailed in the Appendices. These include many of the measurements that have been discussed above, but it should be noted that the tables are, on occasion, taken from studies where different lead systems have been used. In each case, the description of the lead system has been clearly indicated, and details of the different lead systems can be found in ➋ Chap. 11 of *Basic Electrocardiology : Cardiac Electrophysiology, ECG Systems and Mathematical Modeling*. The evolution and normal appearances of the VCG have been discussed in ➋ Sect. 1.6. It must be obvious that the comments relating to age and sex differences of the ECG also apply to the VCG. The variation of the normal limits of the T-vector magnitude with age and sex are shown in ➋ Fig. 1.46. Again, it can be seen that the vector magnitude decreases with increasing age and, in general, is lower for women than men. The maximum T vector in the transverse plane also shifts anteriorly with increasing age, whereas the mean T-vector projection onto the frontal plane tends to be stable around 40° once the adult pattern develops.

The normal limits of maximum spatial velocity are shown in ➋ Fig. 1.47 where a typical normal curve is also contrasted with the curves of spatial velocity in patients with different clinical abnormalities. Sano [87] in particular laid great stress on the value of spatial velocity, although this was never confirmed by others. The work of Macfarlane et al. [88] suggested that although there was undoubtedly variation in spatial-velocity curves between one group of patients and another, these did not lead to improved diagnoses. In other words, since the spatial velocity is a derivative of other leads, the information contained therein should also be available in the original waveforms.

1.7.7 ST-T Wave

The interpretation of the ST-T wave is one of the most difficult aspects of electrocardiography, and it should therefore be based on a thorough knowledge of the normal limits of this component of the ECG. The ST amplitude is normally measured at the end of the QRS complex, although, in certain instances, such as for exercise testing, a point 60 or 80 ms after the end of the QRS is now commonly used. For the purposes of this chapter, however, the ST junction will be regarded as the end of the QRS complex.

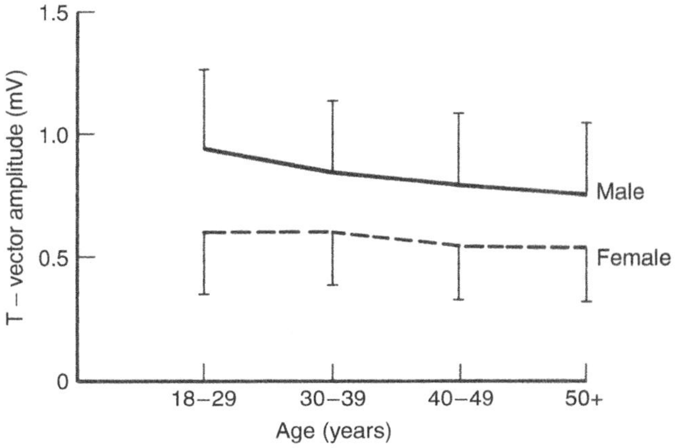

Fig. 1.46
Mean and standard deviation of the T-vector amplitude in males and females in the Glasgow study. There is little variation with age but significant differences with respect to sex

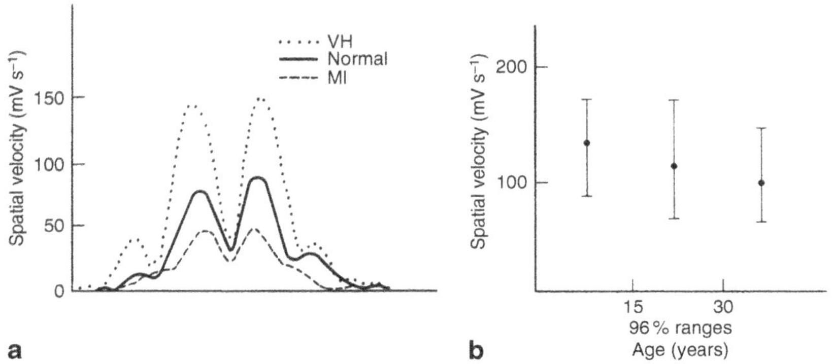

Fig. 1.47
(a) Representative curves of spatial velocity from a patient with ventricular hypertrophy (VH), another with myocardial infarction (MI) contrasted with a normal curve. (b) Means and 96 percentile ranges of spatial velocity from 265 healthy individuals, including 18 under 15 years of age, 94 under 29 years of age, and 153 aged 30 and over (See [88] for further details)

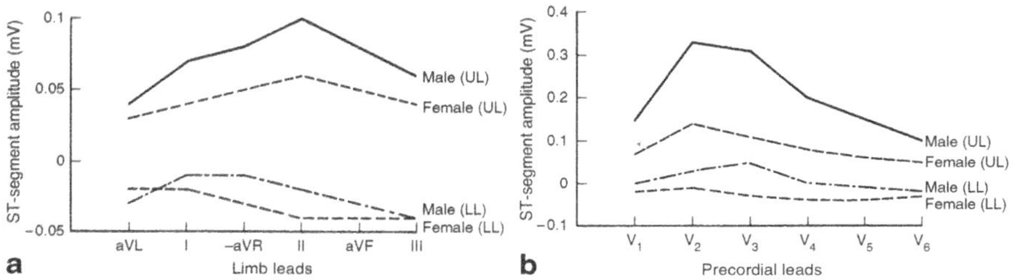

Fig. 1.48
The upper and lower limits of ST amplitude for apparently healthy males and females: (a) limb leads and (b) precordial leads. Note the considerable sex differences in the upper limits (UL) and the more negative lower limit (LL) of ST depression in females, particularly in the limb leads

Data on ST amplitude variation in children is sparse, though our own data in Appendix 2 present tables of normal limits of ST amplitude in this age-group. As expected, the upper normal limit of ST amplitude is generally under 0.1 mV in most leads, though it is higher in some precordial leads.

In general terms, in adults, with the exception of aVR, the ST segment amplitude would be expected to be in excess of −0.05 mV when the heart rate is less than 100 bpm. In the limb leads, there is a small difference of the order of 30 μV in the upper limit of normal ST amplitude between men and women (➋ Fig. 1.48) and a small difference with respect to age (➋ Fig 1.49a). On the other hand, in the precordial leads, there are highly significant differences between men and women and there is a tendency for the ST amplitude to decrease with increasing age particularly for males in the anteroseptal leads V_2–V_4. Some of these changes can be seen in ➋ Fig. 1.49b. The increased ST amplitude in young men in particular is sometimes related to increased vagal tone (vagotonia) and is of no particular significance. It is always associated with a normally shaped ST-T complex in healthy young individuals. There are significant differences between males and females in ST amplitudes in the precordial leads, and also there are significant differences between leads, for example, the upper limit of normal ST amplitude in males in V_1 is twice the upper limit in V_2 both in males (➋ Fig. 1.49c) and females (➋ Fig. 1.49d). This implies that criteria for acute myocardial injury should not be the same in V_1 and V_2.

ST amplitudes of up to 0.1 mV can be found in apparently healthy individuals in the inferior and lateral leads. Sometimes this pattern is referred to as early repolarization. This is often accompanied by a small notch at the end of the QRS complex, particularly in the precordial leads [100]. On occasion, it may be difficult to ascertain whether the ST elevation in a young person is a result of some other abnormality, such as pericarditis, as opposed to being a normal variant.

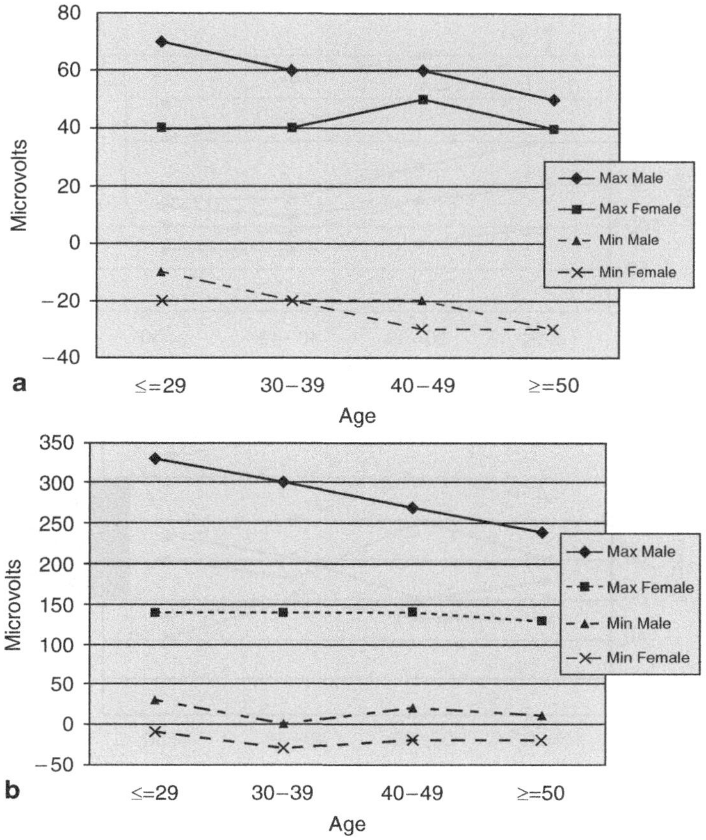

Fig. 1.49a, b
(a) Upper and lower limits of normal ST amplitude in lead I in Caucasian men and women. (b) Upper and lower limits of normal ST amplitude in V_2 in Caucasian men and women. Note the very significant difference in the upper limit of normal between males and females, particularly in the younger age-groups (Reproduced with permission from J Electrocardiol 2001; 34(Suppl): 235–41)

In such situations, the extent of the ST elevation has to be considered, it being generally more widespread when associated with an abnormality such as pericarditis [101].

It should also be noted that race can influence ST amplitude. Our own data on Chinese and Caucasian normals [56, 58] showed minor differences only, but our most recent work together with Dr. Ibraheem Katibi from the University of Ilorin in Nigeria [55] shows that black males have higher mean and maximum STj values than Caucasians particularly in precordial leads such as V_2, while there is a similar but much less marked trend in females (Fig. 1.50). The ST amplitude in lateral leads shows greater similarity.

The normal ranges of ST-segment slope in Caucasians were evaluated for some of the limb and precordial leads and are presented in the Appendices. Of major interest is the fact that on average, ST slope is always higher in males than females in the leads studied (I, aVF, V_2, V_5, and V_6). It also decreases with increasing age. It was highest in V_2 and lowest in aVF though virtually always positive.

The various T-wave amplitudes, normal ranges, and so on are tabulated in the Appendices. The upper and lower limits of T-wave amplitudes in summary form are illustrated in Fig. 1.51. T-wave amplitudes vary considerably with age and sex, as mentioned in Sect. 1.4. Particularly over the early weeks of life, the T-wave amplitudes in the right precordial leads vary considerably. While the T-wave amplitude can remain inverted in V_1 throughout life, the T wave in V_2 becomes

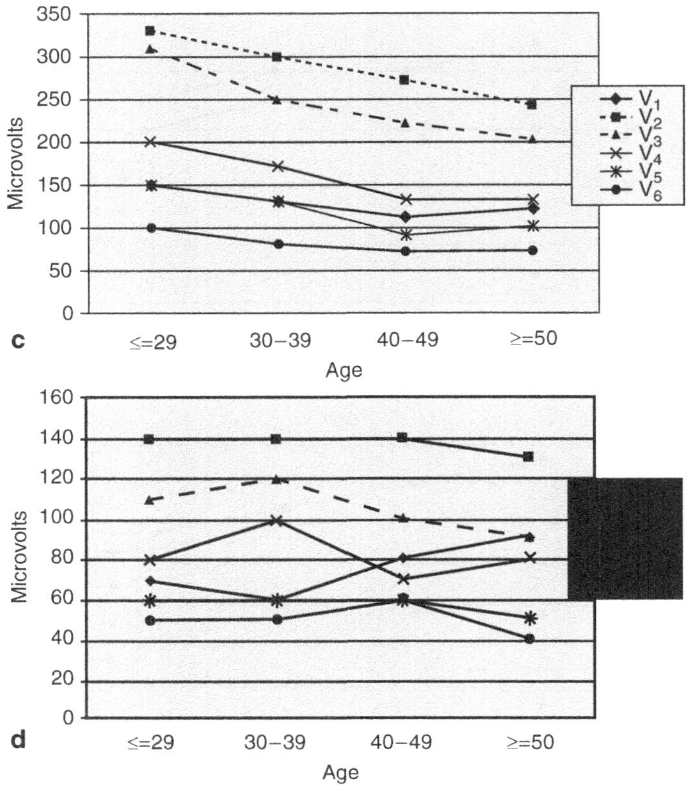

Fig. 1.49c, d
(c) Upper limits of normality for the ST amplitude in the precordial leads for males aged over 18 years. (d) Upper limits of normality for the ST amplitude in the precordial leads for females aged over 18 years (Reproduced with permission from J Electrocardiol 2001; 34(Suppl): 235–41)

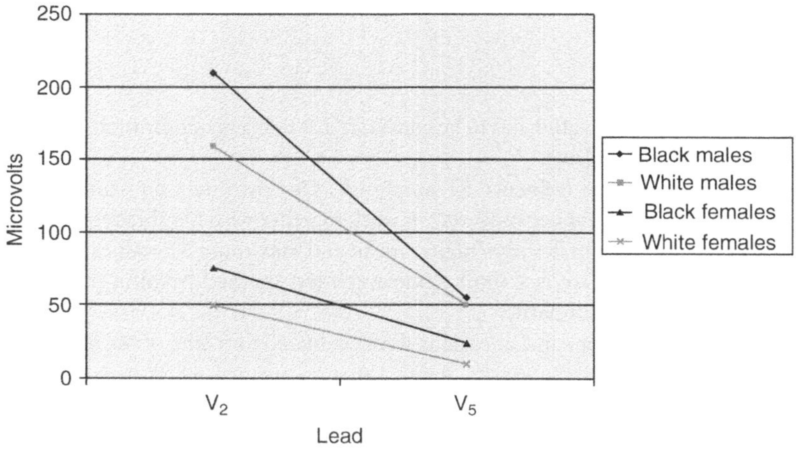

Fig. 1.50
A comparison of the mean ST amplitude for V_2 and V_5 in 123 healthy black males and 97 females aged 18–29 years living in Nigeria versus data from 266 healthy Caucasian males and 317 healthy Caucasian females in the same age range

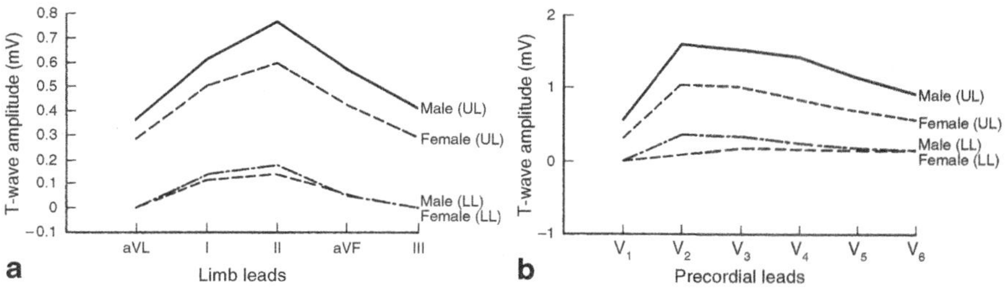

Fig. 1.51
The upper and lower limits (UL and LL, respectively) of normal T-wave amplitude in apparently healthy individuals in the Glasgow study: (a) limb leads and (b) precordial leads. The most obvious difference is in the upper limits of normal that are sex dependent

upright in most people by the age of 12. Nevertheless, T-wave inversion in V_2 particularly in women can often present a diagnostic problem.

In general terms as for the ST segment, the T-wave amplitude in men is much higher than in women, particularly in the precordial leads. Again, however, this difference tends to diminish with increasing age.

From the authors' own data on 601 females, it was found that T-wave inversion in V_2 is indeed an isolated finding and that the lower limit of the normal range for women in this lead is positive. An isolated T-wave abnormality in V_2 in the absence of any other clinical findings should be regarded as equivocal. The range of T-wave amplitudes in V_3 in women shows a similar distribution in that in apparently healthy individuals, the T wave is always positive in this lead. On the other hand, T in V_2 was always positive in men. Similarly, T-wave inversion in the inferior leads, particularly aVF, often presents a diagnostic problem in apparently healthy young men and women.

Our own data in this respect are shown in Fig. 1.52. From this, it can be seen that T-wave inversion up to 0.065 mV occurs in about 4% of healthy women of all ages. This is slightly at variance with the findings of others [3], but may simply be owing to the composition of the different samples. They are, however, in keeping with the data of Simonson [2].

The normal ranges of the T loop are presented in the Appendices. The various comments made for the scalar amplitude also apply to the T-vector loop. In other words, in the frontal plane in women, the T vector may occasionally be superior to 0°, in keeping with shallow inverted T waves in lead Y.

1.7.8 Time Intervals

The advent of simultaneous recording of all 12 leads means that it is possible to compare the apparent onset of the QRS complex in V_6, for example, with the onset in V_1. There can, of course, be only one true QRS onset relating to the start of ventricular activation, but because of the projection of the corresponding electrical activity onto the different lead axes, there can be time delays in the detection of electrical activity in the various leads. Figure 1.53 shows the time intervals measured between the apparent onsets of QRS in V_6 and V_1. It would be expected perhaps that the onset in V_1 would be earlier than in V_6, since septal activation tends to occur from the left to the right of the septum (though anteriorly), thereby giving maximum electrical projection on the V_1 axis and almost zero electrical projection in the direction of V_6. This indeed was found to be the case in the vast majority of ECGs, but nevertheless, there was a sizable group in our normals where electrical activity apparently started earlier in V_6 than in V_1. This, of course, could be a result of measurement error or of a septal activation vector that was essentially directed to the right, that is, oppositely to V_6, producing a small Q wave in V_6 and virtually zero electrical activity in V_1. As yet, few diagnostic criteria have evolved from such simultaneous 12-lead ECG recordings: this is one area of possible development in the future.

The PR interval has diagnostic relevance in relation to the evolution of conduction problems in the heart. In general terms, the PR interval decreases with the increasing heart rate as can be seen particularly in children (see Fig. 1.54). However, at increasingly high rates, it becomes more difficult to determine the precise onset of the P wave, and therefore a degree of uncertainty then enters into the PR-interval estimation. In general terms, PR interval is less than 0.18 ms

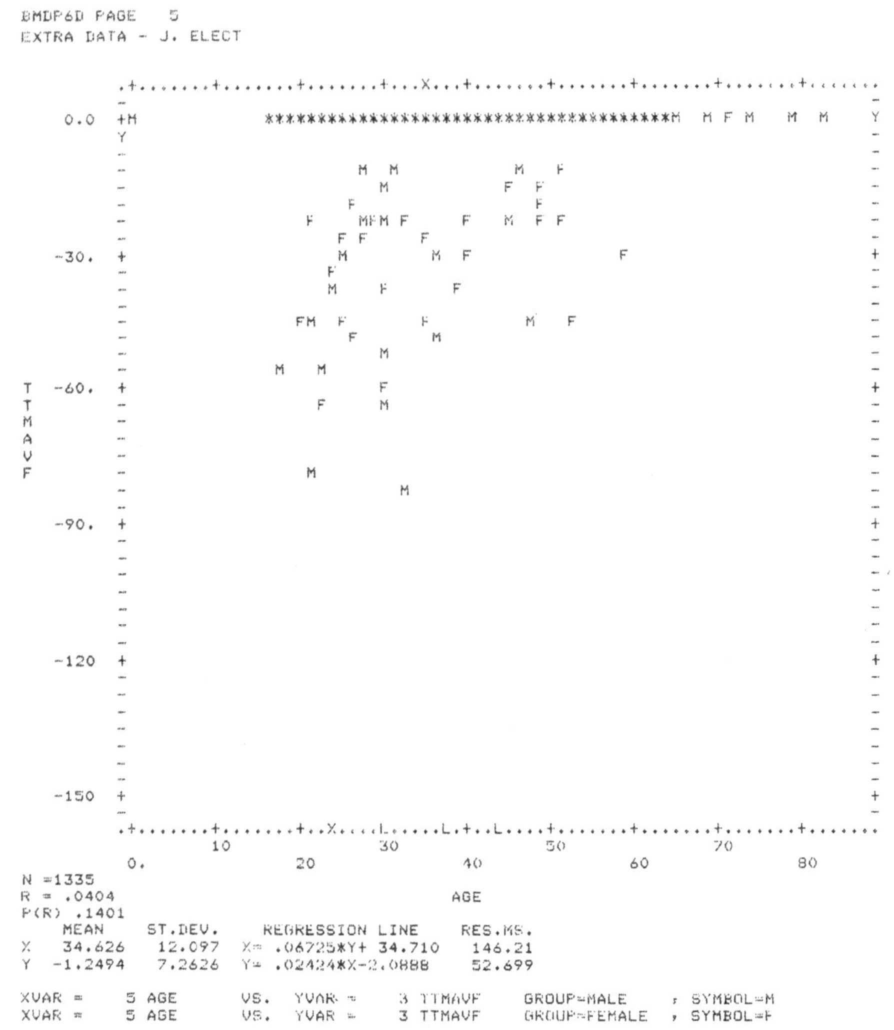

Fig. 1.52
Scattergram of negative T-wave components in a VF with respect to age: *M* male, *F* female. Note that the larger values of negative T amplitude (microvolts) are more often present in young men than young women

in children and young adults. However, the upper limit of normal gradually increases from 150 up to 175 ms as the age increases from 1 to 16 years. On the other hand, considering the variation in the heart rate for a fixed PR interval, it can also be seen from ➋ Fig. 1.54 that the 96 percentile range for the heart rate, when the PR duration is 150 ms, varies from approximately 75 up to 135 bpm. Conversely, at a rate of 140 bpm, the PR varies up to approximately 150 ms. In the adult (➋ Table 1.3), the authors' own data suggests that there is a small but significant difference between the upper limits of normal for males and females, particularly at rates below 80 bpm. The upper limit of normal for males is 210 ms, while for females it is 196 ms. No doubt these very small differences result from the smaller heart size in women.

The QRS duration decreases with increasing age and is shorter in women compared to men. The values are shown in ➋ Table 1.3. Because the upper limit of normal in men is a little higher than in women, some diagnostic criteria for conduction defects take limited cognizance of this finding [64]. The authors' data show 7 ms difference between males

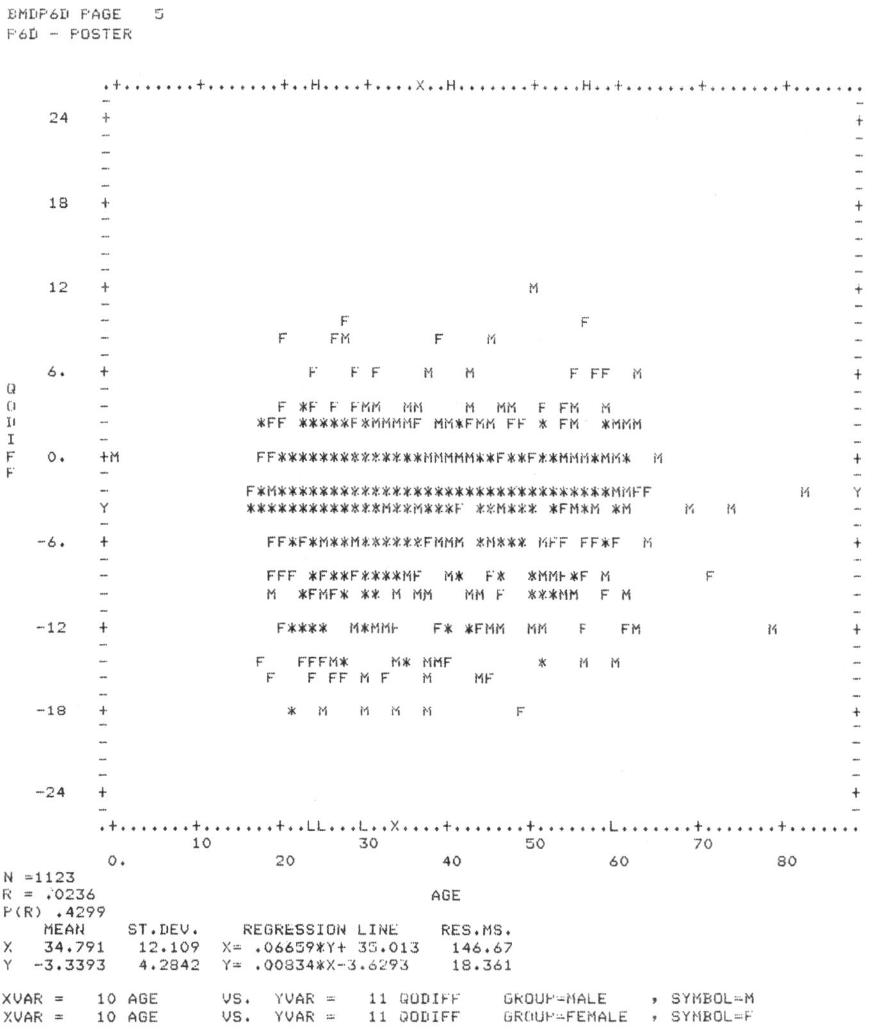

Fig. 1.53

Scattergram of the difference in time between the QRS onset in V_1 and V_6. A negative value denotes a later onset in V_6. The 96 percentile range is from −16 to +4 ms. The vast majority of individuals clearly demonstrate a later onset in V_6 than in VI

and females with respect to the mean normal QRS duration. The data for children are shown in the Appendices where it can be seen that the upper limit of normal QRS duration tends to 0.90 s.

In a comparison of white and black subjects, Pipberger et al. [60] found that on average the QRS duration was 7 ms shorter in black men. In the authors' own comparison of Chinese and Western subjects, no significant difference in QRS durations could be detected. Unless identical methods are used, it is probably not meaningful to compare measurements from different studies. One other QRS interval of some interest is the intrinsicoid deflection or ventricular activation time (VAT). This is the time from the onset of the QRS complex to the peak of the R wave (see Fig. 1.55). This time can be interpreted in a precordial lead as the interval from the onset of ventricular depolarization to the instant that the activation wavefront reaches the area under the electrode. The term more accurately applies to an epicardial electrode. A prolonged intrinsicoid deflection (> 50 ms in V_5) is sometimes used as one of the criteria for LVH.

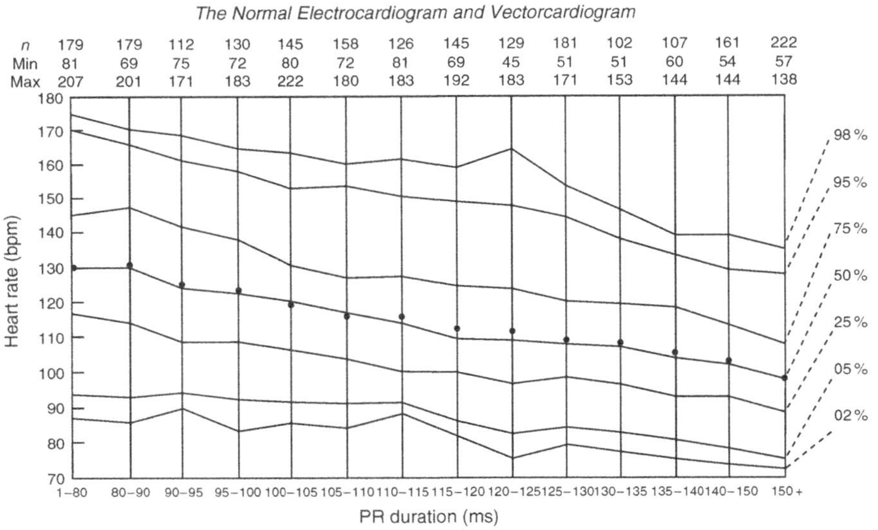

Fig. 1.54
The relationship between PR interval and heart rate. The PR interval decreases with increasing heart rate, from 150 ms and over, to 80 ms as the mean rate increases from approximately 100 to 130 bpm (After Davignon et al. [76]. Springer, New York. Reproduced with permission)

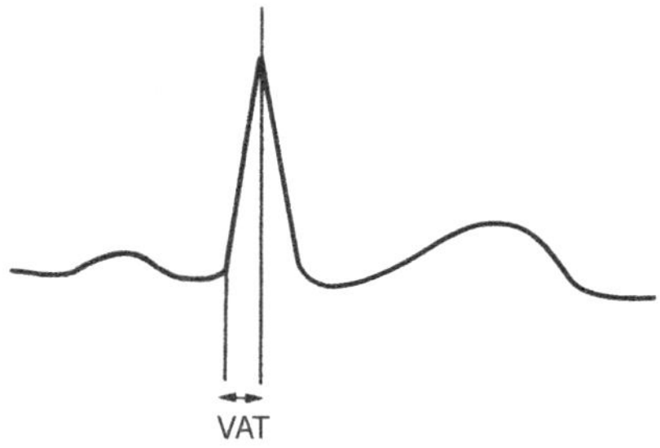

Fig. 1.55
An illustration of the definition of ventricular activation time (VAT), which is the time from the onset of QRS to the peak of the maximum wave

1.7.9 QT Interval

The QT interval has enjoyed something of a renaissance in recent times on account of its susceptibility to change following drug administration and, in certain clinical conditions, for example, following myocardial infarction. Change in the QT interval is also thought to be a precursor of certain arrhythmias, and this too has stimulated considerable research on this variable [102, 103]. The clinical implications associated with the QT interval have been reviewed by Al-Khatib [104] and others. This area of study has grown to such an extent that a separate chapter, Chap. 7, has been devoted to this topic.

Accurate determination of the QT interval, whether it be by computer methods or by manual methods, is difficult. For example, the variation between cardiologists estimating P, QRS, and T reference points in the CSE study [35] was the greatest when they manually estimated the end of the T wave. Likewise, computer programs in the same study also showed the greatest variation when finding the T-wave termination. Furthermore, many researchers wish to monitor QT-interval changes over a period of time by making use of ambulatory monitoring equipment (see Chap. 1 of *Specialized Aspects of ECG*). Older recorders are susceptible to variations in speed over a period of 24 h, although the best have time

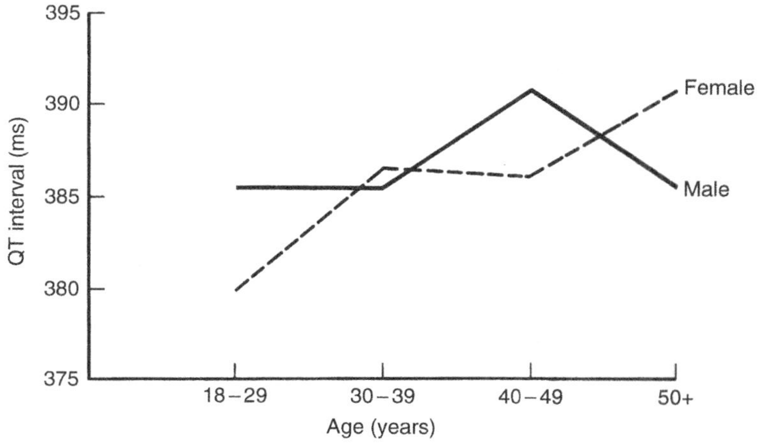

Fig. 1.56
Variation in mean QT interval with age and sex, as derived from the Glasgow data

tracks recorded on the tape. Modern recorders employ digital technology but with varying sampling rates form 128 to 1,000 samples/s which can cause variation in QT measurement, for example.

Notwithstanding these various limitations, the mean QT-interval variation with age and sex is shown with respect to the authors' data in Fig. 1.56. From this it can be seen that, in general, there are no significant differences between men and women, but there is a small increase in the QT interval with age in women.

It is well known that the QT interval varies significantly with the heart rate and a number of formulae have been derived for correcting the QT interval. The most commonly used is that of Bazett [105], where the corrected interval, QT_c, is given by the formula

$$QT_c = QT\left(\frac{\text{rate}}{60}\right)^{1/2}$$

This is a nonlinear correction of the QT interval. Hodges et al. [106] suggested a linear correction, namely,

$$QT_c = QT + 1.75(\text{rate} - 60)$$

The distribution of the corrected QT using these formulae is shown in Fig. 1.57a and b. Hodges et al. showed that the Bazett formula undercorrects the QT interval at heart rates below 60 bpm and overcorrects the QT interval at rates above 60 bpm. Their own formula was said to "reliably" correct the QT interval over the range of heart rates. Furthermore, with the use of this formula, there was no correlation between the linearly corrected QT interval and the heart rate, whereas with the Bazett formula, there was a highly significant correlation between the corrected QT interval and heart rate (see Fig. 1.57a), defeating the purpose of correcting the QT interval. The authors recommend the formula of Hodges et al. in preference to that of Bazett. Although there are no differences between men and women with respect to the QT interval (see Table 1.3), there is a definite increase in the QT_c of women over the whole age range (see Fig. 1.58). This is of the order of 9 ms for QT_c (Hodges) and 16 ms for QT_c (Bazett).

Another formula that has gained increasing popularity recently is that of Fridericia [107]. It has the form

$$QT_c = QT\left(\frac{\text{rate}}{60}\right)^{1/3}$$

Luo et al. [108] compared this with other formulae including those of Bazett and Hodges and concluded that the Bazett formula was most out of line with the others. Bourdillon [109] reviewed several formulae for correcting the QT interval

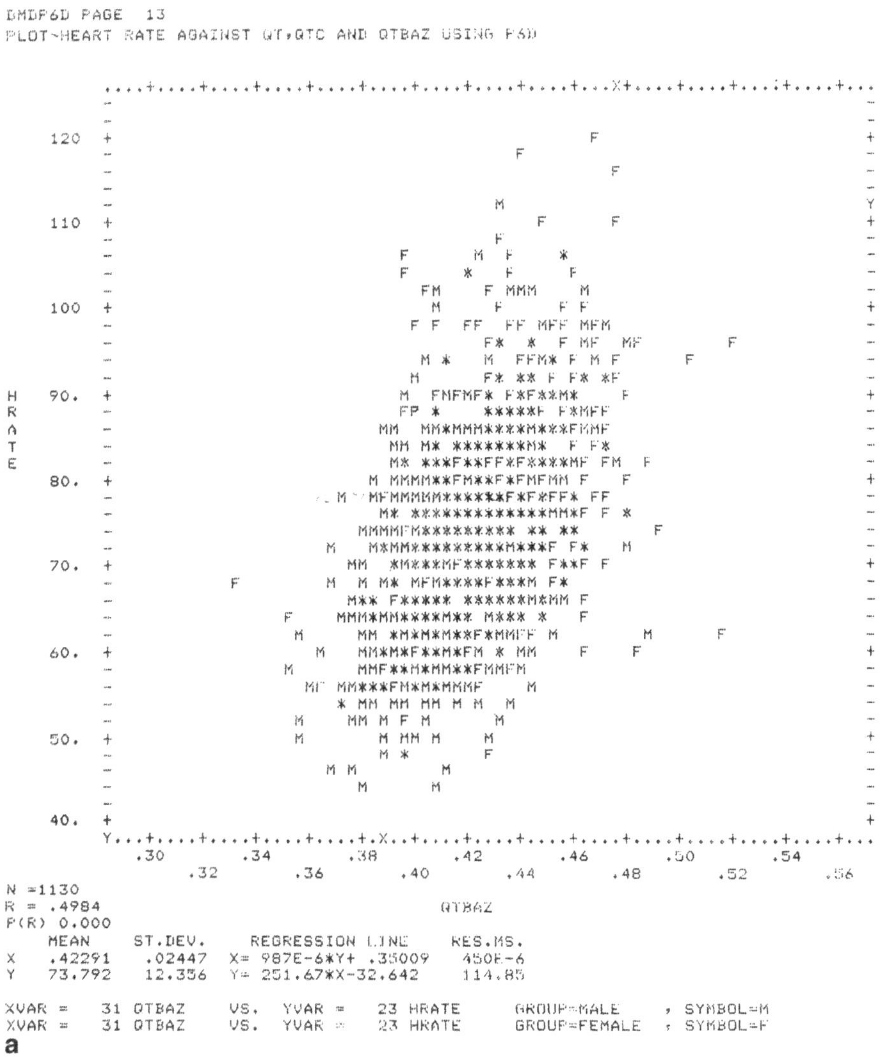

Fig. 1.57a

Scattergram of corrected QT interval versus heart rate. The QT is corrected with respect to the Bazett formula, and the correlation with rate is 0.498, that is, the QT is essentially uncorrected (*M* male, *F* female; *, more than one value at the same point on the plot)

in a study of ECGs incorporated in the CSE project. From this, he showed that the QT interval correlated with the QRS duration so that for a particular rate and QRS duration, the QT interval could be predicted. Hence, a prolonged QT could be detected when the measured QT exceeded the predicted QT by a specified amount. The combination of the R-R interval and QRS duration accounted for 52% of the variance in predicting the QT interval. In some ways, this may in fact be related to Wilson's concept of the ventricular gradient [110] discussed in Chaps. 5 of *Basic Electrocardiology: Cardiac Electrophysiology, ECG Systems and Mathematical Modeling* and 5.

In view of the various factors that impinge on accurate estimation of the QT interval, it is customary for computer programs to utilize a value of at least 460 ms as the upper limit of normal for the corrected QT interval. Some will extend this limit to 470 ms for females. This maintains a high specificity, as is evident from Fig. 1.57b.

```
BMDP6D PAGE  10
PLOT HEART RATE AGAINST QT,QTC AND QTBAZ USING P6D
```

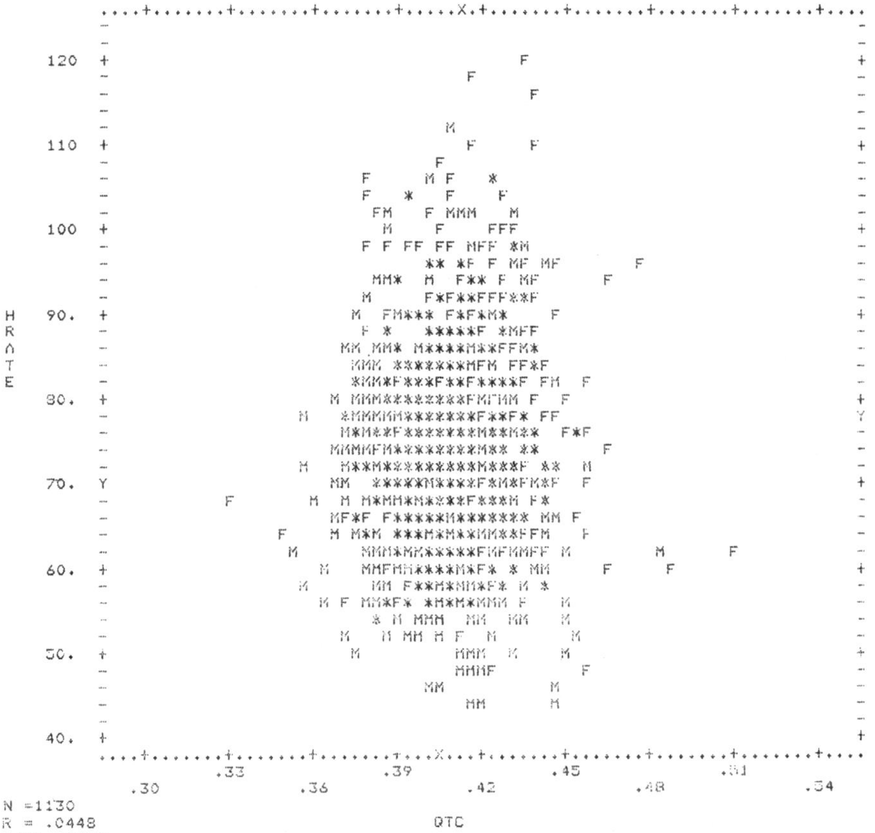


```
N =1130
R = .0448
P(R) .1324
     MEAN      ST.DEV.      RECRESSION LINE     RES.MS.
X    .40855    .01943    X= 704E-7*Y+ .40336    377E-6
Y    73.792    12.356    Y= 28.469*X+ 62.161    152.49

XVAR =    30 QTC         VS.   YVAR =    23 HRATE     GROUP=MALE     , SYMBOL=M
XVAR =    30 QTC         VS.   YVAR =    23 HRATE     GROUP=FEMALE   , SYMBOL=F
```

b

Fig. 1.57b
Scattergram of corrected QT interval versus heart rate. The QT is corrected with respect to the formula of Hodges et al., and there is essentially no correlation with rate, that is, the QT is highly corrected (*M* male, *F* female; *, more than one value at the same point on the plot)

1.8 Coding Schemes

1.8.1 Minnesota Code

It is well known that ECG interpretation may vary from one observer to another (and from one computer program to another). Essentially, for the former reason, a coding scheme was developed in 1960 in the University of Minnesota by Blackburn et al. [20], which ultimately became known as the Minnesota code. This set out to describe various ECG appearances, to which a code number could be ascribed. The first point that must therefore be emphasized with respect to the Minnesota code is that it is, *per se*, not a set of diagnostic criteria but rather a set of descriptors. This code has been used in many studies since 1960, as discussed in detail in ➲ Chap. 8 of *Specialized Aspects of ECG*. More recently,

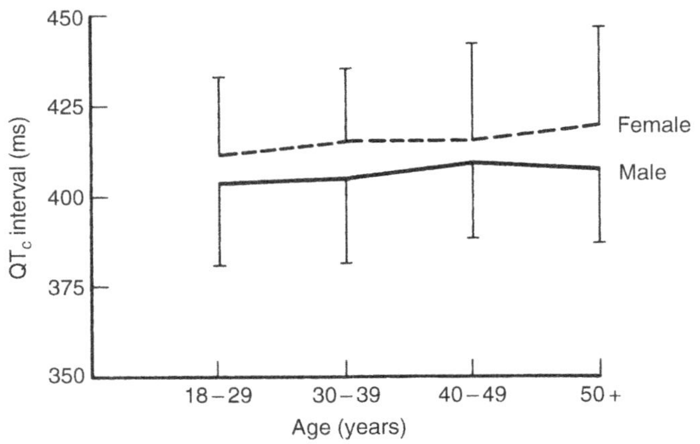

Fig. 1.58
Mean and standard deviation of the QT_c interval (corrected with respect to the formula of Hodges et al. [106]). Note the definite increase in QT_c in women compared to men

the section on serial changes has been revised and expanded, while a new manual of procedures for measurement and classification has been published [22].

The Minnesota code is published in full in the Appendices. From this, it can be seen that no actual diagnoses are included with the possible exception of conduction defects and arrhythmias, where the ECG itself provides the objective evidence upon which the classification can be based (corresponding to type B diagnoses of the American College recommendations [111] on optimal electrocardiography – see Appendix). Thus, code 1-1-1 in relation to an anterolateral site involving leads I, aVL, and V_6 specifies a Q/R amplitude greater than 1/3, together with a Q duration greater than 0.03 s in I or V_6. On the other hand, a 1-1-1 classification in a posterior (inferior) site follows from a corresponding set of criteria applied to lead II. Finally, a positive 1-1-1 code in an anterior lead results from similar criteria being applied to any of V_2–V_5. An ECG exhibiting any of these features would be coded as 1-1-1 and not necessarily as a myocardial infarction although that is the implication.

The code certainly has some shortcomings particularly with respect to the lack of use of age and sex in the various criteria, but nevertheless it has stood the test of time as being one of the few methods available where some standardization of the ECG classification, if not interpretation, can be achieved. A number of computer programs have been developed for automatically coding the ECG [112–114] including one in the authors' own laboratory that also incorporates serial comparison according to the Minnesota code rules [115]. From these studies, it has been shown that the accuracy of programs is similar to that of human coders when compared with an agreed set of codes resulting from a group of experienced Minnesota coders amalgamating their opinions on a set of ECGs [116]. Nevertheless, in the authors' laboratory, for example, in an analysis of over 10,000 ECGs from a cooperative study with London University, both the Minnesota code and conventional 12-lead ECG interpretations are provided, since in some ways they are complementary. The former is required for purposes of international acceptance, while the latter is thought to give a more meaningful interpretation of the ECG that can be returned to the subject's general practitioner.

1.8.2 Washington Code

Pipberger et al. [60] published a classification system relating to the orthogonal-lead ECG. This code honored the late Ernst Simonson who had initiated this particular work shortly before his death in 1974. Use was made of data on black and white subjects gathered by Pipberger and coworkers over a number of years [61, 62]. This code was aimed at producing a simple classification scheme that made use essentially of the scalar amplitudes and durations as well as amplitude ratios of the *X*, *Y*, and *Z* leads. Apart from the unique feature of having different criteria for men and women, black and white, this code also had the novel feature that two different levels of criteria could be established depending on the desired specificity (see ➋ Tables 3.7 and ➋ 3.11, for example). Furthermore, the codes had a definite electrocardiographic diagnosis assigned. Whereas the Minnesota code classification was designated Q and QS patterns, the corresponding Washington code 2 was designated "myocardial infarction."

Pipberger and colleagues carried out an evaluation of this code in comparison with the Minnesota code and showed that, in general terms, the Washington code [50] was more sensitive than the Minnesota code. This would be expected on the basis of greater use of race and sex in the former.

1.8.3 Punsar Code

A less-well-known code is that of Punsar et al. [117] that was used for categorizing the ST-T segment in an attempt to diagnose ischemic heart disease. Punsar was one of the authors of the original 1960 Minnesota code publication. From the various ST-T classifications of the Punsar code as shown in ➋ Fig. 1.59, it can be seen that there are essentially three abnormal categories of ST segment according to this code. In the type labeled ischemic, the ST segment is horizontal or downward-sloping and can be further subdivided into five different grades depending on the degree of ST depression. Grade 1 shows the most depression in excess of 0.2 mV, while Grade 5 shows the least ST depression being less than 0.05 mV. The second category relates to upsloping ST segments where the degree of upslope is somewhat vaguely described as "slowly ascending." Again, further four subdivisions are utilized. The third category relates to upsloping ST segments where there is a more steep slope than in the second category. This group is described as "rapidly ascending" and contains three subdivisions. The fourth and final group of normal ST segments are those where the ST-junction depression is less than 0.05 mV and where the slope is such that the apparent onset of the T wave is above the baseline, that is, it is positive.

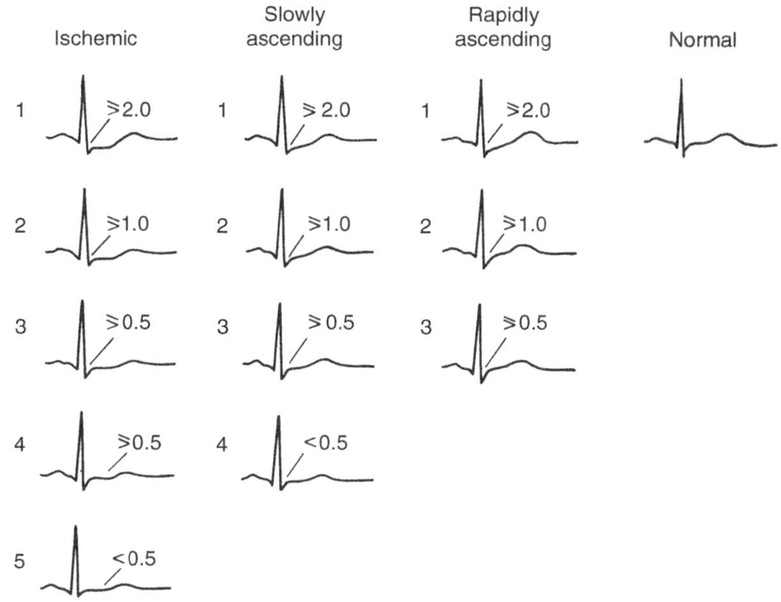

Fig. 1.59
The definitions of the Punsar code for the classification of the ST segment. See text for further discussion (After Punsar et al. [117]. © Finnish Medical Society, Helsinki. Reproduced with permission)

1.8.4 Novacode

Perhaps one of the most complex coding schemes ever to be developed is the Novacode from the lab of Rautaharju [118]. This code is extremely detailed covering all aspects of the ECG and interpretation including progression and regression of ECG changes. Criteria for hypertrophy are in the traditional voltage-based style with some sex dependence but no age dependence. However, the scheme is designed to be applied in clinical trials and in population studies where most individuals would be middle-aged or older. Criteria for pathological Q waves and ST-T abnormalities are based on scoring techniques. The code is structured in a hierarchical way with the aim of identifying a specific abnormality, which can then be further refined if required. For example, code 3.1 defines LBBB, whereas code 3.1.0 defines LBBB without myocardial infarction, and code 3.1.1 defines LBBB with myocardial infarction. The definitions of 3.1.0 and 3.1.1 each require, not surprisingly, that code 3.1 is present. The code has not been used widely in population studies as yet, perhaps due to a perceived complexity and maybe a need for epidemiologists to cling to Minnesota codes from earlier studies to facilitate comparisons.

1.9 The Electrocardiogram and Employment

The normal limits of the ECG have been discussed in detail, and their bearing on the development of diagnostic criteria is clear. A few points remain to be made, however, in relation to employment.

A normal resting ECG does not always imply a normal heart. It is well known to every cardiologist that many patients with ischemic heart disease may have a normal ECG. A normal ECG cannot therefore be used as evidence of cardiovascular fitness in supporting an application for a license to carry out a particular occupation when there may be other clinical signs and symptoms of abnormality.

Conversely, changes in the ECG should not mitigate against the licence when other investigations, including clinical examination, are normal. Various recommendations have been made which would allow an individual with minor ECG abnormalities to continue in employment. For example, for airline pilots, a number of recommendations have been produced [119, 120]. More recently, an excellent review of matters relating to occupational aspects of heart disease has been published [121].

In conclusion, ECG changes must be assessed in the overall context of other investigations before reaching a conclusion on fitness for employment. There are many other techniques for investigating cardiac status which are complementary to the ECG. Nevertheless, the ECG still contains unique information which mandates that it remains a vital rest in many situations relating to fitness for employment.

1.10 Acknowledgement

The authors gratefully acknowledge the statistical advice provided by Mr. Tom Aitcheson, former senior lecturer in Statistics at the University of Glasgow.

References

1. Mason, J.W., D.J. Ramseth, D.O. Chanter, T.E. Moon, D.B. Goodman, and B. Mendzelevski, Electrocardiographic reference ranges derived from 79,743 subjects. *J. Electrocardiol.*, 2007;**40**: 228–234.
2. Simonson, E., *Differentiation Between Normal and Abnormal in Electrocardiography*. St. Louis, MI: Mosby, 1961.
3. Lundh, B., On the normal scalar ECG. A new classification system considering age, sex and heart position, PhD thesis. Lund: University of Lund. *Acta Med. Scand.*, 1984; Suppl. 691.
4. Macfarlane, P.W., J.A. MacLean, M. Low, et al., Revised limits of the normal ECG, in *Advances in Electrocardiology*, P. D'Alché, Editor. Caen: Centre de Publications de l'Université de Caen, 1985, pp. 160–163.
5. Startt/Selvester, R.H., Comprehensive multilead normal ECG data base for the next few decades, in *Computer ECG Analysis: Towards Standardization*, J.L. Willems, J.H. van Bemmel, and C. Zywietz, Editors. Amsterdam: North-Holland, 1986, pp. 221–226.

6. Ostrander, L.D. Jr., Bundle-branch block. An epidemiologic study. *Circulation*, 1964;**30**: 872–871.
7. Anonymous, Unrecognised myocardial infarction. *Lancet*, 1976;**2**: 449–450.
8. Margolis, J.R., W.B. Kannel, M. Feinleib, T.R. Dawber, and P.M. McNamara, Clinical features of unrecognized myocardial infarction-Silent and symptomatic. Eighteen year follow-up: the Framingham study. *Am. J. Cardiol.*, 1973;**32**:1–7.
9. Medalie, J.H. and U. Goldbourt, Unrecognized myocardial infarction: Five year incidence, mortality and risk factors. *Ann. Intern. Med.*, 1976;**84**: 526–531.
10. Schwartz, D., R. Flamant, and J. Lellouch, *Clinical Trials*. New York: Academic Press, 1980.
11. Jain, U. and P.M. Rautaharju, The use of discretized features for classification of electrocardiograms, in *Optimization of Computer ECG Processing*, H.K. Wolf and P.W. Macfarlane, Editors. Amsterdam: North-Holland, 1980 pp. 117–120.
12. Macfarlane, P.W., B. Devine, S. Latif, S. McLaughlin, D.B. Shoat, and M.P. Watts, Methodology of ECG interpretation in the Glasgow program. *Meth. Inform. Med.*, 1990;**29**: 354–361.
13. Macfarlane, P.W., B. Devine, and E. Clark, The University of Glasgow (Uni-G) ECG analysis program. *Comput. Cardiol.*, 2005;**32**: 451–454.
14. McLaughlin, S., T.C. Aitchison, T.-F. Yang, and P.W. Macfarlane, Smoothing techniques for improving the repeatability of the automated diagnosis of inferior myocardial infarction. *J. Electrocardiol.*, 1994;**27**(Suppl): 182–187.
15. McLaughlin, S., T.C. Aitchison, and P.W. Macfarlane, Methods for improving the repeatability of automated ECG analysis. *Meth. Inform. Med.*, 1995;**34**: 272–282.
16. Dudeck, J. and J. Michaelis, Problems in the diagnostic process in electrocardiography, in *Computer Application on ECG and VCG Analysis*, C. Zywietz and B. Schneider, Editors. Amsterdam: North-Holland, 1973, pp. 283–295.
17. Abreu-Lima, C., D.M. Correia, J. Almeida, M. Antunes-Lopes, and M. Cerqueira-Gomes, A new ECG classification system for myocardial infarction based on receiver operating characteristic curve analysis and information theory. *Circulation*, 1983;**67**: 1252–1257.
18. Rautaharju, P.M., H.W. Blackburn, and J.W. Warren, The concepts of sensitivity, specificity and accuracy in the evaluation of electrocardiographic, vectorcardiographic and polarcardiographic criteria. *J. Electrocardiol.*, 1976;**9**: 275–281.
19. Bailey, J.J., Evaluation methodologies, in *Computerized Interpretation of the Electrocardiogram VI*, R. Bonner, Editor. New York: Engineering Foundation, 1982.
20. Blackburn, H., A. Keys, E. Simonson, P. Rautaharju, and S. Punsar, The electrocardiogram in population studies. A classification system. *Circulation*, 1960;**21**: 1160–1175.
21. Kossmann, C.E., D.A. Brody, G.E. Burch, et al., Report of Committee on Electrocardiography, American Heart Association. Recommendations for standardization of leads and of specifications for instruments in electrocardiography and vectorcardiography. *Circulation*, 1967;**35**: 583–602.
22. Prineas, R.J., R.S. Crow, and H. Balckburn, *The Minnesota Code Manual of Electrocardiographic Findings*, 2nd edn., London: Springer, 2010.
23. Pipberger, H.V., R.C. Arzbaecher, A.S. Berson, et al., Report of the Committee on Electrocardiography, American Heart Association. Recommendations for standardization of leads and of specifications for instruments in electrocardiography and vectorcardiography. *Circulation*, 1975;**52**(AHA Suppl): 11–31.
24. Farb, A., R.B. Devereux, and P. Kligfield, Day-to-day variability of voltage measurements used in electrocardiographic criteria for left ventricular hypertrophy. *J. Am. Coll. Cardiol.*, 1990;**15**: 618–623.
25. CSE Working Party, Recommendations for measurement standards in quantitative electrocardiography. *Eur. Heart J.*, 1985;**6**: 815–825.
26. Chung, E.K., *Electrocardiography: Practical Applications with Vectorial Principles*, 2nd edn. Hagerstown, MD: Harper and Row, 1980, pp. 22–25.
27. Chou, T.-C., *Electrocardiography in Clinical Practice*, 2nd edn. Orlando, FL: Grune and Stratton, 1986, pp. 7–10.
28. Holzmann, M., *Klinische Electrokardiographie*, 3rd edn. Stuttgart: Thieme, 1955.
29. Rowlands, D.J., The normal ECG, Section I, *Understanding the Electrocardiogram: A New Approach*. Macclesfield: ICI, 1980, pp. 46–50.
30. Willems, J.L,, E.O. Robles de Medina, R. Bernard, et al., WHO/ISFC Task Force. Criteria for intraventricular conduction disturbances and pre-excitation. *J. Am. Coll. Cardiol.*, 1985;**5**: 1261–1275.
31. Macfarlane, P.W., M. Marriott, M.J. Podolski, D. MacFarlane, and T.D.V. Lawrie, Simultaneous 3-orthogonal and 12-lead hybrid electrocardiogram, in *Computerized Interpretation of Electrocardiograms VIII*, R.H. Selvester and D. Geselowitz, Editors. New York: Engineering Foundation, 1984, pp. 159–169.
32. Draper, H.W., C.J. Peffer, F.W. Stallmann, D. Littmann, and H.V. Pipberger, The corrected orthogonal electrocardiogram and vectorcardiogram in 510 normal men (Frank lead system). *Circulation*, 1964;**30**: 853–864.
33. Willems, J.L., Common Standards for Quantitative Electrocardiography (EEC Concerted Action Project II.2.2). 2nd Progress Report. CSE Ref. 82-11-20. Leuven: ACCO, 1982, pp. 127–227.
34. Macfarlane, P.W., D.K. MacFarlane, M. Podolski, and T.D.V. Lawrie, The ECG analysis program for the MINGOCARE system. *Electromedica*, 1984;**52**: 126–136.
35. Willems, J.L., P. Arnaud, J.H. van Bemmel, et al., Assessment of the performance of electrocardiographic computer programs with the use of a reference data base. *Circulation*, 1985;**71**: 523–534.
36. Willems, J.L., P. Arnaud, J.H. van Bemmel, et al., Establishment of a reference library for evaluating computer ECG measurement programs. *Comput. Biomed. Res.*, 1985;**18**: 439–457.
37. Rose, G.A. and H. Blackburn, *Cardiovascular Survey Methods*. Geneva: WHO, 1968, Monograph Series No.56.
38. Willems, J.L., Common Standards for Quantitative Electrocardiography (EEC Concerted Action Project II.2.2). 4th Progress Report. CSE Ref. 84-11-15. Leuven: ACCO, 1984, pp. 73–152.
39. Willems, J.L., P.F. Poblete, and H.V. Pipberger, Day-to-day variation of the normal orthogonal electrocardiogram and vectorcardiogram. *Circulation*, 1972;**45**: 1057–1064.
40. Simonson, E., J. Brozek, and A. Keys, Variability of the electrocardiogram in normal young men. *Am. Heart J.*, 1949;**38**: 407–422.
41. Cawood, H.T., P.W. Macfarlane, S. Hillis, and T.D.V. Lawrie, Day to day and beat to beat variation in normal 3 orthogonal lead electrocardiograms. *Br. Heart J.*, 1974;**36**: 1225–1230.

42. Simonson, E., The electrocardiogram in coronary heart disease. *Minn. Med.*, 1955;38:871–873.
43. Graybiel, A., Starr, R.S., and P.D. White, Electrocardiographic changes following the inhalation of tobacco smoke. *Am. Heart J.*, 1938;**15**: 89–99.
44. Wilson, F.N. and R. Finch, The effect of drinking iced-water upon the form of the T detection of the electrocardiogram. *Heart*, 1923;**10**. 275–278.
45. Sears, G.A. and G.W. Manning, Routine electrocardiography: postprandial T wave changes. *Am. Heart J.*, 1958;**56**: 591–597.
46. Magendantz, H. and J. Shortsleeve, Electrocardiographic abnormalities in patients exhibiting anxiety. *Am. Heart J.*, 1951;**42**: 849–857.
47. Marriott, H.J.L., *Practical Electrocardiography*, 6th edn. Baltimore, MD: Williams and Wilkins, 1977, pp. 266–269.
48. LaMonte, C.S. and A.H. Freiman, The electrocardiogram after mastectomy. *Circulation*, 1965;**32**: 746–754.
49. Rautaharju, P., L. Park, F.S. Rautaharju, and R. Crow, A standardizes procedure for locating and documenting ECG chest electrode positions. *J. Electrocardiol.*, 1998;**31**: 17–29.
50. Scherer, M.L., T. Aspelund, S. Sigurdsson, R. Detrano, M. Garcia, G.F. Mitchell, L.J. Launer, G. Thorgeirsson, V. Gudnason, and T.B. Harris, Abnormal T-wave axis is associated with coronary artery calcification in older adults. *Scan. Cardiovasc. J.*, 2008;1–9:iFirst Article URL: http://dx.doi.org/10.1080/14017430802471483
51. Tomlinson, D.R., Y. Bashir, T.R. Betts, and K. Rajappan, Accuracy of manual QRS duration assessment: its importance in patient selection for cardiac resynchronization and implantable cardioverter defibrillator therapy. *Europace*, 2009;**11**: 638–642.
52. Littmann, D., Persistence of the juvenile pattern in the precordial leads of healthy adult Negroes, with report of electrocardiographic survey on three hundred Negro and two hundred white subjects. *Am. Heart J.*, 1946;**32**: 370–382.
53. Keller, D.H. and J.B. Johnston, The T wave of the unipolar precordial electrocardiogram in normal adult Negro subjects. *Am. Heart J.*, 1952;**44**: 494–498.
54. Walker, A.R.P. and B.F. Walker, The bearing of race, sex, age, and nutritional state on the precordial electrocardiograms of young South African Bantu and Caucasian subjects. *Am. Heart J.*, 1969;**77**: 441–459.
55. Katibi, I.A., Normal limits of the 12 lead ECG in a healthy Nigerian cohort, MD Thesis. University of Glasgow. In preparation.
56. Macfarlane, P.W., C.Y. Chen, and B.N. Chiang, Comparison of the ECG in apparently healthy Chinese and Caucasians, in *Computers in Cardiology*, K. Ripley, Editor. 1987. Baltimore, MD: IEEE Computer Society Press, 1988.
57. Macfarlane, P.W., M.P. Watts, M. Podolski, D. Shoat, and T.D.V. Lawrie, The new Glasgow system, in *Computer ECG Analysis: Towards Standardization*, J.L. Willems, J.H. van Bemmel, and C. Zywietz, Editors. Amsterdam: North-Holland, 1986, pp. 31–36.
58. Chen, C.Y., B.N. Chiang, and P.W. Macfarlane, Normal limits of the electrocardiogram in a Chinese population. *J. Electrocardiol.*, 1989;**22**: 1–15.
59. Wu, J., J.A. Kors, P.R. Rijnbeek, G. van Herpen, Z. Lu, and C. Xu, Normal limits of the electrocardiogram in Chinese subjects. *Int. J. Cardiol.*, 2003;**87**: 37–51.
60. Pipberger, H.V., E. Simonson, E.A. Lopez Jr., M.A. Araoye, and H.A. Pipberger, The electrocardiogram in epidemiologic investigations. A new classification system. *Circulation*, 1982;**65**: 1456–1464.
61. Pipberger, H.V., M.J. Goldman, D. Littmann, G.P. Murphy, J. Cosma, and J.R. Snyder, Correlations of the orthogonal electrocardiogram and vectorcardiogram with constitutional variables in 518 normal men. *Circulation*, 1967;**35**: 536–551.
62. Nemati, M., J.T. Doyle, D. McCaughan, R.A. Dunn, and H.V. Pipberger, The orthogonal electrocardiogram in normal women. Implications of sex differences in diagnostic electrocardiography. *Am. Heart J.*, 1978;**95**: 12–21.
63. Keys, A., F. Fidanza, M.J. Karvonen, N. Kimura, and H.L. Taylor, Indices of relative weight and obesity. *J. Chronic Dis.*, 1972;**25**: 329–343.
64. Matthes, T., G. Gottsch, and C. Zywietz, Interactive analysis of statistical ECG, diagnosis on an intelligent electrocardiograph—an expert system approach, in *Computer ECG Analysis: Towards Standardization*, J.L. Willems, J.H. van Bemmel, and C. Zywietz, Editors. Amsterdam: North-Holland, 1986, pp. 215–220.
65. Oakley, D.G. and C.M. Oakley, Significance of abnormal electrocardiograms in highly trained athletes. *Am. J. Cardiol.*, 1982;**50**: 985–989.
66. Fagard, R., A. Aubert, J. Staessen, E. van den Eynde, L. Vanhees, and A. Amery, Cardiac structure and function in cyclists and runners. Comparative echocardiographic study. *Br. Heart J.*, 1984;**52**: 124–129.
67. Shapiro, L.M., Physiological left ventricular hypertrophy. *Br. Heart J.*, 1984;**52**: 130–135.
68. Pellicacia, A., F.M. Di Paolo, F.M. Quattrini, C. Basso, F. Culasso, G. Popoli, R. De Luca, A. Spataro, A. Biffi, G. Thiene, and B.J. Marron, Outcomes in athletes with marked ECG repolarization abnormalities. *N. Eng. J. Med.*, 2008;**358**(2): 152–161.
69. Oakley, D., Cardiac hypertrophy in athletes. *Br. Heart J.*, 1984;**52**: 121–123.
70. Lawless, C.E. and T. Best, Electrocardiograms in athletes: interpretation and diagnostic accuracy. *Med. Sci. Sports Exer.*, 2008;**40**: 787–798.
71. Corrado, D., A. Pelliccia, H.H. Bjornstad, L. Vanhees, A. Biffi, M. Borjesson, N. Panhuyzen-Goedkoop, et al., Cardiovascular pre-participation screening of young competitive athletes for prevention of sudden death: proposal for a common European protocol. Consensus statement of the Study Group of Sport Cardiology of the Working Group of Cardiac Rehabilitation and Exercise Physiology and the Working Group of Myocardial and Pericardial Diseases of the European Society of Cardiology. *Eur. Heart J.*, 2005;**26**: 516–524.
72. Wilson, F.N., F.D. Johnston, F.F. Rosenbaum, et al., The precordial electrocardiogram. *Am. Heart J.*, 1944;**27**:19–85.
73. Liebman, J., R. Plonsey, and P.C. Gillette, eds. *Pediatric Electrocardiography*. Baltimore, MD: Williams and Wilkins, 1982.
74. Sreenivasan, V.V., B.J. Fisher, J. Liebman, and T.D. Downs, Longitudinal study of the standard electrocardiogram in the healthy premature infant during the first year of life. *Am. J. Cardiol.*, 1973;**31**: 57–63.
75. Liebman, J., H.C. Romberg, T. Downs, and R. Agusti, The Frank QRS vectorcardiogram in the premature infant, in *Vectorcardiography*, I. Hoffman and R.C. Taylor, Editors. 1965. Amsterdam: North-Holland, 1966, pp. 256–271.
76. Davignon, A., P. Rautaharju, E. Boiselle, F. Soumis, M. Megelas, and A. Choquette, Normal ECG standards for infants and children. *Pediatr. Cardiol.*, 1979;**1**: 123–152.
77. Ziegler, R.F., *Electrocardiographic Studies in Normal Infants and Children*. Springfield, IL: Thomas, 1951.

78. Strong, W.B., T.D. Downs, J. Liebman, and R. Liebowitz, The normal adolescent electrocardiogram. *Am. Heart J.*, 1972;**83**: 115–128.
79. Macfarlane, P.W., E.N. Coleman, E.O. Pomphrey, S. McLaughlin, A. Houston, and T. Aitchisonn, Normal limits of the high-fidelity pediatric ECG: Preliminary observations. *J. Electrocardiol.*, 1990;**22**(Suppl. 1): 162–168.
80. Rijnbeek, P.R., M. Witsenburg, E. Schrama, J. Hess, and J.A. Kors, New normal limits for the paediatric electrocardiogram. *Eur. Heart J.*, 2001;**22**(8): 702–711.
81. Sun, K., F. Li, Y. Zhou, A.M. Dubin, P.M. Rautaharju, J. Liebman, R.E. Gregg, E.D. Helfenbein, J.M. Lindauer, and S.H. Zhou, Normal ECG limits for Asian infants and children. *Comput. Cardiol.*, 2005;**32**: 455–458.
82. Guller, B., F.Y.K. Lau, R.A. Dunn, H.A. Pipberger, and H.V. Pipberger, Computer analysis of changes in Frank vectorcardiograms of 666 normal infants in the first 72 hours of life. *J. Electrocardiol.*, 1977;**10**: 19–26.
83. Chou, T.-C. and R.A. Helm, *Clinical Vectorcardiography*. New York: Grune and Stratton, 1967, pp. 50–63.
84. Cornfield, J., R.A. Dunn, C.D. Batchlor, and H.V. Pipberger, Multigroup diagnosis of electrocardiograms. *Comput. Biomed. Res.*, 1973;**6**: 97–120.
85. Stallmann, F.W. and H.V. Pipberger, Automatic recognition of electrocardiographic waves by digital computer. *Circ. Res.*, 1961;**9**: 1138–1143.
86. van Bemmel, J.H., J.S. Duisterhout, G. van Herpen, L.G. Bierwolf, S.J. Hengeveld, and B. Versteeg, Statistical processing methods for recognition and classification of vectorcardiograms, in *Vectorcardiography*, vol. 2, I. Hoffman, R.I. Hamby, and E. Glassman, Editors. Amsterdam: North-Holland, 1971, pp. 207–215.
87. Sano, T., F. Suzuki, T. Hiroki, and T. Sawanobori, On the spatial velocity electrocardiogram. II. Clinical application. *Jpn. Heart J.*, 1968;**9**: 64–75.
88. Macfarlane, P.W., J. Mitchell, and T.D.V. Lawrle, Spatial velocity of the heart vector, in *Proceedings of the XIIth International Colloquium on Vectorcardiographicum*, P. Rijlant, Editor. Brussels: Presses Academiques Européennes, 1972, pp. 343–346.
89. Morris, J.J. Jr., E.H. Estes Jr., R.E. Whalen, H.K. Thompson Jr., and H.D. McIntosh, P wave analysis in valvular heart disease. *Circulation*, 1964;**29**: 242–252.
90. Cabrera, E., *Électrocardiographie Clinique: Théorie et Pratique*. Paris: Masson, 1959.
91. Sokolow, M. and T.P. Lyon, The ventricular complex in left ventricular hypertrophy is obtained by unipolar precordial and limb leads. *Am. Heart J.*, 1949;**37**: 161–186.
92. Andersen, H.R., D. Nielsen, and L.G. Hansen, The normal right chest electrocardiogram. *J. Electrocardiol.*, 1987;**20**: 27–32.
93. Taha, B., S. Reddy, M.D. Agarwal, and K. Khaw, Normal limits of ST segment measurements in posterior ECG leads. *J. Electrocardiol.*, 1998;**31**(Suppl. 1): 178–179.
94. Macfarlane, P., J. Petryka, and E. Kaczmarska, Influence of age and sex on normal limits of ST-T amplitudes in right-sided and posterior chest leads. *J. Electrocardiol.*, 2006;**39**(Suppl. 1), S129–S130.
95. Wagner, G.S., P. Macfarlane, H. Wellens, et al., AHA/ACCF/HRS recommendations for the standardization and interpretation of the electrocardiogram: Part VI. Acute ischemia/infarction. *JACC*, 2009;**53**: 1003–1011.
96. Grant, R.P. and R.H. Murray, The QRS complex deformity of myocardial infarction in the human subject. *Am. J. Med.*, 1954;**17**: 587–609.
97. Ueda, H., I. Donomae, E. Kimura, et al., The normal value of electrocardiogram in the Japanese. The Report of the Committee on the Criteria of the Heart Disease and Electrocardiogram. *Jpn. Heart J.*, 1963;**4**: 141–172.
98. Hsu, T.S., C.W. Chiang, and Y.S. Lee, A vectorcardiographic study of normal Chinese adults with some relevant echocardiographic and electrocardiographic observation. *Taiwan I Hsueh Hui Tsa Chih*, 1983;**82**: 410–418.
99. Burns-Cox, C.J., L.C. Lau, and B.H. Toh, The electrocardiogram of healthy young Chinese and Malay men. *J. Electrocardiol.*, 1971;**4**: 211–219.
100. Wang, K., R.W. Asinger, and H.J.L. Marriott, ST-T segment elevation in conditions other than acute myocardial infarction. *N. Eng. J. Med.*, 2003;**349**: 22.
101. Ginzton, L.E. and M.M. Laks, The differential diagnosis of acute pericarditis from the normal variant: new electrocardiographic criteria. *Circulation*, 1982;**65**: 1004–1009.
102. Ahnve, S., E. Gilpin, E.B. Madsen, V. Froelicher, H. Henning, and J. Ross Jr., Prognostic importance of QT_c interval at discharge after acute myocardial infarction: a multicenter study of 865 patients. *Am. Heart J.*, 1984;**108**: 395–400.
103. Krapf, R. and M. Gertsch, Torsade de pointes induced by sotalol despite therapeutic plasma sotalol concentrations. *Br. Med. J.*, 1985;**290**: 1784–1785.
104. Al-Khatib SM, LaPointe NM, Kramer JM, Califf RM. What clinicians should know about the QT interval. *J.A.M.A.*, 2003;**289**: 2120–2127.
105. Bazett, H.C., An analysis of the time relations of electrocardiograms. *Heart*, 1920;**7**: 353–370.
106. Hodges, M., D. Salerno, and D. Erlien, Bazett's QT correction reviewed. Evidence that a linear QT correction for heart is better. *J. Am. Coll. Cardiol.*, 1983;**1**: 694. [Abstract.]
107. Fridericia, L.S., Die Systolendauer im Elektrokardiogramm bei normalen Menschen und bei Herzkranken. *Acta. Med. Scan.*, 1920;**53**: 469–486.
108. Luo, S., P. Johnson, K. Michler, and P.W. Macfarlane, A comparison of commonly used Qt correction formulae: the effect of heart rate on the QTc of normal ECGs. *J. Electrocardiol.*, 2004;**37**(Suppl.): 81–90.
109. Bourdillon, P.J. and J.P. Mulrow, QRS duration is an independent predictor of QT duration. Abstracts. *Computer ECG Analysis: Towards Standardization*. Leuven: CSE Working Conference, 1985: 23.
110. Wilson, F.N., A.G. Macleod, P.S. Barker, and F.D. Johnston, The determination and the significance of the areas of the ventricular deflections of the electrocardiogram. *Am. Heart J.*, 1934;**10**: 46–61.
111. Rautaharju, P.M., M. Ariet, T.A. Pryor, et al., Task Force III. Computers in diagnostic electrocardiography. *Am. J. Cardiol.*, 1978;**41**: 158–170.
112. Wolf, H.K., P.J. Maclnnis, S. Stock, R.K. Helppi, and P.M. Rautaharju, The Dalhousie program: a comprehensive analysis program for rest and exercise electrocardiograms, in *Computer Application on ECG and VCG Analysis*, C. Zywietz and B. Schneider, Editors. Amsterdam: North-Holland, 1973, pp. 231–240.
113. Duisterhout, J.S., J.F. May, and G. van Herpen, A computer program for classification of ECGs according to the Minnesota Code, in *Trends in Computer-Processed Electrocardiograms*, J.H.

van Bemmel and J.L. Willems, Editors. Amsterdam: North-Holland, 1977, pp. 345–352.

114. Tuinstra, C.L. and F.H. Bonjer, Validation of a Minnesota Code program, in *Trends in Computer-Processed Electrocardiograms*, J.H. van Bemmel and J.L. Willems, Editors. Amsterdam: North-Holland, 1977, pp. 353–355.
115. Macfarlane, P.W. and S. Latif, Automated serial comparison based on the Minnesota Code. *J. Electrocardiol.*, 1996;**29**(Suppl. 1): 29–34.
116. Tuinstra, C.L., P.M. Rautaharju, R.J. Prineas, and J.S. Duisterhout, Comparison of the operational value of six systems to assess the Minnesota Code, in *New Frontiers of Electrocardiology*, F. de Padua and P.W. Macfarlane, Editors. Chichester: Research Studies Press, 1981, pp. 487–492.
117. Punsar, S., K. Pyoriila, and P. Siltanen, Classification of electrocardiographic S-T segment changes in epidemiological studies of coronary heart disease. *Ann. Med. Intern. Fenn.*, 1968;**57**: 53–63.
118. Rautaharju, P.M., L.P. Park, B.R. Chaitman, F. Rautaharju, and Z.-M. Zhang, The Novacode criteria for classification of ECG abnormalities and their clinically significant progression and regression. *J. Electrocardiol.*, 1998;**31**: 157–187.
119. Joy, M., (ed) The First European Workshop in Aviation Cardiology. *Eur. Heart J.*, 1992;**13**(Suppl. H): 1–175.
120. Joy, M., (ed) The Second European Workshop in Aviation Cardiology. *Eur. Heart J.*, 1999;**20**(Suppl. D): D1–D136.
121. Katritsis, D.G. and M.M. Webb-People, Occupational and regulatory aspects of heart disease. *ESC Textbook of Cardiovascular Medicine*, 2nd edn. Chapter 38, Oxford: Oxford University Press, 2009.

2 Conduction Defects

Fernando de Pádua · Armando Pereirinha · Nuno Marques · Mário G. Lopes · Peter W. Macfarlane

P. W. Macfarlane et al. (eds.), *Electrocardiology*, DOI 10.1007/978-0-85729-874-4_2,

2.1 Introduction

The normal conduction system and the normal electrocardiogram (ECG) (the resultant of normal conduction of the electrical impulse through a normal conduction system) have been previously described in ➋ Chaps. 5 of *Basic Electrocardiology: Cardiac Electrophysiology, ECG Systems and Mathematical Modeling* and ➋ 1.

This chapter deals with conduction defects occurring at the atrial level (intra-atrial or interatrial conduction defects) and at the ventricular level (intraventricular conduction defects). A more particular type of conduction abnormalities – ventricular preexcitation and Brugada syndrome – is dealt with in ➋ Sects. 2.4 and ➋ 2.5. The description of atrioventricular blocks is presented in ➋ Chap. 6 of *Cardiac Arrhythmias and Mapping Techniques.*

For each type of conduction defect, two main sets of problems are analyzed: (1) the correct identification of the ECG pattern and the precise localization of the abnormality within the conduction system and (2) the clinical importance of the conduction defect. With regard to the latter, the following questions must be answered:

(a) Is it a "lone electrical abnormality" or an electrical presentation of a more important anatomic (and/or functional) disease of the heart?
(b) Are there any expected complications (either "electrical," e.g., brady and tachydysrhythmias; or functional, e.g., impairment of the pump performance of the heart)?
(c) Does its presence, by itself, change the prognosis of the patient?

2.2 Intra-Atrial Conduction Defects

Detailed data concerning the sequence of the atrial activation in the human heart are scarce. Three specialized tracts containing Purkinje fibers have been described connecting the sinus node to the atrioventricular (AV) node (anterior, middle, and posterior internodal pathways) (➋ Fig. 2.1a). An interatrial pathway (Bachmann bundle) has also been described between the right and the left atrium. The true role of these specialized pathways (even their existence), in normal atrial activation and conduction, has not been clearly demonstrated. On the contrary, different techniques suggest a radial sequence of activation (➋ Fig. 2.1b) [1–3], similar to that shown in the dog [4, 5]. Although zones with thicker atrial fibers (muscle bands) may have different conduction velocities, this does not imply conduction through individualized special pathways [1, 3, 5, 6].

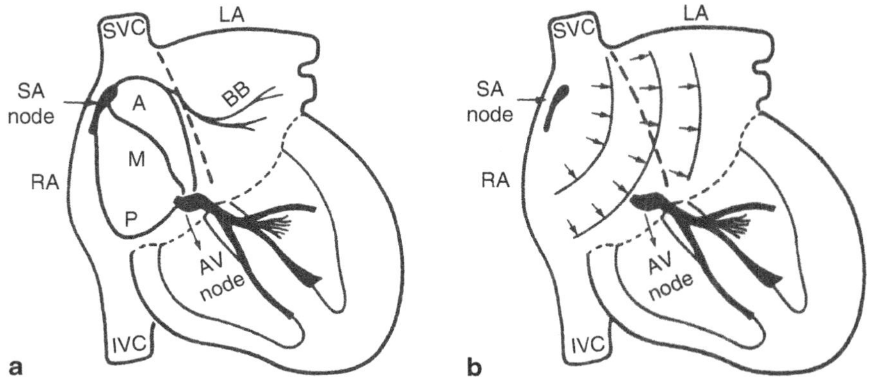

Fig. 2.1
Part (a) is a schematic of the specialized internodal pathways (*A* anterior, *M* middle, *P* posterior) and interatrial Bachmann bundle (BB). Part (b) is a schematic of radial activation of the atria as opposed to conduction through the individualized pathways shown in (a) (*IVC* inferior vena cava, *SVC* superior vena cava, *LA* left atrium, *RA* right atrium)

2.2.1 Electrical Physiopathology and ECG/VCG Patterns

In the normal sinus rhythm, excitation proceeds from the sinus node, localized in the posterior surface of the high right atrium, to the low right and to the high left atrium, and finally to the low left atrium.

While initially only the right atrium is depolarized, the cardiac impulse travels rapidly across the atria. Since the right atrium is anatomically anterior to the left atrium, and the sinus node is located at the right upper portion of the right atrium, the electrical impulse will spread first inferiorly, then leftward, with resultant vectors that rotate progressively more leftward and posteriorly, when the activation wave invades the left atrium.

The normal P-wave pattern (contour, duration, and polarity) is determined by the time course and sequence of the depolarization of the atrial tissue. An increased duration of the P-wave is expected to be present whenever delayed intra-atrial or interatrial activation (intra-atrial or interatrial conduction defect) occurs.

With either left or combined atrial enlargement, a P-wave of longer duration is observed (➋ Fig. 2.2). In the presence of atrial enlargement, stretching or fibrosis of the atrial muscle may justify the intra-atrial conduction defect pattern.

Right atrial enlargement gives rise to peak but not broadened P-waves. The greater duration of right atrial activation in right atrial enlargement does not surpass the time required for left atrial depolarization.

The pattern of left atrial enlargement (wide P-waves, >0.11 s, with terminal negative forces in lead V_1 > 0.04 s, and with amplitude ≥0.1 mV) has been shown to correspond to delayed activation of the lower left atrium [2].

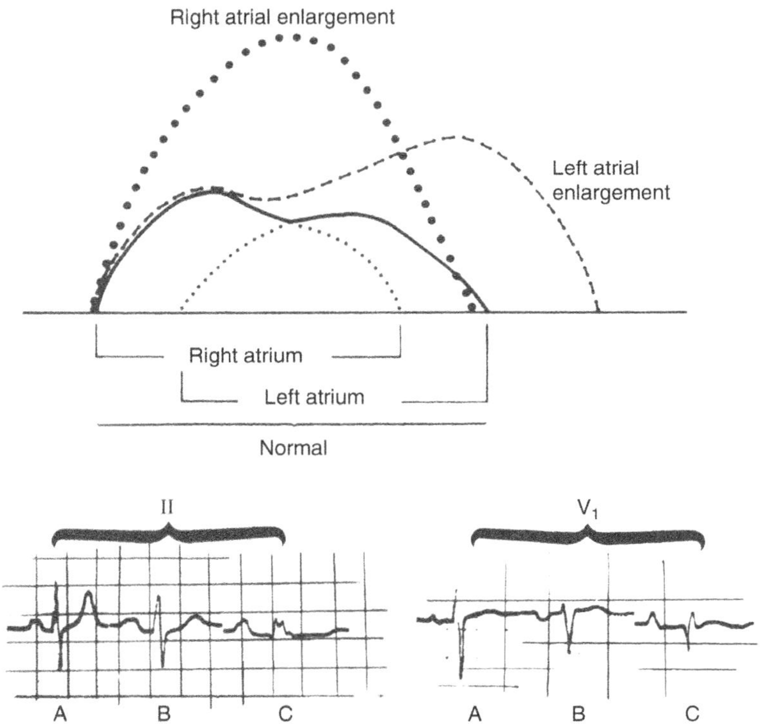

Fig. 2.2
Diagram illustrating left and right atrial contribution to the recorded P-wave, explaining the small notch present in P-waves from some normal individuals. Because right atrial activation is completed before that of the left atrium, right atrial enlargement will cause higher voltage of the P-wave with a normal duration. (Although the right atrial component may become enlarged, it will not surpass the normal left atrial component). With left atrial enlargement, the notching will be accentuated with increased duration of the P-wave. Typical examples of these P-wave patterns in leads II and V_1

It remains uncertain whether local delay (or block) of the atrial activation can result in notching of the P-wave without an increase in its duration. On the other hand, some normal subjects, with no evidence of heart disease, do have a small notch at the peak of the P-wave, which is probably related to the normal asynchronism of activation between both atria. The question remains whether or not by itself notching of the P-wave should be considered evidence of intra-atrial or interatrial conduction defect (usually an interpeak ≥0.04 s is recommended as a criterion for such a conduction defect; however, this usually occurs in cases that also have an abnormal duration of the P-wave).

Another difficult problem is to define the upper limit for normal duration of the P-wave. Several studies of normal populations have been published suggesting an upper limit of 0.10 s [7, 8], 0.11 s [9–11], and 0.12 s [10–12]. It must be remembered, however, that P-wave duration, like other biological values, represents a continuum and consequently, any dividing line will have some normals on the "abnormal" side, as well as some abnormals on the "normal" side. The best cutoff point for the upper limit of normal seems to be 0.11 s.

Besides prolongation of intra-atrial conduction time (first-degree intra-atrial or interatrial block), more advanced degrees of block (second and third degree) have been demonstrated by electrophysiological studies [13–15]. This is also the case for Wenckenbach phenomenon and for dissociated rhythms of the left and right atria or even of a region of one of the atria.

The case of the transplanted heart is a most interesting example, where activation of the remnant auricular tissue can be independent of the activation of the transplanted auricular chambers (➋ Fig. 2.3).

Some cases of apparent first-degree AV block may actually be a result of intra-atrial or interatrial conduction delay with normal conduction through the AV node.

Although the more advanced degrees of interatrial block can be important in the genesis of supraventricular arrhythmias, their identification is not easy using the surface ECG and can only be demonstrated by intracardiac electrophysiological studies.

The Criteria Committee of the New York Heart Association and the World Health Organization/International Society and Federation of Cardiology (WHO/ISFC) Task Force have proposed the following ECG criteria for the diagnosis of intra-atrial (interatrial) conduction defects [8, 16]:

(a) P-wave duration >0.11 s
(b) Notching of the P-wave

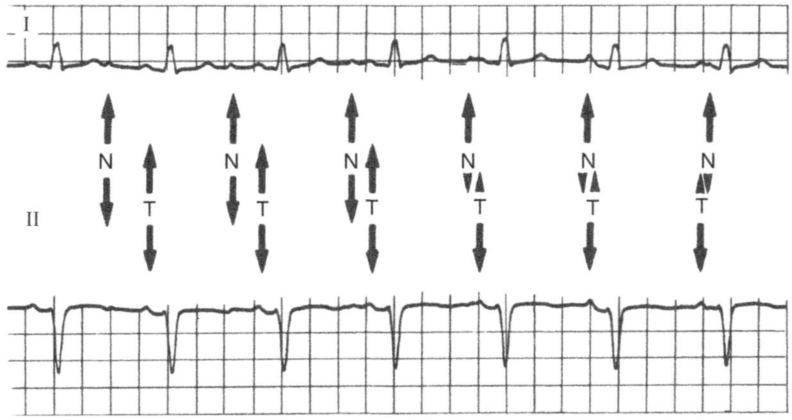

Fig. 2.3
Simultaneous leads (I and II) in a patient with a transplanted heart. Two independent and dissociated atrial rhythms are well identified, one without ventricular conduction (remnant native atrial tissue – N) and the other with normal AV conduction and constant PR interval (transplanted heart-T) (Courtesy of Dr. Queiroz e Melo)

2.2.2 Diagnostic Difficulties

The major diagnostic problem is the identification of left atrial enlargement and distinguishing its ECG from intra-atrial conduction delay alone (without atrial enlargement).

Some of the authors studied 83 hypertensive patients by ECG and echocardiography, correlating the pattern of ECG atrial activity with left atrial dimension by echo [17]. Of 74 patients in normal sinus rhythm, 13 (18%) showed increased terminal negative P-wave forces in V_1 ($\geq$0.04 s and $\geq$0.1 mV) and 20 (27%) had increased duration of the P-wave in lead II (>0.11 s), without increased terminal forces in V_1. The other 41 had normal P-waves.

The former group (increased terminal negative forces in V_1) had a much greater prevalence of left atrial enlargement by echocardiography (62%) than patients with normal P-waves (20%). In our cases, no statistically significant difference was found between patients with enlarged P-waves in lead II and patients with normal P-waves in the same lead, as far as left atrial enlargement prevalence (30% as opposed to 20%) or mean left atrium dimension (38 mm as opposed to 36 mm) were concerned. In our experience, terminal negative P-wave forces in V_1 can be used to identify left atrial enlargement, while P-waves of greater duration, in the absence of increased terminal forces in V_1, do not necessarily imply left atrial enlargement, and more probably correspond to intra-atrial or interatrial conduction defect.

It is suggested that echocardiography should be used to evaluate left atrial dimension in order to decide whether left atrial enlargement is or is not the cause of the abnormal ECG pattern (➋ Fig. 2.2).

2.2.3 Clinical Overview

Intra-atrial and interatrial conduction defects are probably more frequent than is usually recognized. In the presence of an enlarged P-wave, left atrial enlargement should be ruled out (by echocardiography) before the diagnosis of conduction defect is made.

Much is still to be learned about higher degrees of intra-atrial and interatrial block, which need electrophysiological studies to be clearly understood. However, they may play an important role in some cases of supraventricular dysrhythmias [13, 14, 18].

2.3 Intraventricular Conduction Defects

The normal cardiac specialized conduction system has been described in detail in ➋ Chap. 5 of *Basic Electrocardiology: Cardiac Electrophysiology, ECG Systems and Mathematical Modeling.* Normal ventricular activation is summarized here for convenience and to emphasize those aspects of particular relevance to the topic under consideration.

The specialized conduction system consists of the sinoatrial (SA) node, the atrial conduction pathways (whatever their real importance may be), the AV node, the His bundle, the right and left bundle branches (the latter with two main subdivisions – anterosuperior and posteroinferior), and the Purkinje fibers. Occasionally, a third septal subdivision of the left bundle (median or centroseptal) may also be identified [19–21], and in still other cases the branching pattern of the left bundle is not clearly defined (see ➋ Sect. 2.3.1) (➋ Fig. 2.4).

The initial electrical stimulus of the cardiac muscle activity is generated at the SA node. From there, it spreads across the atria and reaches the AV node. Within the AV node, it is physiologically delayed before being propagated rapidly along the His bundle and its right and left divisions and subdivisions, to the Purkinje network. When the wave of activation reaches the myocardial cells, it causes their depolarization and subsequent contraction.

Durrer et al. [1] have investigated the initial ventricular activation in the isolated human heart and found that, normally, three endocardial areas are synchronously excited at the beginning of left ventricular activation:

(a) An area located high on the anterior paraseptal wall, below the attachment of the mitral valve, extending inferiorly to the region of the anterior papillary muscle
(b) A central area in the left surface of the interventricular septum
(c) A posterior paraseptal area at about one-third the distance from the apex to the base

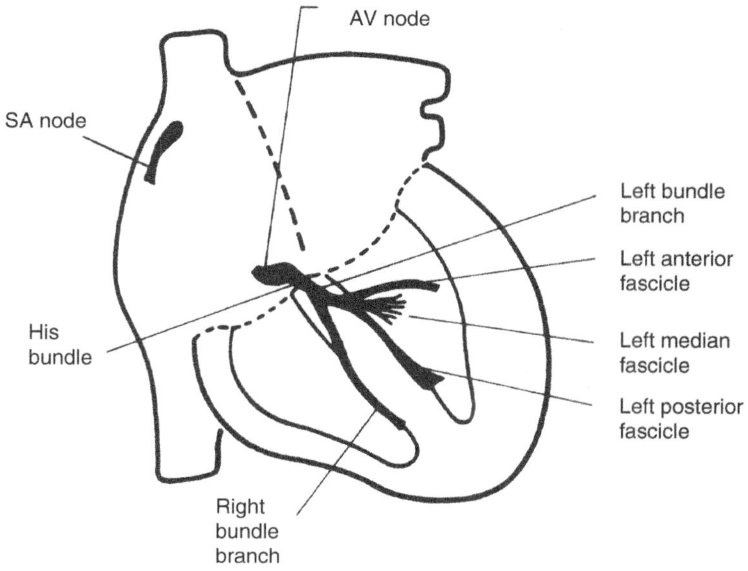

Fig. 2.4
Schematic of the normal IV conduction system. A well-individualized median (or centroseptal) fascicle is represented

Activation of the anterior paraseptal and central areas is mediated by the anterior division of the left bundle branch. The posterior division provides conduction to the posterior paraseptal area (sometimes a less-well-defined subdivision is described providing conduction to the central septum). Since anterior and posterior paraseptal areas are opposite to each other, the direction of the resultant vectors of excitation, during this phase, will be dominated by the potentials of the central area.

After the excitation of the septal areas, the electrical stimulus spreads to the myocardium of the apical and the free wall of both ventricles, which are then activated. As a result of the much larger mass of the left ventricle, the electrical forces produced by its depolarization largely predominate over the right ventricular potentials.

The basal portion of the septum and the posterobasal portion of the free wall of the left ventricle are the latest regions to be depolarized, partly because there is a relative rarity of terminal Purkinje fibers in these areas.

This sequence of ventricular activation can be represented by three basic dominant vectors, as below, occurring sequentially, with their positive extremities inscribing the vectorcardiographic spatial QRS loop.

(a) The initial vector corresponds to the early septal and paraseptal electromotive forces (emfs). The right interventricular septal surface anatomically faces the anterior and right side, either slightly upward or slightly downward (according to the horizontal or vertical positioning of the heart). Since the septum is depolarized from left to right, the initial phase of ventricular depolarization and the subsequent spread of activation across the septum cause the initial vector to be oriented mainly to the right and anteriorly, either upward or slightly downward.
(b) The second vector is the maximal resultant vector related to the activation of the free wall of the ventricles. Left ventricular emfs dominate and give rise to the leftward, inferior and posterior orientation of this vector.
(c) The terminal vector is related to the activation of the basal portions of the ventricles, which results in electrical forces oriented posteriorly, and somewhat superiorly, either slightly to the right or slightly to the left.

These three vectors, when projected upon the axis of the limb and precordial leads, produce, respectively:

(a) A small r in V_1 and a small q in leads I, aVL, and V_6;
(b) A dominant R-wave in I and II as well as V_5 and V_6 with a counterpart in the S-waves of aVR and V_1;
(c) A small s in V_6 and leads I and II, sometimes an r’ in V_1.

The remaining leads will present intermediate patterns, which can be derived from the projection of the QRS spatial loop upon their own axis of derivation. Leads III and aVF on one side, and aVL on the other, will be predominantly positive or negative, in normal subjects, according to their body shape (vertical axis in slim individuals and horizontal in the obese).

Anatomic or functional lesions occur at any point of the very sensitive specialized ventricular conduction system, and may result in delay or interruption of the conduction of the electrical stimulus to the areas forward to the lesion. Since the several divisions and subdivisions of the bundle branches are largely interconnected, conduction will follow across the intact divisions and will result in the activation of the whole ventricular mass. However, the sequence of activation will be different, in each case, from that previously described. Different sequences of activation mean different spatial QRS loops and different ECG patterns.

It must be emphasized from the very beginning that although the electrical patterns will facilitate an approach to the identification of the anatomic location of the conduction defect, different locations and different types of conduction defects may result in similar ECG patterns. For example, a complete left bundle branch block can be caused by a functional lesion within the His bundle, before the bifurcation; by a complete interruption of the main left bundle branch (either anatomic or functional); or by lesions located more distally, either in both the left anterior and the left posterior fascicles, or as a diffuse disease of the more distal ramifications of the left bundle (parietal block). On the other hand, the same pattern can coexist with multiple and diffuse lesions along the conduction system. In pure pathological terms, it can sometimes be very difficult to decide which the most important lesions are. Even the determination of the percentage of injured fibers, in each division or subdivision, by microscopy, has been used to study this problem, although not very conclusively [19, 22]. As a matter of fact, such studies are highly demanding and poorly rewarding.

The understanding of intraventricular conduction-defect patterns has evolved through the years. For instance, during the first decades of electrocardiology, right and left bundle branch block (RBBB and LBBB, respectively) were inversely diagnosed, on the basis of dog experiments. Much was learned, but even today much controversy still exists around some of the criteria used in ECG/VCG classification of conduction disturbances.

Great advances were made owing to the concept of fascicular blocks and its correlation with the anatomic and electrophysiological data, mainly those obtained by endocardial and epicardial mapping, as well as His-bundle electrocardiography. Intermittent or iatrogenic (surgical) conduction disturbances have also been of great help in the understanding of some ECG patterns.

An important effort was made by a WHO/ISFC Task Force [16] who attempted to establish a consensus on international criteria for the diagnosis of intraventricular conduction defects. In this chapter, those criteria will be followed and will occasionally be presented along with other more controversial points of view.

2.3.1 Fascicular Blocks

The correlation of the anatomy of the cardiac conduction system with electrocardiographic and electrophysiological data, leading to the concept of fascicular blocks (so-called "hemiblocks"), has added much to our understanding of the mechanisms of electrical activation and of heart block. Despite some arguments as to its validity, the concept of fascicular blocks has provided a most useful theoretical framework for viewing abnormalities of auriculoventricular and intraventricular conduction.

As previously stated, the left-sided intraventricular conduction system is usually described as a multiple strand of fibers emerging from the His bundle itself, at the septal surface (➋ Fig. 2.4), with two main subdivisions or fascicles: one directed anteriorly and superiorly toward the base of the anterior papillary muscle (the left anterior fascicle) and the other directed inferiorly and posteriorly toward the base of the posterior papillary muscle (the left posterior fascicle). The two main subdivisions have extensive interconnecting anastomoses between them. Occasionally, a group of the left median fibers is more clearly identified, constituting a third septal (median or centroseptal) fascicle [19–21, 23] (➋ Fig. 2.4). This led to a debate around the concept of a bifascicular or trifascicular left-sided conduction system (and trifascicular against a tetrafascicular or quadrifascicular system, for the whole conduction apparatus) [20, 21]. Most probably, the anatomic network of the left-sided conduction system has a variable distribution within the population as happens with other anatomic structures (such as the coronary arterial system). Eventually there exists, for the left main bundle, a continuum from either two or three subdivisions to a nondefined branching type (fanning out as a pencil-like division) of the main left bundle branch.

Indeed, a few cases have also been described where false tendons were found running across the ventricle. These tendons contain conduction tissue, which can therefore alter the activation sequence and contribute to the variation of the normal pattern and hence of electrical axis [24].

In fact, all the above-mentioned structures may be involved, organically or functionally, in the aberrations observed in atrial premature beats, mimicking successively all types of intraventricular conduction disturbances: slight axis deviation, fascicular blocks of any type, complete bundle branch blocks, and trifascicular or tetrafascicular blocks [20, 25].

The concept of a conduction disturbance occurring in one of the two left bundle branch subdivisions has been introduced by Rosenbaum, who used the term hemiblock [26, 27]. For those who accept a trifascicular left-sided conduction system, hemiblock became a misnomer, since there exists three different types of "hemi" blocks – left anterior, left posterior, and left median [20, 21, 28].

"Left fascicular blocks" is probably the best way to refer to these localized conduction disturbances and has become the internationally accepted terminology. Nevertheless, the term hemiblock has stood the test of time and sometimes is used even for the third left subdivision – left median hemiblock (for left median fascicular block) [20, 21, 29, 30].

2.3.1.1 Left Anterior Fascicular Block

(a) ECG/VCG pattern

The hallmark of left anterior fascicular block (LAFB) is marked left axis deviation in the limb leads (➋ Fig. 2.5).

Owing to the organic or functional interruption of the conduction through the left anterior division of the left bundle branch, the electrical impulse must travel through the left posterior division to activate the free wall of the left ventricle. The inferior and posterior portions of the left ventricular free wall are depolarized in the normal way (via the intact left posterior subdivision). The activation of the anterior and lateral regions is delayed (by ≈ 0.02 s) because the stimulus cannot be conducted through the interrupted left anterior division. Consequently, the wave of activation will travel in a retrograde fashion, through the network of the Purkinje system, in order to reach the anterolateral wall. The initial electrical forces (0.02 s) do not have the component of the anterior paraseptal area, thus resulting in the dominance of the forces directed inferiorly and to the right. Subsequently, the inferior wall and the apex are activated (forces directed inferiorly) and only afterward in the anterolateral wall depolarized with a leftward, posterior and superior spread of excitation. The latter QRS forces become more prominent because, being delayed, they are unopposed.

The VCG spatial QRS loop will be of normal magnitude (if there are no associated abnormalities) although with slightly prolonged duration of the QRS (not greater than 0.11 s). The initial vectors point inferiorly and to the right while the body of the spatial QRS loop is superiorly and posteriorly displaced, being located in the left superior and posterior octant.

Typically, in the frontal plane projection, the initial QRS deflection points inferiorly and slight to the right, while the efferent limb is leftward and is inscribed counterclockwise, invading the left superior quadrant. The maximal QRS vector and afferent limb of the spatial QRS loop are oriented superiorly and to the left (the maximal QRS vector can rarely point superiorly and to the right).

As the greater portion of the QRS loop is directed leftward and superiorly, a prominent R-wave is detected in leads I and aVL, while deep S-waves are registered in II, III, and aVF. The initial deflection, pointing inferiorly and slightly rightward, projects itself as a small q-wave in leads I and aVL (qR complexes); if they point anteriorly or slightly leftward, an isolated monophasic R-wave will result in lead I. A small r-wave is always present in leads II, III, and aVF since the initial deflection is always inferior. The superior displacement of the main portion of the loop explains the abnormal axis deviation, between -30° and -90°. Usually ST- and T-waves remain within the normal range, pointing downward and to the left. However, the prominent R-wave in aVL may be accompanied by a slightly negative T-wave.

Criteria for left anterior fascicular block are still debatable [31–40]. Rosenbaum's original criteria [26, 27] were the following:

(a) Frontal plane QRS left axis deviation -45° to -80°
(b) QRS duration ≤0.11 s
(c) Small Q-wave ≤0.02 s in leads I and aVL

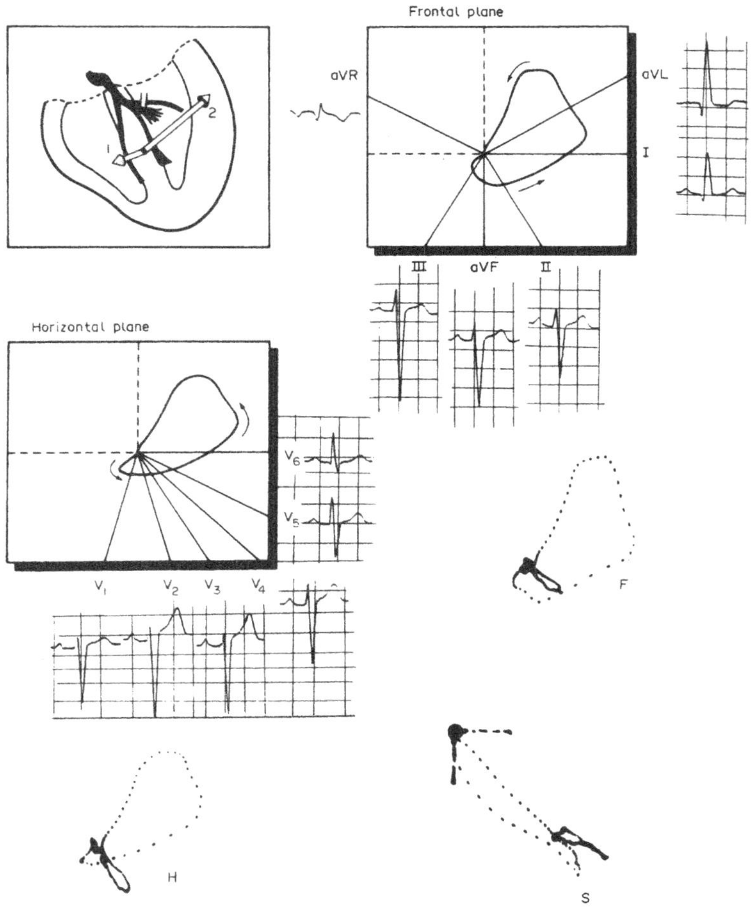

Fig. 2.5
Left anterior fascicular block: schematic of the spatial main vectors of ventricular activation resulting from the interruption of the left anterior fascicle (*top left corner*) and a diagram of the projections of the QRS loop on the frontal and horizontal planes and ECG leads and VCG loops of a typical example (*F* frontal, *H* horizontal, *S* sagittal)

As far as left axis deviation is concerned, there is enough agreement [31, 38, 39] in that left axis deviation alone should not be synonymous with LAFB because this shift of electrical forces to the left and superiorly can be observed with other causes such as extreme obesity, chronic pulmonary disease, thoracic malformations, and inferior and inferolateral myocardial infarction. The limit of −45°, as pointed out by Rosenbaum [26, 27], mostly eliminates those other causes but it also eliminates LAFB of lesser degree (as demonstrated in cases of transient LAFB). Thus the limit of −30° has been used by most groups of investigators [32, 40, 41] although some prefer −40°, unless transient shift is observed. It is possible to demonstrate that the axis deviation occurs during the first 60 ms of the QRS complex (especially in cases with QRS duration beyond 0.11 s, owing to other associated intraventricular conduction disturbances – for instance, RBBB or LBBB).

The small Q-waves in leads I and aVL have also caused some controversy [36, 38, 42–44]. Kulbertus et al. [36] found that the initial 10 ms QRS vectors are almost always directed inferiorly. However, while in 55% they were directed to the right, in 45% they pointed to the left, which in some cases may provoke a QS pattern in V_1. Jacobson et al. [35] and Burchell and Tuna [31] also concluded that a Q-wave in leads I and aVL is not an absolute requirement for LAFB. However, they have been found in most cases of transient or paroxysmal LAFB.

Medrano et al. [45] consider that there should be either slurring of the downstroke of the R-wave with delayed R peak time of at least 45 ms in aVL, or a late slurred terminal R-wave in aVR, or else a slurred S-wave in leads V_5 and V_6.

In fact, although the QRS duration is normal in isolated LAFB, there may be a slight widening of the QRS complex of up to 0.02 s compared to appearances prior to the development of LAFB.

The WHO/ISFC Task Force has proposed the following ECG criteria for diagnosis of LAFB [16]:

(a) Left axis deviation of $-45°$ to $90°$
(b) qR pattern in aVL
(c) R peak time in aVL $\geq$45 ms
(d) QRS duration <0.12 s

When these criteria are present with QRS axis deviation of $-30°$ to $-45°$, the diagnosis of a "possible" LAFB should be made.

Note that the QRS loop in the frontal plane is inscribed counterclockwise – a feature which may be useful in the presence of inferior wall myocardial infarction (the peak of the R-wave in lead III occurs before the peak of the R-wave in lead II).

Lopes [46] has proposed VCG criteria for the diagnosis of LAFB as below:

(a) The QRS duration should be <0.12 s
(b) The frontal plane QRS loop should have the following characteristics:
   (i) Initial vectors directed inferiorly and rightward
   (ii) Counterclockwise inscription
   (iii) QRS axis more superior than $-30°$

   If the major axis of the QRS loop is not directed upward, but the late part of the loop invades the left superior quadrant, "possible LAFB" may be diagnosed.
(c) The horizontal plane QRS loop should have the following features:
   (i) Initial vectors oriented rightward and anteriorly
   (ii) Counterclockwise inscription in general, but about 20–30% may show a predominant anterior loop with clockwise inscription, which can represent associated median or centroseptal fascicular block [29, 30, 47, 48]
   (iii) Terminal vectors may be normal or located predominantly in the right posterior quadrant

(b) Clinical implications

LAFB has been associated with conduction disturbances in the His bundle, anterior ischemia, anterior myocardial infarction, Chagas disease, sclerodegenerative disease, cardiomyopathy [49], hyperkalemia [50], myocarditis, infiltrative and degenerative diseases, and trauma (its association with incomplete RBBB in ostium primum defect is discussed in ➋ Sect. 2.3.2.1). It is usually associated with fibrosis in the anterior fibers, although fibrosis is usually widely distributed over the anterior, mild, and posterior fibers [22].

LAFB unassociated with block in other fascicles is usually considered a benign intraventricular conduction disturbance. Nevertheless, in one angiographic study [51], LAFB was associated with a 50% chance of having 95% or greater occlusion in the left anterior descending artery. However, this was a selected population in which the prevalence of coronary heart disease was high enough to justify a coronary angiographic study. In the Framingham study, the incidence of progression to bifascicular block was 7% and to complete AV block, 3% [52]. In the ambulatory patient, the prognosis of LAFB is exceedingly benign [29, 53, 54]. As will be seen with other types of conduction defects, prognosis depends primarily on the severity of the associated heart disease [55]. In the absence of other cardiovascular abnormalities, LAFB seems not to affect the prognosis, even in old age.

(c) Diagnostic difficulties

LAFB may mimic anteroseptal myocardial infarction (QS in V_1 and/or V_2 and sometimes QR with a negative T-wave in aVL). Sometimes, inferior infarction may also be erroneously diagnosed owing to low voltage of initial R-waves in inferior leads (distinction can be more easily made by the rotation of the frontal plane QRS loop, which is inscribed clockwise in inferior myocardial infarction and counterclockwise in LAFB). The appearance of new initial R-waves in the inferior leads owing to LAFB may hide preexisting inferior myocardial infarction. On the other hand, a recent inferior wall myocardial infarction may abolish the initial R of LAFB in leads II, III, and aVF, so that QS complexes are recorded. All these aspects have been well identified in cases of paroxysmal LAFB. Occasionally, secondary ST–T-wave abnormalities (slight ST depression and negativity of the T-wave in aVL) may also make it difficult to exclude anteroseptal ischemia (➋ Fig. 2.6). R-waves tend to be taller in lead I and aVL when LAFB supervenes; this may occasionally render voltage criteria invalid for left ventricular hypertrophy (false positives).

2.3.1.2 Left Posterior Fascicular Block

(a) ECG/VCG pattern

The hallmark of left posterior fascicular block (LPFB) is the right axis deviation in the limb leads (➋ Fig. 2.7). In fact, in cases of LPFB, either organic or functional, the opposite of LAFB occurs, that is to say, ventricular excitation proceeds through the left anterior division to the anterior paraseptal region and midseptum, and from there to the anterior and anterolateral wall. Activation of the posteroinferior regions of the left ventricle is delayed (proceeding in a retrograde fashion from the anterior fascicle).

Initial QRS forces (10–20 ms) are directed superiorly and leftward (around −45°), with the spatial QRS loop being inscribed clockwise, invading the inferior octants, first the left then the right, either posteriorly or slightly anteriorly.

The main characteristic of LPFB is the inferior and rightward displacement of the spatial QRS loop with an abnormally large portion located in the right inferior and posterior octant. Although there may be slight widening, the duration of the QRS does not exceed 0.11 s. The maximal spatial QRS vector is oriented inferiorly and posteriorly and most of the time to the right.

Initial forces, being leftward, give rise to an initial R-wave in lead I and aVL. Then the rightward displacement of the QRS loop causes deep S-waves in I and aVL while a qR pattern is obtained in II, III, and aVF. The rightward displacement of the loop accounts for the right axis deviation of the QRS.

Rosenbaum [26, 27] first described a QRS deviation $\geq +120°$; later, he accepted $+90°$ as a criterion. Serial observation of the transition to right axis deviation would better support the diagnosis in an individual, more so in cases of intermittent LPFB.

In the horizontal plane, RS complexes in the left precordial leads cause further difficulty in distinguishing LPFB from right ventricular hypertrophy.

In practice, the diagnosis of "pure" LPFB is difficult and needs the clinical exclusion of several conditions which may produce a similar pattern, owing to predominant right ventricular forces, instead of the redistribution of forces within the electrically dominant left ventricle. Examples are right ventricular hypertrophy, chronic obstructive as well as acute pulmonary disease, emphysema, extremely vertical heart (habitus asthenicus), and extensive lateral-wall myocardial infarction. Besides clinical examination, chest x-ray and echocardiography are mandatory. As a result in part of those difficulties, LPFB is rarely recognized [27, 56–58] unless associated with RBBB.

The WHO/ISFC Task Force has proposed the following ECG criteria for the diagnosis of LPFB [16]:

(a) Frontal QRS axis of $+90°$ to $+180°$ (in the absence of other causes of right axis deviation)
(b) rS configuration in leads I and aVL associated with qR pattern in inferior leads (Q-wave is obligatory in leads III and aVF), Q-wave in inferior leads should be ≤ 0.04 s
(c) QRS duration <0.12 s

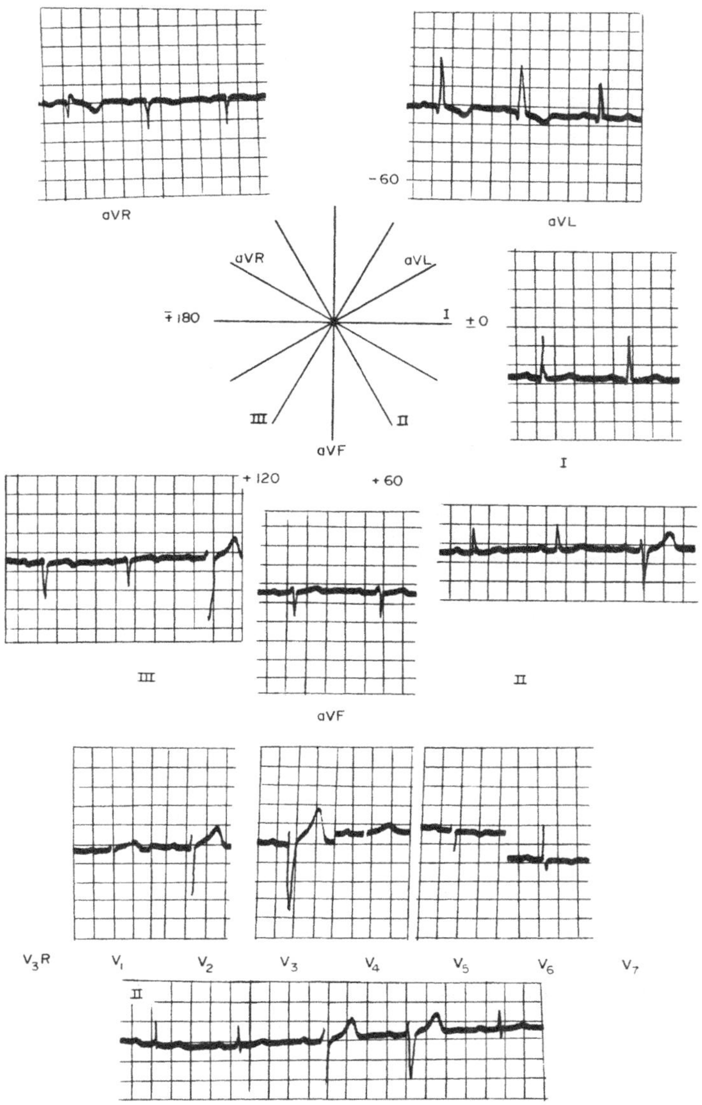

Fig. 2.6
Vectorial display of the 12-lead ECG in a case of paroxysmal LAFB. In aVL, first and second QRS complexes show conduction during LAFB followed by normal IV conduction in the third QRS complex. Note negative T-waves during LAFB become positive during normal conduction. Appearance and disappearance of LAFB is not related to significant R–R interval variation (lead II at the bottom)

Lopes [46] has proposed VCG criteria for the diagnosis of LPFB as below:

(a) The QRS duration should be <0.12 s.
(b) The frontal plane QRS loop should have the following characteristics:
  (i) Initial vectors inscribed superiorly and leftward
  (ii) Clockwise inscription
  (iii) QRS axis more rightward than +90°

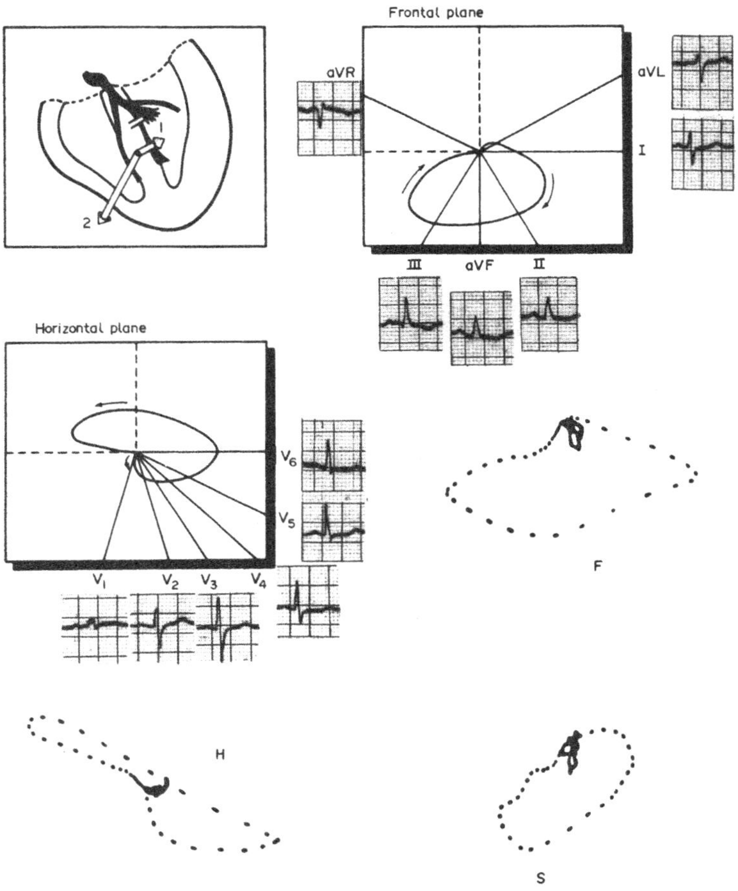

Fig. 2.7
Left posterior fascicular block: schematic of the spatial main vectors of ventricular activation resulting from interruption of the left posterior fascicle together with a diagram of the projections of the QRS loop on the frontal and horizontal planes and ECG leads and VCG loops of a typical case of LPFB (*F* frontal, *H* horizontal, *S* sagittal) (see also Figs. 2.18 and 2.19)

(c) The horizontal plane QRS loop should have the following features:
  (i) Initial vector anterior and leftward
  (ii) Counterclockwise or figure-of-eight inscription generally
  (iii) Rightward and either posterior or anterior maximum QRS vector

(b) Clinical implications

LPFB is much rarer than block of the left anterior fascicle, because the left posterior fascicle is substantially larger and apparently better perfused, and therefore less susceptible to damage. Chronic degenerative or fibrotic processes, ischemic processes affecting this fascicle or the Purkinje system (or the myocardium activated by the fascicle), hyperkalemia, myocarditis, Chagas disease, infiltrative disease, and acute cor pulmonale [59] have been described as associated with LPFB.

(c) Diagnostic difficulties

Isolated LPFB may be difficult to recognize. Obviously, it will be most accurately diagnosed when it occurs as an intermittent pattern. LPFB may mimic an inferior myocardial infarction (inferior q-waves). Abnormal Q-waves (>0.04 s) support the diagnosis of myocardial infarction; history, echocardiography, and radionuclides may help in the differential diagnosis. LPFB may also hide lateral infarction (small r-waves and deep S-waves in lead I and aVL).

When LPFB is associated with positive QRS in V_1 (possibly indicating associated left median fascicular block – see ➋ Sect. 2.3.1.3), right ventricular hypertrophy or even hidden Wolff–Parkinson–White syndrome must be ruled out as a cause of the ECG pattern. In young people, the diagnosis is often difficult owing to the vertical axis, and more so if there is constitutional abnormal anatomical position of the heart (extremely vertical).

The tendency for upright T-waves in leads I and aVL may conceal small or slightly inverted ischemic T-wave changes in these leads. T-waves may become inverted in inferior leads thus mimicking an active ischemic process. Anterolateral myocardial infarction (counterclockwise rotation in the frontal plane) must be ruled out for the identification of LPFB. Acute cor pulmonale, as mentioned above, should also be excluded in clinical terms. The S_IQ_{III} pattern suggestive of pulmonary embolism – the McGinn and White pattern – has been interpreted as representing "functional" LPFB [59].

2.3.1.3 Left Median (Centroseptal) Fascicular Block

As mentioned in ➋ Sect. 2.3.1, left median fascicular fibers do exist and a left median (centroseptal) fascicular block (LMFB) has been produced experimentally [23]. Indeed, in cases of intermittent fascicular or bundle branch blocks, an anterior displacement of the QRS loop, independent of the axis deviation, can be observed and may be a result of the involvement of centroseptal fibers.

(a) ECG/VCG pattern

The ECG pattern is supposed to show prominent R-waves in the right precordial leads ($V_1 - V_2$), similar to those found in "true" posterior myocardial infarction, concomitant with no abnormal axis deviation in the frontal plane (➋ Fig. 2.8). Left median block is rarely identified as an isolated finding (except when paroxysmal – ➋ Fig. 2.9) being confounded with "normal variation." It may explain the anterior displacement of the QRS loop (more prominent R-waves in the right precordial leads) and even the clockwise rotation in the horizontal plane, in cases of left fascicular blocks, RBBB or RBBB associated with either LAFB or LPFB. In relatives of patients with anteriorly displaced loops accompanying more conventional blocks, isolated anterior displacement of the QRS loop has been found. It is uncertain whether this represents normal variation or left median "hemi" block [29, 30, 47, 48].

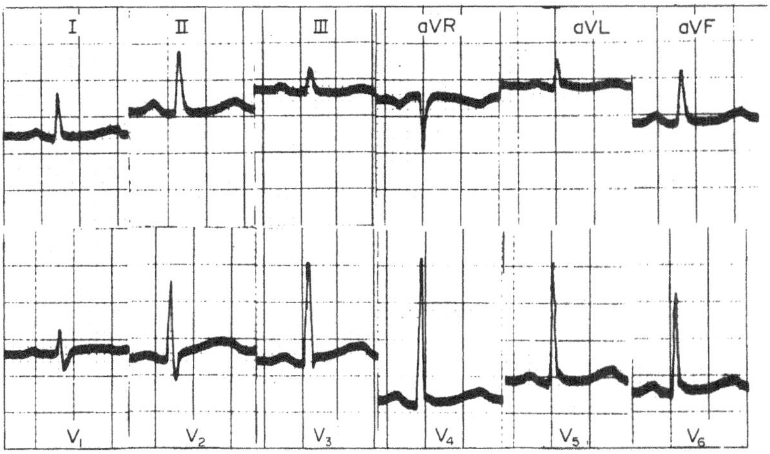

Fig. 2.8

ECG with dominant R-waves in "right" precordial leads (V_1 and V_2) with no other ECG abnormalities. Left median fascicular block would be postulated

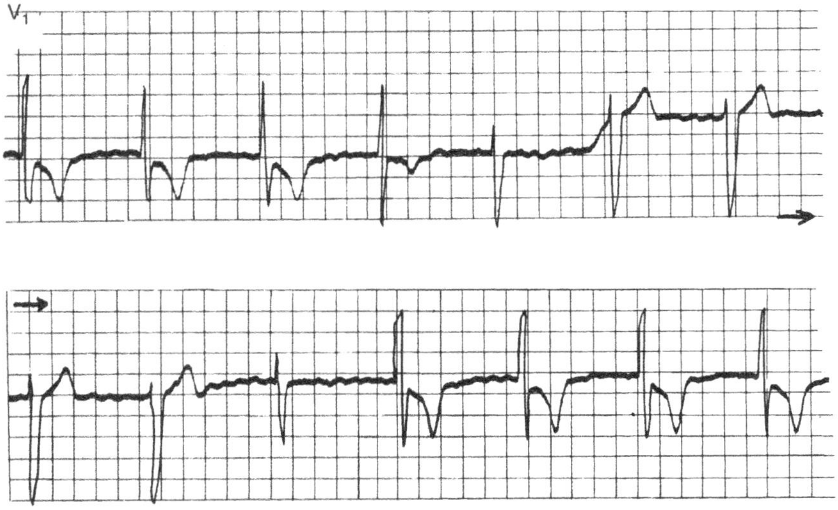

Fig. 2.9
Paroxysmal left median fascicular block: continuous recording of lead V_1 showing the appearance and disappearance of dominant R-waves without increase in QRS duration

(b) Clinical implications
LMFB has been described in patients with ischemic heart disease. It is associated with fibrosis of the corresponding fibers, as well as sclerodegenerative changes of the conduction tissue, although similar lesions can be found simultaneously in the other fascicles [19, 23, 60].

Other etiologies include diabetes mellitus and hypertrophic cardiomyopathy.

(c) Diagnostic difficulties
On the basis of interpreting a single ECG, it is essentially impossible to differentiate LMFB from posterior myocardial infarction, some types of right ventricular hypertrophy or variants of normal.

2.3.2 Incomplete Bundle Branch Block

2.3.2.1 Incomplete Right Bundle Branch Block

(a) ECG/VCG pattern
In incomplete RBBB, the transmission through the right bundle is not totally interrupted but only delayed. ECG/VCG patterns may be similar to complete RBBB (see Sect. 2.3.3.1) but of lesser duration (<0.12 s). Only after the left ventricular septum and free-wall activation is initiated are the right interventricular septum and right ventricular free wall depolarized by impulses which are conducted both through the right and the left bundle branches.

Similar to what will be seen in complete RBBB, only the late part of the activation process is disturbed, on the surface ECG and on the special VCG, with orientation of the terminal electrical vectors rightward, anteriorly and either superiorly or inferiorly. The more the conduction through the right bundle is disturbed (three subdivisions have been described [61] and can be gradually involved in the individual patient), the more prominent these late forces become and the more similar the spatial QRS loop lock to complete RBBB with a more-or-less prominent terminal "fingerlike" appendage. The afferent limb and the terminal deflection of the spatial QRS loop become deviated in the anterior and rightward direction. The T loop is directed leftward and posteriorly.

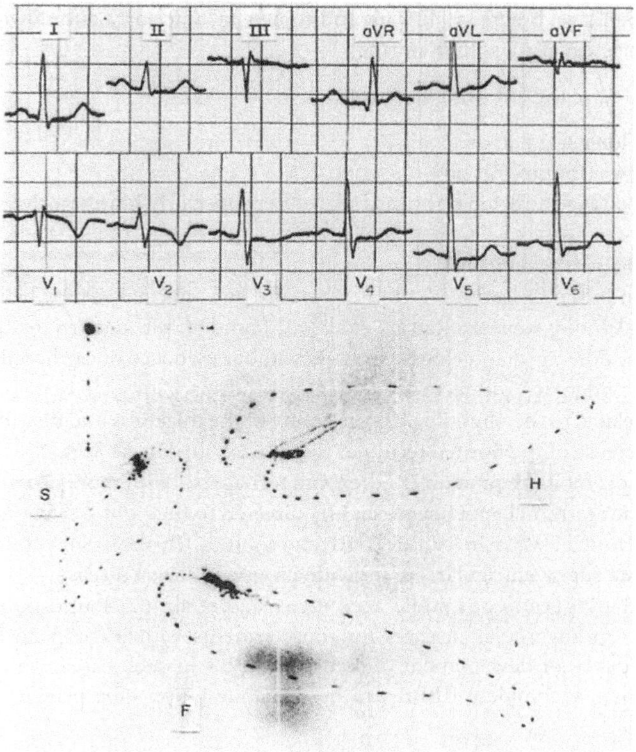

Fig. 2.10
ECG leads and VCG loops of a case of typical incomplete RBBB (compare with terminal appendage in horizontal projection of complete RBBB in Fig. 2.13): *F* frontal, *H* horizontal, *S* saggital

The ECG shows typically an R' wave in lead V_1 and a wider S-wave in lead I and V_6 corresponding to the abnormal anterior and rightward terminal appendage. The amplitude and width of the R′ in V_1 and of the S-wave in leads I and V_6 increase with the degree of conduction delay (Fig. 2.10). By definition, the QRS duration is <0.12 s. T-wave changes arise from the posterior displacement of the spatial T loop. Consequently, the T-wave becomes isoelectric or eventually inverted in the right precordial leads (usually no significant ST–T-wave abnormalities can be identified in the limb and left precordial leads).

The WHO/ISFC Task Force has proposed the following ECG criteria for the diagnosis of incomplete RBBB [16]:

(a) QRS duration <0.12 s
(b) Right precordial pattern rsr′, rsR′, or rSR′ or M-shaped with R′ usually greater than initial R-wave; and
(c) Wide S-wave in leads I and V_5–V_6

The diagnosis is more evident if the condition occurs intermittently.

The VCG criteria for the diagnosis of incomplete RBBB have been recommended as below.

(a) The QRS duration should be <0.12 s.
(b) The spatial QRS loop should have normal overall amplitude but be typically deformed by a small terminal fingerlike appendage, which is oriented to the right.
(c) The transverse plane should have the following characteristics:
   (i) Counterclockwise inscription of the major part of the loop (sometimes figure-of-eight configuration)
   (ii) Initial vector anterior and rightward, with maximal QRS vector leftward and either anterior or posterior

(iii) Small terminal appendage directed rightward and somewhat anteriorly, and slowly inscribed
(iv) Maximal QRS voltage usually less than normal

(d) The frontal plane should have the following features:

(i) The loop generally long and narrow
(ii) Usually clockwise inscription
(iii) Small terminal appendage directed rightward and either superiorly or inferiorly.

(b) Clinical implications and diagnostic difficulties

An incomplete RBBB pattern in the 12-lead ECG can be observed as a "normal variant." Hiss and Lamb [62] reported a prevalence of 2.4% in normal young subjects. Raunio et al. [63] found an rSr′ pattern in V_1 in 2.9% of children, 1.4% of young adults and 0.65% of middle-aged and elderly subjects without evidence of cardiopulmonary disease. Sometimes, these patterns are no longer evident if V_1 in recorded one intercostal space lower [64].

The r′ pattern has been related to the physiological variability of the thickness and distribution of the right ventricular mass [65], with the slight increase of the normal terminal vector described in ➋ Sect. 2.3.

A normal variant QRS loop, more frequent in children and teenagers – with more prominent terminal vectors, giving rise to a posterior and superior terminal appendage, slightly directed to the right – may produce, in the same way, an r′ in V_1 and aVR as well as a terminal S-wave in leads I, II, III, and V_6 [66]. This $S_I S_{II} S_{III}$ pattern may be explained by distal delayed activation of the crista supraventricularis in individuals without heart disease.

In a long follow-up study (20 years) of middle-aged men, Liao et al. [67] found no increased risk of death from coronary heart disease and cardiovascular diseases for those patients with incomplete RBBB pattern. Nevertheless, they observed a higher incidence of development of complete RBBB in such cases, which further supports the concept that in middle-aged men, incomplete RBBB can be a manifestation of a primary abnormality of the cardiac conduction system.

It must be emphasized that the majority of cases diagnosed as incomplete RBBB by ECG alone are not actual examples of a conduction defect. Some of them represent the normal variant just described, while many others correspond to moderate right ventricular hypertrophy. One of the first achievements of vectorcardiography (in the early 1950s) was the demonstration that the so-called "incomplete RBBB pattern" could be caused by right ventricular hypertrophy (in mitral stenosis, for example), with quite different QRS loops in the horizontal plane, although projecting themselves in V_1 and V_6 in a manner similar to RBBB [66, 68] (➋ Fig. 2.11). In fact, subsequently, incomplete RBBB became almost synonymous with moderate right ventricular hypertrophy [66, 68].

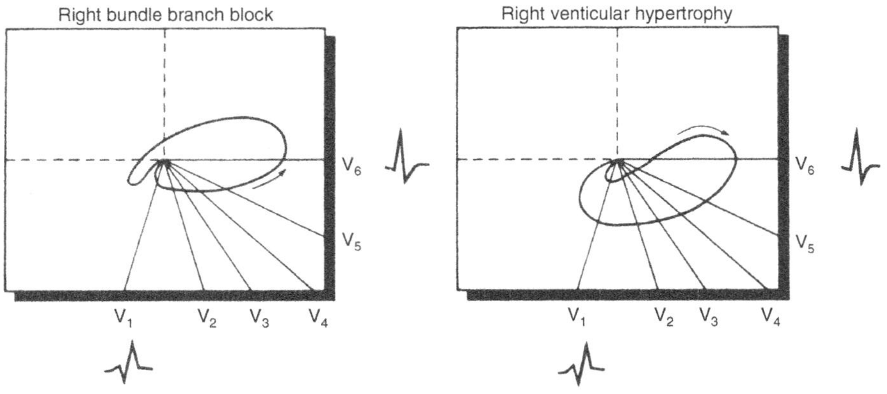

Fig. 2.11

Schematic of the vectorcardiographic loops in the horizontal plane, in cases of RBBB and RVH. Quite different loops, with clockwise and counterclockwise rotation, project themselves as rSR′ in V_1 and qRS in V_6 (see also ➋ Fig. 11.24 of *Basic Electrocardiology: Cardiac Electrophysiology, ECG Systems and Mathematical Modeling*)

Actually, right ventricular hypertrophy, owing to either acquired or congenital heart disease, or even chronic lung disease, may cause the typical ECG pattern of incomplete RBBB. However, the morphology and sense of rotation of the spatial QRS loop, mainly its horizontal planar projection, permit an easy differentiation (see the detailed description in ➋ Sect. 2.3.3.1). In congenital heart diseases, this pattern may be observed in malformations involving hypertrophy of the crista supraventricularis.

Incomplete RBBB can indeed occur as an isolated congenital electrical abnormality. It is associated with the ostium secundum type of atrial septal defect and/or anomalous pulmonary venous drainage. When incomplete RBBB occurs with the ostium primum type of atrial septal defect, especially with endocardial cushion and interventricular septum defects, there is usually an associated left anterior fascicular block (see ➋ Sect. 2.3.4) [69].

Echocardiography [70], as well as radionuclides and angiography, if needed, may help to make the correct diagnosis if the incomplete RBBB pattern is found in a patient with suspected myocardial infarction.

Other clinical factors that may induce an incomplete RBBB pattern are skeletal deformities and LAFB. In the former case, pectus excavatum or straight back syndrome may produce such a pattern. With respect to the latter, sometimes higher degrees of left axis deviation give rise to an r′ in aVR and in V_1–V_2 mainly if registered slightly above the recommended position. On the other hand, leads V_5 and V_6, if recorded lower in the axilla, will exhibit an RS complex instead of R or Rs, recorded slightly above. Both the r′ in V_1–V_2 and/or the S-wave in V_5–V_6, in cases of LAFB, can be erroneously attributed to incomplete RBBB (or right ventricular hypertrophy).

2.3.2.2 Incomplete Left Bundle Branch Block

(a) ECG/VCG pattern

In incomplete LBBB, the conduction of the electrical stimulus through the left bundle branch is not interrupted. However, progression of the wave of excitation should occur at a slower rate and, for this reason (somewhat similarly to complete LBBB – ➋ Sect. 2.3.3.2), the initial activation process will enter through the right bundle. The first area to be depolarized will be located in the right septal surface; from there the activation process spreads across the septum and activates the left septal mass from right to left, at a varying degree, because the impulse traveling through the left branch also arrives. Depolarization of the remaining left ventricular free wall then proceeds in a normal fashion. The spatial QRS loop, somewhat elongated, is oriented posteriorly, to the left and either inferiorly or superiorly. The time of occurrence of the maximal QRS vector may be slight delayed (➋ Fig. 2.12).

Therefore, in incomplete LBBB, the initial QRS pattern may be similar to complete LBBB with absence of normal "septal" Q-waves in the left precordial leads and lead I, and sometimes absence of initial r-wave in V_1–V_2. The conduction during the late activation period is less affected, as is the remainder of the QRS (➋ Fig. 2.12).

The more disturbed the conduction through the left bundle branch, the more the ECG/VCG pattern becomes similar to complete LBBB (with progressive prolongation of QRS and delayed R peak time) in the left precordial leads. ST and

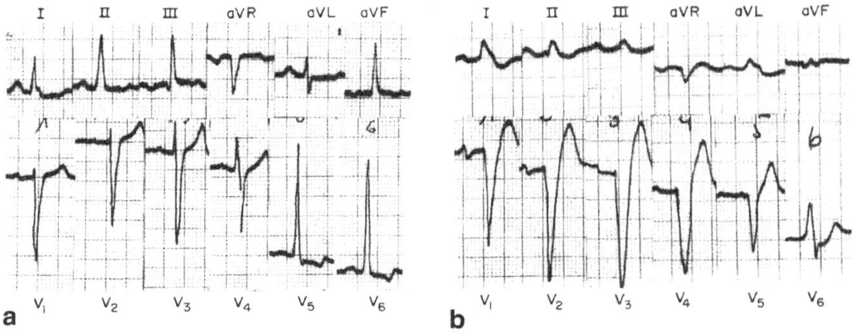

Fig. 2.12
Appearance of complete LBBB (part (b)) in a patient with previous LVH with strain (part (a))

T vectors are usually opposite to the spatial QRS loop thus producing, in the surface ECG, ST-, and T-wave polarities opposite to the main direction of the QRS maximal vector. Surprisingly enough, incomplete LBBB is much more rarely observed than complete LBBB, either as a permanent or as a transient pattern.

A pattern similar to that described for incomplete LBBB can be observed in patients with recognized left ventricular hypertrophy. The question about it being a real conduction defect has been debated [66, 71–74]. Transition within a short time from normal conduction to serial degrees of incomplete and subsequently complete LBBB has been occasionally observed and supports the real existence of incomplete LBBB as a conduction abnormality. Although this evolution would permit a firm diagnosis of conduction defect for the pattern of incomplete LBBB [73], this is only rarely observed and cannot be used for clinical purposes.

The WHO/ISFC Task Force has proposed the following ECG criteria for the diagnosis of incomplete LBBB [16]:

(a) QRS duration >0.10 s but less than the lower limit for complete LBBB (0.12 s);
(b) Prolongation of the R peak time to ≥0.06 s in the left precordial leads
(c) Absence of normal "septal" Q-waves in leads I, V_5, and V_6
(d) Presence of notching, slurring, or both in the ascending limb of the R-wave in the left precordial leads (this is a criteria for increasing the likelihood of the diagnosis of incomplete LBBB).

The VCG criteria for diagnosis of incomplete LBBB have been recommended as follows:

(a) The spatial QRS loop should have the following characteristics:
  (i) Elongated and narrow QRS loop that may be slowly inscribed in the middle and late portion, with a duration <0.12 s
  (ii) Practically, the entire loop oriented posteriorly and to the left
  (iii) Initial vector anterior and leftward
  (iv) Afferent limb superior to the efferent limb
(b) The transverse plane should have the following features:
  (i) Long and narrow loop
  (ii) Clockwise inscription of the majority of the loop
  (iii) Initial vector directed anterior and leftward
  (iv) Afferent limb to the left of the efferent limb
  (v) Slowing on the VCG that may become evident by 40 ms and continues for the entire loop.
(c) The left sagittal plane is characterized by
  (i) A long narrow loop
  (ii) Counterclockwise inscription of the majority of the loop
  (iii) Afferent limb superior to efferent limb
(d) Frontal plane with the following features:
  (i) Small and irregular loop if the spatial QRS loop is almost perpendicular to the frontal plane
  (ii) Counterclockwise inscription of the loop with the afferent limb superior to the efferent limb almost the entire loop on the left

(b) Clinical implications

Incomplete LBBB is associated with the same cardiovascular abnormalities as are usually related to complete LBBB (see ➋ Sect. 2.3.3.2). Actually, it represents an intermediate step, occasionally observed, from normal intraventricular conduction to complete LBBB. Incomplete LBBB is frequently associated with left ventricular hypertrophy [75], and has been used by some authors as a criterion for its presence. Its prognosis is related to the underlying heart disease and to its severity, as in the other types of intraventricular conduction defects.

(c) Diagnostic difficulties

Difficulties with diagnosing incomplete LBBB are greater than those found with complete LBBB because the QRS abnormalities are less specific. The following should be considered:

(a) The pattern in right precordial leads may mimic anteroseptal myocardial infarction.
(b) Inverted T-waves in the left-sided leads may mimic anteroseptal ischemia in the same way that positive T-waves in the right precordial leads may conceal ECG signs of anteroseptal ischemia.

2.3.2.3 Complete Bundle Branch Block

The earliest awareness of importance of the specialized conduction system seems to have been related to the identification of the ECG pattern of complete bundle branch block (BBB) resulting from damage caused in the region of the interventricular septum of the canine heart (Eppinger and Rothberger 1909–1910) [76].

Unfortunately, confusion has resulted from the extrapolation of the patterns identified in the vertical heart of the dog to the more horizontally positioned human heart. Consequently, the pattern of complete LBBB was incorrectly diagnosed as complete RBBB and vice versa. This confusion delayed the correct identification of the conduction defect patterns for at least 25 years.

Bundle branch blocks occur in approximately 0.6% of the population and 1–2% of the population over 60 years of age. Up to 80% of patients with BBB do have organic heart disease (coronary heart disease in 50%) [77]. Bundle branch blocks are associated frequently with pathological conditions in the suspected location [78] and with a higher mortality if significant cardiac disease is present [79, 80].

2.3.2.4 Complete Right Bundle Branch Block

(a) ECG/VCG pattern

The hallmark of RBBB is the appearance of an R′ in V_1 with QRS duration ≥0.12 s (➋ Fig. 2.13). When there is complete interruption of the impulse conduction in the right bundle branch, the activation of the right ventricle is delayed. Left ventricular activation will follow the intact left bundle, as in the normal activation sequence.

During the initial phase of the ventricular depolarization process, the early septal and paraseptal activation takes place, as in the normal activation process, spreading from left to right (and somewhat anteriorly and superiorly according to the usual anatomic position of the interventricular septum). No electrical forces are generated at this time in the right septal surface. The activation front then proceeds to the rest of the left septum, and involves the free wall of the left ventricle. The free-wall electromotive forces dominate, with spatial resultant vectors that are oriented leftward and inferiorly, either slightly anteriorly or slightly posteriorly.

Thus, in RBBB, in spite of the lack of right septal activation, the initial phases of ventricular depolarization give rise to potentials and vectors that are rather similar to the normal activation process.

Only after most of the left ventricular free-wall depolarization has already occurred are the right septum and the right ventricular free wall activated, in a delayed and abnormal fashion (slow fiber to fiber conduction across the septum). The resultant late spatial vectors are then directed to the right and anteriorly and either superiorly or inferiorly. At this time, they are dominant because they are no longer concealed by left ventricular potentials.

According to this sequence of events, the spatial QRS loop can be divided into two distinct major portions – initial and terminal. The initial portions remain essentially similar to the normal and consist of the initial deflection, the efferent limb of the loop, and part of its afferent limb which may, in some cases, be displayed somewhat anteriorly, probably owing to centroseptal fascicular lesions. The terminal portion, which is more slowly inscribed, corresponds to the delayed activation of the right septum and right ventricular free wall. This last portion of the loop takes the configuration of a "fingerlike" appendage, pointing anteriorly and to the right. In fact, this late portion represents the most characteristic feature of complete RBBB.

The duration of the QRS loop is ≥0.12 s, with the terminal appendage slowly inscribed (≥0.03 s).

The abnormal activation sequence is followed by an abnormal repolarization course with ST and T vectors directed leftward and posteriorly, opposite to the terminal QRS forces.

The anterior and rightward initial deflection of the QRS loop, when projected in the horizontal plane, is recorded as a small r-wave in lead V_1 and a small q-wave in I, V_5, and V_6 as in the normal individual. If the initial forces are directed either straight anteriorly or slightly leftward, no Q-wave is recorded in these leads. The body of the loop projects itself as an S-wave in V_1, which will be more evident and deeper when the QRS is posteriorly oriented, and may disappear, giving

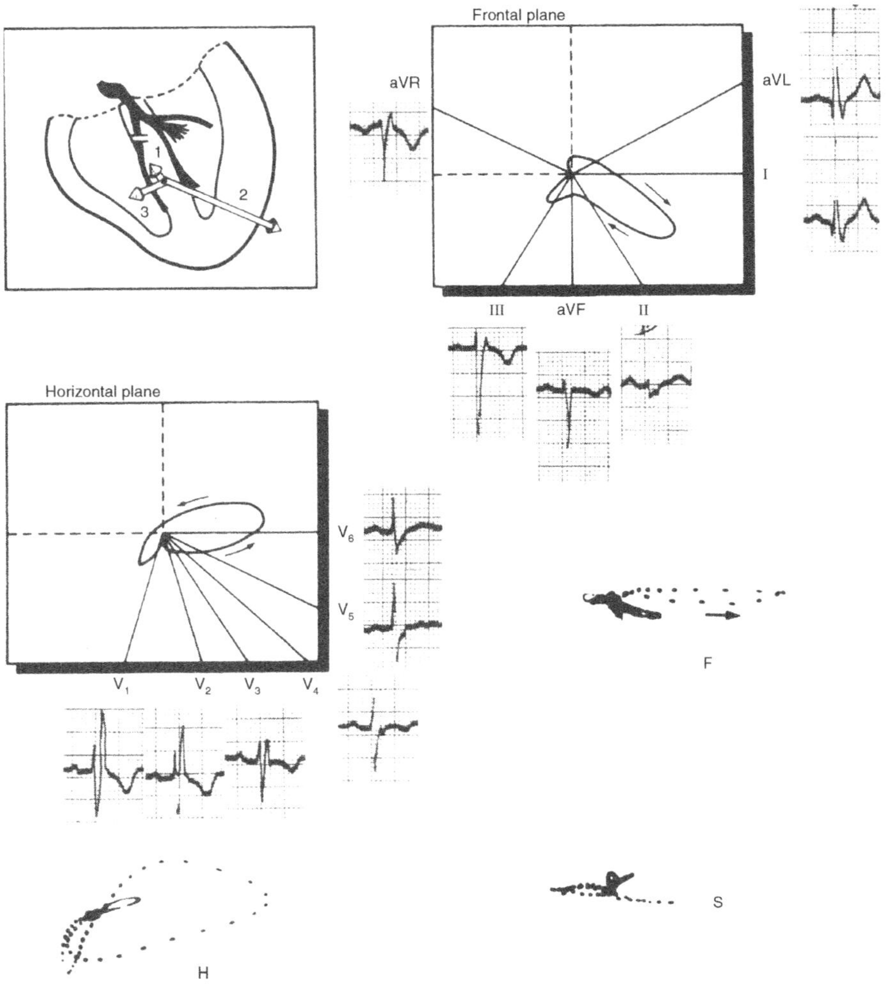

Fig. 2.13
Complete right bundle branch block: schematic of the spatial main vectors of ventricular activation resulting from interruption of the right bundle branch together with a diagram of the projections of the QRS loop on the frontal and horizontal planes and ECG leads and VCG loops of a typical case of complete RBBB (*F* frontal, *H* horizontal, *S* sagittal)

rise to a single broad bifid deflection if it points leftward (see Sect. 2.3.1). The delayed terminal appendage, which points anteriorly and to the right, is inscribed as a wide and slurred R' wave in V_1 and an enlarged S-wave in leads I and V_5–V_6.

ST–T patterns are not used as criteria for RBBB diagnosis. The abnormal repolarization pattern appears in the 12-lead ECG as ST-segment depression, as T-wave inversion (or biphasic − +) in V_1 and V_2, and as upright T-waves in leads I, V_5, and V_6.

Since the delayed activation produces alterations only of the terminal, but not of the initial, ventricular depolarization, the electrical QRS axis keeps its normal orientation provided that it was normal before the appearance of the conduction disturbance. In fact, the coexistence of abnormal left or right axis deviation suggests the coexistence of left anterior or left posterior fascicular block (see Sect. 2.3.4).

The WHO/ISFC Task Force has proposed the following criteria for the diagnosis of complete RBBB [16]:

(a) QRS prolongation to ≥0.12 s
(b) Right precordial patterns should be rsr', rsR', or rSR' or M-shaped with R′ usually greater than initial R-wave (occasionally a wide and notched isolated R pattern may be seen)
(c) Leads I and V_5–V_6 pattern must have a wide S-wave (S duration greater than R-wave or >40 ms in adults)
(d) R peak time >0.05 s in V_1 with normal time in V_5 and V_6 (when a notched dominant R pattern is present in V_1).

Lopes has proposed VCG criteria for the diagnosis of complete RBBB as below [46]:

(a) The spatial QRS loop should have normal overall amplitude but is typically deformed by a terminal fingerlike appendage, which is oriented anteriorly and to the right, and loop duration should be ≥0.12 s.
(b) The transverse plane should show the following characteristics:
    (i) Counterclockwise inscription of the major part of the loop, occasionally figure-of-eight or even clockwise (suspect left median fascicular block – see below)
    (ii) Initial vector anterior and rightward, with maximal QRS vector leftward and either anterior or posterior
    (iii) Terminal appendage directed anteriorly and rightward with duration of slowing from 30 to 85 ms
    (iv) Maximal QRS voltage usually less than normal.
(c) The frontal plane should have the following features:
    (i) In general a long and narrow loop
    (ii) Usually clockwise inscription
    (iii) Terminal appendage directed rightward and either superiorly or inferiorly

(b) Clinical implications

Complete RBBB, like complete LBBB, is most frequently identified in adulthood. However, it has been said that it has a higher prevalence in younger subjects than has LBBB [81]. This has not been confirmed in other series [82].

Besides lesions in the right bundle branch, complete RBBB (once more like LBBB) can also occur as a result of anatomic or functional lesions within the His bundle. RBBB can be part of the presenting features of congenital heart disease or be a consequence of corrective surgery [83–85], particularly for pulmonary stenosis, tetralogy of Fallot or large ventricular septal defect [86]. The surgically induced form of RBBB may regress [87] and has been related to prognosis [88]. In adulthood, complete RBBB frequently coexists with hypertension and/or coronary heart disease (either with or without myocardial infarction) [89, 90]. It may appear transiently after primary coronary angioplasty in acute myocardial infarction [91].

Complete RBBB can also represent a secondary manifestation of several cardiomyopathies, including the hypertrophic obstructive type [92]. In fact, an angiographic study [93] performed in 37 predominantly asymptomatic pilots with newly acquired RBBB showed that some of those without evidence of significant coronary artery disease had hemodynamic evidence of a mild diffuse cardiomyopathy. However, the number of cases of "isolated" intraventricular conduction defect which does represent a mild and "insignificant" cardiomyopathy, including ill-defined processes such as bundle branch fibrosis, remains a matter for speculation.

Fibrosis of the right ventricular conduction system with or without the involvement of the left-sided heart skeleton of conduction tissue (respectively, Lev's and Lenegre's disease) [94, 95] may also be the cause of RBBB either associated with ischemia or not. Complete RBBB pattern may also be associated with hyperkalemia [49] and chest trauma [96–99]. Obstructive pulmonary disease [100] and acute pulmonary embolism [101] often appear with RBBB. In the presence of pulmonary disease, complete RBBB may suggest increased systolic and mean pulmonary pressures, thus indicating significant right ventricular overload. The prevalence of associated relevant heart disease, as well as the prognostic implications of complete RBBB pattern, differs according to the type of population studied.

In military studies, a very low prevalence of the heart disease and a very good prognosis have usually been found [81, 93, 102–105]. In a study of 237,000 airmen, Rotman and Triebwasser [81] identified 394 cases of complete RBBB. One hundred cases were younger than 30 years of age: most of them were asymptomatic (97%) and had an otherwise normal cardiovascular examination (94%), 3% had evidence of coronary heart disease, and 2% were hypertensive (these percentages are significantly lower than the prevalences reported in the same study for cases with LBBB; see Sect. 2.3.3.2). During the follow-up (mean 10 years), only one case needed pacemaker implantation.

In hospital-based populations [106–109], a high prevalence of cardiovascular abnormalities is found, although in all series, subjects with "lone" RBBB are described [108, 109]. The presence of associated left fascicular block (see Sect. 2.3.4) has been described as concomitant with a higher prevalence of heart disease and a worse prognosis, including greater progression to advanced AV block [103, 106–112].

In the Framingham study [52] during a follow-up period of 18 years, 70 new cases of complete RBBB were identified. Hypertension was significantly more common in these cases. In 70%, the identification of the RBBB pattern was preceded by at least one cardiovascular abnormality – hypertension in 60%, cardiac enlargement in 25%, and coronary heart disease in 20%. In patients with RBBB, the development of manifestations of coronary heart disease was twice as frequent and that of congestive heart failure almost four times that in control group. After identification of RBBB, four of the 70 cases (6%) developed high-degree AV block. No prior evidence of cardiovascular abnormalities was found in 20 cases: 75% of them remained free of cardiovascular manifestations while 25% developed coronary heart disease, 5% with evidence of congestive heart failure. Although RBBB were as prone as controls to remain completely free of cardiovascular abnormalities, when heart disease was present there was a higher prevalence of advanced stages of disease (cardiac enlargement, clinical coronary heart disease, and congestive heart failure). The more prolonged the QRS duration, the greater the association with cardiovascular abnormalities as well as cardiovascular mortality.

At each 2-year interval after onset of RBBB, cumulative mortality was three times greater than in the control group. Almost one-third of the patients died within 10 years of onset of RBBB (only 11% for an age-matched population, free from RBBB). As in other studies [110], cardiovascular disease mortality appeared to be highly dependent on whether associated cardiovascular abnormalities were present [113].

In conclusion, it may be stated that in young subjects with otherwise normal change their prognosis. The same cannot be said of other subjects. In the presence of underlying heart disease, the prognosis is mostly related to the severity of the cardiovascular abnormality. Consequently, the identification of an intraventricular conduction defect – RBBB in this case – should be considered a sign of high priority for a complete M-mode and two-dimensional echocardiographic evaluation [30], the most important noninvasive tool for anatomic and functional analysis of the left ventricle as well as prognostic evaluation of the conduction disturbance.

(c) Diagnostic difficulties

There are usually no problems in the identification of the Q-waves of transmural myocardial infarction because initial depolarization is not significantly affected by RBBB. On the other hand, RBBB associated with cor polmunale may exhibit Q-waves in the right precordial leads (perhaps suggesting right ventricular hypertrophy), or Q-waves in the inferior leads that may mimic myocardial infarction.

Voltage criteria for left ventricular hypertrophy have a very low sensitivity in the presence of RBBB. The authors have studied 30 patients with complete RBBB by echocardiography [114]. Contrary to what was found in LBBB with left ventricular hypertrophy (see Sect. 2.3.3.2(c)), the ECG/VCG (Sokolow–Lyon/Pipberger) criteria were not able to identify any of the 21 patients that were found to have left ventricular hypertrophy and/or enlargement by echocardiography. The Sokolow–Lyon index also showed no correlation with left ventricular mass calculated by echocardiography.

Thus, it appears that in the presence of complete RBBB, left ventricular hypertrophy cannot be identified either by 12 leads ECG or by VCG, at least on the basis of the criteria quoted above.

Right ventricular hypertrophy can be a cause of complete RBBB. Actually RBBB can also be observed in acute overload of the right ventricle (pulmonary embolism), possibly owing to the distention of the right bundle.

2.3.2.5 Complete Left Bundle Branch Block

(a) ECG/VCG pattern

When the conduction of the electrical impulse through the main left bundle branch (or through its two or three subdivisions) is interrupted or severely delayed by any type of disease process, the ventricular excitation wave is conducted through the right bundle branch (Fig. 2.14). Activation will then begin low on the right septal surface, in the region corresponding, on the left side, to the base of the anterior papillary muscle. From there, the wave of excitation spreads

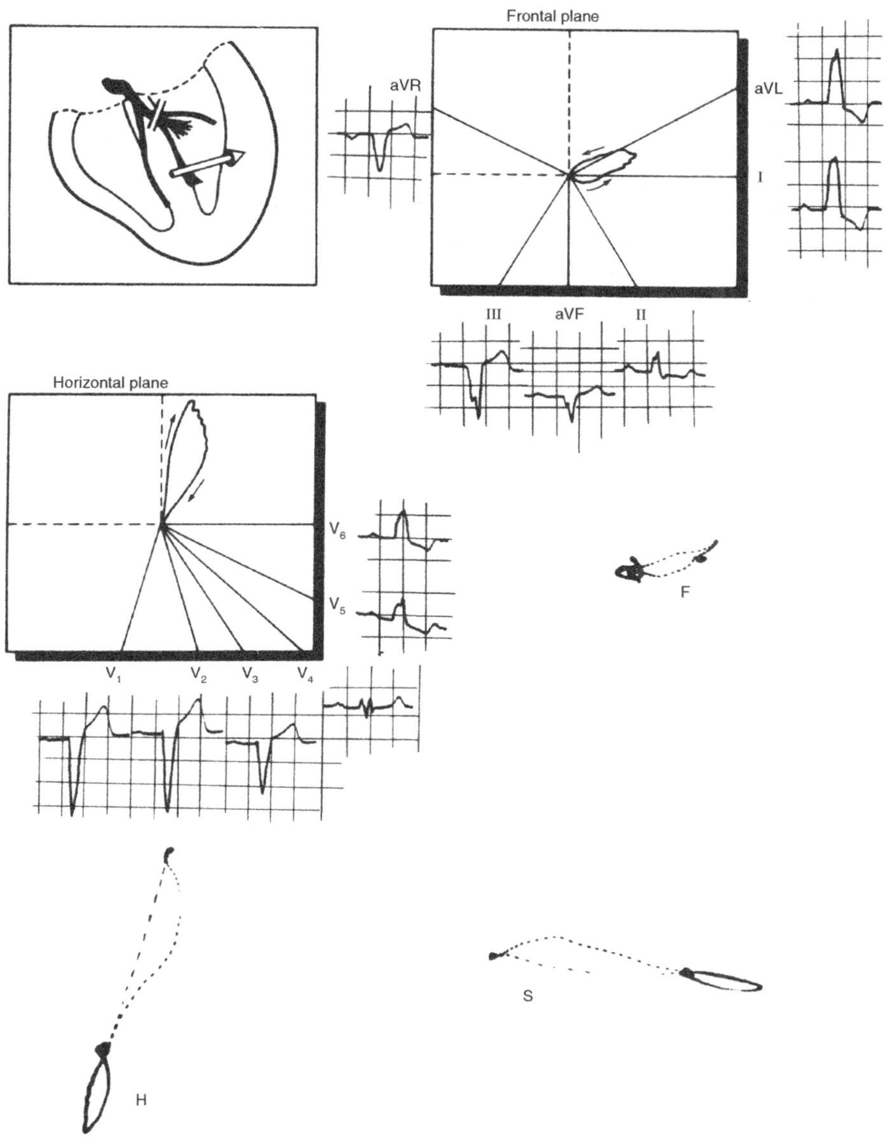

Fig. 2.14

Complete left bundle branch block: schematic of the spatial main vectors of ventricular activation resulting from interruption of the left bundle branch and a diagram of the projections of the QRS loop on the frontal and horizontal planes, and ECG leads and VCG loops of a typical case of complete LBBB (*F* frontal, *H* horizontal, *S* sagittal)

to the right ventricle and transeptally to the left ventricle, which is reached from right to left, at a much lower speed, by conduction from one muscular fiber to another. In this situation, the initial vectors of ventricular activation have their origin on the right side of the septum and are directed mainly to the left, and most often anteriorly and inferiorly, in agreement with the way the activation wave spreads, from right to left, to depolarize the left septal mass. Only afterward does the myocardium of the free wall of the left ventricle begin to be depolarized, either from cell to cell or reutilizing the peripheral fascicles of the subdivisions of the left bundle branch. This late activation of the left ventricular mass generates electrical forces directed toward the left, posteriorly, and inferiorly. The leftward orientation remains until the end of the depolarization process, the last vector being directed, as is usual, posteriorly and somewhat superiorly.

According to the spatial orientation of the electromotive forces of ventricular activation, in LBBB, the major portion of the QRS loop is located posteriorly and to the left, pointing either inferiorly or somewhat superiorly (➋ Fig. 2.14).

The leftward orientation of the initial forces accounts for the absence of the normal "septal" Q-waves in lead I and left precordial leads. The initial forces, being slightly anterior, may or may not inscribe a small r-wave in lead V_1 (posterior orientation of the initial forces is rarely seen). The body of the QRS loop is elongated and oriented mainly posteriorly and so produces increased amplitude of the S-wave in V_1 and somewhat decreased amplitude of the R-wave in V_6.

The slower velocity of left ventricular activation (fiber to fiber) results in a greater duration of the QRS loop being slowly inscribed in the middle portion and in the terminal portion, with broader QRS complexes in all ECG leads, along with slurring and notching which are more evident in the R-waves of the left-sided leads (M-shaped RR′ complexes). The time required to complete the ventricular activation process is obviously greater than usual, the QRS duration being by definition ≥0.12 s.

The altered ventricular depolarization accounts for secondary abnormal repolarization forces, with ST and T vectors directed opposite to the main QRS vector.

In the surface leads, the ST-segment is usually depressed and T-waves are negative in the left-sided leads (V_5, V_6, I, and aVL), in the opposite direction to the widened R-waves. On the contrary, in leads V_1 and V_2, deep S-waves coexist with ST-segment elevation and positive T-waves.

The WHO/ISFC Task Force has proposed the following ECG criteria for the diagnosis of complete LBBB [16]:

(a) QRS duration prolonged to ≥0.12 s;
(b) Left-sided leads (V_5, V_6, I, and aVL) with slurred and broad R-waves
(c) Absence of Q-waves in left-sided leads (possible exception of aVL)
(d) R peak time prolonged to more than 0.06 s in V_5 and V_6 (normal in V_1 and V_2, when it can be determined)
(e) Right precordial leads with very small r-waves followed by deep and broad S-waves (occasionally broad QS complexes in V_1 and V_2, rarely in V_3) and the transition zone in the precordial leads displaced to the left.

Lopes has proposed VCG criteria for the diagnosis of complete LBBB [46] as below:

(a) The spatial QRS loop should have the following characteristics:
    (i) Elongated and narrow QRS loop that is generally larger than without block (slowly inscribed in middle and late portions), duration of the loop ≥0.12 s;
    (ii) Practically the entire loop oriented posteriorly and to the left
    (iii) Initial vector anterior and leftward
    (iv) Afferent limb superior to the efferent limb
(b) The transverse plane should have the following features:
    (i) Long and narrow loop
    (ii) Clockwise inscription of the majority of the loop
    (iii) Initial vector anterior and leftward
    (iv) Afferent limb to the left of the efferent limb
    (v) Slowing on the VCG, usually evident by 40 ms and which continues for the entire loop, being most marked in the midportion
(c) The left sagittal plane is characterized by
    (i) Long narrow loop
    (ii) Counterclockwise inscription of the majority of the loop
    (iii) Afferent limb superior to efferent limb
(d) The frontal plane should show
    (i) A small and irregular loop owing to the spatial QRS loop being almost perpendicular to the frontal plane
    (ii) Counterclockwise inscription of the loop with the afferent limb superior to the efferent limb with almost the entire loop on the left

(b) Clinical implications

Complete LBBB is most frequently identified in adulthood. Its occurrence in "normal" healthy infants may be anecdotal owing to isolated congenital malformation of the conduction system. Besides lesions (either anatomic or functional) of the left bundle branch itself, LBBB can be a result of lesions within the His bundle or of more peripheral lesions (affecting simultaneously the two or three left bundle subdivisions). LBBB has been predominantly associated with hypertensive heart disease, particularly with left ventricular hypertrophy, and with coronary heart disease [115–119] (with or without myocardial infarction). It frequently occurs as a "lone" abnormality as well. It has also been identified in the setting of myocarditis [120, 121], valvular heart disease (particularly aortic valvular disease) and cardiomyopathies, including the obstructive type [92]. Rarely, LBBB can be associated with other conditions such as hyperkalemia [50], bacterial endocarditis [122], and digitalis toxicity [123].

Similar to other types of intraventricular conduction defects, the published prevalence of associated cardiovascular abnormalities, as well as the prognosis, vary largely according to the characteristics of the population under evaluation; for example, hospital populations, asymptomatic ambulatory patients or large community studies. Rotman and Triebwasser [81] published a revision of over 237,000 mostly asymptomatic subjects. Complete LBBB was identified in 125 cases, with a mean age of 40 years; only 12 subjects were younger than 30 years. In their group of 125 LBBB subjects, a low prevalence of coronary heart disease (9%) and hypertension (8%) was found (although greater than that for the subjects with RBBB). Most patients were asymptomatic (95%) and had an otherwise normal cardiovascular examination (89%).

In a study on 67,375 asymptomatic USAF cadets, Lamb [124] found 13 cases with complete LBBB (mean age 35 years) all of them with no demonstrable evidence of cardiovascular disease.

Important information has been published by the Framingham study group [125] concerning the clinical significance of the appearance of LBBB pattern not previously found. During 18 years of follow-up, 55 subjects developed new LBBB; the mean age of appearance of LBBB was 62 years. These patients had a high prevalence of previous hypertension (62%), cardiomegaly by chest roentgenogram (44%), and significant excess of antecedent coronary heart disease.

During the follow-up period, patients who developed LBBB had twice the incidence of coronary heart disease and seven times the incidence of congestive heart failure found in the general population. There was also a highly significant excess of cardiac enlargement by chest x-ray. One-third of the patients free of cardiovascular abnormalities prior to LBBB appearance developed coronary heart disease (more than three times the observed incidence in the control group). Their data suggest that the appearance of new LBBB is usually associated with advanced organic heart disease (and not asymptomatic or milder symptomatic stages of the disease). One-half of those with new LBBB died of cardiovascular disease within 10 years of the onset of LBBB (compared to only 11.6% in an age-matched population free from LBBB). Only 11% of the LBBB subjects remained free of cardiovascular abnormalities for the whole follow-up period (48% in the control group).

These results contrast with those obtained in follow-up studies of newly acquired LBBB in young military populations, which have suggested a relatively benign clinical prognosis [81, 126, 127]. As previously stated, these differences can probably be explained by the high predominance of young men without risk factors found in the military studies (even hypertensive and diabetics were usually excluded).

LBBB in a younger subject with an otherwise normal cardiovascular observation may thus carry a very good prognosis [128, 129]. In older patients with acquired LBBB, careful evaluation and follow-up seems justified because the development of other cardiovascular abnormalities is strongly expected [125]. In the presence of associated organic heart disease, the prognosis is related to the severity of the underlying process [130].

Besides clinical and x-ray evaluation, the identification of LBBB should be considered a high priority for complete M-mode and two-dimensional echocardiography [30].

LBBB and its duration was recently acquired a new clinical importance, particularly in patients with heart failure [131]. In these patients, the duration of LBBB is an important determinant for resynchronization therapy, which consists of the implantation of a bi-ventricular pacemaker which allows improving ventricular performance [132]. This device altered prognosis in patients with advanced heart failure [133].

(c) Diagnostic difficulties

As previously described in ➋ Sect. 2.3.2.2(c), LBBB may mimic or conceal other ECG patterns, namely, myocardial infarction [134–136]. A QS pattern in V_1 (and sometimes V_2 and V_3) is occasionally registered in the presence of LBBB without anteroseptal myocardial infarction (cases of intermittent LBBB are occasionally seen which show a QS pattern in V_1–V_3 with reappearance of normal R-waves when they return to normal conduction). The same may be observed in inferior leads [137] although it may occasionally represent true loss of inferior forces. Havelda et al. [138] indicated that inferior Q-waves in the presence of LBBB were highly specific for myocardial infarction, though not sensitive. On the other hand, anteroseptal or inferior Q- or QS-waves [139] may no longer be seen when LBBB develops [139, 140].

Noninvasive techniques, in particular echocardiography, and isotopic studies can be of great help in identifying localized hypokinesia related to old myocardial necrosis [30, 119, 121]. Single photon emission computed tomography (SPECT) can also be used for differential diagnosis [141, 142].

LBBB by itself has an abnormal repolarization pattern which usually does not enable easy identification of superimposed primary ischemic abnormalities. Nevertheless, serial changing patterns of ST–T, correlated with clinical signs and symptoms, may give important clues concerning myocardial ischemia in the presence of LBBB (sometimes evolving myocardial infarction) [143, 144].

Depending mainly upon leads, the appearance of LBBB may cause a decrease [145] or an increase [146] in voltage, thus making the voltage criteria less accurate for left ventricular hypertrophy.

It is generally recognized that the ECG pattern of LBBB does not allow the differentiation between the presence or absence of left ventricular hypertrophy. However, the authors have found [114], with the help of echocardiography, that voltage criteria may in fact maintain similar accuracy, with similar predictive value, because the negative voltage of the S-wave in V_1 increases, while the positive voltage of the R-wave in V_5 and V_6 correspondingly decreases [114]. Of the patients with left ventricular hypertrophy and/or enlargement detected by echocardiography among 30 patients with LBBB diagnosed by ECG/VCG, the Sokolow–Lyon criteria correctly identified 82% (19/23) with a false-positive rate of 28% (2/7). These percentages are similar to those achieved in a population of hypertensive patients without LBBB [114]. In five cases with transient LBBB the described variation was observed; that is to say, the appearance of LBBB was accompanied by deeper S-waves in V_1 while the amplitude of the R-wave in V_5–V_6 decreases – thus maintaining similar diagnostic accuracy for the Sokolow–Lyon index (➋ Fig. 2.15).

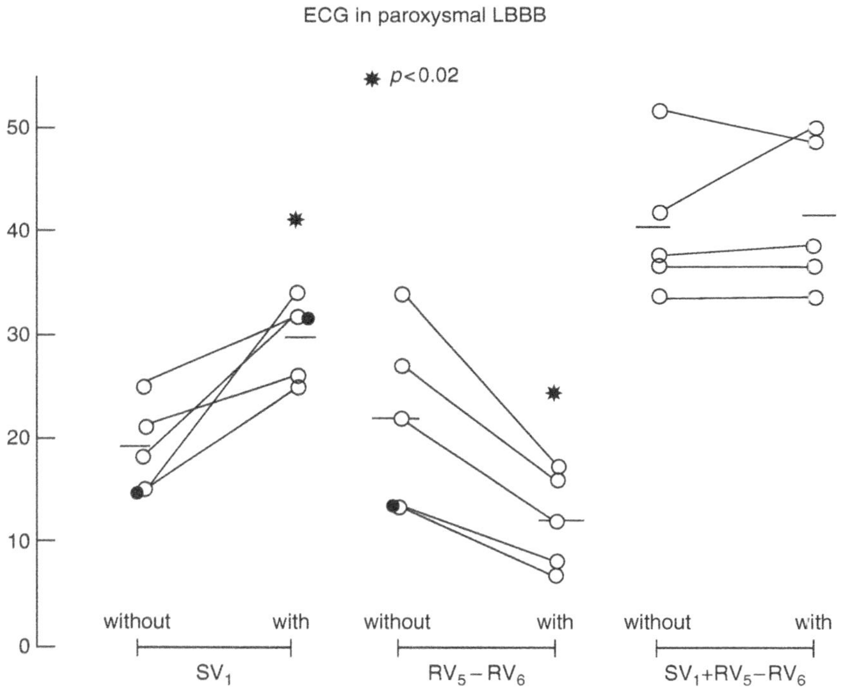

Fig. 2.15
Five cases of paroxysmal LBBB. Graphic representation of the observed increase in S-wave amplitude in lead V_1 and corresponding decrease in R-wave amplitude in leads V_5-V_6, maintaining comparable values for the Sokolow–Lyon index

2.3.3 Bundle Branch Block Associated with Fascicular Block (Bifascicular Block)

According to the fascicular division concept, conduction abnormalities in two of the described fascicles would result in so-called bifascicular block. If LAFB and LPFB occur together, a complete LBBB pattern should result. Some of the cases of complete LBBB may in fact be a result of this type of bifascicular block although, as previously said, the same pattern can also be obtained with other locations of the lesions that cause the block. The combination of RBBB with either left anterior or left posterior block is usually given the designation of bifascicular block. The most common pattern of bifascicular pattern of bifascicular block I that of RBBB with LAFB.

A word must be said about left centroseptal fibers. In some cases of RBBB together with left anterior or posterior fascicular block, the spatial QRS loop is dislocated anteriorly, either counterclockwise or even clockwise in the horizontal plane (➋ Fig. 2.16). In chronic cases, right ventricular hypertrophy or old posterior myocardial infarction may be considered as being the cause of the positive R-waves in the right precordial leads. However, in intermittent blocks (as in the first example that attracted the attention of Rosenbaum, who did not notice this phenomenon) besides the axis deviation in the frontal plane, there can be seen the same anterior displacement that made the authors refer to a third type of "hemi" block, namely, left median fascicular block (see ➋ Sect. 2.3.1.3). Trifascicular block (in a tetrafascicular system) should presumptively be considered in such cases [29, 30, 47, 48].

It is still debatable whether, electrocardiographically, LBBB can coexist with LAFB. However, it is conceivable that, in cases of complete LBBB, when the wavefront reaches the left side of the septum, it may find either the left posterior or the left anterior fascicle accessible. If the activation follows one of these high-speed paths of excitation, the pattern of block in the other, i.e., LAFB or LPFB, can be mimicked. This can be one explanation for the cases with marked, either right or left, axis deviation [147–149].

2.3.3.1 Right Bundle Branch Block and Left Anterior Fascicular Block

(a) ECG/VCG pattern

The ventricular activation in RBBB together with LAFB reflects the combination of the two conduction abnormalities giving rise to the pattern of LAFB, with marked left axis deviation, associated with the characteristic rightward and terminal delay of complete RBBB, with no change of the initial QRS vector, or of the maximal QRS vector and direction of inscription of the QRS loop in the frontal plane (➋ Fig. 2.17).

Owing to the double block (RBBB + LAFB), activation must pass through the noninvolved division (in this case the left posterior fascicle). Initial activation will begin in the posterior paraseptal area of the ventricle (and part of the mild-left septum) with initial forces directed inferiorly, anteriorly, and to the right. The impulse then spreads through the inferior wall and apex with electromotive forces directed inferiorly, leftward and somewhat anteriorly. Subsequently, the activation wave proceeds to depolarize the anterolateral and the posterobasal regions with vectors pointing posteriorly, leftward and superiorly, similar to isolated LAFB. Lastly, the activation of the right septum follows, with late activation of the right ventricle caused by RBBB, with slowly inscribed forces directed anteriorly and to the right.

Thus, there are two distinct portions of the spatial QRS loop (➋ Fig. 2.17):

(a) The main portion is located mostly to the left, superiorly and somewhat anteriorly, with the initial deflection and the efferent limb reflecting the LAFB. However, the afferent limb may be slightly displaced by the associated right bundle branch abnormality (or else by associated lesions on the left middle septum – LMFB) [20, 21, 29, 30].
(b) There is also a slowly inscribed terminal appendage similar to that described for isolated RBBB.

The maximal QRS vector is directed leftward, and superiorly (and somewhat anteriorly) with total QRS duration ≥0.12 s.

ECG leads I and aVL usually have a qRS or RS pattern. The small q-wave is caused by the initial rightward activation while the tall R-wave reflects the superior displacement of the spatial loop owing to the LAFB. The broad and slurred S-wave is related to the terminal delay caused by the RBBB (➋ Fig. 2.17).

ST–T-waves are similar to those observed in isolated RBBB.

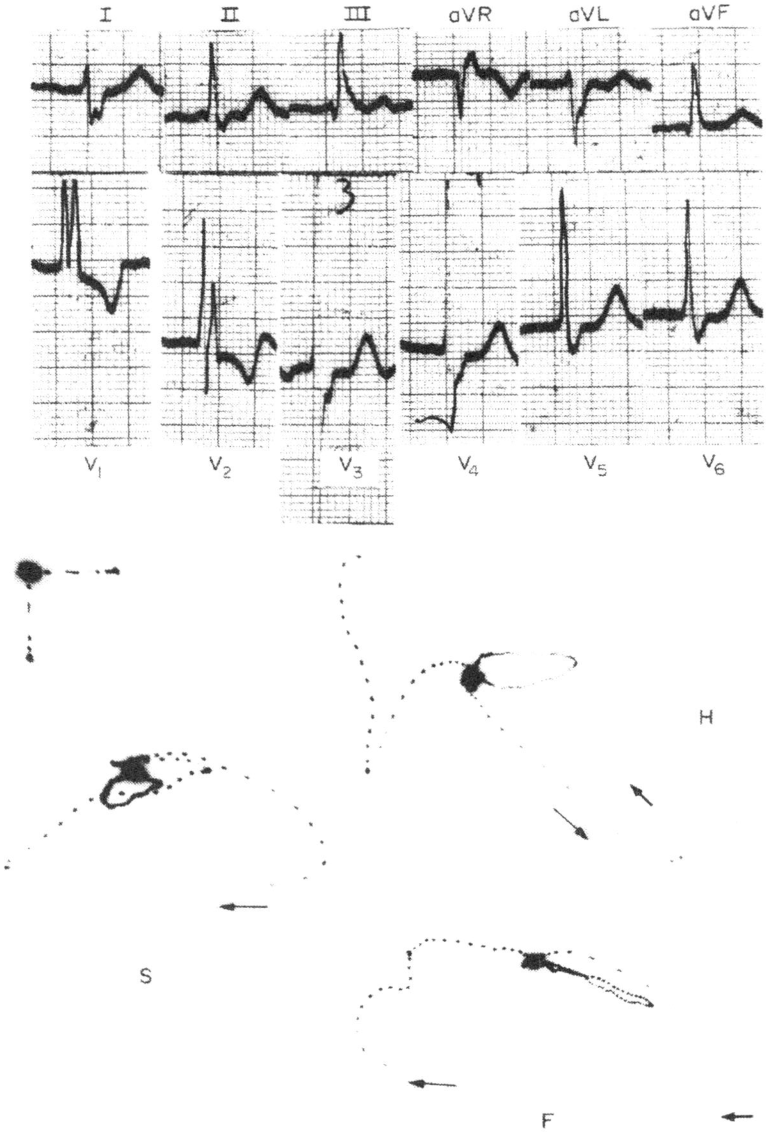

Fig. 2.16
ECG leads and VCG loops of a patient with bifascicular block (RBBB + LPFB). Left median fascicular block (prominent anterior forces) may be postulated

The WHO/ISFC Task Force has proposed the following ECG criteria for the diagnosis of RBBB + LAFB [16]:

(a) QRS prolongation to ≥0.12 s;
(b) Left axis deviation of −45° to −90° (when QRS axis is −30° to −45°, the diagnosis of "possible" associated LAFB should be made)
(c) qR pattern in aVL
(d) rsr′, rsR′, or rSR′ M-shaped right precordial lead pattern with R′ usually greater than initial R-wave (occasionally a wide and notched isolated R pattern may be seen)
(e) Wide S-wave in leads I and V_5–V_6 (S-wave duration greater than R-wave or >40 ms in adults).

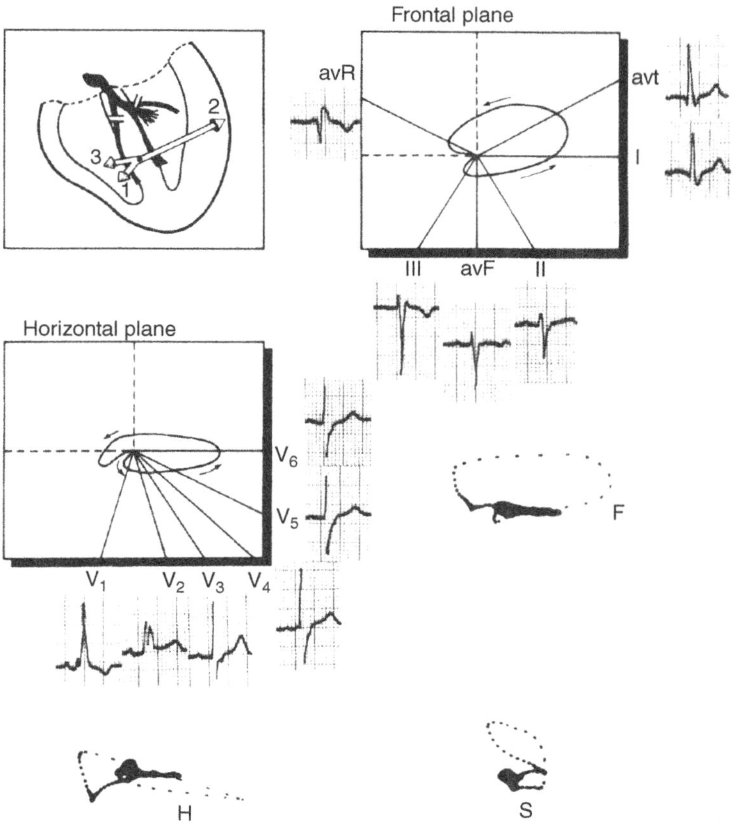

Fig. 2.17
Bifascicular block-RBBB + LAFB: schematic of the spatial main vectors of ventricular activation resulting from interruption of the left anterior fascicle as well as the right bundle branch, together with a diagram of the projections of the QRS loop on the frontal and horizontal planes, and ECG leads and VCG loops of a typical case of RBBB + LAFB (*F* frontal, *H* horizontal, *S* sagittal)

Lopes has proposed VCG criteria for the diagnosis of RBBB + LAFB as below [46]:

(a) The frontal plane should have the following characteristics:
  (i) Initial vectors rightward and inferior
  (ii) Counterclockwise inscription
  (iii) QRS axis more superior than −30°
  (iv) Terminal conduction delay oriented rightward and usually superiorly
(b) The horizontal plane is characterized by
  (i) The initial vector being oriented anterior and rightward
  (ii) Counterclockwise or figure-of-eight inscription
  (iii) The maximal QRS vector being oriented leftward
  (iv) The terminal slowing defect being rightward and anterior

If the body of the QRS loop is anteriorly displaced, the centroseptal fascicle may be involved (associated left main "hemi" block) [21, 28]. Note that accepting three subdivisions of the left bundle branch (tetrafascicular or quadrifascicular conduction system) means that this type of block would actually be trifascicular.

(b) Clinical implications

Most often RBBB + LAFB is associated with sclerodegenerative involvement of the specialized conduction system, mainly in the elderly [26], with or without accompanying hypertension [150] or ischemic heart disease, including myocardial infarction [150, 151]. Pathologically, fibrosis and degenerative changes are usually identified within several zones of the cardiac conduction system [152, 153], including bundle branches and fascicular subdivisions.

RBBB + LAFB may also be a result of a congenital abnormality, either isolated [154, 155] or associated with progressive ophthalmoplegia [156], sometimes being part of a familial disorder associated with syncope and high incidence of sudden death [157–159]. It is routinely part of the electrocardiographic picture of congenital defects in the area of the auriculoventricular canal, namely, ostium primum or cushion defects. Other etiologies include Chagas disease, chest trauma [160, 161], hyperkalemia [50], miocarditis, aortic valvular disease, cardiomyopathy, sarcoidosis [162], and other granulomatous diseases.

RBBB + LAFB may be caused by surgical repair of congenital malformations (namely tetralogy of Fallot or ventricular septal defect). In these cases, LAFB would be related to damage to the conduction system, while isolated RBBB may be produced by involvement of the peripheral Purkinje system [163]. Surgically induced RBBB + LAFB may be a poor risk indicator requiring an artificial pacemaker [164] but may have a long survival if there is no evidence of trifascicular block [165].

As in other fascicular conduction disturbances, the prognosis differs significantly between hospitalized and asymptomatic patients. Asymptomatic patients have a good prognosis [166] but hospitalized patients have a significant risk of sudden death and/or development of complete AV block [85, 151, 167] especially if the His-ventricular (HV) interval is markedly prolonged [168].

In the Framingham study [52], a QRS duration ≥130 ms associated with a QRS axis between -45° and -90° identified those patients most likely to have associated cardiovascular abnormalities.

Studies of young military populations [92, 124] showed a lower prevalence of RBBB with marked left axis deviation than of RBBB with normal QRS axis. In other studies, no difference in the prevalence of associated cardiovascular abnormalities was found. However, in the study of Whinnery et al. [105], a higher prevalence of coronary heart disease was found in patients in whom RBBB was associated with left axis deviation.

(c) Diagnostic difficulties

The diagnostic difficulties are the same as described for each of the two isolated conduction defects (see ➋ Sects. 2.3.1.1 and ➋ 2.3.3.1).

2.3.3.2 Right Bundle Block and Left Posterior Fascicular Block

(a) ECG/VCG pattern

RBBB together with LPFB is manifested as RBBB with otherwise unexplained marked right axis deviation (➋ Figs. 2.18 and ➋ 2.19).

As in isolated LPFB, initial activation of the left ventricle involves the anterior paraseptal area with a vector directed anteriorly, superiorly and leftward, and thereafter progresses to the anterior and anterolateral wall. Then the activation proceeds in a retrograde fashion to the area of the posterior fascicle, that is to say, the inferior and posterobasal areas of the left ventricle, with forces that are inferiorly oriented and to the right. Late terminal forces will be directed anteriorly and to the right, reflecting the delayed activation of the right septum and right ventricular free wall.

Similar to RBBB + LAFB, two main portions of the spatial QRS can be identified (➋ Fig. 2.18).

(a) The main body is located in the inferior left and inferior right octants, with the initial deflection and the efferent limb reflecting the LPFB. The afferent limb is modified by the combined effect of the RBBB (and possibly LMFB).
(b) The terminal appendage is similar to that described for isolated RBBB.

The maximal QRS vector is directed inferiorly, either leftward or rightward, as well as either slightly anteriorly or slightly posteriorly. The total duration of the QRS loop in increased to ≥0.12 s.

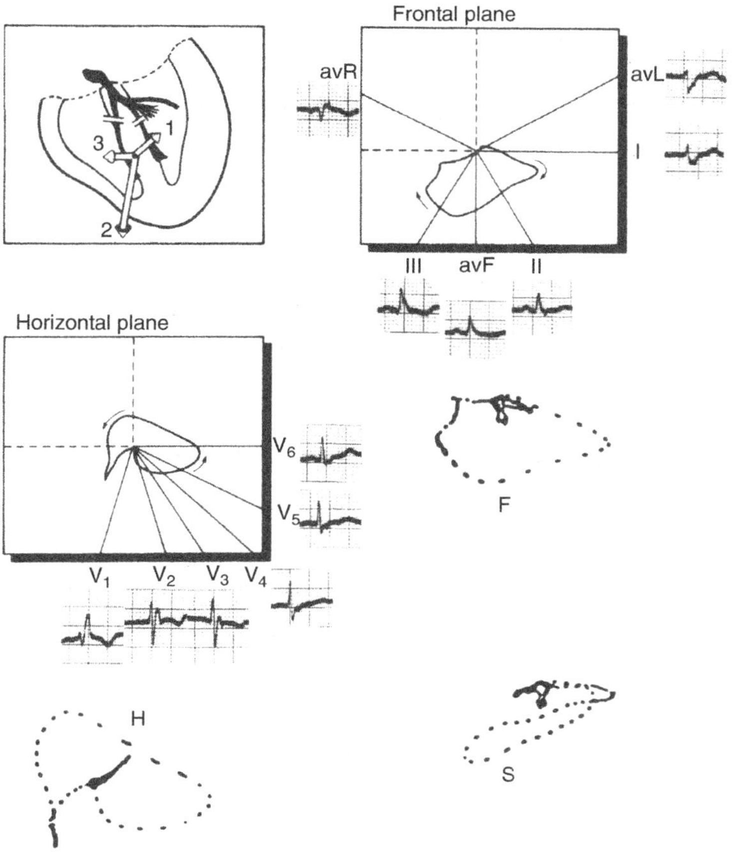

Fig. 2.18
Bifascicular block – RBBB + LPFB: schematic of the spatial main vectors of ventricular activation resulting from interruption of the left posterior fascicle as well as the right bundle branch, together with a diagram of the projections of the QRS loop on the frontal and horizontal planes, and ECG leads and VCG loops of a typical case of RBBB + LPFB (*F* frontal, *H* horizontal, *S* sagittal, same patient as in Figs. 2.7 and 2.19)

ECG leads I and aVL have a small r-wave followed by a deep S-wave which is abnormally broad, with delayed inscription of the late part of the S-wave. In inferior leads, III and aVF, a qR or qRS pattern is present with slurring of the last portion of the R or the S-wave. Abnormal right axis deviation (determined from the first part of the QRS, before the slurring wave) is present. Right precordial leads have an RsR′ pattern (small or absent S-wave). In the left precordial leads, R-wave amplitude is reduced and the S-wave is slurred in its late part (Fig. 2.18).

The WHO/ISFC Task Force has proposed the following ECG criteria for the diagnosis of RBBB + LPFB [16]:

(a) QRS prolongation to ≥0.12 s;
(b) Frontal QRS axis of +90° to +180° (in the absence of other causes of right axis deviation)
(c) rS configuration in leads I and aVL associated with qR pattern in inferior leads (Q-wave obligatory in leads III and aVF) in which Q-wave should be ≤0.04 s
(d) rsr′, rsR′, or rSR′ M-shaped right precordial pattern with R′ usually greater than initial R-wave (occasionally a wide and notched isolated R pattern may be seen)
(e) Wide S-wave in leads I and V_5–V_6 (S-wave duration greater than R-wave or >40 ms in adults)
(f) R peak time >0.05 s in V_1 with normal time in V_5 and V_6 (when a notched dominant R pattern is present in V_1).

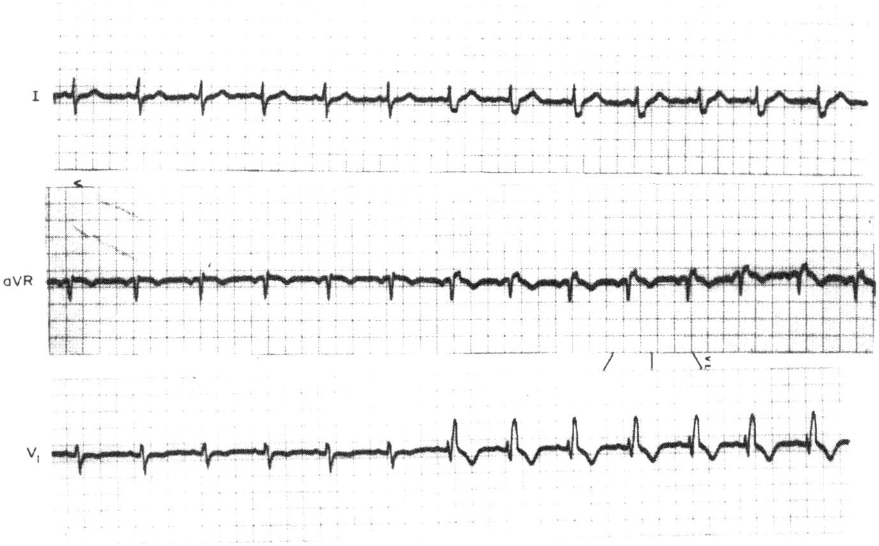

Fig. 2.19
Transition from isolated LPFB to LPFB + RBBB (nonsimultaneous leads). No significant R–R interval variation is observed (same patient as in Figs. 2.7 and 2.18)

Lopes has proposed VCG criteria for the diagnosis of RBBB + LPFB as below [46]:

(a) The frontal plane should have the following characteristics:
  (i) Initial vectors that are leftward
  (ii) Clockwise inscription
  (iii) QRS axis > + 110° (others admit +90°)
  (iv) Terminal slowing directed rightward
(b) The horizontal plane should show the following:
  (i) Initial vectors anterior and leftward
  (ii) Figure-of-eight or clockwise inscription (possible associated LMFB) [30]
  (iii) Maximal QRS vector oriented rightward
  (iv) Terminal slowing oriented rightward and anteriorly

(b) Clinical implications

RBBB + LPFB is usually related to sclerosis of the conduction system most often in the presence of coronary artery disease and/or hypertension. This type of bifascicular block is only about 5% as frequent as the combination of RBBB with LAFB.

It has been said that this association is found more rarely because the left posterior fascicle is broader and so is more resistant. On the other hand, it would have a more ominous prognosis with progression to complete AV block than if the more fragile left anterior fascicle were involved.

(c) Diagnostic difficulties

Difficulties are the same as described for each of the isolated conduction defects (see Sects. 2.3.1.2 and 2.3.3.1).

2.3.3.3 Left Bundle Branch Block with Left Fascicular Blocks

When LBBB is associated with either marked left axis deviation or marked right axis deviation, the suspicion may be raised of associated left fascicular block. The abnormal sequence of septal depolarization owing to the LBBB makes it difficult to identify any type of initial vector alteration. As previously mentioned, the depolarization of the left ventricular free wall may proceed reutilizing the peripheral subdivisions. In this way, it is understandable that block in one of them will alter the sequence of activation in a way similar to isolated fascicular blocks. Some series seem to reflect poorer prognosis when left or right axis deviation is observed in LBBB (corresponding to more extensive lesions either in the conduction system (associated fascicular block) or in the parietal muscle (mural or "distal" block)) [147–149]. Others did not confirm this finding.

2.3.3.4 Progression of Bifascicular Blocks (and Other Intraventricular Conduction Defects) to Advanced AV Block

One particular clinical problem, because of its implications, deserves separate consideration: the possible progression of intraventricular (IV) conduction defects to complete AV block. As a result of the high prevalence of bifascicular blocks, it seems appropriate to include this discussion in this section. However, the conclusions to be reached are relevant to trifascicular blocks as well.

Two different clinical settings must be considered: first, chronic IV conduction defects, and second, IV conduction defects in the setting of acute myocardial infarction.

(a) Chronic IV conduction defects

IV conduction defects are considered to be a risk factor for the development of advanced AV block and eventually prophylactic implantation of a pacemaker is considered. The more advanced the conduction defect (unifascicular block, bifascicular block, or trifascicular block), the larger is the risk of occurrence of complete AV block.

Several studies have demonstrated that a significant number of patients with complete AV block had had prior ECG with patterns of bifascicular block [85, 94, 169–171]. However, quite different risks of progression to advanced AV block have been published – between 10% and 16% for RBBB with LAFB [85, 167, 171–173], but much higher (21–75%) for RBBB + LPFB [85].

In a long-term follow-up study by McAnulty et al. [174], 554 patients with various types of bifascicular or trifascicular blocked were included. The incidence of progression to complete heart block over 5 years was only approximately 1% per year. Most patients with bifascicular block who died suffered ventricular fibrillation rather than complete AV block. An artificial pacemaker was recommended only if symptomatic bradyarrhythmias could be demonstrated.

In the follow up of asymptomatic subjects [81], a very low incidence of advanced AV block was also observed. Other prospective data [52, 125] confirm the low ratios of progression of bundle branch block to complete AV block even for cases with bifascicular block.

Attention has been drawn to the PR interval. Prolongation of the PR interval in the presence of bifascicular block was pointed out as evidence of delay in the other nonblocked fascicle, and thus would represent an indication for pacemaker implantation [175]. Rosen et al. [176] described PR prolongation correlating with His-ventricular prolongation in patients with bifascicular block. However, subsequently, Levites and Haft [177] have shown it to be a poor predictor of trifascicular disease. Denes et al. and Dhingra et al. [178, 179] have also agreed that surface electrocardiographic patterns do not predict high-risk groups.

Scheinman et al. [180] noted that a marked prolongation ($\geq$80 ms) of the HV interval in patients with transient neurological symptoms was a risk indicator of sudden death. However, they later [181] suggested that only patients with moderate or severe congestive heart failure and HV > 70ms were at higher risk of sudden death. It must be remembered that many of their patients had suffered a significant bradyarrhythmia within 3 weeks of admission into the study and thus represent a special subset of patients with transient neurological symptoms.

Dhingra et al. [182] found that an HV $\geq$ 80 ms did not predict high risk of sudden death. McAnulty et al. [174] observed only a trend suggesting that patients with HV > 75 ms were at greater risk of sudden death. Nevertheless, most deaths in this study were not a result of AV block.

A high prevalence of HV prolongation is found in patients with bifascicular block. Although HV prolongation usually indicates more severe heart disease and increase risk of mortality, it has not been proved to be a good predictive sign for complete heart block. Accordingly, in asymptomatic patients with bifascicular block, it cannot be used to decide whether or not prophylactic pacemaker implantation should be undertaken.

Thus, the incidence of advanced AV block in patients with bundle branch block or bifascicular block is relatively small, and BBB or bifascicular block *per se*, without other symptoms (syncope) or signs (dynamic ECG) does not warrant consideration for prophylactic pacemaker implantation [175].

(b) Acute myocardial infarction

In a study by Hindman et al., the prognosis of patients with acute myocardial infarction associated with BBB correlated with the degree of heart failure. The prognosis of anterior and indeterminate myocardial infarction was worse than that for inferior or posterior infarction. RBBB + LAFB [183] developing in the setting of acute anteroseptal myocardial infarction significantly changes the prognosis for surviving the acute episode (especially if the HV interval is prolonged) [184]. It usually corresponds to a large mass of infarcted tissue.

Although AV block may develop, death is usually caused by pump failure and cardiogenic shock. However, in spite of the fact that a prophylactic pacemaker may not change the prognosis, its implication is considered advisable, since it may benefit some individual patients [185]. This strategy has been suggested even in cases in which RBBB existed prior to the myocardial infarction [186]. The same recommendation is also valid for RBBB + LPFB and may be extended for isolated RBBB or LBBB.

The occurrence of isolated fascicular block *per se*, in the setting of acute myocardial infarction, is not an indication for pacemaker implantation [91, 185, 187, 188]. However, if the conduction defect persists and especially if transient second- or third-degree AV block is observed [187, 189, 190] permanent pacing may prolong life [189, 191, 192] and is indicated [175].

2.3.4 Other Associated Intraventricular Conduction Defects

2.3.4.1 Trifascicular Block

Trifascicular block is the term used for the possible combination of complete or incomplete block in the right bundle branch associated with conduction disturbances either in the two main divisions of the left bundle branch or one of them plus a Hisian delay. Usually, this result in one of the bifascicular blocks previously described, associated with first- or second-degree AV block. In order to avoid semantic errors, it has been recommended that each of the individual conduction defects should be listed separately. The existence of three fascicular subdivisions of the left bundle branch only adds to the confusion if this type of designation is to be maintained without clarification of the real defects present.

Simultaneous complete RBBB and block in the main left fascicles will result in complete AV block.

2.3.4.2 Bilateral Bundle Branch Block

The combination of complete BBB on one side (either right or left) with first- or second-degree AV block has been frequently designated "bilateral bundle branch block," assuming that there is incomplete block in the other bundle. However, this is a diagnostic abuse as the block can be located either in the AV node or in the His bundle and not necessary in the contralateral bundle branch. Electrophysiological studies are mandatory for its identification. The designation bilateral BBB should probably be reserved for cases where alternating conduction impairment is observed, with sequential evidence of RBBB and LBBB (➋ Fig. 2.20).

Simultaneous complete RBBB and LBBB would cause complete AV block.

2.3.4.3 Nonspecific IV Block

When the QRS duration is prolonged to ≥0.11 s, without any of the criteria previously described for right or left incomplete or complete bundle branch block, it should be referred to as nonspecific (or unspecified) IV block (or IV conduction delay). Arborization blocks or peri-infarction blocks [66] may fall into this category and the same applies to mural (parietal) blocks.

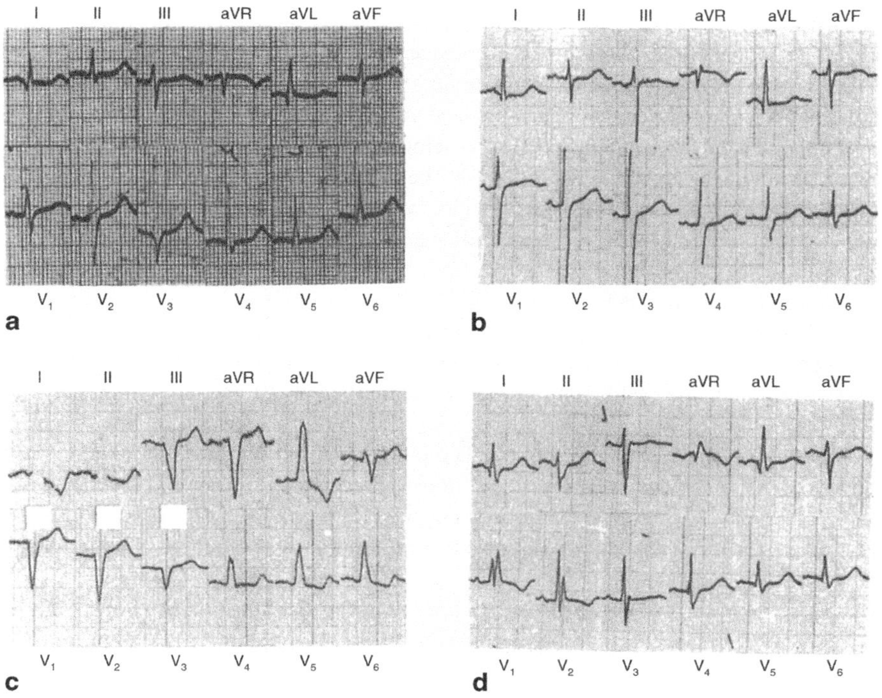

Fig. 2.20
Bilateral bundle branch block: evolution from a normal ECG ((a), 1978) to LAFB ((b), 1985), then to LBBB with normal QRS axis ((c), 1986) and finally to LAFB + RBBB ((d), 1987)

Arborization blocks refer to focal lesions located distally in the conduction system, sometimes related to myocardial necrosis. Castellanos and coworkers, using intracavitary electrograms [61, 193, 194] were able to recognize either further enlargement of "central" RBBB owing to associated peripheral block, or the pattern of complete RBBB without delay in right ventricular apical depolarization. In the latter case, they assumed that the conduction disturbance occurs "distally" after the impulse has emerged from the trunk of the right bundle branch.

Mural or parietal blocks, either left or right sided, correspond to delays either in the more peripheral Purkinje ramifications or in the myocardial fibers. They have been experimentally induced by chemical necrosis [195] and may be a result of, in clinical cases, areas of myocardial necrosis and fibrosis (peri-infarction block), infiltrative granulomatous diseases (such as amyloidosis, Chagas disease or sarcoidosis), myocarditis or cardiomyopathies, hyperkalemia, antiarrhythmic drugs toxicity, and even surgical right ventriculotomy [196].

2.3.5 Clinical Overview of Intraventricular Conduction Defects

Intraventricular conductions defects are among the most frequent ECG abnormalities found in clinical practice. This designation encompasses very different types of abnormalities – anatomic and functional lesions either located in the His bundle or in its main divisions (RBBB and LBBB) or in the subdivisions of the left bundle branch (fascicular blocks – anterior, median, and posterior) or even more peripherally in the Purkinje system or the myocardial cells (arborization blocks, parietal blocks, peri-infarction block). Different degrees of conduction delay in such different locations account for very different paths of electrical activation of the ventricles as well as very different ECG patterns. Although the major types of IV conduction defects are well recognized, many points of controversy still remain to be completely understood.

In spite of representing such a heterogeneous group of abnormalities, all of them can appear either isolated or associated with other cardiac abnormalities (with different prevalence for each type of conduction defect and each type of population studied). Although there are anticipated differences in the prognosis of each conduction defect, they all seem more dependent on the presence and severity of any associated heart disease than on the particular type of conduction defect *per se*. For example, isolated fascicular blocks (LAFB being the most prevalent) have an exceedingly benign prognosis unless associated with an otherwise severe heart disease. Therefore, in the presence of any type of conduction defect, a complete cardiac evaluation must be done and should include, as a priority, a complete echocardiographic study, in order to ascertain accurately and noninvasively the presence and severity of any coexisting cardiac abnormalities as well as their functional significance.

On the other hand, conduction defects frequently make it difficult or impossible to identify other ECG abnormalities, namely, those related to coronary heart disease or hypertrophy of the cardiac chambers. In such cases, once again, a complete cardiac evaluation is mandatory, including a complete echocardiographic study (M-mode, two-dimensional, and Doppler) as well as radionuclide evaluation in order to obtain the correct diagnosis hidden by the ECG pattern of the conduction defect.

For certain IV conduction defects, namely, the so-called bifascicular blocks, an ominous prognosis related with the development of advanced AV block has been described. However, even for bifascicular blocks, the incidence of such a complication (advanced AV block) is very low and does not warrant prophylactic pacemaker implantation or electrophysiological study (unless for the evaluation of the specific symptoms such as syncope or hemodynamically distressing arrhythmias).

On the other hand, in the setting of acute myocardial infarction, the identification of a bundle branch block is a poor risk and warrants pacemaker implantation, although the majority of such patients will die in pump failure.

Much has been learned about IV conduction defects and the cardiac conductions system since the 1950s. However, much is still under debate, mainly concerning the underlying abnormalities that are the basis of many paroxysmal and intermittent conduction defects (some of them rate related) or the more peripheral conduction disturbances at the Purkinje–muscular fiber level, most of them only accessible to electrophysiological studies as well as epicardial and endocardial mapping.

2.4 Ventricular Preexcitation

Preexcitation syndromes – conditions in which the conduction disturbance is characterized by earlier activation of the whole or part of the ventricular myocardium – have been the subject of a huge amount of literature (more dictated by its electrophysiological interest and the multitude of allied tachydysrhythmias than for its known prevalence in the general population). Their study has largely contributed to the elucidation of the pathophysiology of reentrant arrhythmias as well as to the present understanding of the whole conduction system and IV conduction disturbances. Electrophysiological studies as well as endocardial mapping of these conditions are described in other sections of this book.

The Wolff–Parkinson–White (WPW) pattern – short PR interval preceding a wide QRS complex – is by far the most typical and well-known preexcitation ECG pattern. Lately, the term has been extended to include other entities where AV conduction has occurred through other types of anomalous AV connections.

Reference will be made to some cases that have similar anatomic connections (with related arrhythmias) in spite of a normal ECG.

2.4.1 Definition

Ventricular preexcitation can be defined [197] as a condition in which, in relation to atrial excitation, all or some portion of the ventricles are activated by the impulse originating from the atria earlier than would be expected if the impulses were to reach the ventricles by way of the normal conduction pathway.

This "earlier activation" (preexcitation) can only be possible because the electrical stimulus travels through an anomalous "short circuit" that directly conducts it from the atria to an ectopic ventricular site (or that, at least, bypasses the area of normal conduction delay). It appears that a few instances are caused by accelerated conduction within the AV node

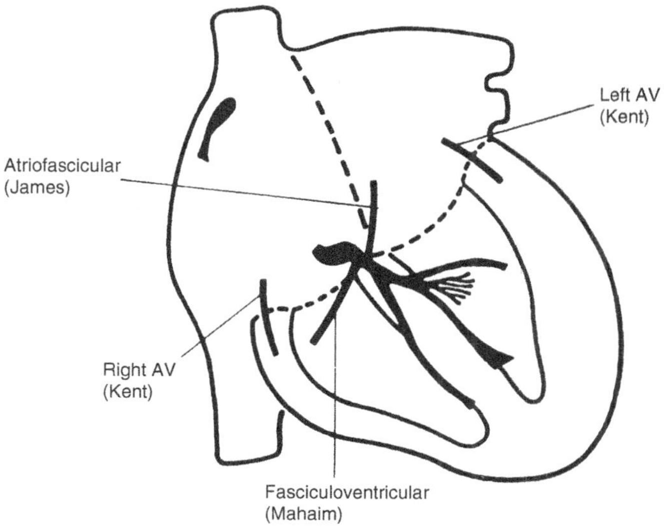

Fig. 2.21
Schematic of the more frequent types of anomalous connections in cases of ventricular preexcitation

itself, without the presence of anomalous conduction pathways (➲ Sect. 2.4.2). Several types of anomalous pathways have been described. The major accessory bypass connections are Kent bundles, James fibers, and Mahaim fibers (➲ Fig. 2.21).

From a histopathological point of view, a distinction between "tract" and "connection" should be made [198]. "Connection" should be used as a general term to describe anomalous conduction pathways that insert into working myocardium while "tract" should be applied to anomalous conduction pathways that insert into specialized conduction tissue. However, the two designations are normally used synonymously.

Preexcitation can be either constant or intermittent, and occasionally can be found on alternate beats. Some patients (particularly those with left-sided accessory pathways) may never show preexcitation in sinus rhythm (be it explained either by enhanced AV conduction or by atrial conduction delay) and only during tachydysrhythmic episodes is the preexcitation pattern observed.

2.4.2 Anatomic Basis

As previously stated, three major types of connection pathways can be described in the human heart [197, 199–204] (➲ Fig. 2.21):

(a) Bundles of Kent are electrically active muscular fibers which directly bridge the atria and the ventricles. Although several locations have been identified for these pathways (actually they can be located almost at any point where the atria and the ventricles are contiguous), they are most frequently identified in a posterior position, connecting the left atrium with the left ventricle [205].
(b) James fibers are presumably continuations of the internodal pathways (connecting the sinus node with the AV node) and connect the atria with the His bundle (atriofascicular accessory pathways) [206]. In this way, they completely bypass the AV node. There is, however, still some dispute on the existence of internodal pathways (see ➲ Chap. 4 of *Basic Electrocardiology: Cardiac Electrophysiology, ECG Systems and Mathematical Modeling*).
(c) Mahaim fibers are accessory pathways between the ventricular muscle on one side and the AV node (nodoventricular) or the His bundle or either of the bundle branches (fasciculoventricular) on the other side. They deviate the electrical impulse from its normal course activating the septal muscle prematurely.

Longitudinal dissociation of the AV node and dual AV nodal pathways have also been described and can present with similar ECG patterns as well as clinical dysrhythmias. Only electrophysiological studies permit the correct diagnosis.

Instead of the above eponyms (Kent, James, Mahaim), which allow some confusion, it is preferable to refer to the several types of connections according to their anatomic location; that is, atrioventricular, nodoventricular, fasciculoventricular, atriofascicular, and intranodal. This is nowadays the accepted classification.

For some cases of preexcitation, an "acquired" theory has been claimed because these syndromes are more frequently identified in adulthood. Nevertheless, it is well known that some accessory pathways remain concealed in sinus rhythm until a precipitating event occurs.

A truly acquired etiology has never been unequivocally demonstrated. However, a case was published by one of the authors [207] in which intermittent WPW, with "concertina" effect (variable shortness of PQ interval as well as a parallel variable enlargement of the QRS [208]) was registered throughout 1 day, in the setting of acute rheumatic fever, to be followed the next day by first-degree AV block (prolonged PR) which later returned to normal.

2.4.3 Wolff–Parkinson–White Syndrome

2.4.3.1 Classification

The classic WPW electrocardiographic pattern was described by Wolff, Parkinson, and White as early as 1930 [204]. It is associated with an AV connection (bundle of Kent) and is estimated to occur in the general population in 0.1–3% depending on the population studied [209]. This estimate is probably low because some pathways do not conduct in the anterograde way and others only have intermittent conduction (see below) and may not be diagnosed [210–214].

Classically, WPW pattern refers to the ECG originally described as consisting of [204]:

(a) Short PR interval <0.12 s during sinus rhythm
(b) The presence of an initial slurring of the QRS ("delta wave") that represents early ventricular activation
(c) An abnormally wide QRS complex ≥0.12 s
(d) Secondary ST-segment and T-wave changes "in healthy young people prone to tachycardia."

Care should be taken to distinguish the WPW pattern and the WPW syndrome [215]. WPW syndrome implies that the patient with the WPW pattern also suffers episodes of tachydysrhytmia.

The QRS pattern will be different according to the specific location of the AV bypass tract, as well as the amount of muscle activated through the accessory pathway. The QRS complexes in preexcitation syndromes can be considered special types of "fusion beats" in which a portion of the activated ventricle is depolarized through the accessory pathways and another portion is activated by the normal pathway. However, if significant delay occurs through the normal pathway, the whole ventricle may be depolarized through the accessory pathway. Some accessory pathways do not conduct anterogradely, either transiently or not, and the whole ventricular activation will always follow the normal pathway. When the "concertina" effect is observed, different types of "fusion beats" will be registered (e.g., nine in the case referred to above [207]) depending upon the gradual increase or decrease of the areas depolarized either normally or through the anomalous pathway. Multiple accessory pathways can coexist in the same patient and give rise to a more complex activation pattern or patterns.

Rosenbaum et al. [216] separated WPW into type A and type B. Type A (➋ Fig. 2.22) was related to a bypass tract between the atria and the posterior left ventricular free wall (left-sided bundle of Kent), which causes an initial anteriorly and rightward delta wave, with an ECG pattern showing predominant or exclusive R-waves in leads V_1 and V_2, in a way similar to RBBB. Conversely, when an anterior bundle of Kent is present, the electrical impulse will pass from the atrium to the anterior right ventricular free wall. In this case (type B WPW) (➋ Fig. 2.23), the delta wave will point posteriorly and to the left and an ECG pattern similar to LBBB (with a dominant S-wave in V_1) will be registered. Other accessory pathways locations (e.g., left septal) were not considered in this classification and were progressively identified. For example, cases with positive delta wave in V_1 trough V_4 but negative in V_5 and V_6 were called type C WPW (related to an abnormal connection on the lateral wall of the left ventricle [217, 218]).

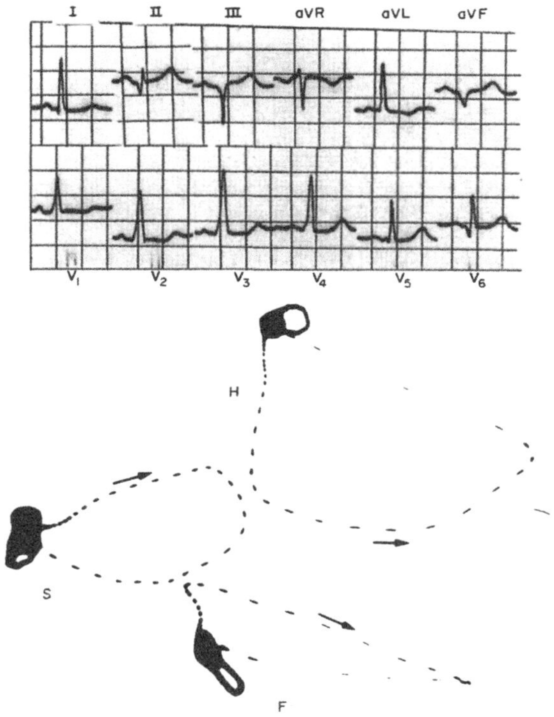

Fig. 2.22
ECG leads and VCG loops of a typical example of the classic WPW pattern type A (*H* horizontal, *S* sagittal, *F* frontal). See text for description

In fact, limb leads contain important data as well. In type A, the delta wave is positive in leads II, III, and aVF and negative in I and aVL. On the contrary, in type B, the delta wave is positive in I and aVL and negative in II, III, and aVF. Using the information contained in the limb leads together with the precordial leads, it is possible to verify that the spatial direction of the initial forces is highly variable.

Fitzpatrick et al. propose an algorithm for accessory atrioventricular pathway localization using a 12-lead ECG (➋ Fig. 2.24) [219]. In this algorithm, if the precordial QRS transition was at or before lead V_1, the pathway had been ablated on the left side. If it was after lead V_2, the pathway had been ablated on the right side. If the QRS transition was between leads V_1 and V_2 or at lead V_2, then if the R-wave amplitude in lead I was greater than the S-wave by ≥1.0 mV, it was right sided; otherwise, it was left-sided (sensitivity 100%, specificity 97%).

The right-sided pathways can be subdivided according to (sensitivity 97%, specificity 95%) the following:

1. If the QRS transition was between leads V_2 and V_3, the pathway was right septal.
2. If after lead V_4, it was right lateral.
3. If it was between leads V_3 and V_4:
   (a) If the delta wave amplitude in lead II was ≥1.0 mV, it was right septal.
   (b) Otherwise, it was right lateral.

Right-sided pathways can be further subdivided (see ➋ Fig. 2.24).

The left-sided pathways can be subdivided according to (sensitivity 100%, specificity 100%):

1. Two or more positive delta waves in the inferior leads or the presence of an S-wave amplitude in lead aVL greater than the R-wave, or both, discriminated left anterolateral pathways.

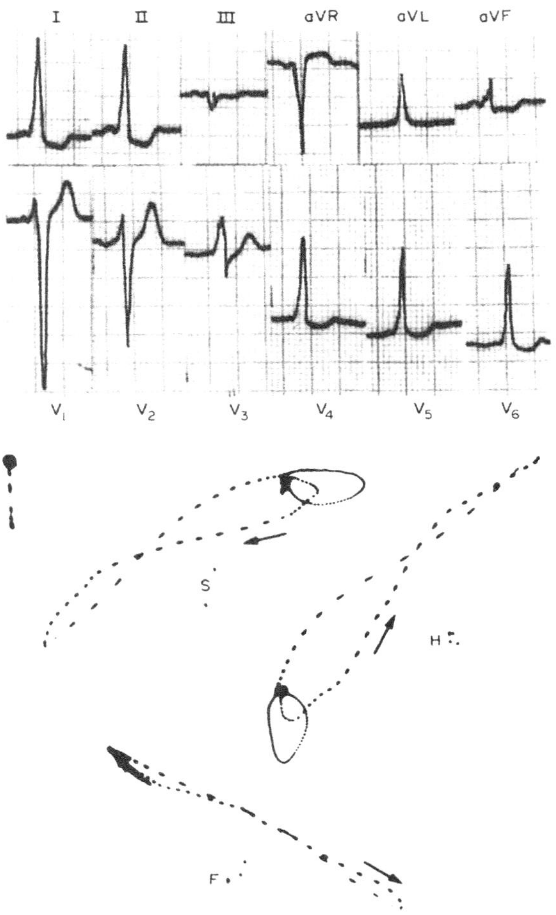

Fig. 2.23
ECG leads and VCG loops of a typical example of the classic WPW pattern type B (*S* sagittal, *H* horizontal, *F* frontal). See text for description

2. If the R-wave in lead I was greater than the S-wave by ≥0.8 mV, and the sum of inferior delta wave polarities was negative, the location was posteroseptal.
3. Otherwise, it was postero-lateral.

However, it must be stressed that any classification of preexcitation pathways based exclusively on standard ECG has important limitations [201] and should be used only as a presumptive clinical approach. The causes of misclassification include [201]:

(a) Coexisting alterations in the QRS complex related to associated congenital or acquired heart abnormalities
(b) The occasional presence of multiple accessory pathways
(c) Variable degrees of "fusion" between normal and accessory conduction
(d) Superimposition of the terminal P-wave with the initial delta wave
(e) Endocardial versus epicardial location of the pathway

With recent advances in the radiofrequency catheter ablation or surgical methods of treatment of refractory dysrhythmias in patients with preexcitation, precise location of the accessory pathways was sought and obtained with special

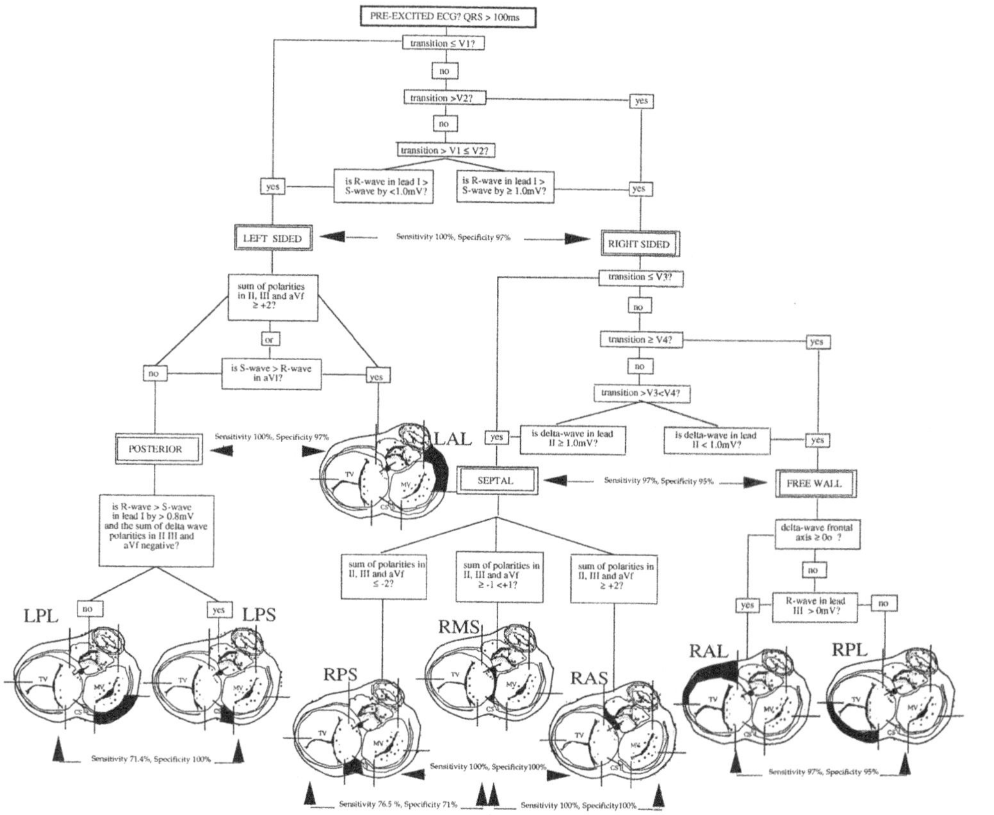

Fig. 2.24

Algorithm for defining location of accessory pathways causing preexcitation of the baseline 12-lead electrocardiogram (ECG). Pathways are initially separated into left and right sided. Right-sided pathways may then be separated into five septal or right lateral locations around the tricuspid valve annulus and left-sided pathways into three septal and lateral locations (reproduced from Fitzpatrick et al. [219])

electrophysiological techniques. These studies have shown a wider variation than expected in the location and functional features of the accessory pathways.

Further discussion on the classification of the WPW pattern using body-surface mapping is given in ➋ Chap. 10 of *Cardiac Arrhythmias and Mapping Techniques.*

2.4.3.2 Associated Arrhythmias

The prevalence of tachyarrhythmias described in patients with WPW is related to the selection of the population studied and recent studies indicated that his frequency augments with age [220]. Values from 4% to 13% have been published [221]. The most typical and frequent arrhythmia in the setting of WPW syndrome is reciprocating (reentrant) tachycardia with anterograde conduction over the AV node and His bundle, and retrograde conduction through the accessory pathway (➋ Fig. 2.25).

As previously stated, during sinus rhythm, conduction spreading normally as well as through the accessory pathway produces two wavefronts which merge to form a ventricular "fusion beat." Most frequently the refractory period of the accessory pathway, during sinus rhythm, is greater than that of the normal conduction system, although conduction time is usually shorter for the anomalous pathway. With the appearance of a premature atrial beat – the usual precipitating

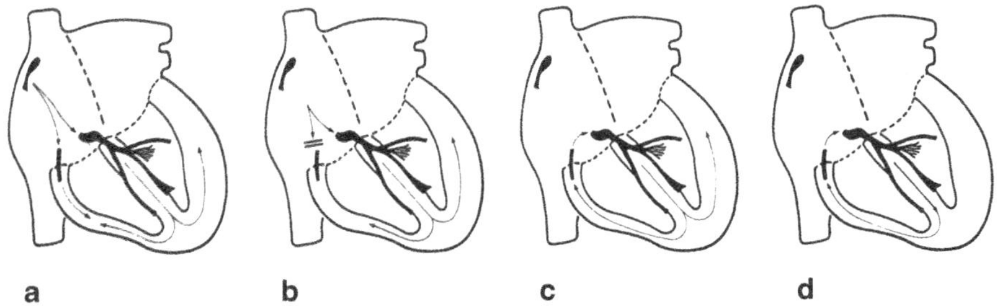

Fig. 2.25
Schematic of initiation of orthodromic tachycardia in patients with WPW. A right-side AV (Kent) pathway is represented. During normal sinus rhythm (a), conduction spreads through the accessory pathway as well as through the normal conduction system, producing a "fusion beat" with the classic WPW pattern. With a premature atrial beat (b), the stimulus may find anterograde conduction through the accessory pathway blocked but is conducted through the normal conduction system. Then, retrograde conduction through the accessory pathway (c) may allow the establishment of a reentry circus rhythm (d) (narrow QRS tachycardia)

factor – the conduction may be blocked anterogradely through the accessory pathway, but be propagated to the ventricle as usual, through the normal conduction system (thus resulting in a normal QRS complex). This dissociation between the refractory period of the normal and the accessory pathways (precipitated by the occurrence of a premature beat) allow reentry to ensue. Conduction through the ventricle will find the accessory pathway excitable in the retrograde direction, allowing the impulse to go back to the atria, thus establishing a circus rhythm: anterograde conduction through the normal conduction system (normal QRS) and retrograde conduction through the accessory pathway (orthodromic AV tachycardia). The precipitating factor is usually a premature beat which arises in the atrium but which can also be generated in the AV junction or in the ventricles.

Some accessory pathways are only capable of retrograde conduction [210–214, 227]. Such pathways are usually classified as concealed pathways. Patients with this abnormality may experience paroxysmal supraventricular tachycardia but have no delta wave on their standard ECG. The tachycardias are usually attributed to reentry within the AV node but they are actually a result of the accessory pathway [211, 214, 222–225]. Only complete electrophysiological studies can disclose the correct cause of tachydysrhythmia in these patients. If such a connection is identified, they should be managed like any other patients with WPW and tachyarrhythmias. Interestingly enough, they are "protected" against life-threatening rapid ventricular response rates in the setting of atrial fibrillation.

The occasional patient with an accessory pathway that conducts only in the anterograde direction [214, 226–228] will not have the classic form of recurrent AV tachycardia with narrow QRS.

In some WPW patients, the reciprocating rhythm can also occur in the reverse direction, termed "antidromic reciprocating tachycardia" [229]. Anterograde conduction is through the accessory pathway (wide QRS, mimicking ventricular tachycardia) and retrograde conduction over the normal conduction system. This appears to be a rare finding but poses special diagnostic problems (see below) [201] (Fig. 2.26).

Atrial fibrillation (although not atrial flutter), in the setting of WPW, is common, occurring in up to 39% of the patients [201, 230, 231] (obviously depending on the selection of the population). The high prevalence of atrial fibrillation in WPW is probably related to the series of predisposing factors given below:

(a) The rate of reciprocating tachycardia in WPW is usually higher than that owing to reentry through the AV node.
(b) There is a possibility that a retrograde impulse arrives at the atria in the vulnerable phase of atrial recovery.
(c) There is nonuniform depolarization of the atria with multiple impulses being conducted at the same time (either from the sinus node or retrogradely from the ventricle). Actually, transition from reciprocating tachycardia to atrial fibrillation has been observed.

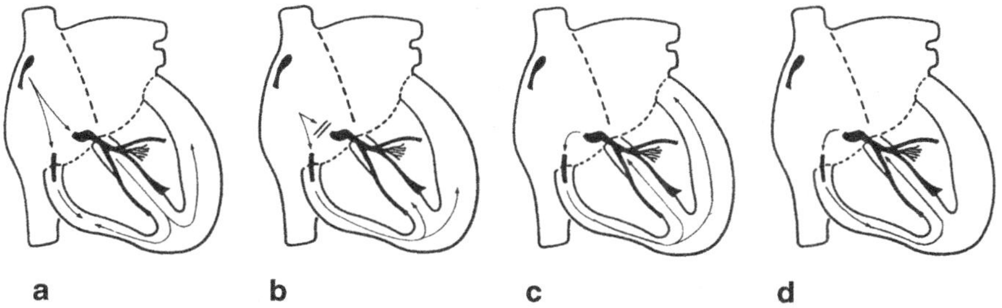

Fig. 2.26
Schematic of the mechanism for initiation of antidromic tachycardia in patients with WPW. A right-side AV (Kent) pathway is represented. During normal sinus rhythm (a), conduction spreads both through the accessory pathway and through the normal conduction system, producing a "fusion beat" with the classic WPW pattern. With a premature atrial beat (b), the stimulus may find anterograde conduction through the AV node blocked but is conducted through the accessory pathway. Then, retrograde conduction through the normal conduction system may ensure (c) and allow the establishment of a reentry circus rhythm (d) (wide QRS tachycardia)

The most important problem concerning atrial fibrillation or flutter associated with WPW is the risk of progression to ventricular fibrillation. Owing to the presence of an accessory pathway with short refractory period, a very rapid ventricular rate of response may be observed. Its degeneration to ventricular fibrillation and sudden death has been described [232–240].

It is important to remember that digitalis will not slow AV conduction in cases of atrial fibrillation in which there is anterograde conduction through the anomalous pathway. In fact, cardiac glycosides may shorten its anterograde refractory period, thereby accelerating ventricular response. For practical purposes, digitalis should be contraindicated in WPW patients with either atrial fibrillation or flutter.

2.4.3.3 Associated Congenital Abnormalities

The association of WPW pattern with congenital heart disease has been frequently reported. The most frequent associations are with Ebstein's anomaly and mitral valve prolapse [201, 241, 242]. It is still debatable whether these associations have an embryological basis [243] or not.

Association has been reported with other congenital and acquired heart diseases as well [201], namely, corrected transposition of the great vessels. A familial form of WPW has been reported and may be associated with congestive or hypertrophic cardiomyopathies [244].

2.4.3.4 Diagnostic Difficulties

Besides the incidence of tachyarrhythmias, preexcitation has interested investigators for a long time because it is a frequent cause for difficult ECG differential diagnosis. First, classic type A WPW (left-sided bundle) has been misdiagnosed as RBBB, true posterior myocardial infarction and right ventricular hypertrophy, while type B WPW pattern (right-sided bundle) may resemble LBBB, anterior myocardial infarction or left ventricular hypertrophy. Second, a PR at the lower limit of normal coexisting with either right or left complete bundle branch block may mimic WPW. Third, preexcitation of the diaphragmatic surface of the heart results in superiorly oriented activation forces thus mimicking inferior myocardial infarction [245]. Fourth, following the abnormal depolarization sequence, the repolarization is also modified. Thus an abnormal ST–T-wave pattern may be falsely diagnosed as ischemic. Fifth, WPW is one of the reported causes of a false positive exercise test [246], even in cases in which the conduction abnormality may disappear with exercise, and finally, as previously stated, the tachydysrhythmias associated with WPW are also a cause of difficult diagnosis.

2.4.3.5 Electrophysiological Evaluation

Electrophysiological examination with intracardiac recording and pacing as well as epicardial mapping, and its full indications and usefulness, is dealt with in ➲ Chaps. 2 and ➲ 3 of *Cardiac Arrhythmias and Mapping Techniques*. Intracardiac recordings provide the only possibilities of diagnosing, for example, concealed WPW as well as most cases of WPW associated with either RBBB or LBBB.

Electrophysiological studies are clearly indicated in WPW patients with distressing symptoms or syncope owing to recurrent attacks of tachycardia, or rapid anomalous pathway conduction during episodes of atrial fibrillation or flutter, and in the evaluation of the acute response to drugs in medically refractory paroxysmal tachycardias, and in the last years the electrophysiological laboratory also makes possible ablation of the anomalous pathway, with great success (>90%) and is now the first line of therapy for WPW syndrome [220]. In patients in whom the surgical therapy is contemplated, electrophysiological study will permit not only the confirmation of the presence of the preexcitation and its functional behavior in the clinically observed tachyarrhythmias, but also the location with certainly of the accessory pathway (and sometimes the identification of multiple accessory pathways).

Asymptomatic or mildly symptomatic patients, as well as those with good clinical response to medical management, will not require an electrophysiological study. Fortunately, they form the majority.

2.4.4 Other Forms of Preexcitation

2.4.4.1 Short PR Syndromes

In cases of atriofascicular accessory pathways (James fibers), the AV node zone of physiological delay is bypassed and the ventricular activation follows its normal path. Thus a short PR interval with normal narrow QRS pattern will be registered [197, 200] (➲ Fig. 2.27).

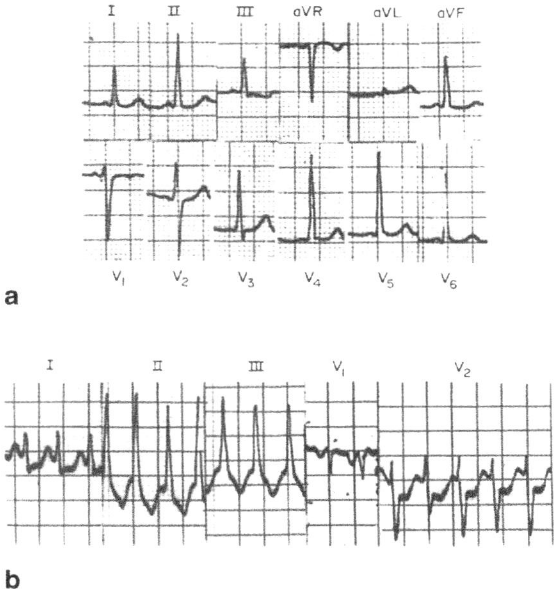

Fig. 2.27
Typical case of LGL syndrome. Part (a) shows an ECG pattern with short PR interval and normal QRS. Part (b) is an ECG during an episode of supraventricular tachycardia

This ECG pattern was first described by Clerc et al. [247] in 1938, but its association with paroxysmal tachyarrhythmias was identified only in 1952 by Lown et al. [248]. The designation of this syndrome (LGL syndrome or short PR syndrome) should be reserved for those cases with tachyarrhytmias associated with the corresponding basal ECG pattern.

Although Lown et al. [248] reported a 9.5% prevalence of paroxysmal tachycardia in patients with short PR interval and normal QRS complex, the actual incidence of supraventricular tachycardia in unselected patients with this ECG pattern remains unknown. Ventricular tachycardia can occur [17, 249]. Actually, two of the patients originally described by Lown et al. with atrial fibrillation died suddenly.

Accelerated conduction through the AV node will give a similar pattern and may represent the electrophysiological substrate of most cases of LGL syndrome. This concept of enhanced AV nodal conduction (EAVN) was proposed for patients found in electrophysiological studies to have little or no prolongation of AV nodal conduction in response to right atrial pacing [201, 250]. EAVN could be explained either by partial bypass of the AV node, or by an underdeveloped or anatomically small AV node, or else by an anatomically normal AV node with rapid conduction properties (functionally or as a consequence of autonomic tone).

2.4.4.2 Nodoventricular Connections

As previously stated, a nodoventricular connection is one of the Mahaim fibers connecting the AV node with the ventricular muscle [198]. The basal PR interval and degree of preexcitation will depend on the relative location of the point where the fiber leaves the AV node to the area (and degree) of AV nodal physiological conduction delay. These fibers can be demonstrated by electrophysiological study. Typically [17], at faster heart rates or with close coupled atrial extrastimuli, the QRS widens and assumes greater degrees of LBBB morphology.

There may be no evidence of ventricular preexcitation in sinus rhythm, becoming manifest only during atrial pacing (because prolonged AV nodal conduction time is produced).

The mechanism of tachycardia involving nodoventricular pathways is not completely understood. Prystowsky et al. [17] suggest that most likely it involves either macroreentry following the nodoventricular fiber, His–Purkinje system and AV node, or AV nodal microreentry with associated anterograde conduction over the nodoventricular connection (● Fig. 2.28).

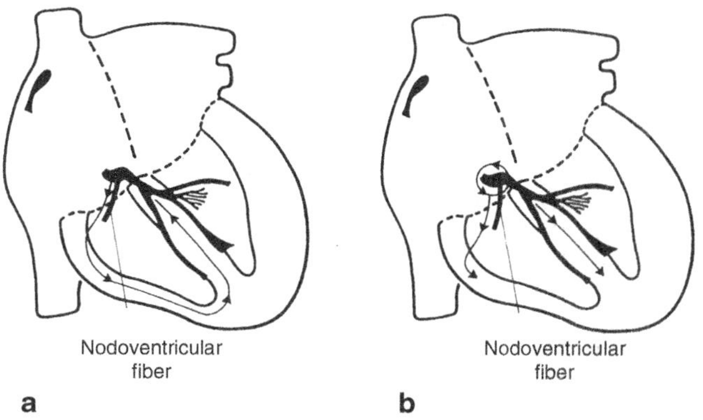

Fig. 2.28
Schematic of the suggested mechanisms for tachycardia initiation in patients with a nodoventricular fiber. Part (a) shows macroreentry using the nodoventricular fiber, His–Purkinje system and AV node. Part (b) shows AV nodal microreentry with associated anterograde conduction through the nodoventricular connection

2.4.4.3 Fasciculoventricular Connections

A fasciculoventricular connection is a type of the Mahaim fibers that arise from the His bundle (or bundle branches) and enters into the ventricle [198].

The PR interval is normal (unless it coexists with EAVN) and usually only minor slurring of the initial QRS forces occurs (because His–Purkinje conduction velocity is rapid with little opportunity for more evident ventricular preexcitation).

In electrophysiological studies, the HV interval is short and during rapid atrial pacing or premature atrial stimulation, the atrial–His (AH) interval lengthens with no change in the HV interval or QRS width [251]. No specific arrhythmias have been causally related to the presence of fasciculoventricular fibers [251].

To conclude the electrical curiosities related to preexcitation, it can be quoted that it is theoretically possible to have an impulse conducted from the atria to the His bundle through James fibers and then to the ventricles by way of Mahaim fibers, thus producing the classic WPW pattern: a short PR interval with a wide QRS complex with delta wave [221].

All the ECG patterns arising from conduction through Mahaim fibers cannot be correctly diagnosed without performing invasive electrophysiological studies.

2.5 The Brugada Syndrome

2.5.1 Classification

In 1992, Pedro and Josep Brugada described a syndrome with an ECG pattern of repolarization and depolarization abnormalities in the right precordial leads that was associated with sudden death in individuals with a structurally normal heart [252]. Brugada Syndrome is suspected to be responsible for 40–60% of what had previously been referred to as "idiopathic ventricular fibrillation" [253]. The criteria for the Brugada Syndrome were presented in a consensus paper [254] which was subsequently followed by a second consensus paper [255] that made some adjustments to the definitions.

The Brugada pattern appears in the ECG as repolarization and depolarization abnormalities in the right precordial leads; three types of repolarization patterns were initially recognized according to the study group of the European Society of Cardiology (➋ Fig. 2.29) [254] but only the first was confirmed as definitively being the Brugada pattern [255]:

- Type 1 prominent coved ST-segment elevation, displaying a J-wave amplitude or an elevated ST-segment ≥2 mm (or 0.2 mV) at its peak, followed by a negative T-wave, with little or no isoelectric separation.
- Type 2 high takeoff ST-segment elevation: in this case the J-wave amplitude ≥2 mm gives rise to a gradually descending ST-segment elevation, remaining ≥1 mm above baseline, followed by a positive or biphasic T-wave, resulting in a saddle back configuration.
- Type 3 ST-segment elevation compromising a <1 mm saddle back or coved configuration (or both).

The PR interval usually is increased and presumably reflects the presence of HV-conduction delay. The QT-interval is either within normal limits or slightly prolonged.

Conduction defects may be specific or nonspecific for any part of the conduction system. Sometimes pronounced broad S in leads I, II, and III, giving rise to an extreme left axis deviation, are encountered. A left axis deviation may indicate left anterior fascicular block. A true RBBB may also be seen. The repolarization pattern type 2 may mimic a RBBB pattern, but the absence of S-waves in the left-lateral leads precludes the true presence of a RBBB.

In Brugada pattern, the ST-segment is dynamic; different patterns may be observed in the same patient sequentially or following the introduction of specific drugs. In the first few hours after DC shock, ECG patterns characteristic of Brugada Syndrome cannot be taken as diagnostic.

This disorder is inherited with an autosomal dominant mode of transmission with incomplete penetrance and an incidence ranging between 5 and 58 per 10,000 [255]. An incidence of 12 per 10,000 was quoted for the Type 1 pattern in Japanese individuals but it was the Type 2 and Type 3 patterns with an incidence of 58 per 10,000 that were much more

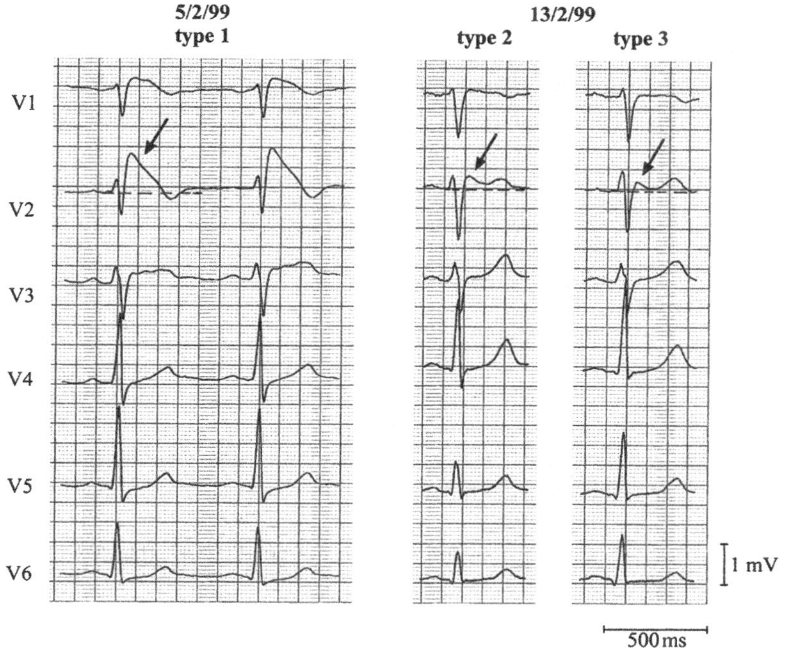

Fig. 2.29
Precordial leads of a resuscitated patient with Brugada syndrome. Note the dynamic course of a couple of days. All three patterns are shown. Arrows denote the J-wave (reproduced from Horan et al. [253]. © American College of Chest Physicians, Northbrook, IL)

common in this population [256]. The only mutations linked to the syndrome appear in the gene that encodes for the sodium channel SCN5A [257].

The second consensus conference revised the initial definition. Brugada syndrome is said to be definitively present when the patient has the Type 1 ECG pattern in the presence or absence of a sodium channel blocking agent and at least one of the following clinical characteristics [255]: documented ventricular fibrillation, polymorphic ventricular tachycardia, a family history of SCD before age 45, coved-type ECGs in family members, electrophysiological inducibility of a ventricular tachycardia, syncope, or nocturnal agonal respiration. The appearance of the ECG features, without these clinical features, is sometimes referred to as an idiopathic Brugada ECG pattern. The second consensus paper stated that Type 2 and Type 3 patterns are not diagnostic of the Brugada pattern.

A diagnosis of Brugada syndrome can also be made if a Type 2 or Type 3 pattern is found in more than one right precordial lead but which changes to a Type 1 pattern after sodium channel blocker administration [255].

2.5.2 Molecular Genetics

Brugada syndrome is often inherited with an autosomal dominant mode of transmission [258].

About 20–25% of Brugada patients have documented SCN5A mutations [258]. Genetic studies have demonstrated that some cases of Brugada syndrome and chromosome 3-linked long-QT syndrome are allelic disorders of the cardiac sodium channel gene (SCN5A, 3p21).

Three types of SCN5A mutations have been identified in the Brugada syndrome: splice-donor, frame-shift, and missense [259]. All of these mutations lead to a reduction in the fast sodium channel current.

2.5.3 Associated Arrhythmias

Brugada syndrome has been associated with sudden death related to arrhythmias like VT or VF. Ventricular tachycardia usually starts with a short coupling interval, and rapid polymorphic VTs are responsible for syncope and sudden cardiac death in a majority.

It has been suggested that there is a higher than normal incidence of supraventricular tachyarrhythmias, including atrial and AV reentrant tachycardias in the Brugada population. Monomorphic VT is rare [260].

2.5.4 Diagnostic Difficulties

There are many conditions that can lead to ST-segment elevation in the right precordial leads. In order to establish a diagnosis of Brugada syndrome, it is necessary to exclude all these conditions, namely, arrythmogenic right ventricular cardiomiopathy (ARVC) and the early repolarization syndrome [257].

ARVC may mimic Brugada syndrome and, in some cases, structural abnormalities may only be found at autopsy. Drug challenge with sodium channel blockers (flecainide, ajmaline, or procainamide) may be useful in discriminating between these two entities.

The early repolarization syndrome may mimic a type 2 or type 3 Brugada ECG pattern. Once again, a drug challenge might provide the clue for a proper diagnosis.

Other causes of ST-segment elevation must be ruled out including epicardial injury, pericarditis, or electrolyte abnormalities.

2.5.5 Drug Challenge

Intravenous administration of certain drugs, like sodium channel blockers (ajmaline, flecainide, or procainamide), unmask or exaggerate the ST-segment elevation. Some discussion exists about the sensitivity and specificity of this test. Procainamide has a very low sensitivity. Reproducibility of the test according to recent studies might be near 100% but is not well established [261].

The patient should be monitored while the drug challenge is performed and a defibrillator should be nearby. Drug administration should be stopped when the test is positive (J-wave amplitude >2 mm in lead V_1 and/or V_2 or V_3 with or without RBBB) and/or when ventricular arrhythmias, including ventricular premature complexes, are evident or QRS widening ≥30%.

Drug challenge is indicated in patients with Brugada syndrome pattern Type 2 or 3 in order to clarify the diagnosis (conversion to Type 1 is considered positive as indicated previously).

The more that sodium channel blockade is needed to elicit Brugada syndrome, the less the patient is at risk under baseline conditions.

2.5.6 Electrophysiological Evaluation

Electrophysiological studies (EPS) may be useful in risk stratification and in establishing the diagnosis [262].

Brugada [263] suggested that an EP study is not required in individuals with the Brugada pattern and syncope or aborted sudden death, i.e., an implanted cardioverter defibrillator (ICD) is required. An ICD is also required for patients with a Brugada ECG and an inducible arrhythmia at EPS, e.g., VF. Asymptomatic individuals (a) without an inducible arrhythmia or (b) with a Brugada ECG which appears only after drug challenge are at low risk and only require follow-up.

EPS is recommended in all symptomatic patients as well in asymptomatic patients when there exists a positive family history for sudden cardiac death. The necessity for EPS is questionable in patients displaying the Brugada ECG pattern, but who are asymptomatic and have a negative family history.

References

1. Durrer, D., R.Th. van Dam, G.E. Freud, M.J. Janse, F.L. Meijler, and R.C. Arzbaecher, Total excitation of the isolated human heart. *Circulation*, 1970;**41**: 899–912.
2. Josephson, M.E., D.L. Scharf, J.A. Kastor, and J.G. Kitchen, Atrial endocardial activation in man. Electrode catheter technique for endocardial mapping. *Am. J. Cardiol.*, 1977;**39**: 972–981.
3. Witting, J.H., M.R. de Leval, and J. Stark, Intraoperative mapping of atrial activation before, during, and after the Mustard operation. *J. Thorac. Cardiovasc. Surg.*, 1977;**73**: 1–13.
4. Puech, P.M., M. Esclavissat, D. Sodi-Pallares, and F. Cisneros, Normal auricular activation in the dog's Herat. *Am. Heart J.*, 1954;**47**: 174–191.
5. Vagueiro, M.C., *Electrocardiografia Hisiana e Estimulação Eléctrica Artificial no Estudo das Alterações da Condução e Ritmo Cardíaco.* Lisboa: Tese de Doutoramento, 1975.
6. Janse, M.J. and R.H. Anderson, Specialized internodal atrial pathways – Fact or fiction? *Eur. J. Cardiol.*, 1974;**2**: 117–136.
7. Sorsky, E. and P. Wood, The use of chest leads in clinical electrocardiography. *Am. Heart J.*, 1937;**13**: 183–196.
8. New York Heart Association Criteria Committee, *Nomenclature and Criteria for Diagnosis of Diseases of the Heart and Great Vessels*, 8th edn., Boston, MA: Little Brown, 1979.
9. Ashman, R. and E. Hull, *Essentials of Electrocardiography*, 2nd edn., New York: Macmillan, 1945.
10. Stewart, C.B. and G.W. Manning, A detailed analysis of the electrocardiograms of 500 R.C.A.F. aircrew. *Am. Heart J.*, 1944;**27**: 502–523.
11. White, B.V., R.C. Parker Jr., and A.M. Master, Disease of the mitral valve: Its effects on the pattern of the electrocardiogram. *Arch. Intern. Med.*, 1944;**74**: 94–99.
12. Shipley, R.A. and W.R. Hallaran, The four-lead electrocardiogram in two hundred normal men and women. *Am. Heart J.*, 1936;**11**: 325–345.
13. Castellanos, A. Jr., R. Iyengar, A.S. Agha, and C.A. Castillo, Wenckenbach phenomenon within the atria. *Br. Heart J.*, 1972;**34**: 1121–1126.
14. Castellanos, A., R.J. Sung, J.L. Aldrich, I.J. Mendoza, and R.J. Myerburg, Alternating Wenckenbach periods occurring in the atria, His-Purkinje system, ventricles and Kent bundle. *Am. J. Cardiol.*, 1977;**40**: 853–859.
15. Castellanos, A., R.J. Sung, S.M. Mallon, M.G. Bloom, and R.J. Myerburg, Effects of proximal intra-atrial Wenckenbach on distal atrioventricular nodal, and His-Purkinje, block. *Am. Heart J.*, 1978;**95**: 228–234.
16. Willems, J.L., E.O. Demedina, R. Bernard, et al., World Health Organization/International Society and Federation of Cardiology Task Force. Criteria for intraventricular-conduction disturbances and preexcitation. *J. Am. Coll. Cardiol.*, 1985;**5**: 1261–1275.
17. Prystowsky, E.N., W.M. Miles, J.J. Heger, and D.P. Ziper, Preexcitation syndromes. Mechanisms and management. *Med. Clin. North Am.*, 1984;**68**: 831–893.
18. Narula, O.S., M. Runge, and P. Samet, Second degree Wenckenbach AV block due to block within the atrium. *Br. Heart J.*, 1972;**34**: 1127–1136.
19. Demoulin, J.C. and H.E. Kulbertus, Histopathological examination of the concept of left hemiblock. *Br. Heart J.*, 1972;**34**: 807–814.
20. de Pádua, F., V.M. Lopes, D.D. Dos Reis, M.G. Lopes, and J.P. Miguel, Hemiblocks. *Adv. Cardiol.*, 1977;**19**: 105–114.
21. de Pádua, F., D.D. Reis, V.M. Lopes, et al., Left median hemiblock – A chimera? in *3rd International Congress on Electrocardiography, (17th International Symposium on Vectorcardiography)*, P. Rijlant and F. Kornreich, Editors. Brussels, 1976.
22. Demoulin, J.-C., L.J. Simar, and H.E. Kulbertus, Quantitative study of left bundle branch fibrosis in left anterior hemiblock: A stereological approach. *Am. J. Cardiol.*, 1975;**36**: 751–756.
23. Uhley, H.N. and L.M. Rivkin, Electrocardiographic patterns following interruption of the main and peripheral branches of the canine left bundle of His. *Am. J. Cardiol.*, 1964;**13**: 41–47.
24. Beattie, J.M., F.A. Gaffney, and C.G. Blomqvist, Transcavitary conduction and the mean frontal QRS axis (abstract), in *14th International Congress on Electrocardiology, (28th International Symposium on Vectorcardiography)*, R.Th. van Dam, Editor. Berlin, 1987, p. 7.
25. Duchosal, P.W. and J.R. Grosgurin, *Atlas D'electrocardiographie et de Vectocardiographie. Étude du Ventriculogramme dans les Conditions Normales et Pathologiques.* Basel: Karger, 1959.
26. Rosenbaum, M.B., The hemiblocks: Diagnostic criteria and clinical significance. *Mod. Concepts Cardiovasc. Dis.*, 1970;**39**: 141–146.
27. Rosenbaum, M.B., M.V. Elizari, and J.O. Lazzari, *The Hemiblocks.* Oldsmar, FL: Tampa Tracings, 1970.
28. de Pádua, F., V.M. Lopes, D.D. Reis, J.M.P. Miguel, and M.G. Lopes, O hemibloqueio esquerdo mediano – Uma entidade discutível. *Bol. Soc. Port. Cardiol.*, 1976.
29. de Pádua, F., Bloqueios fasciculares – Os hemibloqueios em questão. *Rev. Port. Clin. Terapêutica*, 1977;**3**: 199.
30. de Pádua, F., Intraventricular conduction defects – What future? In *New Frontiers of Electrocardiology*, F. de Pádua and P.W. Macfarlane, Editors. Chichester: Research Studies Press, 1981, pp. 181–185.
31. Burchell, H.B. and N. Tuna, The interpretation of gross left axis deviation in the electrocardiogram. *Eur. J. Cardiol.*, 1979;**10**: 259–277.
32. Corne, R.A., R.E. Beamish, and R.L. Rollwagen, Significance of left anterior hemiblock. *Br. Heart J.*, 1978;**40**: 522–527.
33. Das, G., Left axis deviation: A spectrum of intraventricular condition block. *Circulation*, 1976;**53**: 917–919.
34. Horwitz, S., E. Lupi, J. Hayes, W. Frishman, M. Cardenas, and T. Killip, Electrocardiographic criteria for the diagnosis of left anterior fascicular block. Left axis deviation and delay intraventricular conduction. *Chest*, 1975;**68**: 317–320.
35. Jacobson, L.B., L. LaFollete, and K. Cohn, An appraisal of initial QRS forces in left anterior fascicular block. *Am. Heart J.*, 1977;**94**: 407–413.
36. Kulbertus, H.E., P. Collignon, and L. Humblet, Vectorcardiographic study of the QRS loop in patients with left anterior focal block. *Am. Heart J.*, 1970;**79**: 293–304.
37. McHenry, P.L., J.F. Phillips, C. Fish, and B.R. Corya, Right precordial QRS pattern due to left anterior hemiblock. *Am. Heart J.*, 1971;**81**: 498–502.
38. Milliken, J.A., Isolated and complicated left anterior fascicular block: A review of suggested electrocardiographic criteria. *J. Electrocardiol.*, 1983;**16**: 199–211.

39. Perloff, J.K., N.K. Roberts, and W.R. Cabeen Jr., Left axis deviation: A reassessment. *Circulation*, 1979;**60**: 12–21.
40. Rabkin, S.W., F.A.L. Mathewson, and R.B. Tate, Natural history of marked left axis deviation (left anterior hemiblock). *Am. J. Cardiol.*, 1979;**43**: 606–611.
41. Friedman, H.H., *Diagnostic Electrocardiography and Vectorcardiography*. 2nd edn., New York: McGraw-Hill, 1977, pp. 80–55.
42. Cerqueira Gomes, M., F. de Pádua, C. Ribeiro, et al., in *Symposium and Colloquium on the Electrical Field of the Heart*, P. Rijilant, Editor. Brussels: Presses Academiques, 1972.
43. Cerqueira Gomes, M., F. de Pádua, C. Ribeiro, et al., Estudos sobre o desvio esquerdo do eixo médio do QRS (estudo cooperativo). I. Bases experimentais e clínicas. *J. Médico*, 1973;**81**: 345–353.
44. Cerqueira Gomes, M., F. de Pádua, C. Ribeiro, et al., Estudos sobre o desvio esquerdo do eixo médio do QRS (estudo cooperativo). II. Resultados preliminares. *J. Médico*, 1973;**81**: 726–732.
45. Medrano, G.A., C. Brenes, A. DeMicheli, and D. Sodi Pallares, Clinical electrocardiographic and vectorcardiographic diagnosis of the left anterior subdivision block isolated or associated with RBBB. *Am. Heart J.*, 1972;**83**: 447–458.
46. Lopes, M.G., *Seminar in Vectorcardiography*. Stanford University Medical School, Stanford, CA: Stanford University Press, 1974.
47. Miguel, J.M.P., D.D. dos Reis, V.M.M. Lopes, B.B. da Costa, and F. de Pádua, O bloqueio de ramo direito nas suas relações com os hemibloqueios esquerdos. *Livro Resumo Congresso Luso-Espanhol de Cardiologia, Valência*, 1973.
48. Miguel, J.P., D.D. dos Reis, V.M. Lopes, C.M. Pereira, and F. de Pádua, Vectorcardiographic study of right bundle branch block and its associations with the left hemiblocks. *Adv. Cardiol.*, 1976;**16**: 451–464.
49. Lee, S.J., C. McCulloch, I. Mangat, E. Foster, T. DeMarco, and L.A. Saxon, Isolated bundle branch block and left ventricular dysfunction. *J. Card. Fail.*, 2003;**9**(2): 87–92.
50. Cohen, H.C., K.M. Rosen, and A. Pick, Disorders of impulse conduction and impulse formation caused by hyperkalemia in man. *Am. Heart J.*, 1975;**89**: 501–509.
51. Kenedi, P., M.V. O'Reilly, and E. Goldberg, Association between intraventricular conduction defects, coronary artery disease and left ventricular function. *Adv. Cardiol.*, 1976;**16**: 504–506.
52. Schneider, J.F., H.E. Thomas Jr., B.E. Kreger, P.M. McNamara, P. Sorlie, and W.B. Kannel, Newly acquired right bundle branch block. The Framingham study. *Ann. Intern. Med.*, 1980;**92**: 37–44.
53. Lopes, M.G., E. Rocha, V.M. Lopes, D.D. dos Reis, and F. de Pádua, Long-term prognosis of the left anterior hemiblock. *Adv. Cardiol.*, 1977;**19**: 115–119.
54. Lopes, V.M., M. Carrageta, and F. de Pádua, 24-hour continuous electrocardiogram in the diagnosis and the prognosis of the so-called left hemiblock. *Adv. Cardiol.*, 1976;**16**: 469–478.
55. Biagini, E., A. Elhendy, A.F.L Schinkel, et al., Prognostic significance of left anterior hemiblock in patients with suspected coronary artery disease. *J. Am. Coll. Cardiol.*, 2005;**46**: 858–863.
56. Lopes, V.M., J.M.P. Miguel, D.D. dos Reis, B.C.B da Costa, and F. de Pádua, Left-posterior hemiblock. Clinical and vectorcardiographic study of twenty cases. *J. Electrocardiol.*, 1974;**7**: 197–214.
57. Lopes, V.M., D.D. Reis, J.M.P. Miguel, B.B. Costa, and F. de Pádua, Left posterior hemiblock. *Neue Ergeb. Elektrokardiol.*, 1974;**2**: 189.
58. de Pádua, F., V.M. Lopes, and J.M. Pereira-Miguel, Left posterior hemiblock. Good prognosis? *Adv. Cardiol.*, 1975;**14**: 157–175.
59. Scott, R.C., The S_1Q_3 (McGinn-White) pattern in acute cor pulmonale: A form of transient left posterior hemiblock? *Am. Heart J.*, 1971;**82**: 135–137.
60. Nakaya, Y., Y. Hiasa, Y. Murayama, et al., Prominent anterior QRS force as a manifestation of septal fascicular block. *J. Electrocardiol.*, 1978;**11**: 39–46.
61. Castellanos, A. and R.J. Myerburg, *The Hemiblocks in Myocardial Infarction*. East Norwalk, CT: Appleton-Century-Crofts, 1976, p. 4.
62. Hiss, R.G. and L.E. Lamb, Electrocardiographic findings in 122043 individuals. *Circulation*, 1962;**25**: 947–961.
63. Raunio, H., V. Rissanen, C. Jokinen, and O. Penttilä, Significance of a terminal R wave in lead V_1 of the electrocardiogram. *Am. Heart J.*, 1978;**95**: 702–706.
64. Tapia, F.A. and W.L. Proudfit, Secondary R waves in right precordial leads in normal persons and in patients with cardiac disease. *Circulation*, 1960;**21**: 28–37.
65. Moore, E.N., J.P. Boineau, and D.F. Patterson, Incomplete right bundle-branch block: An electrocardiographic enigma and possible misnomer. *Circulation*, 1971;**44**: 678–687.
66. de Pádua, F., *Contribuição Vectocardiográfica para o Estudo das Hipertrofias Ventriculares*, PhD dissertation. Lisbon: Faculty of Medicine, University of Lisbon, 1959.
67. Liao, Y.L., L.A. Emidy, A. Dyer, et al., Characteristics and prognosis of incomplete right bundle branch block: An epidemiologic study. *J. Am. Coll. Cardiol.*, 1986;**7**: 492–499.
68. Grishman, A. and L. Schleris, *Spatial Vectorcardiography*. Philadelphia, PA: Saunders, 1952.
69. Dick, M., D.M. Behrendt, K.E. Jochim, and A.R. Castaneda, Electrophysiologic delineation of the intraventricular His bundle in two patients with endocardial cushion type of ventricular septal defect. *Circulation*, 1981;**63**: 225–229.
70. de Pádua, F., M.G. Lopes, D.D. Reis, A. Pereirinha, V.M. Lopes, and R. Nunes, Deslocamento anterior do complexo QRS – Tentativa de esclarecimento etiológico a partir do estudo ecocardiográfico, in Sociedad Cardiologia de Levante. *Bloqueo Cardíaco*. Barcelona: Cientifico Médica, 1980, pp. 248–252.
71. Barold, S.S., J.W. Linhart, F.J. Hildner, O.S. Narula, and P. Samet, Incomplete left brunche-branch block: A definite electrocardiographic entity. *Circulation*, 1968;**38**: 702–710.
72. Sanchez, C., T.J. Walsh, and E. Massie, The vectorcardiogram in incomplete left bundle branch block. *Am. J. Cardiol.*, 1961;**7**: 629–637.
73. Schamroth, L. and B.A. Bradlow, Incomplete left bundle-branch block. *Br. Heart J.*, 1964;**26**: 285–288.
74. Unger, P.N., M. Greenblatt, and M. Lev, The anatomic basis of the electrocardiographic abnormality in incomplete left bundle branch block. *Am. Heart J.*, 1968;**76**: 486–497.
75. Terasawa, F., M. Kuramochi, Y. Yazaki, et al., Clinical and pathological studies on incomplete left bundle Branco block in the aged. *Isr. J. Med. Sci.*, 1969;**5**: 732–735.
76. Eppinger, H. and C.J. Rothberger, Zur Analyses des Elektrokardiogramms. *Wien. Klin. Wochenschr.*, 1909;**22**: 1091–1098.
77. McAnulty, J. and S. Rahimtoola, Prognosis in bundle branch block. *Annu. Rev. Med.*, 1981;**32**: 499–507.
78. Bharati, S., M. Lev, R. Dhingra, et al., Pathologic correlations in three cases of bilateral bundle branch disease with unusual electrophysiologic manifestations in two cases. *Am. J. Cardiol.*, 1976;**38**: 508–518.

79. Lister, J.W., R.S. Kline, and M.E. Lesser, Chronic bilateral bundle branch block. Long-term observations in ambulatory patients. *Br. Heart J.*, 1977;**39**: 203–207.
80. Singer, R.B., Mortality in 966 life insurance applicants with bundle branch block or wide QRS. *Trans. Assoc. Life Insur. Med. Dir. Am.*, 1968;**52**: 94–114.
81. Rotman, M. and J.H. Triebwasser, A clinical and follow-up study of right and left bundle branch block. *Circulation*, 1975;**51**: 477–484.
82. Ostrander, L.D. Jr., Bundle-branch block: An epidemiological study. *Circulation*, 1964;**30**: 872–881.
83. Gelband, H., A.L. Waldo, G.A. Kaiser, F.O. Bowman Jr., J.R. Malm, and B.F. Hoffman, Etiology of right bundle-branch block in patients undergoing total correction of Tetralogy of Fallot. *Circulation*, 1971;**44**: 1022–1033.
84. Krongrad, E., S.E. Hefler, F.O. Bowman Jr., J.R. Malm, and B.F. Hoffman, Further observations on the etiology of the right bundle branch block pattern following right ventriculotomy. *Circulation*, 1974;**50**: 1105–1113.
85. Scanlon, P.J., R. Pryor, and S.G. Blount Jr., Right bundle-branch block associated with left superior or inferior intraventricular block. Clinical setting, prognosis, and relation to complete heart block. *Circulation*, 1970;**42**: 1123–1133.
86. AbdElRahman, M.Y., W. Hui, M. Yigitbasi, et al., Detection of left ventricular asynchrony in patients with right bundle branch block after repair of tetralogy of Fallot using tissue-Doppler imaging-derived strain. *J. Am. Coll. Cardiol.*, 2005;**45**: 915–921.
87. Mehran-Pour, M., G. Borkat, J. Liebman, and J. Ankeney, Resolution of surgically induced right-bundle branch block. *Ann. Thorac. Surg.*, 1977;**23**: 139–144.
88. Yasui, H., Y. Takeda, S. Yamauchi, et al., The deleterious effects of surgically induced complete right bundle branch block on long-term follow-up results of closure of ventricular septal defect. *J. Thorac. Cardiovasc. Surg.*, 1977;**74**: 210–217.
89. Guerrero, M., K. Harjai, G.W. Stone, et al., Comparison of the prognostic effect of left versus right versus no bundle branch block on presenting electrocardiogram in acute myocardial infarction patients treated with primary angioplasty in the primary angioplasty in myocardial infarction trials. *Am. J. Cardiol.*, 2005;**96**: 482–488.
90. Tomoda, H. and N. Aoki, Right bundle branch block in acute myocardial infarction treated by primary coronary angioplasty and stenting. *Angiology*, 2005;**56**: 131–136.
91. Alfonso, F., Immediate resolution of new right bundle branch block in acute myocardial infarction following primary coronary angioplasty. *Int. J. Cardiol.*, 2005;**105**: 117–118.
92. Chen, C.-H., T. Sakurai, M. Fujita, M. Nobuyoshi, and C. Kawai, Transient intraventricular conduction disturbances in hypertrophic obstructive cardiomyopathy. *Am. Heart J.*, 1981;**101**: 672–674.
93. Lancaster, M.C., E. Schechter, and G.K. Massing, Acquired complete right bundle branch block without overt cardiac disease. Clinical and hemodynamic study of 37 patients. *Am. J. Cardiol.*, 1972;**30**: 32–36.
94. Lenegre, J., Etiology and pathology of bilateral bundle branch block in relation to complete heart block. *Prog. Cardiovasc. Dis.*, 1964;**6**: 409–444.
95. Lev, M., Anatomic basis for atrioventricular block. *Am. J. Med.*, 1964;**37**: 742–748.
96. Harris, L.K., Transient right bundle branch block following blunt chest trauma. *Am. J. Cardiol.*, 1969;**23**: 884–887.
97. Jackson, D.H., Transient post-traumatic right bundle branch block: Report of two cases. *Am. J. Cardiol.*, 1969;**23**: 877–883.
98. Kumpuris, A.G., T.B. Casale, D.M. Mokotoff, R.R. Miller, and R.J. Luchi, Right bundle-branch block. Occurrence following nonpenetrating chest trauma without evidence of cardiac contusion. *J. Am. Med. Assoc.*, 1979;**242**: 172–173.
99. Zinsser, H.F. and G.S. Thind, Right bundle branch block after nonpenetrating injury to the chest wall. *J. Am. Med. Assoc.*, 1969;**207**: 1913–1915.
100. Fedor, J.M., A. Walston, G.S. Wagner, and J. Starr, The vectorcardiogram in right bundle branch block. Correlation with cardiac failure and pulmonary disease. *Circulation*, 1976;**53**: 926–930.
101. Stein, P.D., J.E. Dalen, K.M. McIntyre, A.A. Sasahara, N.K. Wenger, P.W. Willis III, The electrocardiogram in acute pulmonary embolism. *Prog. Cardiovasc. Dis.*, 1975;**17**: 247–257.
102. Froelicher, V.F. Jr., A.J. Thompson, R. Wolthuis, et al., Angiographic findings in asymptomatic aircrewmen with electrocardiographic abnormalities. *Am. J. Cardiol.*, 1977;**39**: 32–38.
103. Johnson, R.L., K.H. Averill, and L.E. Lamb, Electrocardiographic findings in 67375 asymptomatic subjects: VI. Right bundle branch block. *Am. J. Cardiol.*, 1960;**6**: 143–152.
104. Massing, G.K. and M.C. Lancaster, Clinical significance of acquired complete right bundle branch block in 59 patients without overt cardiac disease. *Aerosp. Med.*, 1969;**40**: 967–971.
105. Whinnery, J.E., V.F. Froelicher Jr., A.J. Stewart, M.R. Longo Jr., and J.H. Triebwasser, The electrocardiographic response to maximal treadmill exercise of asymptomatic men with right bundle branch block. *Chest*, 1977;**71**: 335–340.
106. Messer, A.L. and R.P. Johnson, Shreenivas, White P D. Prognosis in bundle branch block: III. A comparison of right and left bundle branch block with a note on the relative incidence of each. *Am. Heart J.*, 1951;**41**: 239–245.
107. Perera, G.A., S.A. Levine, and H. Erlanger, Prognosis of right bundle branch block: A study of 104 cases. *Br. Heart J.*, 1942:**4**: 35–42.
108. Reuch, C.S. and J.R. Vivas, Clinical analysis of right bundle branch block. *Am. Heart J.*, 1959;**58**: 543–546.
109. Shreenivas, M.A.L., R.P. Johnson, and P.D. White, Prognosis in bundle branch block: I. Factors influencing the survival period in right bundle branch block. *Am. Heart J.*, 1950;**40**: 891–902.
110. Bauer, G.E., Development of bundle branch block. *Am. J. Cardiol.*, 1964;**14**: 346–351.
111. Mullins, C.B. and J.M. Atkins, Prognosis and management of ventricular conduction blocks in acute myocardial infarction. *Mod. Concepts Cardiovasc. Dis.* 1976;**45**: 129–133.
112. The Coronary Drug Project Research Group. The prognostic importance of the electrocardiogram after myocardial infarction. Experience in the Coronary Drug Project. *Ann. Intern. Med.*, 1972;**77**: 677–689.
113. Madias, J.E., R. Ashtiani, H. Agarwal, V.K. Narayan, M. Win, and A. Sinha, Stability of the ECG features of complete right bundle branch block over time: A methodological study for implementation in research and clinical practice. *Cardiology*, 2005;**103**: 84–88.
114. Lopes, M.G., A. Pereirinha, and F. de Pádua, The diagnosis of left ventricular hypertrophy in the presence of bundle branch block – An ECG/VCG and echocardiographic correlation, in *Modern Electrocardiology*, Z. Antalóczy, Editor. Amsterdam: Excerpta Medica, 1978, pp. 423–427.
115. Herbert, W.H., Left bundle branch block and coronary artery disease. *J. Electrocardiol.*, 1975;**8**: 317–324.

116. Lev, M., P.N. Unger, K.M. Rosen, and S. Bharati, The anatomic base of the electrocardiographic abnormality left bundle branch block. *Adv. Cardiol.*, 1975;**14**: 16–24.
117. Sugiura, M., R. Okada, S. Ohkawa, and H. Shimada, Pathohistological studies on the conduction system in 8 cases of complete left bundle branch block. *Jpn. Heart J.*, 1970;**11**: 5–16.
118. Li, Z.B., K. Wachtell, P.M. Okin, et al., Association of left bundle branch block with left ventricular structure and function in hypertensive patients with left ventricular hypertrophy: The LIFE study. *J. Hum. Hypertension*, 2004;**18**; 397–402.
119. Jain, A.C. and M.C. Mehta, Etiologies of left bundle branch block and correlations with hemodynamic and angiographic findings. *Am. J. Cardiol.*, 2003;**91**: 1375–1378.
120. Brake, C.M., Complete left bundle branch in asymptomatic airmen. *Aerosp. Med.*, 1969;**40**: 781–782.
121. DeMartino, G., M. Santamaria, Q. Parisi, L. Messano, and F. Crea, Myocarditis as a cause of alternating left bundle branch block. *J. Interv. Card. Electrophysiol.*, 2004;**11**; 19–20.
122. Fenichel, N.M. and F.A. Jimenez, Polachek A A. 2:1 left bundle branch block in acute bacterial endocarditis with septal abscess. *J. Electrocardiol.*, 1977;**10**: 287–290.
123. Singh, R.B., B.V. Agrawal, and P.N. Somani, Left bundle branch block: A rare manifestation of digitalis intoxication. *Acta Cardiol.*, 1976;**31**: 175–179.
124. Lamb, L.E., K.D. Kable, and K.H. Averill, Electrocardiographic findings in 67375 asymptomatic subjects. V. Left bundle branch block. *Am. J. Cardiol.*, 1960;**6**: 130–142.
125. Schneider, J.F., H.E. Thomas Jr., B.E. Kreger, P.M. McNamara, and W.B. Kannel, Newly acquired left bundle-branch block: The Framingham study. *Ann. Intern. Med.*, 1979;**90**: 303–310.
126. Smith, R.F., D.H. Jackson, J.W. Harthorne, and C.A. Sanders, Acquired bundle branch block in a healthy population. *Am. Heart J.*, 1970;**80**: 746–751.
127. Frisella, M.E. and D.H. Spodick, Confirmation of the prevalence and importance of a 12-lead investigation for diagnosis. *Am. J. Cardiol.*, 2005;**96**: 696–697.
128. Dillon, J.C., S. Chang, and H. Feigenbaum, Echocardiographic manifestations of left bundle branch block. *Circulation*, 1974;**49**: 876–880.
129. Wong, B., R. Rinkenberger, M. Dunn, and A. Goodyer, Effect of intermittent left bundle branch block on left ventricular performance in the normal heart. *Am. J. Cardiol.*, 1977;**39**: 459–463.
130. vanHemel, N.M., Left is worse than right: The outcome of bundle branch block in middle-aged men. *Eur. Heart J.*, 2005;**26**: 2222–2223.
131. Ozdemir, K., B.B. Altunkeser, B. Korkut, M. Tokac, and H. Gok, Effect of left bundle branch block on systolic and diastolic function of left ventricle in heart failure. *Angiology*, 2004;**55**: 63–71.
132. Turner, M.S., R.A. Bleasdale, D. Vinereanu, et al., Electrical and mechanical components of dyssynchrony in heart failure patients with normal QRS duration and left bundle-branch block – Impact of left and biventricular pacing. *Circulation*, 2004;**109**: 2544–2549.
133. Abraham, W.T., et al., Cardiac resynchronization in chronic heart failure. *N. Engl. J. Med.*, 2002; **346**: 1845.
134. Goldman, M.J. and H.V. Pipberger, Analysis of the orthogonal electrocardiogram and vectorcardiogram in ventricular conduction defects with and without myocardial infarction. *Circulation*, 1969;**39**: 243–250.
135. Pryor, R., Recognition of myocardial infarction in the presence of bundle branch block, in *Complex Electrocardiography*, vol. 2, Philadelphia, PA: Davis, 1974, pp. 255–271, (*Cardiovasc. Clin.* **6**(1)).
136. Brady, W.J., B. Lentz, K. Barlotta, R.A. Harrigan, and T. Chan, ECG patterns confounding the ECG diagnosis of acute coronary syndrome: Left bundle branch block, right ventricular paced rhythms, and left ventricular hypertrophy. *Emerg. Med. Clin. N. Am.*, 2005;**23**: 999.
137. Timmis, G.C., V. Gangadharan, R.G. Ramos, and S. Gordon, Reassessment of Q waves in left bundle branch block. *J. Electrocardiol.*, 1976;**9**: 109–114.
138. Havelda, C.J., G.S. Sohi, N.C. Flowers, and L.G. Horan, The pathologic correlates of the electrocardiogram: Complete left bundle branch block. *Circulation*, 1982;**65**: 445–451.
139. De Kock, J. and L. Schamroth, Left bundle branch block associated with acute inferior wall myocardial infarction. *S. Afr. Med. J.*, 1975;**49**: 397–398.
140. Nguyen, K., J.E. Cigarroa, R.A. Lange, L.D. Hillis, and E.C. Keeley, Presence and extent of angiographic coronary narrowing in patients with left bundle branch block. *Am. J. Cardiol.*, 2004;**93**: 1426–1427.
141. Demir, H., G. Erbay, K.M. Kir, K. Omurlu, F. Berk, and C. Aktolun, Clinical validation of technetium-99m MEBI-gated single-photon emission computed tomography (SPECT) for avoiding false positive results in patients with left bundle-branch block: Comparison with stress-rest nongated SPECT. *Clin. Cardiol.*, 2003;**26**: 182–187.
142. CandellRiera, J., G. OllerMartinez, O. PereztolValdes, et al., Usefulness of myocardial perfusion SPECT in patients with left bundle branch block and previous myocardial infarction. *Heart*, 2003;**89**: 169–174.
143. Reuben, A.D. and C.J. Mann, Simplifying thrombolysis decisions in patients with left bundle branch block. *Emerg. Med. J.*, 2005;**22**: 617–620.
144. Duncan, A.M., D.P. Francis, D.G. Gibson, and M.Y. Henein, Limitation of exercise tolerance in chronic heart failure: Distinct effects of left bundle-branch block and coronary artery disease. *J. Am. Coll. Cardiol.*, 2004;**43**: 1524–1531.
145. Petersen, G.V. and G. Tikoff, Left bundle branch block and left ventricular hypertrophy: Electrocardiographic-pathologic correlations. *Chest*, 1971;**59**: 174–177.
146. Chung, D.-K., N.M. Panitch, and E.K. Chung, A comparison of the conventional criteria for left ventricular hypertrophy before and after the development of complete left bundle branch block. *Jpn. Circ. J.*, 1969;**33**: 19–24.
147. Blondeau, M., Complete left bundle branch block with marked left axis deviation of QRS. Clinical and anatomical study. *Adv. Cardiol.*, 1975;**14**: 25–38.
148. Flowers, N.C., Left bundle branch block: A continuously evolving concept. *J. Am. Coll. Cardiol.*, 1987;**9**: 684–697.
149. Pereirinha, A., J. Correia, F. de Pádua, and M.G. Lopes, Identificacion de los condicionantes del prognostico en pacientes con bloqueo de rama a partir de la repercusion anatomo funcional valorada por Ecocardiografia (abstract). *Rev. Esp. Cardiol.*, 1982;**35**(Suppl. I): 42.
150. Wei-Min, H. and T. Cheng-Lang, Bilateral bundle branch block. Right bundle branch block associated with left anterior fascicular block. *Cardiology*, 1977;**62**: 35–43.
151. Watt, T.B. Jr. and R.D. Pruitt, Character, cause, and consequence of combined left axis deviation and right bundle branch block in human electrocardiograms. *Am. Heart J.*, 1969;**77**: 460–465.

152. Ohmae, M., Correlative studies on the electrocardiogram and histopathology of the conduction system. I. Right bundle branch block with left axis deviation and prolonged P-R interval. *Jpn. Circ. J.*, 1977;**41**: 677–686.
153. Sugiura, M., R. Okada, K. Hiraoka, and S. Ohkawa, Histological studies on the conduction system in 14 cases of right bundle branch block associated with left axis deviation. *Jpn. Heart J.*, 1969;**10**: 121–132.
154. Husson, G.S., M.C. Blackman, M.S. Rogers, S. Bharati, and M. Lev, Familial congenital bundle branch system disease. *Am. J. Cardiol.*, 1973;**32**: 365–369.
155. Schaal, S.F., J. Seidensticker, R. Goodman, and C.F. Wooley, Familial right bundle-branch block, left axis deviation, complete heart block, and early death. A heritable disorder of cardiac conduction. *Ann. Intern. Med.*, 1973;**79**: 63–66.
156. Morriss, J.H., G.S. Eugster, J.J. Nora, and R. Pryor, His bundle recording in progressive external ophthalmoplegia. *J. Pediatr.*, 1972;**81**: 1167–1170.
157. Brink, A.J. and M. Torrington, Progressive familial heart block – Two types. *S. Afr. Med. J.*, 1977; **52**: 53–59.
158. Evans, W., Familial cardiomegaly. *Br. Heart J.*, 1949;**11**: 68–82.
159. Stéphan, E., Hereditary bundle branch system defect. A new genetic entity? *Am. Heart J.*, 1979;**97**: 708–718.
160. Chuquimia, R., T.S. Ramadurai, W. Towne, and K. Rosen, Bifascicular block due to penetrating wound of the heart: Electrophysiology studies. *Chest*, 1974;**66**: 195–197.
161. Gozo, E.G. Jr., H.C. Cohen, and A. Pick, Traumatic bifascicular intraventricular block. *Chest*, 1972;**61**: 294–296.
162. Gozo, E.G. Jr., I. Cosnow, H.C. Cohen, and L. Okun, The heart in sarcoidosis. *Chest*, 1971;**60**: 379–388.
163. Sung, R.J., D.M. Tamer, O.L. Garcia, A. Castellanos, R.J. Myerburg, and H. Gelband, Analysis of surgically-induced right bundle branch block pattern using intracardial recording techniques. *Circulation*, 1976;**54**: 442–446.
164. Wolff, G.S., T.W. Rowland, and R.C. Ellison, Surgically induced right bundle-branch block with left anterior hemiblock. An ominous sign in postoperative Tetralogy of Fallot. *Circulation*, 1972;**46**: 587–594.
165. Yabek, S.M., J.M. Jermakani, and N. Roberts, Postoperative trifascicular block complicating Tetralogy of Fallot repair. *Pediatrics*, 1976;**58**: 236–242.
166. Kulbertus, H.E., Reevaluation of the prognosis of patients with LAD-RBBB. *Am. Heart J.*, 1976;**92**: 665–667.
167. Lasser, R.P., J.I. Haft, and C.K. Friedberg, Relationship of right bundle-branch block and marked left axis deviation (with left parietal or peri-infarction block) to complete heart block and syncope. *Circulation*, 1968;**37**: 429–437.
168. Gupta, P.K., E. Lichstein, K.D. Chadda, Follow-up studies in patients with right bundle branch block and left anterior hemiblock: Significance of H-V interval. *J. Electrocardiol.*, 1977;**10**: 221–224.
169. Blondeau, M. and J. Lenegre, Bloc de branche et bloc auriculo-ventriculaire complet. *Arch. Mal. Cœur Vaiss.*, 1964;**57**: 1–19.
170. Castellanos, A. Jr., O. Maytin, A.G. Arcebal, and L. Lemberg, Significance of complete right bundle-branch block with right axis deviation in absence of right ventricular hypertrophy. *Br. Heart J.*, 1970;**32**: 85–92.
171. Ranganathan, N., R. Dhurandhar, J.H. Phillips, and E.D. Wigle, His bundle electrogram in bundle branch block. *Circulation*, 1972;**45**: 282–294.
172. Barrett, P.A.,C.T. Peter, H.J. Swan, B.N. Singh, and W.J. Mandel, The frequency and prognostic significance of electrocardiographic abnormalities in clinically normal individuals. *Prog. Cardiovasc. Dis.*, 1981;**23**: 299–319.
173. Kulbertus, H. and P. Collignon, Association of right bundle-branch block with left superior or inferior intraventricular block. Its relation to complete heart block and Adam-Stokes syndrome. *Br. Heart J.*, 1969;**31**: 435–440.
174. McAnulty, J.H., S.H. Rahimtoola, E. Murphy, et al., Natural history of "high risk" bundle-branch block: Final report of a prospective study. *N. Engl. J. Med.*, 1982;**307**: 137–143.
175. American College of Cardiology/American Heart Association – Guidelines for Permanent Pacing. *Circulation*, 2002;**106**: 2145.
176. Rosen, K.M., S.H. Rahimtoola, R. Chuquimia, H.S. Loeb, R.M. Gumar, Electrophysiological significance of first degree atrioventricular block with intraventricular conduction disturbance. *Circulation*, 1971;**43**: 491–502.
177. Levites, R. and J.I. Haft, Significance of first degree heart block (prolonged P-R interval) in bifascicular block. *Am. J. Cardiol.*, 1974;**34**: 259–264.
178. Denes, P., R.C. Dhingra, D. Wu, et al., H-V interval in patients with bifascicular block (right bundle branch block and left anterior hemiblock): Clinical, electrocardiographic and electrophysiologic correlations. *Am. J. Cardiol.*, 1975;**35**: 23–29.
179. Dhingra, R.C., P. Denes, D. Wu, et al., Chronic right bundle branch block and left posterior hemiblock: Clinical, electrophysiologic and prognostic observations. *Am. J. Cardiol.*, 1975;**36**: 867–872.
180. Scheinman, M., A. Weiss, and F. Kunkel, His bundle recordings in patients with bundle branch block and transient neurologic symptoms. *Circulation*, 1973;**48**: 322–330.
181. Scheinman, M.M., R.W. Peters, G. Modin, M. Brennan, C. Mies, and J. O'Young, Prognostic value of infranodal conduction time in patients with chronic bundle branch block. *Circulation* 1977;**56**: 240–244.
182. Dhingra, R.C., P. Denes, D. Wu, et al., Prospective observations in patients with chronic bundle branch block and marked H-V prolongation. *Circulation*, 1976;**53**: 600–604.
183. Gould, L., K. Venkataraman, N. Mohammad, and R.F. Gomprecht, Prognosis of right bundle-branch block in acute myocardial infarction. *J. Am. Med. Assoc.*, 1972;**219**: 502–503.
184. Lie, K.I., H.J. Wellens, R.M. Schuilenburg, A.E. Becker, and D. Durrer, Factors influencing prognosis of bundle branch block complicating acute antero-septal infarction. The value of His bundle recordings. *Circulation*, 1974;**50**: 935–941.
185. Aranda, J.M., B. Beferer, and A. Castellanos Jr., His bundle recordings, bundle branch block, and myocardial infarction. *Ann. Intern. Med.*, 1977;**86**: 106–108.
186. Gann, D., P.K. Balachandran, N.E. Sherif, P. Samet, and J.R. Malm, Prognostic significance of chronic versus acute bundle-branch block in acute myocardial infarction. *Chest*, 1975;**67**: 298–303.
187. Atkins, J.M., S.J. Leshin, G. Blomqvist, and C.B. Mullins, Prognosis of right bundle branch block and left anterior hemiblock: A new indication for permanent pacing (abstract). *Am. J. Cardiol.*, 1970;**26**: 624.
188. Lichstein, E., P.K. Gupta, K.D. Chadda, H.-M. Liu, and M. Sayeed, Findings of prognostic value in patients with incomplete bilateral bundle branch block complicating acute myocardial infarction. *Am. J. Cardiol.*, 1973;**32**: 913–918.

189. Atkins, J.M., S.J. Leshin, G. Blomqvist, and C.B. Mullins, Ventricular conduction blocks and sudden death in acute myocardial infarction. Potential indications for pacing. *N. Engl. J. Med.*, 1973;**288**: 281–284.
190. Godman, M.J., B.W. Lassers, and D.G. Julian, Complete bundle branch block complicating acute myocardial infarction. *N. Engl. J. Med.*, 1970;**282**: 237–240.
191. Resnekov, L., Pacemaking and acute myocardial infarction. *Impulse*, 1978;**11**: 1.
192. Ritter, W.S., J.M. Atkins, C.G. Blomqvist, and C.B. Mullins, Permanent pacing in patients with transient trifascicular block during acute myocardial infarction: Long-term prognosis. *Am. J. Cardiol.*, 1976;**38**: 205–208.
193. Castellanos, A., A.V. Ramirez, A. Mayorga-Cortes, et al., Left fascicular blocks during right-heart catheterization using the SwanGanz catheter. *Circulation*, 1981;**64**: 1271–1276.
194. Mayorga-Cortes, A., J.J. Rozánski, R.J. Sung, A. Castellanos, and R.J. Myerburg, Right ventricular apical activation times in patients with conduction disturbances occurring during acute transmural myocardial infarction. *Am. J. Cardiol.*, 1979;**43**: 913–919.
195. Ribeiro, C.S., *Estudo da activação ventricular nos bloqueios intraventriculares esquerdos (contribuição experimental para o seu diagnóstico clínico)*, PhD dissertation. Lisbon: Faculty of Medicine, University of Lisbon, 1967.
196. Hassan, Z.U., R.A. Mendoza, W.E. Steinke, and D.B. Propert, Multiple conduction defects with markedly prolonged ventricular depolarization in cardiomyopathy. *J. Electrocardiol.*, 1977;**10**: 275–278.
197. Durrer, D., R.M. Schuilenburg, and H.J.J. Wellens, Preexcitation revisited. *Am. J. Cardiol.*, 1970;**25**: 690–697.
198. Anderson, R.H., A.E. Becker, C. Brechenmacher, M.J. Davies, and L. Rossi, Ventricular preexcitation: A proposed nomenclature for its substrates. *Eur. J. Cardiol.*, 1975;3: 27–35.
199. Boineau, J.P., E.N. Moore, J.F. Spear, and W.C. Sealy, Basis of static and dynamic electrocardiographic variations in Wolff-Parkinson-White syndrome. Anatomic and electrophysiologic observations in right and left ventricular preexcitation. *Am. J. Cardiol.*, 1973;**32**: 32–45.
200. Ferrer, M.I., *Pre-Excitation, Including the Wolff-Parkinson-White and Other Related Syndromes*. Mount Kisco, New York: Futura, 1976, pp. 1–274.
201. Gallagher, J.J., E.L.C. Pritchett, W.C. Sealy, J. Kasell, and A.G. Wallace, The preexcitation syndromes. *Prog. Cardiovasc. Dis.*, 1978;**20**: 285–327.
202. Gallagher, J.J., W.C. Sealy, J. Kasell, and A.G. Wallace, Multiple accessory pathways in patients with the pre-excitation syndrome. *Circulation*, 1976;**56**: 571–591.
203. Wellens, H.J.J., Wolff-Parkinson-White syndrome. *Mod. Concepts Cardiovasc. Dis.*, 1983;**52**: 53–74.
204. Wolff, L., J. Parkinson, and P.D. White, Bundle branch block with short P-R interval in healthy young people prone to paroxysmal tachycardia. *Am. Heart J.*, 1930;**5**: 685–704.
205. Boineau, J.P. and E.N. Moore, Evidence for propagation of activation across an accessory atrioventricular connection in types A and B pre-excitation. *Circulation*, 1970;**41**: 375–397.
206. James, T.N., Morphology of the human atrioventricular node, with remarks pertinent to its electrophysiology. *Am. Heart J.*, 1961;**62**: 756–771.
207. de Pádua, F., Interpretação vectocardiográfica das arritmias. *Imprensa Médica*, 1957;**21**: 573.
208. Nakagawa, S., K. Maeda, T. Imamura, H. Kondoh, Y. Koiwaya, and K. Tanaka, Increasing pre-excitation ("concertina effect") during vasospastic angina. *J. Electrocardiol.*, 1986;**19**: 299–302.
209. Rosner, M.H., Electrocardiography in the patient with Wolff-Parkinson White syndrome: Diagnostic and therapeutic issues. *Am. J. Emerg. Med.*, 1999;**17**: 705–714.
210. Neuss, H., M. Schlepper, and J. Thorman, Analysis of re-entry mechanisms in three patients with concealed Wolff-Parkinson-White syndrome. *Circulation*, 1975;**51**: 75–81.
211. Pritchett, E.L.C., J.J. Gallagher, W.C. Sealy, et al., Supraventricular tachycardia dependent upon accessory pathways in the absence of ventricular preexcitation. *Am. J. Med.*, 1978;**64**: 214–220.
212. Sung, R.J., A. Castellanos, H. Gelband, and R.J. Myerburg, Mechanism of reciprocating tachycardia initiated during sinus rhythm in concealed Wolff-Parkinson-White syndrome. Report of a case. *Circulation*, 1976;**54**: 338–344.
213. Tonkin, A.M., J.J. Gallagher, R.H. Svenson, A.G. Wallace, and W.C. Sealy, Anterograde block in accessory pathways with retrograde conduction in reciprocating tachycardia. *Eur. J. Cardiol.*, 1975;**3**: 143–152.
214. Zipes, D.P., R.L. DeJoseph, and D.A. Rothbaum, Unusual properties of accessory pathways. *Circulation*, 1974;**49**: 1200–1211.
215. WHO/ISFC Task Force. Definition of terms related to cardiac rhythm. *Am. Heart J.*, 1978;**95**: 796–806.
216. Rosenbaum, F.F., H.H. Hecht, F.N. Wilson, and F.D. Johnston, The potential variations of the thorax and the esophagus in anomalous atrioventricular excitation (Wolff-Parkinson-White syndrome). *Am. Heart J.*, 1945;**29**: 281–326.
217. Tonkin, A.M., G.S. Wagner, J.J. Gallagher, G.D. Cope, J. Kasel, and A.G. Wallace, Initial forces of ventricular depolarization in the Wolff-Parkinson-White syndrome. Analysis based upon localization of the accessory pathway by epicardial mapping. *Circulation*, 1975;**52**: 1030–1036.
218. Wallace, A.G., W.C. Sealy, J.J. Gallagher, and L.J. Kasel, Ventricular excitation in the Wolff-Parkinson-White syndrome, in *The Conduction System of the Heart: Structure, Function, and Clinical Implications*, H.J.J. Wellens, K.I. Lie, M.J. Janse, Editors. Leiden: Stenfert Kroese, 1976, p. 613.
219. Fitzpatrik, A.P., R.P. Gonzales, M.D. Lesh, G.W. Modin, R.J. Lee, and N.M. Scheinman, New algorithm for the localization of accessory atrioventricular connections using a baseline electrocardiogram. *J. Am. Coll. Cardiol.*, 1994;**23**: 107–116.
220. Zipes, D.P., Specif arrhythmias: Diagnosis and treatment, in *Braunwald's Heart Disease: A Textbook of Cardiocascular Medicine*, 7th edn., D.P. Zipes et al., Editor. Philadelphia, PA: Saunders, 2005.
221. Desanctis, R.W. and J. Ruskin, Disturbances of the cardiac rhythm and conduction, in *Scientific American Medicine*, E. Rubenstein and D. Sederman, Editors. 1987: 1–43.
222. Chung, K.-Y., T.J. Walsh, and E. Massie, Wolff-Parkinson-White syndrome. *Am. Heart J.*, 1965;**69**: 116–133.
223. Barold, S.S. and P. Coumel, Mechanisms of atrioventricular junctional tachycardia: Role of reentry and concealed accessory bypass tracts. *Am. J. Cardiol.*, 1977;**39**: 97–106.
224. Coumel, P. and P. Attuel, Reciprocating tachycardia in overt and latent preexcitation: Influence of functional bundle branch block on the rate of the tachycardia. *Eur. J. Cardiol.*, 1974;**1**: 423–436.

225. Coumel, P., P. Attuel, and D. Flammang, The role of the conduction system in supraventricular tachycardias, in *The Conduction System of the Heart*, H.J.J. Wellens, K.I. Lie, M.J. Janse, Editors. Leiden: Kroese, 1976, pp. 424–452.
226. Hammill, S.C., E.L.C. Pritchett, G.J. Klien, W.M. Smith, and J.J. Gallagher, Accessory atrioventricular pathways that conduct only in the antegrade direction. *Circulation*, 1980;**62**: 1335–1340.
227. Lloyd, E.A., R.N. Hauer, D.P. Zipes, J.J. Heger, and E.N. Prystowsky, Syncope and ventricular tachycardia in patients with ventricular preexcitation. *Am. J. Cardiol.*, 1983;**52**: 79–82.
228. Wellens, H.J. and D. Durrer, Patterns of ventriculo-atrial conduction in the Wolff-Parkinson-White syndrome. *Circulation*, 1974;**49**: 22–31.
229. Fontaine, G., R. Frank, R. Coutte, et al., Rhythme reciproque antidromique dans un syndrome de Wolff-Parkinson-white de type A. *Am. Cardiol. Angeiol.*, 1975;**24**: 59–66.
230. Campbell, R.W.F., R.A. Smith, J.J. Gallagher, E.L.C. Pritchett, and A.G. Wallace, Atrial fibrillation in the preexcitation syndrome. *Am. J. Cardiol.*, 1977;**40**: 514–520.
231. Wellens, H.J. and D. Durrer, Wolff-Parkinson-White syndrome and atrial fibrillation: Relation between refractory period of the accessory pathway and ventricular rate during atrial fibrillation. *Am. J. Cardiol.*, 1974;**34**: 777–782.
232. Ahlinder, S., A. Granath, S. Holmer, et al., The Wolff-Parkinson-White syndrome with paroxysmal atrial fibrillation changing into ventricular fibrillation, successfully treated with external heart massage. *Nord. Med.*, 1963;**70**: 1336–1339.
233. Bashore, T.M., T.D. Sellers, J.J. Gallagher, and A.G. Wallace, Ventricular fibrillation in the Wolff-Parkinson-White syndrome (abstract). *Circulation*, 1976;**54**(Suppl. 2): 187.
234. Castillo-Fenoy, A., A. Goupil, G. Offenstadt, and G.K. Nguyen, Síndrome de Wolf-parkinson-White et mort subite. *Ann. Med. Interne.*, 1973;**124**: 871–875.
235. Dreifus, L.S., H.J. Wellens, Y. Watanabe, D. Kimbins, and R. Truex, Sinus bradycardia and atrial fibrillation associated with the Wolff-Parkinson-White syndrome. *Am. J. Cardiol.*, 1976;**38**: 149–156.
236. Fox, T.T., J. Weaver, and H.W. March, On the mechanism of the arrhythmias in aberrant atrioventricular conduction (Woff Parkinson White). *Am. Heart J.*, 1952;**43**: 507–520.
237. Kaplan, M.A. and K.L. Cohen, Ventricular fibrillation in the Wolff-Parkinson-White Syndrome. *Am. J. Cardiol.*, 1969;**24**: 259–264.
238. Lim, C.H., C.C.S. Toh, and B.L. Chia, Ventricular fibrillation in type B Wolff-Parkinson-White syndrome. *Aust. NZ J. Med.*, 1974;**4**: 515–517.
239. Martin-Noel, P., B. Denis, and D. Grundwald, Buisson Mme. Deux cas mortels de syndrome de Wolff Parkinson White. *Arch. Mal. Cœur Vaiss.*, 1970;**63**: 1647–1656.
240. Okell, B.B., The Wolff-Parkinson-White syndrome: Report of a fatal arrhythmia and autopsy findings of myocarditis, interatrial lipomatous hypertrophy, and prominent right moderator band. *Am. Heart J.*, 1968;**41**: 673–678.
241. Antonelli, G., M. Di Biase, G. Biasco, et al., Prolasso della mitrale e síndrome di pre-eccitazione ventricolare. *G. Ital. Cardiol.*, 1976;**6**: 1365–1377.
242. Devereux, R.B., J.K. Perloff, N. Reichek, and M.E. Josephson, Mitral valve prolapse. *Circulation*, 1976;**54**: 3–14.
243. Lunel, A.A.V., Significance of annulus fibrosis of heart in relation to AV conduction and ventricular activation in cases of Wolff-Parkinson-White syndrome. *Br. Heart J.*, 1972;**34**: 1263–1271.
244. Massumi, R.A., Familial Wolff-Parkinson-White syndrome with cardiomyopathy. *Am. J. Med.*, 1967;**43**: 951–955.
245. Ruskin, J.N., M. Akhtar, A.N. Damato, A.R. Ticzon, S.H. Lau, A.R. Caracta, Abnormal Q waves in Wolff-Parkinson-White syndrome: Incidence and clinical significance. *J. Am. Med. Assoc.*, 1976;**235**: 2727–2730.
246. Chung, E.K., *Electrocardiography. Practical Applications with Vectorial Principles*. Hagerstown, MD: Harper and Row, 1974.
247. Clerc, A., R. Lévy, and C. Cristesco, A propos du raccourcissement permanent de l'espace P-R de l'électrocardiogramme sans déformation do complexe ventriculaire. *Arch. Mal. Cœur Vaiss.*, 1938;**31**: 569–582.
248. Lown, B., W.T. Ganong, and S.A. Levine, The syndrome of short P R interval, normal QRS complex and paroxysmal rapid heart action. *Circulation*, 1952;**5**: 693–706.
249. Benditt, D.G., E.L.C. Pritchett, W.M. Smith, A.G. Wallace, and J.J. Gallagher, Characteristics of atrioventricular conduction and the spectrum of arrhythmias in Lown-Ganong-Levine syndrome. *Circulation*, 1978;**57**: 454–465.
250. Bisset, J.K., N. de Soyza, J.J. Kane, and M.L. Murphy, Altered refractory periods in patients with short P-R intervals and normal QRS complex. *Am. J. Cardiol.*, 1975;**35**: 487–491.
251. Gallagher, J.J., W.M. Smith, J. Kasell, D.W. Benson Jr., R. Sterba, and A.O. Grant, Role of Mahaim fibers in cardiac arrhythmias in man. *Circulation*, 1981;**64**: 176–189.
252. Brugada, P. and J. Brugada, Right bundle branch block, persistent ST segment elevation and sudden cardiac death: A distinct clinical and electrocardiographic syndrome. A multicenter report. *J. Am. Coll. Cardiol.*, 1992;20: 1391–1396.
253. Mattu, A., R.L. Rogers, K. Hyung, A.D. Perron, and W.J. Brady, The Brugada Syndrome. *Am. J. Emerg. Med.*, 2003;**21**(2): 146–151.
254. Wilde, A.A.M., C. Antzelevitch, M. Borggrefe, F. Brugada, R. Brugada, P. Brugada, D. Corrado, R.N.W. Hauer, R.S. Kass, K. Nademanee, S.G. Priori, and J.A. Towbin, Proposed diagnostic criteria for the Brugada Syndrome – Study Group on the molecular basis of Arrhythmias of the European Society of Cardiology. *Eur. Heart J.*, 2002;**23**: 1648–1654.
255. Antzelivitch, C., P. Brugada, M. Borggreffe, J. Brugada, R. Brugada, D. Corrado, et al., Brugada Syndrome: Report of the Second Consensus Conference. *Circulation*, 2005;111: 659–670.
256. Miyasaka, Y., H. Tsuji, K. Yamada, S. Tokunaga, D. Saito, Y. Imuro, N. Matsumoto, and T. Iwasaka, Prevalence and mortality of the Brugada-type electrocardiogram in one city in Japan. *J. Am. Coll. Cardiol.*, 2001;38: 771–774.
257. Naccarelli, G.V., C. Antzelevitch, D.L. Wolbrette, and J.C. Luck, The Brugada syndrome. *Curr. Opin. Cardiol.*, 2002;**17**: 19–23.
258. Rook, M.B., C.B. Alshinawi, W.A. Groenewegen, et al., Human SCN5A gene mutations alter cardiac sodium channel kinetics and are associated with the Brugada syndrome. *Cardiovasc. Res.*, 1999;**44**: 507–517.
259. Antzelevitch, C., J.M. Fish, and J.M. Di Diego, *Cellular Mechanisms Underlying the Brugada Syndrome*. Elmsford, U.K.: Blackwell Publishing, 2005, pp. 52–77.
260. Mills, A.T.D., S. Dasan, and A. Whan, Brugada syndrome: Syncope in the younger patient and the risk of sudden cardiac death. *Emerg Med J.*, 2005;**22**: 604–606.
261. Brugada, R., J. Brugada, C. Antzelevitch, et al., Sodium channel blockers identify risk for sudden death in patients

with ST-segment elevation and right bundle branch block but structurally normal hearts. *Circulation*, 2000;**101**: 510–515.
262. Giustetto, C., S. Drago, P.G. DeMarchi, P. Dalmasso, F. Bianchi, A.S. Masi, et al., Risk stratification of the patients with Brugada type electrocardiogram: A community based prospective study. *Europace*, 2009;11: 507–513.
263. Brugada, P., Amid the fourth lustrum after the description of Brugada syndrome: Controversies over? *Europace*, 2009;11: 412–413.

3 Enlargement and Hypertrophy

Peter W. Macfarlane · Peter M. Okin · T.D. Veitch Lawrie · John A. Milliken†

†Deceased.

P. W. Macfarlane et al. (eds.), *Electrocardiology*, DOI 10.1007/978-0-85729-874-4_3,

3.1 Introduction

Cardiac hypertrophy is an increase in the mass of the heart owing to the enlargement of existing muscle fibers. It may be localized to the apex or septum, for example, or may be diffuse with the latter form being further subdivided into concentric and eccentric hypertrophy depending on whether the chamber size is normal or dilated. Chronic pressure overload as in aortic stenosis or hypertension often results in concentric, diffuse, or global left ventricular hypertrophy (LVH). In contrast, eccentric or dilated hypertrophy is more frequently associated with volume overload, for example, aortic or mitral regurgitation. The terms systolic overload LVH and diastolic overload LVH also have been used as alternatives to pressure and volume overload, respectively [1, 2]. The different types are summarized in ➋ Fig. 3.1.

No single set of electrocardiographic criteria can identify such variable types of hypertrophy. Since electrocardiography relies on electrical phenomena to make inferences about anatomy, it is not surprising that any ECG changes which might occur, such as an increase in QRS voltage, have only a moderate relationship with LV mass [3]. The two most commonly used techniques for defining LV hypertrophy or mass have been assessment of mass at postmortem and echocardiographic determination *in vivo* of cavity and wall dimensions from which mass can be calculated. Each method

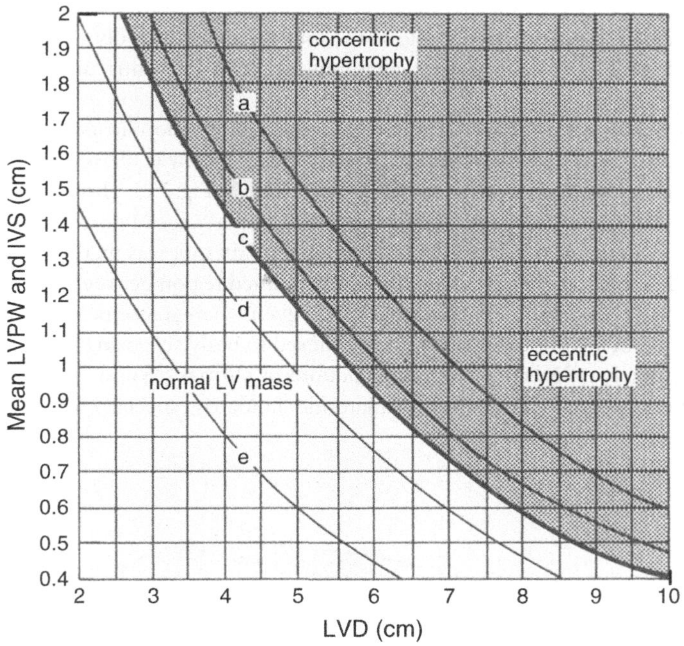

Fig. 3.1
The relationship between concentric and eccentric hypertrophy as illustrated on a nomogram for the determination of LV mass from M-mode echocardiographic (ECHO) measurements. The vertical axis is the mean of LV posterior wall thickness (LVPW) and the interventricular septal thickness (IVS). The horizontal axis is the LV chamber diameter (LVD). The curves represent various LV masses: (a) 400 g, (b) 300 g, (c) 265 g, (d) 200 g, and (e) 100 g. The shaded area above curve c (bold) reflects an abnormally increased ECHO LV mass according to criteria of Woythaler et al. [11]. This value was related by regression analysis to a mass of 225 g at postmortem. At the upper extreme in the shaded area are measurements that suggest concentric LVH, where there is increased thickening of the chamber walls without dilation. Toward the middle and lower portions of the shaded area, there is dilation of the LV chamber in proportion to the thickening of the ventricular walls. These echocardiographic measurements were obtained using the recommendations of the American Society of Echocardiographers rather than the Penn convention (After Woythaler et al. [11]. © American College of Cardiology, Bethesda, MD. Reproduced with permission)

is discussed in turn in view of its relevance to the establishment of ECG criteria for hypertrophy. Although magnetic resonance imaging (MRI) of the heart has also been utilized for this determination of LV mass and hypertrophy [4], it has not as yet played a significant role in the development and/or validation of ECG criteria for LVH.

3.1.1 Anatomic Standards for Hypertrophy

The chamber-partitioning technique of assessing cardiac ventricular weights, which was first introduced in 1888 and reviewed by Bove et al. [5], has been of limited use. Nevertheless, a number of important criteria have been developed and assessed using this approach, which will be outlined briefly.

At postmortem, the heart is first of all stripped of any surface fatty deposits and the atria are then removed. Next, the valve rings and leaflets are dissected out. The remaining ventricular mass is then sectioned serially in a transverse direction with each slice having the appearance shown in ➍ Fig. 3.2. The free right ventricular (RV) wall is dissected away from the septum and the LV wall, as indicated by the dashed line in ➍ Fig. 3.2; in this way, the RV muscle can be weighed separately. The septum is somewhat arbitrarily dissected from the remaining muscle by taking a line at right angles to the septum at its junction with the RV free wall (at both sides). In this way, the septal mass and the LV free wall mass can also be determined separately. This allows the total LV mass to be obtained and various ratios of component masses to be assessed. ➍ Table 3.1 summarizes anatomical criteria for ventricular hypertrophy derived from this technique.

From their study of 100 hearts, Bove et al. recommended several modifications in attempting to classify mild degrees of cardiac hypertrophy not readily recognized at autopsy. Subsequently, Murphy et al. [6, 7] suggested slightly different definitions of right and left ventricular hypertrophy (see ➍ Table 3.1 and ➍ Fig. 3.2). The upper limit of normal was defined by a mean plus two standard deviations or as exceeding the 98 percentile range of normal. Unfortunately, adequate numbers of hearts from normal women were not available. Although an attempt was made to base anatomic criteria on the height of the patient (see ➍ Table 3.1), there remained a poorly defined region between normal and definitely abnormal, leading to descriptions such as "possible LVH" or "mild LVH" even when anatomical details were known. Subsequent study of this area has resulted in anatomic LV mass being indexed to body size using body surface area or height to the 2.7 power, which more accurately reflects the allometric relations of LV mass to body size and obesity [8]. In view of the above, the reader should be aware of the limitations of anatomic standards especially when the specificity and sensitivity of ECG criteria are reported.

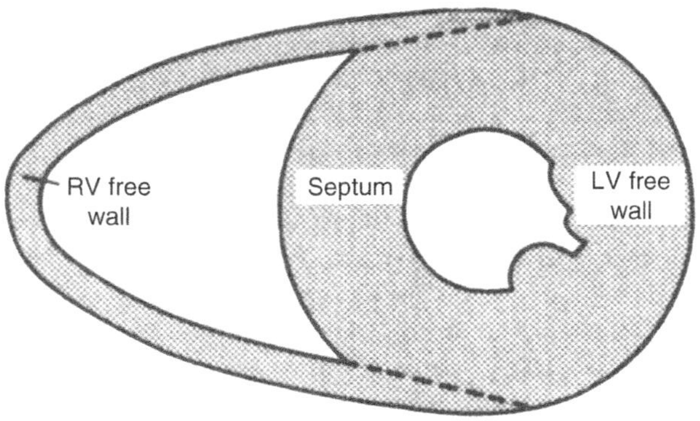

Fig. 3.2
A cross section of the heart showing the method of dissecting the RV free wall from the left ventricle and septum. The septum can be somewhat arbitrarily separated from the LV mass by dissecting it at right angles to the septal surface at its junction with the RV free wall (After Bove et al. [5]. © American Heart Association, Dallas, TX. Reproduced with permission)

Table 3.1

Anatomical cardiac hypertrophy at autopsy[a]

Classification	Bove [4]	Murphy [5]
Normal	Subject < 1.78 m tall	LV + S < 171 g
	LV + S < 176 g	RV < 62 g
	RV < 65 g	
	(LV + S)/RV ratio 2.1–3.6	
	Subject > 1.78 m tall	
	LV < 200 g	
	RV < 75 g	
Left ventricular hypertrophy	LV + S > 200 g	LV + S > 171 g
	RV < 75 g	
	LV/RV ratio > 3.6	Normal RV
Possible LVH or LV preponderance in small hearts	(LV + S)/RV ratio > 3.6	(LV + S)/RV ratio > 3.9
	Weights normal	Weights normal
Right ventricular hyper trophy	RV > 75 g	RV > 62 g
	LV/RV ratio < 2.1	Normal LV
Possible RVH or RV preponderance in small hearts	LV/RV ratio < 2.1	LV/RV ratio < 2.3
	Weights normal	Weights normal
Biventricular hyperrophy	LV + S > 220 g	LV + S > 171 g
	RV > 75 g	RV > 62 g
Mild BVH	LV + S = 175–220 g	
	RV > 60 g	
	Biatrial hypertrophy	

[a] LV, weight of left ventricle; RV, weight of right ventricle; S, weight of septum; all as defined in Fig. 3.2

3.1.2 Echocardiographic Standards for Hypertrophy

Echocardiography (ECHO) is now regarded as the most accurate noninvasive method for estimating LV mass or LVH, correlating well with autopsy measurements, but the aforementioned difficulty of defining standards is now becoming apparent. Two-dimensional echocardiography may be the preferred technique [9, 10], especially in patients with abnormal LV geometry or segmental disease. However, technically adequate M-mode echocardiograms are more easily recorded and may remain the standard for some time. Indeed, Woythaler et al. [11], in a study of 50 hearts examined at post-mortem where both M-mode and two-dimensional echocardiograms had been recorded within 6 months of death, found a much higher correlation between M-mode estimates of LV mass and those at autopsy than between two-dimensional and autopsy values.

There are several different equations used for the estimation of LV mass given either the M-mode echocardiogram or the two-dimensional sector scan. One approach that utilizes the M-mode echocardiogram is to obtain the short-axis internal diameter D of the left ventricle and to assume that the ventricle is a prolate ellipsoid [12] where the major axis is twice the length of each minor axis. It then follows that the semiminor axes each have the same length $D/2$, i.e. half that of the semimajor axis. The volume V is then

$$V = (4/3)\pi\,(D/2)(D/2)D = (\pi/3)/D^3 = 1.047D^3 \sim D^3$$

If the epicardial and endocardial echoes are obtained from the M-mode display, it is possible to calculate a left ventricular mass (LVM) where

$$\mathrm{LVM} = (D_{\mathrm{O}}^3 - D_{\mathrm{I}}^3) \times \text{muscle density}$$

where D_O is the diameter of the outer ventricular shell and D is the internal ventricular diameter. Density is usually given a value of 1.05 g cm^{-3}.

Using a modification of this approach, Devereux and Reichek [13] have validated the method with an anatomic comparison. They found that the optimum equation for LVM was

$$\text{LVM} = 1.04\{(\text{LVID} + \text{PWT} + \text{IVST})^3 - \text{LVID}^3\} - 13.6\,\text{g}$$

where LVID is the LV internal diameter, PWT is the posterior wall thickness, and IVST is the interventricular septal wall thickness. In these measurements, the thickness of the endocardial echo lines was excluded from wall thickness estimates, but the LVID estimate included the thickness of left septal and posterior wall echo lines (the so-called Penn convention). Where a two-dimensional sector scan is available, then a more complex equation can be utilized as follows:

$$\text{LVM} = \left(\frac{4}{3}\right)\pi\left\{\frac{A+2T}{2} \times \frac{B+2T}{2} \times \frac{B+2T}{2} - \frac{A}{2} \times \frac{B}{2} \times \frac{B}{2}\right\} \times \text{density}$$

where T is the thickness of the LV free wall, and A and B are the lengths of the major and minor axes, respectively. Frequently, however, this is simplified to

$$\text{LVM} = (\text{epicardial enclosed volume} - \text{endocardial enclosed volume}) \times 1.05$$

with the result being indexed to body-surface area.

It should be noted that when assessing ECG-echo studies of cardiac hypertrophy, there is some interobserver variation [14] in measuring the echocardiogram, although this has been minimized with the use of two-dimensional methods.

There is little doubt that the estimation of LV mass is a more sensitive indicator of LVH than is the thickness of the posterior wall or septum. Irrespective of body size, an M-mode mass of 215 g [3] or 265 g (LV + septum) [11] has been used to define LVH.

Several investigators have demonstrated that sex differences for increased LV mass (or LVH) are diminished but not eliminated when LV mass is indexed by body-surface area [9, 15, 16]. It has been further suggested that lean body mass be used to eliminate the sex differences [15]. Devereux et al. have defined the indexed M-mode LV mass for LVH as greater than 134 g/m^2 in men and greater than 110 g/m^2 in women or a single limit of 120 g/m^2 [15], and, subsequently, as LVM > 116 g/m^2 in men and 104 g/m^2 in women, based on the ability of these criteria to predict adverse prognosis [17]. Before accepting the sensitivity and specificity of any suggested ECG criteria, the reader should always check the standard used to define an increased ventricular mass. A single cutoff value may underdiagnose LVH in women and overdiagnose it in large athletic men, particularly when unindexed LV mass is being used to define LVH.

The accuracy of the M-mode echocardiogram in assessing RV mass [18] is questionable. Prakash and Matsukubo [19] used RV wall thickness measurements to diagnose RVH. Diastolic thickness had a sensitivity of 90% and a specificity of 94%, while systolic thickness, with a specificity of 100%, had a sensitivity of only 34%. Baker et al. [18] found that an RV internal dimension in diastole greater than 26 mm identified only 36% of those with anatomic RVH, while an RV wall thickness greater than 5 mm correctly identified 67%. They concluded that neither M-mode measurement is accurate enough to use as a standard for increased RV mass. Since anatomic RV wall thickness and anatomic RV mass have a correlation coefficient r of only 0.29, other measurements are required.

In an enlarged right ventricle, the increase in size is more extensive in the direction of the short axis than in the direction of the long axis [20]. Calculation of the RV volume should, therefore, prove a more useful measurement of enlargement than wall thickness alone, there being a good correlation of angiographic and echocardiographic RV volumes: $r = 0.94$ at end diastole and $r = 0.84$ at end systole [20]. Perhaps RV volume derived using a sector scan will prove a better tool for assessing RV mass [21].

While ventricular enlargement includes both dilatation and hypertrophy, the calculation of total mass and surface area are more objective and verifiable than is cavity size or wall thickness [22]. More accurate methods are necessary.

3.2 Factors Affecting ECG Criteria for Ventricular Hypertrophy

Many factors may be related to the presence of high or increased voltage, e.g., sex, obesity, hypertrophy, enlargement, and sympathetic drive and associated disease such as obstructive coronary atherosclerosis.

3.2.1 Age and Sex

Age is one of the principal factors that affect the criteria for LVH. Since ECG voltages decrease with increasing age (see ➋ Chap. 1), the limits of normal voltage should be stratified by age. Although other factors such as body-surface area can be considered, the height and weight of a patient may not be readily available to a cardiologist reporting ECGs. In addition, detailed statistical analysis of over 1,330 normal individuals in the Glasgow database has indicated that age is the most significant factor in explaining voltage variation both in males and females (➋ Chap. 1). The simplest, yet theoretically sound, approach therefore is to utilize age. Likewise, since there are considerable differences between male and female in the limits of normality of ECG measurements, particularly in young adults, criteria should also be sex dependent. This point is discussed further in the Romhilt and Estes scoring technique (➋ Sect. 3.3.1.4) and in the section on Cornell voltage and voltage-duration product (➋ Sect. 3.3.1.6).

3.2.2 Hypertrophy and Dilatation

Antman et al. [23] used LV wall thickness h plotted against the semi-minor radius of the left ventricle R to produce a product hR. A value of this product in excess of 2.6 cm^2 identified all those with LVH by ECG. These authors found that LVH resulting from an enlarged chamber (aortic regurgitation) plays a greater role in augmenting potentials than does a thickened myocardium (aortic stenosis) [23]. In contrast, Devereux et al. concluded that for a given LV mass, ECG voltage criteria of LVH are independent of LV chamber dilatation or other geometric variables. Instead they depend on age, weight, and LV depth in the chest. They suggested that stratification of subjects by these clinical variables might improve the electrocardiographic recognition of LVH [24].

3.2.3 Distance of Heart from Electrodes

Horton et al. [25] found that precordial voltage was strongly influenced by the distance of the left ventricle from the electrodes. They attempted to correct for this by the multiplication of precordial voltage by the square of the distance from the chest wall to the mid-left ventricle. This improved the correlation coefficient of $SV_1 + RV_5$ with LV mass from 0.686 to 0.846.

During an echocardiographic study of ten normal subjects before and after exercise, Feldman et al. [26] noted that there is a direct relationship between R-wave voltage in the left chest leads and LV size. This is true, whether it is measured as LV volume or LV internal dimension. Both LV size and the distance of the heart from V_5 or V_6 seem to interact as determinants of R-wave voltage.

3.2.4 Associated Diseases

The presence of obstructive coronary artery disease may be linked with the development of LVH. Pech et al. [27] showed an increase in LV mass in patients with coronary artery disease compared to those without coronary artery disease. Some muscle fibers became fibrosed with loss of contractility, leading to hypertrophy of the remaining muscle fibers.

3.2.5 Miscellaneous Factors

Other factors influencing voltage in the ECG include the conducting properties of intervening structures and delayed activation in portions of the myocardium. High voltages may commonly occur in young people under the age of 30 (see ➲ Chap. 1), thin elderly women, and emaciated individuals [28]. The influence of race should also be acknowledged. Black individuals have a higher precordial voltage on the ECG than white individuals, while the latter have a higher voltage in the ECG than oriental individuals (see ➲ Chap. 1). The higher precordial voltages in blacks can lead to the overestimation of LVH prevalence due to lower specificity of these criteria [29]. However, amplitudes and performance of Cornell voltage and Cornell product criteria appear to be relatively independent of race [29]. The modest increase in LV mass seen in athletes also produces a high voltage but, unlike pathologic hypertrophy, is not accompanied by slowed LV diastolic filling [30]. Finally, increasing body mass index is strongly and inversely associated with precordial voltage amplitude, leading to higher specificity and lower sensitivity of precordial voltage criteria in overweight and obese individuals [31], with subsequent underestimation of the prevalence of anatomic LVH in the presence of obesity [32]. In contrast, sensitivity and specificity of Cornell voltage and product criteria vary less with body mass index [31] and provide a more accurate measure of the prevalence and severity of LVH in obese and overweight patients [32]. The authors would contend that criteria should take these factors into account in order to minimize false-positive and false-negative ECG interpretations.

3.2.6 Theoretical Considerations

Elsewhere in this book (e.g., ➲ Chaps. 1 and ➲ 5 of *Basic Electrocardiology: Cardiac Electrophysiology, ECG Systems and Mathematical Modeling*), some theoretical considerations on the effect of thoracic inhomogeneities on the electrocardiogram are discussed. It would seem relevant at this point to provide a nonmathematical description of some of these effects and their relationship to the presence or absence of ECG changes in patients with increased LV end diastolic volume or with increased LV wall thickness.

In ➲ Chap. 2 of *Basic Electrocardiology: Cardiac Electrophysiology, ECG Systems and Mathematical Modeling*, the so-called Brody effect is discussed [33]. Essentially, this principle suggests that when there is an increase in blood volume in either ventricle, surface potentials owing to a radial spread of excitation in that ventricle are enlarged and those arising from a more tangential or lateral spread of excitation through the wall muscle are attenuated. This would imply that in patients with aortic regurgitation, for example, there should be an increased voltage in the precordial leads on account of the increased blood volume, even though there may be no increase in muscle thickness. Some quite dramatic changes in voltage can be seen in patients with aortic regurgitation before and after valve replacement (➲ Fig. 3.3), on account of the reduction in blood volume. There have been some apparently contradictory results obtained when low voltages have been found in patients with congestive heart failure [34]. This apparent paradox can be explained on the basis of there being an increase in the conductivity of the lungs owing to the presence of pulmonary edema secondary to heart failure, which then results in an attenuation of surface potentials. Nonetheless, clinical findings with respect to the Brody effect remain conflicting.

Another consideration in the case of a dilated heart is the effect of variation in the generator properties of the muscle. It could be argued that by stretching the myocardium, the electrical sources are more widely available and, therefore, increased. In such a case, Rudy [35] has shown that the voltage increase (82%) is more than double that (35%) in an equally dilated heart where the generator strength remains the same as before dilation.

Other factors that affect the surface voltages have also been discussed fully by Rudy [35] in a theoretical review of the topic. These include the lungs, which tend to reduce the surface voltage as emphasized in patients with chronic obstructive airways disease. The pericardium can also affect surface voltages on account of an increased compression of the heart by an excessive amount of pericardial fluid. The surface muscle layer also contributes to an attenuation of the body-surface potentials on account of a high conductivity so that in any conditions where there is a low muscle conductivity, e.g., Pompe's disease, voltages would be increased.

The final and perhaps most interesting situation is to consider the theoretical effects of increased muscle thickness with a normal ventricular cavity size in comparison to a reduced cavity size. Where the cavity size is normal, but there is an increase in muscle thickness, it can be shown, theoretically, that the surface voltage is increased by 13.6% [35]. The voltage increase, however, is often much greater than this, suggesting that other factors play an important part. On the

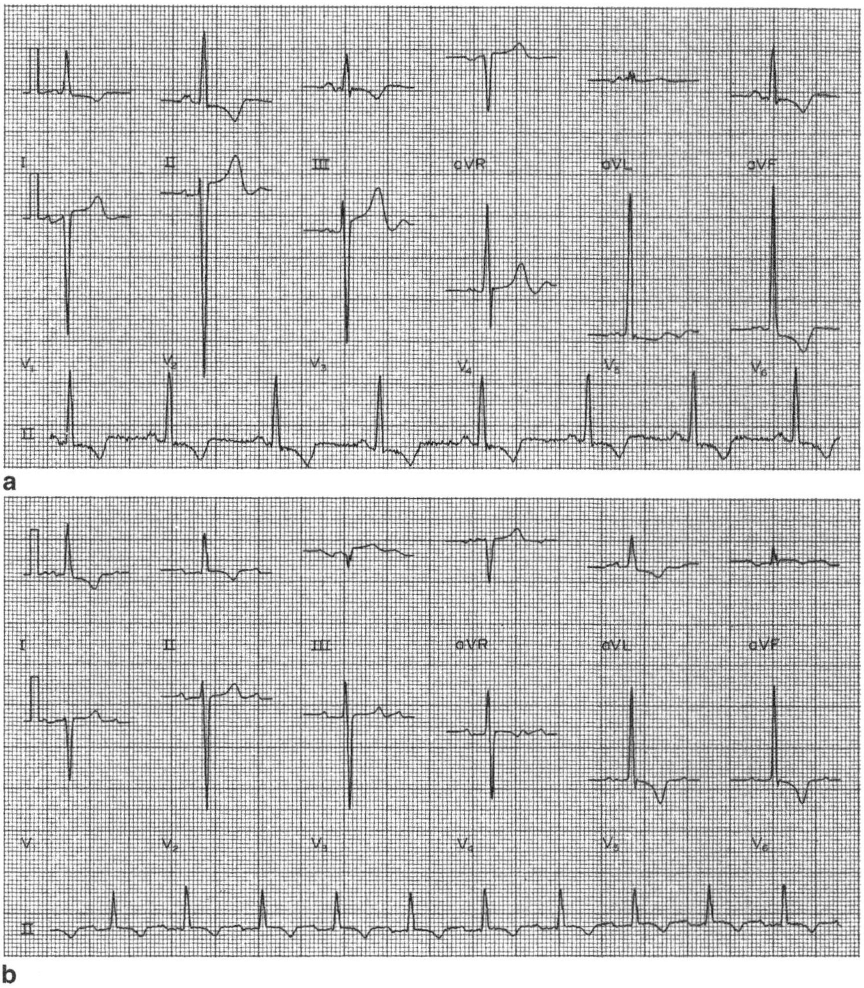

Fig. 3.3
Part (a) shows the ECG from a 49-year-old female with aortic stenosis and incompetence. Part (b) shows the ECG taken 11 days later and following aortic valve replacement. Note the dramatic reduction in the voltage; for example, $SV_2 + RV_6$ has decreased from 7.9 to 5.0 mV. The voltage reduction was most likely related to a reduction in LV volume

other hand, an increased muscle thickness with a reduced cavity size is theoretically associated with a decrease of the same order of magnitude in surface potentials compared to normal. This could explain the not uncommon situation of a grossly thickened heart, such as is found in cardiomyopathy with normal ECG voltages.

3.3 Left Ventricular Hypertrophy (LVH)

3.3.1 ECG Criteria

There are many different criteria for LVH, most of which are presented in ➋ Table 3.2 along with sensitivity and specificity from different studies [36–38]. Some of these criteria are discussed in detail.

Table 3.2
Sensitivity and specificity of commonly used criteria for left ventricular hypertrophy

Criteria/parameters	98% upper limits[a] (mV)	Autopsy study[b]		ECHO-LBBB[c]	
		Sensitivity (%)	Specificity (%)	Sensitivity (%)	Specificity (%)
Limb leads					
RI > 1.3 mV	1.3	11	100	7	94
RI + SIII > 2.5 mV	1.9	11	100	12	100
RaVL > 0.7 mV	0.8	23	96		
RaVL > 1.1	0.8	11	100	24	97
RaVL > 1.3	0.8	8	100	8	100
SaVR > 1.4	1.2	7	100	0	100
RaVF > 1.9	1.4	1.3	99	0	100
Lewis index ⩾ 1.7[d]		18	98	37	78
Left-axis deviation of −30° or more		25	87	32	78
Left-axis deviation of −40° or more				26	94
Chest leads					
$SV_1 \geqslant 3.0$ mV				26	91
$SV_1 \geqslant 2.4$	1.6	19	100	47	56
$SV_2 \geqslant 3.0$ and $SV_3 \geqslant 2.5$				49	90
$SV_3 \geqslant 2.5$				57	88
RV_5 or $RV_6 > 2.6$	2.0	25	98	3	100
$RV_6 > 2.0$	1.5	22	88		
$RV_6 > RV_5$		23	89	74	9
VAT V_5 or V_6 = 0.05+ seconds [4]		29	99		
SV_1 or SV_2 + RV_5 or $RV_6 > 3.5$	3.8	56	88	81	41
$SV_1 + RV_5$ or $RV_6 > 3.5$	3.3	43	95	50	72
$SV_1 + RV_5 > 3.3$ females		40	93	45	67
$SV_1 + RV_5 > 3.6$ males	3.3	40	93	56	73
$SV_2 + RV_5$ or $RV_6 > 4.5$	4.4	35	97	44	84
R + S > 4.5 (largest R + largest S)		45	93	54	81
Point score system[e]		54	97	35	84

[a] After Murphy et al. [6]
[b] After Romhilt et al. [36] (160 patients with LVH and 200 without LVH were studied)
[c] After Kafka et al. [9, 38] (68 patients with LVH and 32 without LVH were studied). Revised using an indexed LV mass for males ⩾ 132 g cm^{-2} and females ⩾ 110 g cm^{-2}
[d] Lewis index = (RI-RIII) + (SIII − SI)
[e] Romhilt and Estes [43]

3.3.1.1 Lewis Index

The index introduced by Lewis [39] in 1914 is still favored by a number of cardiologists in continental Europe. This index is defined as

$$(\mathrm{RI} + \mathrm{SIII}) - (\mathrm{RIII} + \mathrm{SI})$$

A value of 1.7 mV was suggested as a borderline criterion producing a very high specificity of 98% but a low sensitivity of 18%, as shown in ➋ Table 3.2. An illustration of a high Lewis index is presented in ➋ Fig. 3.4, where it can be seen that precordial voltages may well be normal.

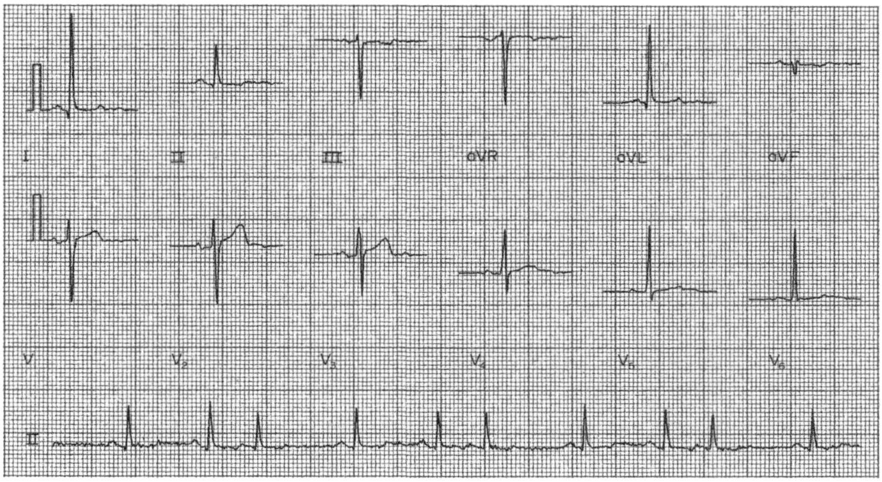

Fig. 3.4
ECG showing voltage evidence of LVH in the limb leads, recorded from a 62-year-old male undergoing surgery for aortic valve replacement. The Lewis index is approximately 3.2 mV, which is well above the upper limit of normal, while it can be seen that the precordial voltages are within normal limits

3.3.1.2 Sokolow and Lyon Index

The voltage criteria of Sokolow and Lyon [40] introduced in 1949 are still used extensively by many cardiologists. These are

(a) $SV_1 + (RV_5 \text{ or } RV_6) \geqslant 3.5$ mV
(b) RV_5 or $RV_6 \geqslant 2.6$ mV
(c) R in aVL $\geqslant 1.1$ mV
(d) R in aVF $\geqslant 2$ mV

Perhaps the most widely used criterion for LVH is $SV_1 + RV_5/V_6 \geqslant 3.5$ mV, sometimes known as the Sokolow–Lyon index, although it was present in only 33% of their 147 patients (➔ Fig. 3.5). Less well known are their ST-T criteria, namely, a depressed ST segment and asymmetric T-wave inversion. In 92% of their cases, ST-T abnormalities were present. Certainly, criterion (a) is too nonspecific for young adults, and the limits should be different for males and females, as demonstrated by Macfarlane and Lawrie (➔ Chap. 1) from their study of 1,330 healthy volunteers (see ➔ Fig. 3.6). In addition, Sokolow–Lyon voltages are significantly greater in blacks than in Caucasians [29], leading to lower specificity and higher sensitivity in blacks if these criteria are not adjusted for race as well as sex [29]. As ➔ Table 3.2 shows, the sensitivity of (a) at 43% and (b) at 22% was less than that of the point score at 54%. The remaining criteria (c) and (d) were highly specific but very insensitive (11% and 1.3%, respectively).

3.3.1.3 McPhie Criterion

McPhie, in 1958, suggested that the tallest R-wave amplitude be added to the deepest S-wave amplitude in any precordial lead [41]. If this total exceeded 4.5 mV, then LVH was present. While this criterion was of little additional value, it did

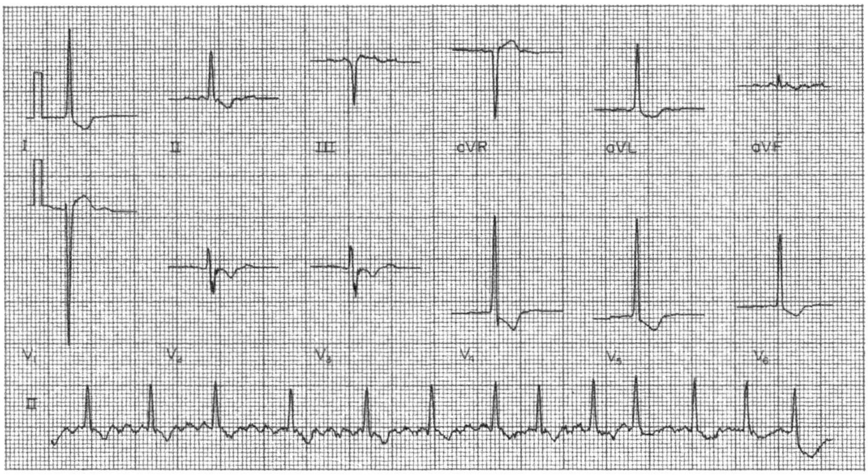

Fig. 3.5
ECG of a 75-year-old lady undergoing aortic valve replacement. The Sokolow and Lyon index is approximately 5.6 mV, which is well beyond the upper limit of normal. Limb-lead measurements are also abnormally high, with the R in aVL exceeding 1.1 mV

recognize that deep S waves in leads V_2 and V_3 may contribute significantly to a diagnosis of LVH. This preoccupation with voltage criteria caused Simonson [42] in 1961 to modify the borderline limit of $SV_1 + RV_5$ slightly to $\geqslant$ 3.3 mV for females and $\geqslant$ 3.6 mV for males. As can be seen from Table 3.2, there was little change in the sensitivity or specificity. Many precordial-lead voltage criteria have subsequently been recommended, with variable results.

3.3.1.4 Romhilt–Estes Point Score System

In 1968, Romhilt and Estes [43] introduced a point-scoring system for the ECG diagnoses of LVH. Although this approach is cumbersome with respect to conventional ECG interpretation, it has been found useful by a number of authors of computer programs for ECG analysis. The scoring system is detailed in Table 3.3. Essentially it gives a high score for an abnormal amplitude of QRS components in either the limb leads or the precordial leads. A single value of 2 mV is used for the limb leads and 3 mV for the precordial leads. A similar high score is obtained for the appearance of the so-called LV strain pattern (Fig. 3.7) although the number of points is reduced if the patient is taking a digitalis preparation. The other items included are left-axis deviation, an increased QRS duration, and a delayed intrinsicoid deflection in V_5 or V_6. An abnormal P terminal force (PTF) in V_1 (see Fig. 3.23) also contributes significantly to the score. The authors obtained a modest sensitivity of about 60% with a high specificity in excess of 95%.

Murphy et al. [7, 44] have modified the point score slightly and also assessed various combinations. The result was a sensitivity value that varied from 57% to 66% and a specificity that ranged from 85% to 93% depending on the cause of the hypertrophy. Their standard for LVH in their 91 subjects was an LV mass greater than 171 g or, if chamber weights were normal, then LV/RV ratio greater than 3.9.

Table 3.4 shows the age-dependent and sex-dependent upper limits of normal for some measurements of the QRS complex that are used by the Glasgow program for computer interpretation of the ECG as part of a modified Romhilt–Estes scoring system. The values in Table 3.4 replace the single precordial-voltage limit of Romhilt and Estes when assessing the number of points to be awarded for high voltage in the precordial leads. Similar considerations apply in the limb leads. In general, sensitivity should be increased in older subjects by the use of lower upper

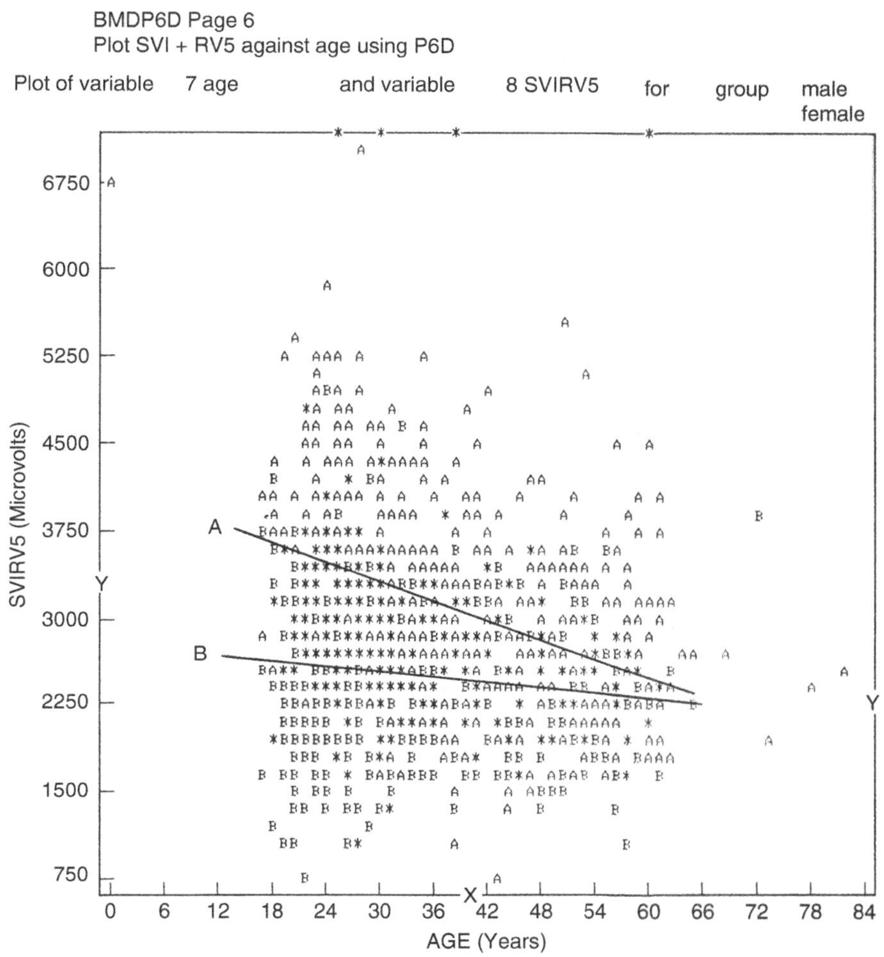

N = 1124
COR = −0.179

	Mean	ST. DEV.	Regression	line	RES. MS.
X	34.811	12.122	X = −0.00257	Y + 42.103	142.37
Y	2837.2	842.46	Y = −12.414	X + 3269.4	687704

Fig. 3.6

Scattergram of $SV_1 + RV_5$ from a subgroup of 1,124 apparently healthy individuals in the Glasgow study (see Chap. 1): A, male; B, female; *, more than one individual. The *y* axis is marked in microvolts. Note the high percentage of individuals who have a Sokolow and Lyon index well in excess of the conventional criterion of 3.5 mV. The regression of voltage with age is also shown where it can be seen that sex differences are most marked at younger age levels

limits of normal, each of which is chosen to be highly specific. Specificity is increased in younger persons by the use of higher limits of normal. Furthermore, the Glasgow scoring system allows an additional point to be scored for each additional 0.5 mV of voltage in excess of the stated values for precordial leads and for each additional 0.3 mV in the limb leads. Note, therefore, that borderline high voltage alone does not constitute ECG evidence of LVH in this system.

Table 3.3
Romhilt–Estes point score system for ECG diagnosis of left ventricular hypertrophy [43][a]

Criteria	Points
Any limb-lead R or S $\geqslant$ 2.0 mV	3
or SV_1 or SV_2 $\geqslant$ 3.0 mV	
or RV_5 or RV_6 $\geqslant$ 3.0 mV	
ST-T is typical of LVH[b]	
No digitalis	3
With digitalis	1
Left atrial involvement[c]	3
P terminal force V_1 > 4 mV ms	
LAD $\geqslant$ −30°	2
QRS duration $\geqslant$ 90 ms	1
Intrinsicoid deflection V_5 or V_6 $\geqslant$ 50 ms	1

[a] 5 points indicate definite LVH, 58% of LVH with 2% false positives. 4 points indicate probable LVH, 62% of LVH with 2% false positives
[b] See Fig 3.7
[c] See Fig 3.24

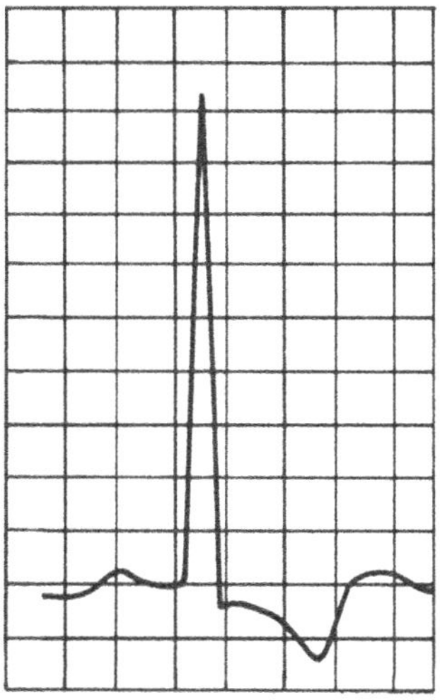

Fig. 3.7
Classic appearances of ST-T changes that are secondary to LVH. These changes are often known as the LV strain pattern that is typified by ST depression and a gently downward sloping ST segment that is convex upward, evolving into an inverted T wave

3.3.1.5 Kansal Criteria

Kansal et al. [45] used a multivariate approach and concluded that the most important ECG variables predictive of LVH are

(a) QRS duration (relative strength F = 27.95)
(b) SV_1 to SV_3 voltage (F = 27.25)
(c) strain in T wave (F = 22.02)
(d) RV_4 to RV_6 voltage (F = 4.03)

Table 3.4

Values used in the Glasgow ECG analysis program as the upper limits of normal voltage for use in the Romhilt–Estes point score system (these values replace those of the first criterion in Table 3.3)

Age (years)	Sex	Lead voltage (mV) RI	RaVL	SV_1/V_2	SV_5/V_6	Lewis index
17–29	Male	1.5	1.1	4.0	4.0	2.5
	Female	1.5	0.9	3.5	2.5	2.0
30–39	Male	1.6	1.2	3.5	3.0	2.5
	Female	1.4	1.0	3.0	2.2	1.8
40–49	Male	1.6	1.3	2.5	2.5	2.0
	Female	1.4	1.2	2.5	2.2	1.8
⩾ 50	Male	1.6	1.3	2.0	2.5	2.0
	Female	1.4	1.2	2.0	2.2	1.8

Table 3.5

Criteria for LVH developed by Casale et al. [46, 49]. Criteria B were published later [49] than criteria A and represent a simplification that makes application easier

Male	Female
Criteria A	
(a) $RaVL + SV_3 > 3.5$ mV or (b) age < 40 years (i) $RaVL + SV_3 > 2.2$ mV (ii) $TV_1 \geqslant 0.0$ mV or (c) age ⩾ 40 years (i) $RaVL + SV_3 > 2.2$ mV (ii) $TV_1 \geqslant 0.2$ mV	(a) $RaVL + SV_3 > 2.5$ mV or (b) age < 40 years (i) $RaVL + SV_3 > 1.2$ mV (ii) $TV_1 \geqslant 0.0$ mV or (c) age ⩾ 40 years (i) $RaVL + SV_3 > 1.2$ mV (ii) $TV_1 \geqslant 0.2$ mV
Criteria B	
$RaVL + SV_3 > 2.8$ mV	$RaVL + SV_3 > 2.0$ mV

They suggest that rescoring these variables in accordance with their correlation with LV mass may improve the ECG sensitivity for LVH.

3.3.1.6 Cornell Multivariate Score and Voltage

Casale et al. have carefully defined LVH using a sex-specific echocardiographic index of LV mass: in men greater than 134 g/m^2 and in women greater than 110 g/m^2 [46]. These values represent approximately the 98th percentile of LV mass index for each sex in two independent normal populations. They demonstrated that the best separation between patients with normal versus increased LV mass at postmortem was obtained using sex-specific LV mass index criteria [47, 48]. The overall accuracy of 83% was better than that for ECHO cross-sectional area (67%) or for indexes of LV wall thickness (39–51%) [48]. They developed new electrocardiographic criteria for the diagnosis of LVH that stratified QRS-voltage and repolarization findings in sex and age subsets (see Table 3.5).

Table 3.6
Multiple logistic regression exponents for detection of left ventricular hypertrophy[a] (After Casale et al. [49])

For patients in normal sinus rhythm
Exponent = 4.558 − 0.092 × ($RaVL + SV_3$) − 0.306 × TV_1 − 0.212 × QRS − 0.278 × $PTFV_1$−0.559 × sex
For patients in atrial fibrillation
Exponent = 5.045 − 0.093 × ($RaVL + SV_3$) − 0.312 × TV_1 − 0.325 × QRS − 0.602 × sex
Partition values of exponent for detection of LVH
In sinus rhythm: LVH < −1.55
In atrial fibrillation: LVH < −1.20

[a]Units of measurement: voltages of RaVL, SV3, and TV1 in millimeters (1 mm = 0.1 Mv); duration in seconds × 100; P terminal force in lead V1 (PTFV1) in millimeter seconds based on area; sex entered as 1.0 for men and 2.0 for women.

They subsequently applied their criteria prospectively to 135 patients at autopsy, achieving a sensitivity of 42% and a specificity of 96%. By means of logistic regression models based on electrocardiographic and demographic variables with independent predictive values for LVH (and separate equations for those in sinus rhythm and atrial fibrillation), they demonstrated a sensitivity of 62% and a specificity of 92% while having an overall test accuracy of 77% [49]. Their new regression criteria (see Table 3.6) are suitable for computer-based analysis of the electrocardiogram. The Cornell voltage criteria (Table 3.5, criteria B) represent a simplification of the multivariate score, with test specificity and sensitivity that are relatively independent of body habitus [31, 32] and race [20].

3.3.1.7 Perugia Score

Schillaci and Verdecchia and their colleagues from Perugia developed an ECG score based on the presence of ECG LVH by Cornell voltage using modified criteria (> 2.4 mV in men), or a Romhilt–Estes point score ⩾ 4, or the presence of the ECG strain pattern [50, 51]. These criteria improved sensitivity of the ECG for the detection of echocardiographic LVH [50] and improved the prognostic value compared with other ECG LVH criteria [51].

3.3.1.8 Voltage-Duration Product and Time-Voltage Area Criteria

Theoretic modeling [52] and observations that the time-voltage integral of the orthogonal-lead vectorcardiographic QRS complex and the time-strength LV dipole derived from the 126-lead multiple dipole ECG can improve ECG correlation with indexed LV mass [53–55], suggest that an ECG representation of the time-voltage integral of ventricular activation should more accurately reflect the presence and severity of LVH than scores that sum QRS voltage and duration. Subsequent study using the orthogonal-lead signal-averaged ECG demonstrated that the time-voltage integral of the horizontal-plane vector complex significantly improved sensitivity of the ECG for detecting echocardiographic LVH [56]. Using sex-specific partitions with 98% specificity, the 81% sensitivity in women and 71% sensitivity in men was significantly greater than the 27–58% sensitivities of sex-specific 12-lead ECG criteria at matched specificity of 98% [56]. Parallel analyses employing time-voltage area criteria derived from the standard 12-lead ECG [57] found the 76% sensitivity of the 12-lead sum of area and 65% sensitivity of Sokolow–Lyon area to be significantly greater than the 46% and 43% sensitivities of the respective simple voltage criteria and than the 54% sensitivity of voltage-duration product criteria (see below) at matched specificity of 98%. Further study and validation of the time-voltage area approach will be required before these criteria can be adapted for use in computerized electrocardiography.

Because time-voltage area criteria are dependent on computerized ECG analyses that are not readily available to all clinicians and have not been well validated, the simple product of QRS duration and voltage, as an approximation of the area under the QRS complex, has been developed and tested [58, 59]. Calculated by simple multiplication of QRS duration in millisecond by the respective ECG voltage criteria, Cornell voltage-duration product criteria in particular have been demonstrated to significantly improve sensitivity for the detection of LVH compared with simple voltage criteria and with the Romhilt–Estes point score [58, 59]. These criteria are gender specific, relatively race insensitive [29], not significantly impacted by increasing body mass index [31, 32], and, as further noted below, can be used to track changes in echocardiographic LV mass [60] and to more accurately assess prognosis [61].

3.3.2 ST-T-Wave Changes

ST-contour changes may be seen in LV leads (I, aVL, V_5, and V_6): the ST segment is depressed, convex upward, and slopes into an inverted T wave (➋ Fig. 3.7). Even in the absence of a significant increase in QRS voltage, such ST-T changes are associated with more marked modifications of echocardiographic parameters. Patients with ST abnormalities arising from LVH (secondary abnormalities – see also ➋ Chap. 5) have a prolonged interval from minimum cavity dimension to mitral valve opening and a reduced rate of early diastolic wall thinning and dimension increase [62]. These ST-T abnormalities, sometimes called LV strain, may be related to impaired early relaxation that is dissociated from cavity dimension, or to the presence of increased mass alone. They are important, however, because their presence worsens the prognosis[51, 63, 64]. Indeed, the strain pattern has been implicated as the strongest standard ECG marker of increased risk when ECG LVH criteria have been utilized for risk stratification [51, 63], and adds significantly to the Cornell product and Sokolow–Lyon voltage for the prediction of cardiovascular mortality and myocardial infarction (MI) in hypertensive patients [64]. They have a sensitivity of 52% and a specificity of 95% according to Devereux and Reichek [65], and are associated with nearly a threefold higher prevalence of echocardiographic LVH in hypertensive patients after controlling for other risk factors for LVH [66]. More recently, continuous computer measurements of ST depression in leads V_5 and V_6 have been shown to be strong independent predictors of increased LV mass and LVH [67].

More prominent larger U waves or even inverted U waves may be found in V_5 and V_6 (see ➋ Chap. 5). When present, other ECG evidence for LVH is usually obvious. LV activation time (the time from QRS onset to R peak) may increase to over 50 ms, but is seen in only a very small percentage of LVH. Finally, LV conduction delay, however, may progress to incomplete left bundle branch block (LBBB) or complete left bundle branch block. In addition, the prolongation of action potential duration and increased inhomogeneity of ventricular repolarization associated with LVH can be manifest as prolongation of the rate-corrected QT interval [68], with increasing QT interval duration seen across quartiles of increasing LV mass and with both concentric and eccentric geometric patterns of LVH [68].

3.3.3 ECG Criteria Summary

Certain 12-lead ECG criteria that may be useful in the diagnosis of LVH in a hospital population where conventional reporting methods are used, may be summarized as follows (where the figures in parentheses under (a) are the upper 98 percentile limits from Murphy et al. [6]).

(a) High voltage as seen in either
  (i) limb-lead voltage (more specific but less sensitive):
    RaVL $\geqslant$ 1.1 mV (0.8 mV) or if axis $< -30°$ then $\geqslant$ 1.3 and SIII $\geqslant$ 1.5 mV,
    RI + SIII > 2.5 mV (1.9 mV),
    RaVF > 1.9 mV (1.4 mV),
    Lewis index $\geqslant$ 1.7 mV; or
  (ii) chest-lead voltage:
    SV_1 + RV_5 or RV_6 > 3.5 mV (3.3 mV) in men and > 3.3 mV in women,
    SV_1 $\geqslant$ 2.5 mV (1.6 mV),
    RV_5 or RV_6 $\geqslant$ 2.5 mV (2.0 mV);
    maximum R + maximum S > 4.5 mV; or
  (iii) combined voltage:
    RaVL + SV_3 > 2.8 mV in men and >2.0 mV in women.

(b) ST contour depressed but convex upward into inverted T waves in LV leads I, aVL, V_5, and V_6 [45].
(c) Left atrial abnormality (LAA, i.e., P terminal force in V1, as defined in Fig. 3.23) is useful but much less specific for LVH.
(d) Left ventricular conduction delay whether incomplete LBBB (usually meets high voltage criteria) or complete LBBB (see Sect. 3.4.4).

The use of multiple criteria to detect LVH is essential when diverse cardiac diseases are considered. A single criterion may have high sensitivity for one disease state only [44]. When more than one criterion is met, the diagnosis becomes more certain ("probable" or "definite") and, in the above criteria, ranges down to "possible" when borderline high voltage in the chest leads is the only abnormality present.

A variety of other miscellaneous criteria for LVH are also included in Table 3.2. While many of them have a low sensitivity, particularly for limb-lead criteria, it should be noted that specificity is high. Therefore, with the use of computer methods, where a number of criteria can be easily checked, different criteria in combination can be very useful.

3.3.4 Orthogonal-Lead and VCG Criteria

As discussed in Chap. 11 of *Basic Electrocardiology: Cardiac Electrophysiology, ECG Systems and Mathematical Modeling*, the orthogonal-lead ECG can be displayed in two ways, namely, a conventional scalar presentation of the *XYZ* leads and the vectorcardiographic presentation of the frontal, sagittal, and transverse planes of the VCG. Diagnostic criteria for LV hypertrophy can be based on a combination of both scalar and vector parameters.

Since there is a certain, though not exact, correspondence between the *XYZ* and the 12-lead ECG, it would be expected that some of the abnormalities found in the 12-lead ECG would similarly occur in the orthogonal-lead ECG. Thus, increased R-wave amplitude in the lateral lead *X* and in the transverse lead *Z* (directed positively to the back) could occur, as might the classical ST-T abnormality pattern in the lateral lead (Fig. 3.7).

The VCG [69, 70] changes are best seen in the transverse-plane QRS loop, which is displaced to the left and posteriorly. It is increased in magnitude, elongated, and inscribed counterclockwise, but occasionally has a figure-of-eight pattern when hypertrophy is severe. The T loop is usually oriented opposite to the QRS, and so is displaced to the right anteriorly (Fig. 3.8). As a result of LVH, there may be a loss of anterior forces, which may simulate an anterior myocardial infarction. The more R*X* exceeds 1.2 mV or R*X* + R*Z* exceeds 2.5 mV, the more likely the diagnosis of LVH [71].

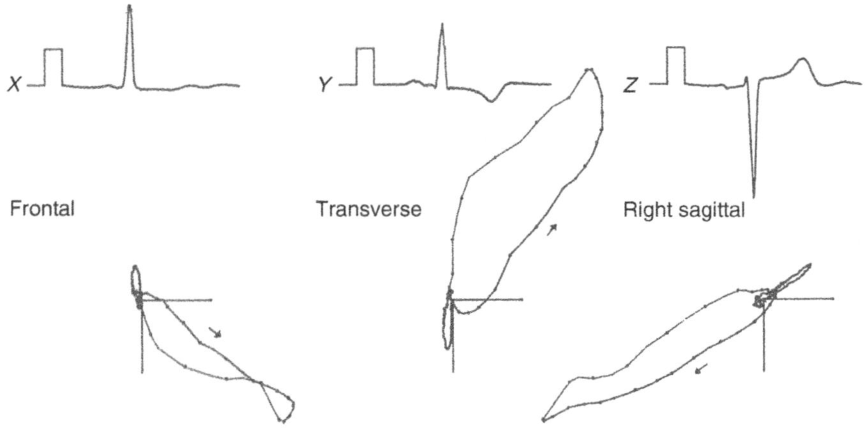

Fig. 3.8
Vectorcardiographic appearances in LVH. Note that the T loop is oppositely directed to the QRS loop, which has the normal direction of inscription in the various planes. The *dots* are printed at 2 ms intervals. Lead *Z* is directed positively anteriorly

Table 3.7
Frank orthogonal-lead criteria for left ventricular hypertrophy [71] (in the absence of ventricular conduction defects)

		White		Black	
		Males	Females	Males	Females
RX amplitude (mV)	A[a]	> 1.9	> 1.4	> 20	> 2.0
	B[b]	> 1.7	> 1.3	> 1.9	> 1.7
RX + *RZ* amplitude (mV)	A	> 2.9	> 2.3	> 3.4	> 2.6
	B	> 2.7	> 2.1	> 3.1	> 2.4
RZ duration (ms)	A	> 70	> 70	> 60	> 70
	B	> 60	> 70	> 60	> 60

[a]Limits in rows labeled A indicate specificity ⩾ 90% associated with relatively low sensitivity
[b]Limits in rows labeled B indicate a specificity of 80–90% associated with higher sensitivity

Several studies have demonstrated that computer analysis of Frank orthogonal leads (see ➋ Chap. 11) improves the detection of LVH [72]. Brohet and Richman [73] found a 26% difference favoring the computer over two physicians (69% versus 43%). Pipberger et al. [74] had earlier demonstrated an even greater advantage, with a difference of 40%. In both of these studies, the greater sensitivity was achieved by means of a Bayesian approach, utilizing prior probabilities and multivariate analysis (see ➋ Chap. 5 of *Basic Electrocardiology*: *Cardiac Electrophysiology, ECG Systems and Mathematical Modeling*).

Using the modified orthogonal-axial-lead system, Macfarlane et al. [75] devised another point score system for diagnosing LVH. Their sensitivity was 65% and their specificity was 91%. Such scoring systems lend themselves to computer applications rather than regular use in the busy heart station.

As can be seen from ➋ Table 3.7, adopted from the Washington code of Pipberger [71] (see ➋ Chap. 1), Frank orthogonal-lead criteria can be relatively simple to use. By combining them with the 12-lead ECG criteria, the diagnosis might be enhanced, as suggested in an earlier study [76]. Others have reported that orthogonal criteria are superior to the 12-lead ECG in detecting LVH [77]. As previously noted in ➋ Sect. 3.3.1.8, the measurement of the time-voltage area of the horizontal-plane vector integral of the signal-averaged VCG can also significantly improve sensitivity of the VCG for detecting LVH [56].

3.4 Miscellaneous LVH Topics

3.4.1 Apical Hypertrophy

When hypertrophic cardiomyopathy is localized to the apex and lower midanterior septum, it can result in a characteristic ECG pattern, namely, giant negative T waves and ST depression in II, III, aVF, and V_4–V_6, as well as negative U waves and a prolonged QT_c. The depth of the negative T wave and ST-segment depression varies from hour to hour or day to day. Coronary angiography is always normal in these patients. This form of hypertrophy is discussed in ➋ Chap. 8 (see ➋ Sect. 8.24.3.2).

3.4.2 Athlete's Heart

As a group, trained athletes will have an increased LV mass with a larger diastolic cavity dimension and/or increased thickness of the posterior wall and septum [78]. Strenuous activity of any kind will produce such physiological hypertrophy appropriate to the body size of the athlete and the degree of activity. For example, the LV wall thickness-to-LV dimension ratio will be increased in weight lifters but remains normal in swimmers. Both will have higher peak rates of LV dimension increase than normals, but when adjusted for larger size, all are within normal limits. In contrast, LV volume or pressure overload with pathologic hypertrophy results in abnormalities of diastolic function or even altered systolic function.

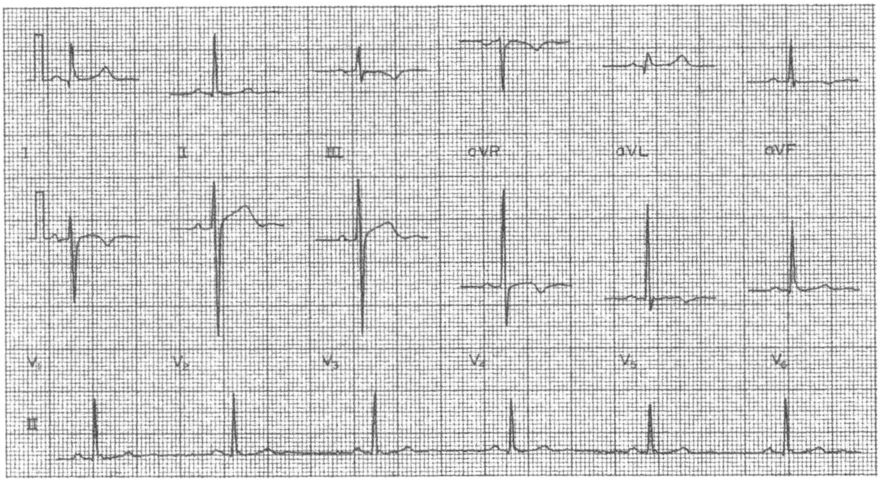

Fig. 3.9
ECG recorded from a 46-year-old runner who was apparently healthy. The LV mass on echocardiography was at the upper end of the normal range. Note the T-wave changes in V_4 and V_5 as well as the interior leads

Highly trained athletes may have ECG criteria for LVH, or have isolated T-wave changes (Fig. 3.9), or other abnormalities [79, 80]. The more extreme changes will cause diagnostic confusion so that exercise electrocardiography and echocardiography may be needed to exclude organic disease. Even left-heart catheterization is justified when doubt still exists. If a positive diagnosis of cardiomyopathy cannot be made and there is no family history of premature sudden death or cardiomyopathy, then such patients should be vigorously reassured that no abnormality is present [81].

3.4.3 Complicating ECG Features

The R waves in V_1 and V_2 may be reduced in amplitude in the presence of LVH with poor R-wave progression, commonly in the right and midprecordial leads. Occasionally, the R is even absent in V_1–V_3 (Fig. 3.10). The resulting QRS complex mimics an anteroseptal infarction. The deeper the S wave in V_1 and V_2, the less likely is anteroseptal infarction and the more likely is LVH.

The absence of septal Q waves in V_5 and V_6 may result from septal fibrosis or incomplete LBBB. On the other hand, Q waves may be produced in the inferior leads in cardiomyopathy.

Some notching of the QRS in midchest leads and an increased QRS duration to 110 ms often accompany increasing degrees of hypertrophy. On the other hand, chronic lung disease, pericardial infusion, or myocardial infarction may all result in reduced R waves masking the voltage criteria for LVH.

3.4.4 Bundle Branch Block and LVH

The diagnosis of LVH is usually considered to be very difficult in the presence of LBBB. However, the occurrence of intermittent LBBB may allow its effects on voltage and axis to be noted, namely, lower voltage in lead I together with a more leftward axis, deeper S waves in V_1 and V_2, and lower R waves in V_5 and V_6 [82]. These changes led Kafka et al. [37, 38] to recommend any one of three criteria for the diagnosis of LVH in the presence of LBBB, namely,

(a) RaVL $>$ 1.1 mV
(b) QRS axis $< -40°$ (RII $<$ SII)
(c) $SV_3 > 2.5$ mV

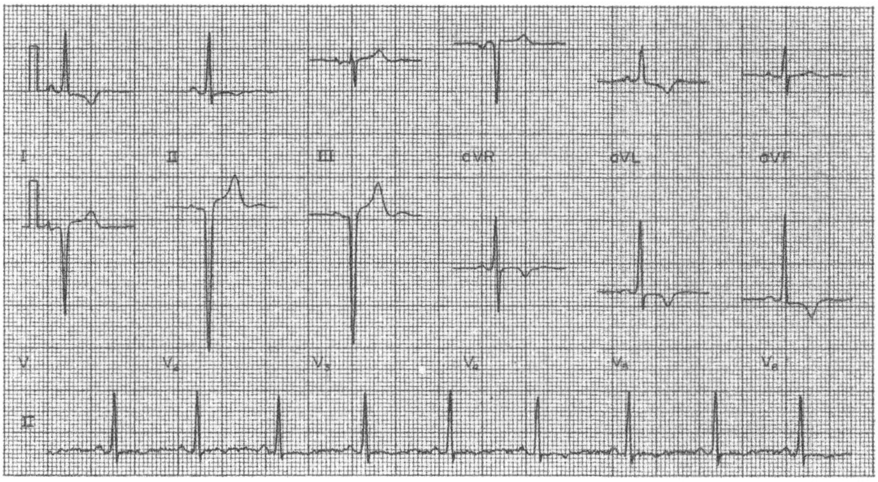

Fig. 3.10
ECG recorded from a 17-year-old girl with a hypertrophic obstructive cardiomyopathy. Note the QS complexes in V_1–V_3 resulting from the severe LVH

From a study of 100 examples of LBBB, Kafka et al. detected 71% with LVH when an indexed LV mass (defined as the M-mode-derived LV mass divided by the body-surface area) exceeded 115g/m^2. Their criteria had a specificity of 90%. Others have also suggested that LVH can be diagnosed in the presence of LBBB [83, 84] (see also Chap. 2).

It should be noted that the incidence of LV enlargement in the presence of LBBB is usually very high. In one series of 1,410 hearts examined at postmortem [85], Havelda et al. found 93% of 70 hearts with ECG LBBB to have LVH. In other words, the diagnosis of LVH in the presence of LBBB can essentially be made by inference alone with a relatively high accuracy.

Since right bundle branch block (RBBB) alters ventricular depolarization markedly, most of the usual criteria for LVH are no longer applicable, but the diagnosis of LVH can still be made (Fig. 3.11). Murphy et al. [86] studied 23 cases of RBBB that at autopsy had LVH by the chamber partition technique (LV mass $\geqslant$ 171 g). They concluded that the use of ECG criteria for left atrial abnormality allows the identification of LVH to rise from 67% to 78% with a false-positive rate of 14–21% depending on the observer.

An echocardiographic study of 47 patients with RBBB revealed 60% with an LV mass greater than 215 g. Vandenberg et al. [87] concluded that limb-lead voltage criteria and the P terminal force in V_1 (see below) are the best detectors of LVH with an "acceptable" specificity of 90%. An R in lead I greater than 1 mV, for example, had a sensitivity of 39% and a specificity of 89%. The specificity might have been higher if they had used the LV mass index as the criterion for LVH.

3.4.5 Regression

Since the introduction of echocardiography (ECHO) for the diagnosis of LVH, measured by LV mass or wall thickness, there have been few properly conducted studies evaluating the correlation between ECG and ECHO markers of LVH. Casale et al. [46] have compared various ECG markers for LVH with M-mode ECHO diagnosis of LVH. The best correlation between ECHO-determined LVH and ECG LVH involved S in V_3 and R in aVL. Hill et al. [88] compared wall thickness to ECG voltages at baseline in an LV regression study in hypertensive patients treated with beta-blockers, but did not find any significant correlation. Wollam et al. [89] assessed the correlation between LV mass and ECG findings in hypertensive patients, treated with a variety of antihypertensive agents, namely, hydrochlorothiazide, methyldopa, and combination therapy. They demonstrated a significant correlation between R-wave amplitude in aVL and LV mass after

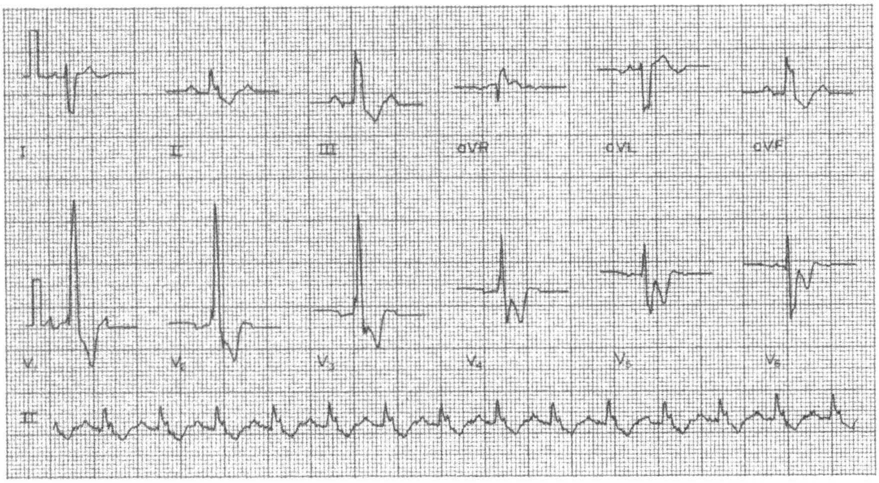

Fig. 3.11

RBBB in a patient with echocardiographic evidence of LVH who underwent aortic valve replacement. The indexed LV mass was 196.9 g/m^2 (using the Penn convention). Note the right-axis deviation (QRS axis = 120°), which might be thought to suggest RVH even in the presence of RBBB. However, there was no evidence of RVH on ECHO, or at operation so that the left posterior fascicular block may be the cause of the right-axis deviation. The ST-T changes in the lateral leads in this case are, most probably, caused by LVH. There is also evidence of left atrial overload in view of the increased P terminal force in V_1 (see Sect. 3.8.1). The QT interval is short because of the heart rate of approximately 120 beats min^{-1} in this patient

6 and 18 months therapy, but no correlation between changes in the Romhilt–Estes score and changes in posterior wall thickness or LV mass index at 6 months. Three other studies [90–92] demonstrated a decrease in LV wall mass as well as precordial QRS voltage, but did not report a correlation between ECHO and ECG. More recently, Okin et al. [60] demonstrated that regression of Cornell product LVH after 1 year of antihypertensive therapy was strongly associated with decreases in LV mass and identified patients who had a greater likelihood of regression of echocardiographic LVH, independent of treatment modality and of changes in systolic and diastolic blood pressure.

These findings might suggest that LV wall mass changes may be reflected in changes in the R-wave amplitude in aVL. Whether computer assessment of the ECG for determining LV mass may yield more information remains to be seen. To this end, Savage et al. and Rautaharju et al. [93, 94] have studied the correlation between ECHO estimates of LV mass and those derived from an ECG model [95].

In valvular disease, Carroll et al. measured the changes in voltage (SV_1 and RV_5–RV_6) after aortic valve replacement and compared these changes to those in LV mass, diagnosed by ECHO [96]. They concluded that after surgical correction of chronic aortic regurgitation, regression of LVH can be assessed by serial ECG data (see Fig. 3.3), which can identify patients with complete, incomplete, or no regression of LVH.

3.4.6 Prognosis of ECG LVH

From a clinical point of view, ECG evidence of LVH with ST-T changes (ECG LVH) indicates a prognosis as serious as ECG evidence of myocardial infarction (ECG MI), at least in asymptomatic persons [97]. In the Framingham study, 1.5% of the original cohort had definite ECG LVH and 45% of all cardiovascular deaths were preceded by its appearance [98].

The 5-year mortality for men with ECG LVH was 35% compared with 15% without ECG LVH. Possible ECG LVH also carried an increased but lower risk of death. Even cardiovascular morbidity, that is, stroke, heart failure, coronary disease, and peripheral vascular disease is increased severalfold in subjects with ECG LVH, while ventricular dysrhythmias are more frequent [99–101].

The diagnosis of ECG LVH with repolarization abnormalities doubles the cardiovascular risk compared to voltage evidence only of LVH [99]. In the British Regional Heart study, it was found that middle-aged men with LVH and secondary repolarization changes had over five times the risk of suffering a fatal or nonfatal myocardial infarction in a 5-year follow-up period compared to men with a normal ECG [102]. Among hypertensive men and women in the LIFE Study [64], the presence of the typical strain pattern was associated with a 1.5-fold greater risk of myocardial infarction or cardiovascular death over a 5-year follow-up period, even after adjusting for baseline severity of ECG LVH and for the substantial decreases in blood pressure during treatment.

More recent data suggest that regression of ECG LVH and prevention of progression of ECG LVH are associated with reduced cardiovascular risk [61, 103, 104]. In an observational study of 524 participants in the Framingham Heart Study with ECG LVH by various criteria at a qualifying exam [103], Levy et al. found that a significant decline in Cornell voltage was associated with a lower risk of cardiovascular disease, whereas a significant increase in Cornell voltage identified individuals at increased risk. In the Heart Outcomes Prevention Evaluation (HOPE) trial [104], the combined endpoint of either regression of ECG LVH or prevention of progression to ECG LVH by Sokolow–Lyon voltage criteria in response to ramipril-based therapy was associated with reduced risk of death, myocardial infarction, stroke, and congestive heart failure. Finally, serial ECG evaluation in the LIFE study [61] found that lower in-treatment measurements of both Cornell voltage-duration product and Sokolow–Lyon voltage were associated with significant reductions in the incidence of major cardiovascular morbidity and mortality, independent of treatment-modality-employed baseline Framingham risk score and of both baseline and in-treatment levels of blood pressure. Taken together, these findings suggest that antihypertensive therapy targeted at regression or prevention of ECG LVH may become an additional goal of therapy beyond that of lowering blood pressure, in order to further decrease the risk of cardiovascular morbidity and mortality [61, 105].

3.4.7 Prevalence

The prevalence of LVH in various population studies has been estimated from the ECG (see ➋ Chap. 8 of *Specialized Aspects of ECG*). On the other hand, as this chapter has pointed out, the sensitivity of ECG criteria is at best around 65% so that there will be considerable underestimation of the true prevalence of LVH using the ECG. Data from the Framingham study have suggested that the prevalence of electrocardiographic LVH increases as the severity of ECHO LV mass index increases [106]. The actual prevalence of LVH as determined by ECHO ranged from 6.6% of younger women to 33% of older females. Corresponding figures for men were 8.6–23.7%. Concentric LVH was most prevalent in the older age-group, and eccentric non-dilated LVH was most common in the younger persons (➋ Table 3.8).

Table 3.8
Prevalence of various forms of electrocardiographic left ventricular hypertrophy in Framingham subjects [106]

Original cohort	Eccentric dilated	Eccentric nondilated	Concentric	Disproportionate septal thickness
Original cohort				
Males (121/510, 23.7%)	24 (20)	38 (31)	54 (45)	5 (4)
Females (282/855, 33.0%)	38 (13.5)	92 (33.5)	136 (48)	16 (6)
Offspring-spouse				
Males (148/1718, 8.6%)	13 (9)	73 (49)	59 (40)	3 (2)
Females (125/1892, 6.6%)	8 (6)	80 (64)	34 (27)	3 (3)

[a] Data expressed as a number, with percent of subjects with ECHO LVH in parentheses.

3.5 Right Ventricular Hypertrophy (RVH)

3.5.1 ECG Criteria

The right ventricular forces are normally masked by the dominant left ventricle. In mild cases of RVH, no apparent change may be noted, whereas when RVH is severe, the precordial leads may show a taller R wave in V_1 than in V_6 (➔ Fig. 3.12).

Since V_1 is closest to the RV mass, it is the lead most sensitive to changes induced by RVH, namely, taller R waves, smaller S waves, and a change in the R:S ratio plus delayed onset of the intrinsicoid deflection (➔ Fig. 3.13). Leads V_3R and V_4R may also be helpful in diagnosing RVH. These leads may show the typical changes usually sought in V_1. Deep S waves in I, V_5, and V_6 also often accompany RVH (➔ Fig. 3.14).

The type of heart disease involved plays a prominent role in the usefulness of various criteria for the detection of RVH. In congenital heart disease for example, the sensitivity of such criteria is generally over 90%. In mitral stenosis, it is approximately 65%, while in chronic cor pulmonale it may be near 30%.

A very extensive study of the sensitivity of the commonly used ECG criteria for RVH is that of Flowers and Horan [107] (see ➔ Table 3.9). They examined 819 hearts using the chamber dissection technique and found 178 with RVH. Criteria based on abnormalities in V_1 are the most specific (>90%) but the least sensitive (2–18%); for example, a QR complex in V_1 (➔ Fig. 3.15) is 8% sensitive but almost 100% specific. The inclusion of criteria involving the left precordial leads decreased the specificity to below 90% but improved the sensitivity to about 30%. The "correctness" of a sign was obtained by dividing the true positives and true negatives by the total group studied. Most of the 18 parameters listed in ➔ Table 3.9 had a "correctness" of 80–89%. The best combination of sensitivity, specificity, and correctness occurs with the constraint that requires the presence of two signs. Adding more only increases specificity at the expense of sensitivity.

Murphy et al. [7] confirmed the relative ineffectiveness of ECG criteria in the diagnosis of RVH. Using any of the four criteria (the first four in ➔ Table 3.10), their sensitivity ranged from 18% to 43% and specificity from 83% to 95%, dependent on patient selection. RVH in the presence of chronic obstructive lung disease proved the most difficult to diagnose, and congenital heart disease with RVH was the easiest to identify. Most of the criteria listed in ➔ Table 3.9 have a much higher sensitivity (24–92%) when primary pulmonary hypertension is present [108]; for example, 79% have an R/S ratio in V_1 > 1.0 and 76% have an SV_5 > 0.7 mV.

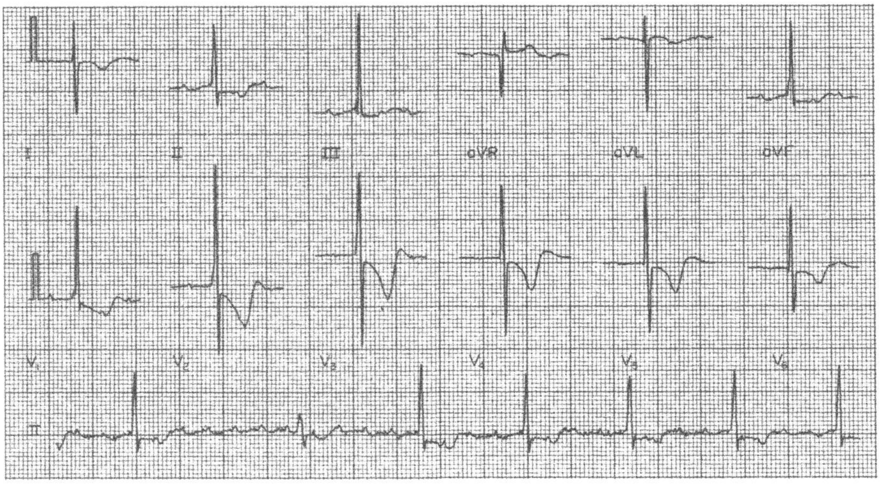

Fig. 3.12
Case of severe RVH in a 57-year-old male with rheumatic heart disease and two previous mitral valvotomies. The R wave in V_1 is taller than in V_6, and widespread secondary ST-T changes are in evidence. The pulmonary artery pressure was 110/50, suggesting severe RVH. There is also atrial flutter

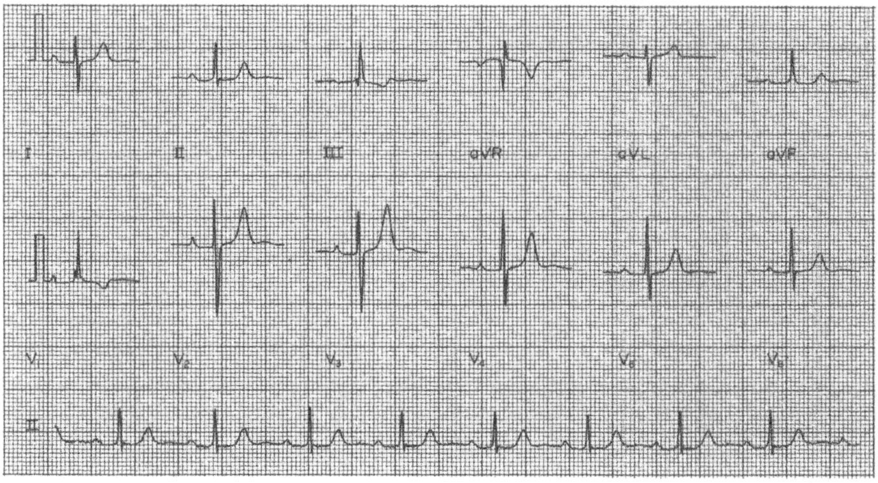

Fig. 3.13
Typical changes of RVH as evidenced by the tall R wave in V_1, with T-wave inversion as well as a deep S wave in lead I giving a QRS axis of 97°. The PR interval was measured as 0.214 s. The ECG was recorded from a 39-year-old female with pulmonary stenosis

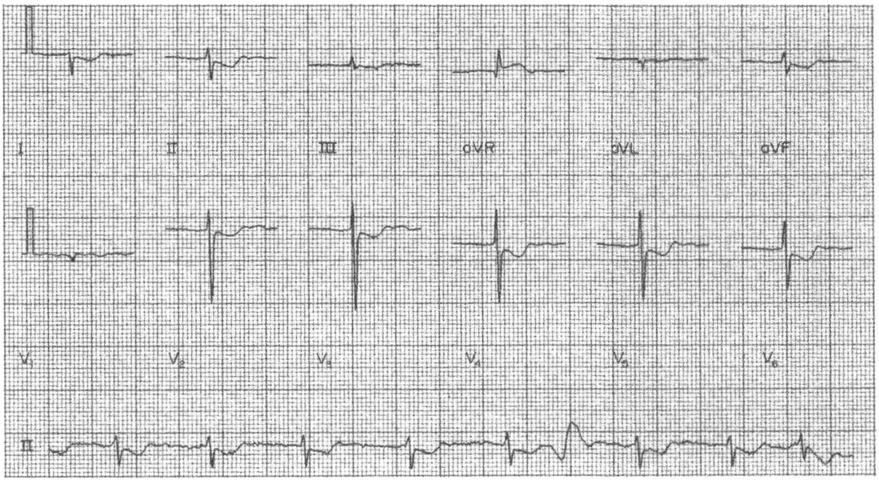

Fig. 3.14
ECG from a 67-year-old female with mitral stenosis and atrial fibrillation. Note the deep S wave in leads I, V_5, and V_6. Widespread ST-T changes are also in evidence

The most useful ECG criteria for RVH are the following. If the QRS duration is less than 0.12 s, then RVH is likely if one or more of the criteria below are present.

(a) Any one of the following:
  (i) Right-axis deviation > 90° (in the presence of disease predisposing to RVH)
  (ii) $RaVR \geqslant 0.5$ mV
  (iii) $RaVR > QaVR$

Table 3.9
Sensitivity and specificity of various ECG parameters for the diagnosis of right ventricular hypertrophy (RVH) or enlargement and chronic obstructive pulmonary disease (COPD) with RVH

	RVH[a]		COPD with RVH[b]	
Parameters	Sensitivity (%)	Specificity (%)	Sensitivity (%)	Specificity (%)
Limb leads				
$S_1S_2S_3$	41	88	36	60
S_1Q_3	31	86	48	90
Right-axis deviation > 110° (> 90°)	19	96	(42)	(95)
R aVR > 0.5 mV	0		6	100
P pulmonale	NS		21	65
Lead V_1				
35 ms ⩽ VAT ⩽ 70 ms	13	94	24	85
R/S ratio > 1.0 and T negative	9	98	9	95
qR pattern	8	99	24	100
S < 0.2 mV (and RV_5 ⩽ 0.4 mV)	6	97	(27)	(85)
R > 0.7 mV	3	99	12	95
R′ < 80 ms	4	98	12	95
rSR′ with R′ > 1.0 mV	0		3	100
Other chest leads				
S in V_5 and V_6	78	55		
RV_5 or RV_6 < 0.5 mV	22	88	27	85
R/S ratio V_5 or V_6 ⩽ 1.0	19	93	30	90
SV_5 or SV_6 > 0.7 mV	18	87	15	100
$RV_1 + SV_5$ or SV_6 > 1.0 mV	13	92	0	
R/S ratio V_5 over R/S ratio V_1 ⩽ 0.4	10	99	0	

[a]Modified from Flowers and Horan [107]. RVH defined as RV weight > 71 g or as relative right ventricular enlargement when RV is > 30% of the total ventricular mass.
[b]After Murphy and Hutcheson [110], using 33 RVH patients and 20 normals. RVH is defined as RV weight > 65 g or ratio (LV + S)/RV < 2.1, or probable RVH if RV weight > 0.34 g cm^{-1} body height and RV weight < 65 g.

(b) Any one of the following in V_1:
 (i) R/S ratio > 1.0 and T negative
 (ii) qR pattern
 (iii) 35 ms ⩽ ventricular activation time < 55 ms
 (iv) R ⩾ 0.7 mV
 (v) S < 0.2 mV
 (vi) rSR′ with R′ > 1.0 mV
(c) In other chest leads, any one of the following:
 (i) $RV_1 + SV_5$ (or SV_6) > 1.0 mV
 (ii) R/S ratio V_5 or V_6 ⩽ 1.0
 (iii) RV_5 or RV_6 < 0.5 mV
 (iv) SV_5 or SV_6 > 0.7 mV
 (v) R/S ratio V_5 over R/S ratio V_1 ⩽ 0.4
(d) ST depression and T inversion in right precordial leads – usually seen in severe RVH, for example, in pulmonary stenosis

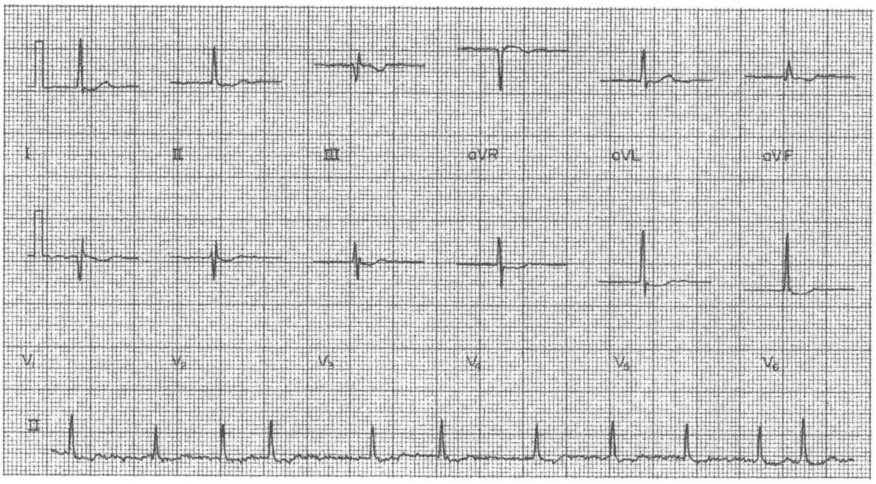

Fig. 3.15
QR complex in V_1 from a 53-year-old female with mitral stenosis and atrial fibrillation. Appearances are strongly suggestive of RVH. Note the absence of other QRS changes of hypertrophy, but the ST-T changes in the inferior leads are often supportive of the diagnosis, although in this case they are also caused by digitalis effect

Table 3.10
Selected ECG criteria for the diagnosis of right ventricular hypertrophy [7]

	Sensitivity[a] (%)	Specificity (%)
R/S ratio V_5 or $V_6 \leqslant 1.0$	44	92
SV_5 or $SV_6 \geqslant 0.7$ mV	26	95
Right-axis deviation > 90°	30	99
P pulmonale or right atrial overload	21	98
Any one of the above criteria	59	86
Any two of first four criteria	40	97
S_1Q_3 pattern	15	92
All others < 10%)		

[a]If BVH is included, then sensitivity falls by ~ 50% for each criterion although specificity is generally similar.

3.5.2 ST-T-Wave Changes

As in LVH, secondary ST-T changes can be found in the right precordial leads in cases of pressure overload of the right ventricle, such as in pulmonary stenosis. The classic appearance is ST depression with a convex upward ST segment merging into a deeply inverted T wave (➋ Fig. 3.16). Since these changes are a direct consequence of the RV hypertrophy, they are often called secondary repolarization abnormalities (or sometimes RV strain).

3.5.3 $S_1S_2S_3$ Syndrome

Although frequently used as a descriptive term by interpreters of electrocardiograms, this type of QRS complex may be seen in normal individuals as well as those with RVH. As a rule, the S waves of smaller amplitude are seen in normals and the deeper S waves are seen in those with RVH. In the latter case, the S wave in lead II is usually larger than the S wave

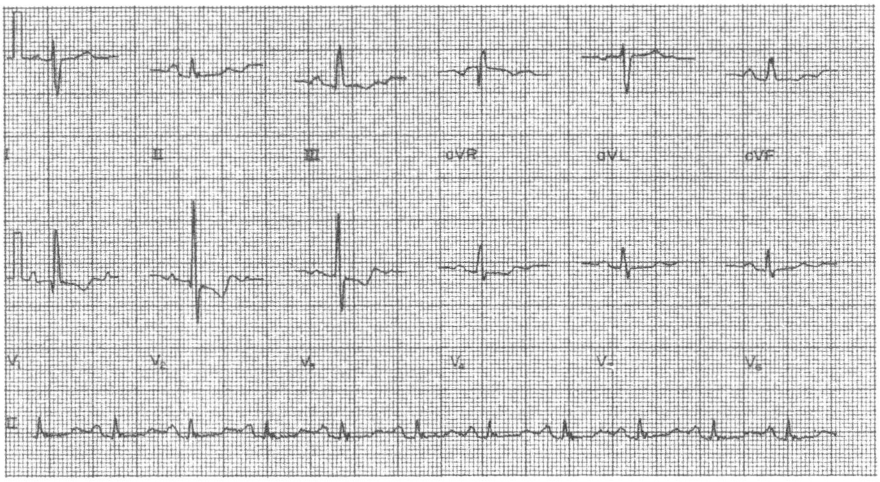

Fig. 3.16
ECG recorded from a 46-year-old male with recurrent thromboembolic disease, gross pulmonary hypertension, and RV failure. The chest x-ray showed cardiomegaly and an enlarged pulmonary artery. Note the QR complex in V_1 with secondary ST-T changes in V_1–V_4 indicating RVH. These ST-T changes constitute the classical RV strain pattern. The P waves suggest right atrial enlargement in addition

in lead III. No definite quantitative definition of the syndrome exists although Chou [109] has suggested the following: an R/S ratio equal to or less than one in each of leads I, II, and III or the S wave exceeds the upper limit of normal for the various age-groups, as defined by Simonson [42] (e.g., in those over 30 years, 0.4 mV in leads I and II and 0.8 mV in lead III).

3.5.4 Chronic Obstructive Pulmonary Disease

The typical ECG changes in patients with chronic obstructive pulmonary disease (COPD) include low voltage P-QRS-T complexes, right-axis deviation, a QS complex in V_1 (Fig. 3.17), and deep S waves in V_5 or V_6, especially when prominent P waves in II, III, and aVF are present. Cor pulmonale should at least be suspected if a subject with known COPD develops any of the following ECG changes:

(a) Rightward shift of the QRS axis by 30° or more
(b) T-wave abnormalities in right precordial leads
(c) ST depression in II, III, and aVF
(d) Transitory RBBB

In general, the diagnosis of RVH (defined as an increased RV mass) superimposed on COPD is difficult. Four suggested criteria [110] for the diagnosis of RVH in the presence of COPD are (a) S_1Q_3 pattern, (b) RAD > 110°, (c) $S_1S_2S_3$ pattern, and (d) an R/S ratio in $V_6 < 1.0$. When any of these four criteria were used, the sensitivity reached 79% but the specificity fell below 60%. The diagnosis of LVH complicating COPD was unreliable since only 30% of 18 such patients had the required ECG criteria.

The vertical position of the heart relative to the chest electrodes in patients with COPD may result in QS complexes in V_1 to V_4, suggesting an anteroseptal infarction. However, the vertical heart, prominent P waves, low voltage, and so on should help identify COPD as the cause. Occasionally, Q waves appear in the inferior leads suggesting an inferior infarction, but the T waves are not inverted.

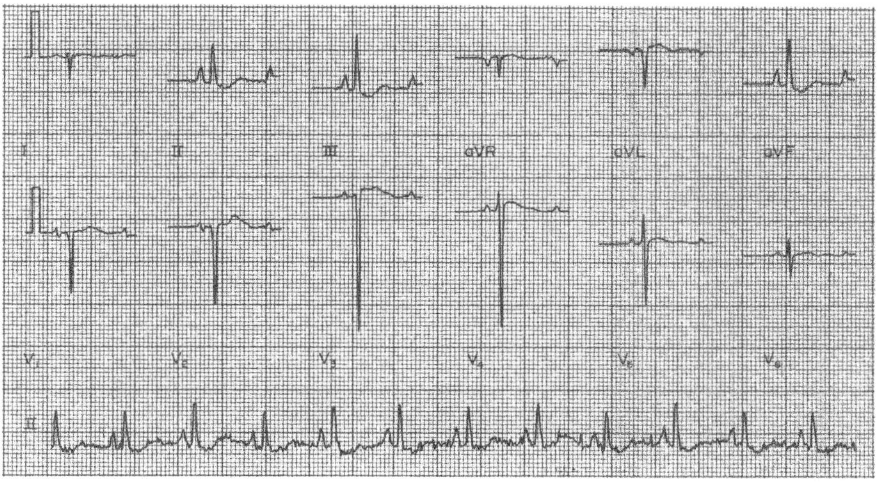

Fig. 3.17
ECG recorded from a 58-year-old male with chronic obstructive airways disease. There is evidence of RVH as exemplified by the deep S waves in the lateral leads I and V_5 together with right atrial enlargement as demonstrated by the tall P waves in the inferior leads

Left-axis deviation may be seen in about 10% of COPD perhaps related to the "axis illusion phenomenon" described by Spodick [111] or even the presence of LVH.

3.5.5 Orthogonal-Lead and VCG Criteria

As with LVH, the orthogonal-lead ECG can contribute to the diagnosis of RVH, using both scalar- and vectorcardiographic measurements. It has been claimed that orthogonal leads can enhance the diagnosis of RVH [77, 112, 113], for instance, in children. Brohet [114] attained a sensitivity of 86% by means of multivariate computer analysis. Scalar criteria, as might be expected, relate to a reduction in the R-wave amplitude in the lateral lead X with a correspondingly low R/S ratio in that lead. In addition, the corresponding scalar orthogonal criterion is an increased Q/R ratio in lead Z (directed positively to the back), analogous to the increased R/S ratio in V_1. In setting out criteria for screening, Pipberger et al. [71] selected the scalar criteria for RVH as illustrated in ➋ Table 3.11. The two levels A and B of criteria relate to different specificities. Note that the criteria are dependent on the race of the subject. Since these criteria were chosen for screening, they are not age dependent in order to make them as simple as possible.

The characteristic VCG changes of RVH may produce three different QRS loops (➋ Fig. 3.18) in the transverse plane, but not all cases of RVH can be classified in this way. The three different loops are as follows:

(a) Type A is a clockwise-inscribed QRS loop located in the right and left anterior quadrants (right anterior area > 30%) or, rarely, a figure-of-eight loop, for instance, as in severe RVH in pulmonary stenosis or severe mitral stenosis. The specificity of this pattern is almost 100%.
(b) Type B is a counterclockwise-inscribed QRS loop, located mainly in the left anterior quadrant, but possibly extending posteriorly to the left and right as in atrial septal defect.
(c) Type C is a counterclockwise-inscribed QRS loop located mainly posteriorly, with over 20% in the right posterior quadrant; for example, it occurs in chronic obstructive lung disease or mitral stenosis and is very specific for pulmonary hypertension (> 90% specificity).

A common occurrence in some of these cases is a frontal-plane QRS axis in excess of +90° (➋ Fig. 3.19) despite an 8% false-positive rate in normals and a 10% false-negative rate in severe pulmonary hypertension [113]. Not all authors

Table 3.11
Frank orthogonal-lead criteria for right ventricular hypertrophy [71] (in the absence of ventricular conduction defects)

		White		Black	
		Males	Females	Males	Females
RX amplitude (mV)	A[a]	< 4.0	< 3.0	< 5.0	< 5.0
	B[b]	< 5.0	< 4.0	< 5.0	< 6.0
(R/S) *X* amplitude ratio	A	< 1.1	< 0.9	< 1.0	< 1.8
	B	< 1.2	< 1.5	< 1.5	< 2.0
(Q/R) *Z* amplitude ratio	A	> 1.5	> 1.6	> 1.5	> 2.1
	B	> 1.3	> 1.5	> 1.3	> 1.5
RZ amplitude (mV)	A	< 3.0	< 2.0	< 4.0	< 2.0
	B	< 4.0	< 4.0	< 4.0	< 3.0

[a]Limits in rows labeled A indicate specificity ⩾ 90% associated with relatively low sensitivity
[b]Limits in rows labeled B have a specificity of 80–90% and are associated with a higher sensitivity than those in A

feel the above classification of types A, B, and C is helpful (see Chap. 9). Cowdery et al. [115] have suggested a specific modification of previous vectorcardiographic criteria for detecting RVH in mitral stenosis. They obtained a sensitivity of 60% and a specificity of 96%.

3.6 Miscellaneous RVH Topics

3.6.1 Complicating ECG Features

Pathological states such as COPD, lateral MI, or left posterior fascicular block, which also cause right-axis deviation, may be suggested by other clinical features.

The differential diagnosis of high posterior MI or other causes of prominent anterior forces (e.g., normal variation, Wolff-Parkinson-White syndrome, IHSS, displaced heart, left median fascicular block, or RBBB) can be difficult. When RVH is severe, it may result in Q waves in the right precordial leads, but with other changes that point to RVH rather than MI. Tall R waves in V_1 and V_2 should not mask a posterior MI since secondary ST changes, namely, negative ST-T waves, usually occur in the presence of RVH while peaked T waves, as are found in posterior infarction, do not occur. Pipberger [71] suggests that if the Q/R amplitude ratio in lead *Y* is greater than 0.25, then posterior MI is likely, especially when the T amplitude in lead *Z* is less than 0.0 (lead *Z* being directed positively to the back). Inferior or lateral MI may also produce an increased R/S ratio in V_1 (Fig. 3.19).

3.6.2 Right Bundle Branch Block and RVH

The diagnosis of RVH in the presence of RBBB (Fig. 3.20) remains a problem despite various criteria for an increased amplitude of R′V_1. None of these is reliable, since such amplitudes occur frequently when RVH is absent [116], that is, there are too many false positives and too few true positives. This is particularly true when biventricular hypertrophy (BVH) is present. In 1959, Del Rio et al. [117] reported that the horizontal loop was directed anteriorly, clockwise, and to the right when RBBB occurred with RVH. In 1978, Brohet [118] quantified these findings as an R/S ratio in lead $X < 2.0$, and a maximum horizontal-plane QRS vector 90° to 270°. These criteria help diagnose RVH, particularly in young subjects. An echocardiographic study of RVH in the presence of RBBB may help to develop new ECG and VCG criteria.

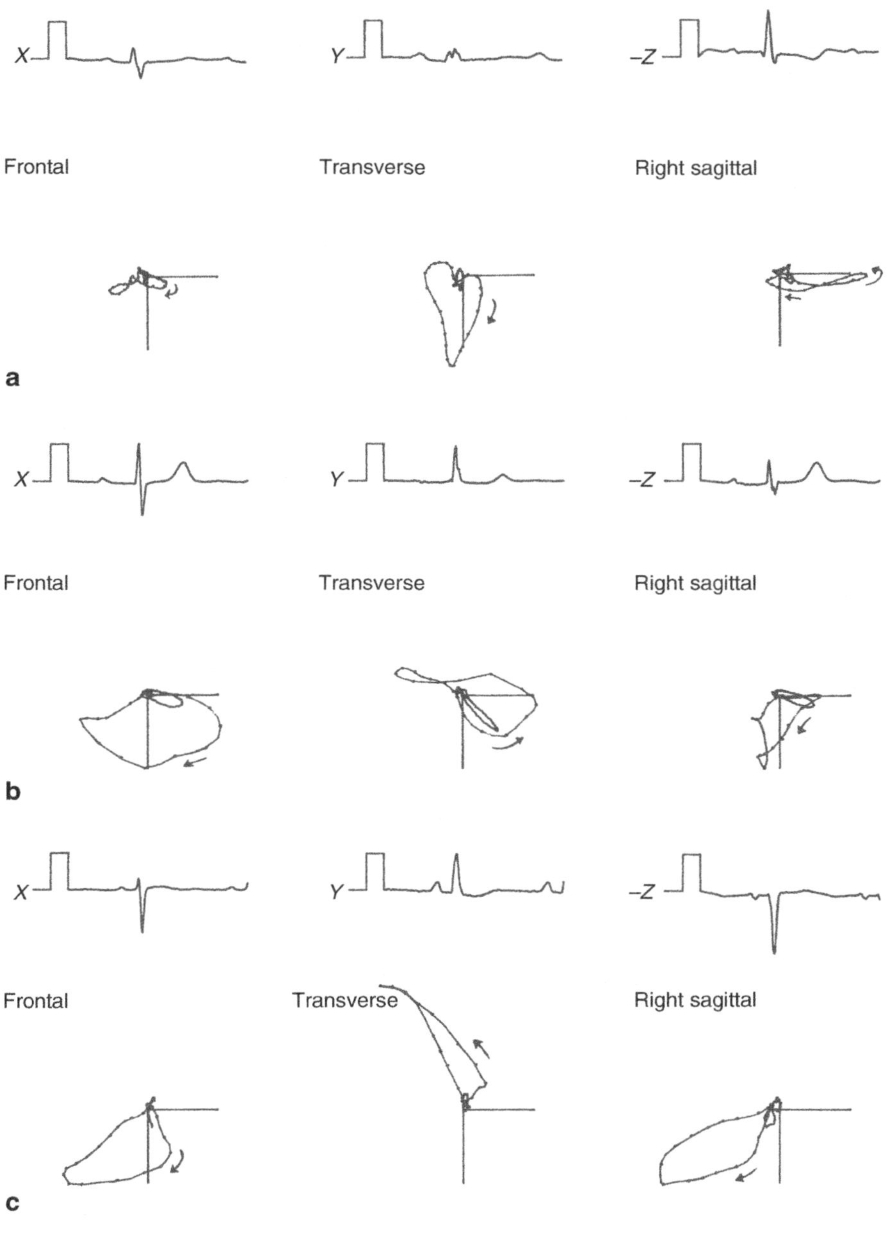

Fig. 3.18
Three types of VCG loops suggestive of RVH: (**a**) the so-called type A RVH, where there is clockwise inscription of the loop in the transverse plane (see Fig. 3.16 for corresponding 12-1ead ECG); (**b**) type B RVH, where there is increased anterior force with counterclockwise inscription of the loop in the transverse plane (see Fig. 3.13 for corresponding 12-lead ECG); and (**c**) type C RVH, which has counterclockwise rotation in the transverse plane with a rightward posterior displacement of the maximum QRS vector (see Fig. 3.17 for corresponding 12-lead ECG). Note that lead Z, shown in scalar form, is directed positively anteriorly, that is, appearances resemble V_1 and V_2

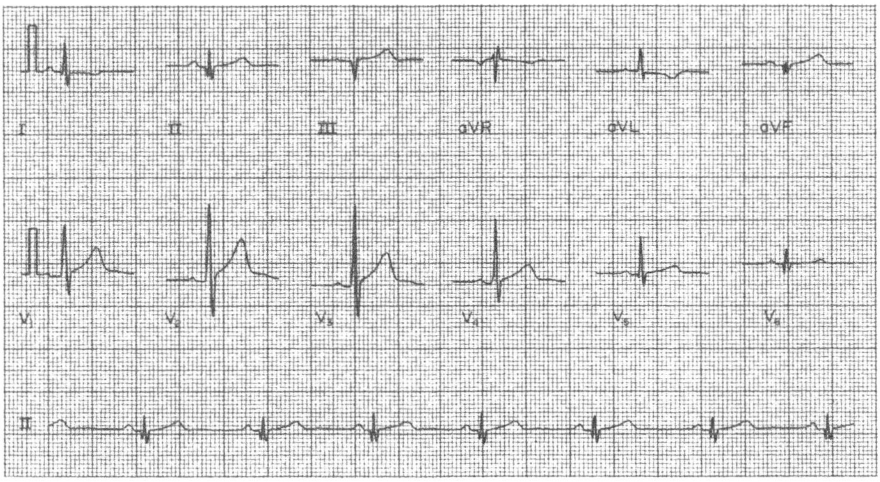

Fig. 3.19
ECG recorded from a 36-year-old male with an infarction involving the inferior/posterolateral wall of the left ventricle. Note the resulting increase in the R-wave amplitude in V_1 and V_2

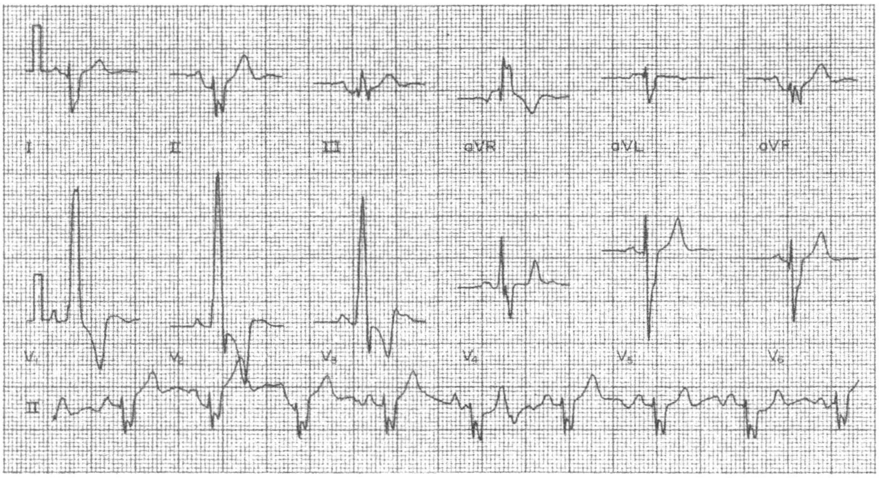

Fig. 3.20
RBBB in a 49-year-old male patient with tetralogy of Fallot. The extreme frontal-plane QRS axis (−172°) together with the tall R wave in V_1 is strongly suggestive of RVH

3.7 Biventricular Hypertrophy (BVH)

3.7.1 ECG Criteria

Combined ventricular hypertrophy or biventricular hypertrophy (BVH) is frequently impossible to identify by means of the electrocardiogram, as marked hypertrophy of one ventricle may mask the hypertrophy of its neighbor. Figure 3.21 shows complementary examples. In Fig. 3.21a, the right ventricular forces in a patient with Eisenmenger's syndrome are dominant, but R in V_5 is 30% above the normal limit suggesting LVH in addition. On the other hand, in Fig. 3.21b,

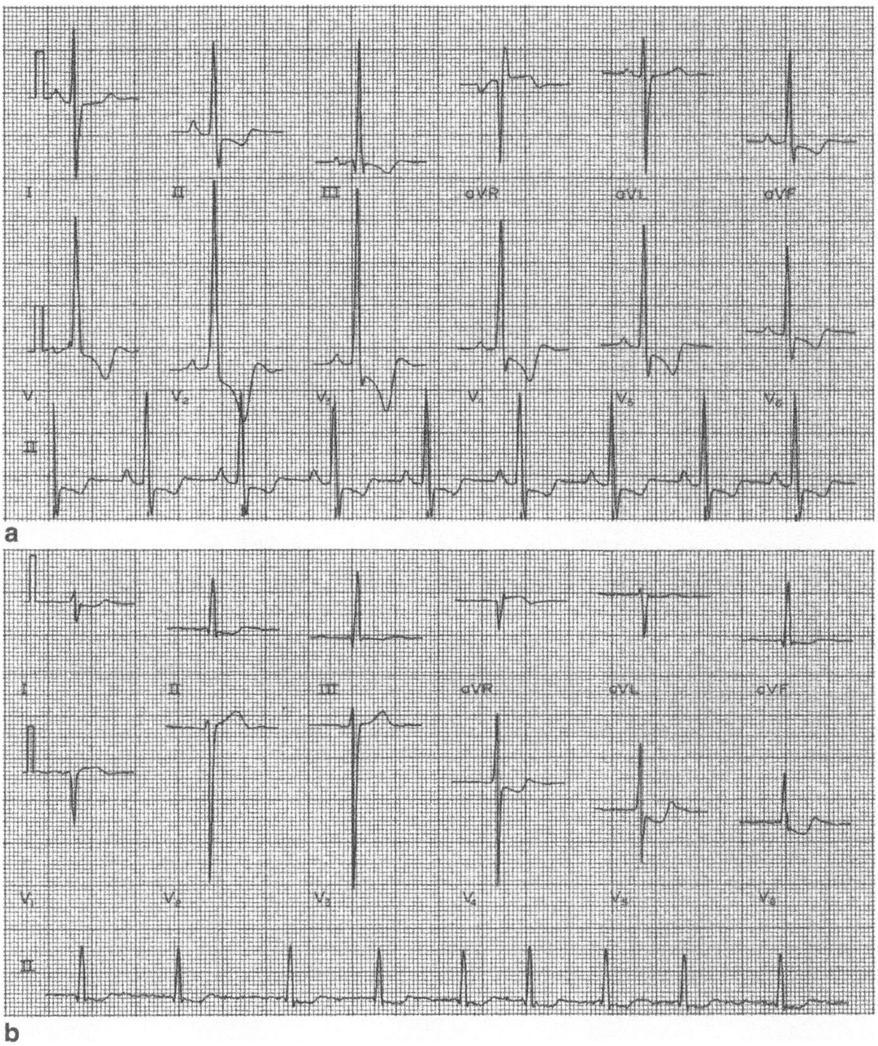

Fig. 3.21

Part (a) is the ECG from a 39-year-old female with Eisenmenger's syndrome. The RV enlargement tends to dominate the pattern, but the tall R wave in V_5, together with the secondary ST-T changes in the lateral leads V_5 and V_6, is suggestive of LVH in addition. Part (b) is the ECG from a 66-year-old female with mitral stenosis and incompetence, as well as aortic incompetence. Aside from the obvious ECG changes of LVH, there is a rightward QRS axis (= 102°), suggesting RV enlargement in addition

from a patient with valvular heart disease, the LVH produces a very deep S in V_2, but there is a rightward QRS axis (102°) suggesting RVH in addition.

Secondary RVH in patients with LVH is frequently masked by the dominant left ventricle, while patients with chronic cor pulmonale may have anatomic LVH that is not detectable on an ECG. If criteria for isolated ventricular hypertrophy are present, signs suggestive of hypertrophy of the other ventricle should be sought since it too is often enlarged. Cancellation of forces can make some ECGs appear entirely normal (pseudonormalization) except perhaps for atrial fibrillation and nonspecific ST abnormalities.

Further support for the concept of overload hypertrophy of one ventricle leading to hypertrophy of the nonstressed ventricle was offered by Gottdiener et al. [119] from an echocardiographic study of 98 patients. Increased RV wall thickness was present in 80% of 49 patients with hypertension and 63% of 16 patients with aortic stenosis. The magnitude of the increase in RV wall thickness was linearly correlated ($r = 0.75$) with LV wall thickness, but was not associated with pulmonary hypertension. The cause of the associated RVH therefore remains elusive.

In the presence of acquired valvular disease producing BVH, the electrocardiographic recognition of LV enlargement is particularly poor. Fortunately, the R/S ratio in $V_1 > 1.0$ remains a sensitive predictor of RV enlargement or severe pulmonary hypertension [120].

Many attempts have been made to develop criteria for the diagnosis of BVH [121–124]. The most reliable criteria are those determined by anatomical standards. By means of a chamber partition technique in an autopsy study of 75 patients, Murphy et al. [7] found that BVH was best diagnosed using left atrial abnormality (indicated by a negative $PV_1 > 0.1$ mV and of a duration > 40 ms) as the sole criterion for LVH, and, in addition, any one of the following three criteria for RVH:

(a) R/S ratio in leads V_5 or $V_6 \leqslant 1$
(b) SV_5 or $SV_6 \geqslant 0.7$ mV
(c) Right-axis deviation > +90°

Even so, the resulting sensitivity was only 20% although the specificity was 94%.

In contrast, Macfarlane et al. [75] studied 26 patients with BVH using the chamber partition technique. Criteria for BVH were developed from the first 14 and tested on the remaining 12 of these patients. Their point score from the modified axial orthogonal-lead system (see Chap. 11 of *Basic Electrocardiology: Cardiac Electrophysiology, ECG Systems and Mathematical Modeling*) had a specificity of 100% and a sensitivity of 64%, which fell to 42% in the test group, while the specificity remained high at 93%.

In 1969, Gamboa et al. [125] described the usefulness of the Frank orthogonal-lead system in diagnosing BVH. They defined anatomic BVH as

(a) Heart weight exceeding 400 g
(b) LV wall thickness > 13 mm and
(c) RV wall thickness > 4 mm

When BVH cases were differentiated stepwise from normals, LVH and RVH and those misclassified eliminated with each step, only 12% remained correctly classified as BVH. However, if the separation were against normal and LVH, or normal and RVH, the percentages of correctly classified cases rose to 43% and 42%, respectively. Using linear discriminant function analysis for separation of BVH and one covariance matrix for the combination of normal LVH and RVH, they correctly classified 69% with 18% false positives. It may be assumed that BVH is present whenever marked hypertrophy of either ventricle occurs. Since no ECG criteria are satisfactory at present [120], the combination of 12-lead ECG and the *XYZ* leads derived therefrom may be more helpful (see Chap. 11 of *Basic Electrocardiology: Cardiac Electrophysiology, ECG Systems and Mathematical Modeling*). In any case, computer assistance is likely to be needed as shown by Brohet [114] who diagnosed 62% of 203 examples of BVH by means of statistical methods applied to Frank orthogonal-lead recordings.

3.7.2 Vectorcardiogram

The vectorcardiograms (Fig. 3.22) of about two thirds of those with BVH have characteristic horizontal-plane loops [126]. In Fig. 3.22a, the transverse loop is inscribed clockwise and lies anteriorly indicating RVH, but has over 50% in the left anterior quadrant, suggesting LVH in addition. In contrast, in Fig. 3.22b, the transverse loop has its maximum QRS vector in the posterior right quadrant, suggesting RVH in addition to the LVH producing the high voltages.

The so-called "pie plate" pattern of the horizontal loop is equivalent to the Katz–Wachtel phenomenon of the standard ECG, namely, large diphasic deflections in the midprecordial leads as in large ventricular septal defects (see Fig. 9.54). In the horizontal plane, the counterclockwise loop has large or equivalent anterior and posterior portions, which are greater than the leftward extension.

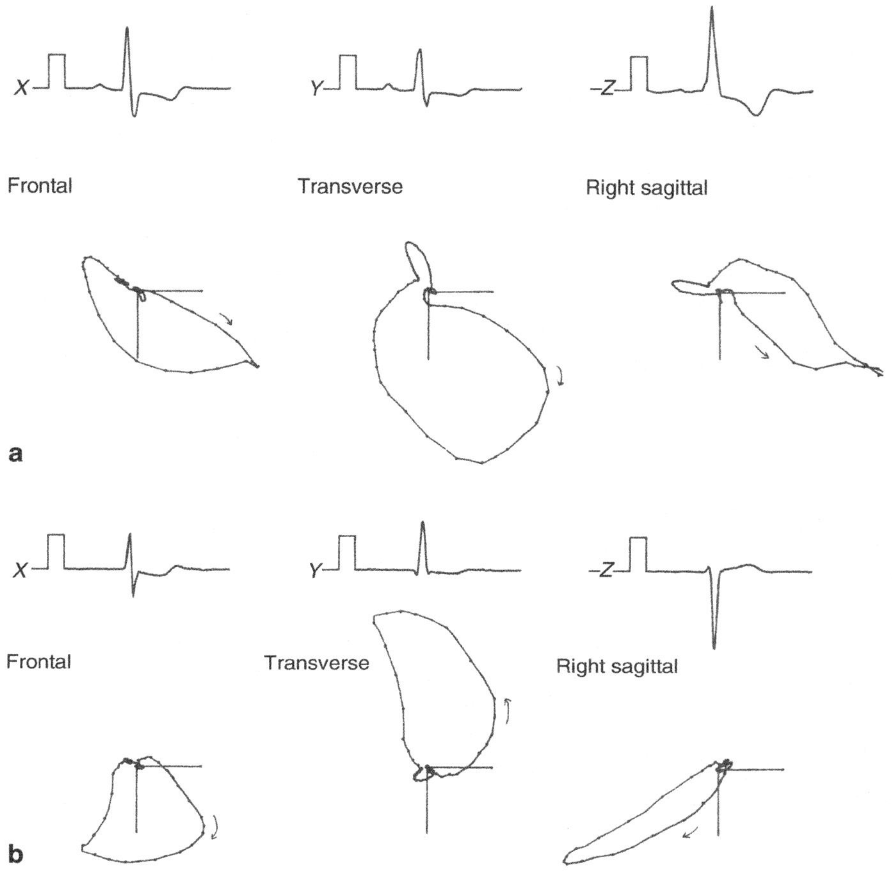

Fig. 3.22
Part (a) shows the vectorcardiogram corresponding to the electrocardiogram of Fig. 3.21a. Note the abnormal inscription of the loop in the transverse plane suggesting RV dominance in this particular patient. Lead *Z* is directed positively anteriorly. Part (b) shows the vectorcardiogram corresponding to the electrocardiogram of Fig. 3.21b

3.7.3 Left Bundle Branch Block and BVH

Right-axis deviation in complete LBBB is a rare occurrence. Tranchesi et al. [127] reported nine patients all of whom had severe congestive failure with marked cardiac enlargement. Usually enlargement of both ventricles was present.

A review by Nikolic and Marriott [128] of the 51 cases reported in the literature indicates it is a rare, insensitive but very specific marker of diffuse myocardial disease, especially idiopathic cardiomyopathy.

3.8 Atrial Enlargement or Overload

The P wave is a neglected area of electrocardiography. Perhaps this is because it is of low amplitude and often has only minor alterations in one or two leads despite a major change in the atrial vector. Furthermore, atrial abnormalities seem to be relatively unimportant as solitary defects because the QRS complexes are frequently obviously abnormal at the same time.

Various terms have been used to describe atrial enlargement or overload. Since an abnormality in atrial conduction may be responsible for a broad notched P wave, it has been suggested that the term left atrial abnormality (LAA) replace left atrial enlargement (LAE) or overload [129–132].

Obviously, better standards for diagnosing atrial enlargement need to be developed. Echocardiography may eventually lead to the development of a standard that includes sex and body-surface area utilizing a 98 percentile normal range as a cutoff rather than a mean plus two standard deviations [133, 134]. Perhaps several-fold amplification of the P wave would enhance its usefulness. Although this was suggested in 1966 [135], there has been little impetus to introduce such a modification in the commercially available computerized ECG systems. Even the simplified bedside method of recording high-gain P waves described by Cristal and Freidberg [136] in 1974 has evoked little enthusiasm.

The early portion of the P wave reflects right atrial depolarization, and the late component largely reflects left atrial depolarization [137]. These components are better visualized in the ECG by increasing the gain fivefold to tenfold [134, 136]. A timed vectorcardiogram was claimed to be over three times as sensitive as the standard ECG [137] in detecting atrial abnormality, while the ordinary VCG was claimed to be more than twice as sensitive [138].

3.8.1 Left Atrial Abnormality

The ECG pattern of left atrial enlargement (LAE) may arise from atrial dilatation, pressure overload [129], atrial pacing, or abnormal intra-atrial conduction [139]. The term left atrial abnormality is therefore preferable although the two terms are used interchangeably. Intra-atrial conduction abnormalities are discussed in ➲ Chap. 2.

Echocardiography provides a simple means of assessing left atrial size, and has now replaced radiographic methods in the detection of LAE [129, 133, 140–144]. The suggested M-mode ECHO criteria for LAE consist of

(a) Left atrial dimension > 40 mm [145]
(b) Left atrial dimension/body surface area > 2.2 cm m^{-2} [145]
(c) Ratio of left atrial (LA) dimension to aortic-root diameter > 1.17 [145, 146]

Waggoner et al. [144] studied 307 normals and patients with varying cardiac abnormalities (see ➲ Table 3.12), all of whom were in sinus rhythm; of these, 108 or 35% had LAE by M-mode echocardiography defined by (a) or (c) as listed above. Only two of 39%, or 5% of the false-positive ECG diagnoses of LAA, were free of organic heart disease. The authors concluded that the usual ECG criteria detect LAA rather than LAE.

Munuswamy et al. [147] used all three of the above criteria as a definition of LAE when reporting the sensitivity and specificity of various ECG parameters in 49 patients (see ➲ Table 3.13). They also tried various combinations of these six parameters with the gain in sensitivity to 90% offset by a loss in specificity to 71%. Since they required all three ECHO

Table 3.12
Sensitivity of commonly used ECG criteria for left atrial enlargement (LAE) of various causes [144] [a]. The total number of patients is 307

	Number of patients	ECHO LAE (%)	Sensitivity (%)	False positive (%)
Normal	55			7
Mitral valve disease	55	67	65	22
Aortic-root disease	52	23	54	31
Left ventricular disease	105	45	58	66
Miscellaneous	40	30	67	11
Left atrial diameter > 40 mm			67	20
Left atrial/aortic-root ratio | > 1.17			59	20

[a] Criteria used: P duration in lead II ⩾ 120 ms, (negative P duration in V_1)/(PR-segment duration) ⩾ 1.0, and terminal force P in V_1 > 3 mV ms. One or more of the criteria are satisfied

Table 3.13
ECG parameters of left atrial enlargement [147]

Criteria	Sensitivity (%)	Specificity (%)
Limb leads		
Notched P with interpeak duration > 40 ms	15	100
P duration > 110 ms	33	88
P duration/PR segment > 1.6[a]	31	64
Lead V_1		
Negative PV_1 duration > 40 ms	83	80
Negative $PV_1 \geqslant 0.1$ mV	60	93
P terminal force > 4 mV ms in V_1	69	93

[a] Macruz index [148]. PR segment is defined as the interval from the end of the P wave to the onset of the QRS complex.

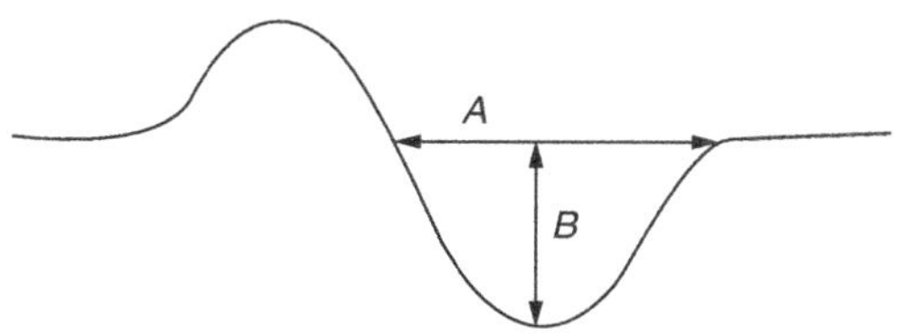

PTF = *A* (ms) x *B* (mV)

Fig. 3.23
Schematic illustration of the P terminal force (PTF) in V_1. It is obtained by multiplying the width (A) of the terminal (inverted) portion of the P wave by the depth (B) of this component. If A is measured in milliseconds and B is in millivolts, then the PTF is AB mV ms

measurements to diagnose LAE, indexing left atrial size to body-surface area would, perhaps, have only improved the specificity.

Macruz et al. [148] introduced an index, namely, P duration/PR segment, which was found to vary between 1 and 1.6 in normal individuals. Note that the PR segment is the interval from the end of P to the QRS onset. A value of the index in excess of 1.6 was said to indicate LAE, but it is a somewhat nonspecific criterion.

Only about 50–65% of patients have the LAE pattern on the ECG when the LA dimension is increased [129, 149]. Nevertheless, the usefulness of a P terminal force (PTF) in V_1 in excess of 4 mV ms has been documented [145, 150]. The PTF was introduced by Morris et al. [151] and is sometimes known as the Morris index. It is defined as the product of the amplitude and duration of the terminal component of the P wave in V_1 (see Fig. 3.23). In the case of LAE, the terminal component may have a negative amplitude (biphasic P wave), and hence the PTF would be negative. An example is shown in Fig. 3.24. It correlates moderately with the pulmonary capillary wedge pressure ($r = 0.67$) and only slightly better with the left atrial tension ($r = 0.72$) [141]. However, a normal PTF excludes a pulmonary capillary wedge pressure of 24 mm or over, while an abnormal PTF excludes one less than 10 mm. For general routine use, Miller et al. [150] found a PTF > 6 mV ms to be superior. Perosio et al. [152] have suggested a new index (duration/voltage of P wave in lead II), which has an excellent correlation with the left atrial size ($p < 0.001$). While the PTF in V_1 is the most frequently observed criterion, it is important to look for other parameters, since any one may be the sole indicator of LAE [153].

In children studied by Maok and Krongrad, a notched terminal P wave in the limb leads with a large negative terminal deflection in lead V_1 had only 40% sensitivity but a predictive value of 85%, although among those with mitral regurgitation, the sensitivity for LAE was 77% [149]. The ECG and echocardiogram frequently disagreed.

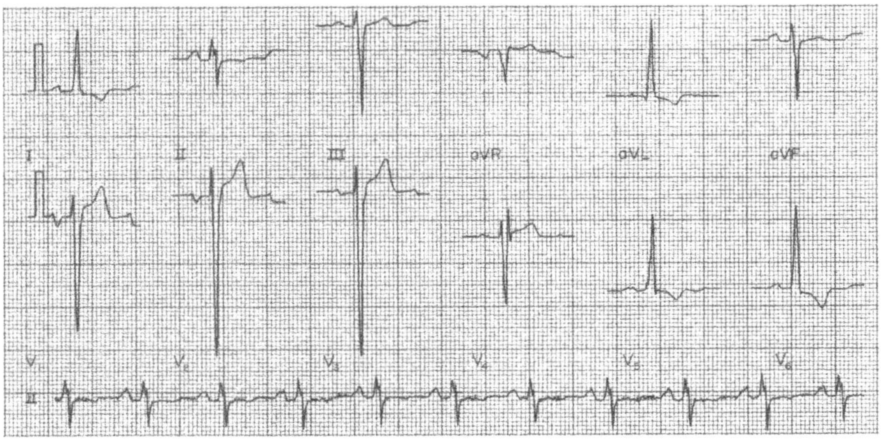

Fig. 3.24
Example of LAE in a 76-year-old male with a history of hypertension and myocardial infarction who was admitted for a suspected recent MI. Note the broad and deeply inverted P waves in V_1

3.8.2 Orthogonal-Lead Criteria for Left Atrial Enlargement

The diagnosis of left atrial enlargement by orthogonal-lead criteria [154, 155] is unlikely to improve the sensitivity obtained using the 12-lead ECG [154–156]. Two possible criteria have been suggested, namely, the sum of the positive amplitudes of PX and $PZ > 0.15$ mV, where Z is directed positively to the back, that is, the P+ in Z compares with the P- in V_1, and $P + Z > 0.1$ mV and P duration > 100 ms. Even so, the best sensitivity obtained was about 30% and the specificity was 92% compared to a PTF V_1 sensitivity of 50% and a specificity of 85% [140].

The time interval between the beginning of the P wave and the second P peak in lead Y in excess of 76 ms was the most useful parameter in identifying LAE in mitral valve disease in one study [155]. It identified only 21% of all cases of LAE, but was correct in 52% of those due to mitral valve disease. Unfortunately, it mislabeled 2% of normals and 7% of right atrial enlargement. Therefore, even a twin-peaked P wave is nonspecific unless qualified carefully.

In a fashion corresponding to the abnormal P terminal force in V_1, the P vector loop in the transverse plane can be displaced mainly posteriorly, with the maximum P vector being at approximately 270°, as shown in ➋ Fig. 3.25.

3.8.3 Right Atrial Abnormality

The electrocardiographic diagnosis of right atrial abnormality (RAA) is often difficult, even in patients with known right atrial overload or enlargement. It is influenced by various factors, such as age, heart rate, adrenergic stimulation, exercise, hypoxia, and RV compliance. Reynolds [157] noted that the positive portion of the P wave in V_1 is largely caused by right atrial depolarization and suggested a P index for V_1 to aid the diagnosis of RAA in children. He found the occasional patient with RAA who had a prominent terminal negative component in V_1. Unlike LAA, the negative P wave is pointed and is less than 40 ms in duration in RAA, while in LAA the terminal component is rounded and is greater than 40 ms in duration. An example of ECG evidence of RAA in a patient with chronic obstructive airways disease is shown in ➋ Fig. 3.17. The criteria for detecting RAA by ECG have been studied many times by radiographic, hemodynamic, or autopsy data to validate right atrial dimensions.

Two-dimensional echocardiography has been used to measure the right atrial size more accurately and test electrocardiographic criteria [7, 158, 159]. Reeves et al. [160] defined RAA as an area greater than 25 cm^2. It was determined after slow-motion, frame-by-frame viewing for maximal right atrial area. P-amplitude criteria alone had little predictive value. RAA was found only in two of 11 with a prominent P in II, and one of five with a prominent $P + V_1$. In contrast, eight out

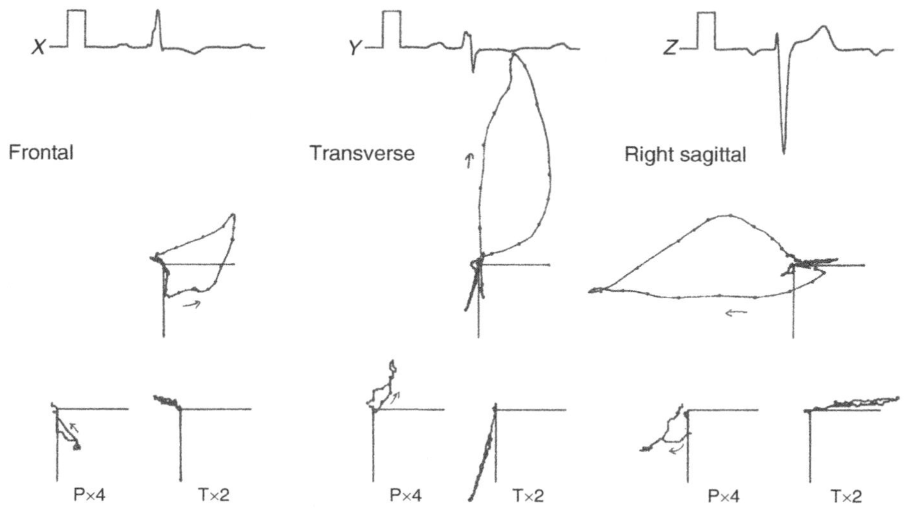

Fig. 3.25
Amplified P vector loop in the transverse plane from a patient whose ECG is shown in Fig. 3.24. The P loop is oriented almost totally posteriorly. Note that in this particular ECG, there is clockwise inscription of the vector loop in the transverse plane, suggesting myocardial infarction in addition, even though there is a prominent R in *Z* (directed similarly to V_2)

Table 3.14
Criteria for right atrial enlargement

Diagnosis	Criteria
Probable RAE	0.25 mV < P amplitude < 0.3 mV in any lead P in $V_1 \geqslant$ 0.5 mV (but less specific if heart rate >100)
Definite RAE	P amplitude > 0.30 mV in any lead qR in V_1 with coronary disease clinically absent

Table 3.15
Frank orthogonal-lead criteria for right atrial enlargement [71]

	White		Black	
	Males	Females	Males	Females
Positive P*Y* amplitude (mV)	> 0.15	> 0.15	> 0.20	> 0.20
Negative P*Z* amplitude (mV)	< −0.05	< −0.05	< −0.05	< −0.1

of eight with a qR in V_1 and no coronary disease had RAA, as did 13 out of 28 whose total QRS amplitude in V_1 was less than 0.6 mV with a ratio of total QRS amplitude in V_2 to total QRS amplitude in V_1 greater than 3.0. No allowance was made for changing the definition of RAA depending on sex or body-surface area (see Tables 3.14 and 3.15). Cacho et al. [158] used a right atrial area greater than 5.0 cm m^{-2} as a criterion for detecting RVH with 100% sensitivity in their 15 test cases. Obviously, echocardiography may offer a new challenge to the development of superior ECG criteria for the diagnosis of RAE.

The term "pseudo P pulmonale" has been used when prominent P waves are found in the absence of RAA. If left-heart disease is present with pseudo P pulmonale, it is suggested that it reflects an increase in the left atrial component [161].

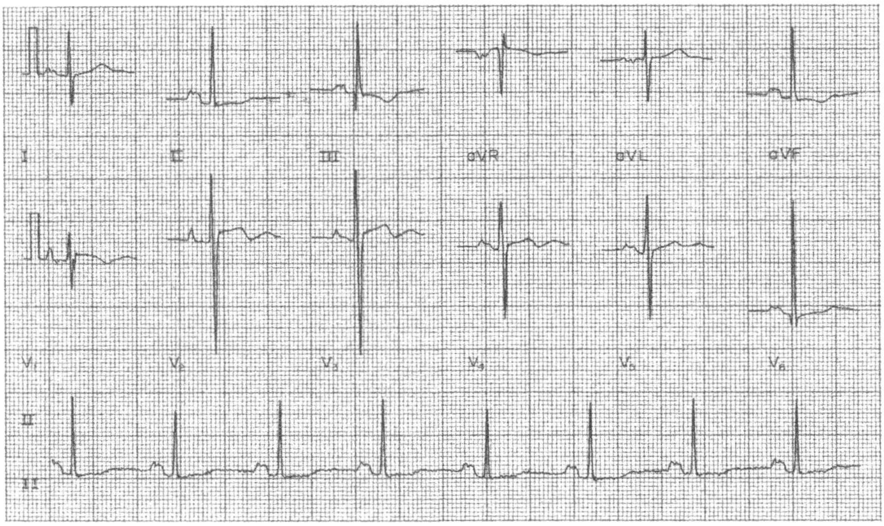

Fig. 3.26
Example of biatrial enlargement in a 30-year-old female with tricuspid and mitral valve disease. The tall P waves in V_1 and V_2 indicate RAE, while the broad bifid P waves seen in leads I, II, and III suggest LAE in addition. There is also a broad, though not excessively deep, terminal component of the P wave in V_1

3.8.4 Orthogonal-Lead Criteria for Right Atrial Abnormality

The orthogonal-lead criteria essentially mirror those of the 12-lead ECG, that is, an increase in P amplitude may be found in lead *Y* as well as in P− in lead *Z* (equivalent to P+ in V_1). P loops are directed inferiorly and anteriorly.

3.8.5 Biatrial Enlargement

The ECG may show features consistent with both RAA (increased P amplitude) and LAA (broad notched P and/or increased PTF V_1), in which case the term biatrial enlargement is appropriate (Fig. 3.26). Usually, however, atrial fibrillation supervenes to prevent its detection. Large fibrillatory waves (>0.2 mV, peak to peak) have been suggested as being indicative of atrial enlargement [162].

References

1. Cabrera, E. and A. Gaxiola, A critical re-evaluation of systolic and diastolic overloading patterns. *Prog. Cardiovasc. Dis.*, 1959;**2**: 219–236.
2. Cabrera, E. and J.R. Monroy, Systolic and diastolic loading of the heart. II. Electrocardiographic data. *Am. Heart J.*, 1952;**43**: 669–686.
3. Reichek, N. and R.B. Devereux, Left ventricular hypertrophy: relationship of anatomic, echocardiographic and electrocardiographic findings. *Circulation*, 1981;**63**: 1391–1398.
4. Grothues, F., G. Smith, J.C.C. Moon, et al., Comparison of interstudy reproducibility of cardiovascular magnetic resonance with two-dimensional echocardiography in normal subjects and in patients with heart failure or left ventricular hypertrophy. *Am. J. Cardiol.*, 2002;**90**: 29–34.
5. Bove, K.E., D.T. Rowlands, and R.C. Scott, Observations on the assessment of cardiac hypertrophy utilizing a chamber partition technique. *Circulation*, 1966;**33**: 558–568.
6. Murphy, M.L., P.N. Thenabadu, L.R. Blue, et al., Descriptive characteristics of the electrocardiogram from autopsied men free of cardiopulmonary disease—a basis for evaluating criteria for ventricular hypertrophy. *Am. J. Cardiol.*, 1983;**52**: 1275–1280.

7. Murphy, M.L., P.N. Thenabadu, N. de Soyza, et al., Reevaluation of electrocardiographic criteria for left, right and combined cardiac ventricular hypertrophy. *Am. J Cardiol.*, 1984;**53**: 1140–1147.
8. de Simone, G., S.R. Daniels, R.B. Devereux, et al., Left ventricular mass and body size in normotensive children and adults: assessment of allometric relations and impact of overweight. *J. Am. Coll. Cardiol.*, 1992;**20**: 1251-1260.
9. Kafka, H., S. Ford, and G. Burggraf, In vitro validation of a two-dimensional echocardiographic method of left ventricular mass estimation using intact postmortem hearts (abstract). *Clin. Invest. Med.*, 1983;**6**(Suppl. I): 44.
10. Reichek, N., J. Helak, T. Plappert, M. St John-Sutton, and K.T. Weber, Anatomic validation of left ventricular mass estimates from clinical two-dimensional echocardiography. Initial results. *Circulation*, 1983;**67**: 348–352.
11. Woythaler, J.N., S.L. Singer, O.L. Kwan, et al., Accuracy of echocardiography versus electrocardiography in detecting left ventricular hypertrophy: comparison with postmortem mass measurements. *J. Am. Coll. Cardiol.*, 1983;**2**: 305–311.
12. Pombo, J.F., B.L. Troy, and R.O. Russell Jr., Left ventricular volumes and ejection fraction by echocardiography. *Circulation*, 1971;**43**: 480–490.
13. Devereux, R.B. and N. Reichek, Echocardiographic determination of left ventricular mass in man. Anatomic validation of the method. *Circulation*, 1977;**55**: 613–618.
14. Ladipo, G.O.A., F.G. Dunn, T.H. Pringle, B. Bastian, and T.D.V. Lawrie, Serial measurements of left ventricular dimension by echocardiography. *Br. Heart J.*, 1980;**44**: 284–289.
15. Devereux, R.B., E.M. Lutas, P.N. Casale, et al., Standardization of M-mode echocardiographic left ventricular anatomic measurements. *J. Am. Coll. Cardiol.*, 1984;**4**: 1222–1230.
16. Wahr, D., Y.-S. Wang, C. Skioldebrand, E. Sehiller, M. Lipton, and N.B. Schiller, Clinical quantitative echocardiography III. Left ventricular mass in a normal adult population. *Clin. Res.*, 1982;**30**: 23A.
17. Koren, M.J., R.B. Devereux, P.N. Casale, D.D. Savage, and J.H. Laragh, Relation to left ventricular mass and geometry to morbidity and mortality in uncomplicated essential hypertension. *Ann. Intern. Med.*, 1991;**114**: 345–352.
18. Baker, B.J., J.A. Scovil, J.J. Kane, and M.L. Murphy, Echocardiographic detection of right ventricular hypertrophy. *Am. Heart J.*, 1983;**105**: 611–614.
19. Prakash, R. and H. Matsukubo, Usefulness of echocardiographic right ventricular measurements in estimating right ventricular hypertrophy and right ventricular systolic pressure. *Am. J. Cardiol.*, 1983;**51**: 1036–1040.
20. Watanabe, T., H. Katsume, H. Matsukubo, K. Furukawa, and H. Ijichi, Estimation of right ventricular volume with two dimensional echocardiography. *Am. J. Cardiol.*, 1982;**49**: 1946–1953.
21. Gibson, T.C., S.W. Miller, T. Aretz, N.J. Hardin, and A.E. Weyman, Method for estimating right ventricular volume by planes applicable to cross-sectional echocardiography: correlation with angiographic formulas. *Am. J. Cardiol.*, 1985;**55**: 1584–1588.
22. Horan, L., N.C. Flowers, and C.J. Havelda, Relation between right ventricular mass and cavity size: an analysis of 1500 human hearts. *Circulation*, 1981;**64**: 135–138.
23. Antman, E.M., L.H. Green, and W. Grossman, Physiologic determinants of the electrocardiographic diagnosis of left ventricular hypertrophy. *Circulation*, 1979;**60**: 386–396.
24. Devereux, R.B., M.C. Phillips, P.N. Casale, R.R. Eisenberg, and P. Kligfield, Geometric determinants of electrocardiographic left ventricular hypertrophy. *Circulation*, 1983;**67**: 907–911.
25. Horton, J.D., H.S. Sherber, and E.G. Lakatta, Distance correction for precordial electrocardiographic voltage in estimating left ventricular mass. An echocardiographic study. *Circulation*, 1977;**55**: 509–512.
26. Feldman, T., R.W. Childers, K.M. Borow, A. Neumann, and R.M. Lang, Relation of ECG R wave amplitude to changes in left ventricular size. *Circulation*, 1984;**70**(Suppl. II): 434.
27. Pech, H.J., J. Witte, R. Romaniuk, R.A. Parsi, and W. Porstmann, Left ventricular mass in coronary artery disease without hypertension. Haemodynamic and angiocardiographic study. *Br. Heart J.*, 1974;**36**: 362–367.
28. Scott, R.C., The correlation between the electrocardiographic patterns of ventricular hypertrophy and the anatomic findings. *Circulation*, 1960;**21**: 256–291.
29. Okin, P.M., J.T. Wright, M.S. Niemienen, et al., Ethnic differences in electrocardiographic criteria for left ventricular hypertrophy: the LIFE Study. *Am. J. Hypertens.*, 2002;**15**: 663–671.
30. Granger, C.B., M.K. Karimeddini, V.E. Smith, H.R. Shapiro, A.M. Katz, and R.L. Riba, Rapid ventricular filling in left ventricular hypertrophy: I. Physiologic hypertrophy. *J. Am. Coll. Cardiol.*, 1985;**5**: 862–868.
31. Okin, P.M., M.J. Roman, R.B. Devereux, and P. Kligfield, Electrocardiographic identification of left ventricular hypertrophy: test performance in relation to definition of hypertrophy and presence of obesity. *J. Am. Coll. Cardiol.*, 1996;**27**: 124–131.
32. Okin, P.M., S. Jern, R.B. Devereux, S.E. Kjeldsen, and F.B. Dahl, for the LIFE Study Group. Effect of obesity on electrocardiographic left ventricular hypertrophy in hypertensive patients: the Losartan Intervention for Endpoint (LIFE) reduction in hypertension study. *Hypertension*, 2000;**35**: 13–18.
33. Brody, D.A., A theoretical analysis of intracavitary blood mass influence on the heart-lead relationship. *Circ. Res.*, 1956;**4**: 731–738.
34. Ishikawa, K., A.S. Berson, and H.V. Pipberger, Electrocardiographic changes due to cardiac enlargement. *Am. Heart J.*, 1971;**81**: 635–643.
35. Rudy, Y., The effects of the thoracic volume conductor (inhomogeneities) on the electrocardiogram, in *Pediatric and Fundamental Electrocardiography*, J. Liebman, R. Plonsey, and Y. Rudy, Editors. Boston, MA: Nijhoff, 1987, pp. 49–73.
36. Romhilt, D.W., K.E. Bove, R.J. Norris, et al., A critical appraisal of the electrocardiographic criteria for the diagnosis of left ventricular hypertrophy. *Circulation*, 1969;**40**: 185–195.
37. Kafka, H., J.A. Milliken, G.W. Burggraf, Improved electrocardiographic diagnosis of left ventricular hypertrophy in left bundle branch block (abstract). *Circulation*, 1984;**70**(Suppl. II): 434.
38. Kafka, H., G.W. Burggraf, and J.A. Milliken, Electrocardiographic diagnosis of left ventricular hypertrophy in the presence of left bundle branch block. An echocardiographic study. *Am. J. Cardiol.*, 1985;**55**: 103–106.
39. Lewis, T., Observations upon ventricular hypertrophy with especial reference to preponderance of one or other chamber. *Heart*, 1914;**5**: 367–402.
40. Sokolow, M. and T.P. Lyon, The ventricular complex in left ventricular hypertrophy as obtained by unipolar precordial and limb leads. *Am. Heart J.*, 1949;**37**: 161–186.
41. McPhie, J., Left ventricular hypertrophy: electrocardiographic diagnosis. *Australas. Ann. Med.*, 1958;**7**: 317–327.

42. Simonson, E., *Differentiation Between Normal and Abnormal in Electrocardiography.* St Louis, MO: Mosby, 1961, pp. 99–101.
43. Romhilt, D.W. and E.H. Estes Jr., A point-score system for the ECG diagnosis of left ventricular hypertrophy. *Am. Heart J.*, 1968;**75**: 752–758.
44. Murphy, M.L., P.N. Thenabadu, N. de Soyza, J. Meade, J.E. Doherty, and B.J. Baker, Sensitivity of electrocardiographic criteria for left ventricular hypertrophy according to type of cardiac disease. *Am. J. Cardiol.*, 1985;**55**: 545–549.
45. Kansal, S., D.I. Roitman, and L.T. Sheffield, A quantitative relationship of electrocardiographic criteria of left ventricular hypertrophy with echocardiographic left ventricular mass: a multivariate approach. *Clin. Cardiol.*, 1983;**6**: 456–463.
46. Casale, P.N., R.B. Devereux, P. Kligfield, et al., Electrocardiographic detection of left ventricular hypertrophy: development and prospective validation of improved criteria. *J. Am. Coll. Cardiol.*, 1985;**6**: 572–580.
47. Devereux, R.B., D.R. Alonso, E.M. Lutas, et al., Echocardiographic assessment of left ventricular hypertrophy: comparison to necropsy findings. *Am. J. Cardiol.*, 1986;**57**: 450–458.
48. Devereux, R.B., P.N. Casale, P. Kligfield, et al., Performance of primary and derived M-mode echocardiographic measurements for detection of left ventricular hypertrophy in necropsied subjects and in patients with systemic hypertension, mitral regurgitation and dilated cardiomyopathy. *Am. J. Cardiol.*, 1986;**57**: 1388–1393.
49. Casale, P.N., R.B. Devereux, D.R. Alonso, E. Campo, and P. Kligfield, Improved sex-specific criteria of left ventricular hypertrophy for clinical and computer interpretation of electrocardiograms: validation with autopsy findings. *Circulation*, 1987;**75**: 565–572.
50. Schillaci, G., P. Verdecchia, C. Borgioni, et al., Improved electrocardiographic diagnosis of left ventricular hypertrophy. *Am. J. Cardiol.*, 1005;**74**: 714–719.
51. Verdecchia, P., G. Schillaci, C. Borgioni, et al., Prognostic value of a new electrocardiographic method for diagnosis of left ventricular hypertrophy. *J. Am. Coll. Cardiol.*, 1998;**31**(2): 383–390.
52. Thiry, P.S., R.G. Rosenberg, and J.A. Abbott, A mechanism for the electrocardiogram response to left ventricular hypertrophy and acute ischemia. *Circ. Res.*, 1975;**6**: 92–104.
53. Uhley, H.N., Study of transmembrane action potential, electrogram, electrocardiogram and vectorcardiogram of rats with left ventricular hypertrophy. *Am. J. Cardiol.*, 1961;**7**: 211–217.
54. Holt, J.H. Jr., A.C.L. Barnard, and M.S. Lynn, A study of the human heart as a multiple dipole electrical source. II. Diagnosis and quantitation of left ventricular hypertrophy. *Circulation*, 1969;**40**: 697–710.
55. Dunn, R.A., H.V. Pipberger, J.H. Holt Jr., A.C.L. Barnard, and H.A. Pipberger, Performance of conventional orthogonal and multiple-dipole electrocardiograms in estimating left ventricular muscle mass. *Circulation*, 1979;**60**: 1350–1353.
56. Okin, P.M., M.J. Roman, R.B. Devereux, and P. Kligfield, Time-voltage area of the QRS for the identification of left ventricular hypertrophy. *Hypertension*, 1996;**27**: 251–258.
57. Okin, P.M., M.J. Roman, R.B. Devereux, T.G. Pickering, J.S. Borer, and P. Kligfield, Time-voltage area of the 12-lead electrocardiogram: detection of left ventricular hypertrophy. *Hypertension*, 1998;**31**: 937–942.
58. Molloy, T.J., P.M. Okin, R.B. Devereux, and P. Kligfield, Electrocardiographic detection of left ventricular hypertrophy by the simple QRS voltage-duration product. *J. Am. Coll. Cardiol.*, 1992;**20**: 1180–1186.
59. Okin, P.M., M.J. Roman, R.B. Devereux, and P. Kligfield, Electrocardiographic identification of increased left ventricular mass by simple voltage-duration products. *J. Am. Coll. Cardiol.*, 1995;**25**: 417–423.
60. Okin, P.M., R.B. Devereux, J.E. Liu, et al., Regression of electrocardiographic left ventricular hypertrophy predicts regression of echocardiographic left ventricular mass: the LIFE study. *J. Hum. Hypertens.*, 2004;**18**: 403–409.
61. Okin, P.M., R.B. Devereux, S. Jern, et al., Regression of electrocardiographic left ventricular hypertrophy during antihypertensive treatment and prediction of major cardiovascular events: the LIFE study. *J.A.M.A.*, 2004;**292**: 2343–2349.
62. Moore, R.B., L.M. Shapiro, and D.G. Gibson, Relation between electrocardiographic repolarisation changes and mechanical events in left ventricular hypertrophy. *Br. Heart J.*, 1984;**52**: 516–23.
63. Kannel, W.B., T. Gordon, and D. Offut, Left ventricular hypertrophy by electrocardiogram: prevalence, incidence, and mortality in the Framingham Study. *Ann. Intern. Med.*, 1969;**71**: 89–105.
64. Okin, P.M., R.B. Devereux, M.S. Nieminen, et al., Electrocardiographic strain pattern and prediction of cardiovascular morbidity and mortality in hypertensive patients. *Hypertension*, 2004;**44**: 48–54.
65. Devereux, R.B. and N. Reichek, Repolarization abnormalities of left ventricular hypertrophy. Clinical, echocardiographic and hemodynamic correlates. *J. Electrocardiol.*, 1982;**15**: 47–53.
66. Okin, P.M., R.B. Devereux, M.S. Nieminen, et al., Relationship of electrocardiographic strain pattern to left ventricular structure and function in hypertensive patients: the LIFE study. *J. Am. Coll. Cardiol.*, 2001;**38**: 514–520.
67. Okin, P.M., R.B. Devereux, R.R. Fabsitz, E.T. Lee, J.M. Galloway, and B.V. Howard, Quantitative assessment of electrocardiographic strain predicts increased left ventricular mass: the strong heart study. *J. Am. Coll. Cardiol.*, 2002;**40**: 1395–1400.
68. Oikarinen, L., M.S. Nieminen, M. Viitasalo, et al., Relation of QT interval and QT dispersion to echocardiographic left ventricular hypertrophy and geometric pattern in hypertensive patients: the LIFE study. *J. Hypertens.*, 2001;**19**: 1883–1891.
69. Abbott-Smith, C.W. and T.-C. Chou, Vectorcardiographic criteria for the diagnosis of left ventricular hypertrophy. *Am. Heart J.*, 1970;**79**: 361–369.
70. Romhilt, D.W. and J.C. Greenfield Jr., Vectorcardiography diagnosis of left ventricular hypertrophy. *Circulation*, 1968;**37**: 15–19.
71. Pipberger, H.V., E. Simonson, E.A. Lopez Jr., M.A. Araoye, and H.A. Pipberger, The electrocardiogram in epidemiologic investigations: a new classification system. *Circulation*, 1982;**65**: 1456–1464.
72. Yankopoulos, N.A., W.K. Haisty, and H.V. Pipberger, Computer analysis of the orthogonal electrocardiogram and vectorcardiogram in 257 patients with aortic valve disease *Am. J. Cardiol.*, 1977;**40**: 707–715.
73. Brohet, C.R. and H.G. Richman, Clinical evaluation of automated processing of electrocardiograms by the Veterans Administration program (AVA 3.4). *Am. J. Cardiol.*, 1979;**43**: 1167–1174.
74. Pipberger, H.V., D. McCaughan, D. Littmann, et al., Clinical application of a second generation electrocardiographic computer program. *Am. J. Cardiol.*, 1975;**35**: 597–608.
75. Macfarlane, P.W., C.Y. Chen, B. Boyce, and R.S. Fraser, Scoring technique for diagnosis of ventricular hypertrophy from

three orthogonal lead electrocardiogram. *Br. Heart J.*, 1981;**45**: 402–410.
76. Macfarlane, P.W., C.Y. Chen, and J.J. Bailey, A comparison of point scoring techniques for the diagnosis of left ventricular hypertrophy, in *New Frontiers of Electrocardiology*, F. de Pádua and P.W. Macfarlane, Editors. Chichester: Research Studies Press, 1981, pp. 353–654.
77. De Backer, G.G., R. Zenner, M. Kornitzer, D.L. Clement, and M.M. Drama, Prevalence of left ventricular hypertrophy in middle-aged men according to various ECG-VCG techniques. *J. Electrocardiol.*, 1983;**16**: 307–311.
78. Shapiro, L.M., Physiological left ventricular hypertrophy. *Br. Heart J.*, 1984;**52**: 130–135.
79. Oakley, D.G. and C.M. Oakley, Significance of abnormal electrocardiograms in highly trained athletes. *Am. J. Cardiol.*, 1982;**50**: 985–989.
80. Magalski, A., B.J. Maron, M.L. Main, M. McCoy, A. Florez, K.J. Reid, H.W. Epps, J. Bates, and J.E. Browne, Relation of race to electrocardiographic patterns in Elite American Football players. *J. Am. Coll. Cardiol.*, 2008;**51**: 2250–2255.
81. Oakley, D., Cardiac hypertrophy in athletes. *Br. Heart J.*, 1984;**52**: 121–123.
82. Cokkinos, D.V., J.N. Demopoulos, E.T. Heimonas, C. Mallios, N. Papazoglou, and E.M. Vorides, Electrocardiographic criteria of left ventricular hypertrophy in left bundle-branch block. *Br. Heart J.*, 1978;**40**: 320–324.
83. Klein, R.C., Z. Vera, A.N. De Maria, and D.T. Mason, Electrocardiographic diagnosis of left ventricular hypertrophy in the presence of left bundle branch block. *Am. Heart J.*, 1984;**108**: 502–506.
84. Noble, L.M., S.B. Humphrey, and G.B. Monaghan, Left ventricular hypertrophy in left bundle branch block. *J. Electrocardiol.*, 1984;**17**: 157–160.
85. Havelda, C.J., G.S. Sohi, N.C. Flowers, and L.G. Horan, The pathologic correlates of the electrocardiogram: complete left bundle branch block. *Circulation*, 1982;**65**: 445–451.
86. Murphy, M.L., P.N. Thenabadu, N. de Soyza, J.E. Doherty, and B.J. Baker, Left atrial abnormality as an electrocardiographic criterion for the diagnosis of left ventricular hypertrophy in the presence of right bundle branch block. *Am. J. Cardiol.*, 1983;**52**: 381–383.
87. Vandenberg, B., K. Sagar, and D. Romhilt, Electrocardiographic criteria for the diagnosis of left ventricular hypertrophy in the presence of complete right bundle branch block. *J. Am. Coll. Cardiol.*, 1985;**5**: 511.
88. Hill, L.S., M. Monaghan, and P.J. Richardson, Regression of left ventricular hypertrophy during treatment with antihypertensive agents. *Br. J. Clin. Pharmacol.*, 1979;**7**(Suppl. 2): 2555–2605.
89. Wollam, G.L., W.D. Hall, V.D. Porter, et al., Time course of regression of left ventricular hypertrophy in treated hypertensive patients. *Am. J. Med.*, 1983;**75**(Suppl. 3A): 100–110.
90. Sonotani, N., S. Kubo, A. Nishioka, and T. Takatsu, Electrocardiographic and echocardiographic changes after one to two years treatment of hypertension. *Jpn. Heart J.*, 1981;**22**: 325–333.
91. Corea, L., M. Bentivoglio, P. Verdecchia, M. Provvidenza, and M. Motolese, Left ventricular hypertrophy regression in hypertensive patients treated with Metoprolol. *Int. J. Clin. Pharm. Ther. Toxicol.*, 1984;**22**: 365–370.
92. Russell, G.I., J.E.F. Pohl, J. Baldwin, et al., Treatment of essential hypertension: changes in blood pressure, echocardiography and electrocardiography on three therapeutic regimes. *Eur. J. Clin. Pharmacol.*, 1985;**28**: 119–124.
93. Savage, D.D., P.M. Rautaharju, J.J. Bailey, et al., The emerging prominence of computer electrocardiography in large population based surveys. *J. Electrocardiol.*, 1987;**20**(Suppl.): 48–52.
94. Rautaharju, P.M., A.Z. laCroix, D.D. Savage, et al., Electrocardiographic estimate of left ventricular mass versus radiographic cardiac size and the risk of cardiovascular disease mortality in the epidemiologic follow-up of the First National Health and Nutrition Examination Survey. *Am. J. Cardiol.*, 1988;**62**: 59–66.
95. Wolf, H., J.W. Warren, P.M. Rautaharju, et al., An electrocardiographic model for prediction of left ventricular mass. *13th Int Congr Electrocardiology* Washington. 1986: 4. [Abstracts.]
96. Carroll, J.D., W.H. Gaasch, S. Naimi, and H.J. Levine, Regression of myocardial hypertrophy: electrocardiographic-echocardiographic correlations after aortic valve replacement in patients with chronic aortic regurgitation. *Circulation*, 1982;**65**: 980–987.
97. Kannel, W.B. and R.D. Abbott, Comparison of ECG-LVH and unrecognized myocardial infarction as predictors of overt cardiovascular events: the Framingham study (abstract). *Circulation*, 1984;**70**(Suppl. II): 434.
98. Savage, D.D., R.D. Abbott, S. Padgett, S.J. Anderson, and R.J. Garrison, Epidemiologic features of left ventricular hypertrophy in normotensive and hypertensive subjects, in *Cardiac Left Ventricular Hypertrophy*, H.E.D.J. Ter Keurs and J.J. Schipperheyn, Editors. Boston, MA: Nijhoff, 1983, pp. 2–3.
99. Kannel, W.B., Prevalence and natural history of electrocardiographic left ventricular hypertrophy. *Am. J. Med.*, 1983;**75**(Suppl. 3A): 4–11.
100. Hamby, R.I., M.N. Prakash, U.A. Wyne, and I. Hoffman, Electrocardiographic left ventricular hypertrophy and coronary artery disease: clinical, hemodynamic, and angiographic correlates. *Am. Heart J.*, 1980;**100**: 794–801.
101. Levy, D., K.M. Anderson, D.D. Savage, S.A. Balkus, W.B. Kannel, and W.P. Castelli, Risk of ventricular arrhythmias in left ventricular hypertrophy; The Framingham heart study. *Am. J. Cardiol.*, 1987;**60**: 560–565.
102. Macfarlane, P.W., British Regional Heart Study; The electrocardiogram and risk of myocardial infarction on follow up. *J. Electrocardiol.*, 1987;**20**(Suppl.): 53–56.
103. Levy, D., M. Salomon, R.B. D'Agostino, A.J. Belanger, and W.B. Kannel, Prognostic significance of baseline electrocardiographic features and their serial changes in subjects with left ventricular hypertrophy. *Circulation*, 1994;**90**: 1786–1793.
104. Matthew, J., P. Sleight, E. Lonn, et al., Reduction of cardiovascular risk by regression of electrocardiographic markers of left ventricular hypertrophy by the angiotensin-converting enzyme inhibitor ramipril. *Circulation*, 2001;**104**: 1615–1621.
105. Gardin, J.M. and M.S. Lauer, Left ventricular hypertrophy: the next treatable, silent killer? *J.A.M.A.*, 2004;**292**: 2396–2398.
106. Savage, D.D., R.J. Garrison, W.B. Kannel, et al., The spectrum of left ventricular hypertrophy in a general population sample: the Framingham Study. *Circulation*, 1987;**75**(Suppl. I): 26–33.
107. Flowers, N.C. and L.G. Horan, Subtle signs of right ventricular enlargement and their relative importance, in *Advances in Electrocardiography*, R.C. Schlant and J.W. Hurst, Editors. New York: Grune and Stratton, 1972, pp. 297–308.

108. Kanemoto, N., Electrocardiogram in primary pulmonary hypertension. *Eur. J. Cardiol.*, 1980;**12**: 181–193.
109. Chou, T.-C., *Electrocardiography in Clinical Practice*. New York: Grune and Stratton, 1979, pp. 22, 23, 77.
110. Murphy, M.L. and F. Hutcheson, The electrocardiographic diagnosis of right ventricular hypertrophy in chronic obstructive pulmonary disease. *Chest*, 1974;**65**: 622–627.
111. Spodick, D.H., Electrocardiographic studies in pulmonary disease. I. Electrocardiographic abnormalities in diffuse lung disease. *Circulation*, 1959;**20**: 1067–1072.
112. Gamboa, R., P.G. Hugenholtz, and A.S. Nadas, Corrected (Frank), uncorrected (Cube) and standard electrocardiographic lead systems in recording augmented right ventricular forces in right ventricular hypertension. *Br. Heart J.*, 1966;**28**: 62–74.
113. Villa, J.G., J. Urbina, J. Sanchez-Dominguez, F. Largo, and A. Menendez, Vectorcardiographic patterns of right ventricular pressure overload, in *New Frontiers of Electrocardiology*, F. de Pádua and P.W. Macfarlane, Editors. Chichester: Research Studies Press, 1981, pp. 357–359.
114. Brohet, C.R., A. Robert, C. Derwael, et al., Computer interpretation of pediatric orthogonal electrocardiograms: statistical and deterministic classification methods. *Circulation*, 1984;**70**: 255–263.
115. Cowdery, C.D., G.S. Wagner, J.W. Starr, G. Rogers, and J.C. Greenfield Jr., New vectorcardiographic criteria for diagnosing right ventricular hypertrophy in mitral stenosis: comparison with electrocardiographic criteria. *Circulation*, 1980;**62**: 1026–1032.
116. Chou, T.-C., *Electrocardiography in Clinical Practice*. New York: Grune and Stratton, 1979, p. 119.
117. Del Rio, R., G. Medrano, V. Rubio, J.P. Olea, J. Soin, and D. Sodi-Pallares, Right bundle branch block with right ventricular hypertrophy. *Am. J. Cardiol.*, 1959;**4**: 294–301.
118. Brohet, C.R., M. Styns, P. Arnaud, and L.A. Brasseur, Vectorcardiographic diagnosis of right ventricular hypertrophy in the presence of right bundle branch block in young subjects. *Am. J. Cardiol.*, 1978;**42**: 602–612.
119. Gottdiener, J.S., J.A. Gay, B.J. Maron, and R.D. Fletcher, Increased right ventricular wall thickness in left ventricular pressure overload: echocardiographic determination of hypertrophic response of the 'non-stressed' ventricle. *J. Am. Coll. Cardiol.*, 1985;**6**: 550–555.
120. Loperfido, F., A. Digaetano, and P. Santarelli, The evaluation of left and right ventricular hypertrophy in combined ventricular overload by electrocardiography: relationship with the echocardiographic data. *J. Electrocardiol.*, 1982;**15**: 327–334.
121. Hiroki, T., Vectorcardiographic diagnosis of combined ventricular hypertrophy in adult patients. *Jpn. Heart J.*, 1974;**15**: 323–336.
122. Lipsett, M.B. and W.J. Zinn, Anatomic and electrocardiographic correlation in combined ventricular hypertrophy. *Am. Heart J.*, 1953;**45**: 86–94.
123. Pagnoni, A. and J.F. Goodwin, The cardiographic diagnosis of combined ventricular hypertrophy. *Br. Heart J.*, 1952;**14**: 451–461.
124. Scoulié, P., J. Laham, I. Papanicolis, and G. Voci, Les Principaux types electrocardiographiques de surcharge ventriculaire combinée. *Arc. Mal. Coeur Vaiss.*, 1949;**42**: 791–810.
125. Gamboa, R., J.D. Klingeman, and H.V. Pipberger, Computer diagnosis of biventricular hypertrophy from the orthogonal electrocardiogram. *Circulation*, 1969;**39**: 72–82.
126. Varriale, P., R.J. Kennedy, and J.C. Alfenito, Vectorcardiogram of combined ventricular hypertrophy: posterior counterclockwise loop (Frank System). *Br. Heart J.*, 1969;**31**: 457–461.
127. Tranchesi, J., P. Moffa, and M. Ebaid, Right axis deviation in left bundle branch block: an electro-vectorcardiographic study, in *Proceedings of the 11th International Symposium on Vectorcardiography 2*, I. Hoffman, R.L. Hamby, and E. Glassman, Editors. Amsterdam: North-Holland, 1971, pp. 283–288.
128. Nikolic, A. and H.J.L. Marriott, Left bundle branch block with right axis deviation: a marker of congestive cardiomyopathy. *J. Electrocardiol.*, 1985;**18**: 395–404.
129. Josephson, M.E., J.A. Kastor, and J. Morganroth, Electrocardiographic left atrial enlargement. Electrophysiologic, echocardiographic and hemodynamic correlates. *Am. J. Cardiol.*, 1977;**39**: 967–971.
130. Saunders, J.L., J.H. Calatayud, K.J. Schulz, V. Maranhao, A.S. Gooch, and H. Goldberg, Evaluation of ECG criteria for P-wave abnormalities. *Am. Heart J.*, 1967;**74**: 757–765.
131. Zoneraich, O. and S. Zoneraich, Intraatrial conduction disturbances: vectorcardiographic patterns. *Am. J. Cardiol.*, 1976;**37**: 736–742.
132. Zoneraich, O. and S. Zoneraich, Electrocardiographic left atrial enlargement versus interatrial conduction defect. *Am. J. Cardiol.*, 1978;**41**: 618–619.
133. Chirife, R., G.S. Feitosa, and W.S. Frankl, Electrocardiographic detection of left atrial enlargement. Correlation of P wave with left atrial dimension by echocardiography. *Br. Heart J.*, 1975;**37**: 1281–1285.
134. Wang, Y.-S., D. Heilbron, J. Outman, D. Wahr, and N.H. Schiller, Clinical quantitative echocardiography. I. End systolic atrial volume in a normal adult population. *Clin. Res.*, 1982;**30**: 23A.
135. Haywood, L.J. and R.H. Selvester, Analysis of right and left atrial vectorcardiograms. Timed records of 100 normal persons. *Circulation*, 1966;**33**: 577–587.
136. Cristal, N. and L. Freidberg, The atriogram. A bedside method for recording high gain P waves. *Chest*, 1974;**65**: 554–555.
137. Selvester, R.H. and L.J. Haywood, High gain, high frequency atrial vectorcardiograms in normal subjects and in patients with atrial enlargement. *Am. J. Cardiol.*, 1969;**24**: 8–17.
138. Benchimol, A., F. Reich, and K.H. Desser, Comparison of the electrocardiogram and vectorcardiogram for the diagnosis of left atrial enlargement. *J. Electrocardiol.*, 1976;**9**: 215–218.
139. Chandraratna, P.A.N. and E. Langevin, On the significance of an abnormal P-terminal force in lead VI. *Am. Heart J.*, 1978;**95**: 267–268.
140. Bosch, X., A. Hayes, J. Doxandabaratz, et al., The value of electrocardiogram and vectorcardiogram in diagnosis of left atrial enlargement. *Adv. Cardiol.*, 1981; **28**: 238–241.
141. Di Bianco, R., J.S. Gottdiener, R.D. Fletcher, and H.V. Pipberger, Left atrial overload: a hemodynamic, echocardiographic, electrocardiographic and vectorcardiographic study. *Am. Heart J.*, 1979;**98**: 478–489.
142. Gutman, J., Y.S. Wang, D. Wahr, and N.B. Schiller, Normal left atrial function determined by 2-dimensional echocardiography. *Am. J. Cardiol.*, 1983;**51**: 336–340.
143. Termini, H.A. and Y.-C. Lee, Echocardiographic and electrocardiographic criteria for diagnosing left atrial enlargement. *South Med. J.*, 1975;**68**: 161–165.

144. Waggoner, A.D., A.V. Adyanthaya, M.A. Quinones, and J.K. Alexander, Left atrial enlargement. Echocardiographic assessment of electrocardiographic criteria. *Circulation*, 1976;**54**: 553–557.
145. Hirata, T., S.H. Wolfe, R.L. Popp, C.H. Helmen, and H. Feigenbaum, Estimation of left atrial size using ultrasound. *Am. Heart J.*, 1969;**78**: 43–52.
146. ten Cate, F.J., F.E. Kloster, W.A. van Dorp, A.T. Meester, and J. Roelandt, Dimensions and volumes of left atrium and ventricle determined by single beam echocardiography. *Br. Heart J.*, 1974;**36**: 737–746.
147. Munuswamy, K., M.A. Alpert, R.H. Martin, R.H. Whiting, and N.J. Mechlin, Sensitivity and specificity of commonly used electrocardiographic criteria for left atrial enlargement determined by M-mode echocardiography. *Am. J. Cardiol.*, 1984;**53**: 829–832.
148. Macruz, R., J.K. Perloff, and R.B. Case, A method for the electrocardiographic recognition of atrial enlargement. *Circulation*, 1958;**17**: 882–889.
149. Maok, J. and E. Krongrad, Assessment of electrocardiographic criteria for left atrial enlargement in childhood. *Am. J. Cardiol.*, 1984;**53**: 215–217.
150. Miller, D.H., R.R. Eisenberg, P.D. Kligfield, R.H. Devereux, P.N. Casale, and M.C. Phillips, Electrocardiographic recognition of left atrial enlargement. *J. Electrocardiol.*, 1983;**16**: 15–21.
151. Morris, J.J. Jr., E.H. Estes Jr., R.E. Whalen, H.K. Thompson Jr., and H.D. McIntosh, P-wave analysis in valvular heart disease. *Circulation*, 1964;**24**: 242–252.
152. Perosio, A.M., L.D. Suarez, A. Torino, J.J. Llera, A. Hallester, and J.M. Roisinblit, Reassessment of electrovectorcardiographic signs of left atrial enlargement. *Clin. Cardiol.*, 1982;**5**: 640–646.
153. Monteiro, A.A., A.C. de Aguiar, and R. Lopes, Mitral stenosis in sinus rhythm: electrocardiographic diagnostic criteria of left atrial enlargement, in *New Frontiers of Electrocardiology*, F. de Pádua and P.W. Macfarlane, Editors. Chichester. *Research Studies Press*, 1981, pp. 360–362.
154. Ishikawa, K., P.M. Kini, and H.V. Pipberger, P wave analysis in 2464 orthogonal electrocardiograms from normal subjects and patients with atrial overload. *Circulation*, 1973;**48**: 565–574.
155. Ishikawa, P. and H.V. Pipberger, Critical evaluation of the twin peaked P wave ("pseudo-P mitrale") in orthogonal electrocardiograms. *J. Electrocardiol.*, 1980;**13**: 181–184.
156. Brohet, C.R., C.-E. Liedtke, and N. Tuna, P wave abnormalities in the orthogonal electrocardiogram: correlation with ventricular overload in pulmonic and aortic valvular heart disease. *J. Electrocardiol.*, 1975;**8**: 103–112.
157. Reynolds, J.L., The electrocardiographic recognition of right atrial abnormality in children. *Am. Heart J.*, 1971;**81**: 748–759.
158. Cacho, A., R. Prakash, R. Sarma, and V.S. Kaushik, Usefulness of two-dimensional echocardiography in diagnosing right ventricular hypertrophy. *Chest*, 1983;**84**: 154–157.
159. Kushner, F.G., W. Lam, and J. Morganroth, Apex sector echocardiography in evaluation of the right atrium in patients with mitral stenosis and atrial septal defect. *Am. J. Cardiol.*, 1978;**42**: 733–737.
160. Reeves, W.C., W. Hallahan, E.J. Schwiter, T.J. Ciotola, E. Buonocore, and W. Davidson, Two-dimensional echocardiographic assessment of electrocardiographic criteria for right atrial enlargement. *Circulation*, 1981;**64**: 387–391.
161. Chou, T.-C. and R.A. Helm, The pseudo P pulmonale. *Circulation*, 1965;**32**: 96–105.
162. Morganroth, J., L.N. Horowitz, M.E. Josephson, and J.A. Kastor, Relationship of atrial fibrillatory wave amplitude to left atrial size and etiology of heart disease: an old generalization re-examined. *Am. Heart J.*, 1979;**97**: 184–186.

4 Myocardial Infarction

Ronald H. Selvester · David G. Strauss · Galen S. Wagner

P. W. Macfarlane et al. (eds.), *Electrocardiology*, DOI 10.1007/978-0-85729-874-4_4,

4.1 General Angiographic and Pathoanatomic Considerations

4.1.1 Essential Principles

Myocardial infarction (MI) by definition *is the process of the death of heart muscle from loss of its blood supply due to occlusion of the nutrient-supplying coronary artery.* Three important points must be taken into account in the functional/angiographic and pathoanatomic consideration of myocardial infarction. First, the location and potential maximum size of the infarct *resulting from this process* is related to the location and extent of the perfusion bed of the occluded coronary artery. Second, the acute electrocardiographic (ECG) changes of ischemia/injury, the ST displacement vectors, are directed outward away from the center of the epicardium in the region of the involved myocardium. The magnitude of this displacement vector is related to both the extent and severity of regional coronary non-perfusion. The direction of this vector in 3D space is a marker for the specific coronary artery or branch occluded when there is typical coronary artery distribution to the myocardium. Third, the death of myocardial cells and the loss of local electric current dipoles from the myocardial excitation wave surface is the *sine qua non* of a completed myocardial infarct. This is seen as loss of ventricular forces (QRS voltage) over time on the electrocardiogram (ECG), that is, loss of local QRS spatial vectors (see ➋ Chap. 2 of *Basic Electrocardiology* : *Cardiac Electrophysiology, ECG Systems and Mathematical Modeling*). The extent of the spatial magnitude and duration (the voltage time integral) of the lost pre-existing local QRS vectors (reflected in loss of localized 12-lead ECG forces), is quantitatively related to the size of the resultant infarct.

The atrioventricular (AV) node sends, via the bundle of His and the branching His-Purkinje conduction system, excitation impulses from the sinus node through the upper chambers of the heart to both the right and left ventricles. Bundle branch fascicles insert into the fine ventricular endocardial peripheral network of this conduction system. This starts the wave of ventricular excitation from endocardium to epicardium in the contractile myocardial cells. Even major myocardial infarction occurs without significant damage to this fine inner endocardial peripheral Purkinje network since it receives its blood supply directly from the cavity blood. However, infarction may produce block of all or part of the thicker proximal left or right bundle branches since these receive their blood supply from intramural septal arteries. Thus proximal coronary artery occlusion can result in a complete right bundle branch block (RBBB), left anterior-superior fascicular block (LAFB), left inferior-posterior fascicular block (LIFB), or complete left bundle branch block (LBBB). Infarction is also seen in the presence of ventricular hypertrophy or dilatation, and with repolarization changes of acute or chronic ischemia. The spatial vector change in the finally recorded ECG is a variable combination of all these effects. The complexity of these interactions precludes the memorization of ECG patterns. A thorough understanding of the three-dimensional (3D) spatial aspects of normal excitation and recovery (➋ Chaps. 4 and ➋ 5 of *Basic Electrocardiology* : *Cardiac Electrophysiology, ECG Systems and Mathematical Modeling*), and that of the conduction defects just described, along with the QRS and ST-T changes tightly linked to them are prerequisites for the rational understanding and interpretation of the ECG. To quote J. Willis Hurst in his 2003 paper [1] on . . . "Suggestions for the Improvement of the Interpretive Process" of clinical ECG, "*The best way to interpret tracings is to learn the basic principles of electrocardiography, including vector concepts, and apply them to each tracing that is being interpreted. Without such an approach, people who memorize are helpless when they see tracings that they have not seen before.*"

This chapter is dedicated to bridging this gap. The local spatial vector changes of acute myocardial infarction lend themselves to quantitative analysis relating to the time from the initial incident into the acute phase, the area at risk, and the potential for myocardial salvage. The loss of local QRS forces from the resultant infarct, in normal and abnormal conduction, can be related quantitatively to the resulting infarct size, functional reserve, and life expectancy.

4.1.2 Historical and Future Perspective

In 1963, Hodgkin and Huxley received the Nobel Prize in medicine for "their discoveries concerning the ionic mechanisms involved in excitation and inhibition in the peripheral and central portions of the nerve cell membrane" [2]. They performed key experiments in 1939 and provided an explanation in 1945 of how the nerve conducts its impulse. Their explanation was that the membrane becomes momentarily very permeable to sodium ions which are positively charged and are much more concentrated outside cells than inside. Later, they came across a paper by Overton, who in 1902, made the same observation in muscle [3]. Overton then repeated the experiment on nerve where he put it in salt-free solution, but the nerve continued to work. He concluded that the nerve is surrounded by a sheath that holds sodium around the fibers.

In 1918, Smith recorded the electrocardiogram in dogs after ligating coronary arteries [4] and, in 1920, Pardee recorded an electrocardiogram of a patient with an acute coronary occlusion [5]. Pardee described the appearance of ST elevation in leads II and III and correctly observed that the ST segment electrical forces were pointing down toward leads II and III. However, at this time it was not understood that the ST vector from transmural ischemia would point away from the heart rather than toward its center.

A number of experiments in the following years showed that electrode location, as well as the size of the ischemic region, affected the magnitude and direction of ST-segment change [6, 7]. In 1933, Frank Wilson applied many of the recently developed electric field theories to the electrocardiogram [8]. Specifically, he developed his central terminal and used the solid angle theorem to evaluate proximity effects [9, 10].

4.1.2.1 The Electrocardiogram to Index the Extent and Severity of Ischemia

In the early 1970s, Braunwald and Maroko proposed that altering myocardial energy supply and demand following coronary occlusion might influence the extent and severity of ischemic injury [11]. They looked to ST-segment elevation on the electrocardiogram as a simple and reproducible means of indexing ischemia. Studies utilizing epicardial electrodes in animals reported that the severity and extent of myocardial ischemia-infarction could be reduced by different therapies including propanolol, nitroglycerin, norepinephrine, mannitol, hypertonic glucose, hyaluronidase, hydrocortisone, cobra venom factor, and others. However, these investigators did not consider the physiologic and theoretical basis of the ST-elevation which had been described decades before by previous investigators. In response, Holland and Brooks performed a series of experiments where they theoretically and experimentally tested the effects of spatial and non-spatial factors on changes in the ST segment in the pig heart [12, 13]. They demonstrated that epicardial ST-segment measurements were not reliable markers of the extent of ischemia, and that increasing size of ischemia could lead to a decrease in the amount of ST-elevation when the electrode was located on the center of the ischemic area. They explained this finding by using solid angle theory.

Following the publications by Holland and Brooks, Braunwald and Maroko published an editorial: "ST-segment mapping: Realistic and unrealistic expectations" [14]. Indeed, direct histological methods to determine infarct size later showed that infarct size expressed as a percentage of the perfusion area was not significantly altered by any of these proposed early therapies [15]. However, this initial work helped stimulate two key fields of research: (1) detailed characterization of the electrophysiology of ischemia and (2) a search for interventions that could limit infarct size.

4.1.2.2 Current and Future Perspective

In the same way as investigators turned to the electrocardiogram when investigations to limit infarct size developed in the 1970s, physicians have recently turned to the electrocardiogram to identify heart failure patients with suspected LV dyssynchrony who might benefit from cardiac resynchronization therapy (CRT) with biventricular pacemakers. This is logical if the patient has a left bundle branch block type electrical activation with considerable delay between contraction of the septum and LV free wall. However, investigators have not used identification of the morphology of LBBB as a criterion for CRT, but rather a QRS duration >120 ms. Not surprisingly, one-third of patients do not respond to CRT. As will be described in this chapter, there are a number of other pathologies that can affect QRS duration which do not have significant asynchrony between the septum and the LV free wall, namely left and right ventricular hypertrophy, left anterior-superior fascicular block, left inferior-posterior fascicular block, right bundle branch block, intra/peri-infarction block, fibrosis, and any combination of these pathologies. Grant and Dodge [16] studied patients with ECGs before and after new onset LBBB and observed that all patients had a QRS duration ≥140 ms with LBBB. Furthermore, as described in this chapter, combinations of fascicular blocks and LVH can cause QRS durations >140 ms that can only be differentiated by QRS morphology. In this chapter, we will make a conscious effort to relate three-dimensional anatomy, electrophysiology, and vector concepts to interpreting ECGs and vectorcardiograms.

4.1.3 Nomenclature and Definitions

The extent of a completed myocardial infarct (MI), defined as the death of myocardial cells from loss of their blood supply, can vary from a few dozen cells replaced by scar, i.e., a microinfarct, to a very large scar from one or more infarcts replacing 50% or more of the heart. Commonly, the term myocardial infarct is used for focal lesions of 1 cm^3 (50–60 million cells) or more caused by major atheromatous and clot occlusion in one or more coronary arteries. *Throughout this chapter, we will use the term* ***acute myocardial infarction*** *for the early process of creating these very large clusters of dead and dying cells and* ***myocardial infarct*** *when the process has been completed, with dead and necrotic cells being, or having been, replaced by a collagen scar.* Microscopic scars that have replaced a few hundred to a few thousand cells can pathologically and etiologically properly be called micro-infarcts, and larger clusters of scar replacing a few hundred thousand cells can properly be called macro-infarcts. However, in order to separate these minute scars that generally occur with peripheral small vessel disease from the larger ones of 1 cm^3 or more, described above, *it is conventional to refer to clusters of small (micro or macro) scars as* ***local, multifocal, or diffuse myocardial fibrosis.***

4.1.3.1 Myocardial Subdivisions

As far as nomenclature of the various myocardial regions is concerned considerable inconsistency and ambiguity exist in the pathology literature, the ECG literature, and in the literature of the various disciplines concerned with imaging the heart. In 1984, the Committee on Nomenclature of Myocardial Wall Segments of the International Society of Computerized Electrocardiography [17] recommended the adoption of a 12-segment left ventricular (LV) subdivision (➋ Fig. 4.1) based on the Ideker 24 LV segment [18] and the Horan et al. 12 LV segment subdivision [19]. The earlier Ideker subdivision was made up of eight circumferential (octant) subdivisions starting with the center of the septum in serial bread-loaf cross sections of the heart as shown in the mid LV cross section, lower right of ➋ Fig. 4.1. Each two adjacent octants were

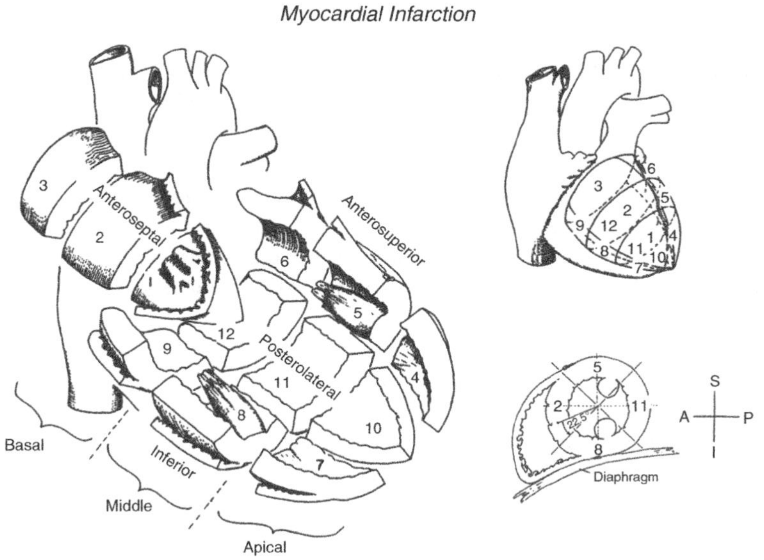

Fig. 4.1
12-segment LV subdivision recommended by the Committee on Nomenclature of Myocardial Wall Segments of the International Society of Computerized Electrocardiography. It is derived from the circumferential octant subdivision of Ideker with 24 LV segments merged to a quadrant subdivision of 12 segments as described in the text. The original octant boundaries are indicated by the *dotted lined* in the *lower right portion* of the figure (*A* anterior, *P* posterior, *S* superior, *I* inferior)

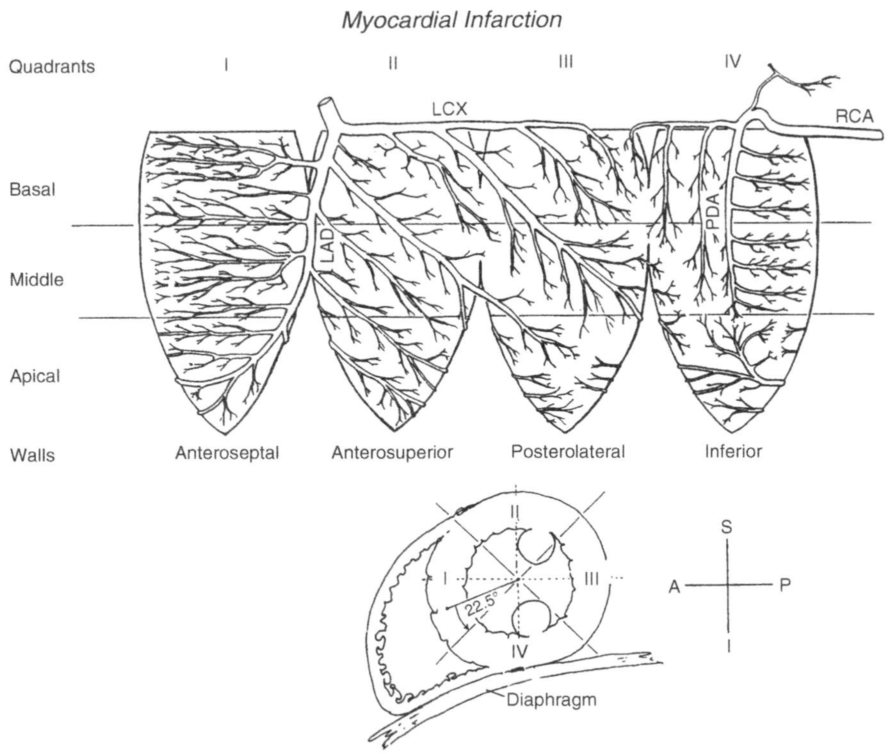

Fig. 4.2
A Mercator projection of the epicardial surface of the left ventricle with a typical distribution of the three major coronary arteries. This specific circumferential quadrant subdivision has the advantage of dividing the left ventricle along the lines of the perfusion beds of the three main arteries. As indicated in the cross section of the heart below, the superior 75–80% of the anteroseptal wall is perfused by septal perforator branches of the left anterior descending (LAD). The inferior 20–25% of the septum is perfused by the shorter septal branches of the posterior (inferior) descending artery (PDA), one of the two distal branches of the right coronary artery (RCA) and is included in the inferior wall. The other distal posterolateral branch of the RCA perfuses the other half of the inferior quadrant via 2–4 marginal branches. As indicated in this diagram, the LAD typically supplies all of the three apical (anteroseptal, anterosuperior, inferior) segments and the distal half of the apical posterolateral segment. It also supplies the remaining anteroseptal and anterosuperior walls. The basal segment of the anterosuperior wall has a dual blood supply. Except for the distal half of the apical segment, the posterolateral wall is supplied by the left circumflex (LCX) coronary artery

combined to provide a quadrant subdivision of four walls: Octant 1 and 2, as anteroseptal, 3 and 4 as anterosuperior, 5 and 6 as posterolateral and 7 and 8 as inferior. Octant 1 was set in the mid septum with the lower anteroseptal boundary dividing the septum, 3/4th for the longer septal arteries from the left anterior descending, and 1/4th for the shorter septals from the posterior descending. The LV was further subdivided from apex to base into three regions (apical, middle, and basal) by passing three planes at right angles to the **internal** long axis of the LV. This internal long axis is divided into three equal parts, thereby producing the final 12 segments of approximately equal volume as shown in ➋ Fig. 4.1. This quadrant subdivision of 4 walls of 3 segments each has the advantage, as shown in ➋ Fig. 4.2, that the boundaries of the perfusion beds of each of the three main coronary arteries usually overlay segmental boundaries. An analogous recommendation appeared at about the same time from the Committee on Nomenclature and Standards of the American Society of Echocardiography [20]. The anatomic landmarks, definition and nomenclature of the 12 LV segments, which are shown in ➋ Fig. 4.1, will be used throughout this chapter.

4.1.3.2 Extent and Sites of Myocardial Infarction and Related Coronary Artery Occlusions

Considerable inconsistency and ambiguity also exists with respect to the labeling of the extent, transmurality, and location of infarcts. The evolution of the labeling of extent/transmurality is as follows: Myocardial infarcts (MIs) with abnormal Q waves have been called transmural and those without were labeled as subendocardial. In later years, a number of investigations [21–23] documented that many of the "transmural" MIs were limited to the subendocardium at autopsy and the absence of abnormal Q waves was noted in a significant number of pathoanatomically large transmural MIs. Thus, in the earlier era of non-reperfusion, descriptive labels "Q-wave MI" and "non-Q MI" gained common usage. In the current early reperfusion era, patients with persistent or unstable resting chest pain and major ST elevation (so called ST elevation MI – or STEMI) have been labeled "acute injury/infarction" with the expectation that a (transmural) Q-wave MI would evolve; those with such chest pain and 1) sub threshold localizing ST elevation or 2) significant ST depression (Non STEMI ECGs) were labeled probable subendocardial infarction. Again, a number of patients with STEMI failed to develop abnormal Q waves and a number with NSTEMI did. The labeling of location and extent of evolving myocardial infarcts has also undergone a similar evolution. The 2007 ACC/AHA guidelines [24] for the management of NSTEMI/UA (Unstable Angina), a subset of Acute Coronary Syndrome, has defined the two major subgroups, (1) and (2) above, of NSTEMI as "High Risk NSTEMI." These groups had a higher in hospital, 30 day and 1 year mortality than acutely revascularized STEMI. These are STEMI equivalents and should be considered for emergency coronary angiography with the intention of performing PCI (percutaneous coronary intervention) or referral to emergency bypass surgery.

The structures and regions in question are all in the human thorax, where the anatomic conventions of the upright human have become widely used: superior, toward the head (cephalad); inferior, toward the feet (caudad); anterior, toward the front of the subject (ventral); and posterior, toward the back (dorsal). The ambiguity in terminology and the plethora of terms, including many hyphenated terms for location (and extent) of MI and cardiac anatomy that have evolved through the last two centuries have arisen from two main sources: (1) the lack of strict adherence to the anatomic conventions of the upright human described above and (2) the fact that the long axis of the heart (and the apex of the LV) is angled forward at about 30° from the frontal plane and downward from the horizontal plane at about the same angle. Three well-defined groups of localized myocardial infarcts can be identified anatomically and angiographically, each being associated with occlusion of one of the three major coronary arteries and/or their branches. Infarcts in each of these arterial distributions range in size from being very small to very large.

Of the ambiguous and at times contradictory terms used to designate location and extent of infarcts, the most contradictory and confusing is "lateral." For infarcts involving the distal LAD and the LV apex with ST elevation and or abnormal Qs in one or more of I, V5, V6, electrocardiographers commonly report "lateral infarct"; if V4 is involved they report "anterolateral" infarct, and when aVL is involved, "high lateral." Early pathoanatomists called the wall between the papillary muscles "lateral," as seen in the LCX distribution in ➋ Fig. 4.2. This wall is still being so labeled by some who are currently imaging the heart. Electrophysiologists dealing with accessory pathways from the atrium to the ventricles tend to call tracts to the base of the right ventricle "anterolateral bypass tracts," and those to the mid basal left ventricle "posterolateral bypass tracts." The inferior wall was labeled posterior by early pathoanatomists, cardiologists and electrocardiographers. It has evolved through diaphragmatic to inferior over the past 60 years. Thanks to earlier AHA guidelines, the most inconsistent of this set is often the basal segment of the inferior wall still being called posterobasal in some recent reports. But this appears to be on the wane. The branch of the RCA supplying the inferior wall is in general called the posterior descending artery (PDA), while there is still reference to the posterior papillary muscle which originates from the inferior wall.

To be simple, brief, and anatomically consistent, the anatomic conventions of the upright human will be used throughout this chapter. For the sake of clear interchange between electrocardiographers, vectorcardiographers and those engaged in the various disciplines that image the heart and thorax, the following nomenclature is strongly recommended.

(a) *Anterior myocardial infarct* (with size modifiers in [f] below) is used for all infarcts resulting from occlusion of the left anterior descending (LAD) coronary artery. This involves both the anteroseptal and anterosuperior walls and usually the inferior apical segment, (see ➋ Fig. 4.2). Anterosuperior myocardial infarct (with size modifiers in [f] below) is used for occlusion of the major diagonal branch of the LAD.

(b) *Posterolateral myocardial infarct* (with modifiers in (f) below) refers to all infarcts resulting from occlusion of the posterior left circumflex (LCX) coronary artery or its branches. This involves mainly the posterolateral wall (see ➋ Fig. 4.2).

(c) *Inferior myocardial infarct* (with modifiers in (f) below) includes all infarcts resulting from occlusion of the usually dominant right coronary artery (RCA) which supplies the posterior (inferior) descending coronary artery (PDA) and its posterolateral branches (as shown in ➋ Fig. 4.2). This usually involves mainly the middle and basal segments of the inferior wall.

(d) *Note*: The term "*posterolateral-inferior myocardial infarct*" (with modifiers in (f) below) will be used in the special case where a combination of (b) and (c) occurs with significant infarction of both the posterolateral wall and the inferior wall of the LV. This commonly occurs from occlusion of a dominant LCX artery, which also has the PDA as its most distal branch. It may also occur from occlusion of a rare dominant RCA with a very large posterolateral branch and a diminutive LCX.

(e) *Apical extension*, with ECG and spatial vector changes in right to left apically oriented leads I, aVR, V4, V5, V6, and X, most commonly occurs with an anterior infarct, in which case the size modifiers below indicate apical extension. A specific notation of "with apical extension" or "anteroapical infarct." while quite appropriate, is redundant. Significant apical extension can occur as a part of local posterolateral or inferior infarct, in which case it is appropriate not only to use the probability and size modifiers but to specify "posteroapical," "inferoapical" or "with apical extension." Because of the ambiguous and variable, often contradictory usage of "lateral" by the many disciplines that describe regional cardiac anatomy [25], the term will be used here only in combination with posterior for the posterolateral wall of the LV.

(f) *Probability modifiers such as* **consider, possible, probable and none** and *Size modifiers such as* **small, moderate, large** and **very large** will be used with each infarct diagnostic category in order to indicate both the ECG reader's confidence in the interpretation and the extent of the infarct. The quantification of extent or size of the infarct linked to size modifiers and the statistical basis for their combination with the probability modifiers are dealt with in more detail in ➋ Sect. 4.3, and ➋ Table 4.3.

4.1.3.3 Myocardial Fibrosis (Multifocal Infarct): Etiology and Common Terms

By definition, infarction is the death of any tissue as a result of disruption of its nutrient blood supply. The resultant myocardial infarct may be a consequence of major atheromatous and clot occlusion in the proximal coronary arteries, or arteriolar micro vascular disease such as in diabetes and hypersensitivity vasculitis, rheumatic disease, collagen disease and so on. In this case, the resultant infarct is very small and multifocal owing to small-vessel occlusion, and may be irregularly scattered throughout the heart or may be uniformly distributed. A similar mechanism can be seen in viral and bacterial vasculitis with intramural and perivascular infiltrate, leading to multifocal local arteriolar occlusion and multifocal infarct. Diffuse fibrosis, by this mechanism, causes excessive fragmentation of the QRS complex as seen on a high-gain high-frequency (1,000 samples/s and signal averaged) ECG. In many patients of this group, there is a mixed inflammatory and hypersensitivity response, but the myocardial consequence is similar, that is, many small-vessel occlusions leading to multifocal infarcts. The changes as a result of myocarditis are discussed in more detail in ➋ Chap. 8 along with the infiltrative diseases of the heart.

The ECG changes produced by these multifocal infarcts depend upon the extent or size of each focal area of necrosis. If these are minute (<0.5 mm across), and diffuse the main consequence will be an overall loss in myocardial substance. The lesions are so small that except for decreased voltage, they produce little discernible local change even in high-gain high-fidelity ECG records. When individual local macro-infarcts are both larger (2–3 mm across) and multifocal, extensive high-frequency notching and fragmentation of the entire QRS in the 150–300 Hz range may occur. While the term "multifocal myocardial infarct" for both micro- and macro- lesions is pathologically and etiologically appropriate, common medical usage has linked the term "myocardial infarct" to larger, more discrete infarcts associated with major coronary artery occlusion. The term "myocardial fibrosis" has gained common usage for these minute infarcts. We will use the term myocardial fibrosis for the usual appropriate modifiers to indicate the severity and extent of the process, and to describe the ECG changes associated with these lesions. They may be either "localized" or "diffuse."

4.1.3.4 High Frequency Signal Averaged ECG Recording

The term "high frequency ECG" has come to be associated with signal averaging and 1,000 samples per second (sps) digitizing rate. This sampling rate covers the upper frequency range of 400 Hz. To make maximal use of these higher frequencies, ECG preamplifiers are adapted to be 2.5–3x the usual upper response rate of 150 Hz of conventional ECG recorders. For the signal averaging process, a typical P QRS T waveform for a specific ECG is chosen as the template for the complete cycle. Each following beat or cycle is compared to the template. Those with a high correlation with the template are time aligned with it to the nearest ms (millisecond) and averaged together. Waveforms that are ectopic, aberrant, or very noisy are excluded by this process. Muscle artifact, electromagnetic noise, and baseline wander that is not systematically related to the ECG waveform are suppressed by the averaging of the time aligned ECG signals. The number of beats that must be averaged together depends on the resolution desired for any application, and the severity of the baseline artifact or noise that needs to be suppressed. This methodology is also used for low amplitude high frequency QRS late potentials and for detailed high resolution digital P wave studies. (see ➋ Chap. 4 of *Specialized Aspects of ECG*).

4.1.4 Regional Distribution of Myocardial Infarcts and Coronary Anatomy

Atherosclerotic occlusive coronary artery disease generally occurs in the proximal third of the coronary tree and involves major branches of this system, often near bifurcations. The posterior descending artery, usually a distal branch of the right coronary artery is the major exception to this rule. The extent of evolving infarction from proximal coronary occlusion in any artery perfusion bed is a function of the size of the area at risk [26]. It is also inversely related to the amount of effective forward collateral circulation that developed around the obstructive lesion and into the area at risk beyond and/or retrograde to collaterals, from well perfused neighboring coronary vascular areas [27]. The size of the associated infarct may vary from none visible angiographically (as in 15–20% of all total occlusions) to all or nearly all of the area at risk in a given perfusion bed (8–10% of all total occlusions). Even though the coronary occlusion is in the proximal few centimeters, in most occlusions smaller infarcts tend to localize to the distal distribution of the involved artery. They are mostly subendocardial consistent with Reimer and Jennings' "wave model of infarction" [28].

4.1.4.1 Left Anterior Descending (LAD) Coronary Artery Occlusion

The resulting infarcts from LAD occlusions, when small, tend to localize at the anterior apex (➋ Fig. 4.3). Moderate-sized infarcts involve the apex and more of the middle segments of the anteroseptal and anterosuperior wall. Large infarcts involve the apex circumferentially and most, or all, of the middle anteroseptal and anterosuperior walls. Very large infarcts involve the same regions and usually extend into the basal segments of the anteroseptal and anterosuperior walls. However, complete involvement of these basal segments even with very large infarcts is uncommon. Four main locations of the LAD coronary artery produce four smaller subsets of these various-sized anterior infarcts as follows:

(a) The mid to distal LAD in most patients, with its "wrap around" onto the distal third of the inferior wall, perfuses the two anteroapical segments of ➋ Fig 4.2, the inferoapical segment and a variable portion of the posteroapical segment. The size of any infarct from distal LAD occlusion thus may vary from small to moderate. In the occasional patient with a very dominant LAD and extension of the "wrap around" well into the inferior middle segment, the infarct may be large. Mid LAD occlusion distal to the first large diagonal may also result in large infarcts.
(b) The proximal main diagonal branch of the LAD perfuses the basal and middle segments of the anterosuperior wall with variable extension to the apical posterolateral segment (see ➋ Fig. 4.2). Any infarct from proximal occlusion of this diagonal branch is usually small, occasionally moderate in size, following the diagonal perfusion bed across the anterosuperior wall.
(c) The proximal first septal perforator branch of the LAD perfuses the basal segment of the anteroseptal wall. Isolated occlusion of this branch is uncommon, and the associated infarct is generally small.

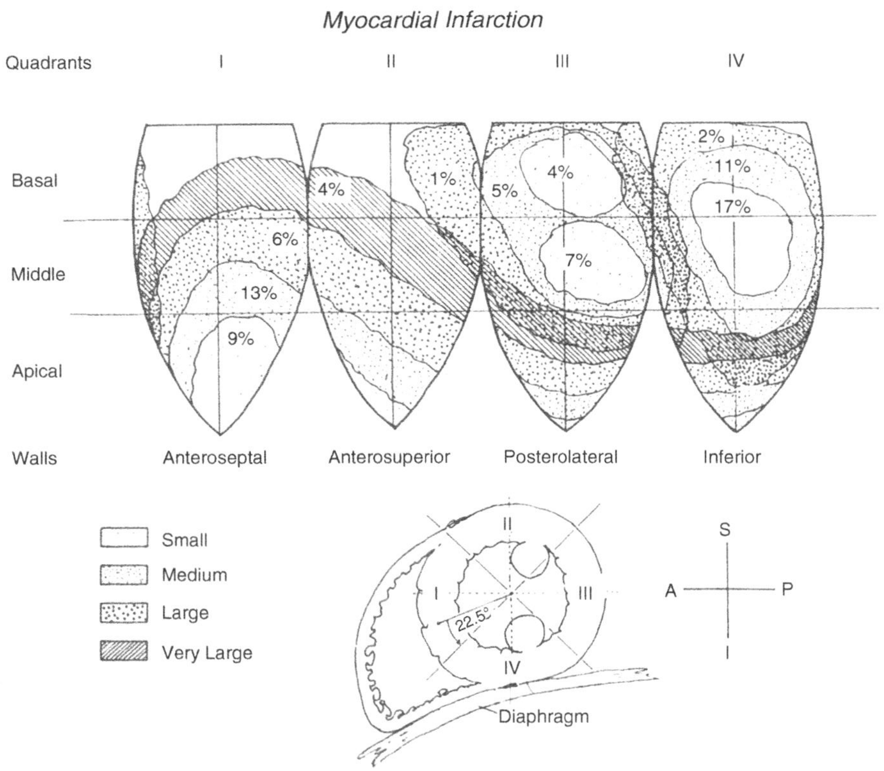

Fig. 4.3
The same mercator projection of the epicardial surface of the left ventricle as shown in Fig. 4.2. Shown here is the regional distribution of the single infarcts seen on biplane ventriculograms (79% of visible infarcts from the Rancho/USC database*). Not included in this figure are the 21% of patients with multiple infarcts. Note that the majority of these single infarcts involve less than half of the potential risk area, and when small tend to localize in the distal distribution of the particular vascular bed. As a result of the smaller areas potentially at risk, posterolateral and inferior infarcts tend to be small to moderate in size. Large to very large anterior infarcts involving more than 25% of the left ventricle, with the concomitant severe dysfunction and ejection fraction below 40% occur in 10% of all of these single infarcts but occurs in only 1% for posterolateral infarcts and 2% for inferior infarcts. By contrast, well over half of the 21% of patients with multiple infarcts have the sum of infarcts as large to very large, severe LV dysfunction and ejection fractions usually well below 40%. * Footnote: Beginning in 1967 the Rancho Los Amigos Medical Center campus of the University of Southern California (Rancho/USC) instituted a post-infarction and chronic angina cardiac rehabilitation program. The coronary angiographic database referred to in this figure, and throughout this chapter, consisted of 701 patients from this program. Biplane ventriculograms of 603 revealed local wall motion abnormalities in the distribution of an occluded coronary artery consistent with myocardial infarct. A single infarct was present in 476/603 (79%). Multiple infarcts were noted in 127/603 (21%). An additional 74 patients had one or more totally occluded coronary arteries and no visible infarct. Another 24 had severe multi-vessel coronary disease and diffuse wall motion abnormality (hypokinesis) with no localization, and a low ejection fraction consistent with severe ischemic myopathy

(d) The LAD perfuses more than 50% of the LV. Occlusion of this artery proximal to the first diagonal and the first septal perforator, produces a sum of all the effects a, b, and c, above. Depending on how late in life this occurred and how aggressive was the formation of collaterals around the obstruction and from the other two major coronary arteries, the infarct size can vary from non existent (15–20% of such occlusions) to very large and lethal.

4.1.4.2 Non-Dominant Left Circumflex (LCX) Occlusion

Three locations of occlusion are found, usually in the proximal third of the LCX distribution. The resultant infarct size varies from none to all of the specific area at risk. The three cases are as follows:

(a) Left obtuse (main) marginal circumflex occlusion usually occurs at or near its origin. The region of perfusion for this artery is mainly the middle segment of the posterolateral wall with variable extension into adjacent regions (➋ Fig. 4.2). Small infarcts are usually localized in the middle posterolateral segment near its junction with the apical posterolateral, middle inferior and apical inferior segments (see ➋ Fig. 4.3). Moderately sized posterolateral infarcts involve most or all of the posterolateral mid-region with extension to the aforementioned adjacent regions as well. Large infarcts are uncommon with occlusion of this branch of the LCX.

(b) Local occlusions also occur in the distal circumflex beyond the branch point of the proximal LCX into the main marginal and distal branch. Total occlusion of the distal non-dominant LCX usually produces small basal posterolateral infarcts (➋ Figs. 4.2 and ➋ 4.3).

(c) Total occlusion of the proximal non-dominant LCX produces a combination of the effects of (a) and (b). Subsequent infarcts may range in size from virtually nothing (15–20% of such occlusions) to moderate or large posterolateral infarction involving most of the posterolateral wall, usually with extension onto some of the inferior wall.

4.1.4.3 Dominant Left Circumflex (LCX) Occlusion

Only 10–15% of subjects have a dominant LCX in which the posterior descending artery is a branch of the circumflex. Under these circumstances, the circumflex perfuses about half of the left ventricle while the LAD perfuses the other half. Very large infarcts occur with total occlusion of such an LCX artery in about the same percentage of patients as with total LAD occlusion. The low incidence of left dominant anatomy, however, accounts for the very low incidence of single-vessel LCX occlusion with very large posterior-inferior infarcts (0.4% of angiographically demonstrable single infarcts) as compared to single-vessel LAD occlusion and very large anterior infarcts of 4%. In 15–20% of cases with proximal total occlusion of a dominant LCX with good collaterals, like other major coronary arteries, there will be no angiographically demonstrable infarct. Small infarcts usually involve the middle posterolateral and inferior regions (➋ Fig. 4.3). Moderately sized infarcts extend into the inferior posterior base and usually somewhat toward the apex. Large infarcts involve most or all of the inferior and posterolateral mid-region and base, and extend into the apex and the inferior anteroseptal wall.

4.1.4.4 Right Coronary Artery (RCA) Occlusion

Most occlusions of the right coronary artery occur in the proximal third, although a significant number of patients have occlusion of this artery in the middle third, or where the posterior descending artery branches off. The proximal occlusions have a significant incidence of right ventricular involvement whereas the distal occlusions do not. The ECG criteria for the diagnosis of this variable right ventricular infarct are presented in ➋ Sect. 4.4.5. The effect on the left ventricle of all three locations of total occlusion of the right coronary artery is similar. One fourth of these occlusions occur with little or no infarction. When present, small infarcts are usually in the inferior mid-region (➋ Fig. 4.3). Moderately sized inferior infarcts will have extended into the basal segments of the inferior and posterolateral walls. Larger inferior infarcts are uncommon and, when present, may extend into the inferior apex, into the lower third of the middle and basal segments of the septum, and into the lower third or more of the entire posterolateral wall. These RCA lesions are associated with a very right dominant coronary artery with a large posterolateral branch and a minimal circumflex. They would be indistinguishable, both anatomically and by ECG, from a mid total occlusion of a dominant LCX artery except in acute infarctions, for the absence of ECG and clinical signs of acute right ventricular infarct in the latter.

In summary, the relationships of size and location of angiographically demonstrable first or single infarct and the percentage distributions of each in the major coronary perfusion beds are shown in ➋ Fig. 4.3. Single local infarcts that are a result of RCA or LCX occlusion are usually small (28% of all infarcts), are occasionally moderate in size (12%) and are only rarely large to very large (3%). On the other hand, anterior infarcts from LAD occlusion are approximately equally distributed between small (10% of all infarcts), moderate (7%), and large to very large (10%). It is prudent to take these prior probabilities as to size and location into account, looking for subtle mid and late (non Q) loss of QRS forces when interpreting ECGs.

4.1.4.5 Multiple-Vessel Occlusion

Multiple lesions from multiple-vessel occlusions account for 21% of all patients with coronary disease and myocardial infarct in the Rancho Los Amigos Hospital, University of Southern California (Rancho/USC) database. While total occlusion of two or three vessels does occur without visible infarct or demonstrable ventricular dysfunction, it is uncommon. In the Rancho/USC series of 45–65 year olds, patients with documented coronary disease, 14% have total occlusion of 1 vessel, 5% have total occlusion of two vessels, and 2% have total occlusion of three vessels without visible infarct on biplane ventriculograms. Not unexpectedly, it is much more usual for multiple-vessel occlusion to be associated with significant infarcts. Three fourths have significant or severe ventricular dysfunction. This is generally because the total extent of infarcts exceeds 30–40% of the LV. The distribution of the extent of damage from multiple occlusions in this dysfunctional subset is as follows: 10% of this group have two small discrete local infarcts that together involve <15%LV; 15% have multiple infarcts with the total extent of damage involving 15–24% LV; 30% of multiple lesions are localized larger infarcts totaling 25–35% LV; and 45% have extensive damage overall of more than 35% of the LV, severe LV dysfunction, and a very poor prognosis. One third of these multiple lesions will not show the "classic changes" of myocardial infarct, but will in general show the extensive QRS slurring and/or notching/splintering, attenuation of R or S, and abnormal R/Q or R/S ratios that will be covered in detail in ➋ Sect. 4.3. In 2–3% of all clinical infarcts, severe diffuse ischemic myopathy occurs without obvious localized or regional wall dysfunction. These patients have diffuse and extensive scarring (ischemic cardiomyopathy) at pathological examination that is often unrelated to the overlying specific coronary occlusive lesions.

4.2 Infarct Anatomy and Related Electrophysiology

4.2.1 Geometry and Anatomy of Typical Myocardial Infarcts

Although occlusion of a proximal coronary artery produces a spectrum of changes, from no pathological change to very large infarcts, there is a rather typical anatomy of these lesions related to their size. Generally, infarcts of increasing size develop along the "wavefront" model of Reimer et al. [28] in any coronary distribution. Small infarcts 2–3 cm in diameter are in general limited to the subendocardial half of the myocardial wall. Moderate 4–6 cm lesions generally extend into the subepicardial half of the wall in their central one third, while their peripheral two thirds are subendocardial. The largest infarcts have a similar geometry, most extending to the epicardium in their central third. The shaggy outer border zone of the moderate healed infarct in ➋ Fig. 4.4 is an example of the typical admixture of interdigitating islands of collagenous scar and viable electrically active myocardium that is the determinant of the local electric field generated from an infarcted region. An understanding of this complex geometry is the prerequisite to the rational interpretation of surface ECG changes. Infarcts of the size shown in the figure usually are not truly "transmural," because they have significant viable subepicardial myocardium surviving over their central region. While not shown here, in infarcts with substantial replacement of necrotic myocardial cells by collagen scar, the scar shrinks with time, producing considerable thinning of the wall of the heart. In section AA in ➋ Fig. 4.4, the effect of the complex border zone where activation fronts must thread their way through and around large pseudopods and islands of scar is clearly evident. The active area of the local electromotive surface changes rapidly, and varies considerably as it moves around the infarct through the viable subepicardium. Since these fronts approach each other as they progress toward the epicardial center over the infarct, they tend to cancel out much of the current fields coming from the "shrinking doughnut" of the excitation wave as it extinguishes itself. This local disruption of the usual continuity of the activation fronts accounts for the remarkable increase in high frequency splintering and notching of the QRS complex. These changes are readily seen in properly

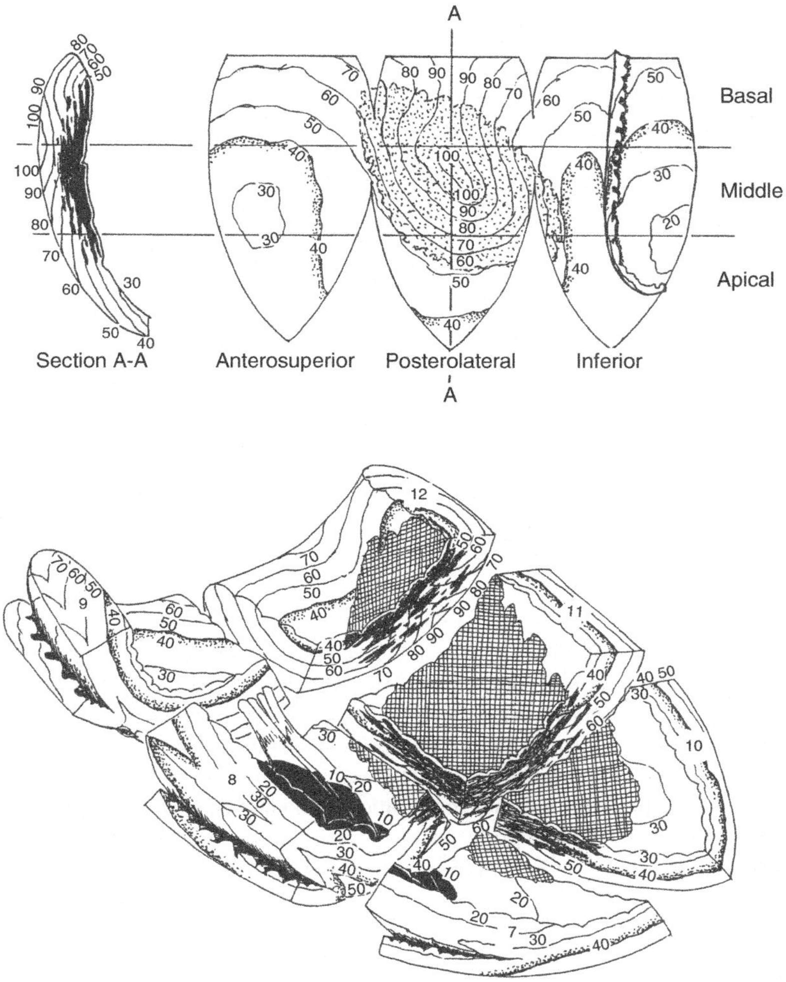

Fig. 4.4
Diagrammatic representation of a small posterolateral infarct in the distribution of the main marginal branch of the LCX, as seen in ➋ Fig. 4.2. It involves mainly the middle segment of the posterolateral wall. Isochrones of activation at 10 ms intervals are indicated beginning, as shown in *black*, at the base of the inferior papillary muscle. The mercator projection of the same unrolled LV, except for the anteroseptal wall, is shown in the upper portion of the figure. The infarct shown is confluent in the subendocardium, extends midway through the wall in a small central portion of the middle segment. As is typical of such lesions it has extensive islands and pseudopods of inactive scar interdigitating with electrically and histologically normal myocardium throughout the border zone of the infarct. As the result of the dense scar, activation can only reach the viable epicardial layers of the LV wall from around the border of the infarct, delaying activation of this part of the heart. In the border zones, the activation fronts encounter many small local scars, producing a significant increase in high frequency components of the signal arising from the region. The main surface ECG changes from this lesion will be noted at 30–100 ms into the QRS. There will be significant loss of posterior forces, notching, slurring of the mid-to-late QRS. The attenuation of these posterior vectors leads to an imbalance in the anterior-posterior forces seen in leads V1, V2, V3, and *Z* as smaller S (post.) and larger R (ant.) waves and increased R/S (ant/post) ratios

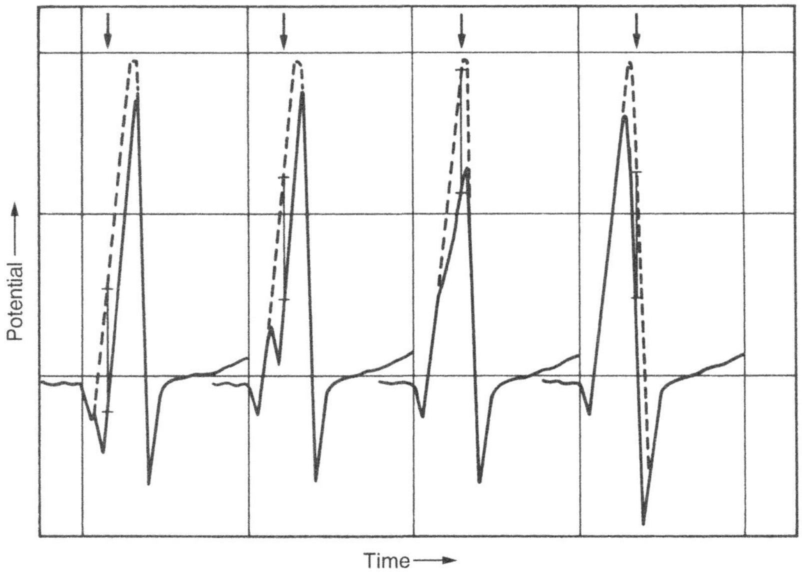

Fig. 4.5

The four panels represent V6 with a small infarct (15 × 7 mm) placed at various levels in the junction of the inferior and posteroapical segment of the propagation model of the heart. The *dotted line* in each case represents the normal activation without infarct as seen in V6. In the *first panel* the lesion is placed in the endocardium. In each of the following panels, the center of the lesion is moved outward by 2.5 mm. The *arrows* represent the time when the activation front passed the center of the small lesion in each instance. In the first case abnormal Q waves were produced only by a very strategically placed lesion. Notched R ("bite out"), attenuated peak R or a change in R/S ratio are equally valid markers of infarction in the wall of the left ventricle. In basal segments in general, and in middle posterolateral segments activated in the mid to later portions of the QRS, only mid to late QRS changes will result from even extensive infarction.

recorded high frequency, high gain unipolar epicardial electrograms and surface ECGs. Changes are most evident in leads perpendicular to the advancing wavefront in the myocardium, and occur, of course, at that time in the QRS when the local region is being activated. Large infarcts (30–35% LV) usually extend to the epicardium in a circular area a few cm across, but in many a 2–3 mm "peel" of normal electrically active myocardium is still present. This phenomenon can account for low amplitude high frequency "after potentials" occurring well beyond the end of the QRS (as usually measured), and into the ST segment (see ➋ Chap. 1 of *Specialized Aspects of ECG*).

It is worth noting that commercially available digital ECG recording systems that digitize at a 4 ms (250 Hz) interval, will significantly attenuate the high frequency signal from the border zones of the infarct as described above. Most current ECG recorders now digitize at 2 ms (500 Hz). A 1 ms or less sampling interval (1,000 Hz) is needed to record accurately this potentially important electrical signal information.

4.2.2 Sensitivity of Conventional ECG Criteria for Infarcts

Well controlled pathology studies noted earlier [21–23] have demonstrated the low sensitivity of conventional ECG criteria for infarct. These data have shown that between 40% and 50% of all confluent healed infarcts 2 cm or larger are not associated with "classic" QRS changes of infarction. The data summarized in ➋ Figs. 4.3 and ➋ 4.5 pinpoint the reason for the poor showing of these criteria. These are as follows:

(a) 15% of all infarcts are limited to the base of the LV and posterolateral wall which is activated during the latter half of the QRS, and thus does not produce initial QRS changes.
(b) 20% of infarcts are small (2–3 cm in diameter) involving less than 10% LV and have only notching, "bite outs," slurring (see ➋ Fig. 4.5 panel 2), and attenuation of R waves, or other non-classic QRS changes (panels 3 and 4).
(c) 7% are multiple and the sum larger in size, with neutralizing (cancellation) effects. For example, a typical anterior infarct is masked by a second inferior posterolateral infarct, or vice versa.
(d) 5% of all infarcts will have had preexisting or new LBBB, or ventricular pacing, and an infarct that would not be diagnosable by classic criteria in the presence of these conduction abnormalities.
(e) 3% are patients with diffuse ischemic myopathy without classic QRS changes of infarct.

The vast majority of these patients will have high frequency notching, mid to late attenuation of QRS vectors, abnormal R/S or R/Q ratios, or other major changes described below in the section on quantification of myocardial infarcts. When prior ECGs are in fact available for comparison, the absence of serial changes is predictive of an unchanged ventriculogram with a remarkable 98% reliability [29]. Furthermore, the magnitude and duration of a change, if present, correlates well ($r = 0.92$) with the size of the new lesion or the change in LV ejection fraction (LVEF) seen on the ventriculogram (see ➋ Figs. 4.13 and ➋ 4.14 part a, with more detail later in the chapter). The classic criteria must then be expanded to include lesser changes such as abnormal notching, slurring or "bite out," abnormal R/S, R/Q ratios, and related changes, in order to diagnose the smaller 2–3 cm infarcts. They must also be expanded to include mid and terminal QRS abnormalities in order to diagnose posterolateral and basal infarction, or to quantify basal extension of infarcts of the mid-region and/or apex. Such expanded criteria have been developed using the computer simulations mentioned above and validated in a series of specificity, nuclear angiographic, and autopsy studies [30–34]. The criteria are described in detail in the ➋ Sect. 4.3 to follow, on quantification of infarcts. Both sensitivity and specificity are significantly improved by incorporating these expanded criteria into the review of serial ECGs, especially using high-gain, high-fidelity recordings.

4.2.3 His-Purkinje Relationship to Coronary Occlusion and Myocardial Infarction

Daniels, Boineau, and Cox made the important observation that because the peripheral Purkinje network is perfused by cavity blood, even with extensive transmural myocardial infarction active Purkinje potentials can be recorded from this network [35, 36]. The timing of the Purkinje excitation is changed very little by the presence of even major transmural infarction over the Purkinje recording site. While the peripheral network is usually not disrupted by infarction, proximal His Purkinje damage does occur in the major fascicles of the left bundle or in the proximal left or right bundle, producing the typical conduction defects described in (➋ Chap. 2). It is estimated that proximal conduction defects of one sort or another occur in about one half of all patients with myocardial infarct. In the remainder, the Purkinje programming of excitation to the endocardium is normal. In this case, very large myocardial infarcts can occur involving the apex or mid region of the left ventricle and produce no prolongation of ventricular activation, i.e. a normal total QRS duration. The QRS duration may in fact be slightly shortened by a septal infarct which removes the part of the heart that produces the first 10 or 15 ms of ventricular activation..

Recent onset left and right bundle branch block in the context of acute myocardial infarction has been reported in a large clinical series by Lie et al., [37]. It was observed that the incidence of recent onset RBBB was 6.6% of all acute myocardial infarcts. In this context, it was associated 20:1 with an evolving acute anterior infarct. In this series, the incidence of recent onset LBBB was 3% and was associated 3:1 with an acute inferior infarct. Persistent left anterior-superior fascicular block occurs in a number of series [38–40] in about 10% of all anterior infarcts, and we present arguments below for our support of the Grant hypothesis [41] that inferior-posterior fascicular (peri-infarction) block occurs in over 85% of all acute inferior infarcts from right coronary occlusion. The ECG changes associated with the various combinations of myocardial infarcts and these conduction abnormalities are delineated in ➋ Sect. 4.5.

4.2.4 Ventricular Activation-Recovery and Myocardial Infarction

As summarized in ➋ Chap. 4 van Dam and Durrer [42–44] have shown that in revitalized human hearts using multipoint intramural plunge electrodes mapping, ventricular activation is consistent from endocardium to epicardium. The activation sequence of the ventricles, as relates to the specific 12-segment LV subdivision of ➋ Fig. 4.1, is initiated by insertion of the middle fascicles of the proximal His Purkinje into the peripheral network on the left septal surface of the middle anteroseptal region near its junction with the apical segment. The adjacent anterior and inferior fascicles insert into their respective papillary muscles and adjacent mural myocardium. This activation sequence has been confirmed by one of the authors, RHS and associates, in a small number of patients at the time of surgery for ventricular pre-excitation, by detailed epicardial mapping and limited intramural plunge electrode recording of the normally conducted beats post-transection of the accessory pathway. An entirely normal surface ECG and body surface potential map was confirmed postoperatively in these patients. Similar data was recorded in more detail in the baboon [45] and chimpanzee. The latter was confirmed by Spach and associates [46]. This normal activation was incorporated into this group's propagation simulation in a 1 mm grid digitized normal human heart from an accident victim, and the 12-segment left ventricular subdivision was used in the development of an ECG infarct-size scoring system which will be considered in detail later (and shown in ➋ Fig. 4.16). This normal heart geometry of the 12-segment left ventricle together with the activation sequences were used to develop a teaching diagram relating this cardiac anatomy and electrophysiology to the ECG (see ➋ Fig. 4.6a). Colored isochrones for each 10 ms are those defined by the expanded color code at the lower right of this figure. Both the propagating active electromotive surface of excitation and the slower broader surface of the sequence of recovery, show effects of the local electrically dead zone of a local myocardial infarct. The details of these effects on the surface ECG will be covered in following sections.

➋ Figure 4.6b depicts the sequence of ventricular recovery in the same 12-segment LV subdivision. It is adapted from the functional refractory period data of Burgess and coworkers [47–52] and from the detailed intramural data of this phase of the cardiac cycle in the chronic closed-chest dog and chimpanzee preparations by Spach, Barr and associates [46, 53]. Recovery occurs more slowly than excitation from epicardium to endocardium as indicated by the action potentials shown at the lower right. The color coding indicates the timing of the peak of the slope of the rapid recovery phase in each region. According to Spach, Barr and associates, as shown here, the earliest recovery potentials appear on the right side of the septum which behaves electrophysiologically like the epicardium of the left ventricle. Recovery proceeds more rapidly at the base as shown in this figure and from the epicardium (B) to endocardium (A) throughout. The latest recovery potentials are seen in the endocardium in the mid regions near the apex, as shown.

4.2.4.1 Computer Simulation of Ventricular Excitation

Excitation velocities in the wall are rather uniform and the electric field is directed outward from the ventricular cavities. All portions of the electromotive surface of excitation from endocardium to epicardium contribute about equally. The wave fronts in the subendocardium are less well organized and thus somewhat less strong than in the mid-wall or subepicardium, but are by no means silent (➋ Fig. 4.7). A model of this propagating electromotive surface was developed by Solomon [45] from multipoint plunge electrode intramural bipolar electrograms of the baboon, chimpanzee, and the limited human data mentioned above. The simulation of this electromotive surface model propagating in myocardium, developed an electric field that generated intramural bipolar electrograms that matched electrograms observed in humans/primates mentioned above. The specific anatomy for the normal human heart used in the simulations was taken from cross sections of the heart of a 25-year-old accident victim digitized at a 1 cubic mm level. The specific activation sequence generated is entirely determined by the geometry of the heart, the Purkinje distribution, the insertion sites of the proximal to peripheral Purkinje network, and the propagation velocities in each. The simulation includes this heart in an inhomogeneous adult male torso, with lungs and intracardiac blood mass. It can generate body surface potential distributions that can be shown as isopotential maps, perspective plots of potential distributions, 12-lead ECGs, or VCGs for any specified lead system. ➋ Fig. 4.8 illustrates the graphic output of this propagating excitation wave in this fine grid heart simulation of normal and fascicular blocks. Part (a) of this figure shows cross sections of the apical, middle and basal myocardial subdivisions defined in ➋ Fig 4.1. In part (b), left anterior (superior) and left inferior (posterior) fascicular blocks (LAFB, LIFB), are simulated by removing the start points for the fan of the left bundle to

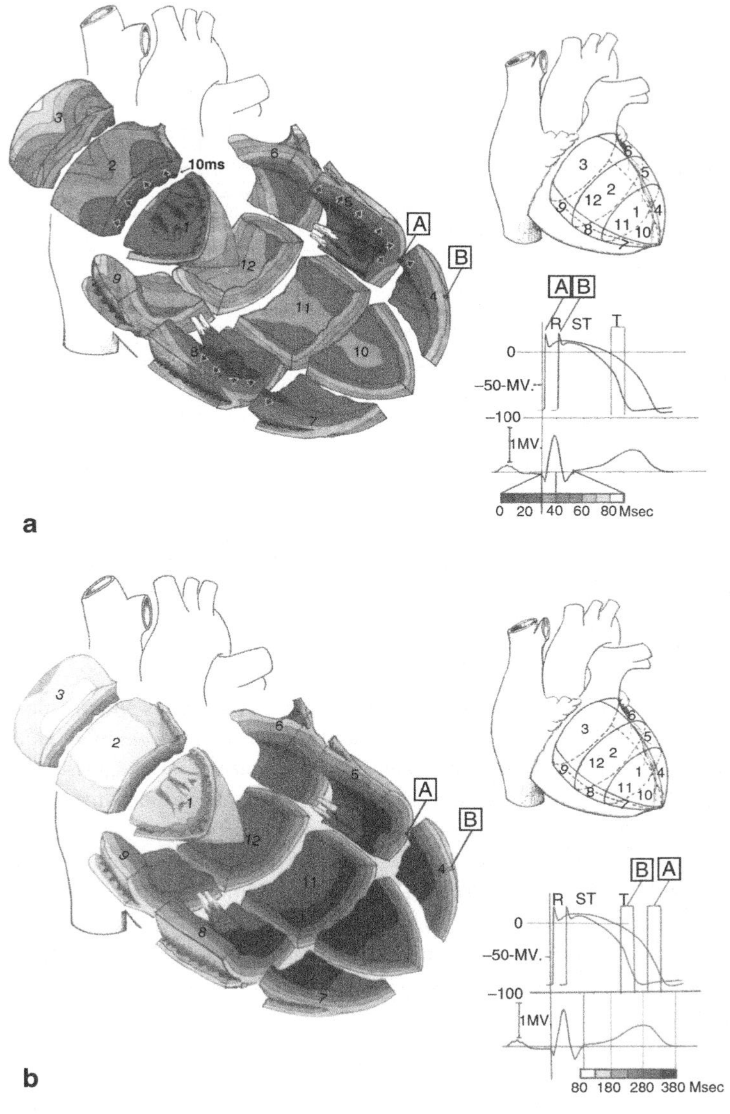

Fig. 4.6
(a) activation, (b) repolarization sequences of the left ventricle (see Sect. 4.2.4 for details)

the distal Purkinje fiber network. The start points for either the anterior (superior) or inferior subdivisions are removed while leaving the start points for the other, and for the middle fascicles. The separation of the initial and terminal 30 ms vectors described by Grant as "peri-infarction block"... "probably due to a block of the superior or inferior fascicles" [16, 41] is produced by the early activation of one wall and late activation of the other. The late and unopposed activation on the side of the blocked fascicle accounts for the shift of the frontal QRS axis toward the blocked fascicle; that is, leftward and superior in LAFB, rightward and inferior in LIFB. The 1 mm grid resolution of the simulation allows for the inclusion of the fine detail of scar interdigitating with normal viable myocardium typical of the border zone of infarcts as shown in Fig. 4.4. The complex interactions of infarcts, conduction abnormalities, including LAFB, LIFB, RBBB,

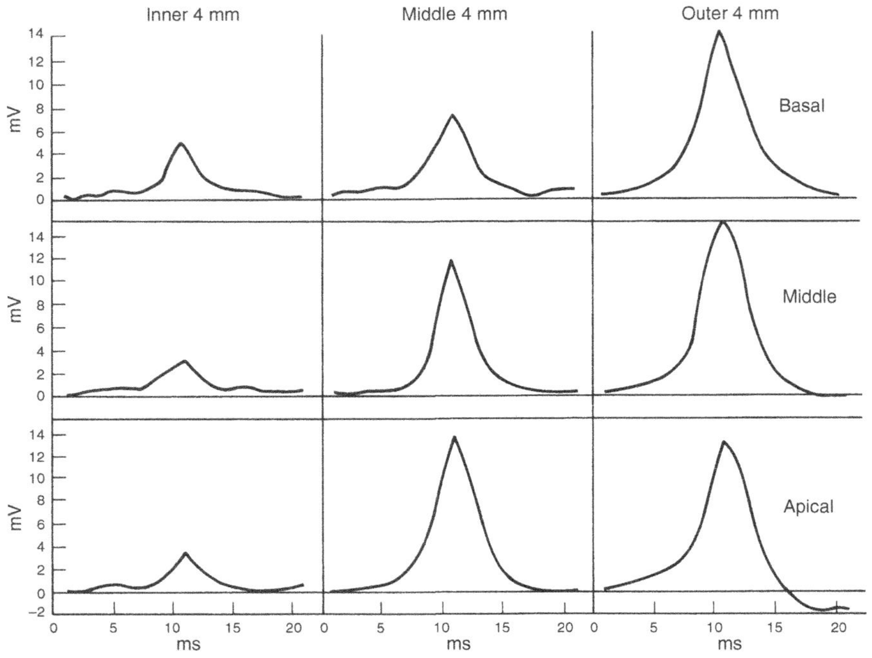

Fig. 4.7

Waveforms recorded in a series of dogs with intramural bipolar plunge electrodes with a 1 mm separation, are shown for the inner, middle and outer 4 mm of the same apical, and basal subdivisions shown in Fig. 4.1. Polarity of the recording system was set so that a wavefront moving from endocardium to epicardium and passing a bipolar pair would record a positive potential. The peak amplitude of the bipolar recording would be proportional to the electric field strength of the local electromotive surface of excitation. Each waveform represents the average of 65 observations in each of the nine regions specified after being digitized at a 1 ms interval and time aligned around the peak voltage in each bipolar pair before averaging. The peak of all the waveforms was set at 11 ms. Time in milliseconds represents the duration of the averaged waveforms and has no relationship to the activation sequence. The averaged waveforms are positive throughout, indicating the propagation is from the endocardium to epicardium in all regions of the heart in these animals. In primates including man, the propagation velocity and local field strength from endocardium to epicardium are more uniform than in dog. In man, therefore, each region contributes about equally to the surface ECG and there are no electrically "silent" regions

LBBB, and ventricular hypertrophies are evaluated in a straightforward manner by this fine-grid computer simulation of the propagating wave of ventricular of excitation and recovery.

For infarcts that localize to the subendocardium, the total extent is usually small. The simulation of such small infarcts introduced into our fine grid (1 cubic mm) model of this ventricular propagating wave in a realistic cardiac geometry and inhomogeneous torso [54–58] was very informative in evaluating the effect on the body surface ECG of these lesions. Small infarcts 20-25 mm across and 3–4 mm thick produce small changes in QRS, i.e., notches, slurs or "bite outs," etc. Only occasionally do such small infarcts produce "classic Q wave" criteria of 30–40 ms for an infarct. They must be strategically placed in that part of the heart activated in the first 15–30 ms of the QRS. These are usually small anterior lesions where proximity effects to the anterior precordial leads are strong. It is also informative to consider a pathological Q wave as loss of normal R wave early in the QRS, as in the first waveform in Fig. 4.5. The same loss of R wave from an area activated a few ms later in the QRS, as shown in the second waveform of this figure, and representing the same size infarct may produce a notch or slur in the upstroke of the R and no abnormal Q waves anywhere in the ECG. An equivalent infarct placed further out in the wall of the left ventricle or in a subendocardial region activated in the mid QRS will produce loss of mid QRS vectors. and may be seen mainly as attenuation of R waves or an increase in S waves or both.

In general, it takes infarcts 3 cm or more in diameter and 5–7 mm thick involving 40% or more of the transmural thickness of a local region of the anterior and inferior left ventricle to produce the 30–40 ms "classic Q wave" abnormalities. These infarcts are located in that part of the heart activated in the initial 40 ms of the QRS needed to produce abnormal Q waves.

Not addressed by these "classic" criteria are those infarcts that occur in the base of all four walls of the heart and the mid posterolateral wall. These regions in general depolarize after 40 ms. Infarcts here produce abnormalities mainly in the terminal half of the QRS. On the other hand, review of ➋ Fig. 4.3 indicates that only about 15% of single first infarcts are limited to these regions. The remaining 85% have significant involvement in mid and/or apical portions of the LV anterior and inferior walls. Thus a definite majority of infarcts have early to mid QRS deformities or loss of spatial vectors. If they are 4 cm or larger in the greatest diameter (12% LV or more), they do in general produce classic initial QRS changes. Nearly one-half of all single infarcts, however, are 3 cm or smaller (9% LV) and many of these fail to develop abnormal Q waves. However, they do have slurred and/or notched or attenuated R or S waves, or abnormal R/S or R/Q ratios. Most large or very large infarcts in any of the three major artery distributions have significant involvement of the base of the heart as well. In order to quantify the total extent of these lesions (see section on sizing of infarct below), mid and late QRS changes must be considered in developing criteria for infarct size.

4.2.4.2 Simulation of Ventricular Excitation and the ECG Infarct Scoring System

Typical examples of the simulation of the propagation wave of normal ventricular excitation, and for left anterior (superior) and left inferior (posterior) fascicular block are shown in ➋ Fig. 4.8. This simulation produced ECGs typical of normal conduction and of fascicular blocks. The location and detailed anatomy of various sized myocardial infarcts documented by both ventriculographic and postmortem anatomic studies in each of the three major coronary artery distributions were simulated; i.e., anterior infarcts (left anterior descending artery); posterolateral infarcts (non-dominant

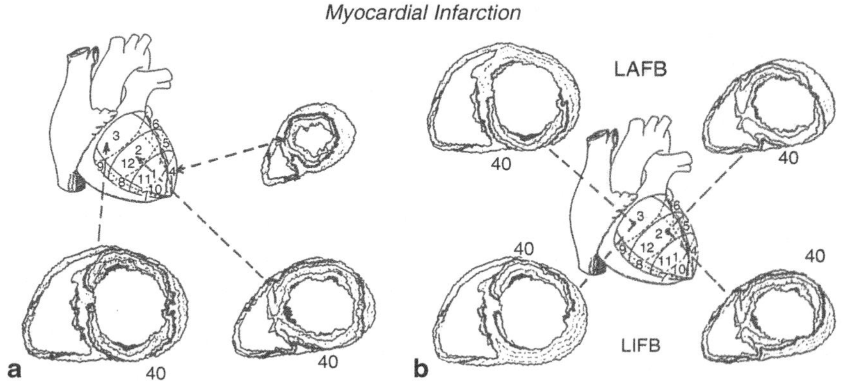

Fig. 4.8
Part (a) Ten millisecond isochrones of the simulated normal ventricular activation sequence is shown in cross sections through the mid regions of the apical, middle, and basal myocardial subdivisions defined in ➋ Fig 4.1. The darkened regions on the left ventricular endocardial surface represent the initial 10 ms isochrone. The computer propagation program generates each time step of the activation as it spreads out from these starting regions. Each line on the diagram represents a 10 ms isochrone. The fourth heavy shaded line is the 40 ms isochrone about midway in the activation. In part 2 (b), left anterior (superior) and inferior (posterior) fascicular blocks (LAFB, LIFB) are simulated by removing the starting points fed by the fan of Purkinje fascicles of the left bundle from one outside subdivision while the starting points of the other remains active as does those fed by the middle fascicles. The early activation of one wall and the late unapposed activation on the side of the blocked fascicle accounts for the significant shift of the frontal QRS axis toward the blocked fascicle, i.e. left anterior superior shift in LAFB and right inferior in LIFB

left posterior circumflex artery); and inferior infarcts (right coronary artery's posterolateral and posterior descending branches). Simulated moderate to large infarcts in these classic locations produced not only the expected abnormal Q waves (or "Q equivalents") in all the expected ECG leads, but mid and late QRS changes as well. Small infarcts in these same locations often failed to produce classic Q wave changes; but instead produced attenuation of R or S waves, notching in the QRS, decreased R/S ratio and mid to late QRS changes, i.e., notched or attenuated S or late R waves in V1, V2, etc., as described earlier in this section.

It became apparent early in these experiments that in any given lead, at right angles to the excitation surface propagating around the local infarct, the amount of QRS change was proportional to the amount of infarct introduced into the simulations. This formed the basis for the Selvester QRS MI Size Scoring System where each point scored was constructed to represent 3% of the left ventricle infarcted (3% LVI). Change in the score was proportional to the volume of the infarct introduced into the simulations. Criteria were devised for all regions of the myocardium. Infarcts in basal regions of the heart, which activate late in the QRS, could be appropriately scored by the criteria for late QRS changes. See ➋ Sect. 4.3.5 below for details of the score and its implementation for normal conduction, and ➋ Sect. 4.5 for conduction defects.

4.2.5 Ventricular Repolarization and Myocardial Injury, Ischemia, and Infarction

Most, if not all, of the extant models of recovery are indebted to some extent to the 1934 ventricular gradient model of Wilson [59] and to a number of studies refining it [60–62]. Schafer and associates in 1943 [63], described the monophasic action potential from the intact heart using suction electrodes, and the intracellular equivalent of this was first recorded by Ling and Gerard in 1949 [64]. Seminal work relating the transmembrane action potential duration and wave shapes to the refractory period of these cells, and to the T wave of the ECG, was done in the 1950s by Hoffman, Kao, Suckling, Cranfield, Brady, and Woodbury [65–68]. Working with Lepeschkin, Surawicz, and Herrlich [69], they demonstrated close correspondence to the intracellular transmembrane action potentials and those recorded from the surface of the heart with suction electrodes. Authenreith et al. [70] demonstrated with suction electrodes that in the intact dog heart, the action potential durations were longer at the apex, intermediate in the mid region and shortest at the base. They also noted that, in mapping action potential durations on the surface, the surface potentials ended well before the end of the T wave indicating that areas not accessible to the surface electrodes depolarized later. From 1952 to 1955 Allan Scher published a series of classic papers [71–73] showing the ventricular excitation in the mammalian ventricle in great detail using multipoint plunge electrodes. This work was also reported at about the same time by Durrer and associates [74], who, with van Dam [75] in the early 1960s, mapped functional refractory periods with intramural electrodes in the open chest dog and showed that the endocardium, while depolarizing first, repolarized last.

In studies noted above, Burgess, Abildskov, Millar, and associates [47–52] reported methodical investigations of functional refractory period in the dog and concluded that there is normally a rather uniform gradient in ventricular recovery times from epicardium to endocardium. The endocardium recovery is longest, the base of the heart has significantly shorter recovery times than the apex, and the right septal side of the interventricular septum behaves like the epicardium of the left ventricle. Finally, Spach and coworkers [46, 53] had recorded bipolar and unipolar electrograms from 300 chronic implanted intramural and epicardial electrodes in dogs and a chimpanzee allowed to recover for several days before measurements were made. The preparations had the advantage that both intramural and epicardial depolarization and repolarization could be mapped in detail in animals that had regained their normal body surface map potential distributions for both QRS and ST-T following chronic electrode implantation. These workers confirmed in this chronic preparation the ventricular activation sequence (depolarization) recorded earlier by Scher, Durrer and van Dam and associates, and by themselves. They also observed that the epicardium at the base of the left ventricle was last to depolarize but first to recover. There was a uniform sequence of recovery from epicardium to endocardium, and that the endocardium in the area at the junction of the mid regions of the left ventricle with the apex was the last to show significant recovery potentials. These data for both normal excitation and recovery in the 12 LV segments of the human heart are shown in ➋ Fig. 4.6a, b. A comprehensive review of "The Origin of the T-wave" by Kootsey and Johnson was published in 1980 [76]. This was expanded in considerable detail in the compilation, "Cardiac Repolarization Bridging Basic Science," by Gussak and Antzelevitch [77]. The reader is encouraged to consult these monographs for details not covered in ➋ Chaps. 3, ➋ 5 of *Basic Electrocardiology : Cardiac Electrophysiology, ECG Systems and Mathematical Modeling*, and this synopsis.

These will form the specific background for interpreting the repolarization (ST-T) changes associated with acute and chronic "injury," ischemia, and infarction along with the depolarization (QRS) changes with which they are so inextricably bound.

In relating ventricular excitation and recovery sequences to myocardial "injury," ischemia, and necrosis or infarction, it has traditionally been depicted that, as the result of a decrease or interruption of the blood supply to the myocardium from progressive coronary stenosis, an area of cardiac necrosis is produced. This central area is seen as surrounded by concentric zones of injury and ischemia. Classically, it has been assumed that the QRS changes result from the central area of necrosis, that injury causes the change in the TQ-ST segment, and ischemia the change in T waves. This concept implies that loss of functional heart muscle is greatest in the central area of necrosis, intermediate in the adjacent zone of injury where "leaky" membranes cause systolic and diastolic currents to flow, and least in the peripheral zone of ischemia where alterations in repolarization produce the "ischemic T wave." Loss of myocardium is considered irreversible in the zone of central necrosis, and potentially reversible in the outer regions of injury and ischemia.

In a well documented critique of the subject, Arnsdorf and Louie [78] conclude that there is little or no direct electrophysiologic or ultrastructural evidence to support the notion that these local regions contribute specific information in a unique way to the three components of the ECG. Indeed, as they point out, Janse et al. [79], by recording transmembrane action potentials with floating microelectrodes from cells within the border zone of myocardial ischemia in the isolated perfused pig heart, found cells with very low intracellular action potentials in close proximity to cells with nearly normal action potentials. In addition, nicotinamide adenine dinucleotide fluorescent staining techniques used by Harken and coworkers [80, 81] suggest that the line between normal and abnormal tissue may be very sharp. Pathoanatomic studies by Ideker in our correlative reports, referred to earlier, demonstrated in general a very complex interdigitation of islands and pseudopods of normal and abnormal tissue at the border of an infarct. This geometric detail is shown graphically in ➲ Fig. 4.4. Cox et al. [82], using dehydrogenase staining techniques to delineate the changing geometry of the infarct border from 18 h to 1 week after infarct, observed that this complex interdigitation of normal and infarcted tissue was generally evident by 24 h.

4.2.5.1 Computer Simulation of Repolarization

While recognizing a conceptual debt to the ventricular gradient model of Wilson [59], Harumi et al. in 1966 [83] were the first to propose relating action potential durations, and functional refractory periods in a quantitative 2-dimensional model of the T wave. The transmural gradient of action potential durations, their amplitudes, and the sequence of recovery shown in ➲ Fig. 4.6b were incorporated into a ventricular cross section, and adjusted so that T vector loops computed by the solid angle theorem conformed to those recorded experimentally. Thiry and Rosenberg [84] were the first to attempt a 3-dimensional multiple dipole model in the form of the cardiac geometry. Miller and Geselowitz in 1978 [85, 86], developed a more realistic simulation that included an external torso boundary still in a homogenous medium and a 4 cubic mm grid to represent the heart. Each 4 cubic mm "cell" was manually assigned action potential wave shapes to conform to those observed experimentally in normal, ischemic, hypoxic, irreversibly injured and dead cells. Both of these latter simplified models, in spite of not taking into account complex internal human torso inhomogeneities, did produce 12 lead ECGs that were quite consistent with normal ECGs. By manipulating regional generator outputs to simulate subendocardial, intramural, subepicardial, and transmural ischemia, and infarction (as shown in a summary form in ➲ Fig. 4.9), ECGs were produced that were entirely consistent with clinically observed changes. ECGs produced by these simulations, read by experienced electrocardiographers who were blinded to the simulation, were interpreted as representing the processes simulated (see ➲ Chap. 7 of *Basic Electrocardiology : Cardiac Electrophysiology, ECG Systems and Mathematical Modeling* for more details). The solid experimental base of a large number of workers of which the foregoing is a very cryptic review, is covered in detail in the Kootsy-Johnson monograph [76]. This review and ➲ Chaps. 6–9 of *Basic Electrocardiology : Cardiac Electrophysiology, ECG Systems and Mathematical Modeling* and this chapter provide the basis for a rational interpretation of the body surface ECG of acute myocardial infarction "injury," ischemia, and chronic healed infarct.

In the mid to late 1980s, the author (RHS) and associates incorporated the complex geometry of regional ischemia and/or infarcts into his validated 1 cubic mm grid propagation model, automating the manually entered local cardiac generator changes reported in the Thiry and Rosenberg [84], and the Miller and Geselowitz [85, 86] models. In addition, this

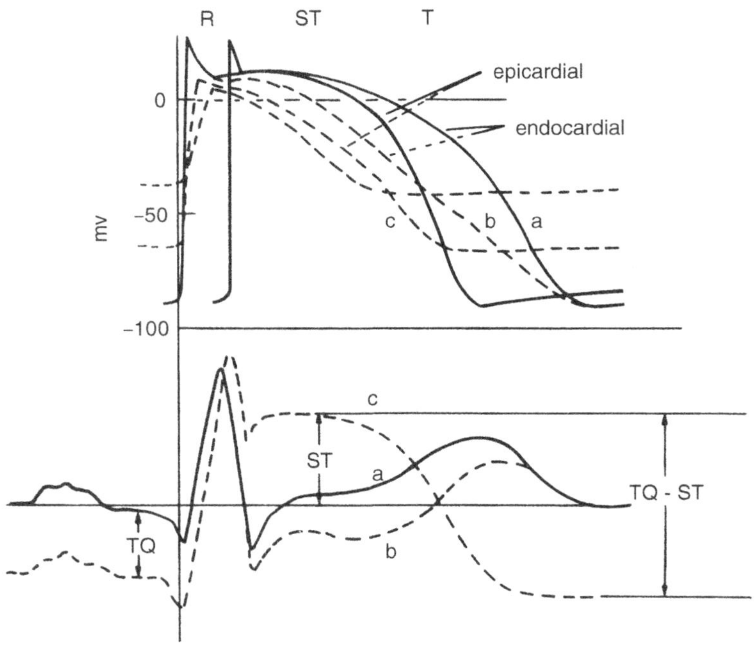

Fig. 4.9
Typical myocardial-cell action potentials (*upper curves*), and body surface ECGs (*lower curves*) that represent various degrees of ischemia (b), injury (c), and cell death (necrosis). Curves (a) represent the normal pattern. These individual action potential waveforms will be used to represent the 1 cubic mm "cell" in the fine-grid propagation model (see Fig. 4.8). This will allow for the simulation of regional subendocardial intramural or transmural ischemia, injury or necrosis. Simulation of the fine detail of infarct anatomy/geometry shown in Fig. 4.4 is incorporated into an interactive system, in an anatomically and electrophysiologically realistic and comprehensive model of the heart and inhomogeneous human torso

simulation also included all the torso and internal boundary effects and inhomogeneities known to influence the surface ECG recordings, and generated as output the total body surface map of which the 12/16 lead ECG is a subset. This allowed us to study in detail the geometrically complex border regions of acute and healed myocardial infarcts for the entire cycle of depolarization and repolarization in subjects with normal conduction (see Fig. 4.10a, b) and those with conduction defects.

The electrophysiologic changes over time of the geometrically complex regions of evolving infarction were included in the simulation. The resulting body surface map, 12 lead ECG, and VCG records integrated the complex boundary effects described above, and the more central loss of QRS forces or vectors from the irreversibly damaged myocardium. Simulations of the local areas of acute ischemia/injury of acute infarction and of chronic subendocardial ischemia [87] produced a major shift in the ST segment that was vectorially related to the local perfusion bed of the coronary artery simulated. The ST field (and vector) for acute ischemia/injury was displaced anteriorly, superiorly and leftward for proximal LAD occlusion, as well as outward from the epicardium via the centroid of the LAD perfusion bed. Similarly there was an inferior, and somewhat rightward and posteriorly directed ST field (and vector) for proximal RCA occlusion, and a posteriorly directed ST for LCX occlusion. There are conflicting data in the clinical literature [88–90], but work by Sederholm et al. [91] using continuous orthogonal lead monitoring suggests that the peak ST elevation of acute injury may occur over a very short time. Both they and Aldrich et al. [92] have demonstrated significant correlation between both the location and extent of the initial ST "injury" currents and the size of the acute infarct that evolved over the next few days, as measured by enzyme methods, the ECG QRS score and radionuclide angiography. The clinical correlates with the simulated acute and evolving infarcts are dealt with in detail later, in Sect. 4.4 of this chapter. These studies confirmed that the simulation projections would be specifically related to the local coronary artery distributions described earlier.

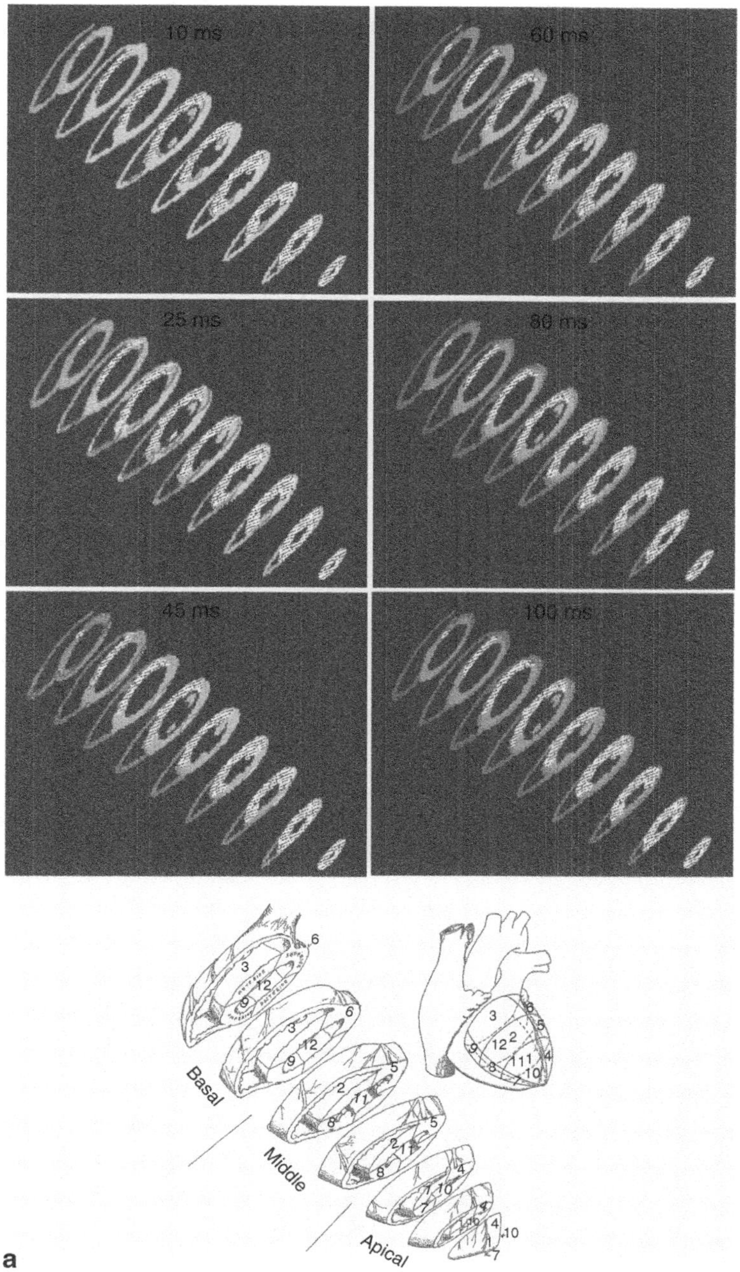

a

Fig. 4.10 (Continued)

In the healed infarct, the direction of the mean T vector away from the local area is a significant predictor of the local area of the infarct [93–95]. The "secondary" ST-T changes of the conduction abnormalities, RBBB, LBBB, ventricular pacing or pre-excitation, and hypertrophy of either ventricle confound these ST-T changes of acute and chronic infarct. Details of dealing with these confounders are also covered in Sects. 4.4 and 4.5 of this chapter.

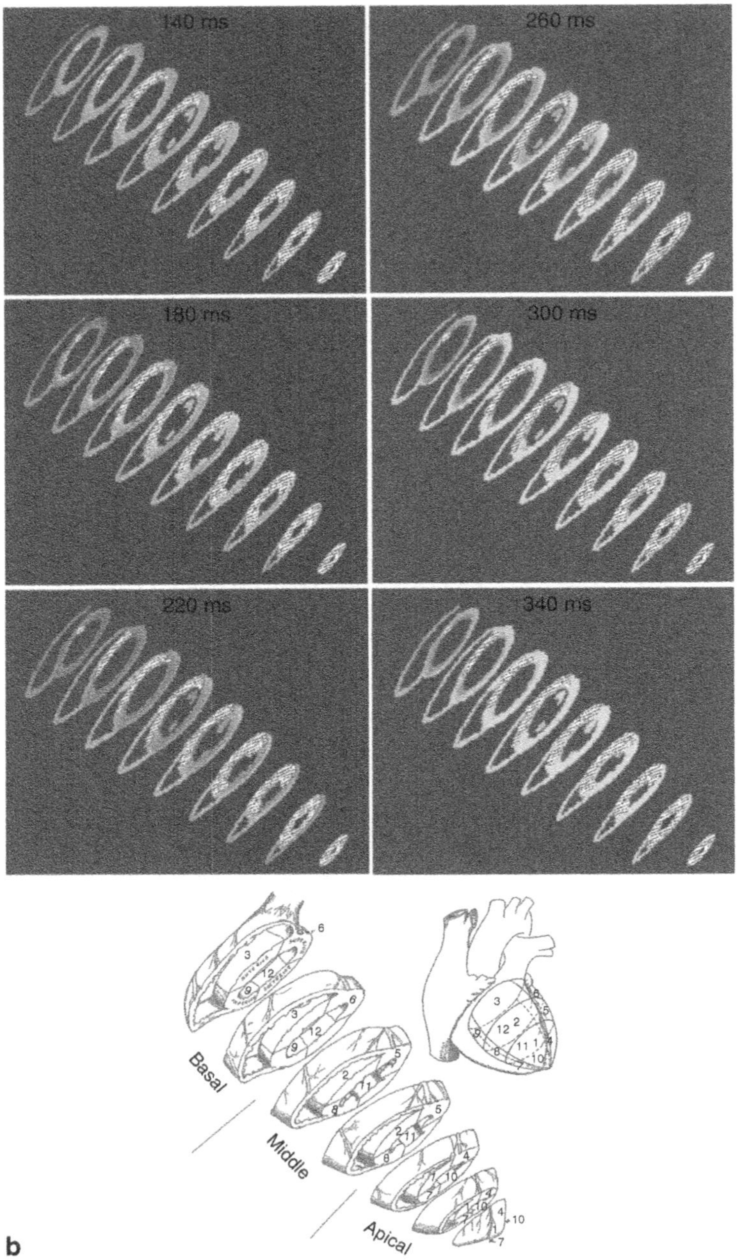

b

Fig. 4.10

(**a**) Anterior view of serial apex-to-base cross-sections of a human heart showing the under-surface of each section as illustrated in the diagram below. Simulated 20–100 ms. excitation sequences (yellow/orange/red to blue) around a large anterior infarct (striated white). (**b**) Anterior view of serial apex-to-base cross-sections of a human heart showing the under-surface of each section as illustrated in the diagram below. Simulated 140–340 ms repolarization sequences (reversing blue to red/orange/yellow), as with the excitation sequences, outlining the large anterior infarct

The simulated local subendocardial ischemia with localizing ECG ST deviation away (inward) from each major coronary artery perfusion bed described above led to the following hypothesis: Subjects with local resting (or exercise induced) ST deviation away (inward) from the centroid of any of the major coronary artery perfusion beds would have high-grade single vessel occlusion of that specific artery. Consider an ancillary hypothesis: Resting (or exercise induced) ST deviation away from the apex (toward the base) would have high-grade distal LAD (left anterior descending), left main or three vessel occlusion. To test this hypothesis, we recorded 16 lead ECGs at rest and with exercise in a preliminary report of some 48 subjects who also had coronary angiograms/angioplasties (96). In no incidence of high-grade single vessel disease was localizing ST deviation maximal away (inward) from the centroid of the perfusion bed of that specific vessel, including distal LAD disease. Likewise, in a 10-year survey of some 3,000 acute myocardial infarctions seen at this large community teaching hospital, 900 of whom had emergent coronary intervention, there was no incident of single vessel occlusive disease with local ST deviation away (inward) from the involved arterial perfusion bed. Noted in this cohort with early intervention was the following: ST depression in anterior-posterior leads V1–V3 was associated with acute occlusive disease of the left circumflex and, ST depression in inferior-superior leads III, aVF, II, and maximal in aVF (a superior ST deviation vector) was seen with acute occlusion of a ramus or a prominent first diagonal. Apically localized ST depression in apex-base oriented leads V4, V5, V6, I, -aVR was associated with high-grade left main and/or proximal multi-vessel disease. These observations strongly support the Ellestad hypothesis (97) that, resting (or exercise induced) subendocardial ischemic ST change is global.

4.3 Quantification of Infarct Size Using ECG and VCG Criteria

4.3.1 Essential Principles

1. Myocardial infarcts develop, of course, in 3-dimensional space; and therefore understanding of their quantitative alteration of ventricular activation and its body surface representation, the QRS complex, requires consideration of a "3-dimensional ECG." Recording of three orthogonal leads (X, Y, and Z) provides the basis for generating this ECG display, termed a "vectorcardiogram" (VCG). The sequential instantaneous points of summation of the propagating ventricular activation (vectors) in the X (direction) lead plotted against those in the Y (direction) lead create the "frontal plane VCG loop"; in the X and Z leads the "transverse plane VCG loop," and in the Y and Z leads the "sagittal plane VCG loop." See ➋ Chap. 11 of *Specialized Aspects of ECG* for a more detailed explanation of the VCG.
2. The QRS deformities between a pre-infarct ECG/VCG and a post-infarct record are a function of infarct size and any change in intraventricular conduction. In patients who maintain normal conduction post-infarct, the degree of QRS deformity, both magnitude and duration, is proportional to the amount of myocardium lost and inversely related to the loss of ventricular function, i.e., to LV ejection fraction (LVEF).
3. Intraventricular conduction defects, when produced, are generally related to a specific coronary artery and a specific local infarct.
4. Once the basic activation sequence (conduction abnormality) is taken into account, the extent of the added QRS change is also proportional to the infarct size and decrease in LVEF.

4.3.2 Infarct Size, Left Ventricular Function, and Prognosis

In recent decades, it has become established that patient prognosis after a myocardial infarct, as well as functional reserve capacity, is related to the amount of the left ventricle (LV) infarcted. Thus, reliable clinical methods, which are able to estimate the extent of both acute and remote myocardial necrosis are needed. The recent interest in the limitation of acute infarct size by therapeutic interventions (clot lysis, coronary atheroma removal, balloon angioplasty, etc.) has prompted the evaluation of many clinical methods aimed at estimating the size of an acute myocardial infarct. In autopsy correlations, Ideker has shown [18] that infarct size and LV ejection fraction (LVEF) are inversely related, with a high correlation ($r = 0.88$). Patients with extensive myocardial losses from one or more infarcts with total extent of infarction approaching 40% LV, and LVEF less than 30%, have an annual mortality rate of more than 20% and major impairment of their functional reserve [98, 99].

For almost a century the ECG has been used to determine the presence and location of myocardial infarcts. Because it is universally available, noninvasive, inexpensive, and easily repeatable, it is important to make optimal use of recent findings regarding the ability to estimate infarct size from ECG/VCG data. The quantitative QRS infarct size scoring system, which was designed from our computer simulations described earlier [54–58], utilizes information in the ECG and VCG to estimate infarct size. It is the purpose of this section to provide enough background information to make the rationale of the method apparent to the reader. We will describe both the 12-lead ECG scoring method and the VCG method in sufficient detail so that the reader can apply the method directly to routinely recorded ECGs and VCGs.

4.3.3 Infarct Size and Left Atrial Overload

LV infarction decreases the diastolic compliance of the LV – in the acute stages by edema and in the chronic stages by scar. Even small infarcts are associated with some stiffening of the wall and increased ventricular filling pressure. Thus ECG/VCG changes of left atrial overload are common in most infarcts. The larger the infarct, the higher the ventricular end-diastolic filling pressure and the more marked is the left atrial overload change. Thus, acute ST, evolving QRS and left atrial P changes are each related to infarct size. Since the left atrium depolarizes during the latter two-thirds of the P-wave with activation fronts directed mainly to the left and posteriorly, four main criteria can be identified where the degree of change relates to the degree of left atrial overload:

(a) Increase in total P duration (> 110ms),
(b) Increased duration of left atrial intrinsicoid deflection (time from peak anterior to peak posterior in V1, V2, or *Z* > 30 ms),
(c) Increased duration posterior (negative P duration) in V1, V2, and *Z* (>45ms).
(d) Increased magnitude of late component posterior (negative P amplitude) in V1, V2, and *Z* (>0.05mV) and/or leftward in V5, V6, and *X* (>0.1 mV).

These relationships, i.e., the extent of these changes as relates to the severity of the left atrial overload, and degree of LV diastolic dysfunction, are defined in ➋ Tables 4.1 and ➋ 4.2. They are more related to left atrial and LV end diastolic pressure than to angiographic or echo left atrial size. This was documented in a well-controlled coronary care unit study by Heikkila et al. [100].

Table 4.1

Score for atrial overload. Criteria and the points given for each for quantifying the degree right and left atrial overload. Those criteria on the top row in each case exceed the 98% upper bounds of normal.

Right atrial overload			Left atrial overload					
P amplitude (mV)			P amplitude (mV)			P duration (ms)		
Anterior	Inferior	Points	Leftward	Posterior	Intr. Def.*	Posterior		Points
V1 (V2, Z)	AVF (Y)	Ea Crit◇	V5 (X)	V1 (V2, Z)	V1 (V2, Z)	V1 (V2, Z)	Total	Ea Crit◇
0.100	0.175	4	0.100	0.075	35	45	120	2
0.125	0.200	8	0.125	0.100	40	50	130	4
0.150	0.225	12	0.150	0.150	45	60	140	6
0.200	0.250	16	0.175	0.200	50	70	150	8
0.250	0.300	24	0.200	0.250	60	80	160	12
0.300	0.350	32	0.225	0.300	70	90	170	16
≥0.400	≥0.400	48	≥0.250	≥0.400	≥80	≥100	≥180	24

*Intr. Def: Intrinsicoid deflection; the duration from peak positive P amplitude to the peak negative.
◇ Ea Crit: (Points for) Each criterion met.

Table 4.2
Diagnostic statements relating to total points accrued in Table 4.1

Total points	Diagnostic statement[a]
4–6	Possible mild RAO/LAO
8–10	Probable mild RAO/LAO
12–18	Moderate RAO/LAO
32–46	Severe RAO/LAO
≥48	Very severe RAO/LAO

[a] *RAO* right atrial overload, *LAO* left atrial overload

4.3.4 Infarct Size and Right Atrial Overload

Patients with right ventricular infarction (see Sect. 4.4.5.1) have right atrial overload, the severity of which is related to the severity of the right ventricular failure. Also, patients with large to very large infarcts or with diffuse ischemic myopathy may have very high left ventricular end diastolic filling pressures and recurrent congestive heart failure. Such patients will have a passive increase in pulmonary pressure to maintain a flow gradient and consequent chronic increase in right ventricular pressure. Such chronic right ventricular overload routinely decreases right ventricular diastolic compliance, producing right atrial overload. The right atrial depolarization from the sinus node region produces activation fronts directed anteriorly and inferiorly. These excitation fronts occur unopposed during the first third of the P-wave at which time leftward and posterior fronts begin to develop in the left atrium. In the adult, a P amplitude >0.1 mV in V1, V2, and *Z* and >0.175 mV inferior in aVF and *Y* exceeds the 98% upper bounds of normal, and are indicative of right atrial overload. The degree of increased anterior and inferior voltage is proportional to the overload of the right atrium as summarized in Tables 4.1 and 4.2. It is a well established clinical axiom that in patients over 50 years of age, the commonest cause of pulmonary hypertension, right ventricular and right atrial overload, is chronic left ventricular failure. It follows from the above that, large to very large infarcts with significant diastolic dysfunction that have not produced chronic left ventricular failure will have moderate to severe left atrial overload but generally normal or minimal right atrial changes. When in addition the ECG/VCG changes of right atrial overload become mild to moderate, associated congestive failure is most likely.

4.3.5 Computer Simulations and QRS Infarct Size Scoring Systems for ECG and VCG

The simulation of ventricular excitation of the human heart formed the basis for an ECG infarct scoring system developed by Selvester, Solomon and co-workers to consider all of the major variables known to influence the surface ECG. These included (1) high resolution (1 cubic mm grid) anatomy of the human myocardium, Purkinje conduction system, and very small to very large infarcts in each of the three major coronary perfusion beds, (2) a simulation of ventricular propagation of excitation at this same resolution, and (3) a simulation of the inhomogeneous volume conductor; including intracardiac blood mass, myocardium, lungs, and an adult torso [55]. It became apparent in the simulation experiments noted earlier in Sect. 4.2.4.2 that in any given lead, at right angles to the propagating excitation surface, the degree of QRS change was proportional to the amount of infarct introduced into the simulations. This led to the ECG scoring system where each point scored was set up to represent infarction of 3% of the left ventricle (LV). Criteria could be devised for all regions of the myocardium, and infarcts in basal regions of the heart which activate late in the QRS could be appropriately scored by the same scoring system, provided late QRS changes were included in the criteria.

A 53-Criteria/32-Point scoring system (representing a total of 96% of the LV) was developed, tested and reported using a learning set of 100 biplane ventriculograms from patients with angiographically proven coronary artery disease [29, 57, 58]. Using the same simulations (Fig. 4.11) and rationale, a nomogram (Fig. 4.12) relating VCG changes (duration and magnitude of a QRS deformity as in Fig. 4.13) was also developed to predict infarct size [29].

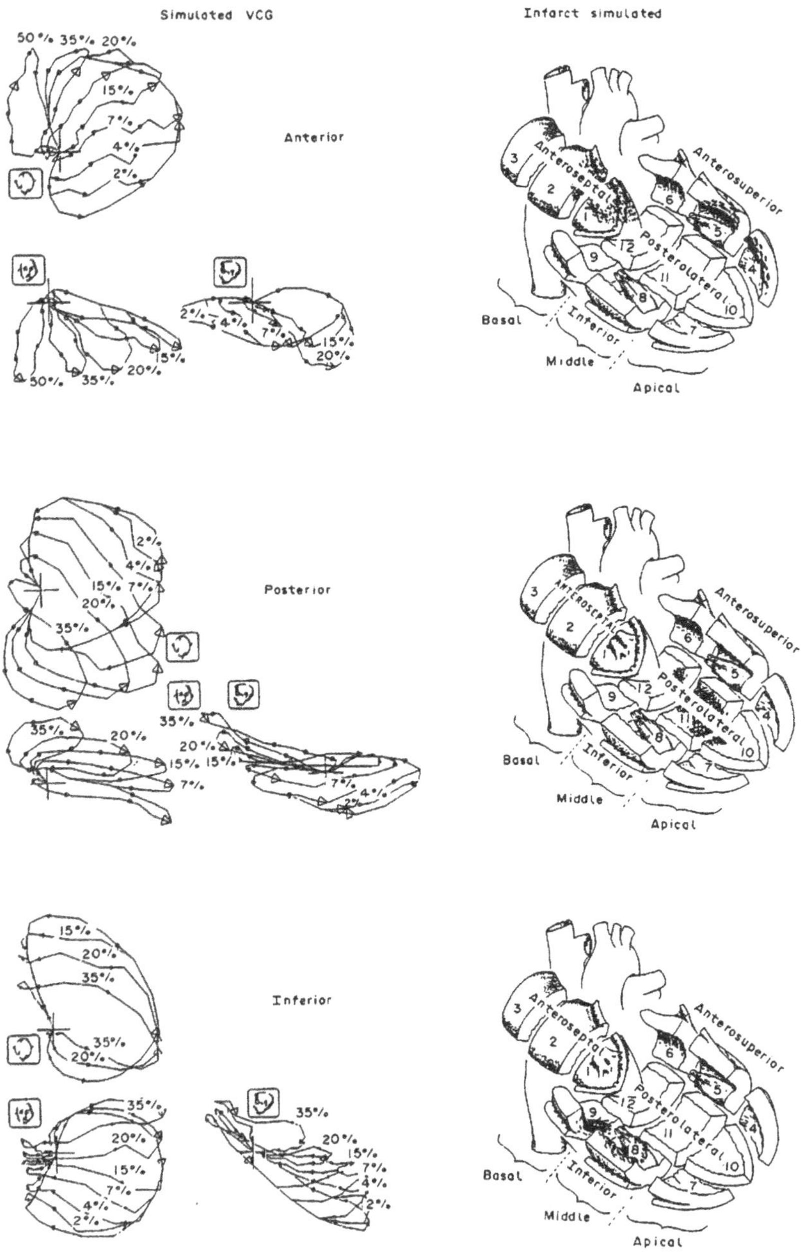

Fig. 4.11
Typical examples of moderately sized infarcts (15% of the LV) in each of the main coronary distributions are shown in the 12-segment LV diagrams at the right of the illustration. The program was directed to plot superimposed vector loops in horizontal, frontal and left sagittal projections when various sizes of infarcts had been simulated in each of these typical locations. The number at each VCG loop represents the percentage LV infarct simulated and ranged from 2% LV to 50% LV. Not shown are body-surface maps and 12-lead ECGs that can be plotted routinely for each run of the simulation program. Normal conduction was simulated for the anterior and posterior infarcts shown, while inferior (posterior) fascicular block was needed in the simulation to produce ECGs and VCGs typical of inferior infarct of various sizes associated with RCA occlusion. Multiple infarcts with various combinations of sizes and locations are readily simulated with this model

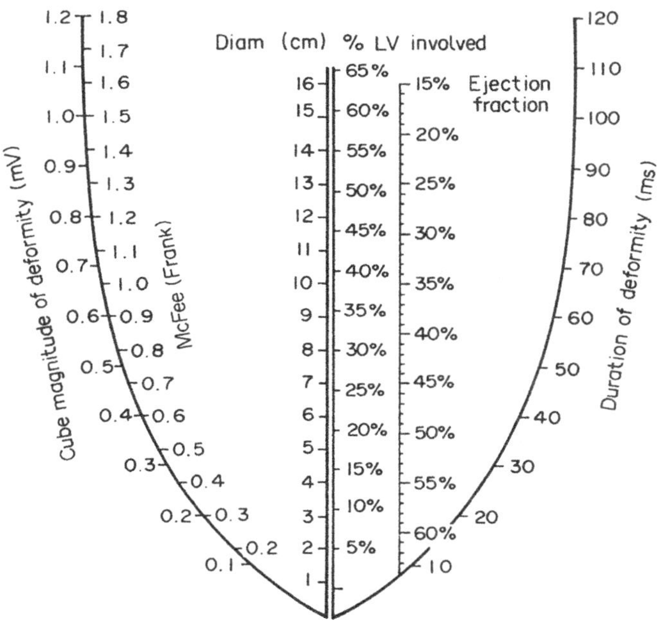

■ **Fig. 4.12**
Nomogram for predicting infarct size from VCG deformities. When preinfarct records are available, as shown in ➤ Fig. 4.13, the peak amplitude of the change (local loop deformity) in records before and after infarct is identified. The amplitude chosen for each lead system is the projection of the loop where the change is greatest. The peak amplitude change for the specific lead system is transferred to the left side of this nomogram, and the duration of that change is transferred to the right side. A line is then constructed through these two points and the point where it crosses the *double line* in the center of the nomogram is used to determine angiographic infarct size. The latter may be represented by (a) diameter in centimeters (i.e., the longest curvilinear dimensions of akinesis in either projection of the biplane ventriculogram); (b) angiographic percentage LV involved (i.e., the percentage of the circumference of either projection that is akinetic); and (c) ejection fraction as computed by the area length method of Dodge, Sandler and Sanmarco. It should be noted that the percentage LV (circumference) involved here is an angiographic determination, and while clearly related to percentage LV infracted at quantitative planometric pathology, it is a quite different measurement. When a preinfarct record is not available and a small local deformity that is outside normal limits for QRS loop is identified (indicating an infarct), a loop is constructed that would be within the limits of normal using the normal portions of the loop for a guide. The magnitude and duration of the deformity is measured from the reconstructed normal and transferred to the nomogram for the estimation of infarct size. When the deformity is large, the mean normal loop for that particular lead system is used to identify the magnitude and duration of the deformity for transfer to the nomogram. ➤ Figure 4.13 is an example of such VCG changes

4.3.5.1 Validation Studies

In a series of 74 patients with serial biplane ventriculograms and serial ECGs and VCGs [29], an unchanged ECG and VCG was predictive of an unchanged ventriculogram with a remarkable 98% reliability. New change in the ECG/VCG (QRS deformity as in ➤ Fig. 4.13) was associated with a change in ventriculogram in 12 out of 14 subjects (Panel a, ➤ Fig. 4.14). The size or extent of new infarction, which in each instance was associated with a proximal coronary occlusion, was correlated with ECG/VCG magnitude-duration criteria for infarct size with a correlation coefficient of 0.90. The major ambiguity was in one patient who had sustained right coronary occlusion and had developed changes of inferior fascicular block in addition to new infarction. When infarct size was recomputed by the criteria discussed below for infarct plus inferior fascicular block, the overall correlation improved to 0.92. The two patients with new ECG/VCG deformities and

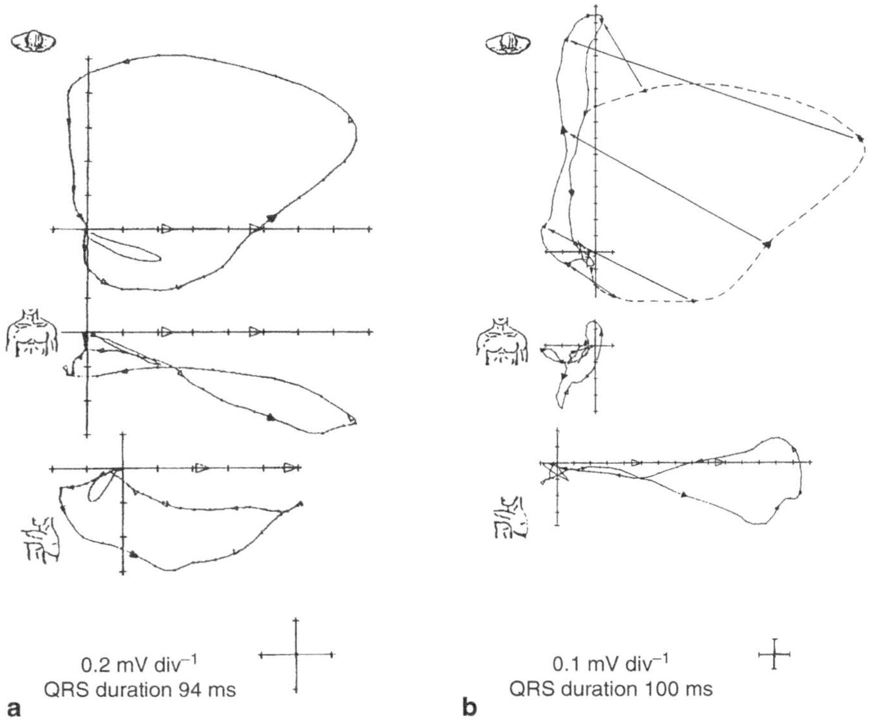

Fig. 4.13

Part (a) shows the McFee lead-system VCG of a 51-year-old white male patient with angina pectoris and single-vessel LAD disease which is entirely normal. Part (b) shows the VCG of the same man at 53, recorded a few weeks after an acute anterior myocardial infarction as a result of total occlusion of the proximal LAD lesion and prior to repeat coronary angiography and ventriculography. A major deformity from 10 to 70 ms was produced with major loss of leftward vectors as shown on the *right*, and a maximal magnitude of 1.5 mV at the 50 ms vector. When the 1.5 mV for 60 ms was transferred to the nomogram (Fig. 4.12), a line constructed between the two values for the McFee VCG crossed the double center line at 12 cm and 45% angiographic LV involvement. It predicted an ejection fraction of 30%. At angiography, a very large akinetic anteroseptal anterosuperior and apical segment was seen as the result of the proximal LAD occlusion and an ejection fraction of 26% was recorded

an unchanged ventriculogram had the ECG/VCG changes of possible small new infarcts (involving 5–10% LV). This suggests that small lesions of this size may produce no discernable wall motion abnormality in the ventriculogram.

Wickline and McNamara [101] reported excellent correlation between infarct size at autopsy in a small number of experimental infarcts in the baboon, and the integral of the change in the vector spatial magnitude compared to the control VCG spatial magnitude in the same animal. Cowan et al. [102] have reported on the integral of the spatial magnitude of initial abnormal depolarization in human subjects in whom control records were not available. She found excellent correlation with quantitative planometric pathoanatomic measurement of infarct size. The correlation was best in anterior infarcts and the correlations with inferior infarcts improved when the integral also included terminal abnormal depolarization [103].

From the authors' data presented above, it follows that carefully recorded high quality multi-lead serial ECGs/VCGs are a simple, inexpensive and effective method to predict the presence or absence of new myocardial damage (98% reliable), and to quantify the degree of damage with more than 90% reliability. WE RECOMMEND, THEREFORE, THAT EVERY YOUNG ADULT ACQUIRE SUCH A HIGH QUALITY BASELINE ECG RECORDING BEFORE AGE 30. A wallet sized photographic and electronic copy could be carried on their person thereafter.

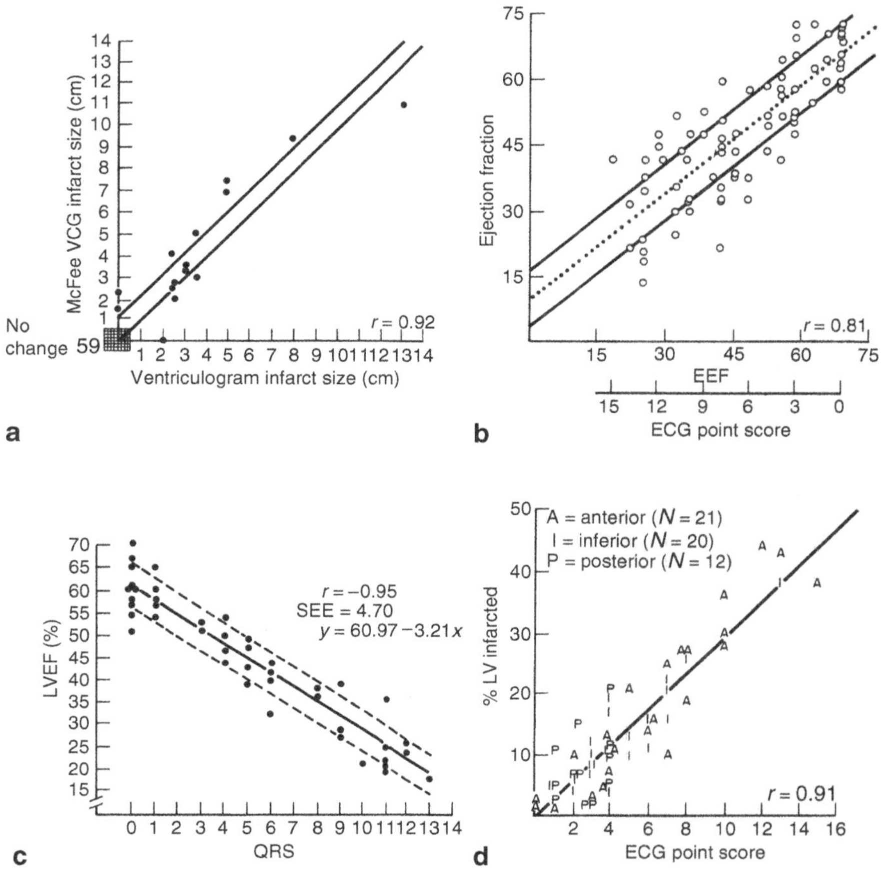

Fig. 4.14

Part (a) plots new infarct size (second study) on serial comparison of VCG change and contrast ventriculograms in 74 consecutive serial coronary angiographic studies [29]. The lower line is the line of unity. The $r = 0.92$ is computed for the 14 subjects where significant VCG change was found. Part (b) shows the correlation between the ECG point score for infarct size, discussed in the text (EEF = estimated ejection fraction), and ejection fraction in a series of 74 consecutive patients with 100% LAD occlusion and less than 75% in the other two coronary arteries [58]. All cases were included regardless of the presence or absence of ECG changes of hypertrophy or conduction abnormality. No case of LBBB was observed in this group. Part (c) compares QRS scores for infarct size and nuclear LV ejection fraction (LVEF) in 43 patients 3 weeks after suffering an acute myocardial infarct [31]. Patients with ECG evidence of conduction abnormalities or ventricular hypertrophy were excluded, but those with history of prior infarct were not. SEE denotes the standard error of the estimate. Part (d) relates the ECG point score to the pathological infarct size at quantitative planometric pathology in the first 53 patients with single infarcts reported by Ideker et al. [18, 32, 33]. Twenty-one of these patients have anterior infarcts, 20 have inferior infarcts and 12 have posterior infarcts

Hindman and associates [108] next evaluated the specificity and intra- and inter-observer agreement of a simplified version of the ECG scoring system proposed by Wagner. The effectiveness of this simplified QRS scoring system for estimating myocardial infarct size was then tested in post-mortem studies involving single infarcts in the anterior [18], inferior [32], and posterolateral [33] quadrants of the left ventricle. Additionally, the simplified scoring system has been found to be of clinical value (see Fig. 4.14 Panel C) in the assessment of left ventricular function after acute myocardial infarction [31, 104, 105].

The simplified system has several potential limitations. Its 29 points are accumulated from 37 criteria which can only indicate infarction in 87% of the LV. There is relative under-representation of the posterior (posterolateral) and basal regions, and it performed suboptimally with infarcts in these locations. Also, minor changes in amplitude and deformities in the QRS (notching) that were apparent in the simulations and in clinical infarcts were not included. The complete quantitative scoring system which includes 20 additional criteria of R and S amplitudes and the presence of notched and late R waves was then evaluated [106, 107]. Fourteen criteria met the 95% specificity standard in normals, three achieved the standard only after modification, and three were excluded. The control population considered at this time was larger and better distributed by age and sex than the original normal population [30]. This study population was composed of 500 consecutively selected Caucasian subjects of both sexes in the five decades between the ages of 20 and 69; there were 50 females and 50 males in each of the decades [107]. Of the 500 subjects, there were 160 healthy volunteers and 340 catheterized patients. The latter underwent diagnostic heart catheterization for the evaluation of chest pain and had totally normal studies including hemodynamics. The resultant 53-criteria/32-point system is presented in ➋ Fig. 4.16.

Age and gender adjustments for the QRS amplitude and duration criteria noted lower left of the scoring worksheet are the result of a review of this normal database and the Macfarlane Western Scotland database of 1339 normals (see Vol. 3), with a similar age and gender distribution.

Studies using this complete scoring system in the first 54 patients of the same postmortem subjects reported above [58], demonstrated that it predicted extent of infarct in each of the three major coronary distributions with good correlation ($r = 0.91$, see ➋ Fig. 4.14, Panel d) when compared to quantitative planometric pathoanatomic findings. It was also demonstrated that, on average, the complete scoring system predicted a distribution of damage in the 12 LV segments that correlated well with the average of the planometric pathology found in those same 12 subdivisions, i.e.: anterior infarcts $r = 0.93$, inferior $r = 0.97$ and posterolateral $r = 0.83$ [34].

4.3.5.2 Comparison of QRS Score to MRI Infarct Quantification

Gadolinium delayed-enhancement magnetic resonance imaging (DE-MRI) has recently emerged as the gold standard to quantify infarction in-vivo. Engblom et al. performed two studies comparing the simplified scoring system to infarct size quantified by DE-MRI [108, 109]. The first study included 25 patients with chronic anterior infarction and found only a moderate correlation of $r = 0.40$ ($P < 0.05$) between ECG and MRI scar size [108]. The reason for this relatively poor correlation is not entirely clear. Of note, the population consisted of chronic ischemic heart disease patients who had significant remodeling and wall thinning that was not taken into account when quantifying infarct size (amount of myocardium lost by necrosis) as had been done in the necropsy studies by Ideker and colleagues [18]. Finally, the accuracy of infarct quantification by MRI in-vivo is confounded by partial volume affects and image quality.

The second study by Engblom et al. in 29 patients with first-time reperfused infarction found a stronger correlation of $r = 0.79$ between ECG and MRI infarct size [108]. They found the best correlation between local QRS score and infarct size in the middle third of the LV. These small ECG-MRI studies will have to be followed by studies in larger populations before definitive conclusions can be drawn.

4.3.6 Methods for the 12 Lead ECG QRS MI Size Scoring System, Manual

In all the studies reported, either 3- or 8-channel recorders were used to obtain standard 12 lead ECGs. The duration and amplitude of each deflection in the QRS complex were measured with hand held micro-adjustable calipers for 10 of the standard 12 leads (I, II, aVL, aVF, and V1–V6). QRS duration measurements (ms) were made horizontally along the PR segment baseline. Amplitude measurements (mV) were made vertically from this baseline even when the ST segment was shifted. From these measurements, a point score was determined from weighted criteria for each ECG. However, when major ST segment shifts are present (1.0 mV or more beyond the 98% normal confidence limits), scoring is less reliable because the injury current usually distorts the appearance of the QRS complex.

Clinical observations of durations and amplitudes of Q, R and S waves on the standard 12 lead ECG are performed routinely by physicians and paramedical personnel. When these observations are required for identifying specific criteria for a quantitative QRS scoring system for estimating infarct size, precise observations of the waveforms are required.

There are several aspects to this precision: (a) adequate ECG recording, (b) rigorous definition of waveforms, (c) accurate waveform measurement, (d) use of simple guidelines for considering relationships among criteria, and (e) a logical format for presenting the scoring system.

4.3.6.1 Adequate ECG Recording

The performance of the ECG recording equipment should be tested at regular intervals to assure proper writing, alignment between channels, amplitude calibration of 10 mm/mV, and appropriate (0.05–150 Hz) frequency response. A minimum of three channel recording with perfect alignment between channels is required for adequate definition of the times of waveform onsets and offsets. This precision is particularly important for the identification of the initial isoelectric portion of a waveform as in (➋ Fig. 4.15). Several commercially available ECG recorders have the ability to display the ECG at double gain and effectively double speed. Such recordings increase the resolution and decrease the variability of measurements for the manual scoring process.

4.3.6.2 Rigorous Waveform Definitions

If the initial deflection of the QRS complex is negative, a Q wave is present. Prior to returning to the baseline, this negative deflection may be either smooth or notched. A "smooth Q" is present (➋ Fig. 4.15) when the initial negative deflection has no reversal in direction equal to or greater than (≥)0.05 mV ("notch"), preceding a positive (R) deflection. The duration of such a Q is measured as the width of the entire initial negative deflection. When the entire complex is a smooth negative deflection, no S wave is present. Therefore the amplitude of the Q wave should also be considered as the "S wave"

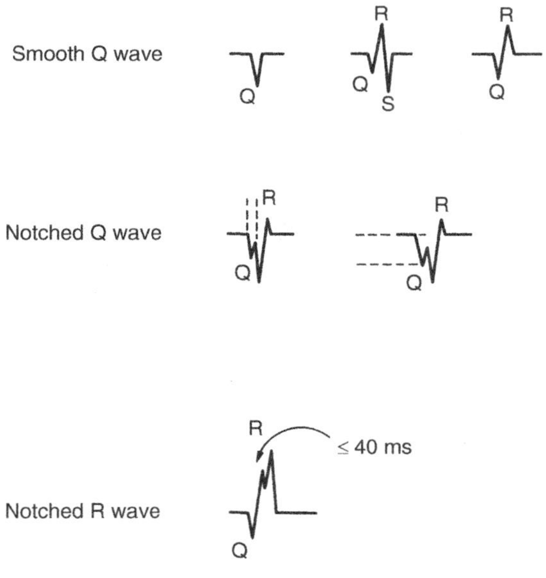

Fig. 4.15
A "smooth Q" is present, if there is no reversal in direction ≥0.05 mV in the first negative deflection (preceding the R wave). A "notched Q" is present when there is a reversal in direction ≥0.05 mV within the initial negative deflection. The duration of the Q, as indicated by the *vertical dashed line*, is taken from the baseline to the point directly above the peak of the notch. The amplitude of the Q, as indicated by the horizontal *dashed lines*, is measured from the nadir of the negative deflection preceding the notch to the PQ-segment baseline. As indicated by the *arrow*, a "notched R" for the purpose of ECG scoring of infarct size is defined as a reversal ≥0.05 mV starting within the first 40 ms of the QRS

amplitude. A "notched Q" is present (➋ Fig. 4.15) if there is any reversal in direction ≥0.05 mV within the initial negative deflection. In this instance, the duration of the Q wave extends along the PR baseline only to the point directly above the peak of the "notch." The amplitude of the Q extends to the nadir of the depression preceding the notch, and when the entire complex is a negative deflection (QS), the amplitude of the S extends to the nadir of the negative deflection following the "notch." When an initial wave is positive an R wave is present. A positive deflection which follows a Q wave is also considered an R wave. For the purpose of the QRS scoring, an "R wave" is considered to be the first positive deflection that appears. It extends until it reaches the baseline to become either an S wave or to complete the QRS complex. A "notched" initial R occurs when there is a reversal in direction ≥0.05 mV beginning within the first 40 ms of the QRS.

Strict and consistent application of the waveform definitions described in detail in this methods section is required to obtain consistent performance of the infarct size criteria. Failure to observe this definition will result in falsely awarding points. For example, an rS complex might be present in lead aVF prior to an infarct. The r wave would then be lost as a result of the infarct, producing an entirely negative deflection. A notch might appear with a peak at 30 ms after the onset. Only three points would be awarded using the above definitions while five points would be awarded if the entire negative deflection were considered a Q wave. A graphic of the waveform definitions of ➋ Fig. 4.15 is present in the lower right of the 53-Criteria/32-Point QRS infarct size scoring worksheet, ➋ Fig. 4.16.

4.3.6.3 Accurate Waveform Measurement

Careful manual measurements of both amplitudes and durations should be made with micro-adjustable calipers using the center of the trace of the inscribed wave form. ECG recorders with double gain, double speed options (some have recording speeds of 250–500 mm/s) would increase the resolution and decrease the variability of measurements for scoring purposes. Only 3-channel, 12-lead ECG tracings recorded at 10 mm/mV and at 25 mm/s paper speed were available on the majority of the tracings used in the validation studies reported. In the presence of major acute ST elevation in any lead, the amplitude measurements will be influenced by the "injury currents." To minimize these effects, the R amplitude should be measured from the PQ segment baseline and the S amplitude from the J point of the ST.

4.3.6.4 Guidelines for QRS Scoring

Two aspects of individual criteria must be considered (➋ Fig. 4.16): weighting and selecting. Weighting refers to the number of points awarded for criteria satisfied (in brackets in ➋ Fig. 4.16). Of the 53 criteria, 37 have a weight of 1, 15 a weight of 2, and 1 a weight of 3. The additional points are awarded when there is increasing magnitude (either amplitude or duration) of the same waveform abnormality. Selecting refers to the process of choosing a single criterion from a group (inside the brackets, ➋ Fig. 4.16). When criteria with multiple weights are included within a bracket, they are ordered by decreasing weights. Therefore, proceeding from the top down within a bracket, one should select only the first criterion satisfied. The total point score for each ECG is the sum of the points accumulated from the criteria satisfied. The significance and appropriate diagnostic statements and probabilities for any given total QRS point score is shown in ➋ Table 4.3. The six steps to be taken to apply the score in general for infarct size are as follows:

(a) Is normal LV conduction present without ECG changes of emphysema, RVH or LVH? *Score ECG for infarct size and location using age and gender criteria adjustments and attach diagnostic statements with modifiers as tabulated in* ➋ Table 4.3.
(b) Are criteria for LVH or conduction defects LAFB, RBBB, LBBB present? If so, they can be QRS scored, with confidence, for infarct size and location using the revised criteria in Appendix and B: ➋ Figs. 4.31a, b, LVH+Anterior MI, ➋ Fig. 4.37a, b RBBB + Posterolateral MI, ➋ Fig. 4.41a, b LBBB + Apical MI and an Inferobasal MI. ➋ Figs. 4.30a, b through ➋ 4.36a, b are examples of typical healed infarcts in each of the three arterial distributions that illustrate the points made above regarding the scoring methodology.

Myocardial Infarction

INFARCT SIZE - ECG SCORE - "HOW TO" WORKSHEET
COMPLETE 53-CRITERIA/32-POINT QRS SCORING SYSTEM

PANEL A: ECG POINTS (3% LV each) — PANEL B: % LV INFARCT IN 12 LV SEGMENTS

Lead	Lead Criteria	Pts. each cri.	Lead max. pts.	LAD ant. 1 2 3	LAD sup. 4 5 6	RCA inf. 7 8 9	CX post 10 11 12
I	Q>=30 MS	1			1 1		1
	{R/Q<=1	1	2		1 1 1		
	{R<=0.2 MV						
II	{Q>=40 MS	2	2			2 2 2	
	{Q>=30 MS	1				2 1	
aVL	Q>=30 MS	1	2		2 1		
	R/Q<=1	1			1 2		
aVF	{Q>=50 MS	3				3 2 2	1 1
	{Q>=40 MS	2				2 2 2	
	{Q>=30 MS	1	5			2 1	
	{R/Q<=1	2				2 3	1
	{R/Q<=2	1				1 2	
V_1 Ant.	any Q	1	1	1 2			
Post.	R/S>=1	1					1 1 1
	{R>=50 ms	2			1	1 1	1 1 1
	{R>=1.0 mV						
	{R>=40 ms	1	4			1	1 1
	{R>0.7 mV						
	Q/S<=0.2 mV	1				1	1 1
V_2 Ant.	{any Q						
	{R<=10 ms	1	1	1 2			
	{R<=0.1 mV						
Post.	R/S>=1.5	1				1	1 1
	{R>=60 ms	2				1 1	1 2 1
	{R>=2.0 mV						
	{R>=50 ms	1	4			1	1 1
	{R>=1.5 mV						
	Q/S<=0.3 mV					1	1 1
V_3	{Q>=30 ms	2		2 2 1	1		
	{R<=10 mS		2				
	{R<=0.2 mv	1		1 1	1		
	{Q>=20 mS						
V_4	Q>=20 ms	1		1 1	1		
	{R/Q<=0.5	2		2 1	1 1	1	
	{R/S<=0.5						
	{R/Q<=1		3				
	{R/S<=1	1		1 1	1		
	{R<=0.5 mV						
	{.04Rnotch						
V_5	Q>=30 ms	1		1 1	1		
	{R/Q<=1	2		2 1	1 1	1	
	{R/S<=1						
	{R/Q<=2		3				
	{R/S<=2	1		1	1 1		
	{R<=0.6 mV						
	{.04Rnotch						
V_6	Q>=30 ms	1				1	2
	{R/Q<=1	2			1	1	2 2
	{R/S<=1						
	{R/Q<=3		3				
	{R/S<=3	1				1	1 1
	{R<=0.6 mV						
	{.04Rnotch						
TOTALS:	Points		32 %LVI→				

If >1 criterion in bracket met, select one with most points.
If >1 criterion in bracket has the same point, score only once.

Age normalize all amplitude criteria to age 55 by increasing them 1%yr age 20−54 and decreasing them 1%/yr for > 55yrs.

For Females further decrease by 10% all QRSdur and QRSamp Criteria.

>= denotes greater than or equal to
<= denoter less than or equal to

INFARCT SIZE - ECG SCORE - HOW TO --

1. CIRCLE EACH ECG CRITERIA MET FROM...PANEL A (If more than one criterion in bracket met, circle one with most points only)
2. CIRCLE POINTS SCORED EACH CRITERIA.. PANEL A (If more than one criterion in bracket has the same point, score only once)
3. CIRCLE %LV INFARCT IN EACH SEGMENT} FOR EACH QRS CRITERIA MET........... PANEL B
4. PLACE ⊗ (FOR EACH 1% LVI) FROM..... PANEL B IN PROPER SEGMENT IN DIAGRAM BELOW

SEGMENT SUBDIVISION

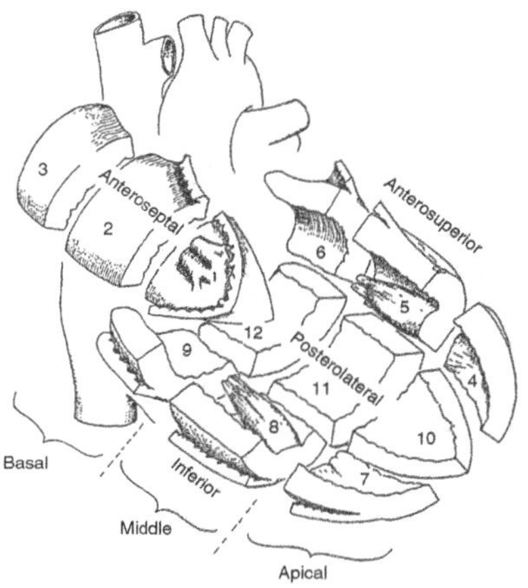

INFARCT SIZE: EJECTION FRACTION:

TOTAL ECG POINTS____x3=% LV INFARCTED (%LVI) ________

65−%LVI = ESTIMATED EJECTION FRACTION (EEF) ________

INFARCT LOCATION: (IN 12 LV SEGMENTS)

EACH ⊗ = 1% OF LV INFARCTED,
8 ⊗ IN A SEGMENT = 100% OF SEGMENT

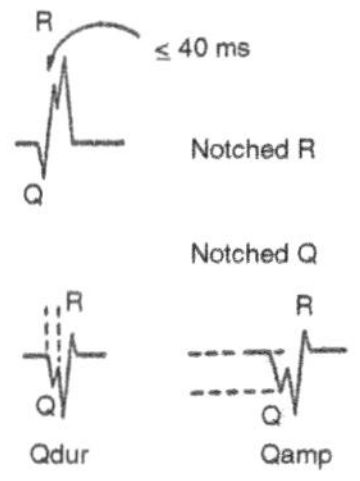

Fig. 4.16
Worksheet that can be copied and used for the routine scoring of an ECG for infarct size. Instructions for scoring are given on the *lower left* and for wave-form definitions of notched R and Q on the *lower right*. Adjustments to the criteria thresholds for age and female gender are defined lower left. *Upper right* are instructions for distributing each 1% of LV infarct in panel B (for each criterion met in panel A) into the 12 segment subdivision on the *middle right*. Also see Sect. 4.3.6.4 for the stepwise use of the score in the presence of hypertrophies or conduction defects

Table 4.3
Diagnostic statements and significance for ECG infarct-size score

ECG points	Diagnostic statement (fill in location ())	Pathology E% LVI[a] (%)	Angiography EEF (%)[b]	Probability (%) CAD[c]	Normal
1[d]	consider small () infarct	3	62	10–24	10–24
2	possible small () infarct	6	59	25–49	5–9
3	probable small: () infarct	9	56	50–94	3–4
4	small () infarct	12	53	95–97	<2
5–7	moderate () infarct	15–21	50–44	98	<1
8–10	large () infarct	24–30	41–35	>99	<1
≥11	very large () infarct	≥33	<33	>99	<1

[a]E% LVI, estimated % left ventricle infarcted
[b]EEF(%), estimated ejection fraction (%)
[c]CAD, coronary artery disease
[d]Diagnostic statement warranted for 1 point from the following highly specific criteria only: Q ≥ 30 ms, I, aVF, V4, V5, V6; R ≥ 40 ms, V1; R ≥ 50 ms, V2. If screening apparently healthy populations where the incidence of CAD is low, accumulate ≥3 points before a diagnostic statement "consider small..." is made, and ≥4 points for "possible small..."

4.3.6.5 Format of Scoring Criteria

The complexity of the criteria characteristics mentioned above requires an innovative format of presentation of the scoring system. The current format (➋ Fig. 4.16) represents a 20-year evolution of attempts to present a simple, logical, and unambiguous approach. As its labeling "INFARCT SIZE – ECG SCORE – 'HOW TO' WORKSHEET" indicates, this worksheet can be readily copied, with enlargement to fill a standard letter copy paper which is the form we have used to good effect for the last several years. The updated worksheets with adjustments for the confounders LVH and conduction defects are in appendices A and B.

4.3.7 Automated ECG Analysis Programs and QRS Score for Infarct Size

The manual method of using the QRS scoring system just described in detail in the preceding section is readily adaptable to automated ECG analysis programs. An automated version of the QRS score that included the distribution of damage into the 12 LV segments as defined in ➋ Fig. 4.16 was originally written by Schussler, adapted by Sharp and Laks, and reported in 1983 at the Engineering Foundation Conference by Madrid et al. [110]. A microprocessor based ECG analysis program in a portable bedside cart system of 12 simultaneous leads with the ECG score incorporated into the cart system was assessed by Madrid et al. in 1984 [106]. It was found, not unexpectedly, that both of these automated measurement and analysis systems were more reproducible than even experienced manual readers. The automated measurement programs were, in general, more accurate in making measurements of both amplitude and duration than manual readers. The bedside cart system of 12 simultaneous leads was also consistently more accurate in measuring QRS onset and offset and in identifying those criteria that depended on these measurements. Programs for the application of the QRS score for infarct size by computer are available as special "research tools" options, or by contact with the individual investigators who developed them.

The well known age, race, and sex differences in QRS amplitudes and durations have an effect on every criterion in the QRS scoring system. In the specificity studies reported by Hindman et al. [107], using only normal Caucasian subjects stratified by age in decades, and by gender, it was observed that the QRS scoring system performed best in the decade of 40–50 for which the original criteria were established. The number of false positives increased in the younger age groups, especially males, due to increased voltages commonly seen in this age group, and in older age groups, particularly the older females due to the lower voltages common in these older subjects. The measurement of a large array of amplitude, duration and wave shape descriptors of each wave of each lead on the ECG for large populations of normals stratified by age, race, and gender, is a near heroic task for the manual reader, but grist for the mill of a modern computer. An important normal database of ECGs from 1,339 ambulatory normal subjects living in Western Scotland recorded using a simultaneous multilead system has been reported by Macfarlane and Lawrie (Vol. 3 of the 1st edition). This database has become widely available for each decades of 1920s–1950s and older, subdivided by gender. A smaller cohort of 503 (255 males, 248 females) normal Chinese was also presented along with a larger cohort of 1,329 Japanese with ECGs recorded earlier on paper and with measurements made by hand. A similar cohort of ambulatory black subjects is not present. Another limitation of this important normal database is the absence of similar data for the older decades, now being seen in chest pain centers with major increased frequency. As comprehensive age, gender and race specific databases become available, the sensitivity and specificity of the ECG diagnosis of the presence, size and location of acute and healed myocardial infarcts in the younger and older decades can be expected to improve significantly. Criteria for the quantification of infarct size can be "fine tuned" to be gender, age, and race specific. Some commercial vendors are now supporting "gender smart" ECG interpretation algorithms and the others appear to be coming online. Enhancements for gender and age are included in our current edition of the QRS MI Size Scoring System presented in ➋ Fig. 4.16.

Based on the presence of important high frequency components as a result of disruption of the activation fronts by the complex geometry at the infarct boundary, and by small multifocal infarcts, the optimal normal digital databases will need to be sampled at rates of at least 1,000 samples per second. This will be necessary in order to identify the limits of these high frequency components in normals before they can be applied with statistical confidence to patient populations suspected of having a myocardial infarction.

Automated ECG/VCG analysis systems with their large database storage capability are also ideally suited to the archiving of digitized ECG/VCGs for later comparison to newly acquired tracings. Detailed wave by wave, lead by lead comparison is a simple task for comparative programs. Automatic gain adjustments are routine to correct for individual ECG preamplifier drift in amplitude. Serial comparison using large high resolution ECG databases of normal controls can readily show when newly measured waveforms are outside the 96% or 98% age-race-sex matched normal ranges, and when similar confidence limits for normal variability of serial comparison records have been exceeded. This kind of detailed comparison to large well validated normal databases is possible by manual means but is so labor intensive that this discourages it being done routinely. Such high resolution and comprehensive comparisons are trivial for a modern computer when validated measurement algorithms are installed and the proper digital data is archived in their electronic files. *We again stoutly reaffirm our earlier recommendation*: **THAT EVERY YOUNG ADULT ACQUIRE SUCH A HIGH RESOLUTION BASELINE ECG RECORD BEFORE AGE 30. A wallet sized photographic and electronic copy can be carried personally thereafter.**

4.4 Principal Areas of Infarction and Typical ECG/VCG Changes

4.4.1 Acute Myocardial Infarction, Evolving Changes of Injury, Ischemia and Necrosis

The evolutionary changes that occur after an acute coronary occlusion and subsequent infarction, when viewed from the vectorial perspective, are the same for each of the arterial perfusion beds. In order to maintain the relationship with part or all of these three main coronary artery perfusion beds, it is important to maintain the separation in nomenclature of the regions, anterior for LAD, posterolateral for LCX and inferior for RCA/PDA as indicated earlier in ➋ Sect. 4.2.3. The direction and amplitude of local electrical field changes over time (mean vector or axis changes) from injury, ischemia and necrosis or infarct, have major reflections in individual leads of a 12-lead ECG (including the 24-view ECG; to be discussed shortly) or the orthogonal *X*, *Y*, and *Z* leads. This corresponds to the orientation of the specific lead to the mean direction of the electric field from the local arterial perfusion bed distal to the obstruction. As discussed in more detail in ➋ Chaps. 2 and ➋ 11 of *Basic Electrocardiology: Cardiac Electrophysiology, ECG Systems and Mathematical Modeling*, if the lead is at right angles to the average direction of the electrical event, that is, on the "null plane" as defined by Grant [41] and others, the particular change, whether it be regional depolarization or repolarization, will be poorly represented in that lead. Likewise, the event will be maximally represented in leads in three-dimensional space that are oriented parallel to the mean axis or vector of the event and perpendicular to the null plane. The orderly sequence (Cabrera) of limb leads used throughout this chapter, including the 24-view 12-lead ECG illustrations, enhance the determination of various axes, i.e., mean P, initial 30 ms, terminal 30 ms and mean QRS, and mean STj and T axes or vectors.

The serial ECG changes of evolving acute myocardial infarction associated with injury/ischemia, necrosis and healing of the infarct can in general be classified into four phases: hyperacute, acute, subacute and completed (chronic healing) (➋ Fig. 4.17). In general, the acute injury/ischemia process is potentially reversible in the hyperacute and early acute phases with progressive infarction occurring throughout the acute phase. The healing phase begins in the subacute and continues with remodeling in the completed or chronic phase. The time course of these phases can vary between individuals. They may be quite rapid as in first infarction occurring early in life with little or no time to have developed collaterals from adjacent normally perfused regions. They may be delayed during gradual or intermittent coronary occlusion in subjects who have developed collaterals. They may be aborted by prompt and sustained reperfusion.

(a) *Hyperacute Phase*: Within seconds after acute coronary occlusion, there is typically a significant increase in amplitude and peaking of the T wave, directed outward from the epicardium of the centroid of the acutely ischemic region. This is commonly called "hyperacute T." Experimental work by Kleber et al. [111] and computer simulation work by Miller and Geselowitz [86] showed that shortening of the action potential is what produces the hyperactue T. Furthermore, more recent work by Shaw and Rudy has suggested that opening of K-ATP channels is what causes the most significant shortening of the ischemic action potential and likely results from shift of excess potassium into the extracellular space [112]. Although this change may persist for some time in a slowly developing process, typically in some seconds to a minute later the ST segment begins to join the hyperacute T as a "current of injury" vector directed outward perpendicular to the epicardium of the centroid of the injured/ischemic region. When these currents of injury/ischemia are large, indicating a large area of severe ischemia, the DC level of the entire baseline (see ➋ Fig. 4.9) becomes negative. The middle and late QRS forces are drawn, with the ST-T, outward from the epicardium of the region at risk.

(b) *Acute Phase*: In the early part of this phase, the terminal portion of the T wave and early QRS forces begin to decrease in amplitude along the axis of the acute injury/ischemia vector that is perpendicular to the epicardium of the risk region. During the early half of this phase, the ischemic process is potentially reversible with consequent salvage of the injured myocardium. The specific QRS changes of the evolving local infarct begin to appear and progress,

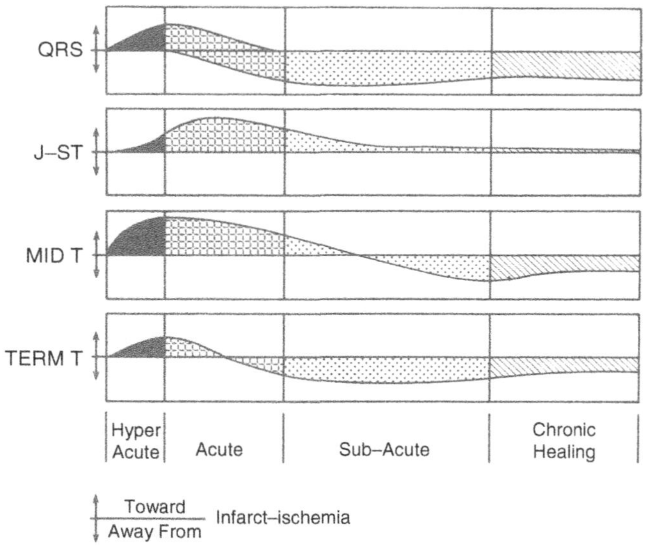

Fig. 4.17
Diagram shows the four ECG phases of acute coronary occlusion. Panels showing the evolution of the acute infarction to its chronic stable phase are indicated at the *bottom*. Each panel illustrates the typical change in direction and amplitude of the QRS complex, J point and ST segment, and mid and terminal T wave. A shift outward toward the ischemic/infarcted area is indicated by an *upward-pointing arrow*; a shift inward away from this area is indicated by a *downward-pointing arrow*

reaching their full extent at the end of the acute phase. As the QRS emerges from the current of injury it shifts away from the region at risk, revealing abnormal Q waves, notched or attenuated R waves, and altered terminal forces. The precise changes depend on the size and location of the infarct. They can be remarkably accelerated following successful early revascularization interventions. In the absence of such interventions, the acute phase typically lasts 6–8 h from the onset of symptoms.

(c) *Subacute (Evolving) Phase*: Over the next day or two, as the infarct evolves through the sub-acute to completed or chronic healing stage, the QRS changes of infarct are fully developed and stable. The ST segments subside toward their normal location, while the mid and terminal T-wave becomes fused with major displacement inward from the infarcted region. The ischemic myocardium has become, in general, irreversibly damaged and healing has begun. T waves are now usually deeply inverted in leads whose positive pole faces the epicardium over the centroid of the infarct. In the 24-lead ECGs of ➲ Figs. 4.22–4.26, this relationship is to be noted for either the positive or negative pole.

(d) *Completed phase*: During the completed or chronic healing phase, the changes on the ECG caused by the infarction have stabilized (see ➲ Fig. 4.17). If there is no recurrence of ischemia, these changes will gradually move toward resolution. The T wave will remain directed inward away from the infarcted region and will gradually decrease in size unless influenced by ischemia elsewhere, or by ventricular hypertrophy, or bundle branch block.

The reader is encouraged to review the serial changes in ➲ Figs. 4.18–4.21 illustrating those changes seen with acute anterior, posterolateral, and inferior infarctions in patients who did not receive revascularization interventions. Scores for

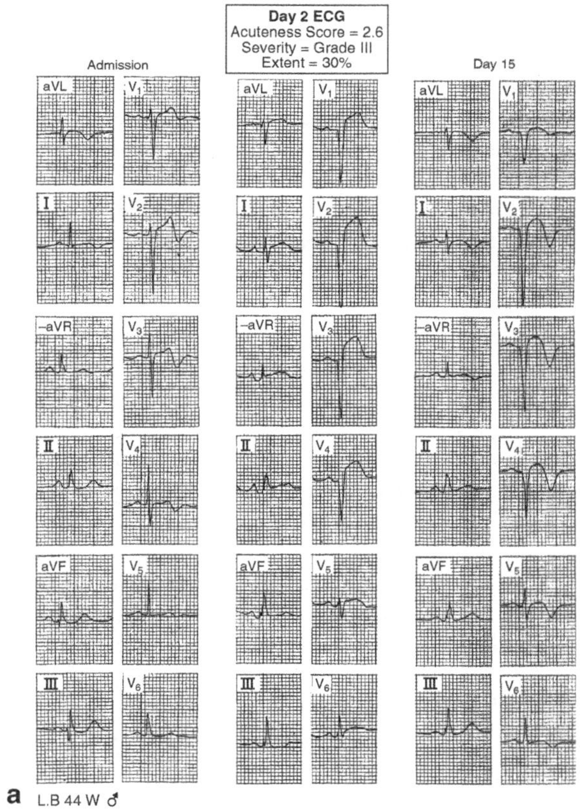

Fig. 4.18 (Continued)

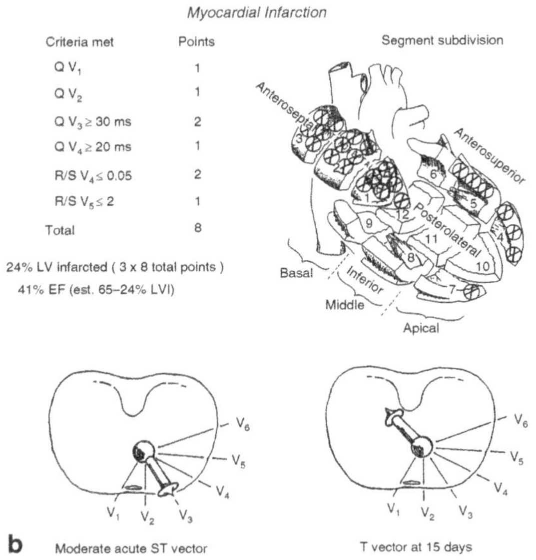

Fig. 4.18
(a) Note limb leads are in the orderly (Cabrera) sequence from the top down, aVL, I, -aVR, II, aVF, III. These serial ECGs are of a 44-year-old man with chest pain who was admitted to the hospital with possible acute myocardial infarction. The slight ST elevation with coving and T inversion in aVL, I, and V1–V5, indicating at most a moderate ischemic risk area (see Sect. 4.4.1 for details). By the next morning he has acute ST elevation changes of acute anterior myocardial infarction and had evolved QRS changes of a moderate sized infarct, see (b). By day 15, the typical evolution of the STT with deeply inverted T waves as noted and the QRS changes of a moderate sized anterior infarct show no further evolution. (b) For the case of (a), the moderate peak acute ST vector was plotted by the method of Grant from the day 2 tracing, as was the T vector at day 15. The scoring criteria met in the day 15 record, the points scored for each, and the total of 8 points are tabulated. As indicated each point represents 3% of the left ventricle infarcted (LVI), the 8 points predict 24% LVI and an estimated ejection (EF) of 41%. The distribution into the 12 LV segments on the *upper right* is derived from panel B of the ECG scoring work sheet, shown in more detail for this specific patient in Fig. 4.16. Angiographic data is not available

the extent, severity and acuteness of ischemia are shown in each of these figures. Detailed descriptions of these acuteness and severity scores are in Sect. 4.4.2.

It follows that major injury, ST-T vectors of acute myocardial infarction or evolving infarct, QRS and T vectors from the anterior or posterolateral wall of the heart, will be seen optimally in anterior-posterolateral oriented leads V1, V2, V3, V4 and *Z*. These changes are usually maximal for either anterior or posterolateral AMI in V2 or V3. Electric field vectors originating in the opposing anterior and posterolateral walls will produce opposite (mirror-image) effects to each other in these same leads. Likewise, anterosuperior or inferior wall injury, ischemia or infarct will produce their main changes in superior-inferior oriented leads aVL, III, aVF, II and Y. As a result of the orientation of the positive end of the leads, III and aVF will generally show mirror-image acute injury/ischemia effects to aVL for acute anterosuperior injury and vice-versa for acute inferior injury. If the lesions also extend toward or localize to the apex (left and 30° inferior) or the left side of the heart, leads with a left-right (base-apex) orientation, i.e., I, -aVR, II, V4, V5, V6, and *X*, will also reflect these changes.

The term "reciprocal changes" which occurs in much of the ECG literature to describe these "mirror image" changes is mainly descriptive. When considered from a vectorial perspective, this term may be misleading and its use should be avoided. It is more anatomically and electrophysiologically correct to assign a direction to these acute ST-T changes, along with a location in the heart, together with size or extent modifiers that denote their significance. When anterior-posterior leads V1–V4 show a prominent anterior ST-T change of acute anterior infarction, the term "with reciprocal changes in

Myocardial Infarction

INFARCT SIZE - ECG SCORE - "HOW TO" WORKSHEET
COMPLETE 53-CRITERIA/32-POINT QRS SCORING SYSTEM

PANEL A — ECG POINTS (3% LV each) / PANEL B — % LV INFARCT IN 12 LV SEGMENTS

Lead	Lead Criteria	Pts. each cri.	Lead max. pts.	LAD ant. 1 2 3	LAD sup. 4 5 6	RCA inf. 7 8 9	CX post. 10 11 12
I	Q>=30 MS	1			1 1		1
	R/Q<=1	1	2		1 1 1		
	R<=0.2 MV						
II	{Q>=40 MS	2	2			2 2 2	
	{Q>=30 MS	1				2 1	
aVL	Q>=30 MS	1	2		2 1		
	R/Q<=1	1			1 2		
aVF	{Q>=50 MS	3				3 2 2	1 1
	{Q>=40 MS	2				2 2 2	
	{Q>=30 MS	1	5			2 1	
	{R/Q<=1	2				2 3	1
	{R/Q<=2	1				1 2	
V1 Ant.	(any Q)	(1)	1	(1)(2)			
Post.	R/S>=1	1					1 1 1
	{R>=50 ms	2			1	1 1	1 1 1
	{R>=1.0 mV						
	{R>=40 ms	1	4			1	1 1
	{R>0.7 mV						
	Q/S<=0.2 mV	1				1	1 1
V2 Ant.	(any Q)						
	{R<=10 ms	(1)	1	(1)(2)			
	{R<=0.1 mV						
Post.	R/S>=1.5	1				1	1 1
	{R>=60 ms	2				1 1	1 2 1
	{R>=2.0 mV						
	{R>=50 ms	1	4			1	1 1
	{R>=1.5 mV						
	Q/S<=0.3 mV					1	1 1
V3	(Q>=30 ms)	(2)		(2)(2)(1)	(1)		
	{R<=10 mS		2				
	{R<=0.2 mV	1		1 1	1		
	{Q>=20 ms						
V4	(Q>=20 ms)	(1)		(1)(1)	(1)		
	(R/Q<=0.5)	(2)		(2)(1)	(1)(1)	(1)	
	R/S<=0.5						
	R/Q<=1		3				
	R/S<=1	1		1 1	1		
	R<=0.5 mV						
	.04Rnotch						
V5	Q>=30 ms	1		1 1	1		
	{R/Q<=1	2		2 1	1 1	1	
	{R/S<=1						
	{R/Q<=2		3				
	(R/S<=2)	(1)		(1)	(1)(1)		
	{R<=0.6 mV						
	{.04Rnotch						
V6	Q>=30 ms	1				1	2
	{R/Q<=1	2			1	1	2 2
	{R/S<=1						
	{R/Q<=3		3				
	{R/S<=3	1				1	1 1
	{R<=0.6 mV						
	{.04Rnotch						
TOTALS:	Points	8	32 %LVI →	6 6 5	3 3	1	

If >1 criterion in bracket met, select one with most points.
If >1 criterion in bracket has the same point, score only once.

Age normalize all amplitude criteria to age 55 by increasing them 1%yr age 20–54 and decreasing them 1%/yr for > 55yrs.

For Females further decrease by 10% all QRSdur and QRSamp Criteria.

>= denotes greater than or equal to
<= denoter less than or equal to

INFARCT SIZE - ECG SCORE - HOW TO --

1. CIRCLE EACH ECG CRITERIA MET FROM...PANEL A (If more than one criterion in bracket met, circle one with most points only)
2. CIRCLE POINTS SCORED EACH CRITERIA.. PANEL A (If more than one criterion in bracket has the same point, score only once)
3. CIRCLE %LV INFARCT IN EACH SEGMENT} FOR EACH QRS CRITERIA MET............ PANEL B
4. PLACE ⊗ (FOR EACH 1% LVI) FROM..... PANEL B IN PROPER SEGMENT IN DIAGRAM BELOW

SEGMENT SUBDIVISION

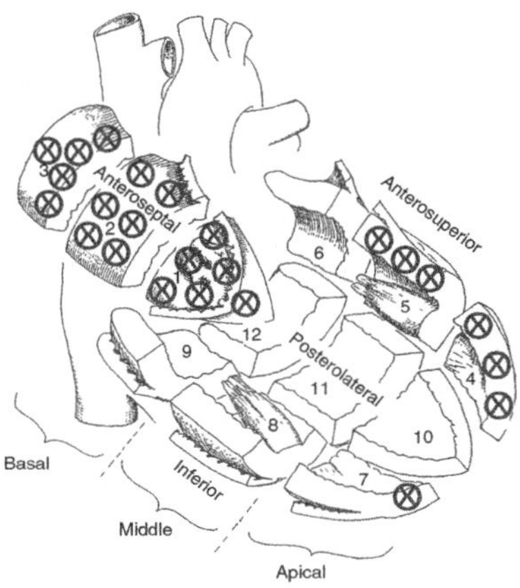

L.B. 44 W. ♂

INFARCT SIZE: EJECTION FRACTION:

TOTAL ECG POINTS **8** x3=% LV INFARCTED (%LVI) **24%**

65–%LVI = ESTIMATED EJECTION FRACTION (EEF) **41%**

INFARCT LOCATION: IN 12 LV SEGMENTS

EACH ⊗ = 1% OF LV INFARCTED,
8 ⊗ IN A SEGMENT = 100% OF SEGMENT

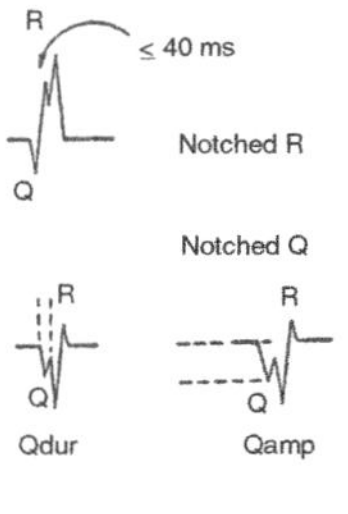

Fig. 4.19

The specific criteria met in the day 15 ECG of the patient in ➋ Fig. 4.18; the distribution into the 12 LV segments for each criterion is indicated in panel A and B. The totals are depicted in each segment in the diagram to the *right*. This is the method of scoring which is used throughout this chapter

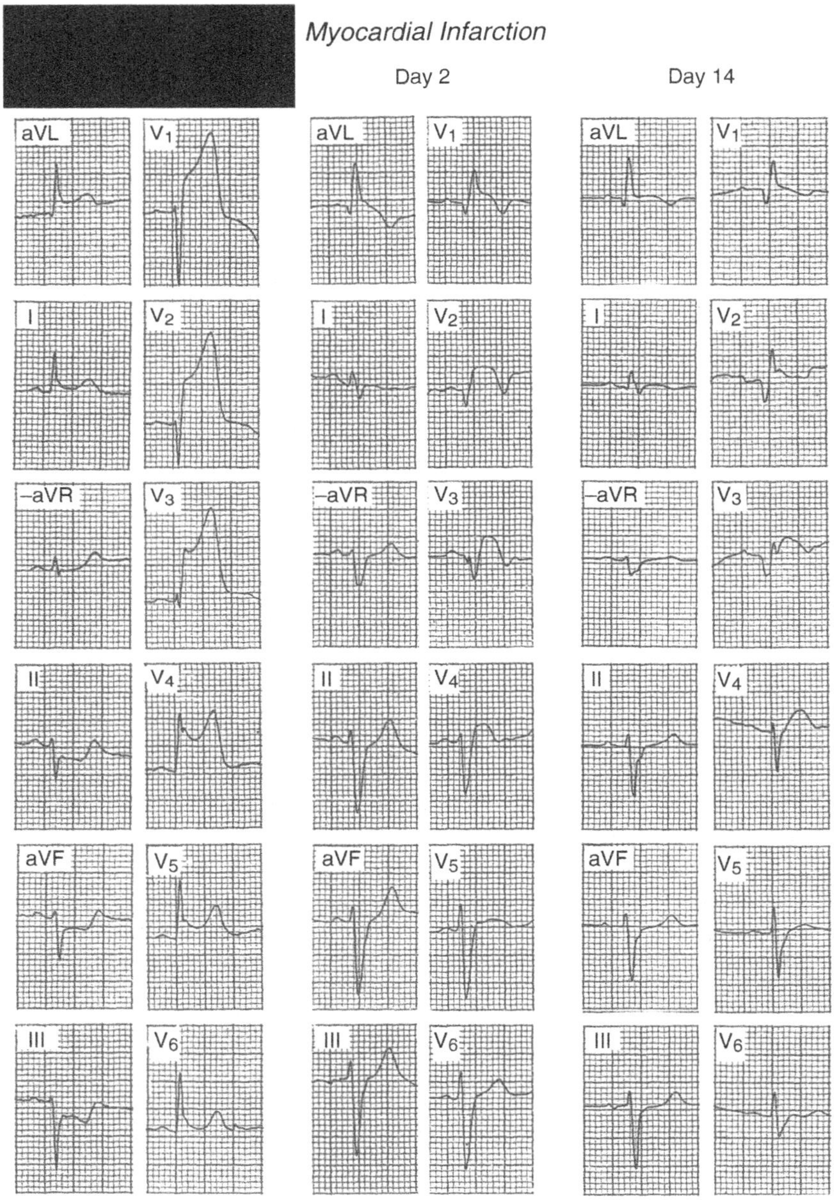

a L.E 53 W ♂

Fig. 4.20 (Continued)

inferior leads" is ambiguous. When an associated superior ST displacement vector is indicated in superior-inferior leads aVL, III, aVF and II, we prefer to use the phrase "with significant anterosuperior involvement" to flag this evidence for a very large area at risk from LAD occlusion proximal to a large first diagonal branch. When the major acute ST changes occur in V1, V2, V3, and V4, and are directed posteriorly, while additionally a lesser degree of acute ST change is directed inferiorly in II and aVF, the label "acute posterolateral infarction with probable inferior extension" is more anatomically and physiologically appropriate. Conversely when major ST-T changes of acute inferior injury and ischemia are present

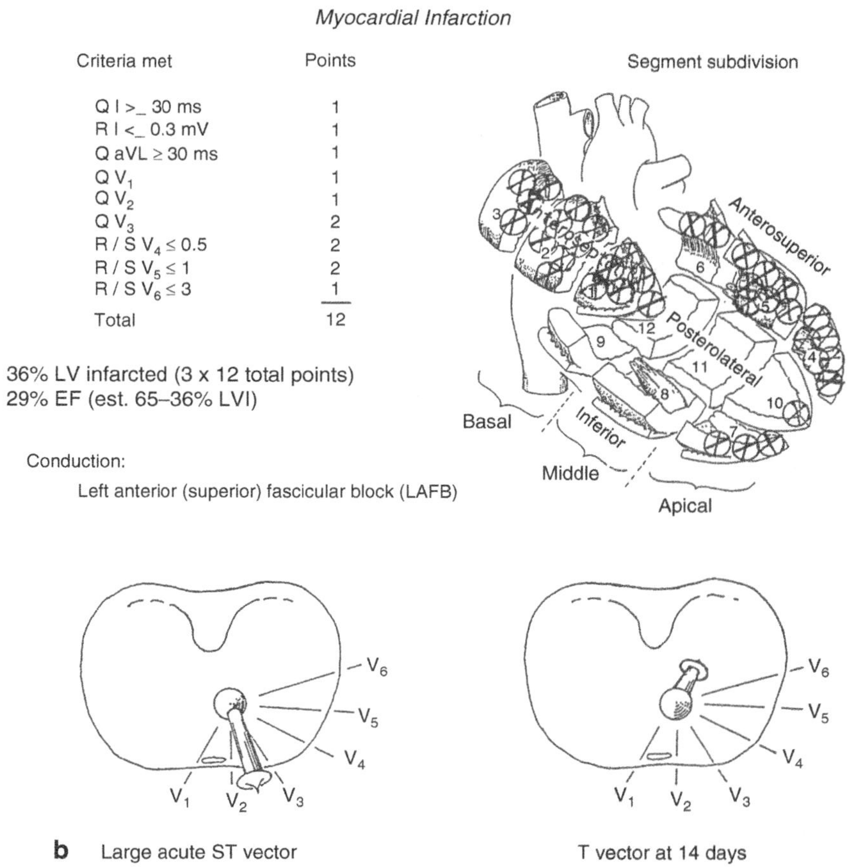

Fig. 4.20

(a) Note limb leads are in the orderly (Cabrera) sequence from the top down, aVL, I, -aVR, II, aVF, III. The admission ECG of a 53-year-old man with severe chest pain shows a large ST-T deviation which is anterior and significantly superior and leftward. This is indicative of a large area at risk in the proximal LAD distribution. The new onset right bundle branch block that appears on day 2 does not influence the QRS infarct size score for anterior infarct as shown in (b). For the case of (a) the large anterior and significantly superior and leftward ST vector on admission is consistent with a large LAD area at risk. The presence of a probable left anterior (superior) fascicular block (LAFB) on admission, and of RBBB by day 2 confirms the large area at risk, as does the QRS MI size score 12 points (estimated %LV I (infarct), 36% and an estimated LV ejection fraction of 29%). The predicted distribution of the infarct in the 12 LV segments is shown on the *right*. Angiographic data was not obtained for this patient

in II, aVF, and III, and posterior changes of a lesser degree are present in V1, V2, and V3, it is more appropriate to diagnose acute inferior myocardial infarction with posterolateral extension, than ascribing the latter to "reciprocal changes." If these local changes extend toward the apex or left border of the heart producing changes in the left-right (apex-base) leads, a notation so indicating would also be consistent, that is, "acute inferior myocardial infarction with probable posterolateral and apical extension." ➋ Table 4.4 provides a summary of the anterior, posterolateral, inferior and apical ST-T changes and the culprit artery responsible for them as well as the probable location in that artery. Details for each of these are provided in the following ➋ Sects. 4.4.3–4.4.9. We have found that these same local primary acute ST-T changes are seen as add-ons to the secondary ST-T changes of ventricular hypertrophies, bundle branch blocks, ventricular pacing and pre-excitation. These are dealt with in detail in ➋ Sect. 4.5.

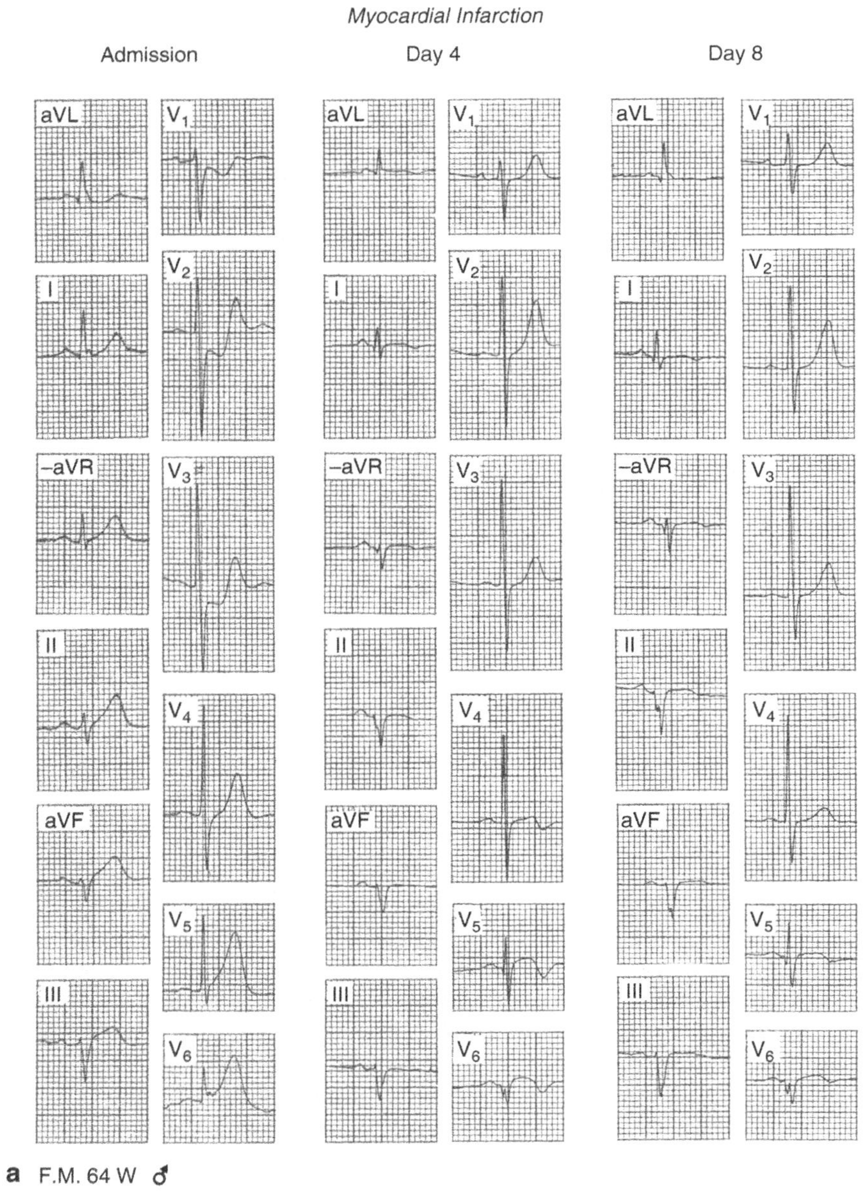

Fig. 4.21 (Continued)

4.4.2 Acuteness, Severity and Extent of Ischemia

Important additions to the ECG evaluation of patients who have acute myocardial ischemia/infarction would be provided by formal indices of the three key aspects of this pathologic process, namely: acuteness, severity and extent. Animal models that incorporated these three variables were able to account for 80% of variability in final infarct size [113], while human studies using the nuclear perfusion agent ^{9}9mTc-Sestamibi were able to account for 70% of the variability in final infarct size [27]. Indeed algorithms for each of these aspects have been developed, and literature regarding their validation has been accumulating for many years. Detailed instructions on how to calculate each of these scores is contained in the text

Criteria met	Points
R / S $V_1 \geq 1$	1
R / $V_1 \geq$ 40 ms	1
R / S $V_2 \geq 1.5$	1
R $V_2 \geq$ 1.5 mV	1
R / S $V_5 \leq 1$	2
Q $V_6 \geq$ 30 ms	1
R / S $V_6 \leq 1$	2
Total	9

27% LV infarcted (3 x 9 total points)
38% EF (est.: 65–27% LVI)

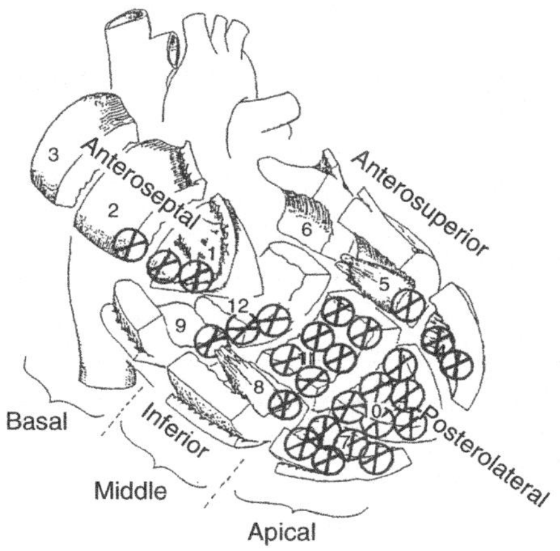

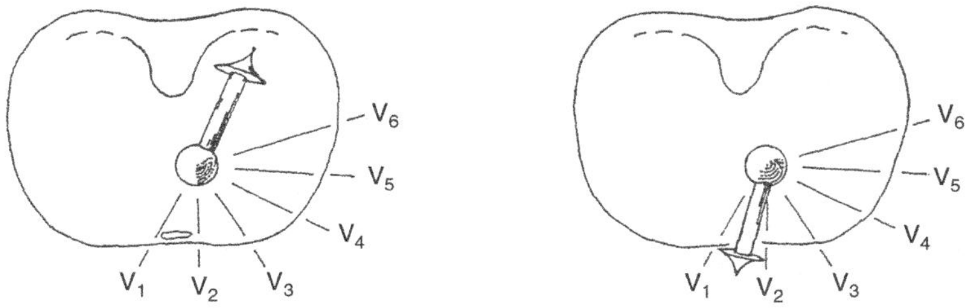

b Moderate to large acute ST vector — T vector at 8 days

Fig. 4.21
(a) Note limb leads are in the orderly (Cabrera) sequence from the top down, aVL, I, –aVR, II, aVF, III. The admission ECG of this 64-year-old man presenting with signs and symptoms of probable acute myocardial infarction had a major acute ST vector directed posterior, and less but significantly leftward. This is diagnostic of a moderate to large area at risk in the LCX distribution. Over the next few days QRS changes of a large posteroapical infarct with inferoapical extension evolved, see (b). (b) The acute ST vector and the evolved T vector at day 8, for the patient of (a), are consistent with a significant posteroapical area of potential infarction. The QRS changes and ECG criteria summarized in the *upper left* and *right* show a large infarct estimated to involve 27% of the left ventricle (estimated EF = 38%). The *upper right* of the figure shows an infarct localized to the distribution of a dominant obtuse marginal branch of the LCX that has significant extension to the inferoapical region. Angiographic data was not available for this patient

to follow. Examples of the scoring systems are shown in ➲ Figs. 4.18–4.20, and ➲ 4.25 for anterior MI, ➲ Figs. 4.22, ➲ 4.28, and ➲ 4.29 for inferior MI, and ➲ Figs. 4.21 and ➲ 4.27 for posterolateral MI.

4.4.2.1 Acuteness of Ischemia

The Anderson-Wilkins score for application on the presenting ECG for estimation of the acuteness of the ischemia/infarction process was introduced in 1995 [114, 115]. It was based on the concept described in ➲ Sect. 4.4.1 of the serial hyperacute, acute, and subacute phases of the ischemia/infarction process (➲ Fig. 4.17). The Anderson-Wilkins score is provided as a continuous scale from 4.0 (hyperacute) to 1.0 (subacute) based on the comparative hyperacute T waves versus abnormal Q waves in each of the leads with ST-segment elevation. ➲ Table 4.4 shows the abnormal

Table 4.4

Limits for abnormal Q waves and tall T waves in different ECG leads, as used for calculating the AW acuteness score. Reproduced from Heden et al. [116]

Leads	Old abnormal Q-wave criterion	New abnormal Q-wave criterion	Tall T-wave criterion
I	≥30 ms	≥20 ms	≥0.50 mV
II	≥30 ms	≥20 ms	≥0.50 mV
III	≥30 ms and abnormal Q in aVF	≥20 ms and abnormal Q in aVF	≥0.25 mV
aVR	–	–	–
aVL	≥30 ms	≥20 ms	≥0.25 mV
aVF	≥30 ms	≥20 ms	≥0.50 mV
V1	Any Q	Any Q	≥0.50 mV
V2	Any Q	Any Q	≥1.0 mV
V3	Any Q	Any Q	≥1.0 mV
V4	≥20 ms	≥20 ms	≥1.0 mV
V5	≥30 ms	≥20 ms	≥0.75 mV
V6	≥30 ms	≥20 ms	≥0.50 mV

Q-duration and T-amplitude criteria. The Q-duration criteria were modified by Heden and colleagues in 2003 to achieve a better distribution of acuteness scores in anterior and inferior MIs [116].

The Anderson-Wilkins ECG timing method considers each standard lead (except aVR) with either 0.1 mV or greater ST elevation or abnormally tall T waves. Acuteness phase is designated for each of these leads on the basis of the presence or absence of a tall T wave or an abnormal Q wave as defined in Table 4.4:

Phase 1A, tall T wave and no abnormal Q wave;
Phase 1B, positive T wave and no abnormal Q wave;
Phase 2A, tall T wave and abnormal Q wave;
Phase 2B, positive T wave and abnormal Q wave.
The Anderson-Wilkins (AW) acuteness score was calculated from the following formula:

$$\frac{4(\#\,\text{leads}\,1\text{A}) \pm 3(\#\,\text{leads}\,1\text{B}) \pm 2(\#\,\text{leads}\,2\text{A}) \pm 1(\#\,\text{leads}\,2\text{B})}{\text{Total}\,\#\,\text{leads with}\,1\text{A},\ 1\text{B},\ 2\text{A or}\ 2\text{B}}$$

The anterior MI acuteness score is derived from all precordial leads (V1–V6), and limb leads aVL, and I. The inferior AMI acuteness score is derived from limb leads II, III, and aVF, and from the following instances in some of the precordial leads: For V1 and V2 to be considered, the ST elevation must be greater in V1 than in V2, indicating right ventricular, rather than anterior left ventricular (left anterior descending artery) involvement. For V4–V6 to be included, the ST elevation must be greater in V6 than in V5 and V4, which would also exclude LAD artery occlusion induced anterior wall involvement [117]. To date, the AW-acuteness score has not been developed for patients with posterolateral MI from LCX occlusion. Future work will look at the relation between ST-depression, T wave inversion and large R waves in V1–V3 to calculate the acuteness.

The Anderson-Wilkins acuteness score is an ECG estimate of the time course of the myocardial infarction that has been shown to be superior to time from symptom onset in predicting myocardial salvage in patients receiving angioplasty for acute MI [118–120]. This is shown in Fig. 4.24 from Sejersten et al. [119] where the Aldrich ECG score was used to estimate the extent of ischemia and Selvester QRS score was used to estimate the final infarct size. This study showed a statistically significant relationship between the AW-acuteness score and 1-year mortality, although the event rate was small. A separate study by Engblom et al. showed a stronger relationship between the AW-acuteness score and myocardial

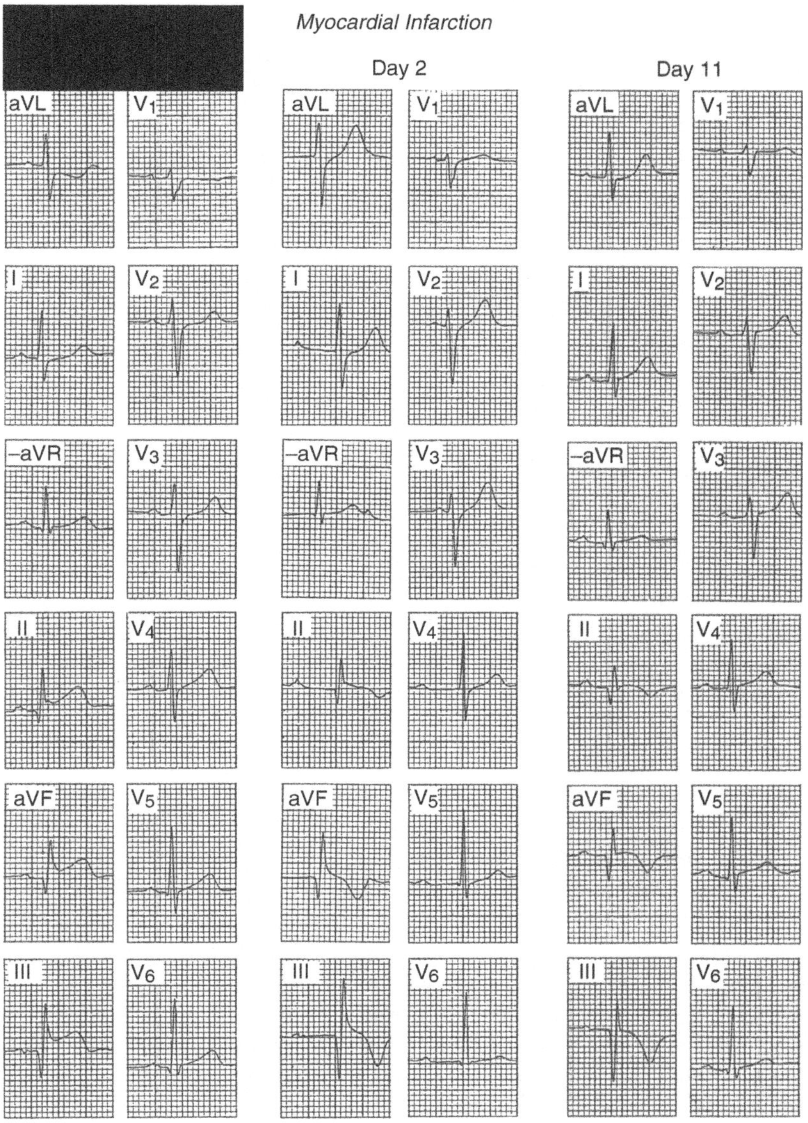

a L.G. 40 W ♂

Fig. 4.22 (Continued)

salvage than time from symptom onset [120]. This study used single photon emission computed tomography (SPECT) to measure the extent of ischemia and MRI to measure final infarct size.

4.4.2.2 The 24-Lead ECG and Acute Myocardial Infarction

The visualization of the spatial 3D ST-T vector and mirror image ("reciprocal") changes associated with acute occlusion of each of the three major coronary arteries or their major branches is facilitated by the use of the 24-lead ECG (which

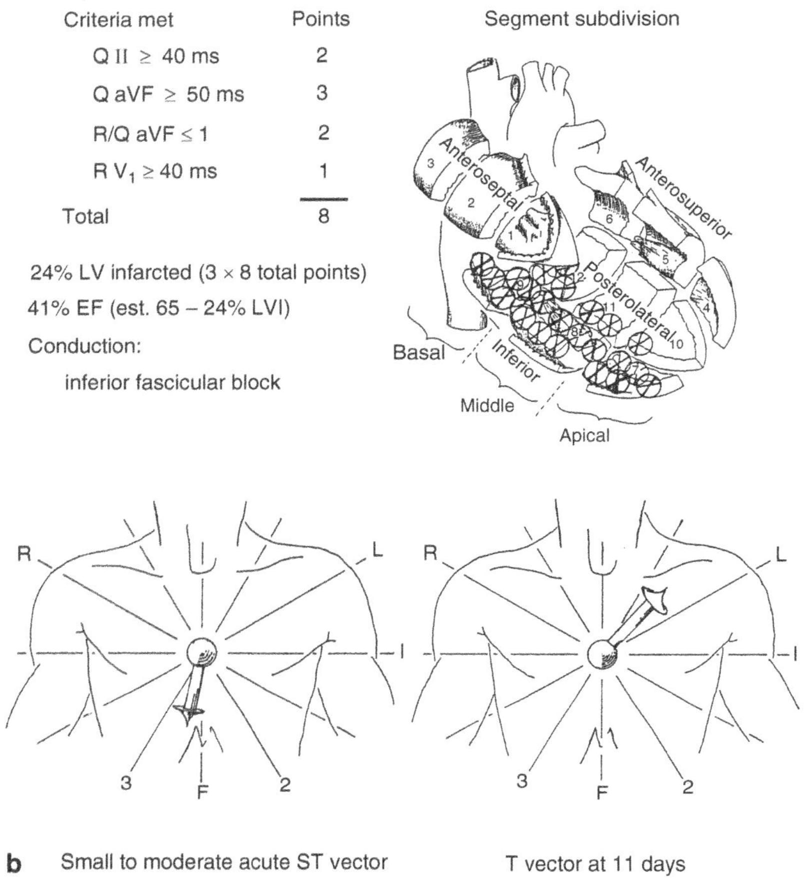

Fig. 4.22

(a) Note limb leads are in the orderly (Cabrera) sequence from the *top down*, aVL, I, –aVR, II, aVF, III. The case of a 40-year-old man seen in the emergency room with indigestion and a possible acute infarct. He had significant inferior Q waves, slightly prolonged QRS (120 ms) with wide separation of initial and terminal 30 ms vectors typical of inferior fascicular (peri-infarction) block as described in the text. Only modest ST elevation is seen with minimal terminal inferior T inversion suggesting (with the Q waves above) that at this time the ST-segment changes are already receding. No evidence of RV infarct (see text) is seen but transient second-degree AV block is present on day 2 that has cleared by day 11. (b) For the patient of (a), by day 11 evidence for minor posterior extension of this inferior infarct has evolved. The infarct is somewhat larger (8 points, 24% LV) than the typical inferior infarct, extending more toward the apex than usual. The acute ST vector and the T vector evolution at 11 days are quite typical. The admission ST vector in this case underestimated the area at risk and the large infarct that, in fact, evolved. The patient had been suffering symptoms for several hours before coming to the emergency room and may have been past his peak ST

includes both poles of the standard 12 leads). This concept was introduced by Pahlm-Webb and colleagues in 2002 [126] to aid in the visual diagnosis of acute occlusion, especially LCX occlusions with ST-segment depression in V1 and V2 but ST elevation in −V1 and −V2 (➋ Fig. 4.29). Cardiac magnetic resonance imaging (MRI) with gadolinium enhancement of the acute ischemic injured area, or the resultant scar when adjusted for wall thinning, provides the basis for a quantitative measure of myocardial infarct. This allows for direct measure of LV and infarct volume, mass, and the percent LV infarcted (%LVI). In the five ➋ Figs. 4.25–4.29, the standard 12-lead electrocardiogram was recorded at 50 mm/s, gain

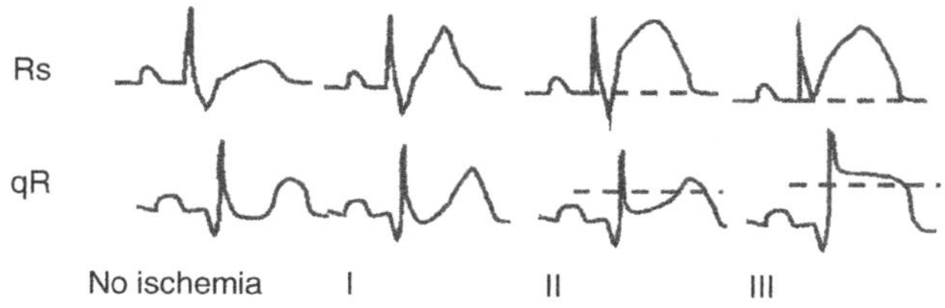

A. Consider only ECGs with (1) no complete RBBB or LBBB, (2) no LVH, (3) no WPW, (4) no ventricular paced or ventricular rhythm, (5) supraventricular QRS morphology, (6) total peak-to-peak QRS amplitude ≥0.4 mV, (7) ST elevation (rounded up to ≥ 0.1 mV) and (8) entirely positive T waves and/or tall positive T waves by Gambill criteria (III and aVL ≥ 0.25 mV; I,II, aVF, V1 and V6 ≥0.5 mV; V5≥0.75 mV; and V2, V3 and V4 ≥1.0 mV)

B. Measure from PR baseline. If there is PR depression consider TP baseline.

C. Assign Grades I,II, or III, to all leads meeting the stated criteria.

For leads I, II, III, aVL, aVF, V4 V5 and V6:

1. Leads with a QR configuration (i.e. R only or QR):
   Grade I tall positive T wave, no ST elevation
   Grade II positive T wave, J point/R wave amplitude ratio <0.5
   Grade III positive T wave, J point/Rwave amplitude ratio =>20 ms

2. Leads with RS or RSR' configuration (i.e. RSR' or QSR'): In leads with terminal S configuration and ST elev; assign grade II because of the presence of S waves.

Leads V4 and V5 in presence of left axis deviation:

- In cases with QRS axis ≤–30° and with S waves in lead V5: If there is ST elevation with out an S wave present in V4, assume that the pre-event ECG had S waves in V4; therefore assign the lead as Grade III.

- In cases with QRS axis ≤–30° and S waves in V6: If there is ST elevation without an S wave in V5, assume that the pre-event ECG had S waves in V5; therefore assign the lead as Grade III.

For leads V1, V2 and V3 regardless QRS configuration

- Grade I tall, positive T wave, no ST elevation.
- Grade II tall, positive T wave, ST elevation with an S wave below the isoelectric line.
- Grade III tall, positive T wave, ST elevation without an S wave below the iso electric line.

Fig. 4.23
Scoring rules for the refined Sclarovsky-Birnbaum [121] Ischemia Severity Grading System. Figure and text reproduced and modified from Billgren et al. [123]

10 mm/mV and displayed as a "24-lead ECG" with 12 views in each of the frontal (above) and transverse (below) planes. The orientation of the x, y, and z axes of each plane is indicated by the perpendicular arrows. The 12 leads in each plane are arrayed as on a clock face around an MRI of the heart within the thorax; as viewed from the front in the frontal plane and from below in the transverse plane. The three dimensional "box" that appears around the heart in situ is expanded on the right of each figure to display the 8 "bread loafed" base to apex slices as viewed from these vantage points. The four quadrants/walls of the LV, (anteroseptal, anterosuperior, posterolateral, and inferior) are defined by the dashed lines on each slice.

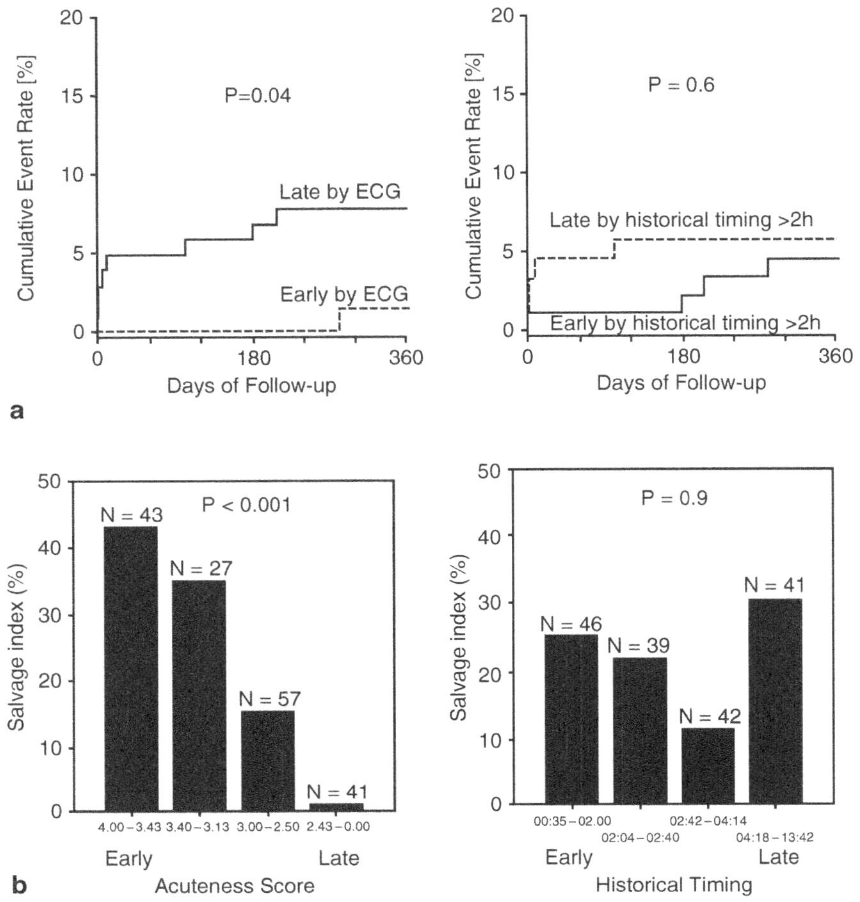

Fig. 4.24
Relation of the Anderson-Wilkens acuteness score versus historical timing with myocardial salvage (*top graphs*) and mortality. Reproduced from Sejersten et al. [124]

4.4.2.3 Severity of Ischemia

The Sclarovsky-Birnbaum ischemia grading system was introduced in 1990 as a clinical tool to estimate severity of first time acute MI [121]. The grading system is based on qualitative assessment of changes occurring in the ST segment and the terminal portion of the QRS complex during the early stages ofischemia-infarction. The ischemia grading system consists of three grades representing increasing severity:

Grade 1 = tall upright T waves without ST segment elevation,
Grade 2 = ST segment elevation in ≥2 adjacent leads without terminal QRS distortion, and
Grade 3 = ST segment elevation in ≥2 adjacent leads with terminal QRS distortion.

Note that different criteria are used for identifying grade 3 of ischemia depending on the presumed baseline QRS morphology (➋ Fig. 4.23). The scoring system is based on the concept that the severity of the ischemia/infarction process

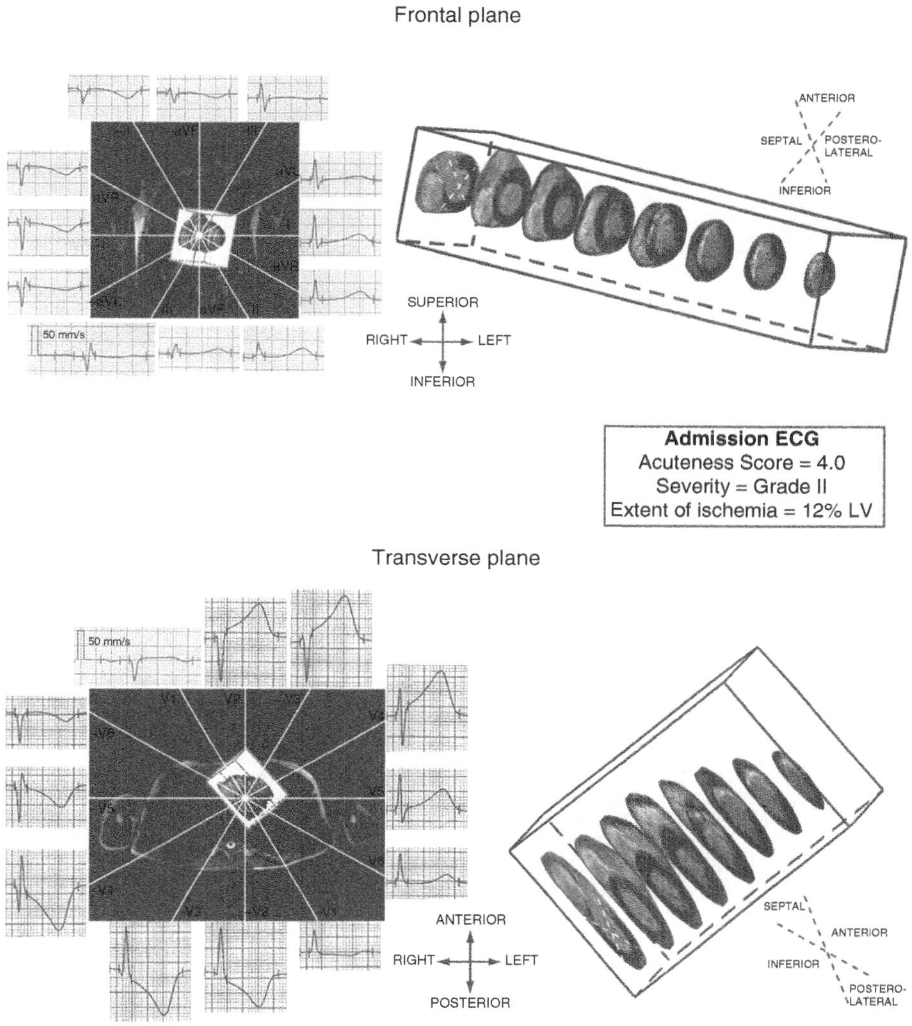

Fig. 4.25
Cardiac MRI and 24-lead ECG (50 mm/s, 10 mm/mV) of a patient with a small to moderate acute MI primarily in the anteroseptal LV wall with some involvement of the anterosuperior LV wall caused by occlusion distal to the major diagonal branch of the left anterior descending coronary artery. The infarct is more extensive at the apex. It involves primarily the apical segment with some extension into the middle segment of the anteroseptal wall, and extends into mid and apical segments of the anterosuperior wall. The ECG manifestation of the acute phase of this MI is anterior ST segment deviation in the chest leads of the transverse plane (*below*) maximal toward leads V3 and V4. There is no apparent ST deviation in the frontal plane limb leads (*above*) because the anteriorly directed ST segment deviation is perpendicular to that plane

is determined by the degree of myocardial protection provided by the combination of collateral vessels and ischemic preconditioning. Studies have shown that patients with grade 3 ischemia have a worse prognosis, larger infarct size, less benefit from reperfusion therapy and less viability in the infarcted zone as compared to patients with grade 2 ischemia [122–124]. Detailed rules for calculation of the score are outlined in Fig. 4.23.

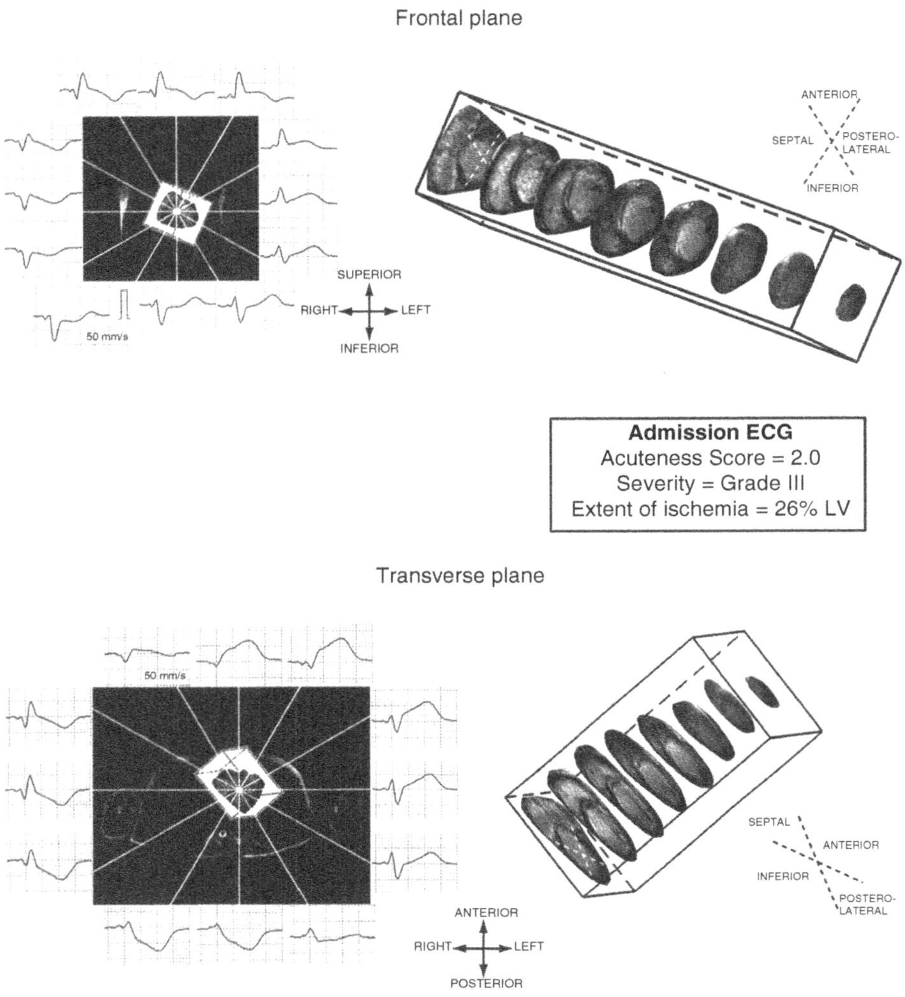

Fig. 4.26
Cardiac MRI and 24-lead ECG (50 mm/s, 10 mm/mV) of a patient with large evolving acute MI in the anteroseptal and anterosuperior LV walls caused by occlusion proximal to the major diagonal branch of the left anterior descending coronary artery. The infarct is circumferential at the apex with extensive involvement of the middle and basal segments of both the anteroseptal wall and the anterosuperior wall. The ECG manifestation of the acute phase of this MI is major anterior ST segment deviation in the transverse plane chest leads (*below*) maximally toward lead V3, and superior deviation in the frontal plane limb leads (*above*) maximally away from lead III (toward lead-III). The QRS changes of a large evolving anterior infarction are already present

4.4.2.4 Extent of Ischemia (Myocardium at Risk)

The Aldrich score for application on the presenting ECG, for estimation of the extent of myocardium at risk of infarction in the absence of successful reperfusion therapy was introduced in 1988 for anterior and inferior MI [93] and in 2005 by Ripa and colleagues for posterolateral MI [125]. It is based on the slope of the relationship between the amount in millimeters of ST segment deviation on the presenting ECG and the QRS score described in this chapter on the predischarge ECG and is expressed as percent LV at risk of infarction.

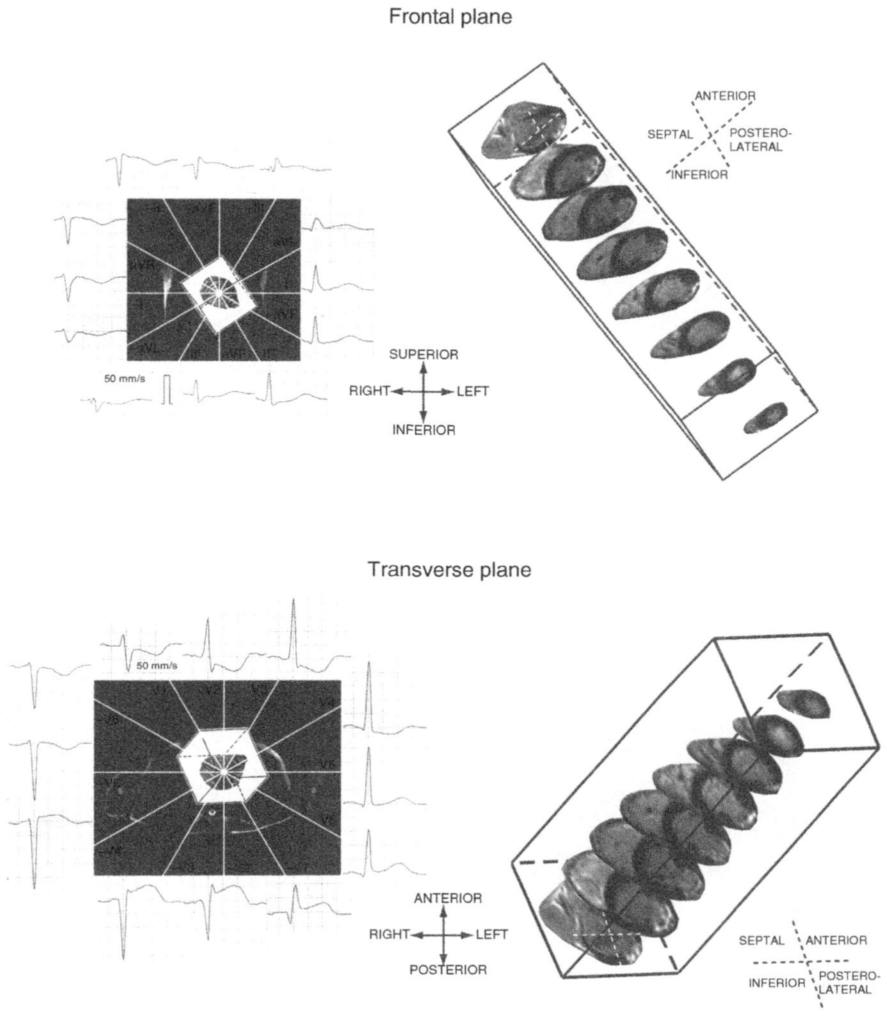

Fig. 4.27

Cardiac MRI and 24-lead ECG (50 mm/s, 10 mm/mV) of a patient with a large acute MI primarily in the posterolateral LV wall caused by left circumflex (LCX) coronary occlusion proximal to the first marginal branch. The infarct is more extensive at the base extending slightly into the anterosuperior segment and tapers toward the apex. It involves the basal and middle segments of the posterolateral LV wall extensively, and extends to about 25% of the apical segment. The ECG manifestation of the acute phase of this MI is posterior ST segment deviation in the transverse plane chest leads (*below*) maximally away from lead V2 (toward lead -V2). There is borderline ST deviation superior in the frontal plane limb leads -aVF, -111, aVL (*above*) indicating a minor extension of the risk area into the basal anterosuperior segment

The formula in anterior ischemia/infarction is

Extent of ischemia (%LV) = 3[1.5(# of leads with ST elevation)−0.4].

The formula in inferior ischemia/infarction is

Extent of ischemia (%LV) = 3[0.6(sum ST elevation in II, III, aVF)+2].

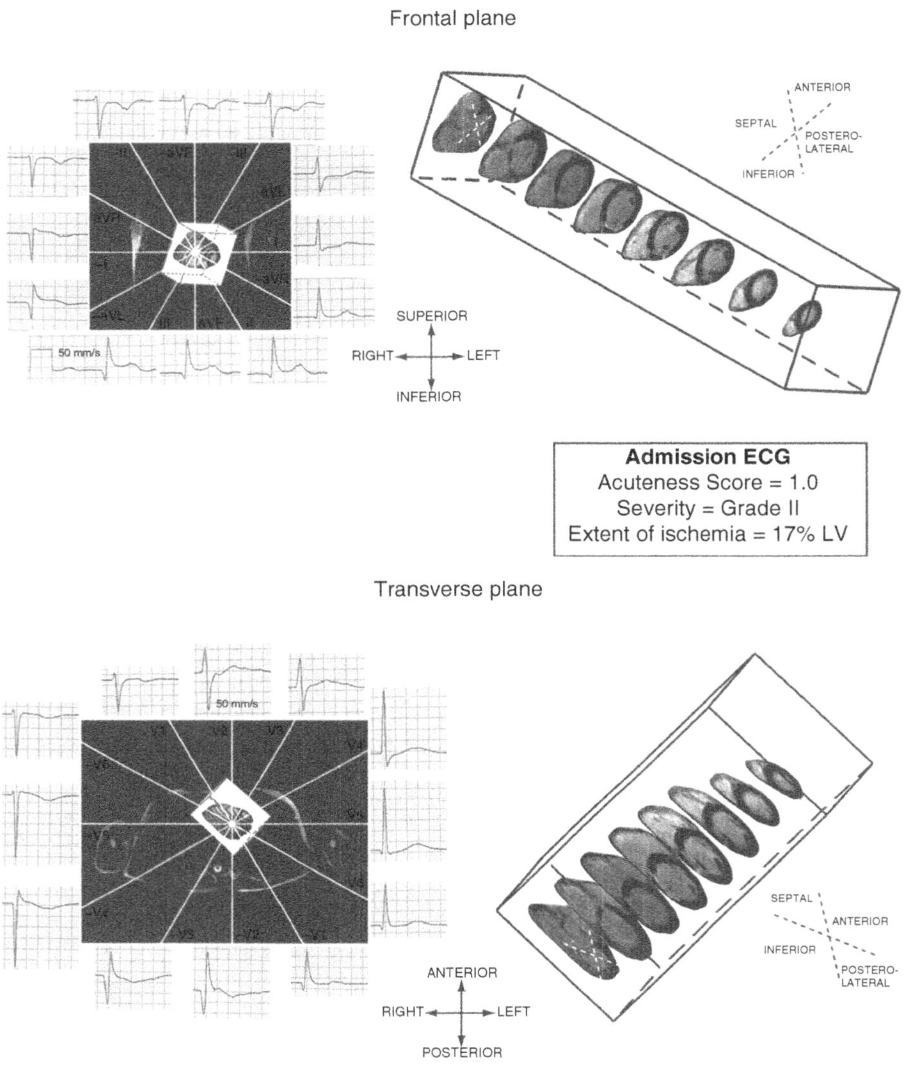

Fig. 4.28
Cardiac MRI and 24-lead ECG (50 mm/s, 10 mm/mV) of a patient with a small acute MI involving primarily the middle segment of the inferior wall with minimal extension into the inferobasal and inferoapical segments. This was caused by occlusion of the PDA proximal to its branching from the distal RCA. The ECG manifestation of the acute phase of this MI is minimal with abnormal inferior ST deviation in the frontal plane leads (*above*) maximally toward lead III

The formula in posterolateral ischemia/infarction is

Extent of ischemia (%LV) = 3[0.22(sum ST elev and ST, dep, all leads)−0.02].

Future work will need to be done to prospectively evaluate the use of all three of these ischemia scoring systems to risk-stratify patients and provide decision support for physicians caring for patients with acute myocardial infarction.

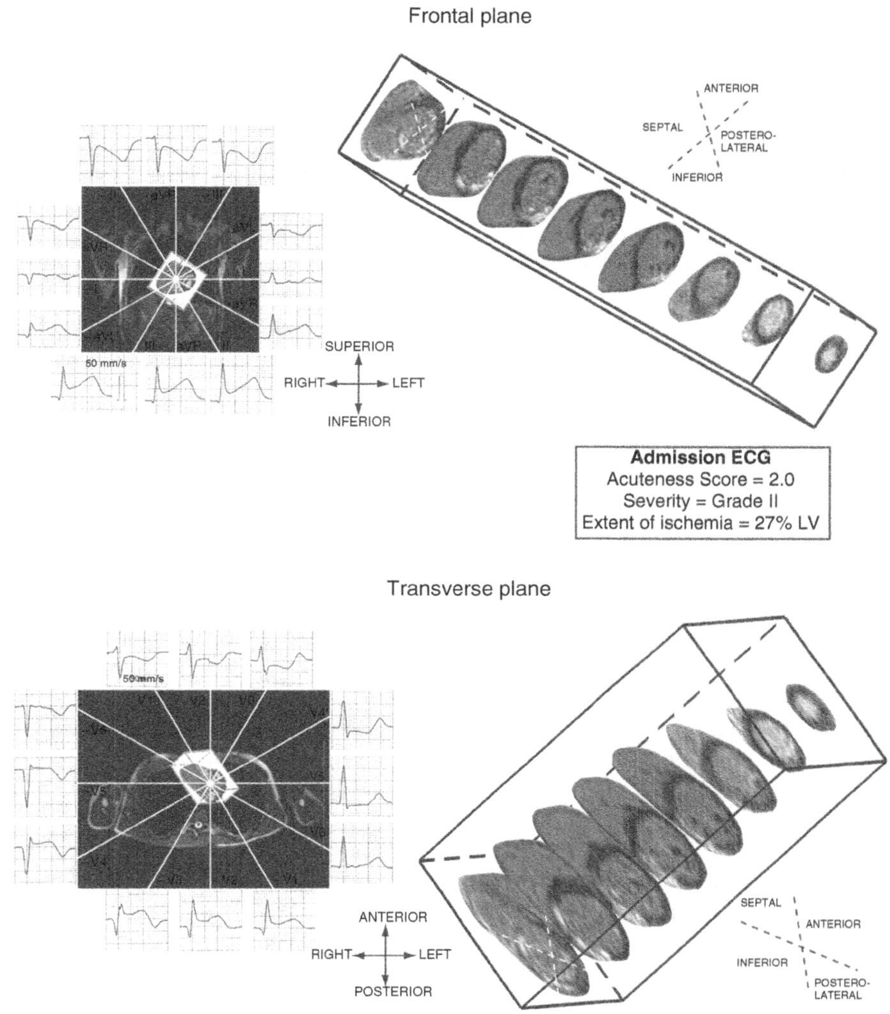

Fig. 4.29

Cardiac MRI and 24-lead ECG (50 mm/s, 10 mm/mV) of a patient with a moderate sized acute MI in the inferior and postero-lateral LV walls, caused by occlusion distal to the major right ventricular branch of a dominant right coronary artery. The infarct is extensive at the base and tapers toward the apex. It involves primarily the middle and basal segments of the inferior wall, extends into middle and basal segments of the posterolateral wall, and also minimally into the basal inferior septum. The ECG manifestation of the acute phase of this MI is inferior ST segment deviation in the frontal plane limb leads (*above*) about equally toward leads III and aVF, and posterior in the transverse plane chest leads (*below*) maximally away from lead V2 (toward lead -V2). The apical involvement is indicated by the inferior directed ST deviation in the frontal plane extending to lead -aVR

4.4.3 Left Anterior Descending Occlusion and Typical Anterior Infarcts

4.4.3.1 Spectrum of ECG/VCG Changes from Acute LAD Occlusion

In most patients, the "wrap-around" of the LAD at the apex onto the inferior apex is quite prominent [127]. Thus ***acute occlusion of the distal LAD*** with acute anteroapical infarction will be associated with ST elevation both in anterior apical directed leads V4, V5, V6, and in apical inferior directed leads –aVR, II, and aVF. The evolving infarct may produce abnormal Q-waves or attenuated/notched R-wave changes in any or all of these leads depending on its size. The differential diagnosis of such changes is covered in more detail in ➍ Sect. 4.4.7.

Infarcts associated with local acute occlusion of a ***major first diagonal branch*** of the LAD system may be limited to the anterosuperior wall or extend into the upper part of the middle and apical segments of the posterolateral wall. These are so-called high lateral, lateral or superior infarctions with abnormal anterior (superior) ST elevation in I, aVL, -III, and -aVF. The evolving infarct is evidenced by loss/notching of R and/or evolving Q waves in I, aVL, and possibly –V2, –V3.

Acute LAD occlusion proximal to the first diagonal adds to the changes mentioned above for the acute ST-T and evolving QRS changes in leads V1–V5, along with many added labels for these infarcts. Terms such as septal, anteroseptal, anterior, strictly anterior, anteroapical, apical and anterolateral are all in wide usage to describe the ECG/VCG changes in V1–V5 that result from LAD occlusion. A combination of these terms is used to indicate extension of the infarct to more than one region, along with additional terms such as large, extensive or massive. A significant simplification occurs when the size modifiers summarized in ➍ Table 4.3, namely, probable small, small, moderate, large and very large, are used along with the simple descriptor "anterior," to describe the spectrum of changes that occurs with occlusion in this arterial system. When major ST-T changes of injury and/or ischemia are also present, modifiers, such as "hyperacute," "acute" or "recent" are appropriate. When there are changes of anteroapical infarct with inferior involvement, then adding the term "with inferior extension" or using "anteroapical inferior" are appropriate but "apical" with size modifiers is simpler. The reader is reminded that to assess the extent of the anatomic change, the ECG/VCG changes considered must include not only ST-T and initial Q-wave vectors, but loss of mid-to-later QRS vectors as well. The interaction of these criteria in the quantification of anterior infarct is discussed in more detail in ➍ Sect. 4.3. Serial ECGs of a typical moderately sized acute anterior infarct are shown in ➍ Fig. 4.18. The QRS MI size, score of the day 15 ECG, the interaction with the individual criteria met and the distribution of the associated infarct in relation to the 12 segment LV of this patient's score worksheet are shown in ➍ Fig. 4.19. The 24-lead ECG and the MRI images of a small acute and large late acute anterior infarct are shown in ➍ Figs. 4.25 and ➍ 4.26. ECG/VCGs of a moderate size and a very large old anterior infarct with angiographic correlations are shown in ➍ Figs. 4.30 and ➍ 4.31.

4.4.3.2 Anterior Infarct with Associated Left Anterior-Superior Fascicular Block, LAFB

Eight percent of the patients in the authors' ventriculographic series with visible anterior infarct and LAD coronary artery occlusion had an associated clear-cut left anterior-superior fascicular block (LAFB), by criteria advocated by the Bethesda Conference Task Forcel on Standardization of terminology [128]. ➍ Figure 4.8 shows a simulation of the sequence of activation seen in these patients. The major difference seen in the ECG/VCGs of these patients in comparison to those with normal conduction and anterior infarct are:

(a) QRS prolonged to 105–110 ms (110–140 ms when evidence of LVH is present);
(b) qR pattern in aVL with wide separation of initial 30 ms vectors from the terminal 30 ms vectors; and
(c) Mean frontal QRS axis −45° to −110°, depending on the size of the infarct.

The important ECG/VCG features for the diagnosis of this combination of fascicular block and infarct are the wide divergence of initial and terminal vectors in the frontal plane. This is particularly evident in the larger infarcts. Grant and Dodge [16, 41] postulated that these changes initially described by First [129] "may be due to a block in the superior division(s) of the left bundle." The important ventriculographic feature which relates to the ECG and VCG is that in no instance in the Rancho Los Amigos Hospital, University of Southern California (Rancho/USC) series of this group was the entire anterosuperior base akinetic (infarcted). It follows that this region, which is activated late and unopposed, will produce prominent late superior posterior vectors. The absence of this vector effectively excludes the diagnosis of left anterior-superior fascicular block. This is unlike left inferior-posterior fascicular block (LIFB), where the inferior base, which produces terminal inferior vectors in this conduction abnormality, is commonly infarcted. A typical clinical example of a patient who developed a left anterior-superior fascicular block (LAFB) and complete RBBB from a very large acute anterior infarct, where the QRS MI size score suggests involvement of 36% of the LV, is shown in ➍ Fig. 4.20.

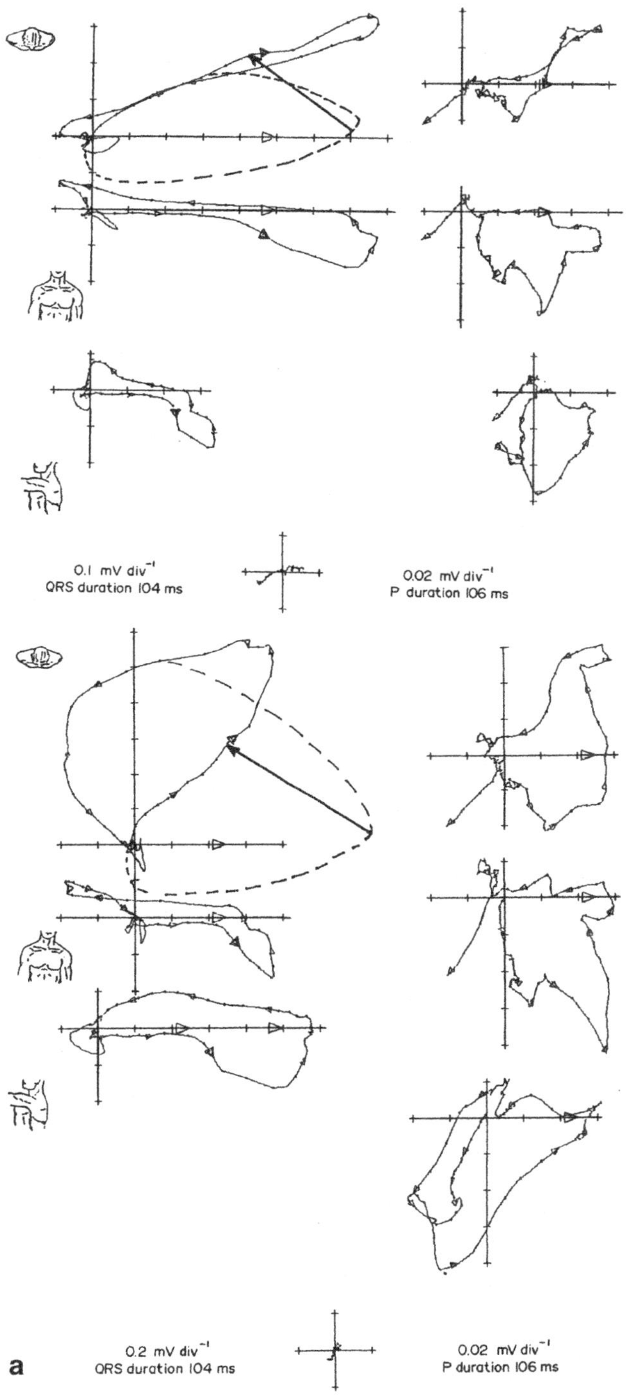

Fig. 4.30 (Continued)

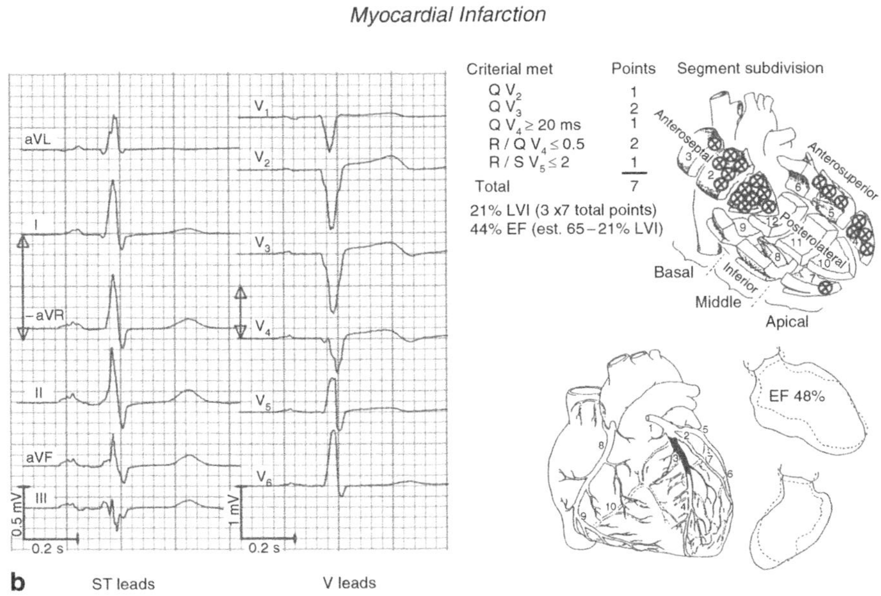

Fig. 4.30

(a) The Cube VCG is the *upper half* of the figure and the McFee in the *lower half*. The horizontal, frontal and left sagittal QRS-T loops are to the *left*; P loops and the initial 10 ms of the QRS at higher gain are to the *right of each set*. Time marks are every 2 ms, the *small arrows* every 10 ms, and the *large arrow* at the 40 ms vector. The calibration is indicated below the Cube and McFee QRS-T VCGs on the *left* and P VCGs on the *right*. This 54-year-old man with a history of a previous infarct shows significant loss of initial anterior and apical forces. The *dotted line* represents the average VCG for each lead system recorded from 97 age-matched normal males. The peak magnitude of this QRS deformity in each is indicated by the *solid line* and *arrowhead*. The peak magnitude and the duration for each lead system, transferred to the nomogram in Fig. 4.12, yields the following: For the Cube, 0.3 mV for 60 ms estimates the infarct size as 6 cm and the ejection fraction (EF) as 47%. For the McFee, 0.9 mV for 50 ms estimates an 8 cm infarct and an EF of 42%. (b) Note limb leads are in the orderly (Cabrera) sequence from the top down, aVL, I, -aVR, II, aVF, III. The ECG here and the VCGs shown in (a) are signal averaged from 1 ms digitized data. The gain is indicated at the bottom of each panel. There are abnormal Qs V2–V4 and further loss of R waves, V4, V5 yielding 7 ECG points as shown above with an estimated infarct size of 21% LV and estimated EF of 44%. These criteria using the autopsy validated distribution from the QRS MI size score shown in Fig. 4.16 yield the prediction of local infarct as shown in the *upper right*. The *lower* figures show the findings of single vessel LAD occlusion at angiography, and the localized anteroapical infarct shown on biplane ventriculograms with an ejection fraction of 48%

4.4.4 Non-Dominant Circumflex Occlusion and Typical Posterolateral Infarcts

The typical serial ECG changes of a large acute posterolateral infarct with apical extension consistent with occlusion of a large obtuse marginal branch of a non-dominant LCX coronary artery are shown in Fig. 4.21. Note that the ST changes in this example reflect predominantly posterior and apical injury and ischemia. The evolving QRS shows major loss of posterior and leftward apical vectors that, by the QRS MI size score, involves 27% of the LV. The activation sequence relating to a similar infarct, but smaller with less apical extension, is shown in Fig. 4.4. ECG/VCGs with angiographic correlations of similar healed small and moderate old posterolateral infarcts from patients in the Rancho/USC CAD database with LCX occlusion are shown in Figs. 4.32 and 4.33. Note that in these two more typical examples of posterolateral infarct, the QRS changes are limited to the mid and terminal QRS. Lesions in this location, as in the example shown in Fig. 4.33b, extend onto the inferior surface (and/or apex) in about one third of cases. They produce acute

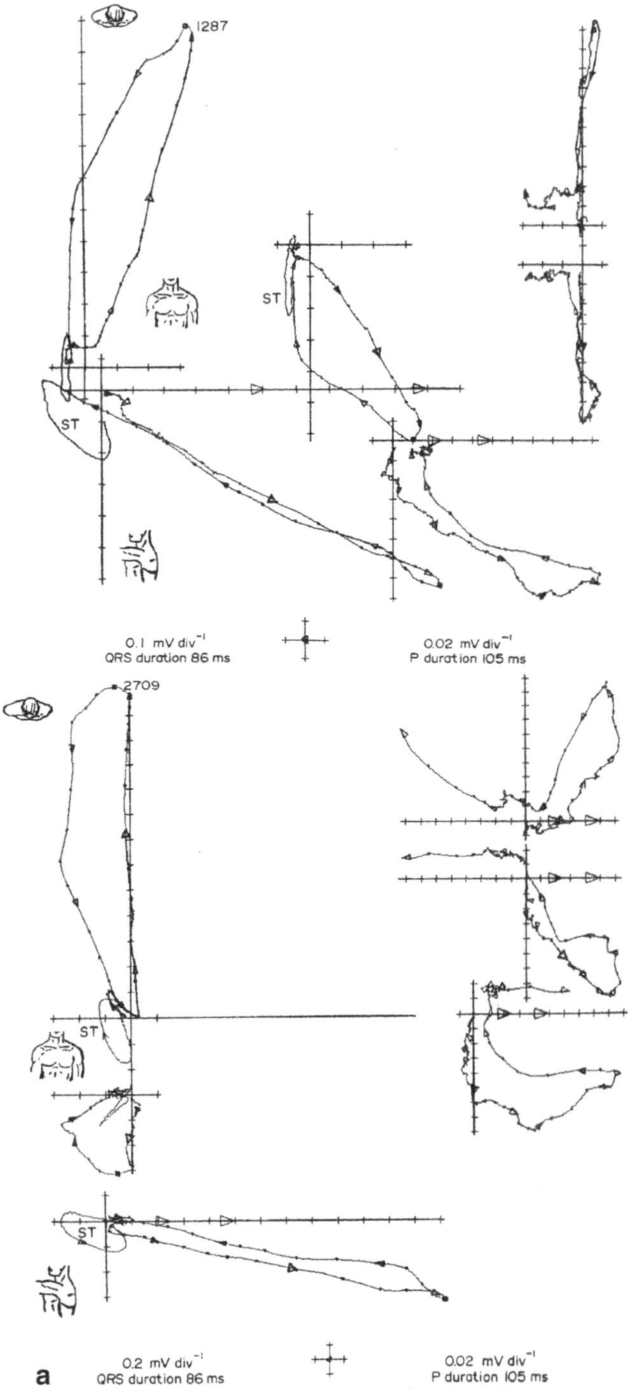

Fig. 4.31 (Continued)

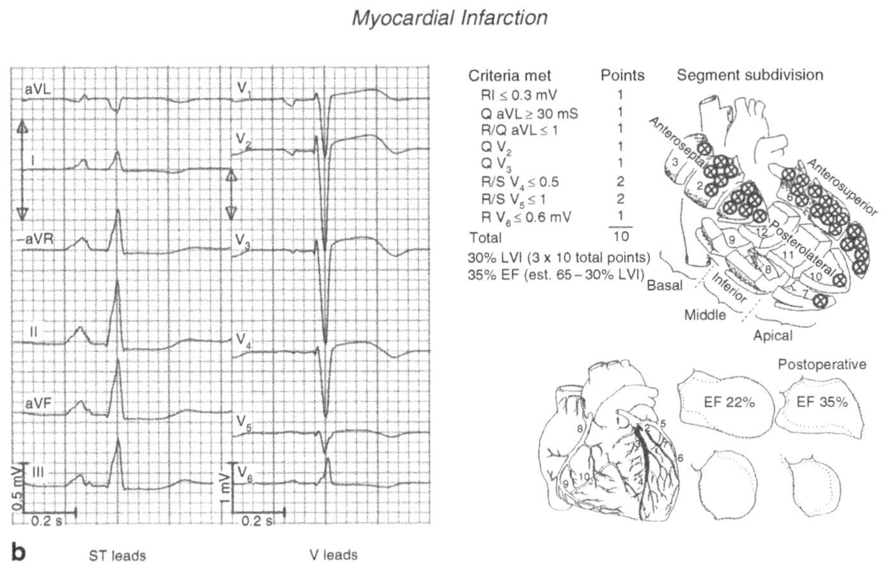

Fig. 4.31

(a) The Cube VCG is the *upper half* of the figure and the McFee in the *lower half*. This 64-year-old man had a history of a single acute myocardial infarct prior to his angiogram. The P loops displayed to the *right* of both lead systems demonstrate major increases in left atrial voltage and activation times indicative of major LV diastolic dysfunction. There is increased posterior QRS voltage of both VCG lead systems consistent with the clinical history of hypertension. The initial right atrial voltages were also mildly increased and the QRS frontal axis is shifted rightward from where it would be expected with LVH. These are consistent with the acute course and the post-infarct period, which had been complicated by congestive heart failure. There is major loss of initial anterior and leftward vectors in both VCGs. Compared to the VCG loops of early LVH, the Cube has lost 0.6 mV for 60 ms and the McFee 1.3 mV for 60 ms. When transferred to the nomogram of ➋ Fig. 4.12 this yields a predicted infarct size of 9 and 11 cm, respectively, and an EF of 38% and 32% respectively. (b) Note limb leads are in the orderly (Cabrera) sequence from the *top down*, aVL, I, -aVR, II, aVF, III. The ECG demonstrates a large anterior infarct and increased posterior voltage suggestive of LVH. There is a rightward shift of the frontal axis to +75 unexpected for LVH, but a common finding in large anterior infarcts with major anterosuperior wall involvement. In this case, as in most, the frontal QRS does not show wide separation of initial and terminal 30 ms vectors and the QRS duration here is 86 ms. Thus inferior fascicular disease is most unlikely and its blood supply is normal. The total ECG score for infarct of 10 would be indicative of 30% LV infarct pathologically, and would predict an EF of 35%. It is noteworthy that no infarct was distributed to the inferior or posterolateral wall at the apex by the observed QRS criteria. A large thin walled anteroapical aneurysm was present with a LV EF of 22%, large LV volumes and high end diastolic pressures. Following resection of the aneurysm there was significant return of inferior wall motion at the apex indicative of "tethering" and improvement in EF to 35%

ST-T changes in inferior (and/or left-sided) leads, and evolve variable small-to-significant Q waves in aVF, II, -aVR, I and V6 (see ➋ Sect. 4.4.9).

4.4.5 Right Coronary Occlusion and Typical Inferior Infarcts

The right coronary artery supplies the AV nodal artery in 85–90% of patients. This artery takes origin from the crux or "U-turn" in the right coronary at the origin of the posterior-inferior descending branch of this artery. This AV nodal artery terminates in a "T," one limb of which supplies the AV node, while the other limb supplies the bundle of His and the first 1–2 cm of the left bundle [130]. Thus, transient AV block is common with right coronary occlusion and in part

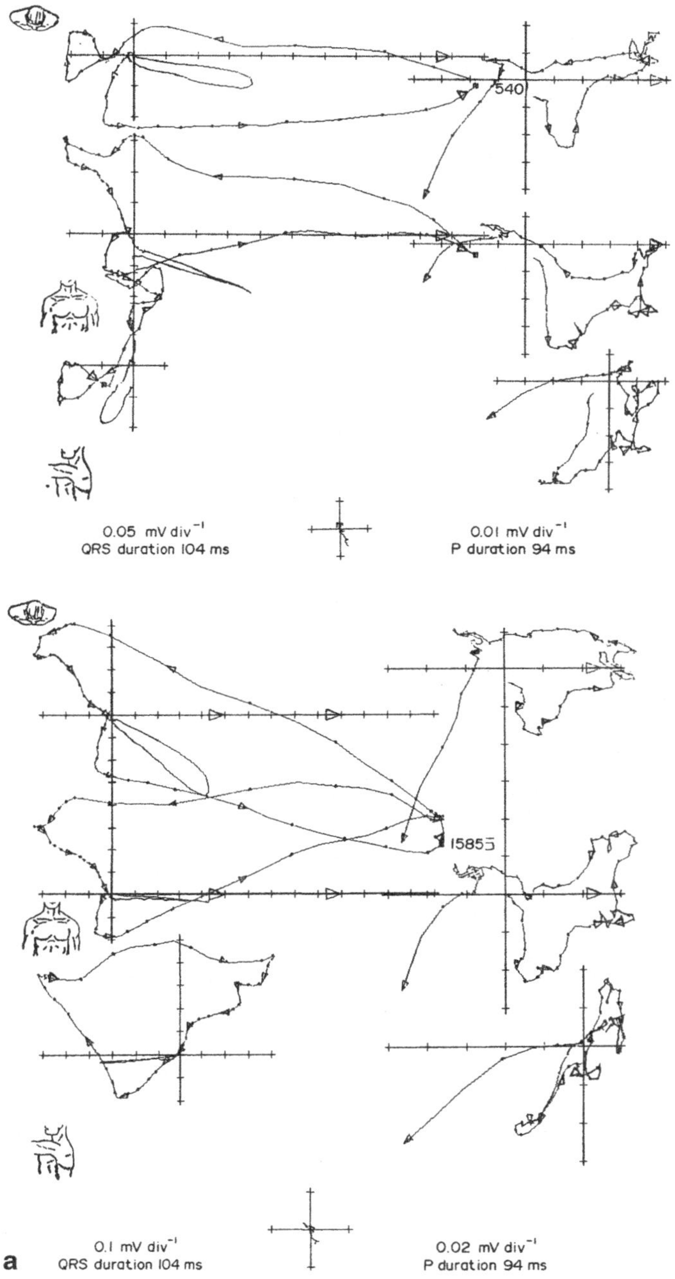

Fig. 4.32 (Continued)

due to the dual and variable blood supply to the region, His bundle and left bundle branch conduction abnormalities are less common. This region has a dual and variable blood supply. The other artery which supplies it is the first septal perforator from the left anterior descending coronary artery. The proximal left bundle is more often supplied by the AV nodal branch of the right coronary. Acute infarction and recent onset left bundle branch block is associated with recent inferior infarct more often than with anterior infarct [37].

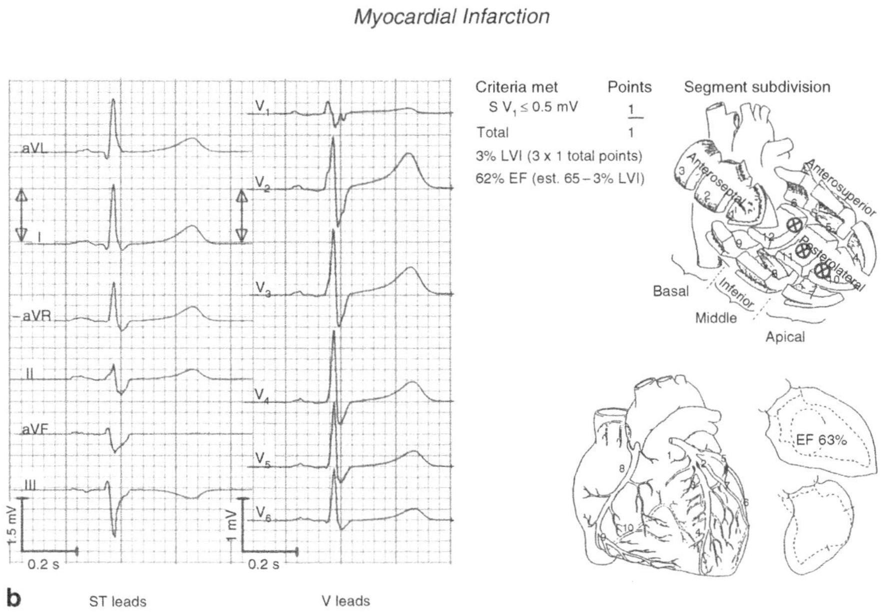

Fig. 4.32

(a) The Cube VCG is the *upper half* of the figure and the McFee in the *lower half*. The main abnormality seen here is a shift of the mid and late QRS vectors superior and anterior to their usual location. The QRS loop in the left sagittal projection is inscribed clockwise particularly evident in the McFee system, and the terminal displacement anterior is clearly abnormal in the Cube. The P vectors for both right and left atria, and the ST-T vectors are normal. The deformity in the Cube is 0.2 mV for 50 ms, and in the McFee is 0.5 mV for 40 ms. From the nomogram (➋ Fig. 4.12) these changes are predictive of a 4 cm and a 5 cm infarct respectively and an EF of 55% and 52%. Both VCG systems have leads on the back and in general are more sensitive to posterolateral infarct from LCX occlusion than the 12-lead ECG. (b) Note limb leads are in the orderly (Cabrera) sequence from the *top down*, aVL, I, -aVR, II, aVF, III. The ECG has abnormal left axis and only 1 point (3% LVI) for posterolateral infarction. There was total occlusion as shown of the LCX just proximal to the obtuse marginal branch and on the LAO ventriculogram a small posterolateral infarct at the junction of the middle and basal segments of the posterolateral wall. Many angiographic laboratories do not routinely report a left anterior oblique (LAO) ventriculogram. Small posterolateral infarcts are easily overlooked in the traditional RAO ventriculogram. Except for a faint double contour on the RAO ventriculogram in this case, there is no reflection of this infarct on the RAO systolic contours. It is also noteworthy that abnormal left axis deviation is seen with little support angiographically for superior fascicular disease. Occlusive arteriographic disease was identified as shown in the proximal LAD, but it was less than 70% and no regional wall motion abnormalities were noted. In this case, the VCG changes which correspond well to the lesion found suggest that the axis change is a straightforward expression of the loss of basal posterior-inferior vectors

The inferior-posterior fascicles of the left bundle through the distal third of their course are supplied from septal branches of the posterior (inferior) descending and the first posterolateral branches of the RCA. The fascicles are variably vulnerable to disruption with right coronary occlusion and inferior infarction. Eighty five percent of patients with inferior MI from RCA occlusion develop the ECG/VCG changes of peri-infarction/inferior fascicular block (LIFB) described below. The changes due to this conduction abnormality must first be reviewed in order to understand the changes seen with right coronary occlusion and inferior infarct. This group of patients has the following evidence of LIFB:

(a) Twenty ms prolongation of QRS to 100–120 ms, which may be intermittent in the early stages of acute inferior infarction.

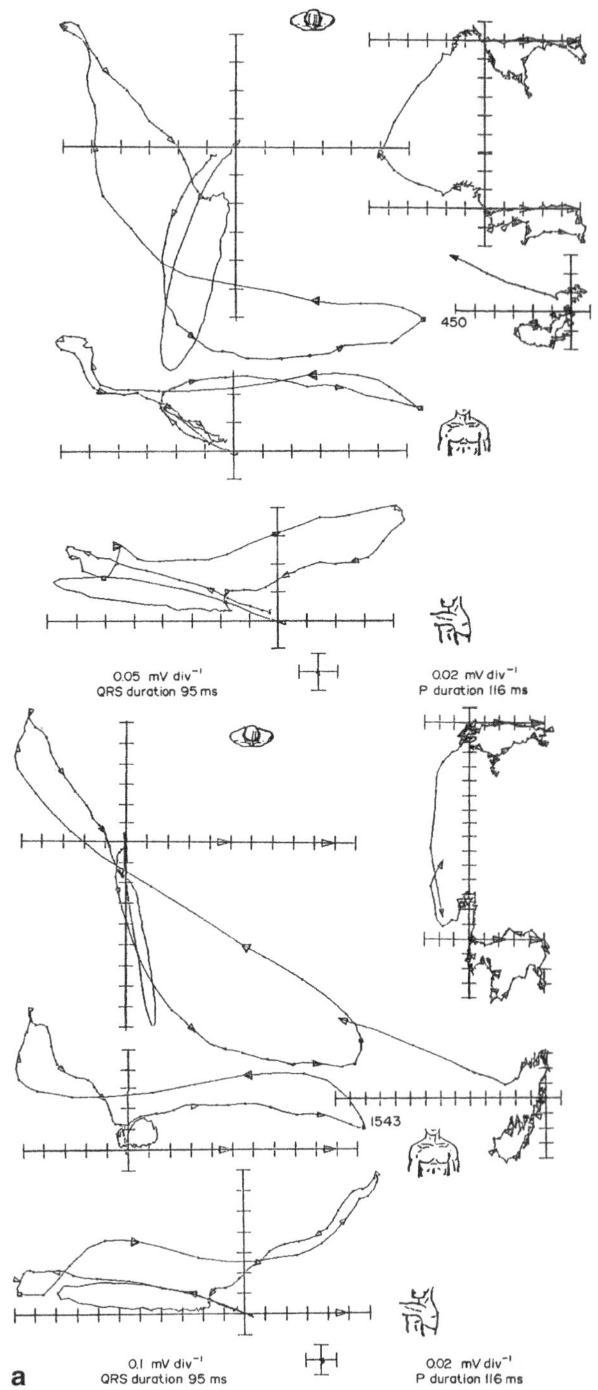

Fig. 4.33 (Continued)

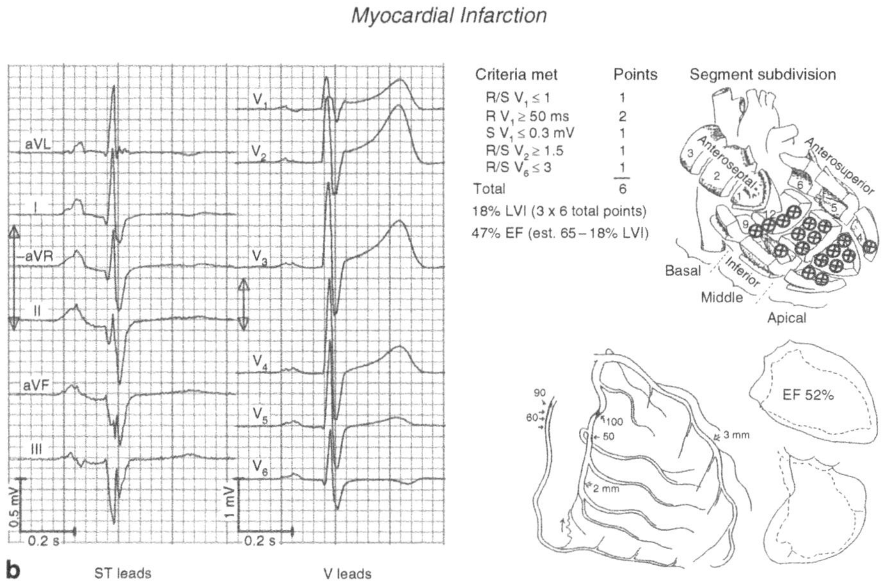

Fig. 4.33

(a) The Cube VCG is the *upper half* of the figure and the McFee in the *lower half*. P vectors here show a modest increase in left atrial activation times (P duration 116 ms) and leftward vectors consistent with mild to moderate LV dysfunction. There is significant loss of posterior and leftward vectors in both lead systems with significant inferior losses from 20 ms onward. The frontal plane is not that of inferior fascicular (peri-infarction) block in that the initial QRS vectors are irregular and terminal vectors are not directed inferior and rightward. The QRS duration is less than 100 ms and is much more suggestive of posterolateral infarct with inferior extension from a codominant LCX occlusion, rather than RCA disease. The large T vector is directed anterior and somewhat rightward and superior predominantly away from the posterolateral wall or LCX distribution. The deformities from the average normal loop are 0.6 mV/50 ms in the Cube and 0.8 mV/50 ms for the McFee. The nomogram of 16.12 predicts an 8 cm lesion for each, and an EF of 42%. (b) Note limb leads are in the orderly (Cabrera) sequence from the *top down*, aVL, I, -aVR, II, aVF, III. The 12 lead ECG in this case above as in the earlier ➋ Fig. 4.32b shows abnormal left axis with a Q in aVL and I that might suggest left anterior fascicular block. The lack of a prominant inferior initial 30 ms vector and of a prominant superior terminal 30 ms vector of 0.8 mV or more in aVF and aVL are inconsistent with this diagnosis as is a QRS duration of <100 ms. In this case the left axis, as in ➋ Fig. 4.32b, is a simple subtraction effect from significant inferior extension of a moderate sized posterolateral infarct from occlusion of codominant LCX, proximal to four prominent marginal branches. The LAD is free of disease and there is little support for the hypothesis that the left axis deviation is due to anterior fascicular conduction delay. Six points are generated by the ECG/QRS score for infarct size, all indicating posterolateral infarct with inferior and apical extension. The predicted infarct size is 18% LV with a predicted EF of 47%

(b) Patients with very small infarcts from right coronary occlusion have the ECG/VCG changes of LIFB, described in ➋ Chap. 3, with an open frontal plane loop as seen in ➋ Fig. 4.34a. They have wide separation of the initial 30 ms and terminal 30 ms of Grant and Dodge's [16, 41] peri-infarction block, which they suggested "was probably due to a block in the inferior fascicles."

(c) The initial vectors are seen as a smooth arc superior and leftward, with no high frequency notches or splintering in the smooth abnormal Q, and are consistent with early unopposed propagation through a normal anterosuperior wall.

(d) The high frequency notching and irregularities are in the mid- and terminal vectors, consistent with activation fronts traversing the areas around the late activated and infarcted inferior wall.

(e) Finally, for years it has been observed that the classic Q wave of inferior infarction occasionally disappears after a typical course of infarction. When this happens, the QRS usually returns to a more normal duration of 80–90 ms,

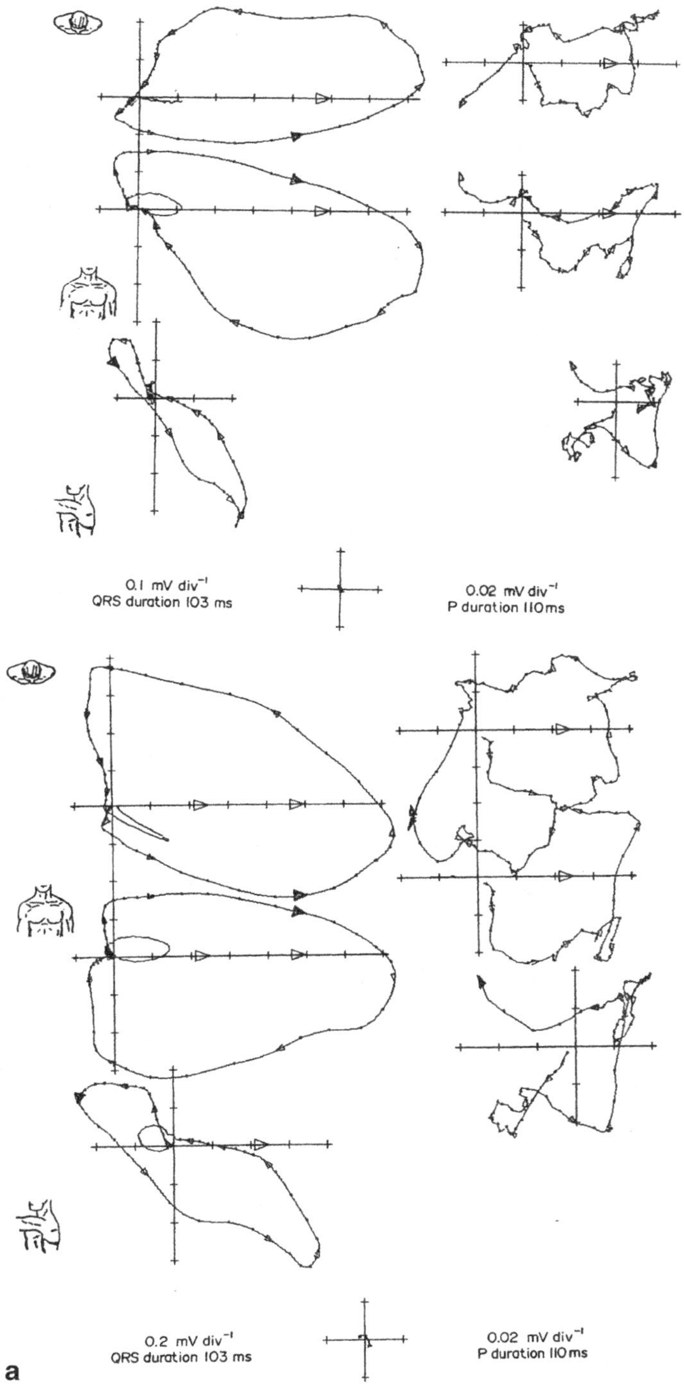

Fig. 4.34 (Continued)

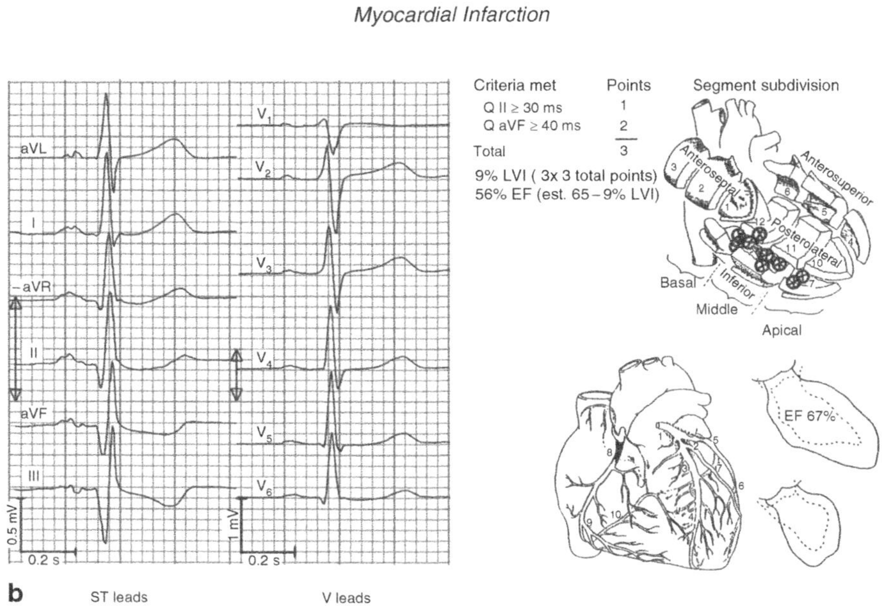

Fig. 4.34

(a) Cube (*top*) and McFee (*bottom*) sets of VCGs from a 60 year old man with the history of prior infarct is typical of a number of patients from the Rancho series with RCA occlusion and small or no visible infarcts. The QRS duration is 103 ms. The frontal plane initial and terminal 30 ms QRS vectors are widely separated in both. In those with no visible wall motion abnormalities, and in simulations of inferior fascicular block, the initial arc superior swings far to the *left*, as is seen here. It crosses the horizontal plane (and the *X* axis in the frontal plane) at 35 ms on the average. The peak left voltage occurs at 40–45 ms. When there is little or no infarction of the inferior base or middle segments, the terminal inferior vectors which arise from this region are well preserved as seen here. The inferior amplitude is 2/3 of the leftward amplitude on the average. This ratio should be used in construction of the non-infarct loop for estimating inferior infarct size in the presence of this conduction abnormality. When this ratio is used for this patient, small infarcts are predicted by both lead systems of 2–3 cm with a predicted EF of 60%. The P vectors are entirely normal, indicating little or no LV diastolic dysfunction. (b) Note limb leads are in the orderly (Cabrera) sequence from the *top down*, aVL, I, -aVR, II, aVF, III. Because the initial and terminal 10 ms are nearly perpendicular to the frontal plane, the QRS duration appears shorter than the 103 ms recorded in the VCG and seen in the precordial leads. Since the electrophysiological variable we look for in measuring QRS duration is total time of ventricular excitation it is important to measure it in the lead where it is longest. In general, ECG analysis from three orthogonal or eight simultaneous standard leads eliminates this ambiguity. The wide separation of initial and terminal 30 ms vectors is also evident in the frontal plane. Three points are accumulated for inferior infarct from the QRS score which represents 9% LV infarcted and 56% EF

and the axis shifts superiorly. These findings support the Grant and Dodge hypothesis that a "block in the inferior fascicles" was transient and has now disappeared. The decrease in QRS duration is due to the return to normal conduction. A significant axis shift to the left, superiorly, would result from the disappearance of the LIFB and a further axis shift superiorly from the inferior infarct. This would be proportional to the infarct size, with loss of late inferior QRS vectors from the base of the inferior LV wall, which activates normally during the late QRS.

The serial ECG changes of a patient with a typical acute inferior infarction from right coronary occlusion, and who evolves the changes of LIFB, described above, is shown in ➋ Fig. 4.22. A 24-lead ECG and MRI image of a small inferior infarct

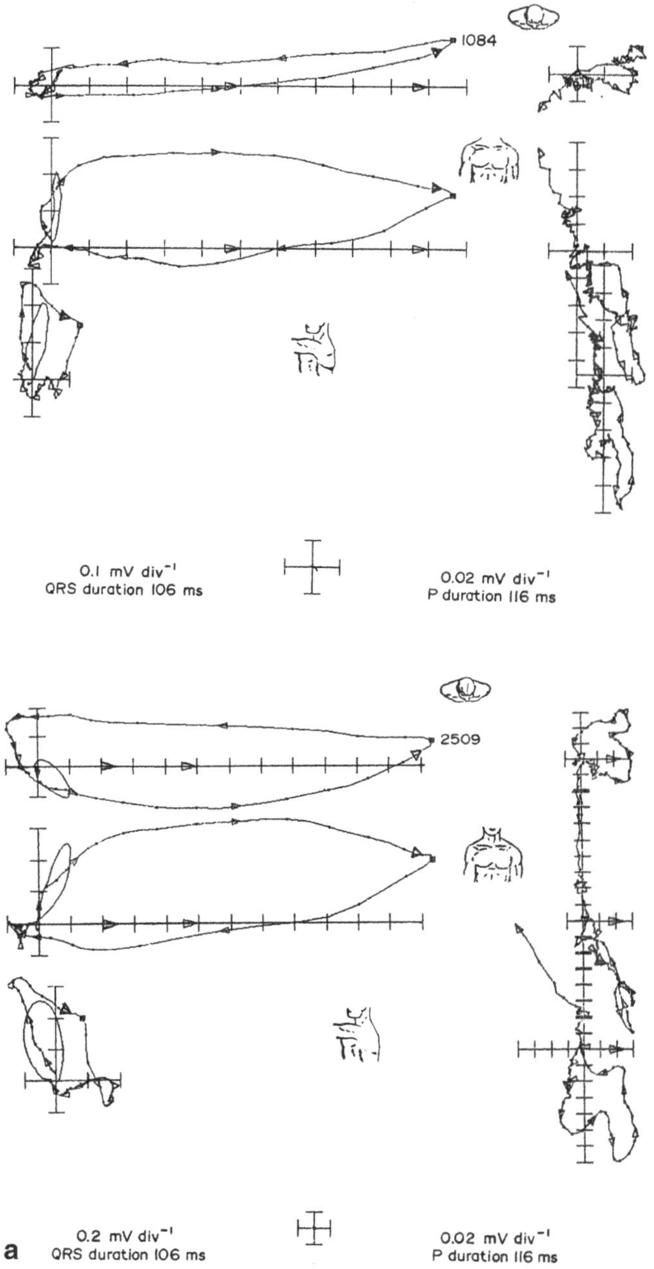

Fig. 4.35 (Continued)

from occlusion of the posterior-inferior descending distal branch of the right coronary artery is shown in Fig. 4.28. A large inferior infarct with significant posterolateral and apical extension is seen in Fig. 4.35. Typical ECG/VCGs of patients with small and large inferior infarcts are presented in Figs. 4.34a and 4.36a, along with the biplane ventriculograms from these same subjects (Figs. 4.34b and 4.36b).

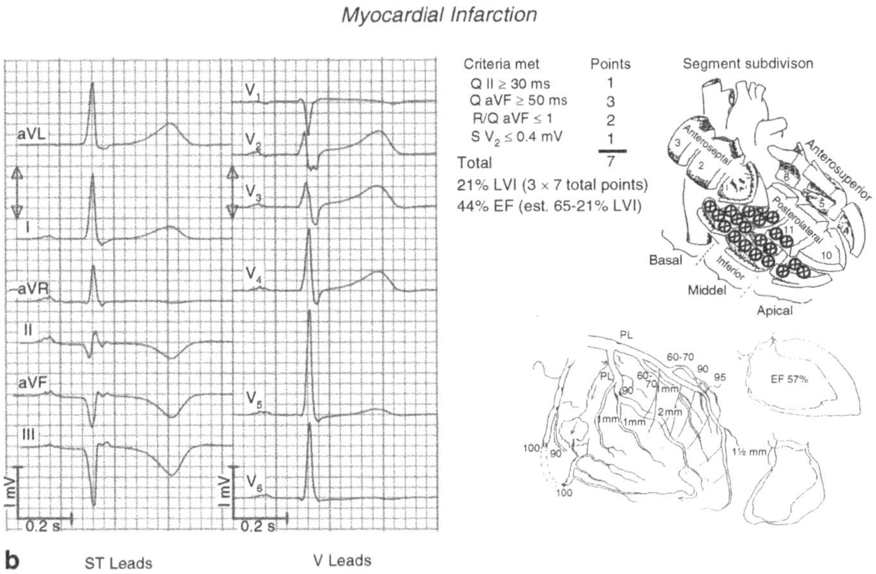

Fig. 4.35
(a) The Cube VCG is the *upper half* of the figure and the McFee in the lower half. This 56-year-old man has Cube and McFee VCG changes typical of the occasional patient with RCA occlusion and large inferior infarct involving most of the inferior wall, with some posterolateral wall and inferior septal extension. There is a slight decrease in initial anterior and terminal posterior vectors resulting in a flattened horizontal plane loop. The QRS duration is 106 ms, initial and terminal 30 ms are widely separated, with the initial vector superior as one would expect with RCA occlusion and inferior fascicular (peri-infarction) block. The terminal inferior rightward vector expected with this conduction, while very diminutive because of the extensive infarction of the segments producing it, is still visible. The initial arc leftward remains superior for 50 and 48 ms respectively and is indicative of significant inferoapical extension. In reconstructing the expected loop for inferior fascicular block by the rule of inferior vectors equal to 2/3 of the maximal leftward vector, it is evident that most of the inferior middle and basal segments are infarcted. Deformities of 0.6,mV/50 ms and 1.4 mV/50 ms yield transferred to the nomogram (➔ Fig. 4.12) estimates of 8 and 10 cm and estimates of EF of 42% and 35%. The left atrial activation times are indicative of mild to moderate left atrial overload, but the voltage is only at the upper limits of normal, which is unusual considering the evidence for large inferior infarct. This suggests that infarct size may be overestimated. (b) Note limb leads are in the orderly (Cabrera) sequence from the *top down*, aVL, I, -aVR, II, aVF, III. The small terminal rightward and inferior 30 ms vector which is widely separated from the initial 30 ms vector is evident in the frontal plane ECG. The QRS infarct size score accumulated 7 points for inferior infarct and distributes them into the inferior wall with significant extension into the apex and onto the posterolateral wall and predicts an EF of 44%. When the systolic and diastolic left ventriculogram center lines were superimposed, there is an akinetic segment involving the same regions predicted by the QRS score. The remaining LV contracted vigorously producing an unusually good ejection fraction (57%) for an infarct of this size

4.4.5.1 Right Ventricular Infarction

Subsequent to proximal RCA occlusion, right ventricular (RV) infarction has been shown [130, 131] to be about as common as LV infarction. The completed infarct in the right ventricle, however, is patchy, macroscopic and multifocal. The lack of confluent localized visible scar probably accounts for the statement in older pathology literature that RV infarct is uncommon. Also, the absence of a large confluent scar can be evoked to account for the fact that, until recently, no QRS changes of RV infarct have been elucidated in the ECG/VCG. Based on the location of RV potentials in body-surface map data, and the proximity of the RV base to the sternum, it was to be expected that both the acute ST-T and evolving QRS changes

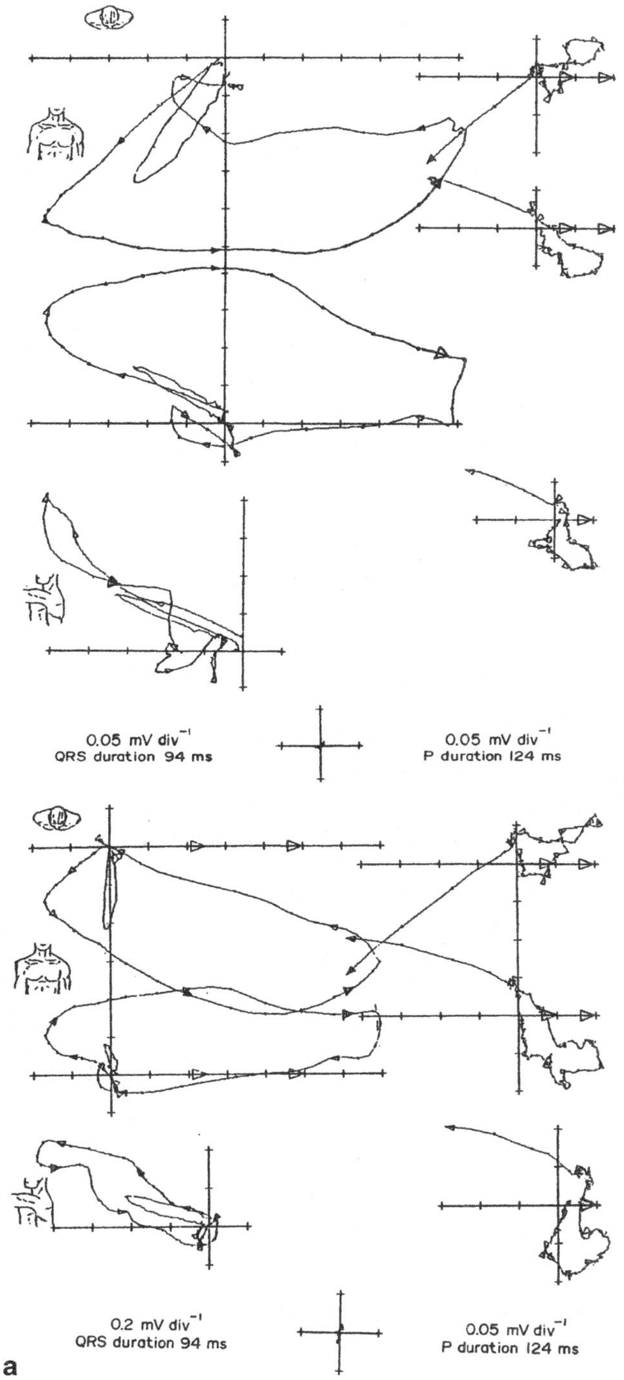

■ **Fig. 4.36** (Continued)

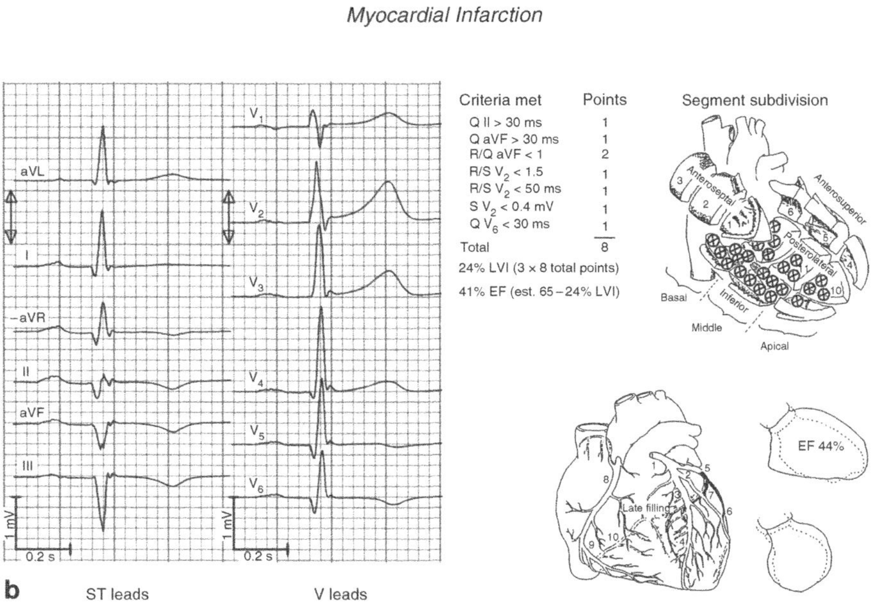

Fig. 4.36

(a) The Cube VCG is the *upper half* of the figure and the McFee in the *lower half*. This VCG combines many of the changes of large posterolateral infarct seen in Fig. 4.33a, b and large inferior infarct of Fig. 4.35a, b. The QRS changes of inferior fascicular conduction delay are less well documented, although much of the small terminal 30 ms vector is opposite the initial 30 ms vector, and the QRS duration is 100 ms. Assuming the basic activation of inferior fascicular block, and reconstructing a non-infarct loop using the 2/3 rule and a normal average left voltage, deformities of 0.5 mV/60 ms and 0.8 mV/50 ms are seen in the Cube and McFee respectively. Infarcts of 8 and 7.5 cm are read from the nomogram (Fig. 4.12) in which case EFs of 42% and 44% would be expected. If normal conduction is assumed, the infarct sizes would be 1–2 cm smaller and the predicted ejection fractions would be 45–50%. (b) Note limb leads are in the orderly (Cabrera) sequence from the *top down*, aVL, I, -aVR, II, aVF, III. The main point of interest in QRS scoring this ECG for infarct size is to note the "notched" Q in F. This leads to a Q duration of only 30 ms when one measures to the point on the baseline directly above the peak of the "notch." Notching this early in the Q is unlikely in inferior fascicular delay where a "smooth" Q is usual in the presence of a normal anterosuperior wall. A "notched" Q in F in normal conduction is usually the result of border effects from inferior extension of anterior or posterolateral infarcts into the apical and middle segments of the inferior wall. In this case 8 QRS points accrued and the criteria distributed the infarct more into the base that was found at ventriculography, and underestimated the apical involvement, although the overall estimate of infarct size and EF were appropriate

of RV infarct would be most marked in V4R, V3R and V1. The abnormal changes of RV infarct are also prominent in lower midchest and right parasternal leads. A series of papers [132–134], which have been reviewed by Kulbertus et al. [135], reported that an ST segment in V4R elevated by as little as 0.05 mV (0.5 mm at a gain of 10 mm = 1 mV) is a highly sensitive and specific marker of acute RV infarction. Carson and associates [136] reported vectorcardiographic changes in the ST-T vectors in seven patients with acute RV infarction in association with inferior infarction. They suggested that a rightward and anterior ST vector of magnitude ≥0.15 mV was a good discriminator between these 7 patients and 20 others with acute inferior infarction and no evidence of RV infarction on cardiac scintigraphic studies. Geft and coworkers [134] also reported that elevated ST segments in precordial leads V1–V3 may be caused by RV, rather than anterior LV infarction. The magnitude of the ST change in this event decreases from right to left and there are no evolving abnormal Q waves in these precordial leads. It is also not surprising that the time-course of the peak amplitude, or even the presence of these acute ST changes, is short and must be looked for attentively to make accurate assessment of the extent of RV infarction.

With the advent of the balloon catheter for right-heart catheterization, the measurement of right-sided hemodynamics has become routinely available in present-day coronary-care units. The clinical evidence for RV infarction is often acute right-heart failure. In the presence of normal left-heart filling pressures and RV failure, there is increased RV diastolic filling pressure, increased right atrial (central venous) pressure and ECG/VCG changes of right atrial overload. Since single inferior infarcts of the left ventricle from an RCA occlusion are rarely large, it follows that LV failure with a high left-atrial filling pressure is, indeed, also rare. The low-cardiac-output state seen in these patients is thus very likely a result of RV failure, not left, and the LV is usually volume-depleted owing to a low output from the right heart. In the adult P wave, 0.1 mV amplitude anteriorly in V1, V2, or Z and 0.175 mV amplitude inferiorly in aVF or *Y* exceeds the 98% upper limits of normal (see ➋ Table 4.1), and should be read as suggesting right-atrial overload. Acute and transient P-wave voltage amplitudes of 0.2 mV in V1, and V2 (and *Z*) and as much as 0.3 mV in aVF (and *Y*) can be seen in this circumstance, from acute right-atrial overload (RAO).

Morgera and coworkers [137] reported on a pathology series of patients with RV infarct in association with inferior infarct in whom right precordial leads V3R-V6R had been recorded serially along with a standard 12-lead ECG. Twenty-one subjects with pathoanatomically confirmed inferior LV infarct and variable degrees of RV infarct were compared to nine patients with necrosis limited to the inferior LV. Specificity studies also included 82 subjects of similar age and sex distribution without clinical evidence of heart disease, for whom V3R-V6R had been recorded in addition to the standard 12-lead ECG. In the normal subjects, an rS complex was seen in V3R in 100% and in V4R in 91% (rSr′ was seen in 6%). On the other hand, QS or Qr in V3R and V4R were specific markers of RV infarct in this small number of autopsy-validated patients (specificity 100%, sensitivity 78%). This group also confirmed that ST elevation ≥0.05 mV in these leads did not occur in the normal subjects, and ST elevation of ≥ 0.1 mV was not seen in the acute stage of the patients with inferior infarction limited to the LV. Zehender and associates [138] in a large clinical series of 200 consecutive patients with acute inferior infarction, confirmed the high sensitivity and specificity of the 0.1 mV of ST elevation in V4R for the diagnosis of acute RV infarction. The relative risk of in-hospital mortality was 7.7 for those with this finding.

In summary, the changes of right atrial overload are seen in conjunction with acute inferior infarction without a history of prior infarct, and suggest RV involvement in the infarct. Prominent ST elevation in V1, especially if accompanied by decreasing or depressed ST amplitude in V2–V4, would further confirm the suspicion of acute RV infarction, even in the absence of a low-output state. If ST amp ≥0.1 mV is seen in V3R and V4R [138], the diagnosis of acute RV infarct is confirmed with a high specificity (88%), sensitivity (78%) and diagnostic accuracy (83%). QS or qR complexes usually evolve in these same leads. Furthermore, the peak ST-segment elevation in these leads, while of short duration, appears to be a reliable measure of the extent of RV involvement.

4.4.6 Dominant Left Circumflex Occlusion and Typical Posterolateral Inferior Infarcts

When the left posterior circumflex supplies the posterior (inferior) descending coronary artery, three locations of infarction occur based on the site of the occlusion as follows:

(a) Acute occlusion of the dominant LCX distal to the main marginal take-off produces acute inferior ST-T changes of LV posterolateral and inferior infarction and evolution of an LIFB pattern indistinguishable from the typical acute distal RCA occlusion described above. On the other hand, the changes in right precordial leads V1, V3R, V4R of acute RV infarction exclude acute LCX occlusion.

(b) Obtuse marginal occlusion produces identical changes to those described earlier for non dominant LCX with infarction of the posterolateral mesial region. In one third of these, there is some extension onto the inferior wall and posterolateral apex.

(c) The group of patients with proximal occlusion of the left dominant posterior circumflex produces a wide range of infarcts from small to very large, involving both the posterolateral and inferior walls.

In the author's (RHS) Rancho/USC database, all of those who had significant infarction met the ECG/VCG criteria for left inferior (posterior) fascicular block (LIFB) described above. A typical ECG/VCG from a patient with these changes is presented in Fig. 4.35.

4.4.7 Differential Diagnosis of Poor R-Wave Progression in Leads V1–V6

Pulmonary emphysema, right or left ventricular hypertrophy, anterior preexcitation (Wolff-Parkinson-White (WPW) pattern) and diffuse infiltrative or myopathic processes are all well-known causes of poor R-wave progression in right precordial leads. In general, consideration of these pathologies sets in motion the differential diagnostic process in the interpretation of the ECG/VCG that will separate out such causes of decreased or absent R waves in V1–V3 from anterior infarction.

In pulmonary emphysema, the generalized low voltage, and in particular the significant attenuation of anterior, leftward and inferior vectors, are volume-conductor effects. Owing to the pulmonary overexpansion, there is an increase in the AP diameter, an elevation of the sternum and ribs anteriorly, a lowering of the diaphragms which "peel off" from the inferior surface of the heart and a downward and posterior displacement of the heart. In addition to these major geometric changes, there is a decrease in the conductivity of lungs resulting from the changes secondary to the emphysema. The displacement of the ribs with their ECG/VCG recording locations upward and anteriorly, along with displacement of the heart downward and posteriorly, significantly increases the distance from the heart to all the precordial recording electrodes. These two factors decrease field strength remarkably to all the usual precordial-lead recording sites. The loss of contact of the heart with the diaphragm decreases the inferior field strength of the ventricles as a result, but the atria, especially the right atrium, have a direct conductor (the vena cava) into the abdomen and to the left-leg recording electrode. The net effect of all of these changes in patients with otherwise normal hearts is to shift the mean P vector so that it is directed inferiorly, while the mean QRS vector is directed posteriorly with generalized low-voltage QRS amplitudes. These are the classic ECG/VCG changes of pulmonary emphysema [139] and rarely lead to a problem in diagnosis. Anteroapical infarct with loss of anterior, leftward and inferior vectors can result in similar or identical QRS changes including generalized low voltage. LV infarct of this degree is generally associated with high-frequency notching of the early to mid-QRS and with significant left atrial overload (LAO) including a leftward shift in the mean frontal-plane P axis. The absence of a vertical frontal P vector and an increase in P duration of $\geq$120 ms effectively excludes emphysematous changes, and the presence of ST-T changes, of anteroapical injury and ischemia, if seen, makes it much more likely that the QRS changes described, together with LAO, are a result of infarction.

Patients with moderate to severe right ventricular hypertrophy (RVH) may have qR changes in right precordial leads without anatomic evidence of an anterior infarct which it mimics. When these changes occur in patients under the age of 25–30, the chance that they are a result of infarction is slight. The presence of moderate to severe right atrial overload (RAO) as defined in Tables 4.1 and 4.2, and the absence of LAO especially when associated with right axis deviation, effectively excludes anterior infarct as a cause of these changes even in the older patients. Conversely, in older patients, when initial and/or mid-QRS notching is widely observed, abnormal Q waves are seen in other leads and definite LAO is seen. Even if the ECG signs of RVH and RAO are noted, it is now highly probable that the q of the qR in V1 and V2 is caused by an anterior infarct.

In 10–15% of patients with left ventricular hypertrophy (LVH), there are decreased or absent initial R waves in V1 and perhaps to V2 and V3, without anatomic evidence of anterior infarct. There is also an increased incidence of infarction in the presence of LVH. It is important, therefore, to assess the presence or absence of each, alone or in combination. Since prognosis is a function of the severity of the LVH and the size of the infarct, it is important to quantify both. If the ECG/VCG signs of LVH (i.e., increased voltage, duration, repolarization changes or LAO) are present, the absence of initial R waves in V1–V3 may not represent anterior infarct, especially in the absence of signs of infarction in other ECG/VCG leads. It has been found appropriate to suppress anterior infarct points from V1 and V2 when scoring for infarct size if the ECG/VCG signs of LVH are present [140]. Notched initial vectors or a qrS pattern is not present in these leads with LVH alone, and when present in V1 or V2, should be tabulated as one point each in the infarct score. For any ECG QRS point score for infarct size of more than three obtained from the rest of the ECG, the probability that absent R waves in V1–V2 are a result of infarct, even if smoothly transcribed, increases to more than 90%, and they should therefore be tabulated.

Anterior pre-excitation can produce absent initial R waves in V1–V3. Since by definition this form of WPW pattern is pre-excitation of the anterior wall (either the septum or right ventricle) via direct accessory pathways from the right atrium, it follows that the PR interval is particularly short and the delta wave from the pre-excitation is unusually prominent, making the diagnosis of WPW pattern straightforward.

The differentiation of the infiltrative and myopathic processes as a cause of poor R-wave progression in right precordial leads is usually made on clinical grounds. These entities should be considered when widespread splintering of the QRS is seen along with significant atrial overload, especially LAO, and increased QRS duration associated with a dilated left ventricle, without the voltage changes of ventricular hypertrophy. When the myopathic process involves the peripheral conduction, as it often does, an atypical wide complex LBBB pattern is commonly seen along with abnormal left or right axis deviation. This is not a confounder in the differential diagnosis of poor R-wave progression.

4.4.8 Differential Diagnosis of Prominent Anterior (and Rightward) Forces

Abnormal initial and/or terminal R waves in V1 or V2, and prominent S waves in V5 and V6 are seen routinely in moderate to severe RVH and quite commonly in posterolateral infarct. Two thirds of the latter do not have inferior or leftward Q waves, and the differentiation of prior posterolateral infarct from RVH cannot be made securely on the basis of QRS changes alone. When the prominent anterior and rightward QRS changes are associated with abnormal inferior or leftward Q waves and abnormal posterior/inferior ischemic ST-T changes, they pose little problem in the differential diagnosis. The case for evolved prior posterolateral infarct becomes quite secure if the mean T vector is anterior, there is no right axis shift in the frontal plane, RAO (right atrial overload) is absent and definite LAO (left atrial overload) is present. In this case, the QRS score for infarct size can be applied with confidence even in the absence of abnormal inferior and leftward Q waves. Conversely, in the presence of even "probable RAO" by the criteria of ➋ Tables 4.1 and ➋ 4.2, the diagnosis of posterolateral infarct is much less reliable and its quantification by the QRS score is unreliable. When the following requirements are satisfied:

(a) Criteria for definite RAO are present,
(b) The QRS axis in the frontal plane is oriented to the right, and
(c) The mean T axis is directed posteriorly,

then the likelihood of RVH is very high and the likelihood of posterolateral infarct very low.

The QRS score is reliable for estimating anterior and inferior infarct size, providing that points from all R/S ratio criteria in V4–V6 are suppressed as well as all posterolateral points in V1 and V2. The probability modifiers as indicated in ➋ Table 4.3 should also be used.

4.4.9 Differential Diagnosis of Abnormal Inferior Q Waves and ST Vectors

Abnormally acute ST-T vectors, together with evolving significant Q waves in II and aVF, and the changes of inferior-posterior fascicular block described earlier, occur in 85% of patients with RCA occlusion and local inferior wall motion abnormalities. These ECG changes also occur in 5% of those with RCA occlusion and no wall motion abnormalities. This is presumed to be a result of small focal lesions disrupting the inferior fascicle. In the latter case, the ST-T change is much less prominent. The Q wave, as it develops, is consistently smoothly inscribed.

Abnormal initial superior QRS vectors evolve in 15% of patients with acute LAD coronary occlusion and anterior infarction. With a mid to distal acute LAD occlusion, the risk area localizes to the apex with the usual "wrap around" of the distal LAD onto the apical third of the inferior wall. This is associated with a variable acute ST vector directed inferiorly and leftward. From a quick review of the spatial relationships of the heart in ➋ Fig. 4.1, it is clear that the apical third of the anterosuperior wall is facing almost entirely left while the inferior apical third faces directly inferiorly. The acute ST change and the evolving QRS changes of infarction are simple subtraction effects. For the evolving infarct, there is a loss of initial inferior QRS vectors because of the loss of activation fronts from the inferior extension of the infarct and dominance of the normal superior activation fronts and their normal superior vectors. The Q waves are usually shallow, irregular, slurred and/or notched and the QRS does not show the wide separation of initial and terminal 30 ms vectors, or the 20 ms increase in QRS duration seen with typical RCA occlusion and the inferior fascicular block pattern.

Acute LCX occlusion and consequent visible posterolateral infarct on biplane ventriculograms is associated with some inferior extension in about one third of cases. This produces abnormal acute inferior, as well as posterolateral, ST-T vectors, while abnormal initial superior QRS vectors with an abnormal left axis evolve. Abnormal Q waves may appear in inferior leads, especially lead III and aVF (but usually not in lead II). This is also a simple subtraction effect, as described above. Typically, the abnormal initial QRS waves in this instance are notched or slurred with a normal QRS duration. They are distinguished from the abnormal but smooth inferior Q waves, wide separation of initial and terminal 30 ms vectors and slightly prolonged QRS of inferior-posterior fascicular block as seen so commonly with the infarcts from RCA occlusion.

4.4.10 Summary of Electrocardiographic Changes Following Acute Coronary Occlusion

In summary for this section, the early minutes of acute coronary occlusion and evolving acute infarction produce a major shift in the ST segment that is vectorially related to the region undergoing acute ischemic injury (➋ Table 4.5). There is:

(a) Prominent superior and slightly leftward and posterior ST vector deviation for proximal occlusion of the first large diagonal branch of the LAD;
(b) Moderate anterior, inferior and leftward ST vector deviation for mid to distal acute LAD occlusion with the usual prominent "wrap around" of the distal LAD onto the inferior apex;
(c) Prominent anterior, superior and leftward ST vector deviation for acute proximal LAD occlusion;
(d) Prominent posterior and moderate leftward (± minimal inferior) ST vector deviation with acute proximal LCX occlusion;
(e) Prominent posterior and moderate inferior ST vector deviation with acute proximal left dominant LCX occlusion. This specific ST change also occurs in acute proximal occlusion of the rare, very right dominant RCA with a large posterolateral branch perfusing most of the posterolateral wall and a diminutive LCX. In this case, local ST amp ≥0.1 mV in V3R and V4R due to RV infarction excludes LCX occlusion. If the occlusion in the RCA is distal, the two are indistinguishable; and
(f) Inferior, ± leftward, and ± posterolateral ST deviation of acute distal RCA occlusion.

The magnitude of the peak ST change is related to the extent of myocardial area at risk. From a review of ➋ Fig. 4.9 and ➋ Chap. 6, the acute injury process of acute infarction can be seen as a continuous process throughout systole and diastole. It follows that the "primary" localized acute injury currents will be superimposed on the "secondary" ST-T changes of RBBB, LBBB, pre-excitation, RVH, and LVH. When adjusted for the secondary ST-T changes of each, the residual ST-T displacement vector of the localized acute injury can still be recovered. This is dealt with in detail for LBBB and ventricular pacing for patients with acute infarction in ➋ Sect. 4.5.5.2.

As the infarction process progresses, if circulation to the affected region is reestablished either spontaneously, by clot lysis, or balloon dilatation, the ST segment returns toward or to normal in a matter of seconds to minutes. The ST-T wave also becomes terminally inverted as the healing infarct evolves. By day 1 post infarction, a large T vector evolves directed away from the infarcted region. In chronic infarct, the T vector tends to decrease in magnitude being

Table 4.5
Summary of local ECG lead ST deviation changes of acute myocardial infarction from occlusion of the Left Anterior Descending, Left Circumflex and Right Coronary arteries

7 Culprit risk areas in the 3 coronary arteries
1. Proximal left anterior descending
Anterior ST deviation V1, ***V2****, ***V3***, V4 and
Superior ST deviation ***-aVF, -III***, aVL, I
2. Main diagonal LAD
Superior ST deviation ***-aVF, -III***, aVL, I
Minor or no anterior ST deviation V1, V2, V3
3. Mid to distal LAD
Anteroapical ST deviation V3 ***V4, V5***, V6 and
Inferoapical ST deviation aVF, ***II, -aVR***, I
4. Non-dominant LCX
Posterolateral ST Deviation V1, ***V2, V3***, V4, V6 and
Less Inferior ST Deviation III, aVF, II
5. Left dominant LCX
Posterior and Inferior ST Deviation about equal
in V1, ***V2, V3***, V4, V6 and aVL, ***III, aVF***, II
6. Proximal RCA
Inferior ST deviation aVL, **V4R**, ***III, aVF***, II
Less or no Posterior ST Deviation V1, V2, V3
7. Distal RCA
Inferior ST deviation aVL, ***III, aVF***, II, None V4R
Less or no posterior ST deviation V1, V2, V3

* ***Italics/Bold*** indicates usual leads with maximum deviation

in general directed posteriorly and rightward in anterior infarct, superiorly and leftward with inferior infarct, and anteriorly with posterolateral infarct. It is important to recognize further that there are effects other than infarction that produce major changes in repolarization. Since repolarization is a passive process linked to depolarization, it follows that any major change in depolarization such as left or right bundle branch block or pre-excitation, for example, has major "secondary" effects on repolarization (➔ Chap. 2). The 3D spatial vector of the ST and T electric fields is directly opposite the late activated terminal half of the QRS in both RBBB and LBBB. Likewise, moderate to severe right and left ventricular hypertrophy have their ST and T vector fields opposite to their mean QRS vector. Electrolyte abnormalities (for specifics see ➔ Chap. 6) also have a major generalized effect on repolarization, as well as variable effects on depolarization.

4.5 Bundle Branch Block and Infarction

4.5.1 Essential Principles

In the consideration of bundle branch block (BBB) and infarction, the following important points should be noted. In the first place, complete disruption of either the right or left bundle from coronary disease produces an uncoupling in time of the excitation of one side of the heart from the other, separating right from left ventricular excitation. Also, a predictable activation sequence occurs with each. Finally, when the activation sequence is taken into account, an associated local infarct produces additional deformities in the resultant surface ECG/VCG which are predictable. The location of an infarct can still be determined, and its size predicted. During an acute infarction, the primary ST-T changes of acute ischemia/injury are add-ons to the secondary effects of the bundle branch blocks. When the secondary effects are adjusted for, the direction and magnitude of residual ST-T deviation is predictive of the location of the acute infarction and its size and/or extent. In the light of the current knowledge of activation, primary and secondary repolarization, coronary anatomy and infarct distribution and size, it is no longer appropriate to say "in the presence of left bundle branch block no statement can be made about the presence or absence of myocardial infarction."

4.5.2 Validation Studies in Bundle Branch Blocks

The pathoanatomic studies correlating infarct size at autopsy and ECG point score for infarct size, reported by the authors [18, 30–34] and described earlier, excluded patients with ECG evidence of conduction defects, ventricular hypertrophy or emphysema. The angiographic correlations did not. For those subjects with complete RBBB and LBBB discussed in this section, the validation consists of coronary and biplane ventricular angiographic correlations from the (Rancho/USC database) databank, as shown in ➋ Figs. 4.30–4.37, and 4.41. The authors are also indebted to the large body of clinical [37, 141–146], epidemiologic [147–150] and anatomic [18, 151, 152] correlations reported in the literature. In pathoanatomic correlations with BBB, the presence of RBBB is generally unambiguous. However, it is difficult to establish from the literature the true incidence of, and therefore the pathoanatomic correlations with, complete LBBB. Most reports in the literature use the original Wilson/NYHA [53] criteria for LBBB which includes a QRS duration of ≥120 ms. On the other hand, Grant and Dodge [16] pointed out that in intermittent LBBB the QRS duration is 140–160 ms in patients with a QRS duration of 80–100 ms in the normally conducted beats. A QRS duration of <140 ms is uncommon in typical LBBB and durations of 170–180 ms occur in many. As these authors point out, those ECGs with intermediate durations of 120–130 ms are often atypical and many have the wide separation of initial and terminal 30 ms vectors typical of the fascicular (or "peri-infarction") blocks. When the published ECG (and VCG) records of LBBB are reviewed, it seems evident that about half of these records with QRS ≥120 ms meet the criteria of fascicular blocks with QRS prolongation. The prolongation appears to be due in part to LVH. The authors estimate the incidence of complete LBBB by the criteria defined by Grant and Dodge (which conform to the authors' data) to be about half that reported in most of the series cited. Horan, Flowers et al. [153] also point out that the reported autopsy correlations of ECG/VCG changes of infarct in patients with so-called LBBB suffer significantly from this admixture of fascicular blocks and complete LBBB. It is not possible from the published data, except in a few instances, to separate out these subgroups and their specific associated pathoanatomic lesions.

In our hands, those patients with an ECG/VCG pattern resembling LBBB with a QRS duration <140 ms, but meeting the Wilson criterion of QRS duration ≥120 ms, usually have LV overload and local infarction which produces the initial and mid-QRS changes reminiscent of LBBB. Indeed, as Grant and Dodge previously observed, it has been found in the patients studied by the authors that even in many of those with LV conduction delay of the left type with QRS duration ≥140 ms, the ECG/VCG will show wide separation of initial and terminal vectors without mid-QRS notching and slowing of transcription. This is atypical for LBBB and more consistent with fascicular block, usually anterior (superior) combined with severe LVH. These patients will have increased LV dimensions at ventriculography. In both subsets, the ECG score and the VCG criteria for infarct size and location, which assume LBBB is not present, will perform well in predicting the angiographic change.

4.5.3 Incidence and Prognosis of BBB in Patients with Coronary Artery Disease

4.5.3.1 Incidence of Preexisting or Recent Onset RBBB

In the series of Hiss and Lamb [154], complete RBBB was found 52 times (0.1%) in 44,213 healthy US Air Force personnel under 25 years of age (whereas LBBB was not seen in this age-group). Acquired RBBB below the age of 50 occurred

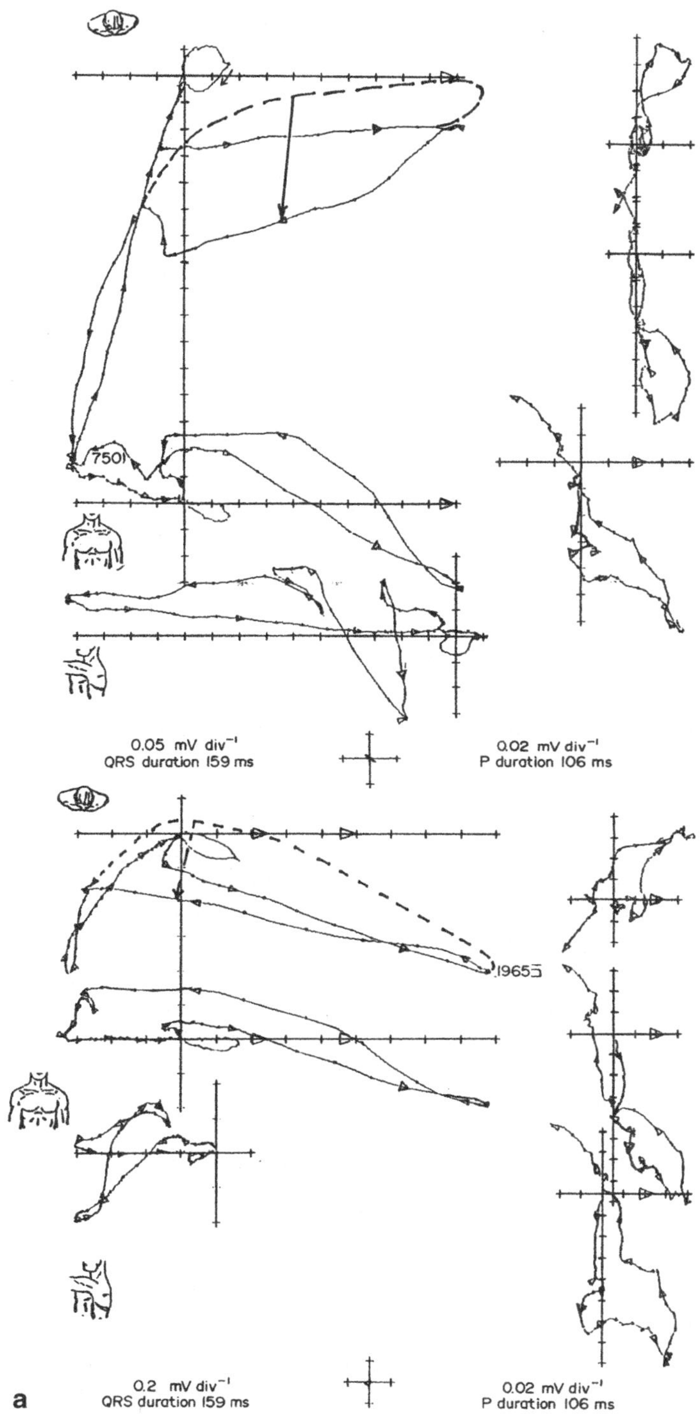

a

■ **Fig. 4.37 (Continued)**

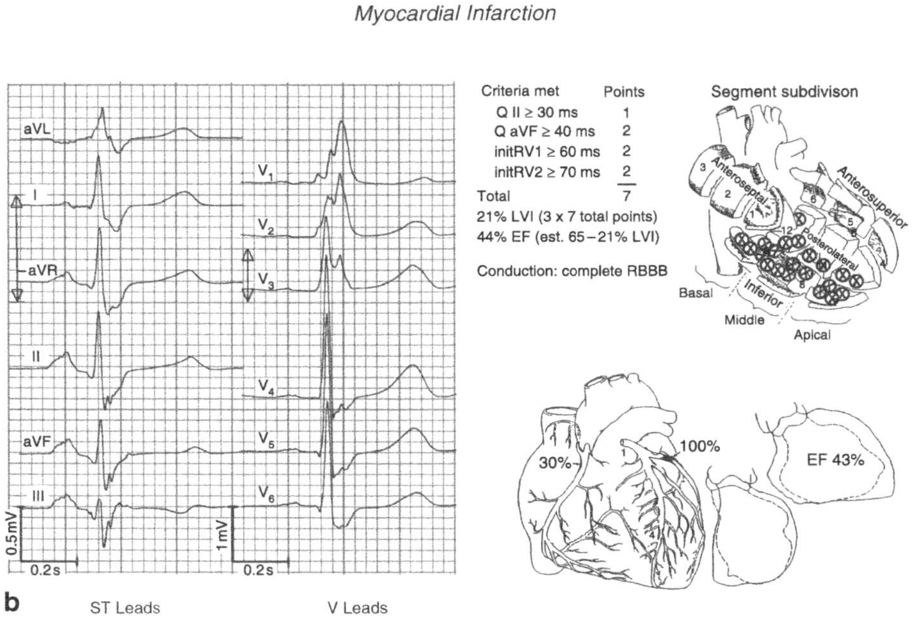

Fig. 4.37
(a) The Cube VCG is the upper half of the figure and the McFee in the lower half. This 55-year-old woman apparently had preexisting right bundle branch block (RBBB). Prior to angiograms done because of angina she had the VCGs recorded. In both lead systems, the VCG inscription is atypical for RBBB in that the 45–80 ms vectors are written in a clockwise fashion in the horizontal and left sagittal planes instead of counterclockwise. The usual VCG change for this interval is shown by the *dotted lines* in both lead systems. It is perhaps more anatomically consistent to say that after the peak leftward vector, i.e., at apical breakthrough of LV activation, the vector fails to swing toward the free posterolateral LV wall before it is overridden by the late RV activation. The latter change is the stereotypical change seen in RBBB even in the presence of severe RV hypertrophy. These subtleties in phase of the surface ECG signal are difficult if not impossible to appreciate from visual inspection of conventional 12 lead ECGs. They can be mathematically defined easily in simultaneous digitized orthogonal lead or 12 lead ECG data. The specific change described and the presence of an abnormal superior initial 34 ms vector are strong VCG evidence for infarction of the posterolateral-inferior wall from this codominant LCX occlusion, as shown on these illustrations the magnitude and duration of the deformities in each lead system, transferred to the nomogram (➜ Fig. 4.12), yielded an estimate of infarct size of 6 cm and an EF of 48%. (b) Note limb leads are in the orderly (Cabrera) sequence from the *top down*, aVL, I, -aVR, II, aVF, III. Since the 1st edition of this book chapter we, the authors, have developed and validated QRS infarct size scores for RBBB. LAFB ± RBBB, LVH and LBBB (see Appendix A). The score for RBBB as shown above, in addition to 3 points for abnormal Qs II, aVF (as noted in 1st edition) gives 2 points each for V1, V2 wide initial R, increasing the points to 7 (21% LVI) for posterolateral-inferior infarct and a 44% EF

in 0.6% of US Air Force pilots [155], and 13% of these (0.08% of the total) were found to have coronary artery disease at angiography. All but a small percent of the remainder had entirely normal angiographic findings and hemodynamics, normal exercise tests and performance, normal electrophysiologic studies, and were returned to flying status. Right bundle branch block is, per se, not incompatible with long life. On the other hand, when it occurs as the result of an acute myocardial infarct, it is usually an ominous sign [37]. The survival rate is reduced to less than one fourth of that expected for acute myocardial infarction as a whole owing to the extensive infarction that usually produces this conduction abnormality. In the setting of acute infarction, RBBB is more common than LBBB. It occurs as a new event in 7% of all patients with acute infarction. In the large majority of cases, it is a result of very proximal LAD coronary artery occlusion with an anterior infarction, which is usually very large, with significant basal septal involvement. Only occasionally (<0.35% of acute infarcts) it is caused by RCA occlusion with inferior and basal septal infarction. Infarction in any of the three arterial distributions can occur in patients with stable long-standing RBBB. Since the presence of the block does not affect prognosis and infarct size does, it becomes very important in terms of management to be able to evaluate infarct size in the presence of this conduction abnormality. Only then can it reasonably be predicted whether the patient has a good prognosis and can be expected to go back to high levels of activity, or whether the patient must expect serious limitation of functional reserve and must plan activity and possible return to gainful employment accordingly.

4.5.3.2 Incidence of Preexisting or Recent Onset Complete LBBB

Hiss and Lamb [154] found 0% incidence of LBBB in 44,231 otherwise healthy US Air Force personnel below the age of 25. Acquired LBBB also occurred much less often in the pilot population below 50 years of age than RBBB [155], namely 0.1% as compared to 0.6%. Significant coronary disease was found at angiography in 22% of subjects with LBBB (0.02% of the total) compared to 13% for RBBB (0.08% of the total). In both groups, all but a small percentage of the remainder were found to have normal angiography, hemodynamics, electrophysiological studies and exercise performance, and were returned to flying status. In patients with angiographically documented coronary artery disease, the incidence of LBBB in the Rancho/USC and Duke University databanks using the Wilson (and NYHA) definition of LBBB was 1.7%. Using the more appropriate criteria from the Grant and Dodge report [16] that include a QRS duration of ≥140 ms, the incidence was 1%.

In earlier reports [37], LBBB was seen as a new event in 2–3% of patients with an acute myocardial infarction. In the current aging populations, 5–6% of patients presenting to chest pain centers who evolve an acute infarction have LBBB on their admission ECG (see ➋ Sect. 4.5.5.2 below).

4.5.3.3 Prognosis

In the US Air Force study, RBBB, while being more common as an incidental finding, was also more common as an acquired finding on follow-up examination. It was four times more often associated with newly diagnosed coronary disease at angiography than acquired LBBB. In both groups, over three fourths of these pilots had normal coronary arteries, normal stress hemodynamics and were allowed to remain on flying status. Long-term survival in epidemiological studies of the general populations of subjects with either RBBB or LBBB is decreased threefold over age-matched cohorts [147–150]. It was concluded that the survival was more closely related to the underlying heart disease and other risk factors than to the presence of the block *per se*.

In asymptomatic subjects, or in those suspected of coronary disease who have preexisting RBBB or LBBB on the ECG/VCG, there is a different admixture of patients with no infarcts or small infarcts with normal LV function, and patients with very large infarcts or ischemic myopathy and very poor LV function. Since prognosis is much more closely related to the severity of the underlying heart disease than to the presence or absence of BBB, it becomes important for both management and prognosis to be able to evaluate the presence, size and location of the infarct. Patients with recent onset LBBB in the setting of acute infarction have, in general, small infarcts, although a few are very large. Such patients have been found to have the same survival rate as age-matched subjects without BBBs [37]. It is not surprising that they have a threefold improved short-term survival rate compared to those with an acute infarct and recent onset of RBBB, most of whom have large anterior infarcts.

4.5.4 Myocardial Infarction and RBBB

In uncomplicated RBBB, the abnormal right ventricular depolarization produces a stereotypic repolarization pattern. These secondary ST-T changes are seen as displacement of the ST segment to the left and posteriorly, directly opposite to the terminal right and anterior QRS of delayed RV depolarization. The prominent T-wave (and vector field) follows the ST segment to the left and posteriorly. The early ST-T changes of acute anterior, posterolateral, or inferior infarction superimposed on the secondary repolarization of RBBB are readily discernible. There are subtle but important changes in the initial 60 ms of the QRS with this abnormality. The most important is a 5–10° shift of the initial forces anteriorly and superiorly owing to loss of normal posteriorly directed vectors from the right septal surface and loss of normal early inferior vectors in the right ventricle. This, however, has no important effect on criteria for quantifying healed anterior infarcts. It does have major effects on criteria for posterolateral infarct and minor, but important, effects for inferior infarct with inferior-posterior fascicular block discussed in ➋ Sect. 4.5.4.4 below.

4.5.4.1 Left Anterior Descending Occlusion, Anterior Infarction and RBBB

When an anterior superior infarct has produced the RBBB, as discussed in the recent onset block described above, the infarct is usually large to very large. On the other hand, when it occurs in a patient with a long-standing congenital or stable RBBB the infarct can be of any size. Thus, the distribution of the size of the infarct is weighted to the end of the scale from large to very large. Nevertheless, the criteria for prior (healed) or acute anterior infarct described in this chapter perform quite well as predictors of the size of this infarct as seen on biplane ventriculograms.

4.5.4.2 Left Anterior Descending Occlusion, Anterior Infarction. RBBB and LAFB

The left anterior-superior fascicles of the left bundle and the right bundle are both supplied by the LAD coronary artery. It is not surprising, therefore, that this combination of blocks and infarction is relatively common. See ➋ Fig. 4.19 for an example of a very large acute anterior infarct in which these conduction abnormalities developed. The left anterior (superior) fascicular block (LAFB) produces changes described in the section on typical anterior infarct. The presence of the additional RBBB does not significantly alter the ability of the ECG and VCG criteria to localize and size anterior infarcts and to predict biplane angiographic change.

4.5.4.3 Circumflex Occlusion, Posterolateral Infarction and RBBB

It is theoretically possible for a very dominant circumflex coronary that also provides a major blood supply to the septum to be etiologically involved in the production of RBBB. Four percent of all recent onset RBBBs are associated with recent inferior infarction. Since 10–15% of all inferior infarcts are the result of total occlusion of a dominant circumflex, it follows that 0.4–0.7% of all recent onset RBBBs would be associated with a recent occlusion of a dominant circumflex and a recent inferior posterolateral infarction. In fact, such a finding has never been documented in the authors' centers, but Grant and Dodge [143] reported a preexisting posterolateral infarct in 6 out of 80 (7.5%) subjects with intermittent RBBB. On the other hand, we have noted that acute chest pain patients with RBBB who have >0.2 mV posterior ST deviation in two leads of V1–V3 have a high probability of having an acute LCX occlusion.

Circumflex occlusion with posterolateral infarction in patients who also have a preexisting RBBB does occur as an isolated lesion. Since initial forces are displaced somewhat anteriorly by the RBBB, a QRS vector loop which is entirely anterior occurs occasionally without any infarction at angiography or autopsy. The changes in QRS described above for RBBB replicate the criteria for posterolateral infarct listed in the ECG score for infarct size, ➋ Fig. 4.16, in the absence of the infarction. Thus, posterolateral points by the ECG QRS score are completely unreliable in the presence of RBBB and should not be used. In patients with large posterolateral infarcts, with apical and inferior extension, the abnormal loss of R and/or Q waves in I, V4, V5 and V6 and in inferior leads may be the most reliable sign of this lesion. Unfortunately, these leads are not usually involved with the more usual small posterolateral infarcts. VCG changes (especially with the Cube lead system – see ➋ Chap. 11 of *Basic Electrocardiology: Cardiac Electrophysiology, ECG Systems and Mathematical Modeling*) are, however, still reliable predictors of infarct size with ventriculographic posterolateral wall motion abnormalities from circumflex occlusion. Irregularities of the 20–60 ms vectors, with anterior displacement that produces a clockwise initial inscription of the horizontal plane VCG (➋ Fig. 4.37), are indicators of localized posterolateral infarction and RBBB. Statistically adequate numbers of these patients to test significance do not exist in the authors' database. Nevertheless, the amount of deformity from the usual counterclockwise initial inscription of the horizontal plane loop has been predictive of the size of posterolateral lesions as seen angiographically in this small number of patients.

4.5.4.4 RCA Occlusion, Inferior Infarction, RBBB and LIFB

In those patients with stable preexisting RBBB (and the few patients with recent onset RBBB) and acute RCA occlusion, the significant ST inferior deviation of acute inferior ischemia/injury (≥0.1 mV) is superimposed on a minor secondary ST elevation (0.05 mV) of RBBB (for a total of ≥0.15 mV). In the evolved/healed inferior infarct, LIFB (inferior-posterior fascicular block), as defined earlier in this chapter, is nearly always present. In these situations, with a normal anterosuperior wall and apex, the criteria for inferior infarct are nearly as effective as if the RBBB were not present. RBBB itself produces early loss of inferior forces (from the absent early activation inferior right ventricle). Thus, there is a slight increase (3%LV) in the inferior QRS MI size score and overestimation of inferior infarct size in the presence of RBBB.

On the other hand, in the somewhat more common situation where the RBBB has been caused by a large anterior infarct, the presence of an inferior infarction is more difficult to deduce and the infarct size is less reliably estimated. The reasons are the same as if the RBBB were not there, namely, inferior Q waves as evidence for inferior infarction, with or without inferior-posterior fascicular block, are dependent upon an intact anterosuperior wall for their production. When a large anterior infarct is also present, there is a major decrease in anterosuperior wall vectors needed to produce abnormal superior vectors. However, the major loss of leftward vectors from the apical involvement of the large anterior infarct is still present. When inferior infarction is present together with a large anterior infarct (with or without RBBB), the anterior infarct is rarely missed by the criteria for infarct size presented in this chapter. Its size, however, may be underestimated. The presence of a separate posterolateral infarct from circumflex occlusion or a significant posterolateral extension of an inferior infarct is suspected in RBBB plus inferior fascicular block by the same criteria described in ➋ Sect. 4.5.4.3 above for RBBB alone.

4.5.5 Myocardial Infarction and LBBB

Recent onset LBBB, when seen, is usually intermittent, rate-dependent, and associated with a high degree of intranodal block. The diagnosis of prior infarct, or the estimation of its size, is rarely a problem in this context because the LBBB is intermittent and the more normal conducted beats are available for analysis. In preexisting or persistent LBBB in patients with chronic angina pectoris or a previously documented infarct, many of the ECG/VCGs exhibiting a LBBB configuration will be atypical. Those with a mild increase in QRS duration of 120–130 ms, small or absent R in V1, V2, notched R in V5 or V6, LVH, and/or with the criteria for superior or inferior-posterior fascicular block, that is, wide separation of initial and terminal 30 ms vectors, are readily analyzed as to presence and size of infarct by the criteria presented in this chapter. In the absence of clinical idiopathic cardiomyopathy in the current aging population, LBBB with QRS ≥ 140 ms will be present in 4–5% of the subset with angina or documented coronary artery disease. Of this subset 40–50% of the "typical" LBBB, as described in detail below, will usually be associated with calcification at the base of the heart around the aortic and mitral rings and/or multiple proximal coronary occlusions involving both the LAD and the right coronary arteries.

4.5.5.1 Secondary ST-T of LBBB Modified by a Local Acute Myocardial Infarction

In the current aging population of patients presenting to chest pain centers, there is an increasing incidence (4–5%) of LBBB, and a similar incidence of ventricular pacing with LBBB type morphology. It has been observed that patients presenting with these LBBB morphologies and signs and symptoms of acute myocardial infarction are significantly less likely to undergo early intervention for coronary reperfusion [156]. The window of opportunity to salvage threatened myocardium is 4–6 h from onset of symptoms [157]. Consequently, a rapid and accurate diagnosis of AMI has become essential. Those with symptoms, normal conduction, and ECG ST deviations of acute myocardial infarction (AMI), in the absence of contraindications, are managed with immediate thrombolytic therapy or percutaneous coronary angioplasty of the acutely occluded artery. However, for those with LBBB morphologies, methodological limitations and conflicting reliabilities of various proposed ECG criteria have resulted in their limited acceptance. This has improved since Sgarbossa et al. and Sgarbossa/Wagner established three electrocardiographic criteria with independent value in the diagnosis of AMI in patients with chest pain and LBBB, which have begun to be more widely utilized. The criteria are (1) STj elevation $\geq$500 μV in any lead and discordant with the QRS complex, and (2) STj depression V1, V2 or V3 $\geq$ 100 μV, (3) STj elevation $\geq$ 100 μV in any lead with upright QRS. A scoring system is utilized.

An improvement in both sensitivity and specificity was found by Polizos and Selvester [156] when they reported a LBBB "10% rule" for the ratio of STj to the |R-S| amplitude. In a control population of 94 chest pain patients documented to be non-ischemia or acute infarction, the STj deviation was 10% of the |R-S| amplitude $\pm 200\ \mu$V in anterior-posterior leads V1, V2, V3 and $\pm 100\ \mu$V in all other leads for 1094/1128 leads giving a specificity of 97%. The sensitivity was 79% (76/96) for the patients with LBBB morphology, QRS $\geq$ 140 ms and documented acute myocardial infarction (AMI) who exceeded the biomarker thresholds confirmatory of the clinical suspicion of possible acute infarction. ➋ Figure 4.38 panel A illustrates the implementation of the 10% rule. There was a reasonable distribution of STj deviations exceeding the 10% ratio consistent with acute anterior, inferior, posterolateral, and apical MIs of the 76 in the following contiguous lead pair(s): Anterior STj deviation beyond the 10% rule in anterior-posterior leads V1, V2, V3 of $\pm 200\ \mu$V in 26 (34%) consistent with anterior AMI, and posterior STj deviations in 11 (15%) consistent with posterolateral AMI; $+100\ \mu$V inferior in inferior-superior leads II, aVF, III, aVL in 21 (27%) consistent with inferior AMI; $-100\ \mu$V base-apex leads I, aVR, V4, V5, V6 in 18 (24%) consistent with acute apical and/or global subendocardial ischemia. Twelve of the 76 did not meet the Sgarbossa-Wagner criteria for acute injury/ischemia. It was also noted that the 10% rule for localizing ST changes of acute MI worked as well for those with single chamber RV pacing which usually has atypical LBBB morphology and a QRS duration $\leq$140 ms.

4.5.5.2 Activation Sequence in LBBB and Regional Healed Infarcts

The incidence of LBBB in the subset of the aging population with angina, history of infarct and documented coronary artery disease is 5–6%. A normal ventriculogram will be seen in 1–2% despite definite angiographic coronary disease, and a diffuse myopathic change will be seen on the ventriculogram in 20–30% of this subset. A typical LBBB with QRS duration $\geq$140 ms ($\geq$130 ms for females) now represents 2–3% of patients with documentable coronary artery disease and either single or multiple local infarcts. The computer simulation of the total-body ECG during depolarization and repolarization was used to unravel the complex interactions of hypertrophy, infarcts (single and multiple) and ischemia and injury, in RBBB and LBBB. The following discussion of ventricular activation in typical LBBB is presented as a basis for the development of the criteria for infarcts in all of the three main coronary distributions.

A better appreciation of this topic can be gained if the activation sequence of LBBB, summarized in 3-plane isochrone maps in ➋ Fig. 4.39, is reviewed along with the distribution of the infarcts associated with LAD, LCX and RCA occlusion shown in ➋ Fig. 4.3. These are the major determinants of ECG/VCG changes of healed infarct plus LBBB. A short review of the activation in LBBB is given here as a basis for understanding these changes. For the first 50 ms of LBBB, the activation fronts are developing simultaneously anteriorly in the right ventricle and posteriorly on the right septal surface in its apical and middle segments as indicated from ➋ Fig. 4.6A and ➋ 4.39. As RV breakthrough of the anterior fronts occurs at about 10 ms, there is a rapid shift of the resultant QRS vector posteriorly since it is dominated by the enlarging posteriorly directed fronts in the anteroseptal wall of the left ventricle. This produces the **first in a series of QRST changes** typical of LBBB, namely a small, short-duration initial vector directed anteriorly and leftward, and sets the stage for all the others.

In the absence of LVH, it requires about 40 ms for this rapidly enlarging posteriorly directed wavefront to traverse the septum in the lower portion. A hole then develops in these septal fronts and remains for next 30–40 ms as the Purkinje

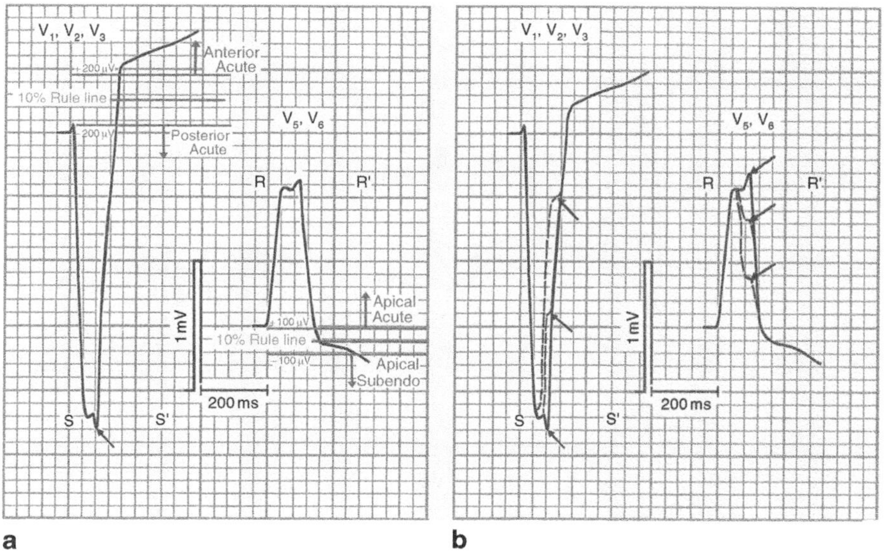

Fig. 4.38

Pane a. For acute myocardial infarction with LBBB the 10% *rule line* represents the expected STJ opposite the absolute value of R-S. The 98% confidence limit is ±200 μV for V1, V2, V3 and ±100 μV in V5, V6, and limb leads. In patients with persistent ischemic chest pain, STJ deviation in 2 or more contiguous leads exceeding these thresholds, the diagnosis of acute myocardial infarction can be made with 97% specificity. The extent of the evolving infarction and its location are a function of the number of leads with ST deviation exceeding thresholds directed outward from the center of the local epicardial region in jeopardy. Pane b. For prior infarct size with LBBB this diagram depicts visually R,R′,S, and S′ used in the QRS scoring system The S in V1 or V2 and the R in V5 or V6 represent change in direction of mean QRS vector (and electric field) at the breakthrough of septal activation on the left septal surface (see Fig. 4.39). This occurs near the first 1/3 of the QRS (at 45–70 ms) when activation fronts propagating through the septum from the *right side* arrive at the *left* and a hole develops in the previously continuous activation front. As the fronts propagate outward in the septum, their area directed posterior remains rather constant (from 70 to 95 ms.) resulting in "slow mid QRS conduction," one of the "classic" criteria for diagnosis of LBBB. It follows that an S′ in V1 or V2 and the R′ in V5 or V6 is the change in direction of the mean QRS vector that occurs near the 2/3 point of the QRS with breakthrough of activation at the apex of the LV. This may show up as a definite S′ or R′, but may be only a slurring of terminal QRS as shown. For the purpose of the infarct size score, any extra notching in the mid QRS between the R and R′ should be ignored. When a definite inflection point does not occur at the 1/3 or 2/3 point in any designated V lead, the time when it occurs in the others is transferred to the lead in question and the R, R′, S, or S′ amplitude is taken at this point

network on the left side is being entered. This produces the **second QRST change typical of LBBB**, that is a slurred notch develops at about 50 ms into the QRS, best seen in anterior leads V1, V2, and Z and in left leads I, V5, V6 and X. Activation progresses outward in the septum enlarging the hole in a ring of active surface of about the same surface area directed from anterior to posterior in the remaining basal, superior, inferior and apical septum. A review of the LBBB activation in Fig. 4.39 with special attention to the 50–80 ms isochrones in the lower left sagittal view will account for the ring of active fronts and their average direction that remain relatively unchanged for this period of time. This adds **the third change of typical LBBB**, namely, mid-QRS slowing of transcription to the notch just described, which is also seen in the same leads as the slurred notch. As the left Purkinje network in the midseptal region is entered, activation spreads rapidly out in the endocardium. At 60–90 ms from the QRS onset, fronts are developing in the subendocardium and mural myocardium of the superior and inferior walls and much of the apex, especially anteriorly. Besides the broad

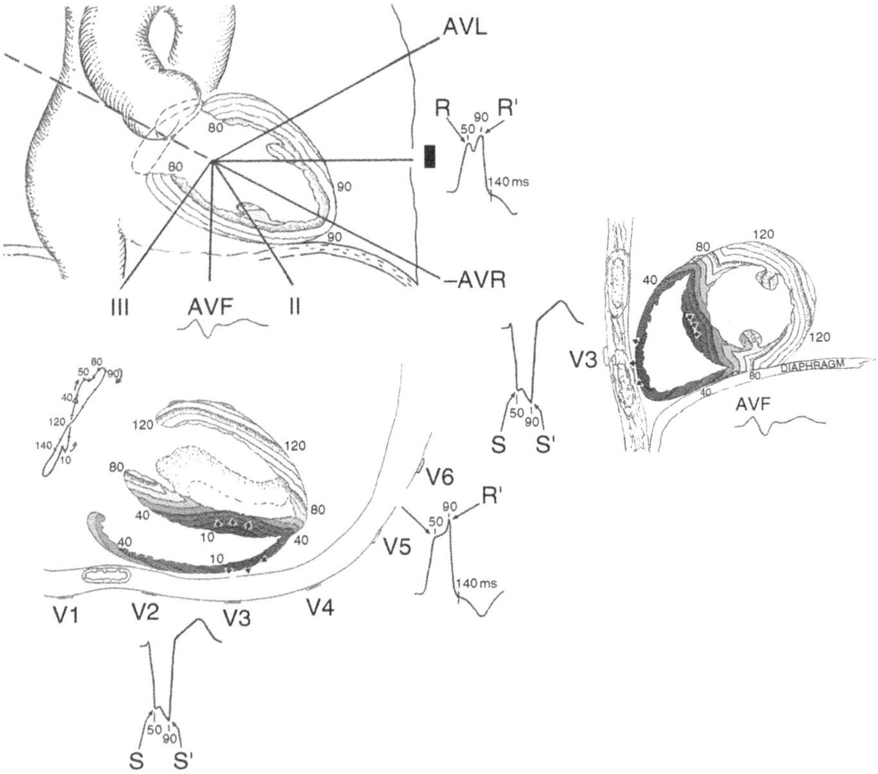

Fig. 4.39
Activation sequences (10 ms isochrones) for LBBB in horizontal, frontal and left sagittal planes with QRS changes of a healed myocardial infarct in any local perfusion bed of the three major coronary arteries and their branches. See Figs. 4.38 and 4.40 for details of the how the typical LBBB QRS complexes shown in this figure are changed of infarction involving infarction in the local regions supplied by the 3 main coronary arteries or thneir branches

fronts propagating in the left ventricle, the only unopposed front at this time is that developing leftward in the apex. This produces a shift leftward in the QRS vector, reaching a peak at about 100 ms, as apical LV breakthrough of activation fronts occurs. This produces the **fourth change typical of complete LBBB**, namely, a second peak in the QRS amplitude, usually higher than the first and following the mid-QRS slowing and notch just described. This change too is best seen in anterior and leftward leads. As this peak is receding, the activation fronts that have been developing on the posterolateral wall are also beginning to decrease in size. The prolated ellipsoid shape of the LV and the smaller diameter of the LV at the mitral valve and adjacent basal segments accounts for the following. Posteriorly directed fronts in the most basal portions of the superior, inferior walls meet and merge on the most basal part of the posterolateral free wall prior to the posterior and leftward directed fronts in the apical and middle posterolateral segments. This produces the **fifth change typical of LBBB**; namely, clockwise inscription of the QRS loop in the horizontal plane. In an LV wall of normal thickness, this activation takes 40–50 ms for a total QRS duration of 140–150 ms (**the sixth classic feature of LBBB**). Since the propagation velocity in human myocardium is 3–4 mm/10 ms, any increase in septal or and posterolateral wall thickness will increase total QRS duration (i.e., for every 2 mm added to the septum and to the posterolateral wall (or 4 mm total), 10–13 ms is added to the total QRS duration).

In uncomplicated LBBB, the balance of superior and inferior wall vectors, where large wavefronts are present throughout much of the QRS, is such that the mean frontal-plane axis is at or near zero degrees with a very narrow frontal-plane

Left bundle branch block QRS MI size score criteria

LBBB QRS-Score

Lead	Criteria	Pts	Max pts
*Anterosuperior wall**			
I	R/Q ≤ 1.5	1	1*
	R/S ≤ 1.5		
aVL	Q ≥ 50 ms	2	4*
	Q ≥ 40 ms	1	
	R/S ≤ 0.5	2	
	R/Q ≤ 0.5		
	R/S ≤ 1	1	
	R/Q ≤ 1		
Inferior wall			
II	Q ≥ 40 ms	2	3
	Q ≥ 30 ms	1	
	R/Q ≤ 0.5	1	
	R/S ≤ 0.5		
aVF	Q ≥ 50 ms	2	3
	Q ≥ 40 ms	1	
	R/Q ≤ 0.5	1	
	R/S ≤ 0.5		
*Anteroseptal wall***			
V1	NCHINIT40	1	3**
	R ≥ 0.3 mV	2	
	R ≥ 30 ms		
	R ≥ 0.2 mV	1	
	R ≥ 20 ms		
V2	NCHINIT40	1	3**
	R ≥ 0.4 mV	2	
	R ≥ 30 ms		
	R ≥ 0.3 mV	1	
	R ≥ 20 ms		
Posterlateral wall			
V1	S/S' ≥ 2.0	3	3
	S/S' ≥ 1.5	2	
	S/S' ≥ 1.25	1	
V2	S/S' ≥ 2.5	3	3
	S/S' ≥ 2.0	2	
	S/S' ≥ 1.5	1	
Apical 4 segments			
I	any Q	1	2
	R ≤ 0.2 mV		
	R/Q ≤ 1	1	
	R/S ≤ 1		
V5	any Q	1	4
	R/R' ≥ 2	2	
	R/R' ≥ 1	1	
	R/S ≤ 2		
	R ≤ 0.5 mV	1	
V6	Q ≥ 20 ms	1	4
	R/R' ≥ 2	2	
	R/R' ≥ 1	1	
	R/S ≤ 2		
	R ≤ 0.6 mV	1	
Total Points _______			33

12 LV Segments

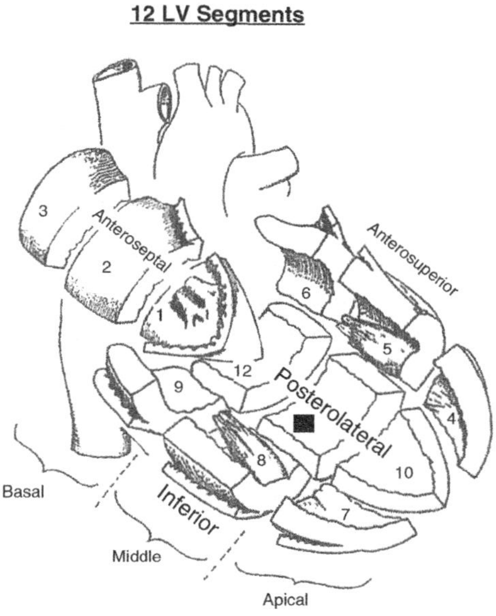

Short-axis View of Middle 4 Segments

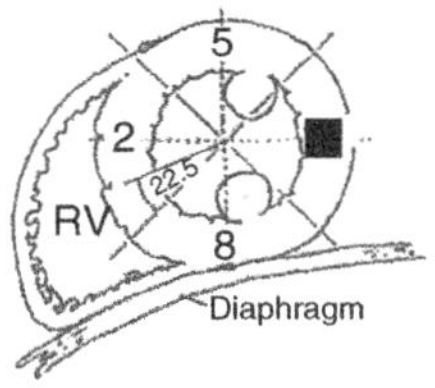

Total QRS points ______ *3 = _______ % LV MI

LBBB QRS Score Instructions

Age normalize all amplitude criteria to age 55 by increasing them 1%/yr age 20-54 and decreasing them 1%/yr for >55 yrs.
For females further decrease by 10% all QRSdur and QRSamp criteria.
Circle each QRS criteria.
If >1 criterion in bracket (box) met, select one with most points.

Criteria Definitions

NCHINIT40 = Notch in initial 40 ms
The definitions of S, S', R and R' are shown below.

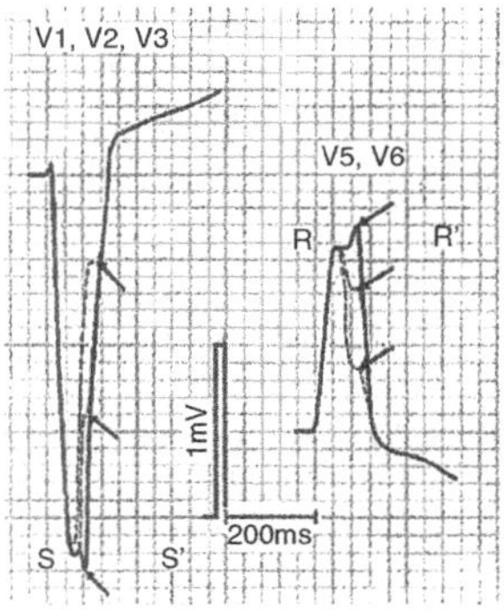

Additional Rules

* Exclude anteroseptal points if right atrial overload (suggesting RVH) is present (P positive amplitude in V1 or V2 P ≥ 0.1 mV or aVF P ≥ 0.175 mV).

** Exclude anterosuperior points if right axis deviation is present (mean QRS axis ≥90°).

Fig. 4.40

projection of the loop. This **is the seventh QRST change typical of uncomplicated LBBB**. Any shift beyond ±20° represents disruption of this balance of vectors, either from missing myocardium or further disruption of the more distal Purkinje conduction. The latter is rare in recent onset LBBB in patients with coronary artery disease, but is common in the congestive cardiomyopathies where the myopathic autoimmune process also extensively involves the peripheral Purkinje system. Marked left axis or right axis shifts have been reported as markers of the process. **The eighth classic change of LBBB** relates to repolarization, which is directly linked to the very abnormal depolarization. ST-T vectors in LBBB are directed opposite to those of QRS in all projections.

In summary, with respect to **superimposed myocardial infarction on LBBB**, the first 50 ms of ventricular depolarization is dominated by the septum and right ventricle (see ➋ Fig. 4.39); the middle 50 ms is dominated by the paraseptal areas of the left ventricle adjacent to the septum, namely, the anterosuperior, anteroapical and inferior walls; and the last 50 ms is made up of activation fronts in the posterolateral wall of the left ventricle. It follows that **anterior infarction** will result in loss of initial posteriorly directed anteroseptal vectors unmasking the early anterior RV forces with the resultant increase in initial anterior vector magnitude and duration. There will also be a significant increase in high-frequency notching and slurring in the initial QRS as the activation fronts encounter the patchy interdigitation of scar and normal myocardium at the border of the infarct. **Anterosuperior extension** of the anterior infarct will deform the early to mid-QRS vectors inferiorly with a mean axis shift inferiorly. Significant **anteroapical extension** of the anterior infarct will result in a loss of leftward vectors and a loss of the second peak of R in I, V5, V6, and *X* with a shift of the mean axis to being almost directly posterior (and/or rightward and inferior if major anterosuperior extension is also present). Details of the QRS MI size score to reflect these changes due to infarct and to quantify infarct size are presented in ➋ Sect. 4.5.5. **Inferior infarction** from posterior-inferior descending artery (PDA) occlusion, usually as the result of RCA occlusion, results in loss of inferior vectors in the early to mid-QRS and significant displacement of these vectors superiorly from their usual location, as seen in typical LBBB. **Posterolateral infarct** from occlusion of a non-dominant LCX, results in an attenuation of the late posterior vectors and a shift of the mid to terminal QRS anterior vectors. **Posterolateral-inferior infarct** from a left dominant LCX, or a rare very dominant RCA occlusion with a large distal posterolateral branch and a diminutive LCX, has a simple combination effect on the QRS of inferior and posterolateral infarct just described. These changes are defined more explicitly for each of the three major coronary distributions in Appendix B, ➋ Fig. 4.39, and in the three sub-sections of the ➋ Sect. 4.5.5 to follow.

4.5.5.3 LAD Occlusion, Anterior Infarction and LBBB

➋ Figure 4.41a, b is an example of a patient who at the time of angiography had two areas of infarction: a large anterior infarct with inferoapical extension from proximal LAD coronary occlusion and a second moderate-sized inferior infarct from RCA occlusion. The ECG/VCG shows changes of atypical LBBB with a QRS duration of 197 ms. In this case, the P vectors seen to the right of the VCG plots show significant abnormalities. The P duration is increased to 133 ms. The initial right atrial vectors are mildly increased in amplitude above normal anterior and inferior component limits, indicative of mildly decreased RV diastolic compliance consistent with mild RV and pulmonary hypertension. The left atrial activation times are significantly increased and voltage amplitude directed leftward and posteriorly is greatly increased (3–4 times normal), which is consistent with a major decrease in diastolic compliance in the left ventricle such as might be seen with severe LV dysfunction from extensive infarction and compensatory hypertrophy.

In the uncomplicated LBBB, all of the QRS except for the first 10–15 ms is directed leftward and posteriorly owing to the posteriorly directed fronts in the septum and the left ventricle. In this case, infarction in the anteroseptal area and apex has two effects. First, notching and slurring is seen especially in V4, V5 and V6 in the initial 50–60 ms, which in uncomplicated LBBB is usually smoothly written. Second, there is increased amplitude and duration of the initial anterior forces or vectors owing to infarction in the septum which allows the anteriorly directed fronts in the right ventricle to dominate. In this case, the first 30 ms are smoothly written with an increased anterior amplitude. This suggests, along with the mild RAO changes, that mild RVH might be responsible for some of this change. Typically, significant septal involvement would produce a broad slurred and notched R wave in V1 and V2 and a prominent, prolonged, irregular initial anterior vector loop in the VCG, in addition to the other features of LBBB. The magnitude and duration of the anterior vectors is related to the size or extent of septal involvement.

The LV apex is extensively infarcted in this patient as it often is in anterior infarcts. There is a significant loss of leftward vectors from 60 to 100 ms when the apex is expected to be activated. This is the usual marker of the presence of

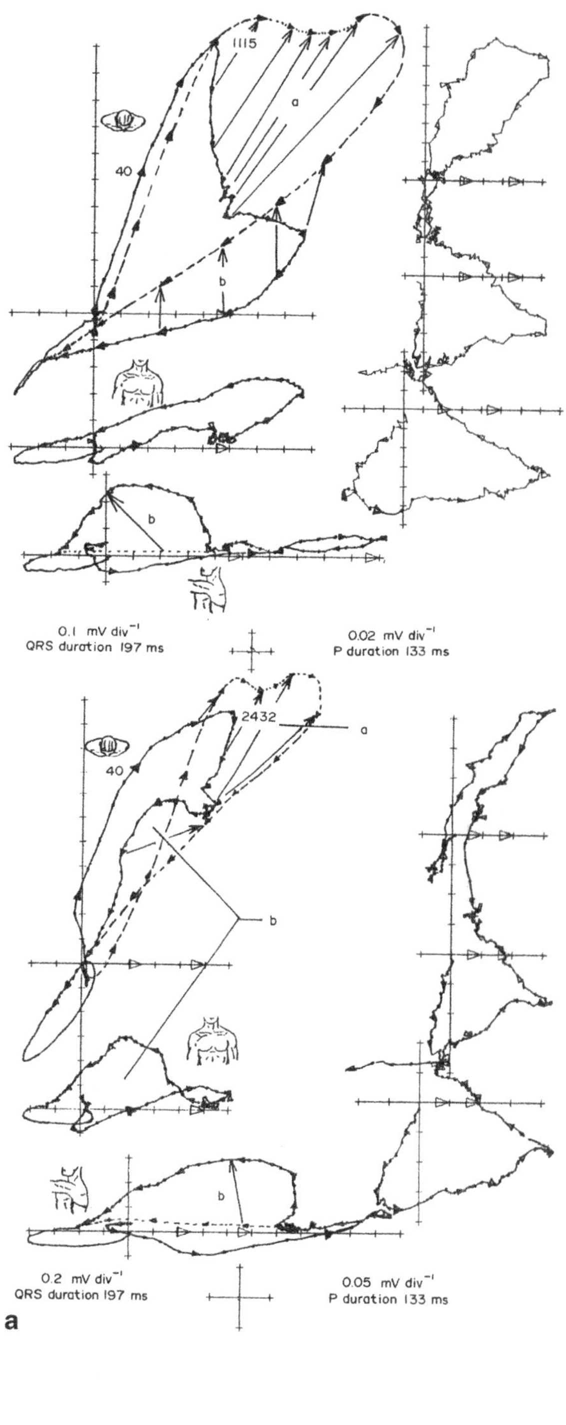

Fig. 4.41 (Continued)

apical extension of this infarct in LBBB. Again, the more extensive the apical involvement, the greater the loss of expected leftward vectors and the longer this deformity lasts. The anterosuperior wall also demonstrates significant involvement. This produces a loss of early superior vectors with a consequent inferior shift of the initial QRS. The two VCGs for this first infarct (see Fig. 4.41a for details) showed major deformities in the early and mid QRS that when transferred to the

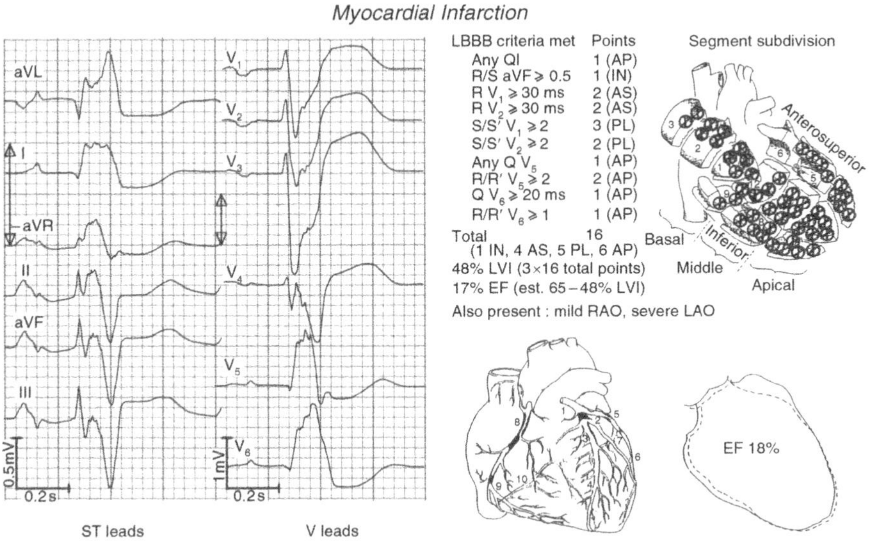

Fig. 4.41

(a) The Cube VCG (*top*) and the McFee (*bottom*) are from a 59-year-old man who had a history of two myocardial infarcts. After the first infarct the ECG and VCG demonstrated a large anterior infarct and normal conduction. Coronary angiograms and biplane Vgrams revealed major 3 vessel disease, 100% LAD, and a large anterior infarct. The patient declined surgery and was symptomatically well controlled on medical management. Three years later he suffered a second infarct and had the VCGs shown here. A second angiogram demonstrated 100% RCA occlusion in the interim and a moderate sized inferior infarct. These VCGs demonstrate a very atypical LBBB with QRS duration of 197 ms. VCGs for typical LBBBs of 197 ms duration are shown in *dotted lines*. The specific changes are discussed in the text in the sections on LAD occlusion, anterior infarct, and LBBB and on RCA occlusion, inferior infarct and LBBB. Infarct #1, shows major deformities (a) of the initial 2/3rds of the QRS in both lead systems, i.e., 0.7 mV/100 ms for the Cube and 1.1 mV/100 ms for the McFee. From the nomogram (➋ Fig. 4.12) a large anteroapical infarct is estimated for both VCGs of 12 cm and 40% involvement of the LV perimeter. Infarct #2 produced deformities (b) in the latter 1/3 of the QRS of 0.3 mV/50 ms and 0.5 mV/50 ms. When transferred to the nomogram (➋ Fig. 4.12) resulted in an estimate for the inferior posterolateral infarct of 6 cm for each VCG and 20% LV involvement angiographically. The sum of 60% of the LV perimeter predicts an LVEF of 18%. (b) Note limb leads are in the orderly (Cabrera) sequence from the *top down*, aVL, I, -aVR, II, aVF, III. Using the version of the LBBB QRS MI size scoring system shown in Appendix B, a total of 16 points or 48% LV infarct is accumulated. As seen in the *upper middle panel* above, this predicted a 17% EF, and distributed the damage into the anterior (septal/superior), apex, inferior, and posterolateral walls as shown. These criteria picked up the anterosuperior and inferior wall involvement seen on the angiogram, and predicted well by the VCGs as shown in (a). A left anterior oblique ventriculogam was not available to evaluate the posterolateral changes predicted by this version of the LBBB QRS MI size scoring system

nomogram (➋ Fig. 4.12) estimated a large anterior infarct of 12 cm and 45% of the LV perimeter. For the second infarct, there is displacement of the terminal 80 ms vectors sharply superiorly and anteriorly from their usual location with LBBB. This is most evident on the Cube lead system and on the 12 lead ECG as prominent S′ in the inferior leads, an abnormal left axis and a broad slurred S" V1–V3. These findings are indicative of a moderately sized basal posterolateral-inferior infarct in addition to the large anterior one described above (see ➋ Fig. 4.41a, b and legends for details). When the magnitude and duration of the VCG changes of both infarcts are transferred to the nomogram, 65% of the perimeter of the LV on the RAO ventriculogram is predicted be involved with infarction and the ejection fraction is predicted to be 14%.

Losses from the septum, apex and superior wall each contribute to the total sum of the criteria for the QRS MI size score for anterior infarct size in LBBB seen here in ➋ Fig. 4.41b and tabulated from Appendix B. A total of 9 points (27% LV) for anteroapical infarction and 7 points (21% LV) for a posterolateral-inferior infarct were scored. The total is 16 points for 48% LV infarcted and an estimated LV ejection fraction of 17%. Appendix B.

4.5.5.4 Differential Diagnosis of LBBB and Prominent Anterior Forces

Left ventricular hypertrophy is often associated with superior fascicular block, and can have a total QRS duration of greater than 140–160 ms. If the fascicular block is associated with or is the result of a moderate anterior apical infarct, as it often is, it may produce a QRS morphology (large notched RR′ V4, V5, V6) quite suggestive of complete LBBB as are small R waves in V1, V2 and Z. A second moderate posterolateral infarct would produce a prominent wide R wave in V1, V2 mimicking a LBBB + anteroseptal infarct. Wide separation of frontal plane (limb leads) initial and terminal 30 ms vectors, as described by Grant and Dodge [91], effectively identifies this combination of changes. The associated infarcts are usually large, and the ECG QRS score and the nomogram for VCG infarct size will give reliable estimates of angiographic regional wall motion abnormalities and global function.

A second major change that mimics some of the changes described above for LBBB and anterior infarct is RVH in the presence of complete LBBB. The increase of anterior, rightward and inferior vectors for the first 70–80 ms from RVH produces a shift in the LBBB vectors. This results in sharp, smooth, and widened initial anterior vectors with increased amplitude in leads V1, V2, and Z similar to those described above for anterior infarct. It also displaces the 20–80 ms vectors to the right and inferiorly. This decreases the initial leftward vector in I, aVL, V5, V6 and *X*. As a result, in some cases Q waves are produced in these leads, again mimicking anterior infarction with apical and superior wall extension. There are two major features that can be used in the differential diagnosis of these changes. First, in right-sided overload, the degree of RAO parallels the degree of RV overload. When even mild to moderate RAO is present, by the criteria described in ➋ Table 4.2, the likelihood increases greatly that the changes described above are in fact caused by RV overload. The second feature that serves as a marker of RV overload in this situation is the presence of a sharp, smooth abnormal initial anterior vector loop of 0.3 mV or more, lasting 20 ms or longer. The magnitude and duration of this deformity, as well as the severity of the RAO, is related to the degree of RV overload. In summary, the presence of RAO and the absence of notching in the initial vectors reasonably exclude anterior infarction as a cause for the changes described above.

Significant confounding can occur with LBBB owing to coronary disease which is associated with extensive infarction, primary or secondary LV overload, left-heart failure, and severe LAO. Significant right-heart failure, RAO and RV overload are then the secondary results which can produce additive effects in the presence of anterior infarct as far as increased amplitude and duration of initial anterior QRS vectors are concerned. However, even so, the information exists in the ECG/VCG, as it did in the case presented in ➋ Fig. 4.41 to provide a reasonable basis for unscrambling each of these effects and in most cases assessing the relative contribution of each to the final ECG/VCG changes observed.

4.5.5.5 Circumflex Coronary Occlusion, Posterolateral Infarction and LBBB

Only in the presence of a dominant circumflex coronary artery would the blood supply to the proximal left bundle be influenced by total occlusion of this vessel. This anatomy occurs in 10–15% of all human hearts. Since a significant percentage of recent onset LBBBs are as a result of inferior infarction, theoretically 8–10% of these (1% of the total) are the result of total circumflex occlusion. These infarcts could be expected to produce a combination of inferior and posterolateral effects as described above. No such combination was identified in the authors' database of single-vessel circumflex occlusions, but an example of such changes is presented in the case shown in ➋ Fig. 4.41. This patient with RCA occlusion appeared to have significant posterolateral extension of the inferior infarct. Appendix B.

4.5.5.6 RCA Occlusion, Inferior Infarct and LBBB

Figure 4.41, discussed earlier, shows an example of a patient who had LBBB and a moderate inferior-posterolateral infarct from total RCA occlusion in addition to a large anterior infarct and total LAD occlusion. The activation of the base of the septum and the base of the inferior and posterolateral walls are separated in time in LBBB from the apical and midseptum. Therefore much of the area perfused by the RCA is activated after that perfused by the LAD, and separate QRS deformities can be identified for each as shown in the figure. In this case, the late deformity, superior and anterior to that seen in typical LBBB, results from local losses, inferiorly and posteriorly. The uncoupling in time of the activation of septal and free wall fronts in LBBB has produced less cancellation and more reliable estimates of multiple infarct size in the presence of this conduction abnormality than in normal conduction.

4.6 Future Advances in ECG Diagnosis and Imaging of Infarction

There are two areas in the ECG/VCG diagnosis of infarction where as yet the possibilities have not been fully exploited: the very early quantification of area at risk in acute infarction and the quantification of infarct size and residual ischemic area at risk in the considerable number of patients with the complex mix of chamber enlargement, BBB and single or multiple infarcts in the various coronary distributions. It is likely that both management and prognosis in these patients will continue to be tightly bound to infarct size and the extent of ischemia or mass of myocardium at risk. The computer simulation of ventricular excitation and recovery is expected to be an important tool in the further clarification of these complex interactions involved in the manifold combinations of regional ischemia, infarction, chamber enlargement and conduction abnormalities (both minor and major).

From reported studies with the model of the authors [159–161], some aspects of which were detailed in this chapter, this exploration is expected to move into larger numbers of simultaneously recorded leads, probably 16–32 with at least two or three of these leads recorded on the back of the thorax. Small multilead ECG recording systems with onboard computer analysis of these 16–32 leads are well within the capability of twenty-first century technology. The computer model, clinical and cardiac MRI, and postmortem validation studies will be used to provide the optimal lead array, digitizing rates, location of these leads and criteria for quantifying regional acute ischemia and chronic infarct size in the presence of normal conduction, various conduction abnormalities, chamber enlargement and variations in torso geometry, conductivity, and heart or coronary anatomy.

With respect to acute coronary care, the future may see more optimal use of three simultaneous quasi-orthogonal monitoring leads with online identification and continuous monitoring of the area of myocardium at risk, including (a) its extent, (b) the size of the evolving infarct in the risk area, and (c) intermittent conduction change and ectopic activity related to the perfusion bed of the area at risk or at a distance. These would all involve straightforward extensions of existing knowledge. The rapid advances in miniaturization of electronic and computer chip components make it realistic to expect this quantitative capability to be resident in online computer monitoring systems, ambulance recorders and highly portable long-term ambulatory physiological monitoring devices.

Noninvasive ECG imaging with inverse isochrone and potential mapping of endocardium, and epicardium from a few centers has appeared [162]. Inverse imaging of the electromotive surface of the propagating wave of excitation using "smart" constraints of the solution is in process in a few centers as well. The three-dimensional color graphic imaging of the heart and infarct geometry for a specific patient, along with direct imaging of the wave of excitation of the atria and ventricles and the recovery process specific for that patient, are also direct extensions of these modeling efforts and automated signal processing and analysis technology. From this type of imaging, it is possible to visualize, directly, regional, and transmural extent of ischemia and infarction, wall thickness and details of local excitation and recovery. This would include delayed or fractionated excitation potentials and areas of slow conduction. Direct visualization of reentrant pathways and their anatomic substrate would also be a direct outgrowth of such developments. The compelling advantage of working first-hand with the heart's own ECG signal is that these noninvasive measurements can be repeated as often as needed with little or no discomfort or risk to the patient. Indeed, continuous monitoring of many ECG leads and algorithmic processing of the information requires only adaptation of existing technology and carefully controlled validation studies.

Suuplemental Data APPENDIX A: QRS-Score Criteria

% LV Scar in 12 LV Segments

For each QRS-score point scored to the left, circle the numbers to the right in the same row which shows the %LV scar in each of the 12 LV segments.

Lead	RBBB Criteria	Pts	LAFB Criteria	Pts	LAFB + RBBB Criteria	Pts	LVH Criteria	Pts	No Confounders Criteria	Pts	Max Pts	Ant-Sep 1	2	3	Ant-Sup 4	5	6	Inf 7	8	9	Postlat 10	11	12
I	Q ≥ 30 ms	1	Q ≥ 30 ms	1	Q ≥ 30 ms	1	Q ≥ 30 ms	1	Q ≥ 30 ms	1	2				1	1					1		
	R/Q ≤ 1 R ≤ 0.2 mV	1	R/Q ≤ 1 R ≤ 0.2 mV	1	R/Q ≤ 1 R ≤ 0.2 mV	1	R/Q ≤ 1 R ≤ 0.2 mV	1	R/Q ≤ 1 R ≤ 0.2 mV	1					1	1	1						
II	Q ≥ 40 ms	2	Q ≥ 40 ms	2	Q ≥ 40 ms	2	Q ≥ 40 ms	2	Q ≥ 40 ms	2	2							2	2	2			
	Q ≥ 30 ms	1	Q ≥ 30 ms	1	Q ≥ 30 ms	1	Q ≥ 30 ms	1	Q ≥ 30 ms	1									2	1			
aVL	Q ≥ 30 ms	1	Q ≥ 40 ms	1	Q ≥ 40 ms	1	Q ≥ 40 ms	1	Q ≥ 30 ms	1	2					2	1						
	R/Q ≤ 1	1	R/Q ≤ 1	1	R/Q ≤ 1	1	R/Q ≤ 1	1	R/Q ≤ 1	1						1	2						
aVF	Q ≥ 50 ms	3	Q ≥ 50 ms	3	Q ≥ 50 ms	3	Q ≥ 60 ms	3	Q ≥ 50 ms	3	5							3	2	2			
	Q ≥ 40 ms	2	Q ≥ 40 ms	2	Q ≥ 40 ms	2	Q ≥ 50 ms	2	Q ≥ 40 ms	2								2	2	2			
	Q ≥ 30 ms	1	Q ≥ 30 ms	1	Q ≥ 30 ms	1	Q ≥ 40 ms	1	Q ≥ 30 ms	1									2	1			
	R/Q ≤ 1	2	R/Q ≤ 1	2	R/Q ≤ 1	2	R/Q ≤ 1	2	R/Q ≤ 1	2									1	3			
	R/Q ≤ 2	1	R/Q ≤ 2	1	R/Q ≤ 2	1	R/Q ≤ 2	1	R/Q ≤ 2	1									1	2			
V1 Ant.	Q ≥ 50 ms	2			Q ≥ 50 ms	2					(2)	2	2	2									
	any Q R ≤ 20 ms	1	any QR	1	any Q	1	any QR (or QS if *) .04S notch	1	any Q	1	1		1	2									
V1 Post.			R/S ≥ 1	1		1	R/S ≥ 1	1	R/S ≥ 1	1	4										1	1	1
	Init R ≥ 60 ms Init R ≥ 1.5 mV	2	Init R ≥ 50 ms Init R ≥ 1 mV	2	Init R ≥ 60 ms Init R ≥ 1.5 mV	2	Init R ≥ 50 ms Init R ≥ 1 mV	2	Init R ≥ 50 ms Init R ≥ 1 mV	2							1	1	1		1	1	1
	Init R ≥ 50 ms Init R ≥ 1.0 mV	1	Init R ≥ 40 ms Init R ≥ 0.7 mV	1	Init R ≥ 50 ms Init R ≥ 1.0 mV	1	Init R ≥ 40 ms Init R ≥ 0.7 mV	1	Init R ≥ 40 ms Init R ≥ 0.7 mV	1								1			1	1	
Exclude if ** :			Q&S ≤ 0.2 mV	1			Q&S ≤ 0.2 mV	1	Q&S ≤ 0.2 mV	1										1		1	1
V2 Ant.	Q ≥ 50 ms	2			Q ≥ 50 ms	2					(2)	2	2	2									
	any Q R ≤ 10 ms R ≤ 0.1 mV	1	any QR R ≤ 10 ms R ≤ 0.1 mV	1	any Q R ≤ 10 ms R ≤ 0.1 mV	1	any QR (or QS if *) .04S notch	1	any Q R ≤ 10 ms R ≤ 0.1 mV	1	1		1	2									
V2 Post.			R/S ≥ 1.5	1			R/S ≥ 1.5	1	R/S ≥ 1.5	1	4									1		1	1
	Init R ≥ 70 ms Init R ≥ 2.5 mV	2	R ≥ 60 ms R ≥ 2 mV	2	Init R ≥ 70 ms Init R ≥ 2.5 mV	2	R ≥ 60 ms R ≥ 2 mV	2	R ≥ 60 ms R ≥ 2 mV	2								1	1		1	2	1
	Init R ≥ 50 ms Init R ≥ 2.0 mV	1	R ≥ 50 ms R ≥ 1.5 mV	1	Init R ≥ 50 ms Init R ≥ 2.0 mV	1	R ≥ 50 ms R ≥ 1.5 mV	1	R ≥ 50 ms R ≥ 1.5 mV	1									1		1	1	
Exclude if ** :			Q&S ≤ 0.3 mV	1		1	Q&S ≤ 0.3 mV	1	Q&S ≤ 0.3 mV	1									1			1	1
V3	Q ≥ 30 ms R ≤ 10 ms	2	Q ≥ 30 ms R ≤ 10 ms	2	Q ≥ 30 ms R ≤ 10 ms	2	QR+Q ≥ 30 ms .04S notch	2	Q ≥ 30 ms R ≤ 10 ms	2	2	2	2	1		1							
	Q ≥ 20 ms R ≤ 20 ms	1	Q ≥ 20 ms R ≤ 20 ms	1	Q ≥ 20 ms R ≤ 20 ms	1	any QR (or QS if *)	1	Q ≥ 20 ms R ≤ 20 ms	1		1	1			1							
V4	Q ≥ 20 ms	1	Q ≥ 20 ms	1	Q ≥ 20 ms	1	Q ≥ 20 ms	1	Q ≥ 20 ms	1	3	1	1		1								
	R/Q ≤ 0.5 R/S ≤ 0.5	2	R/Q ≤ 0.5 R/S ≤ 0.5	2	R/Q ≤ 0.5 R/S ≤ 0.5	2	R/Q ≤ 0.5 R/S ≤ 0.5	2	R/Q ≤ 0.5 R/S ≤ 0.5	2		2	1		1	1		1					
	R/Q ≤ 1 R/S ≤ 1 R ≤ 0.5 mV .04R notch	1	R/Q ≤ 1 R/S ≤ 1 R ≤ 0.5 mV .04R notch	1	R/Q ≤ 1 R/S ≤ 1 R ≤ 0.5 mV .04R notch	1	R/Q ≤ 1 R/S ≤ 1 R ≤ 0.5 mV .04R notch	1	R/Q ≤ 1 R/S ≤ 1 R ≤ 0.5 mV .04R notch	1		1	1		1								
V5	Q ≥ 30 ms	1	Q ≥ 30 ms	1	Q ≥ 30 ms	1	Q ≥ 30 ms	1	Q ≥ 30 ms	1	3	1	1		1								
	R/Q ≤ 1 R/S ≤ 1	2	R/Q ≤ 1 R/S ≤ 1	2	R/Q ≤ 1 R/S ≤ 1	2	R/Q ≤ 1 R/S ≤ 1	2	R/Q ≤ 1 R/S ≤ 1	2		2	1		1	1		1					
	R/Q ≤ 2 R/S ≤ 2 R ≤ 0.6 mV .04R notch	1	R/Q ≤ 2 R/S ≤ 1.5 R ≤ 0.6 mV .04R notch	1	R/Q ≤ 2 R/S ≤ 1.5 R ≤ 0.6 mV .04R notch	1	R/Q ≤ 2 R/S ≤ 2 R ≤ 0.6 mV .04R notch	1	R/Q ≤ 2 R/S ≤ 2 R ≤ 0.6 mV .04R notch	1		1			1	1							
V6	Q ≥ 30 ms	1	Q ≥ 30 ms	1	Q ≥ 30 ms	1	Q ≥ 30 ms	1	Q ≥ 30 ms	1	3							1			2		
	R/Q ≤ 1 R/S ≤ 1	2	R/Q ≤ 1 R/S ≤ 1	2	R/Q ≤ 1 R/S ≤ 1	2	R/Q ≤ 1 R/S ≤ 1	2	R/Q ≤ 1 R/S ≤ 1	2					1			1			2	2	
	R/Q ≤ 3 R/S ≤ 3 R ≤ 0.6 mV .04R notch	1	R/Q ≤ 3 R/S ≤ 2 R ≤ 0.6 mV .04R notch	1	R/Q ≤ 3 R/S ≤ 2 R ≤ 0.6 mV .04R notch	1	R/Q ≤ 3 R/S ≤ 3 R ≤ 0.6 mV .04R notch	1	R/Q ≤ 3 R/S ≤ 3 R ≤ 0.6 mV .04R notch	1								1			1	1	
Total	Points		Points		Points		Points		Points		32												

QRS Score Instructions

1. Select column with appropriate conduction (tan highlights show differences in criteria between conduction types).
2. Age normalize all amplitude criteria to age 55 by increasing them 1%/yr age 20-54 and decreasing them 1%/yr for >55 yrs.
3. For females further decrease by 10% all QRSdur and QRSamp criteria.
4. Circle each QRS criteria met; if >1 criterion in a box met, select one with most points.

Waveform Definitions

Init R = Initial R

.04R notch = notch in initial 40 ms

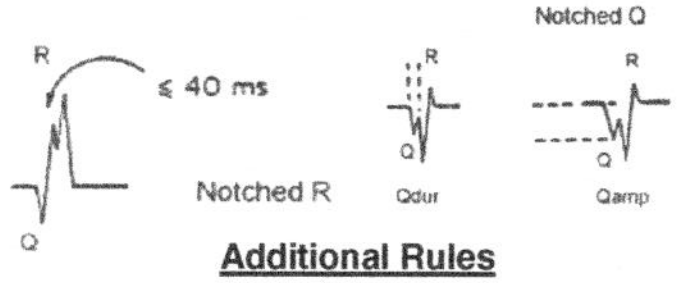

Additional Rules

*(for LVH) if ≥ 4 anterior/apical QRS points present (other than QS), then count QS in V1-V3.

**(for posterolateral criteria) exclude if right atrial overload present (suggesting RVH) if P positive amplitude in V1 or V2 P≥0.1 mV or aVF P≥0.175 mV.

12 LV Segments

For each 1% scar place an X in corresponding LV segment to right to show scar location

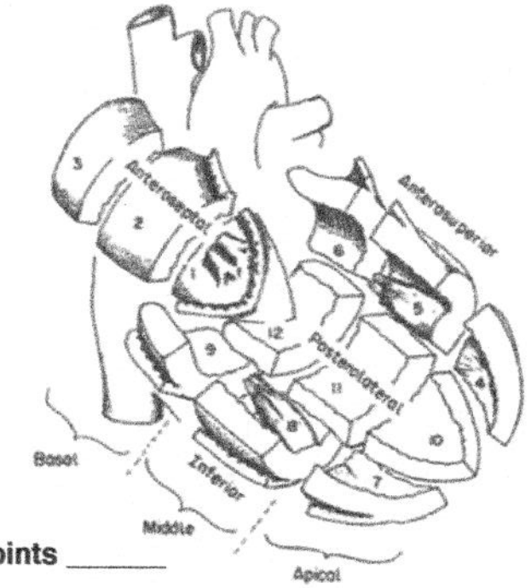

Total QRS points ______

***3 = ______ % LV scar**

References

1. Hurst, J.W., Current status of clinical electrocardiography with suggestions for the improvement of the interpretive process. *Am. J. Cardiol.*, 2003;**92**: 1072–1079.
2. Foundation, T.N., The Nobel Prize in Physiology or Medicine 1963. 2007 [cited January 7, 2008]; Available from: http://nobelprize.org/nobel_prizes/medicine/laureates/1963/.
3. Overton, E., The general muscle- and nerve physiology - Second Notice - The indispensability of natrium (or lithium) ions for muscle contraction. *Arch. Ges. Physiol.*, 1902; **92**: 346.
4. Smith, F.M., The ligation of coronary arteries with electrocardiographic study. *Arch. Int. Med.*, 1918;**22**: 8–27.
5. Pardee, H.E.B., An electrocardiographic sign of coronary artery obstruction. *Arch. Int. Med.*, 1920;**26**: 244–257.
6. Otto, H.L., The ventricular electrocardiogram. An experimental study. *Arch. Int. Med.*, 1929;**43**: 335–350.
7. Barnes, A.R., Study of the R-T interval in myocardial infarction. *Am. Heart J.*, 1929;**5**: 142–171.
8. Wilson, R.N., A.G. MacLeod, and P.S. Barker, The distribution of action and injury displayed by heart muscle and other excitable tissues. *Scientific Series*, vol. X. Ann Arbor, MI: University of Michigan Press, 1933.
9. Wilson, F.N, F.D. Johnston, A.G. MacLeod, et al., Electrocardiograms that represent the potential variations of a single electrode. *Am. Heart J.*, 1933;**9**: 447–471.
10. Wilson, F.N., F.D. Johnston, F.F. Rosenbaum, et al., Einthoven's triangle, the theory of unipolar electrocardiographic leads, and the interpretation of the precordial electrocardiograms. *Am. Heart J.*, 1946;**32**: 277–310.
11. Braunwald, E. and P.R. Maroko, The reduction of infarct size – an idea whose time (for testing) has come. *Circulation*, 1974;**50**: 206–209.
12. Holland, R.P. and H. Brooks, Precordial and epicardial surface potentials during Myocardial ischemia in the pig. A theoretical and experimental analysis of the TQ and ST segments. *Circ. Res.*, 1975;**37**: 471–480.
13. Holland, R.P., H. Brooks, and B. Lidl, Spatial and nonspatial influences on the TG-ST segment deflection of ischemia. Theoretical and experimental analysis in the pig. *J. Clin. Invest.*, 1977;**60**: 197–214.
14. Braunwald, E. and P.R. Maroko, ST-segment mapping. Realistic and unrealistic expectations. *Circulation*, 1976;**54**: 529–532.
15. Janse, M.J., ST segment mapping and infarct size. *Cardiovasc. Res.*, 2000;**45**: 190–193.
16. Grant, R.P. and H.T. Dodge, Mechanisms of QRS complex prolongation in man; left ventricular conduction disturbances. *Am. J. Med.*, 1956;**20**: 834–852.
17. Wagner, G.S., M.J. Cowan, N.C. Flowers, L.E. Ginzton, R.E. Ideker, M.M. Laks, R.H. Selvester, and S.R. Swiryn, Nomenclature of myocardial wall segments. Committee report. Computerized Interpretation of the ECG VIII. *Proceedings of the Engineering Foundation Conference*, vol. 222, R.H. Selvester, Editor. New York, 1983.
18. Ideker, R.E., G.S. Wagner, W.K. Ruth, et al., Evaluation of a QRS scoring system for estimating myocardial infarct size. II. Correlation with quantitative anatomic findings for anterior infarcts. *Am. J. Cardiol.*, 1982;**49**: 1604–1614.
19. Horan, L.G., N.C. Flowers, and J.C. Johnson, Significance of the diagnostic Q wave of myocardial infarction. *Circulation*, 1971;**43**: 428–436.
20. Henry, W.L., A. DeMaria, H. Feigenbaum, R. Kerber, N. Nanda, R.L. Popp, D. Sahn, N.B. Schiller, A.I. Tajik, and A.E. Weyman, Identification of myocardial wall segments: Report of the ASE Committee on Nomenclature and Standards, Raleigh, NC: American Society of Echocardiography, 1982.
21. Zinn, W.J. and R.S. Cosby, Myocardial infarction; a re-evaluation of the diagnostic accuracy of the electrocardiogram. *Am. J. Med.*, 1950;**8**: 177–179.
22. Johnson, W.J., R.W. Anchor, H.B. Burchell, and J.E. Edwards, Unrecognized myocardial infarction; a clinicopathologic study. *AMA Arch. Intern. Med.*, 1959;**103**: 253–261.
23. Woods, J.D., W. Laurie, and W.G. Smith, The reliability of the electrocardiogram in myocardial infarction. *Lancet*, 1963;**2**: 265–269.
24. Anderson, J.L., Chair Writing Committee, ACC/AHA 2007 guidelines for the management of patients with Unstable Angina/Non-ST-Elevation myocardial infarction. A report of the American College of Cardiology/American Heart Association task force on practice guidelines (Writing Committee to revise the 2002 guidelines for managing UA/NonSTEMI). *JACC*, 2007;**50**(No 7): el–157.
25. Selvester, R.H., Nomina anatomica contradicta. Especially as relates to the heart and electrocardiology. *J. Electrocardiol*, 1992;**25**: 157–162.
26. Reimer, K.A. and R.B. Jennings, The "wavefront phenomenon" of myocardial ischemic cell death. II. Transmural progression of necrosis within the framework of ischemic bed size (myocardium at risk) and collateral flow. *Lab. Invest*, 1979;**40**: 633–644.
27. Christian, T.F., R.S. Schwartz, and R.J. Gibbons, Determinants of infarct size in reperfusion therapy for acute myocardial infarction. *Circulation*, 1992;**86**: 81–90.
28. Reimer, K.A., J.E. Lowe, and M.M. Rasmussen, The wavefront phenomenon of ischemic cell death. 1. Myocardial infarct size vs. duration of coronary occlusion in dogs. *Circulation*, 1977;**56**: 786–794.
29. Selvester, R.H. and M.E. Sanmarco, Infarct size in hi-gain, hi-fidelity VCGs and serial ventriculograms in patients with proven coronary artery disease, in *Modern Electrocardiology*, Z. Antaloczy, Editor. Amsterdam: Exerpta Medica, 1978, pp. 523–528.
30. Wagner, G.S., C.J. Freye, S.T. Palmeri, S.F. Roark, N.C. Stack, R.E. Ideker, F.E. Harrell Jr., and R.H. Selvester, Evaluation of a QRS scoring system for estimating myocardial infarct size. I. Specificity and observer agreement. *Circulation*, 1982;**65**: 342–347.
31. Palmeri, S.T., D.G. Harrison, F.R. Cobb, K.G. Morris, F.E. Harrell, R.E. Ideker, and R.H. Selvester, A QRS scoring system for assessing left ventricular function after myocardial infarction. *N. Engl. J. Med.*, 1982;**306**: 4–9.
32. Roark, S.F., R.E. Ideker, G.S. Wagner, D.R. Alonso, S.P. Bishop, C.M. Bloor, D.A. Bramlet, J.E. Edwards, J.T. Fallon, G.J. Gottlieb, D.B. Hackel, H.R. Phillips, K.A. Reimer, W.J. Rogers, W.K. Ruth, R.M. Savage, R.D. White, and R.H. Selvester, Evaluation of a QRS scoring system for estimating myocardial infarct size.

III. Correlation with quantitative anatomic findings for inferior infarcts. *Am. J. Cardiol.*, 1983;**51**: 382–389.
33. Ward, R.M., R.D. White, R.E. Ideker, et al., Evaluation of a QRS scoring system for estimating myocardial infarct size. IV. Correlation with quantitative anatomic findings for posterolateral infarcts. *Am. J. Cardiol.*, 1984;**53**: 706–714.
34. Ideker, R.E., G.S. Wagner, and R.H. Selvester, Anatomic validation of computer model ECG criteria for infarct size and location, in *Computeized Interpretation of ECG VII, Proceedings of the Engineering Foundation Conference*, M.M. Laks, Editor. New York: Engineering Foundation, 1982, pp. 147–152.
35. Daniel, T.M., J.P. Boineau, and D.C. Sabiston Jr., Comparison of human ventricular activation with a canine model in chronic myocardial infarction. *Circulation*, 1971;**44**: 74–89.
36. Cox, J.L., T.M. Daniel, and J.P. Boineau, The electrophysiologic time-course of acute myocardial ischemia and the effects of early coronary artery reperfusion. *Circulation*, 1973;**48**: 971–983.
37. Lie, K.I., H.J. Wellens, and R.M. Schuilenburg, Bundle branch block and acute myocardial infarction, in *The Conduction System of the Heart: Structure, Function, and Clinical Applications*, H.J. Wellens, K.I. Lie, and M.J. Janse, Editors. Philadelphia, PA: Lea and Febiger, 1976, p. 666.
38. Mullins, C.B. and J.M. Atkins, Prognoses and management of venticular conduction blocks in acute myocardial infarction. *Mod. Concepts Cardiovasc. Dis.*, 1976;**45**: 129–133.
39. Marriott, H.J. and P. Hogan, Hemiblock in acute myocardial infarction. *Chest*, 1970;58: 342–344.
40. Rosenbaum, M.B., The hemiblocks: diagnostic criteria and clinical significance. *Mod. Concepts Cardiovasc. Dis.*, 1970;**39**: 141–146.
41. Grant, R.P., *ClinicalElectrocardiography, the Spatial Vector Approach*, New York: McGraw-Hill, 1957.
42. Durrer, D., R.T. Van Dam, F.L. Meijler, R.C. Arzbaecher, E.J. Muller, and G.E. Freud, Electrical activation and membrane action potentials of the perfused normal human heart. *Circulation*, 1966;**34**: 412–422.
43. Durrer, D., R.T. van Dam, G.E. Frued, F.L. Meijler, and J.P. Roos, Excitation of the human heart, in *Electrical Activity of the Heart*, C.C. Thomas, Editor. Springfield: C.C. Thomas, 1969, p. 53.
44. Durrer, D., R.T. van Dam, G.E. Freud, M.J. Janse, F.L. Meijler, and R.C. Arzbaecher, Total excitation of the isolated human heart. *Circulation*, 1970;**41**: 899–912.
45. Selvester, R.H. and J.C. Solomon, Optimal ECG electrode sites and criteria for detection of asymptomatic coronary artery disease at rest and with exercise. *USAFSAM Technical Report*, 1984;**85–47**: 80–98.
46. Spach, M.S., R.C. Barr, C.F. Lanning, and P.C. Tucek, Origin of body surface QRS and T wave potentials from epicardial potential distributions in the intact chimpanzee. *Circulation*, 1977;**55**: 268–268. *of IEEE. Computer Society*, 1982, pp. 87–90.
47. Burgess, M.J., K. Millar, and J.A. Abildskov, Cancellation of electrocardiographic effects during ventricular recovery. *J. Electrocardiol.*, 1969;**2**: 101–107.
48. Burgess, M.J., K. Millar, and J.A. Abildskov, The geometry of ventricular repolarization boundaries. *Am. Heart J.*, 1970;**79**: 524–530.
49. Burgess, M.J., L.S. Green, K. Millar, R. Wyatt, and J.A. Abildskov, The sequence of normal ventricular recovery. *Am. Heart J.*, 1972;**84**: 660–669.
50. Abildskov, J.A., M.J. Burgess, K. Millar, R. Wyatt, and G. Baule, The primary T wave – a new electrocardiographic waveform. *Am. Heart J.*, 197;**81**: 242–249.
51. Abildskov, J.A., A.K. Evans, R.L. Lux, and M.J. Burgess, Ventricular recovery properties and QRST deflection area in cardiac electrograms. *Am. J. Physiol.*, 1980;**239**: H227–31.
52. Abildskov, J.A., L.S. Green, A.K. Evans, and R.L. Lux, The QRST deflection area of electrograms during global alterations of ventricular repolarization. *J. Electrocardiol.*, 1982;**15**: 103–107.
53. Spach, M.S. and R.C. Barr, Ventricular intramural and epicardial potential distributions during ventricular activation and repolarization in the intact dog. *Circ. Res.*, 1975;**37**: 243–257.
54. Selvester, R.H., R. Kalaba, C.R. Collier, R. Bellman, and H. Kagiwada, A digital computer model of the vectorcardiogram with distance and boundary effects: simulated myocardial infarction. *Am. Heart J.*, 1967;**74**: 792–808.
55. Selvester, R.H., J.C. Solomon, and T.L. Gillespie, Digital computer model of a total body electrocardiographic surface map. An adult male-torso simulation with lungs. *Circulation*, 1968;**38**: 684–690.
56. Solomon, J.C. and R.H. Selvester, Simulation of measured activation sequence in the human heart. *Am. Heart J.*, 1973;**85**: 518–524.
57. Selvester, R.H., J.C. Solomon, and D. Sapoznikov, Computer simulation of the electrocardiogram, in *Computer Techniques in Cardiology*, L.D. Cady, Editor. Washington, DC: Marcel Decker, Inc., 1979, pp. 417–453.
58. Selvester, R.H., M.E. Sanmarco, J.C. Solomon, and G.S. Wagner, Methods of determining infarct size, ECG: QRS change, in *Myocardial Infarction: Measurement and Intervention*, G.S. Wagner, Editor. Hague: Martinus Nijhoff, 1982, p. 23.
59. Wilson, F.N., A.G. Macleod, P.S. Barker, and F.D. Johnston, The determination and the significance of the areas of the ventricular deflections of the electrocardiogram. *Am. Heart J.*, 1934; **19**: 46.
60. Wilson, F.N., A.G. Macleod, and P.S. Barker, The potential variations produced by the heart beat at the apices of Einthoven's triangle. *Am. Heart J.*, 1931;**7**: 207–211.
61. Burger, H.C., A theoretical elucidation of the notion ventricular gradient. *Am. Heart J.*, 1957;**53**: 240–246.
62. Fruehan, C.T., B. Crain, M.J. Burgess, K. Millar, and J.A. Abildskov, Observations concerning the validity of the ventricular gradient concept. *Am. Heart J.*, 1969;**78**: 796–801.
63. Schafer, H., A. Pena, and P. Scholmerich, Der Monophasische Aktionsstrom von Spitze und Basis des Warmbluterherzens und die Theorie der T-Welle des EKG. *Pflugers Arch.*, 1943;**246**: 728–745.
64. Ling, G. and R.W. Gerard, The normal membrane potential of the frog Sartorius fibers. *J. Cell. Comp. Physiol.*, 1949;**34**: 383–395.
65. Hoffman, B.F. and E.E. Suckling, Relationship between cardiac cellular potentials and the deflections of the electrogram. *Am. J. Physiol.*, 1952;**171**: 737.
66. Hoffman, B.F., C.Y. Kao, and E.E. Suckling, Refractoriness in cardiac muscle. *Am. J. Physiol.*, 1957;**190**: 473–482.
67. Hoffman, B.F. and P.F. Cranefield, *Electrophysiology of the Heart*, New York: McGraw-Hill, 1960.
68. Brady, A.J. and J.W. Woodbury, Effects of sodium and potassium on repolarization in frog ventricular fibers, in *The Electrophysiology of the Heart*, H. Hecht, Editor. Ann. N.Y. Acad. Sci., 1957, p. 687.

69. Hoffman, B.F., P.F. Cranefield, E. Lepeschkin, B. Surawicz, and H.C. Herrlich, Comparison of cardiac monophasic action potentials recorded by intracellular and suction electrodes. *Am. J. Physiol.*, 1959;**196**: 1297–1301.
70. Autenrieth, G., B. Surawicz, and C.S. Kuo, Sequence of repolarization on the ventricular surface in the dog. *Am. Heart J.*, 1975;**89**: 463–469.
71. Scher, A.M. and A.C. Young, The pathway of ventricular depolarization in the dog. *Circ. Res.*, 1956;**4**: 461–469.
72. Scher, A.M. and A.C. Young, Ventricular depolarization and the genesis of QRS. *Ann. N.Y. Acad. Sci.*, 1957;**65**: 768–778.
73. Scher, A.M., A.C. Young, A.L. Malmgren, and R.R. Paton, Spread of electrical activity through the wall of the ventricle. *Circ. Res.*, 1953;**1**: 539–547.
74. Durrer, D. and L.H. Van Der Twell, Spread of activation in the left ventricular wall of the dog. I. *Am. Heart J.*, 1953;**46**: 683–691.
75. van Dam, R.Th. and D. Durrer, Experimental study on the intramural distribution of the excitability cycle and on the form of the epicardial T wave in the dog heart in situ. *Am. Heart J.*, 1961;**61**: 537–542.
76. Kootsey, J.M. and E.A. Johnson, The Origin of the T wave. *CRC Crit. Rev. Bioeng.*, 1980;**4**: 233–270.
77. Gussak, I. and C. Antzelevitch, Editors. *Cardiac Repolarization, Bridging Basic and Clinical Science*. Totowa, NJ: Humana Press, 2003.
78. Arnsdorf, M.F. and E.K. Louie, The ECG: spatial and non spatial determinants of the extracellularly recorded potential with emphasis on the TQ-ST segment, in *Myocardial Infarction, Measurement and Intervention*, G.S. Wagner, Editor. The Hague: Martinus Nijhoff, 1980, p. 51.
79. Janse, M.J., J. Cinca, H. Morena, J.W. Fiolet, A.G. Kleber, G.P. de Vries, A.E. Becker, and D. Durrer, The "border zone" in myocardial ischemia. An electrophysiological, metabolic, and histochemical correlation in the pig heart. *Circ. Res.*, 1979;**44**: 576–588.
80. Harken, A.H., C.H. Barlow, W.R. Harden, and B. Chance, Two and three dimensional display of myocardial ischemic "border zone" in dogs. *Am. J. Cardiol.*, 1978;**42**: 954–959.
81. Simson, M.B., W. Harden, C. Barlow, and A.H. Harken, Visualization of the distance between perfusion and anoxia along an ischemic border. *Circulation*, 1979;**60**: 1151–1155.
82. Cox, J.L., V.W. McLaughlin, N.C. Flowers, and L.G. Horan, The ischemic zone surrounding acute myocardial infarction. Its morphology as detected by dehydrogenase staining. *Am. Heart J.*, 1968;76: 650–659.
83. Harumi, K., M.J. Burgess, and J.A. Abildskov, A theoretic model of the T wave. *Circulation*, 1966;**34**: 657–668.
84. Thiry, P.S. and R.M. Rosenberg, On electrophysiological activity of the normal heart. *J. Franklin Inst.*, 1974;**297**: 377.
85. Miller, W.T. and D.B. Geselowitz, Simulation studies of the electrocardiogram. I. The normal heart. *Circ. Res.*, 1978;**43**: 301–315.
86. Miller, W.T. 3rd and D.B. Geselowitz, Simulation studies of the electrocardiogram. II. Ischemia and infarction. *Circ. Res.*, 1978;**43**: 315–323.
87. Selvester, R.H., J.C. Solomon, and G.D. Tolan, Fine grid computer simulation of QRS-T and criteria for the quantitation of regional ischemia. *J. Electrocardiol.*, 1987;**20**(Suppl. 1–8).
88. Maroko, P.R., P. Libby, J.W. Covell, B.E. Sobel, J. Ross Jr., and E. Braunwald, Precordial S-T segment elevation mapping: an atraumatic method for assessing alterations in the extent of myocardial ischemic injury. The effects of pharmacologic and hemodynamic interventions. *Am. J. Cardiol.*, 1972;**29**: 223–230.
89. Akiyama, T., M. Hodges, T.L. Biddle, B. Zawrotny, and C. Vangellow, Measurement of S-T segment elevation in acute myocardial infarction in man. Comparison of a precordial mapping technique and the Frank vector system. *Am. J. Cardiol.*, 1975;**36**: 155–162.
90. Wikswo, J.P. Jr., S.C. Gundersen, W. Murphy, A.K. Dawson, and R.F. Smith, Sequential QRS vector subtractions in acute myocardial infarction in humans. Time course and relationship to serial changes in serum CK-MB concentration. *Circ. Res.*, 1981;**49**: 1055–1062.
91. Sederholm, M., P. Grottum, L. erhardt, and J. Kjekshus, Quantitative assessment of myocardial ischemia and necrosis by continuous vectorcardiography and measurement of creatine kinase release in patients. *Circulation*, 1983;**68**: 1006–1012.
92. Aldrich, H.R., N.B. Wagner, J. Boswick, A.T. Corsa, M.G. Jones, P. Grande, K.L. Lee, and G.S. Wagner, Use of initial ST-segment deviation for prediction of final electrocardiographic size of acute myocardial infarcts. *Am. J. Cardiol.*, 1988;**61**: 749–753.
93. Friedman, H.H., *Diagnostic Electgrocardiography and Vectorcardiography*. San Francisco, CA: McGraw-Hill, 1971.
94. Benchimol, A., *Vectorcardiography*. Baltimore, MD: Wilkins & Wilkins, 1973.
95. Eisenstein, I., M.E. Sanmarco, W.L. Madrid, and R.H. Selvester, Electrocardiographic and vectorcardiographic diagnosis of posterior wall myocardial infarction. Significance of the T wave. *Chest*, 1985;**88**: 409–416.
96. Selvester, R.H., J.C. Solomon, K. Baron, H.A. Saetre, and M.H. Ellestad, Optimal electrode sites and crriteria for detection of asymptomatic coronary artery disease detection: update 1990. *USAF Armstrong Laboratory Technical Report*, 1991:0029: 8–48.
97. Ellestad, M.H., Personal communication.
98. Nelson, G.R., P.F. Cohn, and R. Gorlin, Prognosis in medically-treated coronary artery disease: influence of ejection fraction compared to other parameters. *Circulation*, 1975;**52**: 408–412.
99. Coronary artery surgery study (CASS): a randomized trial of coronary artery bypass surgery. Survival data. *Circulation*, 1983;**68**: 939–950.
100. Heikkila, J., P.G. Hugenholtz, and B.S. Tabakin, Prediction of left heart filling pressure and its sequential change in acute myocardial infarction from the terminal force of the P wave. *Br. Heart J.*, 1973;**35**: 142–151.
101. Wickline, S.A. and J.J. McNamara, Vectorcardiographic quantification of infarct size in baboons. *Circulation*, 1978;**57**: 910–920.
102. Cowan, M.J., D.D. Reichenbach, R.A. Bruce, and L. Fisher, Estimation of myocardial infarct size by digital computer analysis of the VCG. *J. Electrocardiol.*, 1982;**15**: 307–316.
103. Cowan, M.J., R.A. Bruce, and D.D. Reichenbach, Estimation of inferobasal myocardial infarct size by late activation abnormalities of the QRS complex. *Am. J. Cardiol.*, 1984;**54**: 726–732.
104. Anderson, C.I., D.G. Harrison, N.C. Stack, N.B. Hindman, R.E. Ideker, S.T. Palmeri, R.H. Selvester, and G.S. Wagner, Evaluation of serial QRS changes during acute inferior myocardial infarction using a QRS scoring system. *Am. J. Cardiol.*, 1983;**52**: 252–256.
105. DePace, N.L., A.S. Iskandrian, A.H. Hakki, S.A. Kane, and B. Segal, Use of QRS scoring and thallium-201 scintigraphy to assess left ventricular function after myocardial infarction. *Am. J. Cardiol.*, 1982;**50**: 126–128.

106. Madrid, W.L., M.M. Laks, and R.H. Selvester, Evaluation of the performance of a Hewlett Packard program for myocardial infarct size determination. Computerized Interpretation of the Electrocardiogram, in *Engineering Foundation Conference*, Santa Barbara, CA, 1983.
107. Madrid, W.L., N.B. Hindman, G.S. Wagner, and R.H. Selvester, Infarct size by on-line computer analysis of ECG in a bedside microprocessor ECG cart, in Computers in Cardiology, *Proceedings of the IEEE Computer Society*, Los Angeles, CA, 1984, pp. 325–328.
108. Hindman, N.B., D.D. Schocken, M. Widmann, W.D. Anderson, R.D. White, S. Leggett, R.E. Ideker, T. Hinohara, R.H. Selvester, and G.S. Wagner, Evaluation of a QRS scoring system for estimating myocardial infarct size. V. Specificity and method of application of the complete system. *Am. J. Cardiol.*, 1985;**55**: 1485–1490.
109. Engblom, H., G.S. Wagner, R.M. Setser, R.H. Selvester, T. Billgren, J.M. Kasper, C. Maynard, O. Pahlm, H. Arheden, and R.D. White, Quantitative clinical assessment of chronic anterior myocardial infarction with delayed enhancement magnetic resonance imaging and QRS scoring. *Am. Heart J.*, 2003;**146**: 359–366.
110. Engblom, H., E. Hedstrom, E. Heiberg, G.S. Wagner, O. Pahlm, and H. Arheden, Size and transmural extent of first-time reperfused myocardial infarction assessed by cardiac magnetic resonance can be estimated by 12-lead electrocardiogram. *Am. Heart J.*, 2005;**150**: 920.
111. Kleber, A.G., M.J. Janse, F.J. van Capelle, and D. Durrer, Mechanism and time course of S-T and T-Q segment changes during acute regional myocardial ischemia in the pig heart determined by extracellular and intracellular recordings. *Circ. Res.*, 1978;**42**: 603–613.
112. Shaw, R.M. and Y. Rudy, Electrophysiologic effects of acute myocardial ischemia: a theoretical study of altered cell excitability and action potentialduration. *Cardiovasc. Res.*, 1997;**35**: 256–272.
113. Reimer, K.A., R.B. Jennings, F.R. Cobb, et al., Animal models for protecting ischemic myocardium: results of the NHLBI Cooperative Study. Comparison of unconscious and conscious dog models. *Circ. Res.*, 1985;**56**: 651–665.
114. Anderson, S.T., M. Wilkins, W.D. Weaver, R.H. Selvester, and G.S. Wagner, Electrocardiographic phasing of acute myocardial infarction. *J. Electrocardiol.*, 1992;**25**(Suppl. 3–5).
115. Wilkins, M.L., A.D. Pryor, C. Maynard, et al., An electrocardiographic acuteness score for quantifying the timing of a myocardial infarction to guide decisions regarding reperfusion therapy. *Am. J. Cardiol.*, 1995;**75**: 617–620.
116. Heden, B., R. Ripa, E. Persson, Q. Song, C. Maynard, P. Leibrandt, T. Wall, T.F. Christian, S.C. Hammill, S.S. Bell, O. Pahlm, and G.S. Wagner, A modified Anderson-Wilkins electrocardiographic acuteness score for anterior or inferior myocardial infarction. *Am. Heart J.*, 2003;**146**: 797–803.
117. Wagner, G., T. Lim, L. Gettes, A. Gorgels, M. Josephson, H. Wellens, S. Anderson, R. Childers, P. Clemmensen, P. Kligfield, P. Macfarlane, O. Pahlm, and R. Selvester, Consideration of pitfalls in and omissions from the current ECG standards for diagnosis of myocardial ischemia/infarction in patients who have acute coronary syndromes. *Cardiol. Clin.*, 2006;**24**: 331–342.
118. Corey, K.E., C. Maynard, O. Pahlm, M.L. Wilkins, S.T. Anderson, M.D. Cerqueira, A.D. Pryor, M.H. Raitt, R.H. Selvester, J. Turner, W.D. Weaver, and G.S. Wagner, Combined historical and electrocardiographic timing of acute anterior and inferior myocardial infarcts for prediction of reperfusion achievable size limitation. *Am. J. Cardiol.*, 1999;**83**: 826–831.
119. Sejersten, M., R.S. Ripa, C. Maynard, P. Grande, H.R. Andersen, G.S. Wagner, and P. Clemmensen, DANAMI-2 Investigators. Timing of ischemic onset estimated from the electrocardiogram is better than historical timing for predicting outcome after reperfusion therapy for acute anterior myocardial infarction: a DANish trial in Acute Myocardial Infarction 2 (DANAMI-2) substudy. *Am. Heart J.*, 2007;**154**(61): e1–8.
120. Engblom, H., B. Heden, E. Hedstrom, G. Wagner, and H. Arheden, ECG Estimate Of Ischemic Acuteness and Time from Pain Onset for Predicting Myocardial Salvage in Patients Undergoing Primary Percutaneous Coronary Intervention. *Circulation*, 2007;**116**: II 528 (abstr).
121. Sclarovsky, S., A. Mager, J. Kusniec, E. Rechavia, A. Sagie, R. Bassevich, and B. Strasberg, Electrocardiographic classification of acute myocardial ischemia. *Isr. J. Med. Sci.*, 1990;**26**: 525–531.
122. Birnbaum, Y., R.A. Kloner, S. Sclarovsky, C.P. Cannon, C.H. McCabe, V.G. Davies, B.L. Zaret, F.J. Wackers, and E. Braunwald, Distortion of the terminal portion of the QRS on the admission electrocardiogram in acute myocardial infarction and correlation with infarct size and long-term prognosis (Thrombolysis in Myocardial Infarction 4 Trial). *Am. J. Cardiol.*,1996;**78**: 396–403.
123. Birnbaum, Y., I. Herz, S. Sclarovsky, B. Zlotikamien, A. Chetrit, L. Olmer, and G.I. Barbash, Prognostic significance of the admission electrocardiogram in acute myocardial infarction. *J. Am. Coll. Cardiol.*, 1996;**27**: 1128–1132.
124. Sejersten, M., Y. Birnbaum, R.S. Ripa, C. Maynard, G.S. Wagner, and P. Clemmensen, ;ANAMI-2 Investigators. Influences of electrocardiographic ischaemia grades and symptom duration on outcomes in patients with acute myocardial infarction treated with thrombolysis versus primary percutaneous coronary intervention: results from the DANAMI-2 trial. *Heart*, 2006;**92**: 1577–1582.
125. Ripa, R.S., L. Holmvang, C. Maynard, M. Sejersten, P. Clemmensen, P. Grande, B. Lindahl, B. Lagerqvist, L. Wallentin, and G.S. Wagner, Consideration of the total ST-segment deviation on the initial electrocardiogram for predicting final acute posterior myocardial infarct size in patients with maximum ST-segment deviation as depression in leads V1 through V3. A FRISC II substudy. *J. Electrocardiol.*, 2005;**38**: 180–186.
126. Pahlm-Webb, U., O. Pahlm, S. Sadanandan, R.H. Selvester, and G.S. Wagner, A new method for using the direction of ST-segment deviation to localize the site of acute coronary occlusion: the 24-view standard electrocardiogram. *Am. J. Med.*, 2002;**113**: 75–78.
127. Engelen, D.J., A.P. Gorgels, E.C. Cheriex, E.D. De Muinck, A.J. Ophuis, W.R. Dassen, J. Vainer, V.G. van Ommen, and H.J. Wellens, Value of the electrocardiogram in localizing the occlusion site in the left anterior descending coronary artery in acute anterior myocardial infarction. *J. Am. Coll. Cardiol.*, 1999;**34**: 389–395.
128. Surawicz, B., H. Uhley, R. Borun, et al., Task Force 1: Standardization of terminology and interpretation. *Am J Cardiol.*, 1978: **41**: 130–45
129. First, S.R., R.H. Bayley, and D.R. Bedford, Peri-infarction block; electrocardiographic abnormality occasionally resembling bundle branch block and local ventricular block of other types. *Circulation*, 1950;**2**: 31–36.

130. Isner, J.M. and W.C. Roberts, Right ventricular infarction complicating left ventricular infarction secondary to coronary heart disease. Frequency, location, associated findings and significance from analysis of 236 necropsy patients with acute or healed myocardial infarction. *Am. J. Cardiol.*, 1978;**42**: 885–894.
131. Ratliff, N.B, and D.B. Hackel, Combined right and left ventricular infarction: Pathogenesis anc clinicalpathologic correlations. *Am. J. Cardiol.*, 1980;**45**: 217–221.
132. Cohn, J.N., N.H. Guiha, M.I. Broder, and C.J. Limas, Right ventricular infarction. Clinical and hemodynamic features. *Am. J. Cardiol.*, 1974;**33**: 209–214.
133. Klein, H.O., T. Tordjman, R. Ninio, P. Sareli, V. Oren, R. Lang, J. Gefen, C. Pauzner, E. Di Segni, D. David, and E. Kaplinsky, The early recognition of right ventricular infarction: diagnostic accuracy of the electrocardiographic V4R lead. *Circulation*, 1983;**67**: 558–565.
134. Geft, I.L., P.K. Shah, L. Rodriguez, S. Hulse, J. Maddahi, D.S. Berman, and W. Ganz, ST elevations in leads V1 to V5 may be caused by right coronary artery occlusion and acute right ventricular infarction. *Am. J. Cardiol.*, 1984;**53**: 991–996.
135. Kulbertus, H.E., P. Rigo, and V. Legrand, Right ventricular infarction: Pathophysiology, diagnosis, clinical course, and treatment. *Mod. Concepts Cardiovas. Dis.*, 1985;**54**: 1.
136. Carson, W., Y.Z. Tseng, P.J. Huang, C.D. Tseng, and T.L. Wu, Vectorcardiographic features of acute right ventricular infarction. *J. Electrocardiol.*, 1984;**17**: 253–261.
137. Morgera, T., E. Alberti, F. Silvestri, C. Pandullo, M.T. Della Mea, and F. Camerini, Right precordial ST and QRS changes in the diagnosis of right ventricular infarction. *Am. Heart J.*, 1984;**108**: 13–18.
138. Zehender, M., W. Kasper, E. Kauder, M. Schonthaler, A. Geibel, J. Olschewski, and H. Just, Right ventricular infarction as an independent predictor of prognosis after acute inferior myocardial infarction. *N. Engl. J. Med.*, 1993;**328**: 981–988.
139. Selvester, R.H. and H.B. Rubin, New criteria for electrocardiographic diagnosis of emphysema and cor pulmonale. *Am. Heart J.*, 1965;**69**: 437–447.
140. Freye, C.J., N.B. Wagner, C.M. Howe, N.C. Stack, R.E. Ideker, R.H. Selvester, and G.S. Wagner, Evaluation of a QRS scoring system for estimating myocardial infarct size. VIII. Specificity in a control group with left ventricular hypertrophy and proposal of a new scoring system for use with this confounding factor. *J. Electrocardiol*, 1992;**25**: 19–23.
141. Norris, R.M. and M.S. Croxson, Bundle branch block in acute myocardial infarction. *Am. Heart J.*, 1970;**79**: 728–733.
142. Bauer, G.E., Development of bundle branch block. *Am. J. Cardiol.*, 1964;**14**: 346–351.
143. Dodge, H.T. and R.P. Grant, Mechanisms of QRS complex prolongation in man; right ventricular conduction defects. *Am. J. Med.*, 1956;**21**: 534–550.
144. Scott, R.C., Left bundle branch block–a clinical assessment. III. *Am. Heart J.*, 1965;**70**: 813–829.
145. Scott, R.C., Left bundle branch block–a clinical assessment. II. *Am. Heart J.*, 1965;**70**: 691–712.
146. Scott, R.C., Left bundle branch block–a clinical assessment. I. *Am. Heart J.*, 1965;**70**: 535–566.
147. Ostrander, L.D. Jr., Bundle branch block: an epidemiological study. *Circulation*, 1964;**30**: 872.
148. Edmands, R.E., An epidemiological assessment of bundle-branch block. *Circulation*, 1966;**34**: 1081–1087.
149. Schneider, J.F., H.E. Thomas Jr., B.E. Kreger, P.M. McNamara, and W.B. Kannel, Newly acquired left bundle-branch block: the Framingham study. *Ann. Intern. Med.*, 1979;**90**: 303–310.
150. Schneider, J.F., H.E. Thomas, B.E. Kreger, P.M. McNamara, P. Sorlie, and W.B. Kannel, Newly acquired right bundle-branch block: The Framingham Study. *Ann. Intern. Med.*, 1980;**92**: 37–44.
151. Rhoads, D.V., J.E. Edwards, and R.D. Pruitt, The electrocardiogram in the presence of myocardial infarction and intraventricular block of the left bundlebranch block type. A clinical pathologic study. *Am. Heart. J.*, 1961;**62**: 735–745.
152. Haft, J.I., M.V. Herman, and R. Gorlin, Left bundle branch block: etiologic, hemodynamic, and ventriculographic considerations. *Circulation*, 1971;**43**: 279–287.
153. Horan, L.G., N.C. Flowers, and W.J. Tolleson, Thomas JR: The significance of diagnostic Q waves in the presence of bundle branch block. *Chest*, 1970;**58**: 214–220.
154. Hiss, R.G. and L.E. Lamb, Electrocardiographic findings in 122,043 individuals. *Circulation*, 1962;**25**: 947–961.
155. Hickman, J.R. and G.M. McGranahan Jr., Clinical aerospace cardiology, in *Fundamentals of Aerospace and Flight Medecine*, R.L. DeHart, Editor. Philadelphia, PA: Lea & Febiger, 1985, p. 421.
156. Polizos, G. and R.H. Selvester, Left bundle branch block and acute myocardial infarction: Diagnosis and location. abstract in AHA Scientific Sessions. *Circulation*, 2003.
157. Rogers, W.J., L.J. Bowlby, N.C. Chandra, W.J. French, J.M. Gore, C.T. Lambrew, R.M. Rubison, A.J. Tiefenbrunn, and W.D. Weaver, Treatment of myocardial infarction in the United States (1990 to 1993). Observations from the National Registry of Myocardial Infarction. *Circulation*, 1994;**90**: 2103–2114.
158. Sgarbossa, E.B., S.L. Pinski, A. Barbagelata, D.A. Underwood, K.B. Gates, E.J. Topol, R.M. Califf, and G.S. Wagner, Electrocardiographic diagnosis of evolving acute myocardial infarction in the presence of left bundle-branch block. GUSTO-1 (Global Utilization of Streptokinase and Tissue Plasminogen Activator for Occluded Coronary Arteries) Investigators. *N. Engl. J. Med.*, 1996;**334**: 481–487.
159. Tolan, G.T., R.H. Selvester, and J.C. Solomon, Optimal ECG electrode sites and criteria for detection of asymptomatic coronary artery disease. Computer ECG Analysis: towards Standardization, in *3rd International Conference on Common Standards for Quantitative Electrocardiography*, Amsterdam: North Holland Publ. Co. 1985.
160. Selvester, R.H., J.C. Solomon, and R.B. Pearson, ECG body surface map criteria for quantifying infarct, as derived from computer simulations, in *3rd International Symposium on Body Surface Mapping*. Dordrecht: Martinus Nijhoff, Publ. Co., 1985.
161. Solomon, J.C., R.H. Selvester, and G.T. Tolan, *Forward ECG simulation. Proceedings of the Society for Computer Si006Dulation. in 5th Annual Multiconference, Society for Computer Simulation*, San Diego, 1986.
162. Ramanathan, C., R.N. Ghanem, P. Jia, K. Ryu, and Y. Rudy, Noninvasive electrocardiographic imaging for cardiac electrophysiology and arrhythmia. *Nat. Med.*, 2004;**10**: 422–428.

5 Ventricular Repolarization: Theory and Practice in Non-Ischemic Myocardium

Borys Surawicz

P. W. Macfarlane et al. (eds.), *Electrocardiology*, DOI 10.1007/978-0-85729-874-4_5,

5.1 Introduction

Of all components of the electrocardiogram (ECG), the ST segment and the T wave are subject to the greatest potential misinterpretation because the line dividing normal from abnormal is not sharp, and because the patterns of abnormal repolarization resulting from structural derangements and functional disturbances are similar to each other. The amplitudes of ST and T deflections can be measured accurately, but the normal ranges are wide and the absolute values are not meaningful unless related to the QRS amplitude. Also, a meaningful interpretation of the direction of the T wave vector in one or more planes requires correlations with the mean QRS vector or the vector of one of the QRS components; for example, terminal slurred portion of QRS in right bundle branch block. The greatest difficulties of interpretation may be caused by problems related to the timing, and involve the following questions:

1. When does the ST segment end and the T wave begin?
2. Where does the T wave end and the U wave begin?
3. How does one differentiate the terminal dip of the T wave from a depressed TU junction or a negative TU segment?

Electrocardiography is abundant in descriptive terms. The depression of the ST segment is pictured as trough-, sickle-, claw-, plane-, or wing-like. Various forms of T waves bear such designations as notched, diphasic, coved, saddlelike, blunted, dimpled, cloven, tent-shaped, and so on [1]. It is apparent that the evaluation of the ST segment and the T wave is frequently based on descriptive rather than measurable properties, and that the electrocardiographic diagnoses are frequently made on the basis of visual impressions rather than detailed measurements.

Cellular electrophysiology has made an important contribution to the understanding of the processes controlling ventricular repolarization. The uniform changes in the shape and duration of the ventricular action potential can adequately explain most of the metabolic and pharmacological effects on repolarization [2]. However, other types of ST segment and T wave changes are caused predominantly by the changes in the sequence of repolarization. Such changes may be either primary or secondary to the changes in the sequence of depolarization. The latter may not involve changes in the shape and duration of the ventricular action potential. Accordingly, assumptions underlying the interpretation of T wave changes concern the basic shape of the ventricular action potential, the local difference between action potential durations and the sequences of activation.

➋ Figure 5.1 shows the electrocardiogram (ECG) and the right ventricular endocardial monophasic action potential (MAP), recorded with a suction electrode in man. It can be seen that the MAP ends near the end of the T wave, that the ST segment corresponds to the early slower phase of repolarization, and that the T wave corresponds to the more

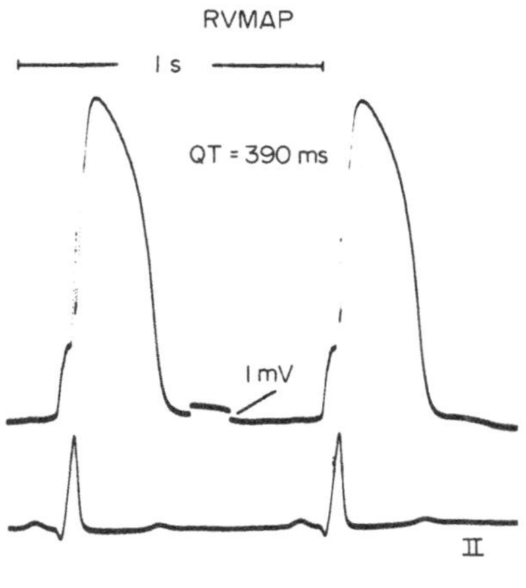

Fig. 5.1
Normal right ventricular monophasic action potentials (RVMAP) and normal electrocardiogram (ECG) in a patient with mitral stenosis. (After Shabetai et al. [3]. © American Heart Association, Dallas, Texas. Reproduced with permission)

rapid terminal portion of repolarization. More detailed correlations between the morphology of repolarization in the ECG and in the single fibers have been performed in isolated perfused rabbit hearts. With the exception of a shorter QRS duration (i.e., 35 ms as opposed to 80 ms), the morphology of the ECG complex in the rabbit and man is similar [4, 5]. Our correlations of simultaneously recorded ventricular transmembrane action potentials (TAPs) and ECGs in isolated perfused rabbit hearts showed that action potentials (APs) of varying shape and duration terminated near the end of the T wave. A shorter duration of the AP was accompanied by a shorter QT interval, and a longer duration of the AP was accompanied by a longer QT interval in the ECG. A prolonged plateau was associated with a longer duration of the ST segment, and a shorter plateau with a shorter duration of the ST segment. The increased velocity of the initial portion of repolarization was associated with a deviation of the ST segment from the baseline, and a steeper slope of terminal repolarization with a more abrupt descent of the T wave; that is, "peaking." A slower slope of repolarization, approaching a straight line, was associated with a wide, poorly defined T wave of low amplitude; a prolongation of the terminal portion of repolarization was accompanied by the appearance of a prominent U wave and fusion of T and U waves [2]. Such abnormalities were induced by changes in heart rate, body temperature, electrolyte imbalance, and drugs, and were reversible when the underlying metabolic or pharmacological abnormality disappeared. It follows that an accurate interpretation of the ECG requires information regarding the metabolic status and the drug intake of the patient.

5.2 ST Segment

5.2.1 Duration

The isoelectric course of the ST segment is caused by the relatively long flat slope of ventricular repolarization during phase 2 (plateau) of the AP. The duration of the ST segment tends to parallel the duration of ventricular AP, and the rate-dependent changes in the duration of the ST segment reflect the rate-dependent changes in the duration of the plateau of the ventricular AP [6]. The parallel relation between the durations of the ST segment and the plateau of ventricular AP is exemplified by the effects of the extracellular calcium concentration. Both the plateau of the AP and the ST segment lengthen during hypocalcemia and shorten during hypercalcemia. However, the T wave remains unchanged, provided the slope of terminal repolarization and the sequence of repolarization are not changed. ➋ Figure 5.2 shows a simultaneous recording of the MAP and ECG in a patient with hypocalcemia due to hypoparathyroidism. Both the amplitude and the polarity of the T wave remain unchanged when the ST segment shortens after the administration of calcium. It can be seen that the ST segment shortening is associated with shortening of the plateau but without change in the slope of phase 3 (see ➋ Chap. 3 of *Basic Electrocardiology : Cardiac Electrophysiology, ECG Systems and Mathematical Modeling* for definitions). As a rule, hypocalcemia and hypercalcemia do not change the polarity of the T wave, but a few exceptions have been found in patients in whom severe hypocalcemia caused flattening or inversion of the T wave in the leads with an upright QRS complex [7–9].

Aside from the effects of heart rate, catecholamines, calcium, and several class III antiarrhythmic drugs the changes in the duration of the ventricular AP are seldom a result of, solely or predominantly, changes in the duration of the plateau. Under most other conditions that alter the duration of the AP, changes in the duration of the plateau are associated with a concomitant change in the slope of the plateau, and usually with the changes in the slope of phase 3. For example, digitalis and hypokalemia shorten phase 2 and prolong phase 3, while class 1A antiarrhythmic drugs, e.g., quinidine and disopyramide, prolong both the phase 2 and the phase 3 of the ventricular AP.

5.2.2 Deviations from the Baseline

Theoretically, the absence of ST segment deviation from the baseline implies an absence of significant potential differences during phase 2 of ventricular repolarization. Even under normal circumstances, this condition is not always fulfilled, particularly at the onset of repolarization. ➋ Figure 5.3 is a schematic diagram in which the ECG is derived from the potential difference between two APs hypothetically attributed to the first and the last ventricular fiber depolarized during recording of a single QRS complex. In the derived ECG, the configuration of the ST segment and T wave is determined

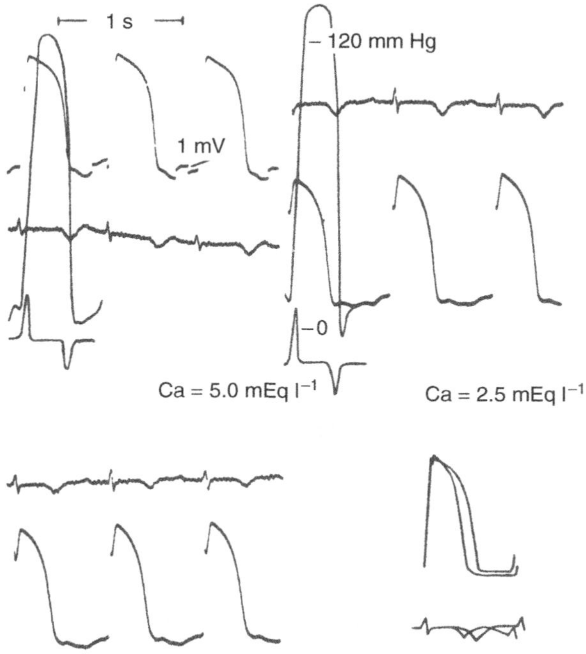

Fig. 5.2
Effect of the administration of $CaCl_2$ to a patient with hypoparathyroidism (*top left*). Plasma calcium is 2.5 mEq l^{-1}. Phase 2 of the right ventricular MAP and the ST segment in lead II are prolonged. Retouched tracings of left ventricular pressure and its first derivative are superimposed on the first complex (*top right*). After intravenous administration of 0.7 g of $CaCl_2$, plasma calcium concentration is 5.0 mEq l^{-1}. Note shortening of phase 2 of the right ventricular MAP and of the ST segment and increased left ventricular pressure and first derivative (After Shabetai et al. [3]. © American Heart Association, Dallas, Texas. Reproduced with permission)

by the potential difference during repolarization. The diagram shows that after the end of depolarization, some potential differences do exist before the onset of uniform depolarization to the level of the plateau. This interval is short but it may cause deviation of the junction (J depression) and of the early portion of the ST segment. As a result of this, measurements of ST segment deviation are usually made about 60–80 ms after the end of the QRS complex when all ventricular fibers are expected to be depolarized (discharged) to the same membrane potentials indicated by two superimposed segments of repolarization (phase 3) before the onset of rapid repolarization. Mapping studies have shown that the ST segment may be appropriately modeled as a single current dipole directed toward the apex of the heart, unaltered by the heart rate [10]. The potential difference between the rapid repolarizations (phase 3) is responsible for the T wave. Afterward, all fibers are "at rest" (charged) and potential differences are absent [11].

5.2.2.1 ST Deviations in the Absence of Ischemia (Secondary Repolarization Changes)

The two diagrams in ➲ Fig. 5.3c explain why the entire ST segment or its major portion may deviate from the baseline in the absence of myocardial ischemia. The diagram on the left shows the mechanism of repolarization abnormalities secondary to conduction delay, indicated by a prolonged interval between the upstrokes of the first and the last APs. The longer conduction time lengthens the QRS complex and enhances the potential differences during the entire repolarization. This happens because some of the early depolarized fibers begin to pass through the rapid phase 3 repolarization while the late depolarized fibers will be still at the level of the plateau. In the diagram, potential differences (arrow) persist throughout the entire repolarization phase and therefore the entire ST segment deviates from the baseline. Secondary ST segment changes are usually accompanied by secondary T wave changes.

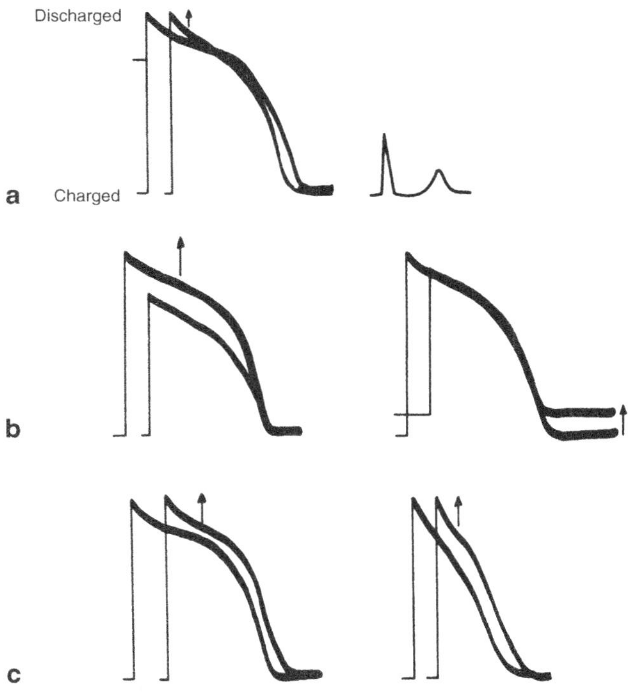

Fig. 5.3
Schematic diagrams: (a) the normal electrocardiogram is derived from the potential differences between two ventricular APs; (b) the potential differences responsible for systolic and diastolic currents of injury; (c) potential differences responsible for secondary repolarization abnormalities to the left and changes in the repolarization slope (e.g., digitalis effect) to the right (After Surawicz and Saito [11]. © Yorke Medical Group, Magazine Division, New York. Reproduced with permission)

5.2.2.2 ST Deviations Arising from Primary Repolarization Abnormalities in the Absence of Ischemia

The diagram on the right in Fig. 5.3c shows the mechanisms of primary repolarization abnormalities caused by APs in which potential differences persist during most or all of repolarization because the slope of repolarization during phase 2 is steeper than normal. This mechanism will cause deviation of the ST segment from the base line in the absence of ischemia or any changes in the sequences of depolarization. The short ventricular AP with a steep slope of repolarization shown in this diagram depicts changes induced by digitalis or tachycardia. This may be one of the mechanisms of ST segment depression during exercise-induced tachycardia in the absence of myocardial ischemia.

5.2.2.3 Depression of the ST Segment

ST depression in precordial leads reflects a posteriorly directed deviation of the ST-segment vector. Several mechanisms of such deviation are shown in schematic diagrams in Fig. 5.4. In the upper left diagram, the crosshatched area represents a region of subendocardial ischemia or infarction that causes a systolic and a diastolic current of injury; the former results in depression of the ST segment (solid arrow) and the latter in elevation of the baseline (dashed arrow). It has been shown that ST segment depression during ischemia correlated well with the decrease in subendocardial blood flow and presence of perfusion defects in scintigrams as well as wall motion abnormalities in the echocardiogram (see Chap. 6).

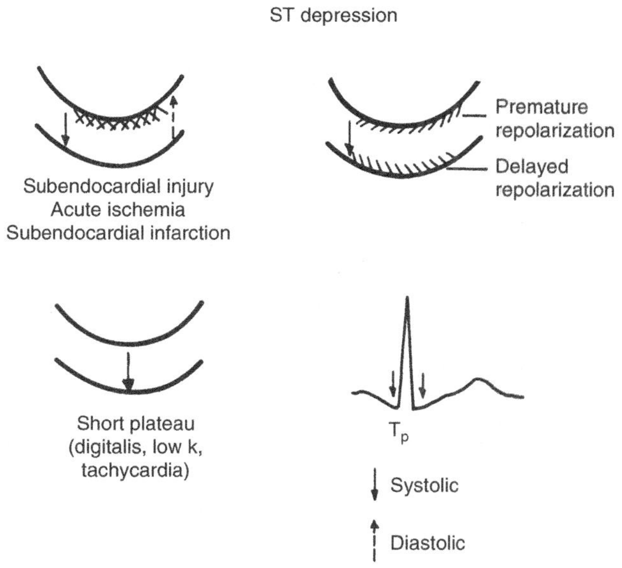

Fig. 5.4
Diagram of several mechanisms of ST-segment depression. The direction of the arrows indicates the flow of current and not the ST-segment vector. See text for explanation (After Surawicz and Saito [11]. © Yorke Medical Group, Magazine Division, New York. Reproduced with permission)

In the upper right diagram, secondary ST segment depression is a result of delayed repolarization in the subepicardial region, or alternatively because of premature repolarization in the subendocardial region. In the lower left diagram, ST segment deviation occurs in the absence of injury or conduction delay, because of the uniform shortening of phase 2 (plateau) of the ventricular AP; owing to the effect of digitalis, hypokalemia, or tachycardia, for example.

Finally, the lower right diagram shows that the depression of ST segment may be caused by atrial repolarization represented by a negative T wave of the P wave (T_P), which is inscribed during the interval between the two arrows. Note that the ST depression is relative to P onset and would not be measured as such by a computer program using QRS onset as a baseline reference. The inscription of atrial repolarization during the ST segment has been documented in man during the recording of atrial MAP using suction electrodes [3] (Fig. 5.5). In Fig. 5.5, the negative T_P wave causes an upsloping course of the PR segment. This pattern helps to recognize false positive ST depression, even though it may be caused not only by a negative T_P wave but also by a P wave superimposed on a U wave.

5.2.2.4 Elevation of the ST Segment

ST elevation in precordial leads reflects an anteriorly directed deviation of the ST segment vector. Several mechanisms of such deviation are shown in the schematic diagrams in Fig. 5.6. In the diagram on the left, the crosshatched region represents a region of subepicardial injury, infarction, pericarditis [12], cardiac tumor [13], or transient ischemia during variant angina pectoris. The resulting systolic and diastolic currents of injury will cause elevation of the ST segment (solid arrow) and depression of the baseline (dashed arrow). In the diagram on the right, secondary ST segment elevation is a result of either delayed repolarization in the subendocardial region, or alternatively from premature repolarization of the subepicardial region. The latter phenomenon is the commonly assumed mechanism of a normal male pattern in young males Another cause of ST segment elevation is an abnormal atrial repolarization; that is, an upright Ta wave [14].

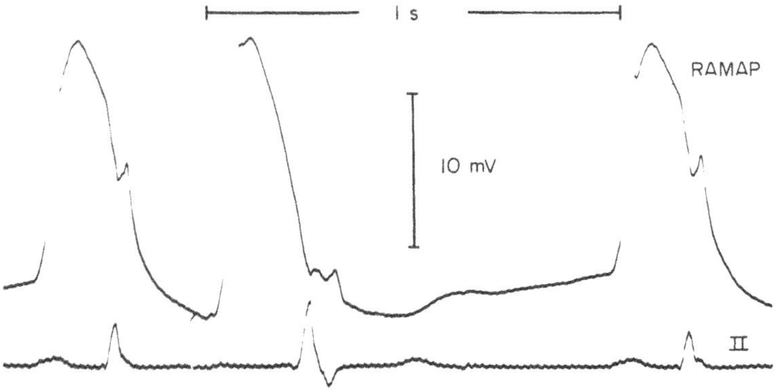

Fig. 5.5
Effect of rate on the right atrial monophasic action potential (RAMAP). The duration of the RAMAP cannot be accurately measured because the QRS artifact distorts phase 3. However, phase 2 is not distorted. Phase 2 is longer in the sinus beats (first and third potentials) than in the atrial premature beat (second potential) with aberrant ventricular conduction. The tracing shows also that atrial repolarization continues during the inscription of the QRS complex and ST segment (After Shabetai et al. [3]. © American Heart Association, Dallas, Texas. Reproduced with permission)

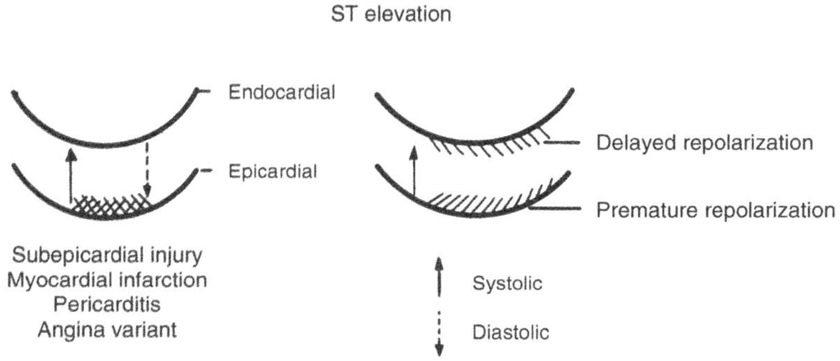

Fig. 5.6
Diagram of several mechanisms of ST-segment elevation. The direction of the arrows indicates the flow of current and not the ST-segment vector. See text for explanation (After Surawicz and Saito [11]. © Yorke Medical Group, Magazine Division. Reproduced with permission)

5.2.2.5 ST Segment Depression-Normal Variant

A slightly downsloping or horizontal ST segment depression may occur as an apparent normal variant in the absence of myocardial ischemia, digitalis, hypokalemia, or secondary repolarization abnormalities. At rest, in the routine ECG, this occurs more commonly in women than in men [15–17]. However, during ambulatory monitoring, transient ST segment depression from 0.1 to 0.4 mV, lasting from 30 s to 2 h was recorded in 15 of 50 normal male volunteers who were 35–59 years old [18].

5.2.2.6 ST Segment Elevation-Normal Variant and Acute Pericarditis

In some individuals, particularly young men, ST segment elevation occurs as a normal variant [19–23]. The term early or premature repolarization is frequently applied to this pattern [22, 23] although in most cases this is a normal male pattern (see below). The latter term implies that the ST segment shift is attributed to the shortening of ventricular APs in some epicardial regions. A rapid early repolarization in these regions may be expected to produce potential differences resulting in a "current of injury" and a consequent elevation of the ST segment. In partial support of this theory are the observations that exercise and isoproterenol [23, 24] abolish the ST segment elevation presumably as a result of diminished difference between ventricular AP durations [25]. However, mapping studies have not substantiated the rationale for the term "early repolarization" because in normal young volunteers, the overlap between the onset of ventricular repolarization and the end of QRS ranged from 4 to 16 ms. Further, there was no significant correlation between these values and ST segment deviation in the precordial leads [26].

The pattern of "early repolarization" may simulate the early pattern of acute pericarditis, possibly because both may be caused by a similar mechanism. In both patterns, the inscription of the ST segment begins before QRS forces have returned to baseline [12, 22] but the ST elevation in pericarditis is usually present in both limb and precordial leads, while in the pattern of "normal variant," ST elevation is confined more frequently to only the precordial leads [23]. Also, the T-wave amplitude in the left precordial leads tends to be greater in persons with "normal variant" than in patients with acute pericarditis [27].

5.2.2.7 ST Segment: Effect of Gender and Age

Anecdotal differences between ventricular repolarization in males and females have been observed for a long time, but only recently quantitatively defined. The typical male pattern prevails in young males and the typical female in ca 80% of women of all ages and in elderly males [28, 29]. The pattern is usually best expressed in the precordial lead with the tallest T wave, and the measurable descriptors are the level of J point and the angle of the ascent of the ST segment. In the male pattern, which is often labeled as premature or early repolarization variant (see above), the J point is situated more than 0.1 mV above the baseline, and the ST segment ascends at an angle > 20°. In the female pattern, the J point is situated less than 0.1 mV above the baseline, most often on the baseline, and the angle of the ST ascent is < 20°, most often close to 0°. The indeterminate patter, present in about 10–20% of men and women is characterized by J point as in male and the ST segment as in female pattern. Typical patterns are shown in ➋ Fig. 5.7 and the distribution of patterns in both genders from childhood to old age is shown in ➋ Fig. 5.8.

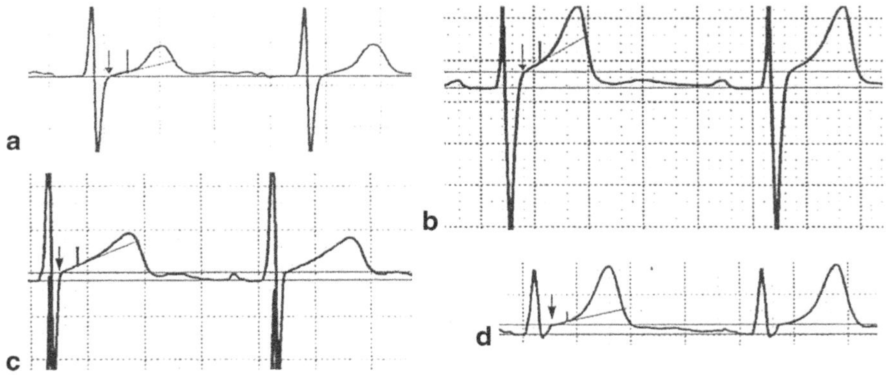

Fig. 5.7
Method of pattern determination in representative ECG complexes of lead V3. The two horizontal lines represent the Q–Q line and the line parallel to the Q–Q line at the level of the J point, respectively. The *arrow marks* the J point; the short ventricle line marks the point 60 ms after the J point; the *oblique line* connects the J point with the above point (see text). (a) Female pattern: the J point is at the level of the Q–Q line, and the ST angle is 19°. (b) Male pattern: the J point is > 0.1 mV above the Q–Q line, and the ST angle is 36°. (c) Variant of the male pattern in which the T wave ascends at the J point; the J point is > 0.1 mV above the Q–Q line, and the angle between the line parallel to the Q–Q line at the level of the J point and the ascent of the T wave is 29°. (d) Indeterminate pattern: the J point is > 0.1 mV above the Q–Q line, and the ST angle is 15° (From Surawicz et al., 2002 [29]. © *J. Am. Coll Cardiol*. Reproduced with permission)

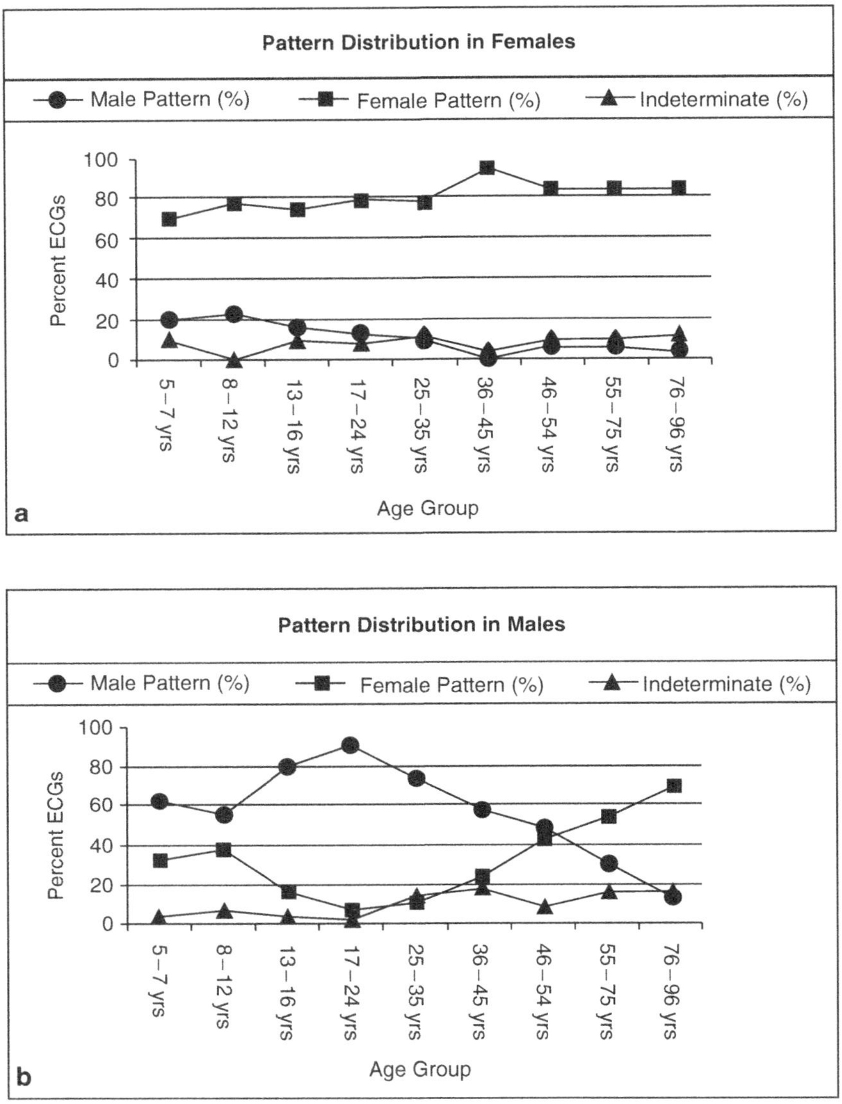

Fig. 5.8
Pattern distribution in different age groups of females and males (From Surawicz et al., 2002 [29]. © J. Am. Coll. Cardiol. Reproduced with permission)

5.2.2.8 Alternans of the Depressed and the Elevated ST Segment

Alternans of the ST segment is known to occur both in experimental animals and in man. The alternans pattern may consist of an alternating depth of ST segment depression, or an alternating amplitude of ST segment elevation. To the best of the author's knowledge, an alternation of ST segment depression and elevation has not been reported.

The most common cause of the alternans of the ST segment is myocardial ischemia [30–34]. Alternans of an elevated ST segment was observed also in man during hyperkalemia [35] and in a cyanotic infant [36]. Alternation in the degree of ST segment depression was observed following critical decrease of flow in the left main coronary artery in dogs, in association with alternation of blood pressure, stroke volume, and occasionally with alternation of T wave [31]. In the pig,

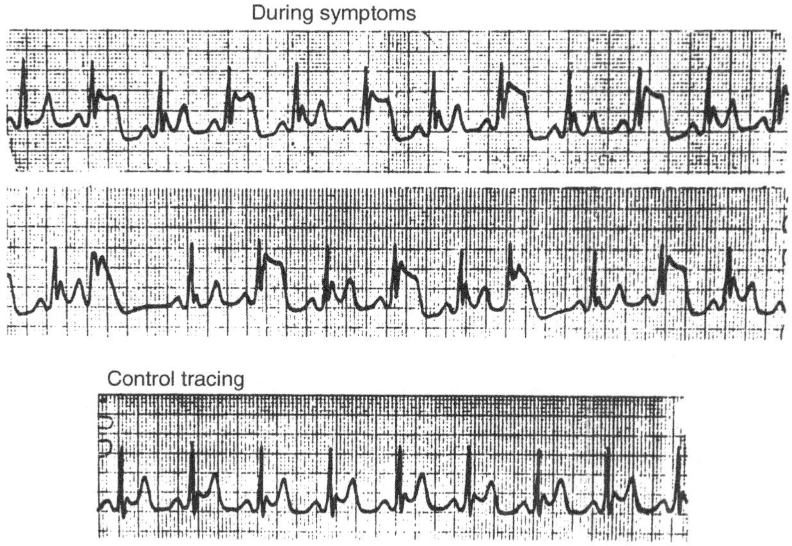

Fig. 5.9
Electrocardiogram of a patient recorded from a continuous coronary-care unit monitor lead during an episode of Prinzmetal angina. Note the striking 2:1 electrical alternans involving the ST segment. A control tracing (for comparison) was taken with the same leads immediately after the pain subsided (After Williams et al. [32]. © American College of Physicians, Philadelphia, Pennsylvania. Reproduced with permission)

ST segment alternans was observed not only after coronary artery ligation but also during reperfusion [37]. The alternans of the ST segment elevation in man is not uncommon during attacks of vasospastic angina pectoris (➋ Fig. 5.9), but has not been reported in the presence of ST segment elevation resulting from myocardial infarction [38].

More than one hypothetical mechanism can be postulated to explain the alternans of the ST segment elevation or depression in association with the alternans of contractile force. However, the most plausible mechanism appears to be an alternans of the slope of phase 2 (plateau) of the ventricular AP. Such an alternans has been observed in the records of MAPs registered simultaneously with electrograms during ST segment alternans produced by occlusion of the left anterior descending coronary artery (LAD) artery in dogs [31]. In some cases, the alternans appeared to occur also at the level of resting membrane potential [33].

5.3 T Wave

5.3.1 General Considerations: Ventricular Gradient

The T wave represents the uncanceled potential differences of ventricular repolarization. Since most of the electromotive forces generated during cardiac activity undergo cancellation, the area of the T wave is estimated to represent only 1–8% or less of the total time–voltage product of the heart [39, 40]. As will be discussed later in this section, the normal sequences of ventricular repolarization and the anatomic sites of the uncanceled potential differences responsible for the T wave in the normal heart are still not known.

The analysis of the T wave may be approached by relating the T-wave area to the QRS area. Wilson et al. pointed out that if all ventricular action potentials had the same magnitude and the same duration, the net area of the ventricular complex (QRS and T) should be zero [41]. However, in the normal heart, the mean QRS vector and the mean T vector form a narrow angle, and the area of the ventricular complex has a positive value. This indicates that in some parts of the ventricles, the intensity, or the duration of activity, must be greater than in others. This difference of activity was designated as the ventricular gradient. The ventricular gradient points from the parts of the ventricle with greater duration of activity toward the parts with the lesser duration [41, 42]. The main source of the ventricular gradient is the nonhomogeneous duration of recovery; that is, the difference in duration of action potentials in different parts of the ventricles [41–44]. Several other sources of expected differences between the QRS area and the T area in the surface ECG (changes in the position or orientation of cardiac fibers during activity, and the nonlinear relation between the source of potentials and the surrounding field) appear to play only a negligible role in the genesis of the ventricular gradient [39, 45].

The concept of ventricular gradient developed by Wilson et al. applied only to a small unit of two adjacent fibers with different AP durations [41]. Subsequently, Gardberg and Rosen extended the validity of the concept to a strip of turtle ventricle [46]. In this preparation, the area of the electrogram was determined by differences in the rate of repolarization, but was not dependent on the path of excitation [46]. The presence of ventricular gradient in the entire heart can be demonstrated after an application of a brief and very strong electric shock that depolarizes simultaneously all ventricular elements. This shock causes a T wave without a QRS complex, and the area of this T wave represents the pure ventricular gradient [47]. The application of such shocks to dogs produced a large, upright T wave in leads II and III, and suggested an overall direction of repolarization from the apex to the base of the heart [47]. The principle of the independence of ventricular gradient of the sequence of activation has been reaffirmed in a study of QRST isoarea maps utilizing 192 electrodes [48] The same conclusion was reached by the mathematical analysis of a theoretical model in which propagation occurred under uniform isotropic conditions and the action potentials were identical except for possible variations in the duration of plateau [49].

It has been shown that compared to depolarization, repolarization generates more dipolar electrical fields [50]. However, our present knowledge of the spatial and temporal characteristics of the normal recovery process is still very incomplete. Studies of local electrograms and local effective refractory periods indicate that the general order of recovery is approximately the same as the order of activation [41, 45, 47, 51]. However, the QRST area in the local electrograms is seldom zero, even when the records are made with very closely spaced bipolar electrodes [63]. This indicates that inhomogeneities of repolarization occur within very small distances over the entire surface of the heart, and most probably within the entire ventricular wall [2].

Studies utilizing suction electrodes to record MAPs on the ventricular surface in dogs suggested a complex and geographically nonuniform sequence of ventricular repolarization [52], which had a tendency to shorten progressively in progressively later activated areas. This shortening appeared to be determined by the time of activation rather than by the site of activation [76] (➋ Table 5.1.). Accordingly, the relation of the. MAP duration on the ventricular surface agreed with the direction of ventricular gradient [52]. Several studies utilizing refractory periods to estimate the sequence of repolarization reported similar recovery properties [53, 54]. It was shown that the sequence of recovery at the epicardial level was similar to the sequence of normal activation, but the sequence of excitation and recovery differed at the endocardium with some basal areas recovering excitability earlier than the apex in spite of later activation [55–57]. Also, in humans, body-surface mapping utilizing 192 electrocardiographic leads showed that the normal sequences of ventricular excitation and recovery were similar, and that the potential-difference boundaries with stable locations were widely distributed during later portions of the T wave [54].

With regard to the transmural sequence of excitation, early studies showed that the functional refractory period in the canine ventricle was approximately 15 ms longer in the subendocardial than in the subepicardial layers [58] (➋ Fig. 5.10). Subsequently, more detailed studies confirmed that the normal sequence of recovery proceeded from epicardium to

Table 5.1

Relation between the duration of the monophasic action potential (MAP) expressed as a percentage of longest MAP in each dog and the activation time on the ventricular surface

Group	Activation time (ms)	Number of dogs	Number of APs	Duration average ± SD	Differences between groups
I	8–20	14	46	95.1 ± 3.4	III*
II	21–30	17	97	94.4 ± 4.5	III**
III	> 31	21	41	92.5 ± 4.7	I*, II**

*$p < 0.01$; **$p < 0.05$

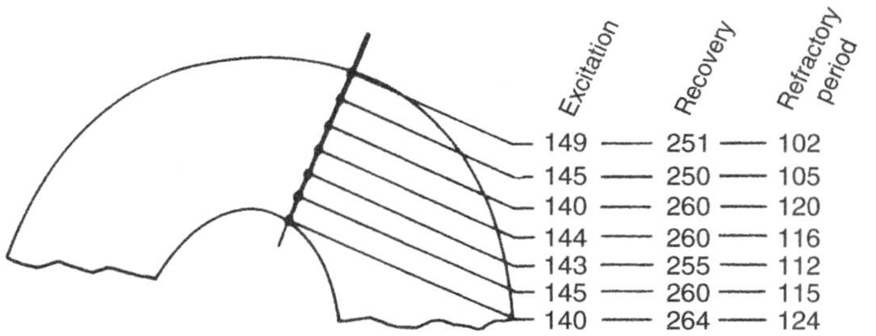

Fig. 5.10
Excitation times, recovering times, and refractory period on the endocardial–epicardial axis in the posterolateral left ventricular wall. The times shown are in milliseconds after atrial stimulation. Findings are representative of five experiments in which comparable measurements were made shortly after thoracotomy and without pericardial incision over the ventricles. Excitation was earliest at the endocardium, and endocardial refractory periods were longer than those near the epicardium, as has been previously established (After Abildskov [55]. © American Heart Association, Dallas, Texas. Reproduced with permission)

endocardium [55, 59]. It has been shown that action potentials from scattered myocytes, assumed to represent mainly the intramural action potentials, were longer than both the subendocardial or the subepicardial action potentials, and approximated more closely than the latter, the QT duration in the guinea pig heart [60].

The mechanisms responsible for the differences between the duration of repolarization in different regions of the ventricles remains to be identified. Wilson et al. considered two possible explanations: first, the inherent characteristics of the fibers; or second, the effects created by different environmental influences; for instance, differences in innervation, blood supply, or temperature [51]. In the canine and human ventricle, the temperature on the epicardial surface exceeds the temperature of the endocardium by 0.5–0.7°C [61, 62]. However, several studies have shown conclusively that the ventricular gradient cannot be attributed entirely, or even predominantly, to these temperature differences [61–63]. It has also been shown that ventricular gradient is not caused by increased pressure in the subendocardial regions because, in patients with severe hypertension, marked and rapid lowering of blood pressure with hexamethonium did not alter the ventricular gradient [2].

The magnitude of the ventricular gradient depends on factors that still remain unknown [63]. The inhomogeneous behavior of repolarization may represent an inherent property of the myocardium, because an upright T wave and a high gradient are present even in isolated papillary muscles or muscle strips [45]. It appears likely that some of the "inherent" AP duration differences in the ventricular myocardium result from electrotonic interactions during ventricular repolarization. An attempt to estimate these influences by comparing refractory periods during repeated stimulation (drives) at single ectopic sites, and during fusion drives from two ectopic sites, showed that refractory periods were as much as 10 ms shorter when a fusion occurred within 1 mm of the test site; an effect probably arising from electrotonic interactions [64].

Another factor proposed as an explanation of the differences in AP duration in different portions of ventricular myocardium is the difference in the thickness of the ventricular wall in different portions of the ventricles and the septum [65].

Numerous studies have demonstrated that local changes in the duration of recovery can alter the amplitude, duration, and polarity of the T wave without changes in the QRS complex. Regional changes in the duration of recovery produced by cooling and warming have resulted in predictable deviations of the T-wave vector from the area with the longer duration toward the area with the shorter duration of the recovery period [41, 46, 47, 66–69]. Calculations based on experimental data have shown that small alterations in the local form of the AP may cause large percentile changes in the configuration of the T wave [39]. This means that the ventricular gradient is very sensitive to local differences in the duration of repolarization and that the T wave may be considered as "some kind of special detector for differences in repolarization of the various parts of the ventricle" [39].

Experimental and clinical studies in our laboratory have provided certain estimates of the magnitude of repolarization changes required to alter the T-wave morphology or the T vector. Isoproterenol (2 mcg ml^{-1}) administered into four different vessels of anesthetized open-chest dogs induced T-wave changes without QRS changes. By correlating these

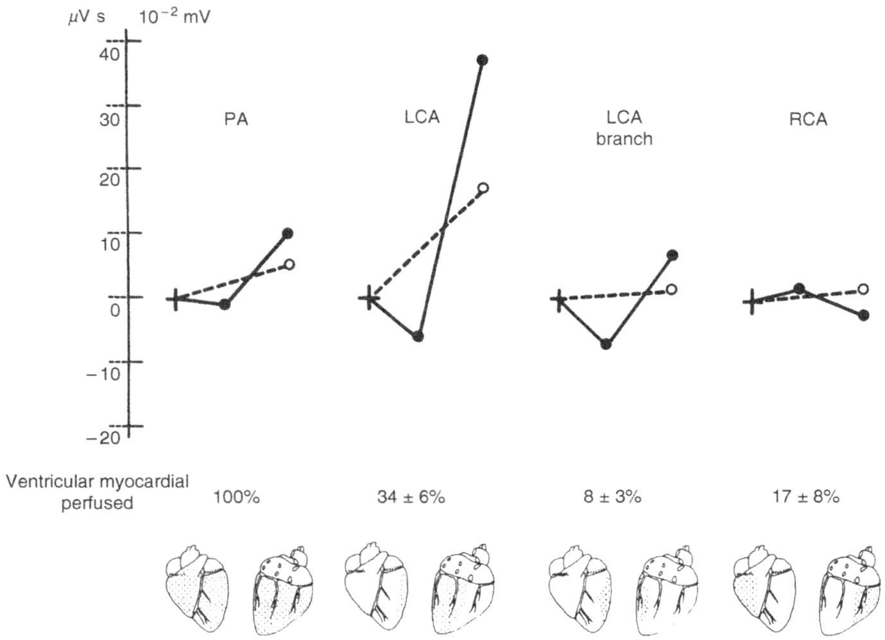

Fig. 5.11
Late (steady-state) effect of isoproterenol (ISP) on T-wave amplitude in 10^{-2} mV (*solid line*) and T-wave area in μVs (*broken line*) in four groups of experiments. The points represent average change from control values. In each panel, the proximal *solid dot* represents the a_1T amplitude and the distal *solid dot* the a_2T amplitude; a_1 and a_2 refer apices of a bifid T wave. The lower part shows the percentage of the ventricular myocardial mass perfused with ISP. The ISP-perfused area of the ventricles is indicated by the *dotted area* in the diagram under each number. In each panel, the anterior surface of the heart is shown on the left and the posterior surface on the right. *PA* pulmonary artery (group I), *LCA* left circumflex coronary artery (group II), *LCA branch* left circumflex coronary artery branch (group III), and *RCA* right coronary artery (group IV) (After Autenrieth et al. [69]. © American Heart Association, Dallas, Texas. Reproduced with permission)

T-wave changes with the changes in the duration of MAPs recorded with suction electrodes and with the tissue mass perfused with isoproterenol, it was possible to demonstrate that a significant change in T-wave amplitude in orthogonal leads occurred when MAP shortened by 18:+/−8 ms in the portion of left ventricular wall comprising about 8% of ventricular myocardium [25]. As expected, T-wave changes were greater when MAP shortening of similar magnitude extended over a mass comprising about 34% of ventricular myocardium (➔ Fig. 5.11). However, other results from the same study showed that the magnitude of T-wave change was not proportional to the mass of tissue with the uniformly shortened repolarization. Some of these discrepancies were attributed to cancellation, and some to an uneven contribution of different repolarization regions to the T wave [25]. Subsequently, changes in the duration of MAP on the anterior and posterior walls of the dog ventricle were correlated with changes in T-wave polarity and duration of the QT interval after:

1. Left stellate-ganglion transection,
2. Right stellate-ganglion stimulation, and
3. Administration of isoproterenol before or after these procedures.

Left stellate-ganglion transection and right stellate-ganglion stimulation produced similar changes in T-wave polarity, but the former prolonged and the latter shortened the QT interval. All procedures changed the duration of the MAP and the QT interval in the same direction [25]. The reversal of T-wave polarity induced by left stellate-ganglion transection, right stellate-ganglion stimulation, or the administration of isoproterenol after left stellate-ganglion transection was associated with an average change of 13–17 ms in the difference between the MAP durations on the anterior and posterior ventricular walls. Isoproterenol restored to normal the neurogenic T-wave abnormalities produced by left stellate-ganglion transection and right stellate-ganglion stimulation. The drug shortened the previously prolonged MAP more than the normal MAP, and the normal MAP more than the previously shortened MAP. This study confirmed that the T wave is a sensitive indicator of relatively small changes (<20 ms) in the sequence of ventricular repolarization, and also explained the mechanism by which isoproterenol "normalized" the primary T-wave abnormalities [25].

In a parallel clinical study, the effects of isoproterenol on the T wave were compared with the effects of atropine or pacing at the same rate [70]. In 37 patients, isoproterenol reversed the T-wave polarity from negative to positive, while the T-wave abnormality persisted after atropine or pacing following an identical rate increase. The average QT shortening with isoproterenol was 20 ms greater than that with atropine or pacing. This suggested that a lengthening of repolarization by 20 ms in some portion of ventricular myocardium might have been responsible for the inversion of T wave. A similar value was obtained in a different manner in 29 patients with left ventricular hypertrophy (LVH) pattern and negative T waves in the left precordial leads. In 18 of these patients, the negative T wave persisted after the administration of isoproterenol and in 11, the T wave became upright. In the patients in whom the T wave became upright, the QRS duration averaged 85 ms and in patients in whom the T wave remained negative, the QRS duration averaged 106 ms. Since QT shortening produced by isoproterenol was the same in both groups, it was concluded that conduction delay by 21 ms was responsible for the secondary T-wave inversion in the left precordial leads [70].

5.3.2 Normal Configuration and Direction

The configuration of the normal T wave is largely determined by the asynchrony of the phase 3 of ventricular repolarization duration of ventricular TAPs. In the theoretical model deriving ventricular complex in the ECG by the algebraic subtraction of 2 APs in ➋ Fig. 5.3, the T wave would be upright when the terminal AP ends before the initial AP, isoelectric when both APs end simultaneously and inverted when the initial AP ends before the terminal AP. Notwithstanding the obvious limitations of such a simplistic model, it proved to be applicable in the derivation of T-wave polarity in local bipolar electrograms. The study of Taggart et al. [71] showed an excellent correlation between T-wave polarity in the local electrogram in the intact pig heart in vivo and the T wave of the ECG-like waveform derived by the subtraction of 2 MAPs recorded at the sites of the corresponding electrode. The successful reproduction of T-wave configuration in this model appears to reflect two general properties of ventricular repolarization, i.e., the simple dipolar nature of the generated electrical fields and the smooth electrotonic modulation of the AP duration during impulse propagation.

In our two studies, the average maximum differences of the MAP duration on the ventricular surface in dogs were 22 ± 9 ms [72] and 27 ± 10 ms [72]. The reported differences of MAP durations on the surface of the isolated cat heart averaged 25 ms [73]. These values suggest that the differences of AP durations on the entire surface may be greater than the transmural differences of refractory period [58].

Some indication of the approximate maximum differences between AP durations in an individual dog can be obtained from the relation between the timing of the T-wave apex and the repolarization slope of the MAP. The T wave results from many simultaneous local gradients between APs during repolarization. The peak of the T wave is expected to coincide with the maximum of these local gradients. The maximum local gradient between two APs during repolarization may be expected during the inscription of the steepest repolarization slope of the AP, which terminates earlier. If this consideration is applied to the entire heart, the peak of the T wave should not occur before the onset of rapid repolarization in some portion of the ventricle. This, in turn, suggests that the duration of the interval between the peak of the T wave (aT) and the end of the T wave (eT) bears a certain relation to the dispersion of repolarization in the entire heart. In our study, the interval between aT (second peak if the T wave was bifid) and eT in leads II or *Y* averaged 33 ± 12 ms. The precise relation between the dispersion of repolarization and the aT–eT interval is not known, but, knowing the repolarization slope of the individual MAP, the probable upper limits of dispersion in an individual case were calculated. An example of such a calculation is illustrated in ➋ Fig. 5.12, which shows one ventricular complex from ➋ Fig. 5.13.

In ➋ Fig. 5.13, the MAP at the anterior base ends 17 ms before the end of the T wave, and the MAP at the posterior base ends 33 ms before the end of the T wave. Thus, the dispersion of repolarization between these two MAPs was 16 ms. The shape of the T waves was derived from the plot of "potential differences" produced by superposition of these two MAPs

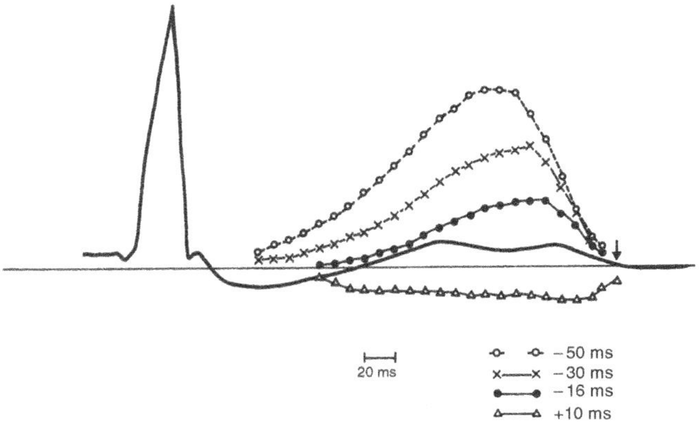

Fig. 5.12
Magnified ventricular complex from Fig. 5.13 (solid trace) with an additional four different T waves derived from the "potential differences" between two superimposed MAPs illustrated in Fig. 5.13. The *solid circles* mark the T wave derived from the MAPs superimposed in the same sequence as they occurred in the experiment (MAP at the anterior base ends 17 ms and MAP at the posterior base 33 ms before the end of the T wave). Other T waves represent "potential differences" between MAPs of the same configuration but after shortening or lengthening, phase 2 of the MAP at the posterior base. The T wave marked by crosses was constructed after the MAP at the posterior base was shortened by 14 ms; this increased the eMAP–eT difference (e denotes end) between these two MAPs from 16 to 30 ms. The T wave marked by *empty circles* is constructed after the MAP at the posterior base was shortened by 34 ms; this increased the eMAP–eT difference between these two MAPs to 50 ms. The T wave marked by *triangles* was constructed after the MAP duration at the posterior base was increased by 26 ms; this altered the eMAP–eT sequence between these two MAPs and produced a negative T wave. Note that the aT–eT interval (second peak) of the recorded T wave is 40 ms, and that the aT–eT intervals of the derived T waves are 44 ms (dispersion 16 ms), 55 ms (dispersion 30 ms), and 75 ms (dispersion 50 ms) (After Autenrieth et al. [52]. © Mosby, St Louis, Missouri. Reproduced with permission)

when the dispersion of repolarization was unchanged (16 ms) and when the dispersion was shortened or prolonged by "shortening" or "lengthening" the MAP at the posterior base. Fig. 5.12 shows that, unlike the recorded T wave, the derived T waves had only one peak. The timing of this peak is within the observed range of aT–eT intervals when the dispersion of repolarization is 10, 16, or 30 ms, but it occurs earlier than observed in any experiment when the dispersion is 50 ms. This suggests that the dispersion of repolarization in dogs is less than 50 ms; that is, less than the duration of the QRS complex [75].

In the study of Yanowitz, Preston, and Abildskov [74], unilateral stellate-ganglion stimulation was followed by an apparent lengthening of the QT interval. This suggested that certain APs terminate after the end of the T wave but do not generate deflections, because they end simultaneously and undergo cancellation [74]. Fig. 5.14 shows that in our study of dogs, there was no evidence to support such "silent repolarization" on the ventricular surface, since all MAPs terminated during the inscription of T wave. The same results were obtained from studies on the rabbit and man [76].

The normal T wave in humans is always positive in lead I, nearly always positive or isoelectric in lead II, and positive, negative, or diphasic in leads III and a VF. The normal angle between the T-wave axis and QRS axis seldom exceeds 80°. The angle tends to be more narrow in persons with a vertical QRS axis, and wider in persons with horizontal QRS axis [42]. Immediately after birth and during the first few days of life, the T wave is usually upright in the right precordial leads but afterward it becomes negative in the leads extending from V_4R to V_2, and sometimes to V_3. The gradual change from a negative to positive T wave in these leads occurs during childhood and adolescence. In the majority of the normal adults, the T wave is upright in the leads V_2 to V_6. A "juvenile pattern" is an ECG with negative T waves in the right precordial leads occur in young adults without heart disease. The term implies a failure of normal evolution from the childhood pattern to the adult pattern. Several studies of normal persons below age 40 have shown that negative T waves in leads V_2 and V_3 occur more frequently in black than in white persons. In young, healthy black persons, negative T

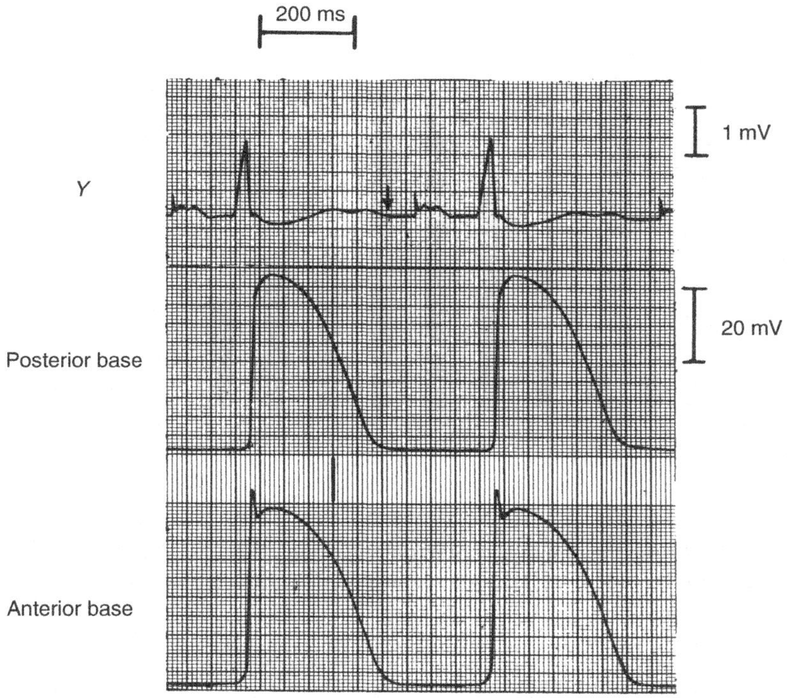

	Activation time ms	Duration ms
Anterior base	29	274
Posterior base	35	252

Fig. 5.13
Typical example of the differences between two MAPs from two different sites. The T wave is upright and bifid. The *arrow marks* the end of the T wave. Heart rate is kept constant by atrial pacing (After Autenrieth et al. [52]. © Mosby, St Louis, Missouri. Reproduced with permission)

waves may occasionally be present even in the leads V_4 and V_5. However, in persons above age 40, the negative T waves in the right precordial leads rarely indicate a juvenile pattern.

Another rare normal variant is an isolated negative T wave in the midprecordial leads V_3 and/or V_4. In such cases, the T wave tends to be diphasic rather than frankly negative. In cases of isolated negative or biphasic T wave in the midprecordial leads occurring in the absence of heart disease, the area of the T wave abnormality over the precordium is small, and shifting the electrodes downward will usually reveal an upright T wave.

Consistent with the smooth course of phase 3 of the ventricular AP, the T wave is smooth and rounded, and contains little frequency content in excess of 10 cycles s^{-1}. The apex of the T wave is reached after an interval amounting to 68–84% of the QT interval [6]. As a rule, the ascent of the normal T wave is longer than the descent, whereas the ascent of the U wave is shorter than its descent (➋ Fig. 5.15, see below). The apex configuration of the T wave helps to differentiate between the T wave and the P wave, which usually displays notches that are indicative of higher frequency components. However, when the T wave is notched in the precordial leads, a second summit may be as pointed as a P wave.

The duration of the Q–aT interval depends on the heart rate in the same manner as the QT interval, but the duration of the interval from the apex to the end of the T wave (aT–eT interval) changes normally only slightly with changes in

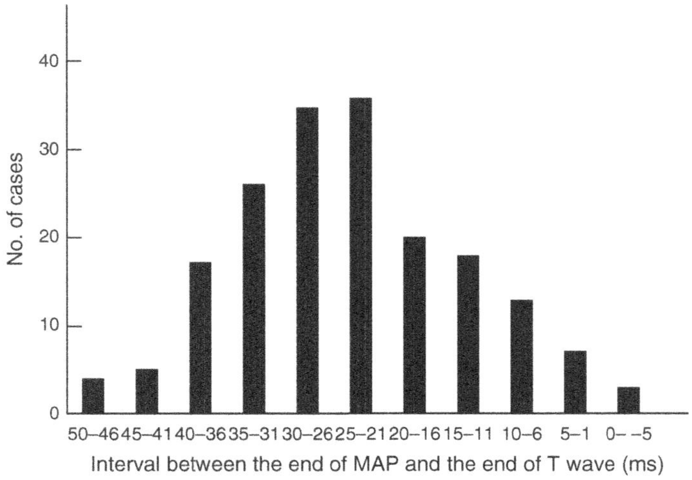

Fig. 5.14
Distribution of the intervals between the end of the monophasic action potential (MAP) and the end of the T wave in 178 tracings (After Autenrieth et al. [52]. © Mosby, St Louis, Missouri. Reproduced with permission)

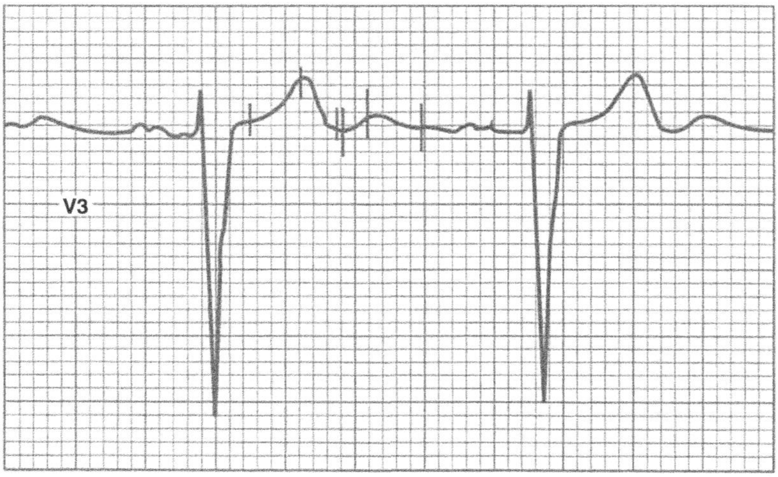

Fig. 5.15
The difference between the configuration of the T wave and the U wave in a normal ECG. The consecutive vertical lines from left to right show the beginning, apex, and end of the T wave, followed by the beginning, apex, and end of the U wave. Note that the ascent of the T wave is longer than its descent – that is, similar to the course of repolarization of ventricular and Purkinje fibres – whereas the ascent of the U wave is shorter than its descent. The duration of the QT interval is 420 ms; the duration of the QU interval is 680 ms (Reproduced from Surawicz: U wave: facts, hypotheses, misconceptions, and misnomers. *J. Cardiovasc. Electrophysiol.* 1998;9: 1117–1126, © Wiley, Reproduced with permission)

rate [4]. Thus, the difference between the intervals at a rate of 50 min^{-1} and at a rate of 100 min^{-1}, averaged 70 ms for the end of the QRS–aT interval and 15 ms for the aT–eT interval [4].

Vectorcardiography is a major alternative way of expressing electrical activity during repolarization. Vectorcardiography may have certain advantages over the ECG because it can record the sense of rotation, the speed of inscription, and the form of the T loop expressed by Chou et al. [75] as length–width ratio (L/W ratio).

The studied characteristics of the T loop have included:

1. The direction of the maximal vector in the frontal, horizontal, and right sagittal planes,
2. The magnitude of the maximal vector in each plane,
3. The L/W ratio,
4. The rotation of the T loop in each plane,
5. The speed of inscription, and
6. The QRS/T angle.

The normal T loop [75] in adults is a long ellipse with the L/W ratio of >2.6 (average 7.16 ± 4.18). The amplitude of the maximal vector lies in the range 0.2–0.75 mV (mean 0.5 mV in frontal and horizontal planes, and 0.4 mV in the right sagittal plane). The normal T-wave loop is directed to the left, anteriorly, and inferiorly. In the horizontal plane, the T-loop inscription is characteristically counterclockwise, occasionally not definable because of a very narrow loop, and rarely clockwise. In the right sagittal plane, it is clockwise and very rarely counterclockwise with a narrow loop. In the frontal plane it is either clockwise or counterclockwise. As a rule, the inscription of the efferent portion of the loop is slower than that of the afferent portion of the loop. The QRST angle shows marked variation in horizontal and right sagittal planes but is usually < 28° in the frontal plane. The spatial QRST angle ranges from 26 to 134° [75].

5.3.3 Classification of T-Wave Abnormalities

The concept of ventricular gradient allows one to define the primary and the secondary T-wave abnormalities according to their independence or dependence on changes in the QRS complex [41, 76, 77]. A "secondary" T wave is a deflection, which would follow a given QRS complex if ventricular recovery properties were uniform. Therefore, the area of primary T wave is equal to ventricular gradient and the primary T wave describes variations of the ventricular gradient as a function of time [54]. The concept was tested in a theoretical model consisting of 1,675 elements of left ventricular myocardium [78]. The satisfactory feature of this model was that the derived secondary T waves under zero-gradient conditions were independent of the sequence of activation. However, in another series of correlations the derived primary T wave was compared with the T wave generated by means of total instantaneous depolarization. The two waveforms were closely related but by no means identical. Calculations of this type suggest that although the concept of primary and secondary T waves may be clinically applicable, the accurate quantitative analysis of the components of repolarization is difficult to perform.

➋ Table 5.2 shows that primary abnormalities may be caused first, by a uniform alteration in the shape or duration of all ventricular APs without a change in the sequence of repolarization [60]; and second, nonuniform changes in shape or duration of the ventricular APs resulting in an altered sequence of repolarization [79]. Abnormal T waves may also be caused by various combinations or primary and secondary mechanisms, as presented in ➋ Table 5.2.

Certain types of primary T-wave abnormalities are labeled as "functional" or "nonspecific." Neither of these two categories can be precisely defined. Functional T-wave abnormalities are usually aggravated by hyperventilation and corrected by reassurance, potassium [80], and isoproterenol administration. Functional abnormalities reportedly occur more frequently in blacks and in young persons with anxiety or psychiatric disorders [81, 82]. The present criteria for separating "functional" from "organic" T-wave abnormalities are based more on the results of clinical evaluation rather than on any particular electrocardiographic characteristics [2].

Table 5.2
Classification of T-wave abnormalities

Sequence of depolarization	Shape and duration of ventricular AP	Sequence of repolarization	Type of abnormality
Abnormal	Normal	Abnormal	Secondary
Normal	Uniformly abnormal	Normal	Primary
Normal	Nonuniformly abnormal	Abnormal	Primary

The term nonspecific implies an abnormality of unknown cause. This term is popular among electrocardiographers, but is usually unsatisfactory to the physician who receives the report [84]. The use of the term nonspecific abnormalities should decline with increasing recognition of various specific causes of T-wave abnormalities. In practice, it is helpful to follow the term nonspecific by some clarifying descriptor, e.g., minor, slight, compatible with myocardial ischemia, etc.

The term "rapidly reversible primary T-wave abnormality" has been introduced to characterize a category of primary T-wave abnormalities, which disappear spontaneously with changes in posture or heart rate, or within minutes after the administration of certain drugs. Rapidly reversible T-wave abnormalities are not synonymous with "labile" T-wave abnormalities, which only represent cases of spontaneous variability. The category of rapidly reversible primary T-wave abnormalities includes most cases with functional and nonspecific T-wave abnormalities, but does not exclude T-wave abnormalities in patients with documented heart disease or with abnormalities caused by known extracardiac factors.

5.3.4 Secondary T-Wave Abnormalities

In theory, secondary T-wave abnormalities can be recognized by measuring ventricular gradient planimetrically, or by correlating the sequence of depolarization with the sequence of repolarization in the maps of local MAPs on the body torso. Neither method is practical. Haws and Lux [83] have shown that the time from the onset of activation to the V_{max} of T wave in the unipolar electrograms in dogs correlated with the duration of APs with an accuracy of up to 24 ms. This method of estimating APD simplifies the interpretation of precordial mapping in humans. Yamaki et al. [84] applied this method to differentiate between secondary and primary T-wave changes using an array of unipolar body surface leads. Secondary T-wave abnormalities can be expected under any condition of altered sequence of depolarization. In practice, the recognition of secondary T-wave abnormalities is not difficult when the T-wave vector deviates in a direction opposite to that of the main QRS vector in the presence of ventricular hypertrophy, or left bundle branch block patterns. Also, a secondary T-wave is directed opposite to the slow terminal QRS component in the presence of right bundle branch block, and opposite to the delta wave in the presence of a ventricular preexcitation pattern. However, the recognition of the secondary T-wave abnormalities may be difficult in the presence of conduction disturbances accompanied by independent primary T-wave abnormalities such as peri-infraction block, hyperkalemia, or quinidine-like antiarrhythmic drugs. An illustrative example of secondary T-wave changes is shown in ➋ Fig. 5.16 from a subject with Wolff–Parkinson–White syndrome and varying degree of preexcitation. Planimetric measurement showed that in all complexes the QRST area was approximately the same.

In the typical "left ventricular strain pattern," the T wave is inverted and the ST segment is depressed in leads in which the QRS area is positive; that is, usually in left precordial leads, and limb leads I and II. If the QRS complex is upright in lead III, the T wave is inverted in all three limb leads ("concordant left ventricular strain pattern"). In some cases, the T wave is upright in lead I but inverted only in one or more of the left precordial leads and in lead aVL. The secondary T wave abnormalities caused by left ventricular hypertrophy reflect an abnormally wide QRST angle in both the frontal and the horizontal planes in the presence of an unchanged ventricular gradient. During typical evolution of the left ventricular strain pattern, the phase of T wave lowering precedes the stage of inversion. When the T wave is low but upright, the

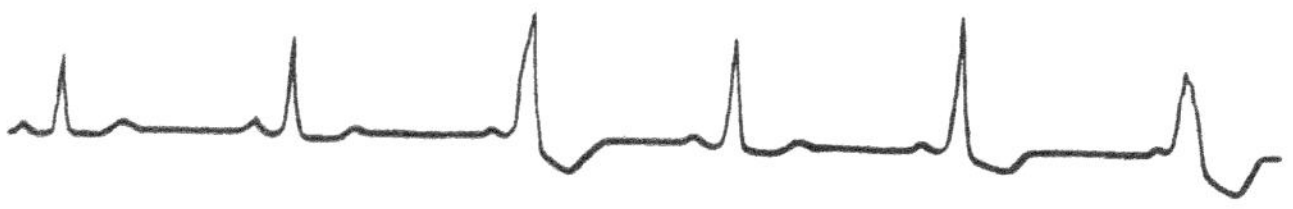

Fig. 5.16

Example of secondary T-wave changes caused by ventricular preexcitation. The consecutive ventricular electrocardiographic complexes represent conduction without preexcitation (*first complex*), during presumed maximal preexcitation (*last complex*), and varying degrees of fusion complexes. Note widening of the QRS/T angle and association of T-wave changes with depression of ST segment whereas the QRST area is approximately the same in all complexes (Reproduced with permission from Suracwicz, B., *Electrophysiological Basis of Electrocardiogram and Cardiac Arrhythmias*. Williams & Wilkins, Baltimore, MD, 1995, p. 584)

secondary abnormalities of T wave amplitude should be suspected when the QRST angle is abnormally wide or when the T wave amplitude is less than about 10–15% of the R-wave amplitude. In patients with arterial hypertension, the changes in the magnitude of secondary T wave abnormalities sometimes correlate with the efficacy of hypertension treatment.

In patients with aortic valve disease, the evolution of the secondary T-wave abnormalities tends to parallel the progression of left ventricular hypertrophy and dilatation. However, in young patients with uncomplicated aortic regurgitation, T waves may remain upright in the leads with increased amplitude of R wave. The same may be observed in other conditions associated with the so-called left ventricular diastolic overload pattern; for example, ventricular septal defect with a large left-to-right shunt, or patent ductus arteriosus.

In a typical pattern of "right ventricular hypertrophy and strain," for example, in patients with pulmonary valvular stenosis, tetralogy of Fallot, or severe pulmonary hypertension, T wave inversion and ST segment depression are present usually in leads in which the QRS area is positive – leads II, III, and right precordial leads. In such cases the QRST angle is wide, and the T wave is upright in the leads in which the QRS area is negative – lead I, and the left precordial leads. In the presence of acute cor pulmonale (pulmonary embolism, for example), transient T-wave changes are probably primary and not secondary. In patients with chronic lung disease and deep S waves in the limb and left precordial leads, the T wave tends to be in an opposite direction to the main QRS axis.

In the presence of right bundle branch block, the T-wave vector is oriented opposite to the vector of the terminal wide QRS component. The constancy of QRST area in many cases of intermittent right bundle branch block, or during progression from incomplete to complete right bundle branch block, has generally validated the concept of ventricular gradient.

In the presence of left bundle branch block, the T wave is usually directed oppositely to the main QRS axis. Therefore, the negative T waves in the leads with a deep S wave are indicative of additional primary T-wave abnormalities (➋ Fig. 5.17). However, the persistence of an upright T wave in leads with a tall R wave-lead I or V_6 does not have the same implication since it may simply result from lowering of a T wave that had been taller in the absence of left bundle branch block, or other unexplained factors. Secondary T-wave inversion owing to left bundle branch block is usually associated with a depressed ST segment and the ascending limb of the inverted T wave being steeper than the descending limb [42].

In the vectorcardiogram of a left ventricular hypertrophy pattern, the T loop shifts rightward, inferiorly, and either anteriorly or posteriorly; the spatial QRST angle increases, the T loop becomes wider and therefore the L/W ratio decreases. The T-loop inscription in the frontal plane is counterclockwise in approximately one-third of all patients. In 75% of patients with clockwise horizontal T loops, the T loop is located within the 90–180° quadrant although only 40% of T loops located within this quadrant are inscribed clockwise. Left bundle branch block produces changes in T loops similar to those in left ventricular hypertrophy. In right ventricular hypertrophy (RVH), the T-loop vector shifts posteriorly but maintains the leftward orientation; it becomes wider and the L/W ratio decreases [85]; the rotation in the horizontal plane is frequently clockwise and in the right sagittal plane, counterclockwise. The T-loop changes in right bundle branch block [86, 87] are also similar to those in right ventricular hypertrophy.

5.3.5 Primary T-Wave Abnormalities

5.3.5.1 Ventricular Transmembrane Action Potentials

T-wave abnormalities caused predominantly by uniform changes in the shape or duration of ventricular transmembrane action potentials include abnormalities of ventricular repolarization induced by drugs or abnormal electrolyte concentrations. The majority of such abnormalities can be attributed to changes in the slope of phase 3 alone, or to combined changes in the slope of phase 2 and 3 of the ventricular AP.

5.3.5.2 Cardiac Glycosides

The principal abnormalities of ventricular repolarization produced by digitalis are the result of shortening of phase 2, decreased slope of phase 3, and absolute shortening of the ventricular AP. The earliest ECG change in repolarization

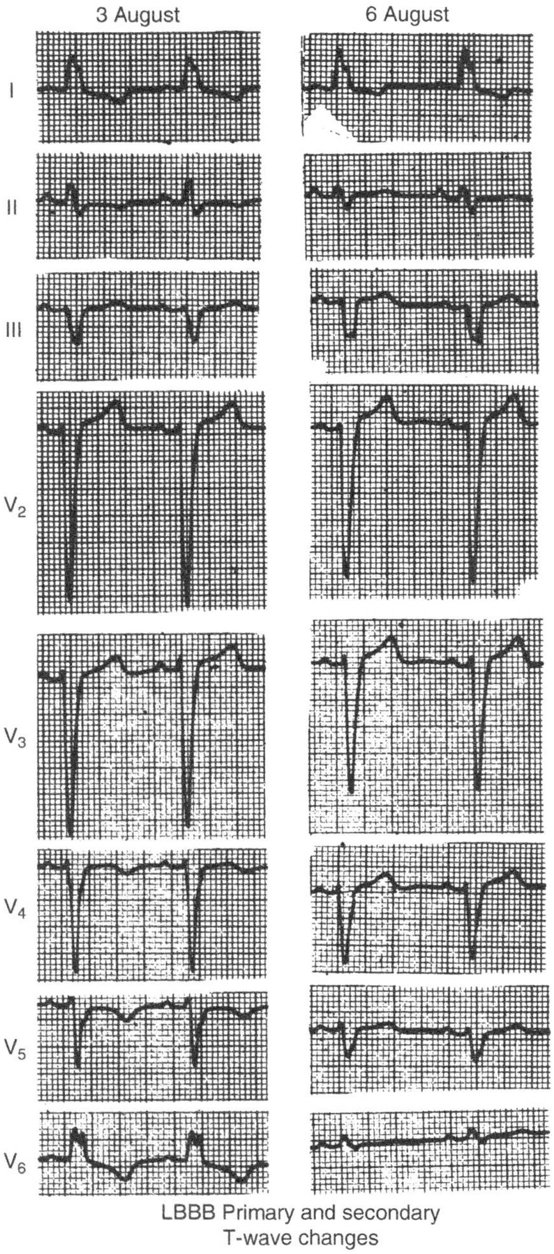

Fig. 5.17
Electrocardiograms of a patient with left bundle branch block (LBBB) and myocardial infarction. The negative T waves in V_4–V_5 on August 3 represent primary T-wave abnormalities that are no longer present on August 6

produced by digitalis consists of a decrease in T-wave amplitude and shortening of the QT_c interval. These changes are followed by the depression of the ST segment, decrease in the ventricular gradient, and inversion of the T wave. Although lowering of the T wave can occur without the depression of the ST segment, the inversion of the T wave is nearly always associated with ST depression. Initially, the entire ST segment is slightly depressed, but later the terminal portion becomes more depressed, making an angle of about 90° with the ascending limb of the T wave (Fig. 5.18).

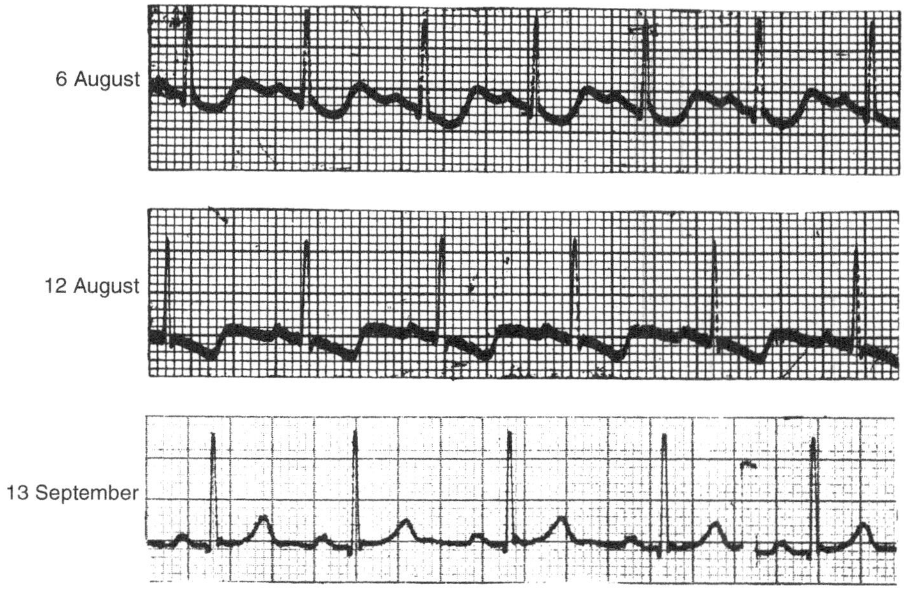

Fig. 5.18
Electrocardiograms of a patient who received a last maintenance dose of 0.1 g of digitalis leaf on August 6. Note diphasic T wave and depression of ST segment, which makes an angle of almost 90° with ascending limb of T wave in the first two tracings. Digitalis effect on the ECG disappeared within 6 weeks (bottom trace) (Reproduced from Surawicz and Lasseter [90]. © Grune and Stratton, New York. Reproduced with permission)

Later the ST segment has a steep downward course and the T wave appears diphasic (negative–positive). These changes are usually most pronounced in leads that have the highest QRS complex [42].

The effects of digitalis on ventricular repolarization may simulate the patterns of left ventricular hypertrophy, acute ischemia, and various nonspecific repolarization abnormalities. The abnormalities of repolarization produced by digitalis are frequently more pronounced at rapid rather than at slow heart rates, possibly because phase 2 of the AP is shortened more at rapid heart rates [86, 87]. The ST abnormalities produced by digitalis during exercise-induced tachycardia are similar to changes attributed to acute myocardial ischemia. Thus, digitalis may cause a false positive exercise test.

In addition to the usual T-wave abnormalities, digitalis may produce two atypical patterns: pointed inverted T waves [42] and peaking of the terminal T-wave portion [90]. The pointed inverted T wave is similar to the T wave arising from myocardial ischemia or pericarditis, but is associated with shortened QT_c interval. This interval is usually normal in pericarditis and prolonged in myocardial ischemia. Peaking of the terminal portion of the T wave was observed in about 10% of patients receiving digitalis and was sometimes, but not always, related to increased plasma K^+ concentration [88, 89].

Although in an individual patient digitalis administration usually produces progressive ECG changes, there is no satisfactory correlation between the dose and such changes. The individual variations depend on the underlying ECG pattern and the rhythm. In some patients, the effects of digitalis on repolarization cannot be recognized even in the presence of toxicity manifested by nausea, vomiting, or ectopic complexes [90]. With the advent of routine measurements of blood digoxin concentrations there has been an appreciable decline in digitalis toxicity and marked ECG abnormalities.

5.3.5.3 Class IA Antiarrhythmic Drugs

Increasing doses of quinidine progressively increase the QRS duration. The most pronounced ECG changes are produced by quinidine, the use of which has markedly declined, but the ECG effects are most characteristic for a type 1A drug.

Typically, the entire QRS complex widens uniformly, but sometimes the widening predominantly affects the terminal portion. In the absence of QRS widening, quinidine produces primary T-wave changes but in the presence of a wide QRS, the T-wave abnormalities may be a result of a combination of primary and secondary changes. Quinidine prolongs the duration of the T wave and QT_c interval. In leads with upright T waves, the T wave initially becomes lower and later becomes notched or slightly inverted; in leads with inverted T waves, the T wave becomes less deeply inverted. These T-wave alterations usually occur without concomitant depression or elevation of the ST segment, but are accompanied by an increased U-wave amplitude [42, 91]. When QRS widening becomes pronounced, the secondary T-wave changes may alter the T-wave vector; usually the T-wave vector moves in the direction opposite the wide portion of the QRS complex. The peak effect of quinidine on the ECG occurs within about 2–4 h after the oral administration of the drug. This effect is reduced by about 50% after 12 h.

The T-wave changes produced by quinidine and other antiarrhythmic drugs in class 1A category can be attributed to the prolongation and decreased slope of phase 3 in ventricular AP [5]. The latter effect also explains the increase in the U-wave amplitude, although lowering of plasma K^+ concentration, which may be produced by quinidine, can contribute to this effect [92].

Abnormalities of ventricular repolarization produced by doses of quinidine that result in plasma-quinidine concentrations of less than about 5.0 mgl^{-1} are difficult to distinguish from various nonspecific T wave abnormalities. However, the combination of the QRS, T- and U-wave changes produced by higher doses results in a fairly specific ECG pattern. Digitalis exaggerates quinidine-induced abnormalities of repolarization by lowering the T-wave amplitude and increasing the U-wave amplitude. In addition, digitalis shortens phase 2 of the ventricular AP and causes depression of the ST segment. Therefore, the combination of digitalis and quinidine produces an ECG with a depressed ST segment, low T wave, and a prominent U wave. This pattern is indistinguishable from the pattern produced by severe hyperkalemia [93]. It has been mentioned earlier that quinidine does not depress the ST segment, probably because phase 2 of the ventricular AP is not appreciably altered by the drug. In contrast to digitalis, quinidine may prevent the appearance of ST depression during exercise and thus may contribute to a false-negative response to exercise [94].

Procainamide and ajmaline alter the ECG in the same manner as quinidine, but the effect of the customary maintenance dosages is usually less pronounced. In patients treated with 1–2 g of procainamide per day, the QRS interval becomes wider, the QT_c is prolonged, the T wave becomes notched, and the U-wave amplitude may be increased [95–97]. Like quinidine, the combination of procainamide with digitalis produces an ECG pattern simulating hypokalemia. Procainamide is a shorter-acting drug than quinidine; therefore, its effect on the ECG appears earlier and persists for a shorter time.

Disopyramide prolongs QRS and QT intervals and causes primary and secondary T-wave changes similar to those produced by quinidine and procainamide.

5.3.5.4 Class III drugs

Class III action prolongs T-wave duration most often by blocking one of the potassium channels, but it may be produced by other mechanisms, such as increased inward sodium current. Some of the potassium channel–blocking drugs in this category are sotalol, amiodarone, bretylium, dofetilide [98], ibutilide [99], sematilide [100], and almokalant [101]. On the ECG, these drugs prolong the QT and JT interval without QRS prolongation (with the exception of amioadorone) and exhibit the property of reversed use dependence.

5.3.5.5 Phenothiazines

The effects of phenothiazines on ventricular repolarization are very similar to those of quinidine. Studies of the phenothiazine effect on the canine ventricular AP have shown that these drugs prolong the duration of phase 3 and either do not change or shorten the duration of phase 2 [102]. These effects explain the quinidine-like repolarization abnormalities in the ECG induced by therapeutic doses of chlorpromazine and thioridazine.

Several phenothiazine derivatives produce dose-dependent reversible abnormalities of ventricular repolarization. These abnormalities occur most commonly after the administration of thioridazine. They are apparently less pronounced after chlorpromazine and even less so after trifluoperazine [103]. The earliest ECG change produced by phenothiazines consists of lengthening of the QT_c interval, and widening, blunting, and notching of the T wave. Higher doses produce lowering and inversion of the T wave in the standard limb and precordial leads [104, 105]. The effects may be more pronounced in the right than in the left precordial leads. Sometimes, lengthening of the QT_c interval may occur in the absence of appreciable T-wave abnormalities. The U-wave amplitude is frequently increased, but ST changes are usually absent.

5.3.5.6 Hyperkalemia

Peaking of the T wave is the earliest electrocardiographic manifestation of hyperkalemia (➲ Fig. 5.19). Peaking occurs when the plasma K^+ concentration exceeds 5.5 $mEql^{-1}$, usually before the ECG shows any measurable alteration of the QRS complex [106–108]. The diagnosis of hyperkalemia cannot be made with certainty on the basis of T-wave changes alone. The characteristic tall, steep, narrow, and pointed T wave was found in only 22% of patients with hyperkalemia [109]. In the remainder of patients, the tall T waves were very similar to tall T waves in patients with bradycardia, psychiatric disorders, cerebrovascular accidents, left ventricular diastolic overload, subendocardial ischemia, and in some individuals with no apparent abnormalities. When the tall, peaked T wave is the only electrocardiographic abnormality produced by hyperkalemia, and the duration of the QRS complex and of the ST segment is normal, the QT_c interval is either normal or decreased. In the presence of a pattern of advanced hyperkalemia with a wide QRS complex, the T wave may lack its characteristic peaked and narrow configuration, probably because the T-wave abnormalities secondary to intraventricular conduction disturbances obscure the primary T-wave changes caused by the increased steepness of phase 3 of the AP.

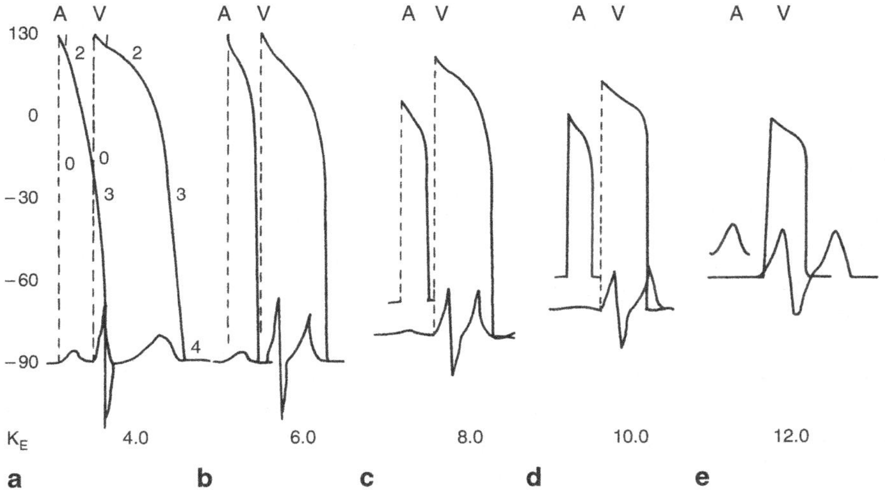

Fig. 5.19
Diagram of an atrial (A) and a ventricular (V) action potential (AP) superimposed on the electrocardiogram. The numbers on the left designate the transmembrane potential in millivolts (mV) and the numbers at the bottom, the extracellular concentration of potassium (K_E) in milliequivalents per liter ($mEq\ l^{-1}$). In tracings (a) and (b), the resting membrane potential (RMP) is −90 mV, whereas the total amplitude of the AP is 130 mV because the upstroke overshoots the 0 potential by +40 mV. Note the shortening of the AP, the increased velocity of phase 3, the progressive decrease in RMP, and in the amplitude of the AP with increasing K_E. The most rapid upstroke of the AP is shown as a line interrupted by wide spaces ((a) and (b)); the slowest upstroke is shown as a continuous line (atrial AP in (d) and ventricular AP in (e)). Note the decreasing upstroke velocity and the increasing duration of the QRS complex with increasing K_E. In (a) and (b), the atrial and the ventricular AP have the same RMP and the same amplitude, whereas in (c) and (d), the RMP of the atrial AP is less negative than the RMP of the ventricular AP, and the amplitude of the atrial AP is lower than that of the corresponding ventricular AP. See text for further discussion (After Surawicz [9]. © Mosby, St Louis, Missouri. Reproduced with permission)

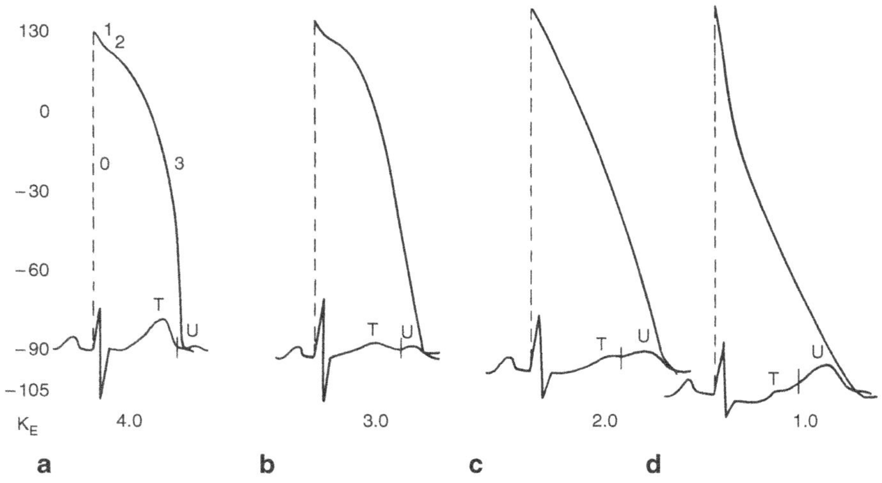

Fig. 5.20
Diagram of the ventricular AP superimposed on the electrocardiogram for extracellular concentration of potassium (KE) of (a) 4.0, (b) 3.0, (c) 2.0, and (d) 1.0 ml^{-1}. The numbers on the left designate the transmembrane potential in millivolts, as in Fig. 3.18. The RMP, the amplitude of the AP, and the overshoot in the control tracing (a) are the same as for the ventricular AP in Fig. 5.19. Note the progressively increasing velocity of phase 2, decreasing velocity of phase 3, and increasing duration of the AP. Furthermore, note the progressive increase in the RMP (more negative), and the increasing amplitude of the AP. The electrocardiographic changes are described in the text (After Surawicz [9]. © Mosby, St Louis, Missouri. Reproduced with permission)

5.3.5.7 Hypokalemia

The changes in the shape of the AP (Fig. 5.20) are reflected in the ECG as a progressive depression of the ST segment, a decrease in the T-wave amplitude and an increase in the U-wave amplitude in the standard limb and precordial leads. As long as the T wave and the U wave are separated by a notch, the duration of the QT interval is unchanged [93, 110] In more advanced stages of hypokalemia, the T wave and the U wave are fused and an accurate measurement of the QT interval is not possible.

It has been suggested that in hypokalemia, the U wave is superimposed on the gradually increasing diastolic potential produced by the prolonged duration of the ventricular repolarization [111]. If this assumption is correct, then the progressive increase in U-wave amplitude in hypokalemia may be more apparent than real. This concept finds some support in the observations that the intervals from the onset of the QRS complex to the apex and the end of the U wave (Q–aU and Q–eU. intervals) are not altered during the development and regression of the pattern of hypokalemia [9].

5.3.5.8 Combination of Abnormal Potassium and Calcium Concentration

In patients with hypokalemia and hypocalcemia, the ECG shows a prolonged ST segment and a prominent "repolarization" wave, which consists of T + U waves. This is owing to a prolongation of both phase 2 and phase 3 of the AP [4] (Fig. 5.21). The recognition of the hypokalemia pattern in the presence of hypocalcemia may be facilitated by the administration of calcium, which shortens the ST segment and separates the T wave from the U wave [93]. The combination of hypocalcemia and hyperkalemia, which frequently occurs in patients with uremia, can be recognized by the presence of a prolonged ST segment and a peaked, narrow T wave.

An increased extracellular concentration of calcium decreases the duration of phase 2 and the ventricular AP becomes similar to the normal atrial AP [112]. In patients with hypercalcemia, the ST segment is short or absent, and the QT_c

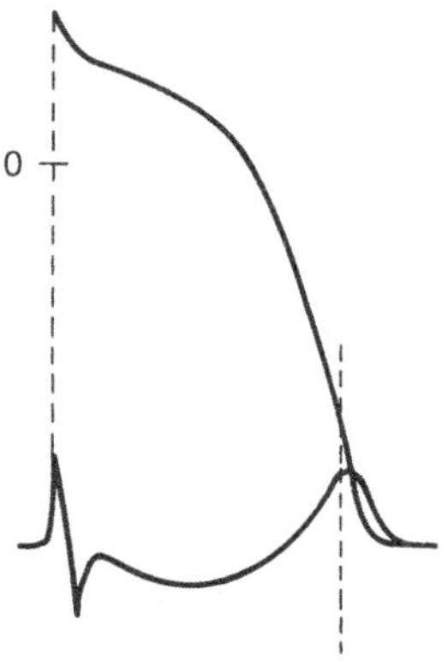

Fig. 5.21
Ventricular AP and electrocardiogram from isolated perfused rabbit heart (retraced) during perfusion with low-calcium, low-potassium Krebs–Henscleit solution. Note the prolonged duration of phase 2 and slow slope of phase 3. The corresponding ECG changes are prolonged and depressed ST segment, and wide repolarization T + U wave. The interrupted *vertical line* bisecting the apex of the T wave represents the end of mechanical systole

interval is shortened. However, the U-wave amplitude is either normal or increased. In patients with hypercalcemia and hypokalemia, the ECG shows a short ST segment and a prominent repolarization wave, which consists of T + U waves (9).

5.3.6 T-Wave Abnormalities Caused by Nonhomogeneous Repolarization

This category of primary T-wave abnormalities [113] accounts for the largest number of structural and functional disturbances of ventricular repolarization. Characteristically, these abnormalities affect only the T wave and do not alter either the course or the duration of the ST segment. In the normal ECG, the apex of the T wave is reached at the time corresponding to 68–84% of the entire QT interval [6]. The duration of the Q–aT interval depends on the heart rate in the same manner as that of the QT interval, but the duration of the interval from the apex to the end of the T wave (aT–eT interval) is similar in all normal persons and changes only slightly with changes in rate [6]. Thus, the difference between the intervals at a rate of 50 min^{-1} and at a rate of 100 min^{-1} averaged 70 ms for the end of the QRS–aT interval and 15 ms for the aT–eT interval [6].

T-wave abnormalities owing to asynchronous repolarization may be associated with a prolonged or normal QT_c interval. The QT_c lengthening is usually attributed to some regional increase in the AP duration. Primary T-wave abnormalities as a result of nonhomogeneous repolarization are frequently associated with an increased duration of the aT–eT interval. This suggests that the regional alterations of AP duration may arise from differences in the duration of phase 3.

5.3.6.1 Syndrome X

The label of syndrome X has been pinned to several different groups of patients who have in common angina-like chest pain and no evidence of obstructive disease in the large coronary artery branches. In some of these groups there is evidence of either myocardial ischemia induced by stress or abnormal vasomobility of coronary microvessels. Some individuals with this syndrome have inverted T waves in many leads. In one study of such patients, the presence of symmetrical inverted T waves at rest was associated with a coronary vasoconstrictor response to cold pressor test [114]. In other studies, evidence of myocardial ischemia was present in some but not in all patients with syndrome X and abnormal T waves. Also, presence of stress-induced ST segment depression in patients with syndrome X occurs with and without myocardial ischemia. Lactate metabolism, oxygen saturation in the coronary sinus, regional myocardial perfusion, and left ventricular wall motion abnormalities in these patients may be or may be not abnormal [114–119].

5.3.6.2 Pericarditis

The T-wave vector in patients with pericarditis is usually directed to the right and superiorly. In typical cases, the T wave becomes inverted in all standard leads with the exception of leads aVF and V_1. The T-wave inversion usually persists after the disappearance of ST abnormalities and is attributed to superficial myocarditis (epicarditis). Unlike myocardial infarction, the interval between the nadir of the negative T wave and its end is usually not prolonged, and the duration of the QT_c interval is normal [12]. The direction of the T-wave vector in pericarditis suggests prolongation of activity in the damaged fibers. Histological studies suggest that the damage is limited to a thin subepicardial layer of myocardium. Accordingly, pericarditis appears to represent an example of a large T-wave abnormality produced by a relatively small mass of abnormal myocardium extending over a wide surface area.

5.3.6.3 Other T-Wave Abnormalities Attributed to Myocardial Damage

The primary "coronary" or "postischemic" T-wave pattern with a normal ST segment, abnormal T vector, pointed T wave, and prolonged QT interval may appear in patients with various types of pathologic processes, including, among others, pulmonary embolism, acute cor pulmonale, myocardial tumor, abscess, and acute myocarditis caused by diphtheria, brucellosis, malaria, trichinosis, rheumatic fever, mumps, measles, scrub typhus, and various other infections [42, 120]. Similar T-wave changes may be caused by acute and chronic cardiomyopathy of obscure etiology [121], Friedreich's ataxia [122, 123], chest trauma [124], lightning stroke [125], various poisons, e.g., phosphorus [126], carbon monoxide [127], venoms, adder bite [128], scorpion sting [129], and certain drugs e.g., emetine, chloroquine, plasmoquin, antimony compounds, lithium, and arsenicals [66, 110]. These abnormalities are probably caused by transient or permanent prolongation of repolarization in certain regions of the heart. They usually regress slowly after the recovery from the disease or after the elimination of the noxious agent from the body. Some of these T-wave abnormalities may not be a result of organic myocardial damage but may arise from functional, neurogenic repolarization changes precipitated by the disease. For instance, in one patient with abnormal T waves attributed to myocardial damage produced by scorpion sting, autopsy did not reveal cardiac abnormalities and the ECG changes were thought to be a result of excessive catecholamine liberation [129]. T-wave abnormalities in patients with primary myocardial disease are usually secondary to QRS abnormalities produced by hypertrophy. However, in some patients, primary T-wave abnormalities precede the appearance of changes in duration, amplitude, or axis of the QRS complex [121, 130–132]. The mechanism of such T-wave abnormalities is unknown. A study by Coltart and Meldrum [133] demonstrated that the ventricular AP from a muscle band excised in a patient with hypertrophic cardiomyopathy had a slow slope of phase 3. The duration of this AP was 498 ms as compared to an average duration of 302 ms in eight control human subjects. This observation would adequately explain the primary T-wave abnormalities and prolonged QT_c interval in patients with hypertrophic obstructive cardiomyopathy.

Primary T-wave abnormalities frequently occur also in patients with mitral insufficiency owing to mitral valve prolapse [134] and with mitral insufficiency owing to a floppy mitral valve in patients with Marfan's syndrome [133]. In the majority of patients with mitral insufficiency owing to the former, the T waves are flat or inverted in leads II and III, and the QT_c interval is prolonged [135–137]. The mechanism of these T-wave abnormalities is obscure. Myocardial ischemia is unlikely because these changes frequently occur in children and in young adults. In two young patients with such T-wave abnormalities and atypical chest pain, coronary arteriograms were normal [138]. It is possible that the T-wave abnormalities in this syndrome are caused by the similar factors that produce T-wave abnormalities in familial cardiomyopathy. This is because the mitral valve prolapse is associated with localized dysfunction of the left ventricular myocardium. On the other hand, it is conceivable that T-wave abnormalities are a result of prolonged repolarization in the abnormal left ventricular ridge described in this syndrome [136].

5.3.6.4 ECG Pattern of Cerebrovascular Accident

In 1954, Burch et al. identified a specific electrocardiographic pattern peculiar to certain patients with cerebrovascular accident (CVA) [139]. This pattern occurs most frequently in patients with intracranial hemorrhage [139–145] but has been also found in patients with other intracranial lesions, such as cerebral venous thrombosis, acute cerebral infarction [144], head injuries [145], neurosurgical procedures, and cryohypophysectomy [2].

Patients with the typical ECG pattern (➋ Fig. 5.22) have one or more of the following abnormalities:

1. Prolongation of the QT_c interval by 20% or more,
2. T-wave amplitude exceeding 0.5 mV, and
3. U-wave amplitude exceeding 0.15 mV.

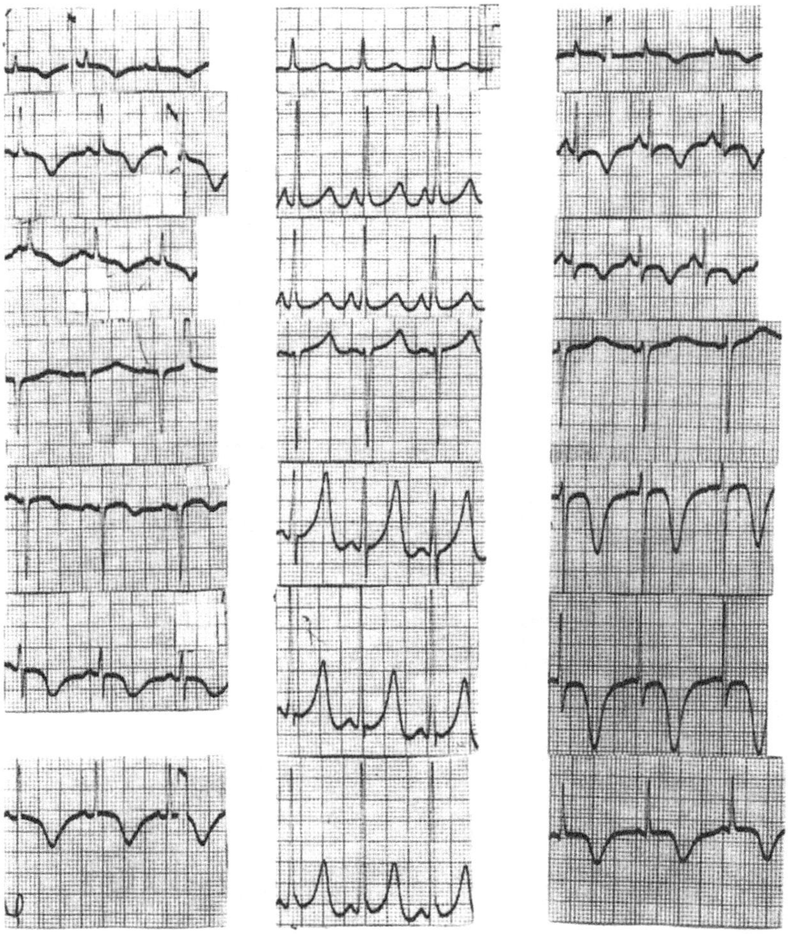

Fig. 5.22
Three examples of ECG pattern in patients with subarachnoid hemorrhage. Note, prolonged QT and increased amplitude of negative (*left and right*) upright (*middle*) T wave

ECGs with these abnormalities can be classified into five types:

1. Type I – QT_c is prolonged and T-wave amplitude is increased,
2. Type II – QT_c is prolonged and U-wave amplitude is increased,
3. Type III – only the QT_c interval is prolonged,
4. Type IV – T-wave and U-wave amplitudes are increased, and
5. Type V – the QT_c interval is prolonged and both T-wave and U-wave amplitudes are increased.

All of these patterns, particularly the "giant" T waves or "massive T inversion" may be caused by many other factors, such as electrolyte imbalance, hypertrophy, intraventricular conduction disturbances, myocardial infarction or ischemia [146–148], bradycardia, second- or third-degree atrioventricular (AV) block [147–149], and acute disease of abdominal viscera [150]. After the elimination of all patients with the above disorders, a CVA pattern was found in 60 of among approximately 45,000 ECGs recorded during the 4-year period 1965–1969 [151]. Of these, 48 patients with this pattern had intracranial lesions; in three patients, the pattern was attributed to hypothermia, and in one patient, to myxedema coma. In one patient, the pattern was recorded 1 day prior to a hypertensive crisis secondary to pheochromocytoma; in six patients without heart disease, the cause of CVA pattern was not established. The combination of long QT and increased T-wave amplitude (type 1) occurred in 78% of patients with the "CVA pattern" while other types were less common [2].

Schindler and Surawicz [151] also studied the prevalence of the CVA in various central nervous system (CNS) disorders. The CVA pattern was present in 32% of patients with intracranial hemorrhage, in 10% of patients with primary intracranial neoplasm, and in 7% of patients with acute cerebral thrombosis and increased intracranial pressure. The pattern was found only in one patient with hypertensive encephalopathy and in one of 32 patients with brain metastases. In two patients, the pattern appeared after cryohypophysectomy (➋ Fig. 5.23). In these patients, the procedure also produced a transient diabetes insipidus. The CVA pattern and the diabetes insipidus regressed in both patients within a few weeks. Subsequently, the appearance of the CVA pattern after cryohypophysectomy in several other patients was observed. These observations suggest that the CVA pattern may arise from the injury of the hypothalamus. This hypothesis would explain

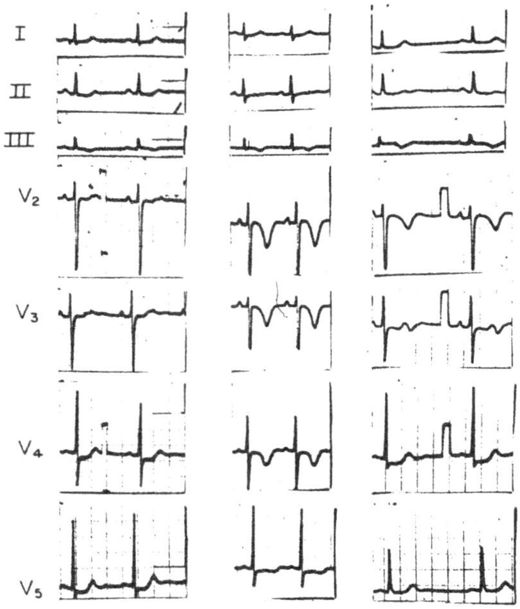

Fig. 5.23
Electrocardiogram of a 52-year old woman, receiving 0.25 mg maintenance dose of digoxin, before (*left*) 3 days (*middle*), and 18 days (*right*) after cryohypophysectomy (After Surawicz [2]. © Grune and Stratton, New York. Reproduced with permission from: Surawicz B, Knoebel SK. Long QT: good, bad and indifferent? J Am Coll Cardiol 1984;4: 398)

the relatively high prevalence of this pattern in patients with subarachnoid hemorrhage because hypothalamic lesions occur frequently after the rupture of aneurysms of the anterior and posterior communicating arteries. In the study of Crompton, hemorrhagic lesions in the hypothalamus were present in 22 of 32 patients with a ruptured anterior communicating artery and in 19 of 27 patients with a ruptured posterior communicating artery [152]. Studies by Jenkins et al. demonstrated functional disturbances of hypothalamic function in the majority of patients with ruptured intracranial aneurysm [153].

Millar and Abildskov have shown that minor repolarization abnormalities (low or notched T waves, prolonged QT_c interval, and ST depression) occur more frequently in patients with various CNS disorders than in a control population [154]. In another study, T-wave inversion without prolongation of the QT_c interval occurred in 15% of patients with meningitis and intracranial space-occupying lesions [153]. These two studies suggest that many patients with CNS disease have less distinct T-wave abnormalities than the typical pattern described by Burch et al. [139].

5.3.6.5 Other T-Wave Abnormalities Associated With an Apparent Dysfunction of the Autonomic Nervous System

T-wave abnormalities in patients with various dysfunctions of the autonomic nervous system are probably caused by the effects of nonhomogeneous sympathetic stimulation on ventricular repolarization [2]. Such a mechanism may explain T-wave abnormalities preceding hypertensive crisis owing to pheochromocytoma, or abnormalities arising from adrenal and pituitary insufficiency [2]. Typically, the T waves in patients with endocrine disorders become normal after the correction of the hormonal deficiency. In patients with pituitary insufficiency, the correction of T-wave abnormalities may require several months of hormone replacement therapy. However, transient reversal to normal can be achieved by small doses of intravenously administered isoproterenol (➋ Fig. 5.24).

Visceral reflexes are thought to be responsible for the rapidly reversible T-wave changes present in some patients with acute abdominal processes (cholecystitis, peritonitis, appendicitis, pancreatic necrosis, and ileus) [42]. These ECG abnormalities may simulate myocardial ischemia in patients without pathologic abnormalities of the heart and coronary vessels [155, 156].

T-wave abnormalities occur frequently in patients with acute and subacute pancreatitis [157]. This may be caused in some cases by pericarditis or myocardial necrosis induced by circulating enzymes from the damaged pancreas [158–161]. Also, a T-wave pattern resembling the CVA pattern, namely a wide, deeply inverted T wave and prolonged QT_c interval, was recorded in 10 of 106 patients after transabdominal truncal vagotomy for the treatment of peptic ulcer disease [162]. The authors of this report suggested that the ECG abnormalities could be a result of vagal reflex causing central autonomic stimulation or to catecholamine release in response to the parasympathetic stimulation [162].

Other neurogenic T-wave abnormalities have been reported with spinal cord injury [163] and in association with electroconvulsive therapy [164].

5.3.6.6 Giant and Global Negative T Waves

The designation of negative T wave as giant or global is based on impression rather than on specific measurements of the depth and with of the T wave. The term "global" was used by Walder and Spodick [165] who found such pattern in 100 cases among approximately 30,000 consecutive routine ECGs they interpreted. Eighty two of these patients were women. The QTc interval was prolonged. The most common causes were myocardial ischemia and central nervous system disorders. Other conditions included pericarditis, myocarditis, apicalhypertrophic cardiomyopathy (➋ Fig. 5.25), cardiac metastases, carotid endarterectomy, cocaine abuse, and pheochromocytoma. In some cases, no associated condition was apparent. After following these patients for up to 11 years, the authors [166] concluded that their long-term prognosis depended on the underlying or associated disease, and that the striking diffuse T-wave changes per se do not imply poor prognosis. Brsic et al. [167] reported a series of 17 patients (all women) with "global" T-wave inversion with "ischemic" chest pain, normal coronary arteriograms, and intact left ventricular function [168]. In another series of nine patients (all women), the pattern was associated with acute cardiogenic but nonischemic pulmonary edema [169]. The ECG changes gradually resolved within 1 week and had no immediate prognostic implications. Another cause of "global" T inversion

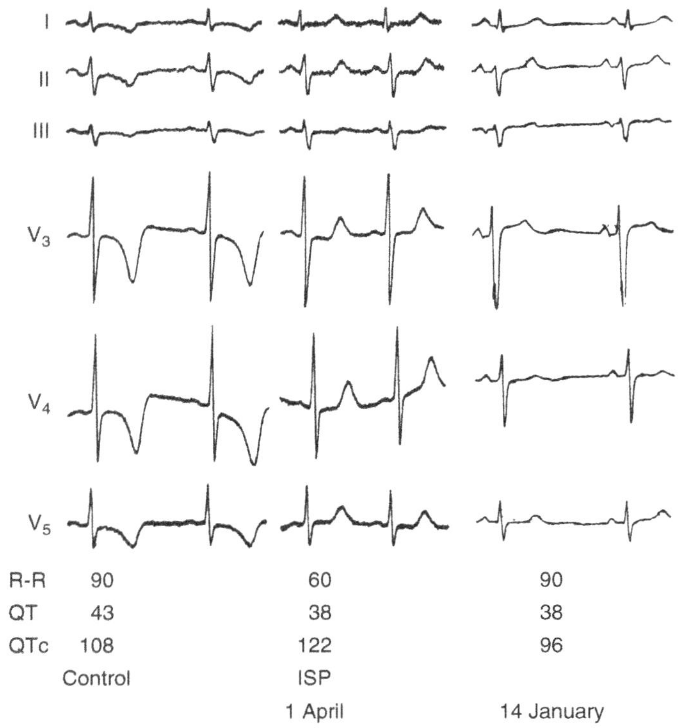

Fig. 5.24
Electrocardiogram of a 43-year old man with pituitary insufficiency and no evidence of heart disease. In the control tracing on April 1, the T wave is inverted before, and upright after the administration of 1.5 μg of isoproterenol (ISP). The T wave became upright within 9.5 months after the onset of treatment with prednisone and thyroid (January 14, following year). At the latter date, the heart rate is the same as in the control electrocardiographic tracing of April 1, but the QT interval is 0.05 s shorter. The QT interval on January 14 is the same as the QT interval after the administration of ISP on April 1 (After Daoud et al. [70]. © Yorke Medical Group, Magazines Division, New York. Reproduced with permission)

is the presence of complete A-V block. In patients with hypertrophic cardiomyopathy, reports from Japan [170] indicate that patients with giant negative T waves have hypertrophy confined to the left ventricular apex, mild symptoms, and few adverse prognostic features. The study of Alfonso et al. [171], however, showed that patients in the West with giant negative T waves have a wider clinical spectrum and that their prognosis is not different from that of patients without such T waves.

5.3.6.7 Isolated T-Wave Inversion of Adults

Another rare variant is an isolated negative T wave in the midprecordial leads V_3 and V_4. In such cases the T wave tends to be diphasic rather than frankly negative. This pattern occurs sometimes in the absence of heart disease. Under these circumstances the region in which the T wave is abnormal over the precordium is small, and a slight downward shift of the electrode usually reveals an upright T wave. In a series of 86 consecutive patients with isolated T-wave inversion reported by Okada et al. [172], 23 had no symptoms and represented a normal variant [172]. The remaining 63 patients had chest pain, and most of them had coronary artery disease. The presence or absence of structural heart disease could be differentiated by recording additional precordial leads. In the absence of heart disease, the area of negative T waves extended downward and rightward and in patients with heart disease, leftward and upward [172].

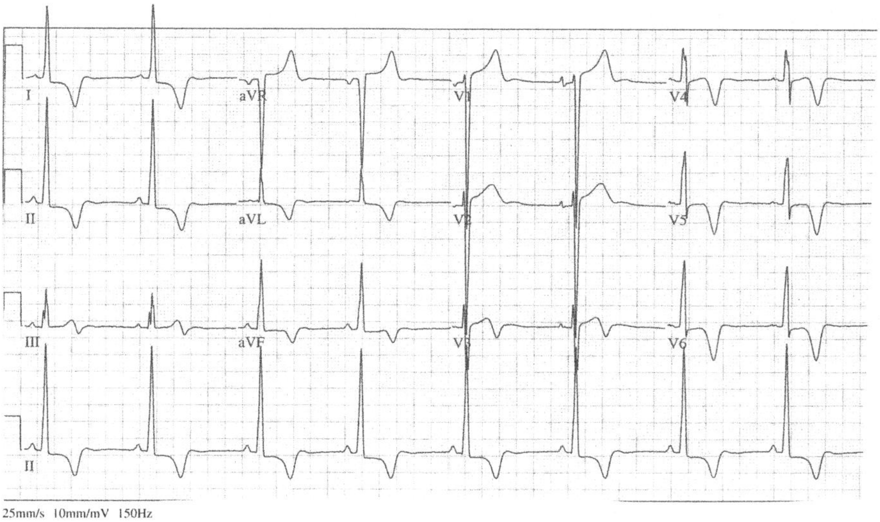

Fig. 5.25
Electrocardiogram of a 40-year old woman with apical hypertrophic cardiomyopathy and normal coronary arteries

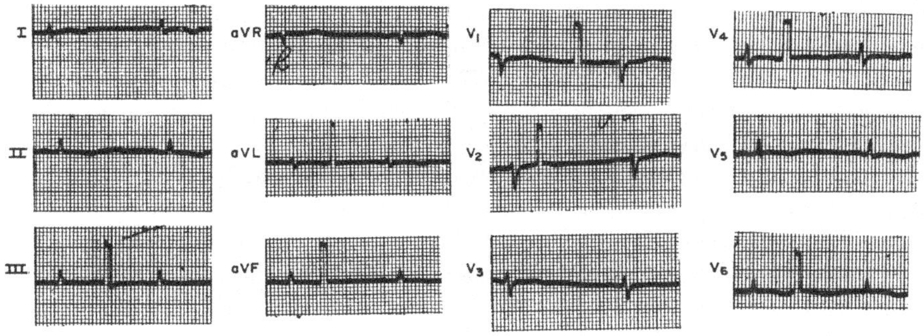

Fig. 5.26
Typical ECG pattern of a patient with untreated myxedema (After Surawicz and Mangiardi, The electrocardiogram in endocrine and metabolic disorders, in *Clinical Electrocardiographic Correlations*, J.E. Rios, Editor. Philadelphia, PA: © Davis, 1977, pp. 243–66. Reproduced with permission)

5.3.6.8 Hypothyroidism

Hypothyroidism usually causes a decrease of T-wave amplitude attributed to the low voltage caused by myxedema (➋ Fig. 5.26). T-wave inversion can also occur, probably owing to pericarditis [42]. The T-wave abnormalities regress within weeks or months after start of specific treatment [42, 173, 174]. Sometimes, however, the abnormalities subside within days or even within 24 h [174]. Rapid regression suggests that at least in some cases, the T-wave abnormalities in hypothyroidism may be related to abnormal function of the autonomic nervous system rather than to the effect of myxedema on the myocardium or to pericarditis.

5.3.6.9 T-Wave Abnormalities Attributed to Fear, Anxiety, and Nervous Tension

Fear, especially fear of operation [175], anxiety, worry, or longing suggested by hypnosis, and other emotional factors may produce T-wave abnormalities in persons without heart disease. Berman et al. found lowering or inversion of the T wave in 5 of 14 normal persons in an anxiety fear situation induced by hypnotic suggestion [176]. These abnormalities have usually been associated with tachycardia. Ljung attributed T-wave abnormalities induced by "fright" to hyperventilation [177]. Others ascribed the T-wave changes produced by fear and anxiety to sympathetic stimulation [175] or to abnormal "sensitivity" of the myocardium to adrenaline [178]. It has been shown that T-wave abnormalities in anxious patients may disappear after reassurance and rest, even without change in heart rate [179].

Several studies reported T-wave abnormalities in a vaguely defined syndrome of neurocirculatory asthenia (NCA) characterized by tachycardia, hyperventilation, labile blood pressure, and low effort tolerance. However, it has been shown conclusively that NCA is not associated with a characteristic ECG pattern [180–184]. In many patients with NCA, abnormal T waves are associated with tachycardia and therefore may arise from excessive sympathetic stimulation [185], but sometimes T-wave abnormalities appear when the heart rate is slow and disappear when the rate increases following the administration of nitrates and atropine, or when the subject is in an upright position [105].

5.3.6.10 Transient T-Wave Abnormalities Arising from Extracardiac Factors

This category of T-wave abnormalities includes changes attributed to transient asynchrony of repolarization produced by a variety of factors acting on a normal or an abnormal heart.

Hyperventilation

In the author's study, hyperventilation (HV) produced T-wave inversion in at least one of several simultaneously recorded ECG leads in 73% of randomly selected healthy students. In some of the author's subjects, T-wave abnormalities were more pronounced after 20 s than after 60 s of HV (➋ Fig. 5.27). Others reported similar observations [186, 187]. The study of Biberman et al. suggests that the true incidence of T-wave abnormalities during HV may be underestimated unless multiple ECG leads are monitored during the HV [188].

The study of Biberman et al. showed that the T-wave abnormalities produced by HV could not be attributed to alkalosis [188], changes in plasma sodium, potassium, calcium, or magnesium concentrations, or changes in heart position. The T-wave abnormalities produced by HV were always accompanied by tachycardia but could not be attributed solely to a critical increase in heart rate. This conclusion is in agreement with previous studies in which the T wave became inverted after HV but remained upright when tachycardia was induced by exercise [189, 190], intravenous administration of propantheline [190], or breathing air containing 5% CO_2 [191, 192].

The transient T-wave inversion that occurs during HV was similar to the transient T-wave abnormalities produced by isoproterenol infusion [190]. The T-wave abnormalities produced by HV were attributed to an asynchronous shortening of ventricular repolarization during the early phase of sympathetic stimulation [190]. In keeping with this hypothesis are the observations that T-wave abnormalities produced by HV can be prevented by pretreatment with propranolol [193, 194], and that the suppression of T-wave abnormalities by propranolol is not attributable to the prevention of tachycardia because after the administration of atropine with propranolol, the heart rate increased but the T wave remained upright [195].

Orthostatic Abnormalities

In the upright position, ventricular gradient decreases, QRST angle widens [193], and T-wave changes occur in the majority of normal young individuals [194]. However, the incidence of unequivocal orthostatic T-wave abnormalities varies in different patient groups. Lepeschkin and Surawicz found an abnormal orthostatic ECG only in 3% of individuals with a negative exercise test but in 30% of persons with junctional ST depression and in 23% of patients with ischemic heart disease and positive exercise tests [41]. In patients with NCA, orthostatic T-wave abnormalities occurred in 63% of women and 30% of men [185].

Transient orthostatic T-wave abnormalities have been attributed to increased sympathetic activity [184]. This hypothesis is supported by the observation that adrenergic blockade increases the ventricular gradient and decreases the QRST

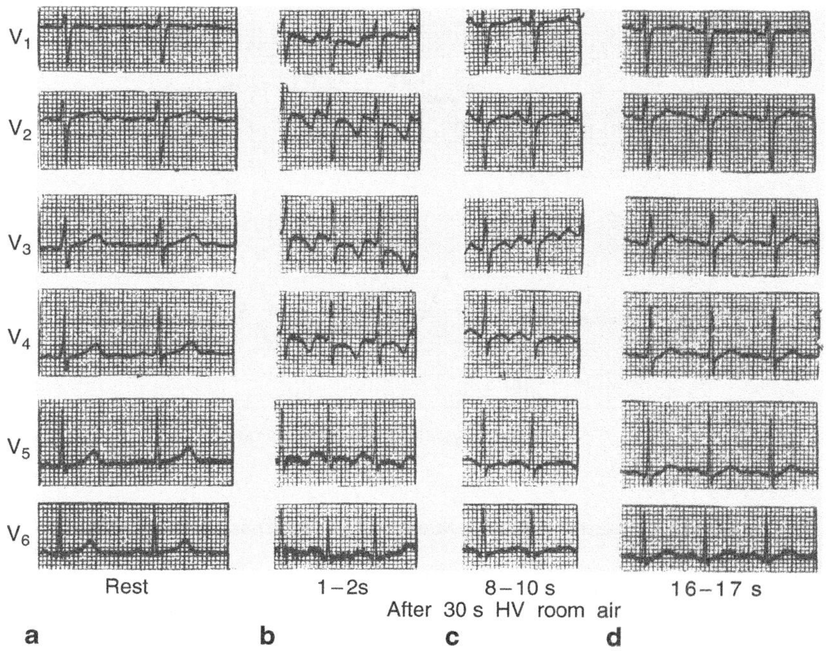

Fig. 5.27
Simultaneously recorded ECG leads V_1–V_6 (paper speed 25 m ms^{-1}) in a 21-year old student. (a) control, before hyperventilation (HV): R–R = 85, QT = 38, QT_c = 41; (b) during first 2 s after 30 s of HV: R–R = 44, QT = 32, QT_c = 48; (c) during 8th and 10th second: R–R = 44, QT = 30, QT_c = 45; (d) during 16th to 17th second: R–R = 56, QT = 32, QT_c = 43. Note that the R–R intervals in (b) and (c) are the same, but in (c) the QT and QTc intervals are shorter and the T waves less inverted (After Biberman et al. [188]. © Mosby, St Louis, Missouri. Reproduced with permission)

angle in the upright position [193]. Similarly, intravenous administration of propranolol prevents orthostatic T-wave abnormalities [196–198]. Propranolol blocks an increase in heart rate that occurs after standing up, but the suppression of the orthostatic T-wave changes is apparently not solely a result of the decrease in heart rate [196].

Postprandial Abnormalities

A decrease in T-wave amplitude or T-wave inversion in leads I, II, V_2–V_4 occurs frequently within 30 min after a meal of about 1,200 calories [199]. Postprandial T-wave abnormalities occurred in 3.9% of 2,000 young healthy airmen [200]. These abnormalities may arise from lowering of plasma K^+ concentration, tachycardia, and possibly sympathetic stimulation. It has been shown that various nonspecific T-wave abnormalities frequently disappear when the ECG is recorded after fasting [201].

Postextrasystolic Abnormalities

The cause of occasional primary T-wave changes in the first and sometimes also in the second or third postextrasystolic beats is not known (➋ Fig. 5.28). Asynchrony of repolarization has been suggested as the cause in a case of postextrasystolic T-wave inversion associated with prolongation of QT interval [202]. The postextrasystolic T-wave changes apparently occur more frequently in patients with heart disease than in normal persons [202–204], but the reason for this association is not obvious.

Post-tachycardia Abnormalities

In about 20% of patients with paroxysmal tachycardia, the normal T wave becomes inverted for hours or days after the termination of the attack [42] or interruption of tachycardia by ablation. This may occur after ventricular [205] or

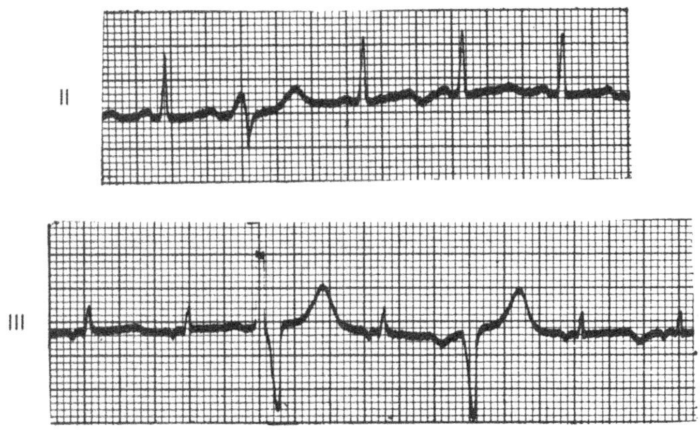

Fig. 5.28
Postextrasystolic T-wave inversion in a person with no evidence of heart disease and a normal ECG except for ventricular premature complexes

supraventricular tachycardias [206], and is unrelated to the age of the patient or to the presence or absence of heart disease. In a 21-year-old patient with normal hemodynamic findings and a normal coronary arteriogram, T-wave inversion in leads II, III, and V_3–V_6 persisted for 19 days after termination of a tachycardia [206]. The cause of the long duration of the "post-tachycardia syndrome" is not clear, but the abnormalities usually persist longer than would be expected on the basis of physiological adjustment to the new rate.

Induced and Accidental Hypothermia: Cooling of the Posterior Wall of the Heart

Profound hypothermia alters depolarization and repolarization, but moderate hypothermia may produce T-wave abnormalities without appreciable QRS changes. Homogeneous cooling of the entire heart causes the expected increase in the T-wave duration without change in polarity. Such patterns have been observed in patients with accidental hypothermia [207]. Cooling the posterior wall of the heart by drinking iced water usually produces deviation of the T-wave vector anteriorly and superiorly with the resulting T-wave inversion in leads II and III [42]. This effect is a result of the local prolongation of repolarization in the cooled area of the ventricle.

Abnormalities Produced by Injection of Contrast into Coronary Arteries

Injection of ionic contrast into coronary arteries produces transient prolongation of the QT_c interval and changes in the T-wave morphology. These T-wave changes are sometimes associated with prolongation of the QRS complex, but in most cases they are primary. As a rule, the T-wave vector is directed away from the area perfused by the contrast [208, 209]. These T-wave changes have been attributed to the regional prolongation of repolarization caused by the high sodium concentration in the contrast medium [210], or the medium's calcium-binding properties [211]. The author and coworkers have shown that transient T-wave abnormalities, which occur during injection of the contrast into the right coronary artery, were associated with prolongation of the ventricular MAP in the right ventricle without changes in the MAP in the left ventricle [3] (➔ Fig. 5.29).

Abnormalities Produced by Ventricular Pacing

Ventricular pacing frequently produces T-wave inversion in the nonpaced sinus impulses. These T-wave changes occur without changes in the QRS duration. The T-wave abnormalities increase with increased duration of pacing and the amount of energy used for pacing [212, 213]. The site of stimulation determines the vector of the T wave. After pacing the endocardial surface of the right ventricle or the epicardial surface and the apex of the left ventricle, abnormal T waves appear predominantly in leads II, III, and V_3–V_5 but after pacing the right ventricular outflow tract, the T-wave inversions

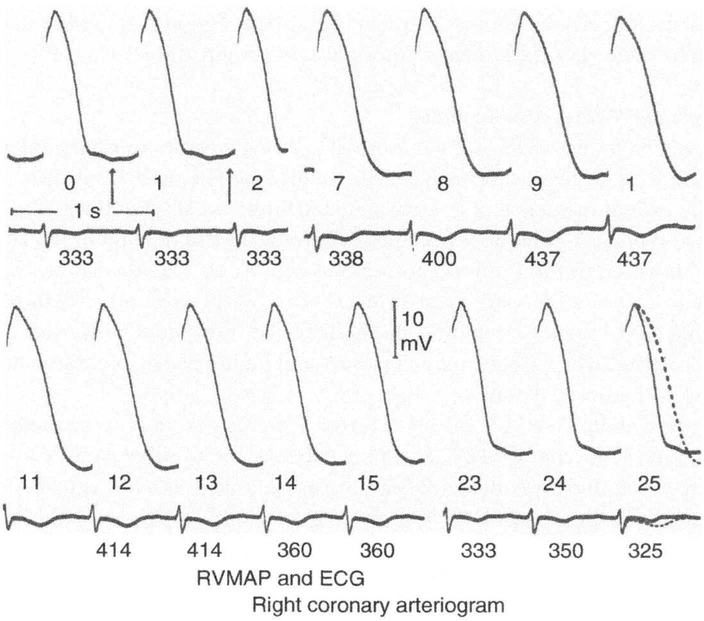

Fig. 5.29
Right ventricular monophasic action potential (TVMAP) and lead II recorded during injection of 4 ml of 75% Hypaque (diatrizoate) into the right coronary artery. Arrows mark the onset and end of the injection. The consecutive 25 beats after the injection are numbered. The numbers under the T wave represent the QT intervals in milliseconds. See text for further discussion. The MAP and electrocardiogram of the tenth beat are superimposed on those of the 25th beat (After Shabetai et al. [3]. © American Heart Association, Dallas, Texas. Reproduced with permission)

occur mainly in leads V_1 and V_2 [212]. Recently, Shvilkin et al. [214] reported that a combination of positive T wave in aVL, positive or isoelectric T wave in lead I, and maximal T-wave inversion in precordial leads greater than T-wave inversion in lead III was 92% sensitive and 100% specific for postpacing T-wave changes. The duration of the T-wave abnormalities after pacing depends on the duration of pacing. In some cases, T-wave abnormalities persisted for 1 or 2 years after the termination of pacing. T-wave changes do not appear after atrial pacing or after ventricular pacing during the ventricular refractory period [214]. Thus, the T-wave abnormalities appear to be related to the presence of abnormal depolarization in the stimulated area. It may be assumed that T-wave abnormalities are produced by prolongation of repolarization in the vicinity of the pacing electrode, but the mechanism of such prolongation is unknown. It has been reported that T-wave abnormalities produced by pacing are not reversible after oral administration of potassium or after an increase in heart rate with isoproterenol.

Abnormalities Following Preexcitation and Left Bundle Branch Block. Cardiac "Memory"

Transient T-wave abnormalities have been found in patients with intermittent preexcitation [215–217] and intermittent left bundle branch block [218, 219]. These abnormalities apparently persist for a variable amount of time after the disappearance of the left bundle branch block or preexcitation pattern respectively. Similar abnormalities have not been recorded in patients with intermittent right bundle branch block. The most consistent and conspicuous T-wave abnormality after disappearance of a left bundle branch block pattern has been recorded in right precordial leads [219–221], but in one study [219], abnormalities in the limb leads were present also in approximately 50% of patients. The natural history of this phenomenon has not been studied adequately and the clinical significance of such T-wave abnormalities is debatable [219]. The appearance of primary T-wave abnormalities following cessation of pacing, normalization of intraventricular conduction, and disappearance of secondary T-wave abnormalities has been considered by Rosenbaum et al. as a possible manifestation of repolarization "memory" [213]. This hypothesis implies that the abnormal sequence of activation is "remembered" following the return of a normal activation pattern.

Normal Variants and Unexplained T-Wave Abnormalities

T-wave abnormalities have been found in 0.5–4.2% of normal persons in various population groups [82, 221, 222]. The largest group of individuals without heart disease has been studied by Hiss and Lamb [82]. In their study of 122,043 men, aged 16–50 years, the overall incidence of T-wave abnormalities was 11.5/1,000 with the highest incidence in the youngest and the oldest age groups. T-wave abnormalities occurred most frequently in the lateral precordial leads and least frequently in lead I. However, in the studies reported by Fisch, ST or T abnormalities were absent in 776 normal individuals below the age of 25 years but were present in 15.7% of 671 persons older than 65 years [223]. A study of 12 asymptomatic men, aged 18–19 years, selected on the basis of flat, notched, or inverted T waves in the precordial leads, showed that this group had higher systolic blood pressure and higher plasma noradrenaline concentration than an age-matched control group with normal T waves [224].

Major unexplained T-wave abnormalities – deeply inverted T waves – were observed in about 2 out of 1,000 [225], and 7 out of 1,000 patients [84] in two large groups of hospital patients, and in about 4 out of 1,000 in a large group of life-insurance applicants. Pruitt et al. found no evidence of heart disease in 3 of 62 patients with deeply inverted (at least 5 mm) T waves [226]. Life-insurance statistics report a 226% increase in mortality in persons with major T-wave abnormalities and a 166% increase in mortality in persons with minor T-wave abnormalities [85]. This increased mortality suggests that a group of persons with isolated T-wave abnormalities may represent a mixture of persons with abnormalities unrelated to heart disease and persons with clinically silent or "atypical" ischemic heart disease [83].

5.3.6.11 Tests Employed in the Recognition of Rapidly Reversible T-Wave Abnormalities

This discussion will be limited to the methods used in the differential diagnosis of primary T-wave abnormalities attributed to nonhomogeneous repolarization. These abnormalities may be arbitrarily divided into three types:

1. Rate-dependent abnormalities associated with normal or slow heart rate,
2. Rate-dependent abnormalities associated with rapid heart rate, and
3. Abnormalities independent of heart rate.

Detection of T-Wave Abnormalities Associated with Normal or Slow Heart Rate

In certain patients without heart disease, primary T-wave abnormalities appear only at normal or slow heart rates and disappear after a certain critical increase in rate. Several patients have been observed in whom primary negative T waves became upright after a certain critical increase of heart rate with exercise, hyperventilation, pacing, and administration of atropine or isoproterenol. This type of purely rate-dependent T-wave abnormality can be identified most conclusively with atrial pacing while the effects of exercise, hyperventilation, and isoproterenol may be attributed to the sympathetic stimulation, and the effects of atropine on the vagolytic action of the drug. It has been suggested that T-wave abnormalities, which disappear after the administration of vagolytic drugs, are caused by vagal reflex [227, 228]. However, the suppression of T-wave abnormalities by atropine or Pro-Banthine is more likely to be a result of a nonspecific increase in heart rate rather than to the specific vagolytic action of the drug. The vagolytic drugs do not exert a specific effect on normal repolarization. In persons with normal T waves, atropine decreases the T-wave amplitude [229], but this decrease is proportional to the increase in heart rate [230] and, therefore, is probably caused by tachycardia. Although in some patients with nonspecific T-wave abnormalities atropine may reverse the abnormality, in the majority of patients atropine either does not change or may even exaggerate the abnormal T-wave pattern [70, 231].

Detection of T-Wave Abnormalities Associated with Rapid Heart Rate

Various nonspecific T-wave abnormalities are frequently associated with tachycardia and disappear when the heart rate becomes slower. The effect of sympatholytic drugs on the T wave may be in part owing to the slowing of heart rate. Numerous studies have shown that certain T-wave abnormalities may be abolished by the administration of ergotamine, dihydroergotamine, or propranolol. It has been reported that the intravenous administration of 10–20 mg propranolol abolishes ST and T abnormalities at rest and prevents the orthostatic and exercise-induced changes in patients without heart disease but not in patients with T-wave abnormalities arising from myocardial ischemia or myocarditis [199]. Beta-blocking agents decrease heart rate but their effect on the orthostatic and hyperventilation-induced T-wave abnormalities is apparently not exclusively owing to the slowing of the heart rate [193, 195].

Detection of Rapidly Reversible Rate-Independent T-Wave Abnormalities

Administration of Potassium Salts

A moderate increase in the concentration of potassium can change an abnormally low or a negative T wave into an upright T wave without change in heart rate. Several investigators have administered about 10 g of potassium salts orally in order to differentiate the T-wave abnormalities produced by structural heart diseases from various functional and nonspecific abnormalities. This procedure may be diagnostically useful because oral administration of potassium does not alter the angle between the mean spatial QRS and T-wave vector in persons with a normal T wave and in patients with myocardial infarction or left ventricular hypertrophy. However, potassium restores to normal the QRST angle in persons with T-wave abnormalities, which are not a result of heart disease. The administration of potassium salts in order to differentiate functional abnormalities from abnormalities arising from organic disease is apparently not safe because ventricular tachycardia, ventricular fibrillation, and asystole have been reported to follow such tests [2].

Administration of Isoproterenol

In persons with normal T waves, isoproterenol (ISP) administered at a rate of 3–6 mcg min^{-1} for 4–6 min produced a biphasic effect [188]. During the early phase of the infusion, the T-wave amplitude decreased in all subjects, and in 10 of 11, the previously upright T wave became negative in one or more of leads I, II, or V_3–V_6. The maximum T-wave inversion usually occurred 30–40 s after beginning the ISP infusion. Subsequently, the T wave became upright and the U-wave amplitude increased. After approximately 2 min of ISP infusion, the T-wave amplitude was similar to the control and in some cases even greater than before the ISP infusion. The initial decrease of T-wave amplitude was always associated with an increase in heart rate but without an appreciable change in QT interval. As a result, the QT_c interval was increased. The subsequent increase of T-wave amplitude was associated with a significant decrease in QT and QT_c intervals but an insignificant decrease in the R–R interval. Accordingly, the T-wave inversion was associated with the hysteresis of the QT interval (➲ Fig. 5.30). This was attributed to an asynchronous shortening of ventricular repolarization.

The effect of ISP on the sequence of normal repolarization suggested to Daoud et al. that it may be of interest to study the effect of the drug on the abnormal T wave. Isoproterenol was administered at the rate of 2–6 μg min^{-1} for 30–90 s to 80 patients with various types of T-wave abnormalities. The ISP infusion increased the heart rate by 27–55 (average 37) beats min^{-1} [70]. In patients with secondary T-wave abnormalities arising from hypertrophy and bundle branch block and in patients with primary T-wave abnormalities after myocardial infarction or pericarditis, administration of ISP altered only the amplitude and not the polarity of the T wave. In these patients, the ISP effect was similar to the effect of tachycardia produced by atropine or pacing [93]. However, in patients with various primary T-wave abnormalities and a normal QRS complex, ISP transiently shifted the abnormal T-wave vector to the left and anteriorly by 60–180° and "normalized" the ECG (➲ Fig. 5.31).

Our studies favor the hypothesis that ISP reverses the primary T-wave abnormalities by an asynchronous shortening of the AP. The effect of ISP on ventricular repolarization is probably a result of beta adrenergic stimulation because it can be blocked by pronethalol without any changes in heart rate [232]. Our studies suggest that the rapidly reversible primary T-wave abnormalities probably result from some regional deficiency of sympathetic stimulation and that ISP has a greater absolute shortening effect on AP in the areas with deficient stimulation than in the areas with normal responses to sympathetic stimulation. This hypothesis is supported by our studies in dogs, which showed that ISP changed T-wave polarity and restored the control T-wave configurations after both left stellate-ganglion transection and right stellate-ganglion stimulation. In each case, ISP produced unequal shortening of the MAP on the anterior and posterior walls of the ventricle and thereby restored the normal relation between their durations. After left stellate-ganglion transection, ISP shortened the previously prolonged MAP more than it did the control MAP; after right stellate-ganglion stimulation, ISP shortened the control MAP more than the previously shortened MAP [25] (➲ Fig. 5.32).

If the results of our experiments in dogs are applicable to man, normalization of the T wave after the administration of ISP may be expected in all cases of primary T-wave changes induced by regional shortening of ventricular APs or regional lengthening of ventricular APs provided that the latter are susceptible to the shortening effect of the drug. We assume that

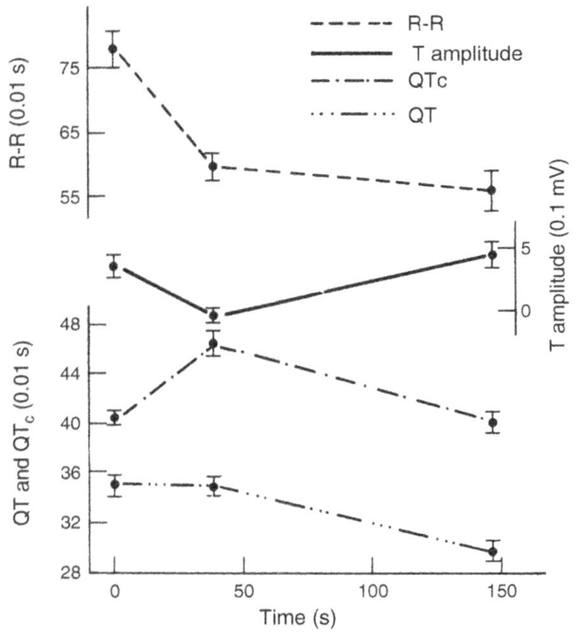

Fig. 5.30
Changes in R–R, T amplitude, QT, and QT_c during isoproterenol administration to 11 healthy volunteers. Each point designates the mean value, and each vertical bar, the standard error (After Biberman et al. [188]. © Mosby, St Louis, Missouri. Reproduced with permission)

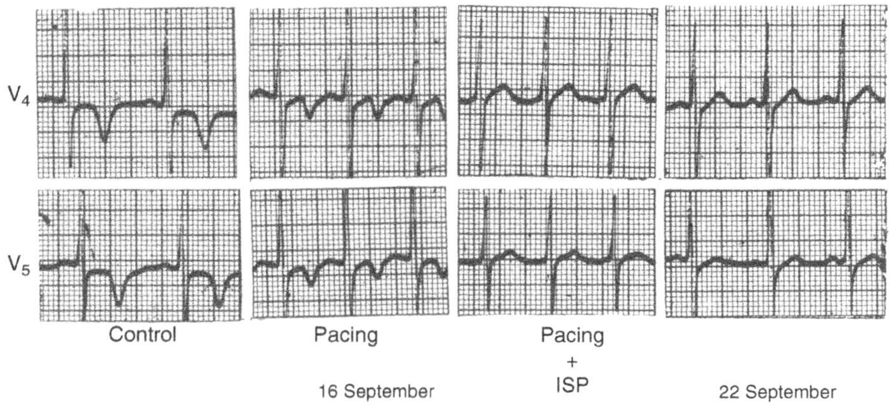

Fig. 5.31
Electrocardiogram of a 55-year old man with diabetes mellitus, increased left ventricular end-diastolic pressure, and normal coronary arteriogram, before (control), during atrial pacing, and during pacing and isoproterenol (ISP) infusion. Note the effect of ISP on the T wave. The QT interval during pacing with isoproterenol is 34, and without isoproterenol is 32 (After Daoud et al. [70]. © Yorke Medical Group, Magazine Division, New York. Reproduced with permission)

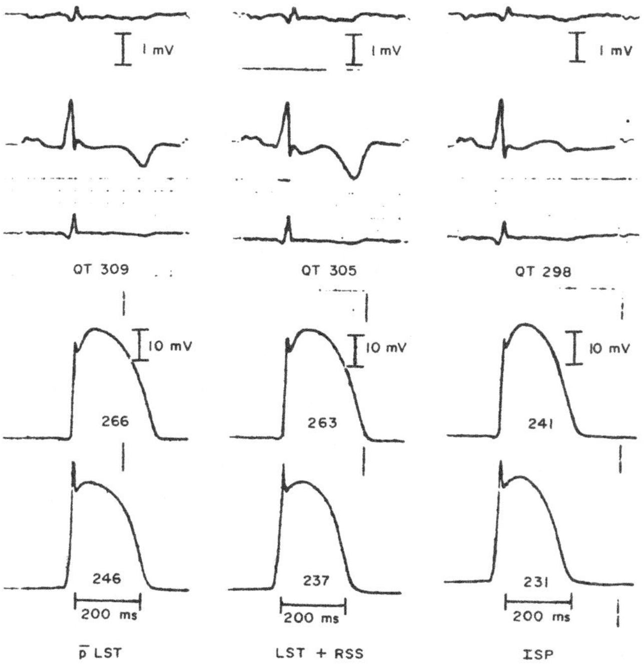

Fig. 5.32
From *top to bottom*, leads *X*, *Y*, and *Z* and MAP on the posterior and anterior walls of the left ventricle. Effects of left ventricular stellate-ganglion transection (LST) alone (*left panel*), subsequent right stellate-ganglion stimulation (RSS) (*middle panel*), and the administration of isoproterenol (ISP) (3 μg) after right stellate-ganglion stimulation (*right panel*). See text for further discussion (After Kuo and Surawicz [76]. © Yorke Medical Group, Magazines Division, New York. Reproduced with permission)

one or both of these two mechanisms account for the high incidence of isoproterenol-induced T-wave normalization in persons with T-wave abnormalities of diverse origins and with different QT intervals [70].Conversely, the lack of T-wave normalization in patients after myocardial infarction or pericarditis [70] may be attributed to an inadequate shortening effect of isoproterenol on the abnormally prolonged APs [232]. The effect of sympathetic stimulation on reversal of T-wave polarity from negative to positive is not limited to isoproterenol. It is seen often during exercise, e.g., during stress tests in the absence of myocardial ischemia. Similarly during dobutamine infusion T-wave normalization is reported to indicate viable myocardium in patients after recent myocardial infarction [233].

5.3.7 T Wave Alternans

Electrical and mechanical alternans may be concurrent or dissociated from each other. At the cellular level, mechanical alternans in the ventricular myocardium is usually accompanied by an alternating shape of the ventricular action potential. T-wave alternans is usually associated with a long QT interval [234–237]. In the majority of published cases, the alternating T wave occupied nearly the entire diastolic interval [234–239].

Also, T-wave alternans experimentally produced by stellate-ganglion stimulation in anesthetized and vagotomized cats [235], or by hypocalcemia in dogs [240, 241], was associated with prolonged QT interval.

Lepeschkin suggested that T-wave alternans was a result of the alternans of ventricular AP associated with alternation of the diastolic intervals [242]. A close proximity to preceding repolarization exerts a shortening effect on AP duration [243]. Consequently, the diastolic interval after a short AP increases and the AP becomes longer. In the author's laboratory, T-wave alternans occurred simultaneously with ventricular AP alternans in the isolated perfused rabbit heart when the

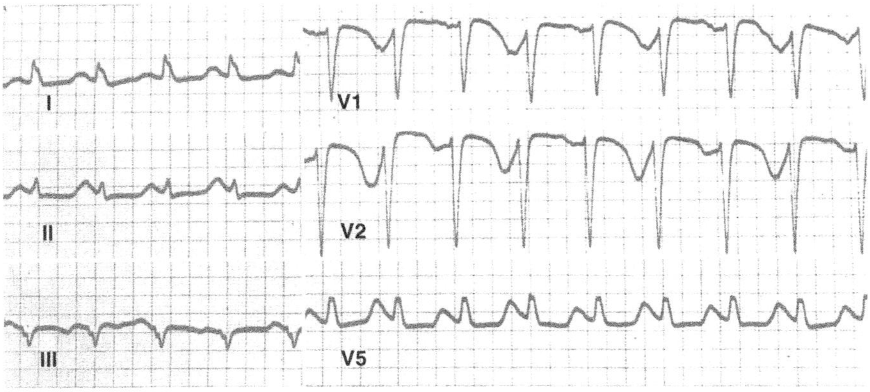

Fig. 5.33
T-wave alternans in a 60-year old woman with severe hypocalcemia and history of hypocalcemic tetany (From Aravindakshan and Surawicz B et al. [246] © Elsevier, Inc. Reproduced with permission)

AP duration was prolonged by cooling quinidine or a combination of hypocalcemia and hypokalemia. In each case, the mechanism suggested by Lepeschkin [241] could account for the T-wave alternans. However, this may not be the only mechanism of T-wave alternans since experimental T-wave alternans can occur in the absence of appreciable QT lengthening, and conversely, alternans of the AP duration cannot always be explained by alternans of the diastolic intervals (personal observations and examples given by Kleinfeld et al. [244].

T-wave alternans depends on critical shortening of the diastolic interval when the duration of the ventricular AP exceeds the cycle length. Therefore a QT interval occupying nearly the entire cycle length can be seen in many cases of repolarization alternans associated with a long QT interval (Fig. 5.33). T-wave alternans with a long QT has been reported in some of the following conditions: congenital long-QT syndrome, hypocalcemia, treatment with quinidine, hypokalemia, hypokalemia with hypocalcemia, and hypomagnesemia and after defibrillation. It may also be unexplained.

In addition to the manifest alternans, on the ECG, subtle alternans forms may become detectable by digital processing techniques. It has been shown that these subtle forms of alternans are associated with increased susceptibility to inducible ventricular tachyarrhythmias in patients with coronary artery disease and nonischemic cardiomyopathy and therefore may represent a noninvasive marker of electrical instability [245].

5.3.8 ST–T Abnormalities

As a result of the differences in the underlying mechanisms, the behavior of the ST segment and of the T wave differ under a variety of conditions discussed earlier. For example, hypocalcemia usually causes lengthening of the ST segment without T-wave changes. Conversely, moderate hyperkalemia causes T-wave changes without appreciable change of ST segment duration. Although myocardial ischemia frequently produces both ST segment and T-wave changes, our studies have shown that during exercise, the behavior of the T wave bears no relation to the behavior of the ST segment [246].

In spite of the fundamental differences in the genesis of the ST segment and the T wave, electrocardiographers frequently use the expression ST–T changes to describe the patterns associated with the alterations of these two repolarization components. One of the reasons for using this definition is the lack of a distinct point of demarcation between the end of the ST segment and the onset of T wave. Another reason is a common occurrence of concomitant ST and T-wave abnormalities associated with either the secondary repolarization abnormalities such as left ventricular hypertrophy or left bundle branch block (Fig. 5.3c), or the primary repolarization abnormalities caused by shortening of the plateau of the ventricular AP; for example, tachycardia, digitalis, or hypokalemia (Fig. 5.3c). Nevertheless, it is the author's opinion that in many cases the electrocardiographic diagnosis gains in precision when the ST segment, the T wave, and also the U wave are analyzed as separate components rather than as an expression of an integrated process of "repolarization."

5.3.9 Prognostic Value of the Descriptors of T-Wave Morphology

Numerous studies in the recent literature have explored the prognostic value of various computerized descriptors of T-wave characteristics, e.g., morphology analysis [246], heterogeneity of ventricular repolarization [247], principal components of the T-wave vector loop [248], and spatial T-wave deviation [249, 250]. The clinical usefulness of these analyses will depend on their comparison with more conventional electrocardiographic and clinical parameters.

5.4 U Wave

The purpose of this section is to review briefly some concepts of U-wave genesis and the clinical significance of this ECG deflection, which owes its designation to Einthoven. Compared to other components of the ECG, the U wave has been less intensely investigated and its mechanism is still poorly understood [251]. Some of the reasons for this are its low amplitude, the difficulty of separating it from the T wave and/or the P wave, particularly at rapid rates, and its uncertain clinical significance. The experimental animal models are also difficult to interpret because various diastolic deflections recorded in local electrograms do not necessarily have the same timing as the U wave recorded in the human surface ECG.

5.4.1 Identification of the U Wave

This discussion will be limited to a deflection, which is usually detectable at slow or moderate heart rates in the surface ECG [252]. It is inscribed during protodiastole; that is, it coincides with the isovolumic relaxation. The interval between the end of the T wave and the apex of the U wave is usually about 100 ms. It is of interest that this interval is little affected by the heart rate [6].

The distinction between the U wave and the T wave may become difficult when the T wave is notched, diphasic, or prolonged. In such cases, various degrees of fusion between the T wave and the U wave may occur. In hypokalemia, the initial portion of ventricular repolarization (phase 2) is shortened and the terminal portion (phase 3) is prolonged. These changes result in the disappearance of the isolelectric ST segment, obliteration of the apex of the T wave, and a shift of the major repolarization deflection toward early diastole. It appears that the U wave proper becomes fused with this repolarization component and evolves into the largest deflection during repolarization. If the notch between T and U persists, the QT interval is not prolonged. A complete fusion results in a large T+U complex. In cases with true QT prolongation caused by delayed repolarization in certain portions of the myocardium, the T wave also merges with the U wave but the resulting T–U deflection has a different configuration from the T–U complexes during hypokalemia. This occurs because instead of lifting the U wave to prominence, the T wave tends to encroach upon the U wave, which becomes less distinct or unrecognizable. Thus, differences in the morphology of the T+U complex reveal the differences in the pathogenesis. However, in most cases in clinical electrocardiography, the T wave can be distinguished from the U wave using published and suggested maneuvers [253]. Among these, timing the apices of the waves in question, correlation with the second sound, or incisura of the arterial pulse, and in some cases, the administration of calcium salts intravenously, tend to be most helpful [253].

5.4.2 Relation Between the U Wave and Other Deflections of the ECG

In a number of patients with left ventricular hypertrophy, the U wave is inverted in the left precordial leads. Frequently, when the blood pressure of these patients is lowered, the U wave becomes upright; this is usually associated with a decrease in the QRS amplitude. Similarly, in acute myocardial ischemia during exercise, an increase in QRS amplitude and U-wave inversion frequently occur simultaneously. In these cases, the common cause of increased QRS amplitude and the U-wave inversion may be the increase in the intracardiac blood volume

In both left and right ventricular hypertrophy (LVH and RVH, respectively), the axis of the U wave tends to be directed opposite to the main QRS axis; that is, the U wave is negative in the left precordial leads in LVH and negative in the right precordial leads in RVH. Typically, in such cases, the U-wave vector parallels that of the T wave. In some cases of LVH, the U wave is inverted in the leads where the T wave is upright. The independent behaviors of the T wave and U wave also become obvious during transient changes in T-wave polarity associated with myocardial ischemia or changes in systemic vascular resistance.

5.4.3 ST Segment

Ordinarily, the U wave shows no correlation with the ST segment but during acute ischemia or development of the left ventricular "strain" pattern, ST depression and U-wave inversion may occur concomitantly.

5.4.4 U-Wave Amplitude

The U-wave amplitude tends to be inversely proportional to the R–R interval. At heart rates exceeding about 90–100 min^{-1}, the U wave becomes indistinct [252]. Its amplitude is increased by interventions associated with positive inotropic effect, such as catecholamines, hypercalcemia, and digitalis. As mentioned above, a prolonged phase 3 of the ventricular AP, e.g., during hypokalemia or quinidine administration, increases the U-wave amplitude. Presumably, this is by superposition of the U wave on the repolarization potentials inscribed during the late portion of the prolonged AP. The U-wave amplitude is diminished during tachycardia and hyperkalemia. A negative inotropic effect appears to cause a decrease in U-wave amplitude. In hypocalcemia, the U wave is not detectable but the cause is difficult to determine because of the prolonged QT interval.

5.4.5 The Negative U Wave

The negative U wave seldom occurs in the absence of heart disease or other electrocardiographical abnormalities. Holzmann and Zurukzoglu [254] found that 197 of 200 patients with a negative U wave had heart disease. Of 100 patients reported by Ameur-Hendrich et al. [255], 99 had heart disease and 1 had anemia.

In the study of Kishida et al. of 488 patients with a negative U wave, this was the only electrocardiographic abnormality in 25 (5.1%) of patients [256]. In an additional 34 (7%) of the patients, the electrocardiogram was normal at rest and became abnormal after exercise. In the study of Holzmann and Zurukzoglu [254], the U wave was the only abnormality in 19.5% of their patients, most of whom had hypertension. In patients with hypertension, a negative U wave was the only abnormality in 9 out of 45 patients in the study of Georgopoulos et al. [257], and in 1 out of 66 in the study of Kemp et al. [258]. The above studies refer to patients with purely negative U waves only. Lambert included patients with a depressed T–U junction and diphasic U wave but this apparently did not decrease the specificity of the pattern since all but 3 of 245 patients had organic heart disease [259].

U-wave inversion has also been reported during attacks of variant angina [260]. In a study of 38 patients in whom angina was induced by ergonovine maleate, transient U-wave inversion was apparent in 17 with ST elevation in the precordial leads but only 3 of 21 with ST elevation in the inferior leads. In the 17 subjects who had spasm of the LAD coronary artery, the lead that most frequently exhibited U-wave inversion was V_4 (94%), which also showed ST elevation in 82%. In this study, negative U waves frequently occurred without ST elevation. This caused the authors to suggest that such a finding may be a result of ischemia in areas marginal to the central ischemic zone or of recovery from temporary ischemia.

With respect to exercise testing, it was shown that U-wave inversion could be induced in patients with stenosis of the LAD coronary artery [261]. The sensitivity was low at 21% but the specificity was high, being 93%.

In the study of Kishida et al. [256], systemic hypertension was the primary diagnosis in the largest number of patients (➋ Table 5.3).

Previous studies have shown that, in patients with hypertension, the regression of U-wave inversion was associated with lowering of blood pressure [257, 258]. Kishida et al. [256] reviewed the records of 130 patients in whom the U wave changed polarity from negative to positive or vice versa in the same lead within a period of less than 1 year (➋ Fig. 5.34). In 107 patients, the change from a negative to a positive U wave occurred during the course of medical treatment, and in 23 patients, the change in polarity occurred after a surgical procedure; in 9 within 1 week after kidney transplantation; in

Table 5.3
Primary clinical diagnosis of 488 patients with a negative U wave

	Total[a]	Percentage
Valvular heart disease	75 (48)	15.4
Pure aortic	43 (25)[b]	
Pure mitral	15 (12)[c]	
Combined aortic and mitral	17 (11)[d]	
Congenital heart disease	12 (9)	2.5
Coronary artery disease	162 (33)	33.2
Myocardial infarction; acute	7 (0)	
Old	61 (20)	
Angina pectoris	94 (13)	
Hypertension	193 (28)	39.5
Chronic renal failure	43 (14)	
Cerebrovascular disease	8 (0)	
Peripheral vascular disease	23 (1)	
Without above complications	119 (13)	
Primary cardiomyopathy	4 (3)	0.8
Hyperthyroidism	7 (0)	1.4
No manifest heart disease	35 (0)	7.2
	488 (121)	100

[a]Number of patients on digitalis are shown in parentheses
[b]Predominant aortic regurgitation – 35
[c]Predominant mitral regurgitation – 11
[d]Aortic + mitral regurgitation – 10

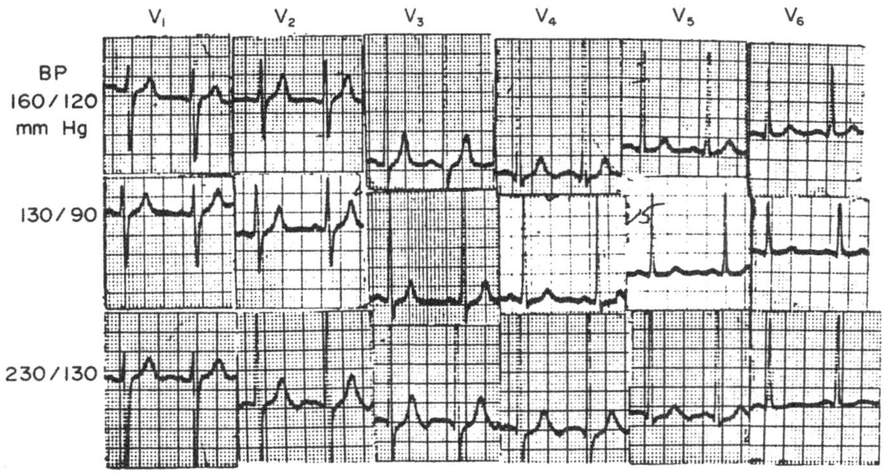

Fig. 5.34
An example of reversible U-wave inversion related to blood-pressure changes in an adult with hypertension. The U wave is negative in leads V_3 and V_4 in the upper row and in leads V_2–V_5 in the lower row. In the middle row, the U wave is isoelectric or positive in all leads, and the QRS amplitude is lower in most leads compared to that in the upper and lower rows. BP denotes the blood pressure (After Kishida et al. [256]. © Yorke Medical Group, Magazines Division, New York. Reproduced with permission)

6 within 1 week after insertion of aortic or mitral valve prosthesis; and in 8 within 1 month after coronary artery-aorta saphenous bypass graft.

In 29 patients with systemic hypertension and a normal QRS duration, the change in U-wave polarity occurred more than once in the course of a follow-up period of less than 1 year. Each appearance of the negative U waves in these patients was associated with a significant increase in systolic and diastolic blood pressure without significant changes in heart rate, QRS duration, or the duration of QT_c, Q–aU_c (aU denotes the U-wave apex), and QU_c intervals.

No consistent change was found in the pattern of T wave or ST segment changes associated with the change in U-wave polarity. These results suggest that changes in U-wave polarity are independent of electrophysiological processes that control the level of the ST segment and the morphology of the T wave. However, these conclusions do not apply to U-wave inversion associated with transient exercise-induced myocardial ischemia since such patients were not included in this group.

The decrease in QRS amplitude accompanying the change from a negative to upright or isoelectric U wave is a consistent finding in patients with hypertensive and valvular heart disease [256]. Fu et al. [262] recorded echocardiograms in hypertensive patients in whom handgrip caused inversion of the U wave as well as an increase in QRS amplitude. They showed that these changes were associated with an increase in left ventricular dimension. These observations implicate left ventricular dilatation as the possible cause of the U-wave inversion and the associated increase in the QRS amplitude. The increase in QRS amplitude in the dilated ventricle may be attributed to the Brody effect resulting from the increase in intracavitary blood volume at the end of diastole. The association between the negative U wave and the increased diastolic dimension or volume of the left ventricle implicates stretch as a possible cause of U-wave inversion [256]. It has been shown that left ventricular relaxation was prolonged in patients with hypertension [263] and either prolonged or incomplete in patients with myocardial ischemia [264]. Abnormalities in ventricular relaxation have also been reported in patients with aortic and mitral regurgitation [265].

5.4.5.1 Timing of the Negative U Wave

Watanabe suggested that the longer duration of the T–aU interval in patients with left bundle branch block favored the Purkinje fiber repolarization theory of U-wave genesis [255]. In our opinion, the delayed appearance of the U wave in relation to ventricular repolarization is of no help in establishing the mechanism of the U wave, because the finding could be owing to either delayed repolarization of the Purkinje fibers in the left ventricle or to delayed relaxation of the left ventricle. The role of prolonged QT_c in the absence of QRS prolongation has been examined. It was observed that patients with a LVH pattern and negative T waves in leads I, aVL, and V_4–V_6 tended to have greater QRS amplitude and a longer QT interval than patients with a less wide QRS–T angle. In this group of patients in whom QRS duration was normal, the U wave appeared later when the QT_c interval was longer. This finding suggests that the timing of the U wave is influenced by the total duration of ventricular repolarization and not by the pattern or duration of ventricular depolarization as suggested by Watanabe [266]. Similar conclusions can be drawn from the study of Ferrero and Maeder [267] who found that the T–aU intervals in patients with right bundle branch block were significantly longer in patients with RVH than in those without hypertrophy or with LVH. This suggests that the delayed U-wave timing was caused by some factors directly related to myocardial hypertrophy, rather than to the delayed activation of the Purkinje fibers.

5.4.6 Theories of U-Wave Genesis

5.4.6.1 Repolarization of Purkinje Fibers

Since the AP duration in the Purkinje fibers is longer than in the ventricular muscle fibers, it has been suspected that the U wave may be caused by the repolarization of Purkinje fibers. One of the difficulties with this concept is the small mass of the conducting tissue. Lepeschkin [268] listed the following observations, which would be difficult to reconcile with the Purkinje fiber theory:

1. Amphibia have U waves but no Purkinje fibers;
2. The configuration of the normal U wave does not conform to the Purkinje fiber repolarization pattern because the descent is longer than the ascent; (➋ Fig. 5.15) and
3. Dependence on mechanical events as exemplified by the relation of the U wave to the preceding P wave during atrioventricular dissociation, bradycardia, postextrasystolic pauses, exercise, digitalis, and catecholamines.

Additional arguments against the Purkinje fiber theory are as follows:

1. The time difference between the end of the T wave and apex of the U wave is nearly constant within the range of heart rates between 60–90 min^{-1}; in this range, the AP duration differences between Purkinje and ventricular fibers should be greater when the rate is slower;
2. In patients with right bundle branch block, the timing of the U wave correlated better with the presence of RVH than with intraventricular conduction [267]; and
3. The results of Kishida et al. [256] showed no consistent difference between the direction of the U-wave vector in the presence of right bundle branch block and left bundle branch block.

5.4.6.2 Ventricular Repolarization Theory

If it is assumed that the U wave arises from a delay in repolarization in some portion of the ventricle, e.g., the papillary muscle, then the corresponding deflection must be designated as a part of the T wave rather than a U wave. However, if the terminal repolarization is prolonged, the U-wave amplitude may be increased owing to superposition of the T wave and U wave. In these cases, the deflection corresponding to the timing of the U wave may become the most prominent component of ventricular repolarization.

5.4.6.3 Mechanoelectrical Coupling

This is the most likely cause of a U wave of normal amplitude. It has been shown that stretch prolongs terminal repolarization in single fibers [269] and therefore may be expected to produce an ECG deflection after the T wave. Its vector may be determined by the sequence of ventricular relaxation. Changes in U-wave polarity may be attributed to changes in the sequence of relaxation. This would explain the mechanism of U-wave inversion in patients with hypertension or aortic regurgitation. In patients with acute ischemia, changes in U-wave polarity may be explained by an abnormal relaxation pattern during protodiastole known as protodiastolic shortening or "aftercontraction."

Recently, further support for a mechanoelectrical mechanism as the cause of inverted U waves has come from Choo and Gibson [270]. They studied the relationship between ECG hypertrophy and ventricular function using M-mode echocardiography and apex cardiography in 73 patients with LVH. Thirty eight of these cases had secondary ST–T changes together with U-wave inversion, 20 had LVH with ST–T changes, and 15 had LVH without ST–T or U-wave changes. The main findings were that U-wave inversion was related to a prolonged isovolumic relaxation period, delayed mitral valve opening relative to minimum cavity dimension, and reduced diastolic wall thinning rate. In the absence of U-wave inversion, LVH with secondary ST–T changes was weakly related to diastolic abnormalities. The authors noted that when U-wave inversion was present, a significant increase in transverse dimension occurred (almost one-third of the total for diastole) during the period between minimum dimension and left ventricular filling. Since the volume was constant during this period, other dimensions must have reduced, "implying the presence of incoordinate relaxation." Thus U-wave inversion appears to be linked to a mechanical event, the latter being thought by Choo and Gibson to be the more likely primary cause, if indeed there is a mechanoelectrical coupling.

Recently, Di Bernardo and Murray explored the hypotheses of U-wave genesis in a computer model of left ventricular repolarization, which exhibited an afterdepolarization. They investigated separately the effect of the amplitude of the afterpotential, dispersion of repolarization, and the timing of the afterpotential relative to the principal component on the 12-leadelectrocardiogram. They found that delaying repolarization in different regions of the heart could not explain the U wave. However, U-wave polarity and other characteristics of the U wave could be explained by the presence of afterpotentials. In their model, U-wave inversion correlated with an abnormal afterpotential timing [271].

Further studies are needed to clarify the genesis of normal and abnormal U waves.

References

1. Surawicz, B., Primary and secondary T wave changes. *Heart Bull.*, 1966;**15**: 31–35.
2. Surawicz, B., The pathogenesis and clinical significance of primary T wave abnormalities, in *Advances in Electrocardiography*, R.C. Schlant and J.W. Hurst, Editors. New York: Grune and Stratton, 1972, 377–421.
3. Shabetai, R., B .Surawicz, and W. Hammill, Monophasic action potentials in man. *Circulation*, 1968;**38**: 341–352.
4. Surawicz, B., E.Lepeschkin, H.C. Herrlich, and B.F. Hoffman, Effect of potassium and calcium deficiency on the monophasic action potential, electrocardiogram and contractility of isolated rabbit hearts. *Am. J. Physiol.*, 1959;**196**: 1302–1307.
5. Gettes, L.S., B. Surawicz, and J.C. Shiue, Effect of high K, low K, and quinidine on QRS duration and ventricular action potential. *Am. J. Physiol.*, 1962;**203**: 1135–1140.
6. Lepeschkin, E. and B. Surawicz, The duration of the Q-U interval and its components in electrocardiograms of normal persons. *Am. Heart J.*, 1953;**46**: 9–20.
7. Ljung, O., The electrocardiogram in hypocalcemia, with special reference to the T wave. *Acta Med. Scand.*, 1949;**136**: 56–70.
8. Reynolds, T.B., H.E. Martin, and R.E.Homann, Serum electrolytes and the electrocardiogram. *Am. Heart J.*, 1951;**42**: 671–681.
9. Surawicz, B., Relationship between electrocardiogram and electrolytes. *Am. Heart J.*, 1967;**73**: 814–834.
10. Mirvis, D.M. and J. Marin-Garcia, Effects of tachycardia with normal and ectopic ventricular activation on S-T segment potential and patterns in the dog. *J. Electrocardiol.*, 1985;**18**: 223–231.
11. Surawicz, B. and S. Saito, Exercise testing for detection of myocardial ischemia in patients with abnormal electrocardiograms at rest. *Am. J. Cardiol.*, 1978;**41**: 943–951.
12. Surawicz, B. and K.C. Lasseter, Electrocardiogram in pericarditis. *Am. J. Cardiol.*, 1970;**26**: 471–474.
13. Harris, T.R., G.D. Copeland, and D.A. Brody, Progressive injury current with metastatic tumor of the heart. Case report and review of the literature. *Am. Heart J.*, 1965;**69**: 392–400.
14. Puletti, M., M. Curione, F. Pozzar, G. Righetti, and G. Jacobellis, Atrial repolarization: its role in ST elevation. *J. Electrocardiol.* 1979;**12**: 321–324.
15. Gubner, R., Determinants of ischemic electrocardiographic abnormalities and chest pain. Part II – The exercise electrocardiogram test. *J. Occup. Med.*, 1961;**3**: 110–120.
16. Surawicz, B., QRS, ST segment, T wave and U-wave specificity for myocardial ischemia and infarction, in *Clinical Strategies in Ischemic Heart Disease*, E. Corday and H.J.C. Swan, Editors. Baltimore, MD: Williams and Wilkins, 1979, pp. 160–165.
17. Lepeschkin, E. and B. Surawicz, Characteristics of true-positive and false-positive results of electrocardiographic Master two-step exercise test. *N. Engl. J. Med.*, 1958;**258**: 511–520.
18. Armstrong, W.F., J.W. Jordan, S.N. Morris, and P.L. McHenry, Prevalence and magnitude of S-T segment and T wave abnormalities in normal men during continuous ambulatory electrocardiography. *Am. J. Cardiol.*, 1982;**49**: 1638–1642.
19. Shipley, R.A., and W.R. Hallaran, The four lead electrocardiogram in two hundred normal men and women. *Am. Heart J.*, 1936;**11**: 325–345.
20. Goldman, M.J., RS-T segment elevation in mid- and left precordial leads as a normal variant. *Am. Heart J.*, 1953;**46**: 817–820.
21. Wasserburger, R.H. and W.J. Alt, The normal RS-T segment elevation variant. *Am. J. Cardiol.*, 1961;**8**: 184–192.
22. Kambara, H. and J. Phillips, Long-term evaluation of early repolarization syndrome (normal variant RS-T segment elevation). *Am. J. Cardiol.*, 1976;**38**: 157–161.
23. Spodick, D.H., Differential characteristics of the electrocardiogram in early repolarization and acute pericarditis. *N. Engl. J. Med.*, 1976;**295**: 523–526.
24. Morace, G., L. Padeletti, M.C. Porciani, and F.Fantini, Effect of isoproterenol on the "early repolarization" syndrome. *Am. Heart J.*, 1979;**97**: 343–347.
25. Kuo, C.S. and B. Surawicz, Ventricular monophasic action potential changes associated with neurogenic T wave abnormalities and isoproterenol administration in dogs. *Am. J. Cardiol.*, 1976;**38**: 170–177.
26. Mirvis, D.M., Evaluation of normal variations in S-T segment patterns by body surface isopotential mapping: S-T segment elevation in absence of heart disease. *Am. J. Cardiol.*, 1982; **50**: 122–128.
27. Ginzton, L.E. and M.M. Laks, The differential diagnosis of acute pericarditis from the normal variant: new electrocardiographic criteria. *Circulation*, 1982;**65**: 1004–1009.
28. Bidoggia, H., J.P. Maciel, N. Capalozza, S. Mosca, E.J. Blaksley, E. Valverede, G. Bertran, P. Arini, B.S.C. Biaggetti, and R.A. Quinteiro, Sex differences on the electrocardiographic pattern of cardiac repolarization: possible role of testosterone. *Am. Heart J.*, 2000;**140**: 678–683.
29. Surawicz, B. and R.S. Parikh, Prevalence of male and female patterns of early ventricular repolarization in the normal ECG of males and females from childhood to old age. *J. Am. Coll. Cardiol.*, 2002;**40**: 1870–1876.
30. Hellerstein, H.K. and I.M. Liebow, Electrical alternation in experimental coronary artery occlusion. *Am. J. Physiol.*, 1950;**60**: 366–374.
31. Roselle, H.A., R.S. Crampton, and R.B.Case, Alternans of the depressed S-T segment during coronary insufficiency: its relation to mechanical events. *Am. J. Cardiol.*, 1966;**18**: 200–207.
32. Williams, R.R., G.S. Wagner, and R.H. Peter, ST segment alternans in Prinzmetal's angina: a report of two cases. *Ann. Intern. Med.*, 1974;**81**: 51–54.
33. Nakashima, M., H. Hashimoto, M. Kanamaru, T. Nagaya, M. Hashizume, and H. Oishi, Experimental studies and clinical

report on the electrical alternans of ST segment during myocardial ischemia. *Jpn. Heart J.*, 1978;**19**: 396–408.
34. Puletti, M., M. Curione, G. Righetti, and G. Jacobellis, Alternans of the ST segment and T wave in acute myocardial infarction. *J Electrocardiol.*, 1980;**13**: 297–300.
35. Levine, H.D., S.H. Wanzer, and J.P. Merrill, Dialyzable currents of injury in potassium intoxication resembling myocardial infarction or pericarditis. *Circulation*, 1956;**13**: 29–36.
36. Chung, E.K., Principles of cardiac arrhythmias. Baltmore, MD: Williams and Wilkins, 1971, pp. 385–395.
37. Liechti, M., M. Gertsch, A. Kleber, and U. Althaus, Experimenteller Myokardinfarkt beim Schwein: Einfluss von, Probeligatur und Revaskularisierung auf die ST -Strecke im epikardialen Ekg. und auf die Haufigkeit von Kammerflimmern. *Schweiz. Med. Wochensch.*, 1977;**107**: 1552–1554.
38. Rozanski, J.J. and M. Kleinfeld, ST segment alternans in Prinzmetal's angina and associated ventricular arrhythmias. *Circulation*, 1976;**53/54** (Suppl. 2): 77.
39. Schaefer, H. and H.G. Haas, Electrocardiography, in *Handbook of Physiology*, vol. 1, section 2: Circulation, W. F. Hamilton and P. Dow, Editors. Washington, DC: American Physiological Society, 1962, pp. 323–415.
40. Burgess, M.J., K. Millar, and J.A. Abildskov, Cancellation of electrocardiographic effects during ventricular recovery. *J. Electrocardiol.*, 1969;**2**: 101–107.
41. Wilson, F.N., A.G. Macleod, and P.S. Barker, The *T* deflection of the electrocardiogram. *Trans. Assoc. Am. Physicians*, 1931;**46**: 29–38.
42. Lepeschkin, E., *Modern Electrocardiography*. Baltimore, MD: Williams and Wilkins, 1951, pp. 307, 420.
43. Harumi, K., M.J. Burgess, and J.A. Abildskov, A theoretic model of the T wave. *Circulation*, 1966;**34**: 657–668.
44. Ashman, R. and E. Byer, The normal human ventricular gradient. I. Factors which affect its direction and its relation to the mean QRS axis. *Am. Heart J.*, 1943;**25**: 16–57.
45. Haas, H.G., Ein Beitrag zur Theorie des Ventrikelgradienten. *Cardiologia*, 1960; **36**: 321–336.
46. Gardberg, M. and I.L. Rosen, Monophasic curve analysis and the ventricular gradient in the electrogram of strips of turtle ventricle. *Circ. Res.*, 1959;**7**: 870–875.
47. Van Dam, R. and D. Durrer, The T wave and ventricular repolarization. *Am. J. Cardiol.*, 1964;**14**: 294–300.
48. Abildskov, J.A., P. Urie, R. Lux, J. R. Burgess, and R.Wyatt R, Body surface distribution of QRST area. *Adv. Cardiol.*, 1978;**21**: 59-64.
49. Plonsey, R., A contemporary view of the ventricular gradient of Wilson. *J. Electrocardiol.*, 1979;**12**: 337–341.
50. Brody, D.A., D.M. Mirvis, R.E. Ideker, et al., Relative' dipolar behavior of the equivalent T wave generator: quantitative comparison with ventricular excitation in the rabbit heart. *Circ. Res.*, 1977;**40**: 263–268.
51. Wilson, F.N., F.F. Rosenbaum, and F.D. Johnston, Interpretation of the ventricular complex of the electrocardiogram. *Adv. Intern. Med.*, 1947;**2**: 1–63.
52. Autenrieth, G., B. Surawicz, and C.S. Kuo, Sequence of repolarization on the ventricular surface in the dog. *Am. Heart J.*, 1975;**89**: 463–469.
53. Burgess, M. J., L.S. Green, K. Millar, R. Wyatt, and J.A. Abildskov, The sequence of normal ventricular recovery. *Am. Heart J.*, 1972;**84**: 660–669.
54. Abildskov, J.A., M.J. Burgess, R.L. Lux, R. Wyatt, and G.M. Vincent, The expression of normal ventricular repolarization in the body surface distribution of T potentials. *Circulation*, 1976;**54**: 901–906.
55. Abildskov, J.A., The sequence of normal recovery of excitability in the dog heart. *Circulation*, 1975;**52**: 442–446.
56. Franz, M.R. et al., Monophasic action potential mapping in human subjects with normal electrocardiograms: direct evidence for the genesis if the T wave. *Circulation*, 1987;**75**: 379–386.
57. Cowan, J.C. et al., Sequence of epicardial repolarization and configuration of the T wave. *Br. Heart J.*, 1988;**60**: 424–433.
58. van Dam, R.Th. and D. Durrer, Experimental study on the intramural distribution of the excitability cycle on the form of the epicardial T wave in the dog heart in situ. *Am. Heart J.*, 1961;**61**: 537–542.
59. Spach, M.S. and R.C Barr, Ventricular intramural and epicardial potential distributions during ventricular activation and repolarization in the intact dog. *Circ. Res.*, 1975;**37**: 243–257.
60. Watanabe, T., P.M. Rautaharju, and T.F. McDonald, Ventricular action potentials, ventricular extracellular potentials, and the ECG of guinea pig. *Circ. Res.*, 1985;**57**: 362–373.
61. Engelking, R. and W Bienroth, Untersuchungen tiber den intramuralen Temperaturgradienten des Herzens und seinen Einfluss auf das Elektrokardiogramm. *Cardiologia*, 1959;**34**: 147–163.
62. Reynolds, E W. Jr.and P.N. Yu, Transmyocardial temperature gradient in dog and man: relation to the polarity of the T wave of the electrocardiogram. *Circ. Res.*, 1964;**15**: 11–19.
63. Abel, H., I. Briske, R. Engelking, W. Gartner, and H. Schaefer, L'action des gradients de temperature de la paroi du ventricule sur Ie gradient ventriculaire dans l'electrocardiogramme. *Acta Cardiol.*, 1958;**13**: 278–298.
64. Toyoshima, H. and M.J. Burgess, Electrotonic interaction during canine ventricular repolarization. *Circ. Res.*, 1978;**43**: 348–356.
65. Abel, H. and H. Loeper, Transverse sections of myocardial fibers and the T wave. *Z. Kardiol.*, 1973;**62**: 380–387 (article in German).
66. Burgess, M.J., K. Hammi, and J.A. Abildskov, Application of a theoretic T wave model to experimentally induced T wave abnormalities. *Circulation*, 1966;**34**: 669–678.
67. Hoff, H.E. and L H. Nahum, The factors determining the direction of the T wave: the effect of heat and cold upon the dextro- and levocardiogram. *Am. J. Physiol.*, 1941;**131**: 700–709.
68. Toyoshima, H., M. Prinzmetal, M. Horiba, et al., The nature of normal and abnormal electrocardiograms. *Arch. Intern. Med.*, 1965;**115**: 4–16.
69. Autenrieth, G., B. Surawicz, C.S. Kuo, and M. Arita, Primary T wave abnormalities caused by uniform and regional shortening of ventricular monophasic action potential in dog. *Circulation.* 1975;**51**: 668–676.
70. Daoud, F,S., B. Surawicz, and L.S. Gettes, Effect of isoproterenol on the abnormal T wave. *Am. J. Cardiol.*, 1972;**30**: 810–819.
71. Taggart, P, et al., Interplay between adrenaline and interbeat interval on ventricular repolarisation in intact heart in vivo. *Cardiovasc. Res.*, 1990;**24**: 884–895.
72. Kuo, C-S., J.P. Amlie, K. Munakata, C.P. Reddy, and B. Surawicz, Dispersion of monophasic action potential durations and activation times during atrial pacing, ventricular pacing, and ventricular premature pacing stimulation in canine ventricles. *Cardiovasc. Res.*, 1983;**17**: 152–161.

73. Sarachek, N.S, J. Roberts, and J.J. Leonard, A new method to measure non-uniformity in the intact heart. *J. Electrocardiol.*, 1972;**5**: 341–348.
74. Yanowitz, F., J.B. Preston, and J.A. Abildskov, Functional distribution of right and left stellate innervation to the ventricles: production of neurogenic electrocardiographic changes by unilateral alterations of sympathetic tone. *Circ. Res.*, 1966;**18**: 416–428.
75. Chou T C, Helm R A, Lach R, The significance of a wide TsE loop. *Circulation*, 1964; **30**: 400-410.
76. Kuo, C.S. and B. Surawicz, Relationship of transmembrane action potential form to the T wave and T loop, in *Vectorcardiography 3*, B.F. Hoffman and R.I.Hamby, Editors. Amsterdam: North-Holland, 1976, pp.67–74.
77. Wilson, F.N, F.D. Johnston, and I.G.W. Hill, The form of the electrocardiogram in experimental myocardial infarction. IV. Additional observations on the later effects produced by ligation of the anterior descending branch of the left coronary artery. *Am. Heart J.*, 1935;**10**: 1025–1041.
78. Horan, L.G., R.C. Hand, J.C. Johnson, M.R. Sridharan, T.B. Rankin, and N.C. Flowers, A theoretical examination of ventricular repolarization and the secondary T wave. *Circ. Res.*, 1978;**42**: 750–757.
79. Hecht, H H., Some observations and theories concerning the electrical behavior of heart muscle. *Am. J. Med.*, 1961;**30**: 720–746.
80. Wasserburger, R.H. and R.J. Corliss, Value of oral potassium salts in differentiation of functional and organic T wave changes. *Am J. Cardiol.*, 1962;**10**: 673–687.
81. Hiss, R.G. and L.E. Lamb, Electrocardiographic findings in 122,043 individuals. *Circulation*, 1962;**25**: 947–961.
82. Friedberg, C.K. and Zager A, "Nonspecific" ST and T wave changes. *Circulation*, 1961;**23**: 655–661.
83. Haws, C.W. and R.L. Lux, Correlation between in vivo transmembrane action potential durations and activation-recovery intervals from electrograms. *Circulation*, 1990;**81**: 281–288.
84. Yamaki, M., et al., Relation between recovery sequence estimated from body surface potentials and T wave shape in patients with negative T waves and normal subjects. *Circulation*, 1992;**85**:1768–1774.
85. Hamby, R.I., I. Hoffman, and E. Glassman, The T loop in right ventricular hypertrophy. *Dis. Chest*, 1969;**55**: 105–109.
86. Rubler, S., I. Hoffman, W.D. Franklin, and R.C. Taymor, The T loop in right bundle branch block: a vectorcardiographic study of 82 cases. *Am. Heart J.*, 1968;**76**: 217–226.
87. Hoffman, B.F., Effects of digitalis on electrical activity of cardiac fibers, in *Digitalis*, C. Fisch, and Surawicz B, Editors. New York: Grune and Stratton, 1969 pp. 93–109.
88. Levine, H.D. and E.T. Angelakos, Late peaking of the T wave as a digitalis effect. *Am. Heart J.*, 1964;**68**: 320–324.
89. Tandowsky, R M., N. Anderson, and J.K. Vandeventer, An electrocardiographic and clinical study of various so-called cardiac drugs. *Am. Heart J.*, 1944;**28**: 298–310.
90. Surawicz, B. and K C Lasseter, Effect of drugs on the electrocardiogram. *Prog. Cardiovasc. Dis.* 1970;**13**: 26–55.
91. Sagall, E.L., C.D Horn, and J.E.F. Riseman, Studies on the action of quinidine in man. I. Measurement of the speed and duration of the effect following oral and intramuscular administration. *Arch. Intern. Med.*, 1943;**71**: 460–473.
92. Lee, Y.C., Quinidine intoxication: an experimental study of the effect of molar sodium lactate and potassium chloride. *Am. Heart J.*, 1960;**60**: 785–798.
93. Surawicz, B, Lepeschkin, E, The electrocardiographic pattern of hypopotassemia with and without hypocalcemia. *Circulation*, 1953;**8**: 801–828.
94. Freedberg A S, J.E.F. Riseman, and E.D. Spiegl., Objective evidence of the efficacy of medicinal therapy in angina pectoris. *Am. Heart J.*, 1941;**22**: 494–518
95. Kayden, H.J., B.B. Brodie, J.M. Steele, Procaine amide: a review. *Circulation*, 1957;**15**: 118–126.
96. McCord, M.C, J.T. Taguchi, A study of the effect of procaine amide hydrochloride in supraventricular arrhythmias. *Circulation*, 1951;**4**: 387–393.
97. Zapata-Diaz J, E. Cabrera, and R. Mendez, An experimental and clinical study on the effects of procaine amide (Pronestyl) on the heart. *Am. Heart J.*, 1952;**43**: 854–870.
98. Rasmussen, H.S., M.J.Allen, K.J. Blackburn, G.S. Butrous, and H.W. Dalrymple, Dofetilide, a novel class III antiarrhythmic agent. *J. Cardiovasc. Pharmacol.*, 1992;**20** (Suppl. 2): S96–105.
99. Di Marco, J.P., The ibutilde for atrial arrhythmias study group cardioversion of atrial flutter by intravenous ibutilide: a new class III antiarrhythmic agent. *J. Am. Coll. Cardiol.*, 1991;**17**: 324A.
100. Wong, W., H.N. Pavlou, U.M. Birgesdorfer, D.E. Hilleman, S.M. Mohuddin, and D.M. Roden, Pharmacology of the class III antiarrhythmic agent sematilide in patients with arrhythmias. *Am. J. Cardiol.*, 1992;**69**: 206–212.
101. Carmeliet, E., Use-dependent block and use-dependent unblock of the delayed rectifier K+ current by almokalant in rabbit ventricular myocytes. *Circ. Res.*, 1993;**73**: 857–868.
102. Arita, M. and B. Surawicz, Electrophysiologic effects of phenothiazines on canine cardiac fibers. *J. Pharmacol. Exp. Ther.*, 1973;**184**: 619–630.
103. Kelly, H.G., J.E. Fay, and S.G.Laverty, Thioridazine hydrochloride (Mellaril): its effect on the electrocardiogram and a report of two fatalities with electrocardiographic abnormalities. *Can. Med. Assoc. J.*, 1963;**89**: 546–554.
104. Alexander, S., R. Shader, and L. Grinspoon, Electrocardiographic effects of thioridazine hydrochloride (Mellaril). *Lahey Clin. Found. Bull.*, 1967;**16**: 207–215.
105. Wendkos, M.H., The influence of autonomic imbalance on the human electrocardiogram. I. Unstable T waves in precordial leads from emotionally unstable persons without organic heart disease. *Am. Heart J.*, 1944;**28**: 549–567.
106. Butcher, W.A., K.G. Wakim, H.E. Essex, R.D. Pruitt, and H.B. Burchell, The effect of changes in concentration of cations on the electrocardiogram of the isolated perfused heart. *Am. Heart J.*, 1952;**43**: 801–814.
107. Levine, H.D., J.P. Vazifdar, B. Lown, J.P. Merrill, 'Tent-shaped" T waves of normal amplitude in potassium intoxication. *Am. Heart J.*, 1952;**43**: 437–450.
108. Winkler, A.W., H.E. Hoff, and P.K. Smith, Electrocardiographic changes and concentration of potassium in serum following intravenous injection of potassium chloride. *Am. J. Physiol.*, 1938;**124**: 478–483.
109. Braun, H.A., B. Surawicz, and S.T. Bellet, waves in hyperpotassemia: their differentiation from simulating T waves in other conditions. *Am. J. Med. Sci.*, 1955;**230**:147–156.
110. McAllen, P.M., The electrocardiogram associated with low levels of serum potassium. *Br. Heart J.*, 1951;**13**: 159–166.

111. Sjostrand,T., The electrocardiogram in hypopotassemia. *Acta Med. Scand.*, 1955;**151**: 73–83.
112. Hoffman, B.F. and E.E. Suckling, Effect of several cations on transmembrane potentials of cardiac muscle. *Am. J. Physiol.*, 1956;**186**: 317–324.
113. Abildskov, JA., M.J. Burgess, K. Millar, R.Wyatt, and G. Baule, The primary T wave – a new electrocardiographic waveform. *Am. Heart J.*, 1971;**81**: 242–249.
114. Montorsi, P., F. Fabbiochi, A. Loaldi, L. Annoni, A. Polese, N. De Cesare, and M. Guazzi, Coronary adrenergic hyperactivity in patients with syndrome X and abnormal electrocardiogram at rest. *Am. J. Cardiol.*, 1991;**68**: 1698–1703.
115. Camici, P.G, P. Marraccini, R. Lorenzoni, G. Burrigoli, N. Pecori, and A. Perissonotto, E. Ferrannini, A. L'Abate, and M. Marzilli, Coronary hemodynamics and myocardial metabolism in patients with syndrome X response to pacing stress. *J Am. Coll. Cardiol.*, 1991;**171**: 1461–1470.
116. Cannon, R.O., P.G. Camici, and S.E. Epstein, Pathophysiological dilemma of syndrome X. *Circulation*, 1992;**85**: 883–892.
117. Niboyannopoulos, P., J.C. Kaski, and A. Crake Maseri, Absence of myocardial dysfunction during stress in patients with syndrome X. *J. Am. Cardiol.*, 1991;**18**:1461–1470.
118. Tousoulis, D., T. Crake, D.C. Lefroy, A.R. Galassi, and A. Maseri, Left ventricular hypercontractility and ST segment depression in patients with syndrome X. *J. Am. Coll. Cardiol.*, 1993;**22**: 1607–1613.
119. Tweddel, A.C., W. Martin, and I. Hutton, Thallium scans in syndrome X. Br. Heart J., 1992;**68**: 48–50.
120. Levine, H.D., Non-specificity of the electrocardiogram associated with coronary artery disease. *Am. J. Med.*, 1953;**15**:344–355.
121. Stapleton, J.F., J.P. Segal, and W.P.Harvey, The electrocardiogram of myocardopathy. *Prog. Cardiovasc. Dis.*, 1970;**13**: 217–239.
122. Evans, W. and G. Wright, The electrocardiogram in Friedreich disease. *Br. Heart J.*, 1942;**4**: 91–102.
123. Nadas, A.S., M.M. Alimurung, and L.A. Sieracki, Cardiac manifestations of Friedreich's ataxia. *N. Engl. J. Med.*, 1951;**244**: 239–244.
124. Dolara, A., P. Morando, and M. Pampaloni, Electrocardiographic findings in 98 consecutive non-penetrating chest injuries. *Dis. Chest*, 1967;**52**: 50–56.
125. Burda, C.D., Electrocardiographic changes in lightning stroke. *Am. Heart J.*, 1966;**72**: 521–524.
126. Diaz-Rivera, R.S., F. Ramos-Morales, M.R. Garcia-Palmieri, and E A. Ramirez, The electrocardiographic changes in acute phosphorous poisoning in man. *Am. J. Med. Sci.*, 1961;**241**: 758–765.
127. Cosby, R.S. and M. Bergeron, Electrocardiographic changes in carbon monoxide poisoning. *Am. J. Cardiol.*, 1963;**11**: 93–96.
128. Chadha, J.S., D.W. Ashby, and J.O. Brown, Abnormal electrocardiogram after adder bite. *Br. Heart J.*, 1968;**30**: 138–140.
129. Gueron, M., J. Stern, and W. Cohen, Severe myocardial damage and heart failure in scorpion sting. Report of five cases. *Am. J. Cardiol.*, 1967;**19**: 719–726.
130. Bahl, O.P., T.J. Walsh, and E. Massie, Electrocardiography and vectorcardiography in idiopathic hypertrophic subaortic stenosis. *Am. J. Med. Sci.*, 1970;**259**: 262–271.
131. Bowers, D., An electrocardiographic pattern associated with mitral valve deformity in Marfan's syndrome. *Circulation*, 1961;**23**: 30–33.
132. Braudo, M., E.D. Wifle, and J.D. Keith, A distinctive electrocardiogram in muscular subaortic stenosis due to ventricular septal hypertrophy. *Am. J. Cardiol.*, 1964;**14**: 599–607.
133. Coltart, D.J. and S.J. Meldrum, Hypertrophic cardiomyopathy. An electrophysiological study. *Br. Med. J.*, 1970;**4**: 217–218.
134. Barlow J B, Bosman C K, Pocock W A, Marchand P, Late systolic murmurs and non-ejection ("mid-late") systolic clicks. Analysis of 90 patients. *Br. Heart J.* 1968; **30**: 203–18.
135. Bittar, N. and J.A. Sosa, The billowing mitral valve leaflet: report on fourteen patients. *Circulation*, 1968;**38**: 763–770.
136. Ehlers, K.H., M.A. Engle, R. Levin, H.Grossman, and R.J. Fleming, Left ventricular abnormality with late mitral insulficiency and abnormal electrocardiogram. *Am. J. Cardiol.*, 1970;**26**: 333–340.
137. Hancock, E.W. and K.Cohn, The syndrome associated with midsystolic click and late systolic murmur. *Am. J. Med.*, 1966;**41**: 183–196.
138. Stannard, M., J.G. Sloman, W.S.C.Hare, and A J. Goble, Prolapse of the posterior leaflet of the mitral valve: a clinical, familial, and cineangiographic study. *Br. Med. J.*, 1967;**3**: 71–74.
139. Burch G E, R. Meyers, and J.A. Abildskov, A new electrocardiographic pattern observed in cerebrovascular accidents. *Circulation*, 1954;**9**: 719–723.
140. Abildskov, J.A., K. Millar, M.J. Burgess, and W Vincent, The electrocardiogram and the central nervous system. *Prog. Cardiovasc. Dis.*, 1970;**13**: 210–216.
141. Cropp, G.J. and G.W. Manning, Electrocardiographic changes simulating myocardial ischemia and infarction associated with spontaneous intracranial hemorrhage. *Circulation*, 1960;**22**: 25–38.
142. Fentz, V. and J. Gormsen, Electrocardiographic patterns in patients with cerebrovascular accidents. *Circulation*, 1962;**25**: 22–28.
143. Hersch, C., Electrocardiographic changes in subarachnoid haemorrhage, meningitis, and intracranial space-occupying lesions. *Br. Heart J.*, 1964;**26**: 785–793.
144. Levine, H.J. and N.W. White, Unusual ECG patterns in rupture of vertebral artery aneurysm. *Arch. Intern. Med.*, 1962;**110**: 523–525.
145. Shuster, S., The electrocardiogram in subarachnoid haemorrhage. *Br. Heart J.*, 1960;**22**: 316–320.
146. Fisch, C, Giant negative T wave. *J. Indiana State Med. Assoc.*, 1961;**54**: 1664–1665.
147. Ippolito, T.L., J.S. Blier, and T.T. Fox, Massive T wave inversion. *Am. Heart J.*, 1954;**48**: 88–94.
148. Jacobson, D. and V.Schrire, Giant T wave inversion. *Br. Heart J.*, 1966;**28**: 768–775.
149. Szilagyi, N. and S L. Solomon, Variations in the form of the T wave in a case of partial heart block. *Am. Heart J.*, 1959;**8**: 637–644.
150. Dolara, A. and L.Pozzi, Electrical alteration of T wave without change in QRS complex. *Br. Heart J.*, 1971;**33**: 161–163.
151. Schindler, S.C. and B. Surawicz, Clinical significance of the ECG pattern with prolonged Q- T c interval, and increased T or U amplitude (CVA pattern). *Am. J. Cardiol.*, 1967;**19**: 148. [Abstract.]
152. Crompton, M.R., Hypothalamic lesions following the rupture of cerebral berry aneurysms. *Brain*, 1963;**86**: 301–314.
153. Jenkins,J.S., M. Buckell, A.B. Carter, and S. Westlake, Hypothalamic-pituitary-adrenal function after subarachnoid haemorrhage. *Br. Med. J.*, 1969;**4**: 707–709.
154. Millar, K. and J.A. Abildskov, Notched T waves in young persons with central nervous system lesions. *Circulation*, 1968;**37**: 597–603.

155. Averbuck,S.H., Acute generalized postoperative peritonitis simulating coronary artery occlusion. *J. Mt. Sinai Hosp.(NY)*, 1942;**8**: 335–340.
156. Fulton, M.C. and H.J.L. Marriott, Acute pancreatitis simulating myocardial infarction in the electrocardiogram. *Ann. Intern. Med.*, 1963;**59**: 730–732.
157. Gottesman. J., D. Casten, and A.J Beller, Changes in the electrocardiogram induced by acute pancreatitis. *J. Am. Med. Assoc.*, 1943;**123**: 892–894.
158. Kiessling, C.E., R.S. Schaaf, and A.M. Lyle, A study of T wave changes in the electrocardiograms of normal individuals. *Am. J. Cardiol.*, 1964;**13**: 598–602.
159. Lieberman, J.S., A. Taylor, and I.S. Wright, The effect of intravenous trypsin administration on the electrocardiogram of the rabbit. *Circulation*, 1954;**10**: 338–342.
160. Pollock, A.V., C.A. Bertrand, Electrocardiographic changes in acute pancreatitis. *Surgery*, 1956;**40**: 951–960.
161. Spritzer, H.W, C.R. Peterson, R.C. Jones, and E.L. Overholt, Electrocardiographic abnormalities in acute pancreatitis: two patients studied by selective coronary arteriography. *Mil. Med.*, 1969;**134**: 687–693.
162. Gallivan, G.J., H. Levine, and A.J. Canzonetti, Ischemic electrocardiographic changes after truncal vagotomy. *J. Am. Med. Assoc.*, 1970;**211**: 798–801.
163. Lehmann, K.G., A.H. Shandling, A.U. Yusi, and V.F Froelicher, Altered ventricular repolarization in central sympathetic dysfunction associated with spinal cord injury. *Am J. Cardiol*, 1969;**63**:1498–1504.
164. O'Brien, K.E, N. Pastis, and J.B.Conti, Diffuse T wave inversions associated with electroconvulsive therapy. *Am J. Cardiol.*, 2004;**93**: 1573–1574.
165. Walder, L.A. and D.H. Spodick, Global T wave inversion. *J. Am. Coll. Cardiol.*, 1991;**17**:1479–1485.
166. Walder, D.A. and D.H. Spodick, Global T wave inversion: long-term follow-up. *J. Am. Coll. Cardiol.*, 1993;**21**: 1652–1656
167. Brscic, E., A. Brusca, P. Presbiterio, F. Orzan, R. Conte, and E. Rosettoni, Ischemic chest pain and global T wave inversion in women with normal coronary arteriograms. *Am. J. Cardiol.*, 1997;**80**: 245–247.
168. Littmann, L., Large T wave inversion and QT prolongation associated with pulmonary edema: a report of nine cases. *J. Am. Coll. Cardiol.*, 1999;**34**: 1106–1110.
169. Suzuki, J., R. Shimamoto, J. Nishikawa, et al., Morphological onset and early diagnosis in apical hypertrophic cardiomyopathy: a long-term analysis with nuclear magnetic resonance imaging. *J. Am. Coll. Cardiol.*, 1999;**33**: 146.
170. Sakamoto, T., K. Amano, Y. Hada, et al., Asymmetric apical hypertrophy: ten year's experience. *Postgrad. Med. J.*, 1986;**62**: 567–570.
171. Alfonso, F., P. Nihoyannopolous, J. Stewart, S. Dickie, R. Lemery, and W.J. McKenna, Clinical significance of giant negative T waves in hypertrophic cardiomyopathy. *J. Am. Coll. Cardiol.*, 1990;**15**: 965–971.
172. Okada, M., M.Yotsukara, T. Shimada, and K. Ishikawa, Clinical implications of isolated T wave inversion in adults: electrocardiographic differentiation of the underlying causes of the phenomenon. *J. Am. Coll. Cardiol.*,1994;**24**: 739–745.
173. Urschel, D.L. and G.E. Gates, Mean spatial vectorcardiography: the T vector changes in hypothyroidism. *Am. Heart J.*, 1953;**45**: 611–622.
174. Zondek, H., The electrocardiogram in myxoedema. *Br. Heart J.*, 1964;**26**: 227–232.
175. Mainzer, F., L'influence de l'anxiete sur l'electrocardiogramme: son importance dans l'ectrocardiographie pratique. *Cardiologia*, 1958;**32**: 362–374.
176. Berman, R., E. Simonson, and W. Heron, Electrocardiographic effects associated with hypnotic suggestion in normal and coronary sclerotic individuals. *J. Appl. Physiol.*, 1954;**7**: 89–92.
177. Ljung, O., Alterations in the electrocardiogram as a result of emotionally stimulated respiratory movements especially with reference to the so-called "fright electrocardiogram." *Acta Med. Scand.*, 1951;**141**: 221–229.
178. Mitchell, J.H. and A.P. Shapiro, The relationship of adrenalin and T wave changes in the anxiety state. *Am. Heart J.*, 1954;**48**: 323–330.
179. Magendantz, H., and J. Shortsleeve, Electrocardiographic abnormalities inpatients exhibiting anxiety. *Am. Heart J.*, 1951;**42**: 849–857.
180. Kannel ,W.B., T.R. Dawber, and M.E. Cohen, The electrocardiogram in neurocirculatory asthenia (anxiety, neurosis or neurasthenia): a study of 203 neurocirculatory asthenia patients and 757 healthy controls in the Framingham study. *Ann. Intern. Med.*, 1958;**49**: 1351–1360.
181. Logue, R.B., J.F. Hanson, and W.A. Knight, Electrocardiographic studies in neurocirculatory asthenia. *Am. Heart J.*, 1944;**28**: 574–577.
182. Wendkos, M.H. and R.B. Logue, Unstable T waves in leads II and III in persons with neurocirculatory asthenia. *Am. Heart J.*, 1946;**31**: 711–723.
183. Wheeler, E.O., Emotional stress: cardiovascular disease and cardiovascular symptoms. in *The Heart*, 2nd edn., J.W. Hurst and R.B. Logue, Editors. New York: McGraw-Hill, 1970, pp. 1414–1422.
184. White, P.D., M.E. Cohen, and W.P.Chapman, The electrocardiogram in neurocirculatory asthenia, anxiety neurosis, or effort syndrome. *Am. Heart J.*, 1947;**34**: 340–344.
185. Levander-Lindgren, M., Studes in neurocirculatory asthenia (Da Costa's syndrome). I. Variations with regard to symptoms and some pathophysiological signs. *Acta Med. Scand.*, 1962;**172**: 665–676.
186. Lewis, B.I., Mechanism and management of hyperventilation syndromes. *Biochem. Clin.*, 1964;**4**: 89–96.
187. Crede, R.H., N.C. Chivers, and A.P. Shapiro, Electrocardiographic abnormalities associated with emotional disturbances. A case report. *Psychosom. Med.*, 1951;**13**: 277–288.
188. Biberman, L., R.N. Sarma, and B. Surawicz, T wave abnormalities during hyperventilation and isoproterenol infusion. *Am. Heart J.*, 1971;**81**: 166–174.
189. Salvetti, A., P.L. Cella, P. Arrigoni, and D. Biancalana, Comportamento della fase di ripolarizzazione ventricolare dopo sforza e dopo iperventilazione volontaria in giovani sani. *Cuore Circ.*, 1964;**48**: 192–208.
190. Yu, P.N., B.J.B. Yim, and C.A. Stanfield, Hyperventilation syndrome. *Arch. Intern. Med.*, 1959;**103**: 902–913.
191. Christensen, B.C., Studies on hyperventilation. II. Electrocardiographic changes in normal man during voluntary hyperventilation. *J. Clin. Invest.*, 1946;**25**: 880–889.
192. Christensen, B.C., Variations in the carbon dioxide tension in the arterial blood and the electrocardiogram in man. *Acta Physiol. Scand.*, 1946;**12**: 389–396.

193. Schweitzer, P., T. Hildebrand, H. Klvanova, S. Simko, E. Galajdova, and J. Gregorova, Der Einfluss der adrenergen Blockade auf die orthostatischen Veriinderungen der Integralvektoren von QRS. T sowie des Ventrikelgradienten bei Patienten mit neurozirkulatorischer Asthenie und Thyreotoxikose. Z. *Kreislaufforsch.*, 1967;**56**: 316–325.
194. Hiss, R.G., G.B. Smith Jr., and L.E. Lamb, Pitfalls in interpreting electrocardiographic changes occurring while monitoring stress procedures. *Aerosp. Med.*, 1960;**31**: 9–18.
195. Furberg, C. and C.F. Tengblad, Adrenergic beta receptor blockade and the effect of hyperventilation on the electrocardiogram. *Scand. J. Clin. Lab. Invest.*, 1966;**18**: 467–472.
196. Pentimone, F., A. Pesola, A. L'Abbate, A. Smorfa, and C. Siusti, Effetto del propanolol sulle modificazioni elettocardiografiche secondarie alla prova da iperventillazione volontaria ed alla prova ortostatica. *Cuore Circ.*, 1967;**51**: 79–93.
197. Furberg, C., Adrenergic beta-blockade and electrocardiographical ST-T changes. *Acta Med. Scand.*, 1967;**181**: 21–32.
198. Nordenfelt, O., Orthostatic ECG changes and the adrenergic beta-receptor blocking agent, Propanolol (Inderal). *Acta Med. Scand.*, 1965;**178**: 393–401.
199. Simonson, E. and C.A. McKinlay, The meal test in clinical electrocardiography. *Circulation*, 1950;**1**: 1006–1016.
200. Sears, G.A and G.W. Manning, Routine electrocardiography: postprandial T wave changes. *Am. Heart J.*, 1958;**56**: 591.
201. Sleeper, J.C. and E.S.Orgain, Differentiation of benign from pathologic T waves in the electrocardiogram. *Am. J. Cardiol.*, 1963;**11**: 338–347.
202. Mann, R.H. and H.B. Burchell, The significance of T wave inversion in sinus beats following ventricular extrasystoles. *Am Heart J.*, 1954;**47**: 504–513.
203. Paparella, N., F. Ouyang, G.Fuca, K.H. Kuch, R.Cappalo, and P.Alboni, Significance of newly acquired negative T wave after interruption of paroxysmal reentrant supraventricular tachycardia with narrow QRS complex. *Am. J. Cardiol.*, 2000;**85**: 261–263.
204. Levine, H.D., B. Lown, and R.B.Streeper, The clinical significance of postextrasystolic T wave changes. *Circulation*, 1952;**6**: 538–548.
205. Meyer, P. and C. Schmidt, Troubles postextrasystoliques de la repolarisation. *Arch. Mal. Coeur Vaiss.*, 1949;**42**: 1175–1180.
206. Graybiel, A. and P.D. White, Inversion of the T wave in lead I or II of the electrocardiogram in young individuals with neurocirculatory asthenia with thyrotoxicosis, in relation to certain infections, and following paroxysmal ventricular tachycardia. *Am. Heart J.*, 1935;**10**: 34–54.
207. Kernohan, R.J., Post-paroxysmal tachycardia syndrome. *Br. Heart J.*, 1969;**31**: 803–806.
208. Trevino, A., B. Razi, and B.M. Beller, The characteristic electrocardiogram of accidental hypothermia. *Arch. Intern. Med.*, 1971;**127**: 470–473.
209. MacAlpin, R.N., W.A.Weidner, A.A. Kattus Jr., and W.N. Hanafee, Electrocardiographic changes during selective coronary cineangiography. *Circulation*, 1966;**34**: 627–637.
210. Smith, R.F., J.W. Harthorne, and C.A. Sanders, Vectorcardiographic changes during intracoronary injections. *Circulation*, 1967;**36**: 63–76.
211. Wolf, G.L. and J.W. Hirshfeld Jr., Changes in QTc interval induced with Renografin-76 and Hypaque-76 during coronary arteriography. *J. Am. Coll. Cardiol.*, 1983;**1**: 1489–1492.
212. Chatterjee, K., A. Harris, G. Davies, and A. Leatham, Electrocardiographic changes subsequent to artificial ventricular depolarization. *Br. Heart J.*, 1969;**31**: 770–779.
213. Rosenbaum, M.B., H.H. Blanco, M.V. Elizari, J.O. Lazzari, and J.M. Davidenko, Electrotonic modulation of the T wave and cardiac memory. *Am. J. Cardiol.*, 1982;**50**: 213–222.
214. Shvilkin, A., K.L. Kalon, M.R. Rosen, and M.E. Josephson, T-vector direction differentiates postpacing from ischemic T wave inversion in precordial leads. Circulation, 2005; **111**: 969–974.
215. Nicolai, P., J.L. Medvedowsky, M. Delaage, C. Barnay, E. Blache, and A. Pisapia, Wolff-Parkinson-White syndrome: T wave abnormalities during normal pathway conduction. *J. Electrocardiol.*, 1981;**14**: 295–300.
216. Kalbfleisch, S.J., J. Sousa, R. El Atassi, et al., Repolarization abnormalities after catheter ablation of accessory atrioventricular connections with radiofrequency current.*J. Am. Coll. Cardiol.*, 1991;**18**: 761.
217. Surawicz, B., Transient T wave abnormalities after cessation of ventricular pre-excitation. Memory of what? *J. Cardiovasc. Electrophysiol.*, 1996;**7**: 51–59.
218. Engel, T.R., R.Shah, L.A. DePodesta, W.S. Frankl, and R.L. Krause, T wave abnormalities of intermittent left bundle branch block. *Ann. Intern. Med.*, 1978;**89**: 204–206.
219. Denes, P., A. Pick, R.H. Miller, R.J. Pietras, and K.M. Rosen, A characteristic precordial repolarization abnormality with intermittent left bundle branch block. *Ann. Intern. Med.*, 1978;**89**: 55–57.
220. Surawicz, B., Transient T wave abnormalities in intermittent bundle branch block. *Am. J. Cardiol.*, 1982;**50**: 363–364.
221. Stewart. C.B and G.W. Manning, A detailed analysis of the electrocardiograms of 500 R.C.A.F. aircrew. *Am. Heart J.*, 1944;**27**: 502–523.
222. Viscidi, P.C. and A.J. Geiger, Electrocardiographic observations on 500 unselected young adults at work. *Am. Heart. J.*, 1943;**26**: 763–768.
223. Fisch, C., The electrocardiogram in the aged, in *Geriatric Cardiology*, R.J. Noble and D.A. Rothbaurn, Editors. Philadelphia, PA: Davis, 1981, pp. 63–74 (Brest, A.N. Editor, *Cardiovasc. Clin.*, **12**).
224. Atterhog, J.H., K. Eliasson, and P. Hjemdahl, Sympathoadrenal and cardiovascular responses to mental stress, isometric handgrip and cold pressor test in asymptomatic young men with primary T wave abnormalities in the electrocardiogram. *Br. Heart J.*, 1981;**46**: 311–319.
225. Littmann, D., Abnormal electrocardiograms in the absence of demonstrable heart disease. *Am. J. Med.*, 1948;**5**: 337–350.
226. Pruitt, R.D., C.H. Klakeg, and L.E Chapin, Certain clinical states and pathologic changes associated with deeply inverted T waves in the precordial electrocardiogram. *Circulation*, 1955;**11**: 517–530.
227. Kaufman, J.M. and R. Lubera, Preoperative use of atropine and electrocardiographic changes. Differentiation of ischemic from bilary-induced abnormalities. *J. Am. Med. Assoc.*, 1967;**200**: 197–200.
228. Wasserburger, R.H. and T.H. Lorenz, The effect of hyperventilation and pro-banthine on isolate RS-T segment and T wave abnormalities. *Am. Heart J.*, 1956;**51**: 666–683.
229. Leitner, St. J. and H. Steinlin, Untersuchungen iiber den Einfiuss des vegetativen Nervensystems auf das Elektrocardiograrnrn. *Arch. Kreislaufforsch.*, 1943;**13**: 62–96.

230. Dauchot, P. and J.S. Gravenstein, Effects of atropine on the electrocardiogram in different age groups. *Clin. Pharmacol. Ther.*, 1971;**12**: 274–280.
231. Sparks H V Jr, Hollenberg M, Carriere S, Funkenstein D, Zakheim R M, Barger A C, Sympathomimetic drugs and repolarization of ventricular myocardium of the dog. *Cardiovasc. Res.* 1970; **4**: 363–70.
232. Kuo, C.S., D.F. Butler, C.M. Chen, and B. Surawicz, Pathogenesis of post-ischemic T wave abnormalities. *Am J. Cardiol.*, 1974;**33**: 149. [Abstract.]
233. Salustri, A., P. Garyfallidis, A. Elhendy, M. Ciavatti, J.H. Cornel, A. Gemelli, F.J. Ten Cate, J.R.T.C Roelandt, and P.M. Fioretti, T wave normalization during dobutamine echocardiography for diagnosis of viable myocardium. *Am. J. Cardiol.*, 1995;**75**: 505–507.
234. Hiejima, K. and T.Sano, Electrical alternans of TU wave in Romano-Ward syndrome. *Br. Heart J.*, 1976;**38**: 767–770.
235. Schwartz, P.J. and A. Malliani, Electrical alternation of the T wave: clinical and experimental evidence of its relationship with the sympathetic nervous system and with the long Q-T syndrome. *Am. Heart J.*, 1975;**89**: 45–50.
236. Saitoh, H., J.C. Bailey, and B. Surawicz, Alternans of action potential after abrupt shortening of cycle length: differences between dog Purkinje and ventricular muscle fibers. *Circ Res.*, 1988;**62**: 1027.
237. Surawicz, B. and C. Fisch, Cardiac alternans: diverse mechanisms and clinical manifestations. *J. Am Coll. Cardiol.*, 1989;**20**: 483–499.
238. Sharma, S, K.G. Nair, and H.A. Gadekar, Romano-Ward prolonged QT syndrome with intermittent T wave alternans and atrioventricular block. *Am Heart J.*, 1981;**101**: 500–501.
239. Fisch C, Edmands R E, Greenspan K, T wave alternans: An association with abrupt rate change. *Am. Heart J.* 1971; **81**: 817–821.
240. Navarro-Lopez, F., J. Cinca, G. Sanz, J. Magriiia, and A. Betriu, Isolated T wave alternans elicited by hypocalcemia in dogs. *J. Electrocardiol.*, 1978;**11**: 103–108.
241. Surawicz B., Effect of Ca on duration of Q-T interval and ventricular systole in dog. *Am. J. Physiol.*, 1963;**205**: 785–789.
242. Lepeschkin, E., Electrocardiographic observations on the mechanism of the electrical alternans of the heart. *Cardiologia*, 1950;**16**: 278–287.
243. Gettes,L.S., N. Morehouse,and B. Surawicz, Effect of premature depolarization on the duration of action potentials in Purkinje and ventricular fibers of the moderator band of the pig heart: role of proximity and the duration of the preceding action potential. *Circ. Res.*, 1972;**30**: 55–66.
244. Kleinfeld, M., E. Stein, and C.E. Kossmann, Electrical alternans with emphasis on recent observations made by means of single-cell electrical recording. *Am. Heart J.*, 1963;**65**: 495–500.
245. Surawicz, B., in *Chou's Electrocardiography in Clinical Practice*, B. Surawicz and T. Knilans, Editors. Philadelphia, PA: WB Saunders, 2001, p.562.
246. Aravindakshan, V., B. Surawicz, and R.D. Allen, Electrocardiographic exercise test in patients with abnormal T waves at rest. *Am. Heart J.*, 1977;**93**: 706–714.
247. Zabel, M., A. Burak, T. Klingenheben, M.R. Franz, S.H. Hohenloser, and M. Malik, Analysis of 12-lead T wave morphology for risk stratification after myocardial infarction. *Circulation*, 2000;**102**:1252–1572.
248. Zabel, M., M. Malik, K. Hnatkova, V. Papademetriou, R.D. Fletcher, and M. R. Franz, Analysis of T wave morphology from the 12-lead electrocardiogram for prediction of long-term prognosis in male US veterans. *Circulation*, 2002;**106**; 1066–1070.
249. Okin, P.M., R.B. Devereux, R.R. Fabsitz, E.T. Lee, J.M. Galloway, and B.V. Howard, Principal component analysis of the T wave and prediction of cardiovascular mortality in American Indians. The Strong Heart Study. *Circulation*, 2002;**105**: 714–719.
250. Rautaharju P M, Nelson J C, Kronmal R A, Zhang Z M, Robbins J, Gottdiener J S, Furberg C D, Manolio T, and Fried L, Usefulness of T-axis deviation as an independent risk indicator for cardiac events in older men and women free from coronary heart disease (The cardiovascular health study). *Am J Cardiol* 2001; **88**: 118–123.
251. Surawicz. B., Is the U wave in the electrocardiogram a mechano-electric phenomenon? in *Cardiac Mechano-Electric Feedback and Arrhythmias. From Pipette to Patient*, P. Kohl, F. Sachs, and M.R. Franz, Editors. Philadelphia, PA: Elsevier, pp. 179–190.
252. Surawicz, B., U-wave: facts, hypotheses, misconceptions and misnomers. *J. Cardiovasc. Electrophysiol.*, 1999;**8**: 1117–1126.
253. Lepeschkin, E. and B. Surawicz,. The measurement of the Q-T interval of the electrocardiogram. *Circulation*, 1952;**6**: 378–388.
254. Holzmann, M. and W. Zurukzoglu, Die klinishe Bedeutung der negativen und diphasischen U-Wellen in menschlichen Ekg. *Cardiologia*, 1955;**27**: 202–214.
255. Ameur-Hendrich, C., G. Cordier, F. Hessel, J.P. Chemouny, and G. Laval, Onde U negative a valeur diagnostique et pronostique. A propos de 100 cas. *Ann. Cardiol. Angeiol.*, 1976;**25**: 103–110.
256. Kishida, H., J.S. Cole, and B. Surawicz, Negative U wave: a highly specific but poorly understood sign of heart disease. *Am. J. Cardiol.*, 1982;**49**: 2030–2036.
257. Georgopoulos. A.J., W.L. Proudfit, and I.H. Page, Relationship between arterial pressure and negative U waves in electrocardiograms. *Circulation*, 1961;**23**: 675–680.
258. Kemp, R.L., B. Surawicz, J.C. Bettinger, H. Gottlieb, and S. Bellet, Prognostic significance of negative U waves in the, electrocardiogram in hypertension. *Circulation*, 1957;**15**: 98–101.
259. Lambert, J., Clinical study of the abnormalities of the terminal complex TU-U of the electrocardiogram. *Circulation*, 1957;**15**: 102–104.
260. Miwa, K., T. Murakami, H. Kambara, and C. Kawai, U wave inversion during attacks of variant angina. *Br. Heart J.*, 1983;**50**: 378–382.
261. Gerson, M.C., J.F. Phillips, S.N. Morris, and P.L. McHenry, Exercise-induced U wave inversion as a marker of stenosis of the left anterior descending coronary artery. *Circulation*, 1979;**60**: 1014–1020.
262. Fu, L.T., N. Takahashi, M. Yamamoto, M. Kuboki, and S. Koyama, Handgrip induced negative U-wave in electrocardiogram of hypertensive subjects. *Jpn. Heart J.*, 1981;**22**: 59–73.
263. Hanrath,P., D.G. Mathey, R. Siegert, and W. Bleifeld, Left ventricular relaxation and filling pattern in different forms of left ventricular hypertrophy: an echocardiographic study. *Am. J. Cardiol.*, 1980;**45**: 15–23.
264. Mann, T., S. Goldberg, G H. Mudge Jr., and W.Grossman, Factors contributing to altered left ventricular diastolic properties during angina pectoris. *Circulation*, 1979; **59**: 14–20.
265. Rousseau, M.F., H. Pouleur, J.M.R Detry, and L.A. Brasseur, Impaired left ventricular relaxation in patients with aortic or mitral regurgitation *Am. J. Cardiol.*, 1982;**49**: 990. [Abstract.]

266. Watanabe, Y. and I.M. De Azevedo, Electrocardiographic correlation of bundle branch block and the U wave. *J. Electrocardiol.*, 1979;**6**: 215–220.
267. Ferrero, C. and J. Maeder, Bloc de branche droite: diagnostic de l'hypertrophie ventriculaire droite par la chronologie de l'onde V. *Schweiz. Med. Wochenschr.*, 1970;**100**: 190–192.
268. Lepeschkin, E., Physiologic basis of the U wave, in *Advances in Electrocardiography*, R.C. Schlant and J.W. Hurst, Editors. New York: Grune and Stratton, 1972, pp. 431–447.
269. Dudel, J. and W. Trautwein, Das Aktionspotential und Mechanogramm des Herzmuskels unter dem Einfluss der Dehnung. *Cardiologia*, 1954;**25**: 344–362.
270. Choo, M.H. and D.G.Gibson, U waves in ventricular hypertrophy: possible demonstration of mechano-electrical feedback. *Br. Heart J.*, 1986;**55**: 428–433.
271. Di Bernardo, D. and A. Murray, Origin of the electrocardiogram of U-waves and abnormal U-wave inversion. *Cardiovasc Res.*, 2002;**53**: 202–208.

6 Ventricular Repolarization in Myocardial Ischemia and Myocardial Infarction: Theory and Practice

Borys Surawicz

P. W. Macfarlane et al. (eds.), *Electrocardiology*, DOI 10.1007/978-0-85729-874-4_6,

6.1 Physiologic and Biochemical Processes Responsible for the Electrocardiographic Alterations During Myocardial Ischemia and Myocardial Infarction

The dominant effects of ischemia during the first few minutes are cellular K^+ loss, extracellular K^+ accumulation, and acidosis, resulting in rapid depolarization, inexcitability, and loss of active tension development. After a latency period of several minutes, there is a second phase of K^+ loss, increase in free cytosolic Ca^{2+}, electrical cell-to-cell uncoupling, and development of ischemic contracture [1].

Normally, the cell maintains a balance between influx and efflux of K^+. The influx occurs mainly through the Na^+/K^+ pump that has been assumed to function normally within the first 10–15 min of ischemia [2, 3]. Thus, the increase in extracellular K^+ must be attributed to an increased K^+ efflux taking place passively as a consequence of the K concentration gradient and through gated K^+ channels. One of the suggested causes of K^+ loss is the intracellular acidosis causing efflux of inorganic phosphate and lactate and carrying K^+ out of the cells [4, 5]. Increased K^+ efflux contributes to shortening of the action potential (AP) [6–8]. There is evidence that the K_{ATP} channel plays an important role in the K^+ loss during myocardial ischemia [9].

The resting membrane potential (RMP) decreases within minutes after experimental coronary occlusion [10–12]. During acute global ischemia in the perfused guinea pig heart, the RMP decreased within 15 min from −82 to −49.5 mV. This degree of depolarization could be accounted for by an extracellular K^+ level of 15 mM. This means that RMP approached the estimated K equilibrium potential [4].

Along with depolarization, the upstroke velocity of the AP decreases. A frequent precursor of the loss of excitability (when the RMP falls below about −60 mV) in the ischemic myocardium is electrical alternans.

During the healing phase of myocardial infarction (MI), encompassing the first 2 weeks, the fibers in the surviving epicardial muscle are arranged in closely packed fascicles but an increase in fibrous tissue sometimes separates individual muscle fibers. The RMP and AP amplitudes are frequently decreased, but in most surviving fibers RMP is more negative than −60 to −70 mV, implying that the slow conduction depends on the depressed sodium current rather than on calcium current [9]. Conduction velocity in the epicardial zone overlying the infarct is decreased as a result of the abovementioned depressed Na channel and altered anatomical fiber arrangement [13]. At most sites, within the infarcted region, the effective refractory period is prolonged with depressed excitability and increased dispersion of both excitability and refractoriness [14, 15].

The characteristics of APs of the surviving endocardial cells from human infarcts have been studied in tissues resected during cardiac surgery. In all aspects, the APs, the extracellular electrograms, and the structural abnormalities have resembled the respective counterparts from the experimental animal models [9].

6.2 Systolic and Diastolic Currents of Injury

➋ Figure 5.3b in the preceding chapter shows two mechanisms of ST segment displacement encountered in myocardial ischemia: first, the shortening and decreased amplitude of the AP, and second, depolarization, i.e., less negative resting membrane potential. The shortening and decreased amplitude causes potential differences during repolarization that is electrical systole, and this results in a systolic current of injury. The depolarization causes potential differences during electrical diastole and results in a diastolic current of injury. The left arrow in ➋ Fig. 5.3b shows that the potential difference produced by the systolic current of injury displaces the ST segment and the right arrow shows that the potential difference produced by the diastolic current of injury displaces the baseline. Both effects influence the ECG in the same manner (see below).

6.3 ST Segment Deviations Arising from Epicardial or Endocardial Injury

➋ Figure 6.1 is a diagrammatic representation of the effects of epicardial and endocardial injury on the ST segment in the standard limb or anterior precordial leads of the ECG. Epicardial injury may cause elevation of the ST segment and depression of the baseline, whereas subendocardial injury may cause the depression of the ST segment and the elevation

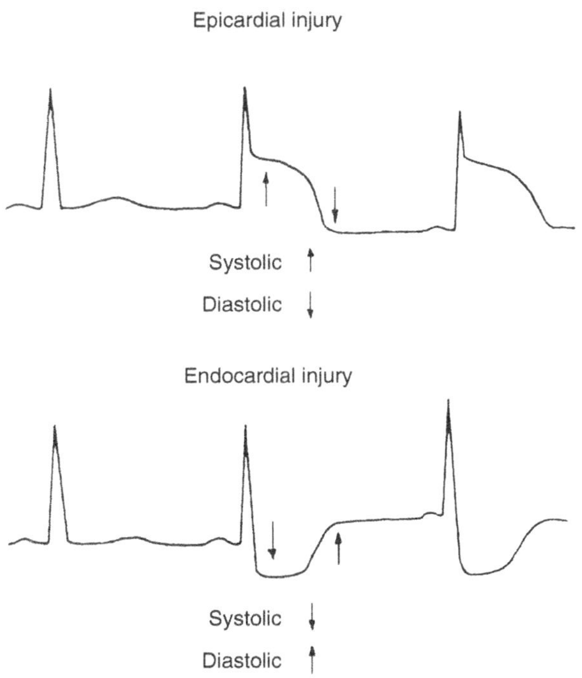

Fig. 6.1
Diagram illustrating the effects of subepicardial and subendocardial injury on the ST segment and the baseline of the electrocardiogram. The direction of the arrows indicates the flow of the injury current and not the direction of the ST segment vector. For explanation see text. With permission from Surawicz B and Saito S: Exercise testing for detection of myocardial ischemia in patients with abnormal electrocardiograms at rest (*Am. J. Cardiol.*, 1978;41: 943–951)

of the baseline. The conventional ECG recorded with alternating current (ac)-coupled amplifiers does not reveal displacement of the baseline and therefore does not differentiate between the ST segment displacement caused by the systolic and that caused by the diastolic current of injury [16].

Studies using the magnetocardiogram which records the same currents as the ECG but, unlike the ECG, responds to direct current, have been helpful in separating the systolic from the diastolic "current of injury" [17]. The magnetocardiogram also showed that ST depression during exercise-induced ischemia is a result of baseline shift, produced by a steady injury current which flows during the entire cardiac cycle but is interrupted during the ST interval [18].

Several studies have shown that the major change after coronary occlusion in dogs is the "diastolic injury current" owing to depolarization in the ischemic areas, while the shortening of AP during acute ischemia makes only a small contribution to the ST segment displacement. In the isolated perfused pig heart, TP (baseline) depression occurred within 1.5 min and ST elevation within 4 min after occlusion of the left anterior descending (LAD) coronary artery [3, 19]. It has been shown that the injury current arises at the ischemic border [20] which in the study of Coronel et al. [19] consisted of interdigitated normal and ischemic zones sharply demarcated from each other. Potential gradients at the "electrical border" between the ischemic and normal myocardium in the dogs during LAD coronary artery occlusion measured 12–20 mV [21].

In patients with acute myocardial infarction, isopotential body-surface mapping has shown early appearance of repolarization potentials, i.e., −21.3+/−:4.6 ms before the end of the QRS complex in patients with anterior infarction and 34.6:+/−12.4 ms before the end of the QRS complex in patients with inferior infarction [3]. The topographic configuration of the isopotential maps was relatively simple, and in patients with both types of infarction, the pattern was compatible with a single-dipole equivalent cardiac generator [22]. For additional discussion of the systolic and diastolic injury currents, see ➋ Chap. 5.

Acute injury pattern is an electrocardiographic term that defines an abnormal ST segment elevation in 2 or more adjacent standard 12 leads except lead aVR. The term is derived from an injury current flowing between an injured, i.e., depolarized tissue and a normally polarized tissue (see above). The most common cause of injury current and the corresponding injury pattern is acute myocardial ischemia, e.g., during thrombotic, embolic, or spastic coronary occlusion. It needs to be emphasized that acute injury is not synonymous with acute myocardial infarction (MI). An acute injury pattern may appear as a precursor of MI, concomitantly with a pattern of acute MI, or in the presence of pre-existing MI pattern. Transient injury current producing a similar ECG injury pattern may result from pressure exerted by the pericardial fluid during acute pericarditis.

As a rule, the vector of the deviated ST segment is directed toward the site of ischemia. Thus, ischemia or infarction of the anterior wall causes ST segment elevation in the anterior precordial leads, whereas ischemia or infarction of the inferior wall causes ST segment elevation in the "inferior leads" (see below).

An ST segment depression in the anterior precordial leads usually indicates a subendocardial or nontransmural ischemia or infarction unless it is reciprocal to ST segment elevation in leads II, III and aVF (see below).

Kornreich et al. [23] used 120 leads to construct body-surface potential map in 131 patients with acute myocardial infarction. They found that the most abnormal ST segment elevations and depressions at each location of myocardial infarction were localized outside the standard precordial lead positions. This study supports the prevailing notion that larger numbers of electrodes such as employed during mapping of the torso can improve the diagnostic accuracy of the ECG.

6.4 Localization of the Site of Ischemia

6.4.1 Anterior Wall Myocardial Infarction and Occlusion of Left Anterior Descending (LAD) Coronary Artery

In patients with acute injury associated with anterior MI, ST segment elevation is usually present in leads I, aVL, variable number of precordial leads (usually 2–6), and occasionally in lead II. Examples of various types of anterior MI, i.e., anterior, anterior-superior, anterolateral, and anterior-inferior are shown in ➲ Figs. 6.2–6.8. Differences in type depend to some extent on the site of left anterior descending (LAD) coronary artery occlusion.

Birnbaum et al. [24] attempted to predict the level of obstruction of the LAD artery in patients with acute anterior infarction. The culprit lesions were proximal to the first diagonal branch of the artery in 59 patients and distal to that artery in 38 patients. When the ST segment was elevated in the anterior precordial leads, the presence of ST segment elevation in leads I and aVL was predictive of a proximal lesion in 87% of cases; its absence was predictive of a distal lesion in 73%. The presence of reciprocal ST segment depression in the inferior leads was also suggestive of a proximal lesion (➲ Figs. 6.2–6.4, ➲ 6.6, and ➲ 6.7). In agreement with the above observations, unpublished studies from the author's laboratory showed that the ST segment elevation after the LAD occlusion distal to the takeoff of the first septal perforator and the first diagonal artery usually involves leads V_{2-4} (➲ Fig. 6.8), whereas a more proximal obstruction involves, in addition, leads aVL and/or V_{5-6} (➲ Figs. 6.2–6.7).

In patients with an anterior MI, ST segment elevation in lead V_1 occurs less frequently than in leads V_2 and V_3. The presence of ST segment elevation in lead V_1 suggests that the conal branch of the right coronary artery is either absent or small and therefore does not reach the intraventricular septum [25]. Conversely, the absence of ST segment elevation in lead V_1 during acute anterior MI suggests the presence of a large conal branch of the right coronary artery protecting the septum from a transseptal MI [25].

Occlusion of the LAD artery "wrapped" around the apex could be recognized by the presence of ST segment elevation and Q wave in the "inferior" leads during the early stage of infarction [25] (➲ Fig. 6.5).

In patients with anterior MI, reciprocal ST segment depression is present usually in leads III and aVF (➲ Figs. 6.2, ➲ 6.3, ➲ 6.6, and ➲ 6.7) and often in lead aVR (➲ Figs. 6.4, ➲ 6.7, and ➲ 6.9). Reciprocal ST segment depression tends to be absent in lead aVF when the LAD coronary artery is occluded distally [26].

Occlusion of the first diagonal branch of LAD coronary artery causes ST elevation mainly in leads I and aVL and fewer changes in the precordial leads [28–30] (➲ Fig. 6.9).

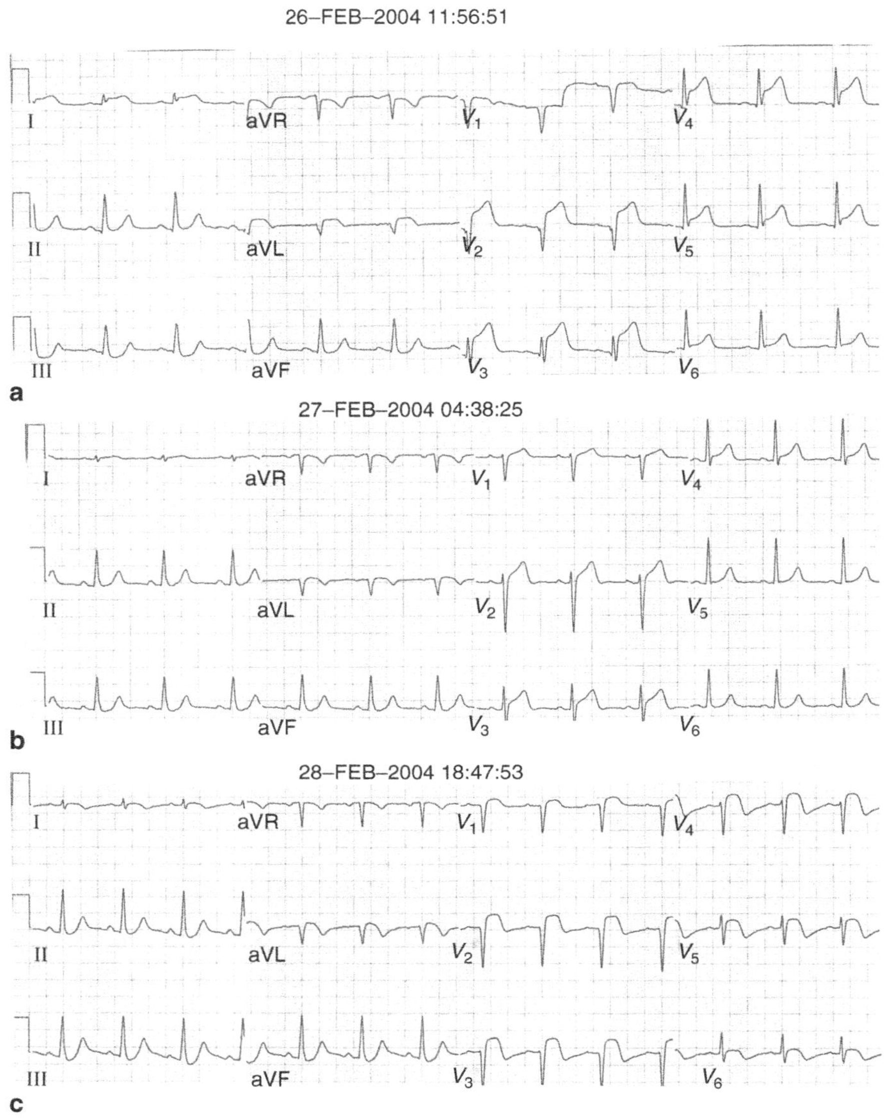

Fig. 6.2

Electrocardiogram of a 51-year-old man with acute anterior-superior myocardial infarction caused by total occlusion of left anterior descending coronary artery proximal to the first septal perforator and the first diagonal branch; there was also 40% occlusion of the first obtuse marginal branch of the left circumflex artery and 70% occlusion of the right coronary artery. Kinesis involved large portion of the anterior wall and the apex. with an estimated left ventricular ejection fraction of 15%. In (**a**): ST elevation in leads aVL and V_{1-6}, with reciprocal ST depression in leads III and aVR. In (**b**): one day later "pseudonormalization" with slight ST elevation in the leads V_{2-3} and T wave inversion in lead aVL as the only abnormalities. In (**c**): on the following day when chest pain resolved. ST elevation and T wave inversion in leads I, aVL and V_{1-6} with reciprocal ST depression in the leads III, aVF compatible with the evolution of the infarction pattern. Incipient T wave inversion in leads a VL, V_{2-6}

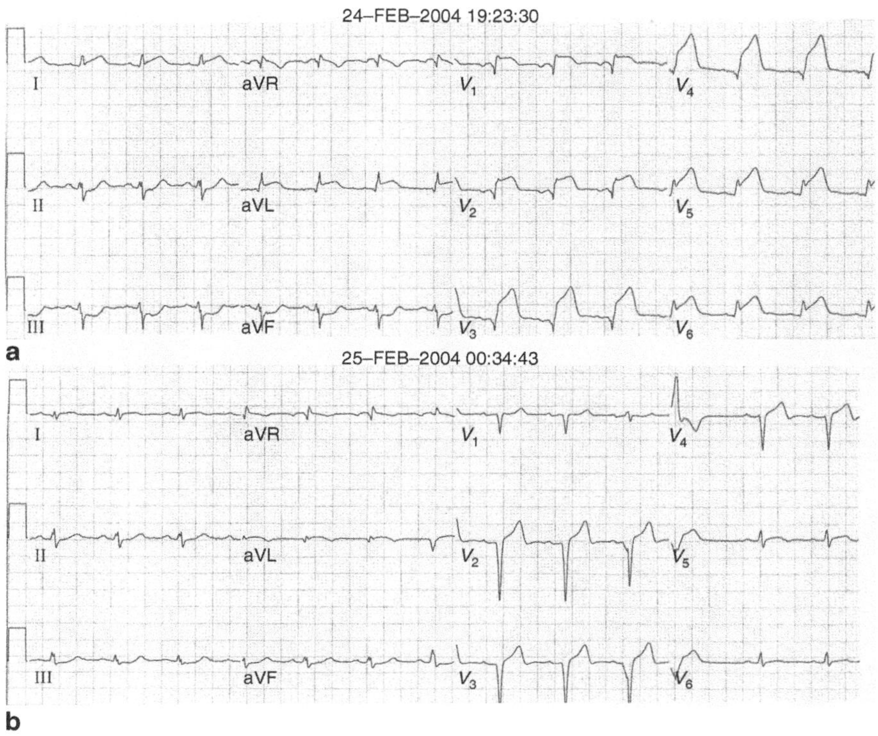

Fig. 6.3
Electrocardiogram of a 52-year-old man with acute anterior-superior myocardial infarction caused by "very proximal" total occlusion of left anterior descending coronary artery before first septal perforator. Other lesions included: 60% occlusion of the proximal left circumflex artery and 50% proximal occlusion of the right coronary artery., Large portion of the anterior wall including apex was akinetic with an estimated left ventricular ejection fraction of 25%. In (a): Q waves in leads aVL, V_{1-4}, ST elevation in I, aVL and V_{1-6} with reciprocal ST-depression in leads II, III, aVF. In (b), 5 h later after percutaneous intervention: Q waves in aVL, V_{1-3}, slight residual ST deviation with an incipient T wave inversion in lead V_4

Occlusion of the main septal branch causes ST elevation in leads V_1 and V_2 and reciprocal ST segment depression in leads II, III, aVF, V_5, and V_6. Assali et al. [27] observed that persistent ST segment depression in leads V_{5-6} in survivors of anterior MI was associated with increased left ventricular filling pressure and a restrictive left ventricular filling pattern.

6.5 Inferior Wall MI

In the presence of acute injury associated with inferior MI, ST segment is elevated in leads II, III, aVF, and, occasionally, in leads V_{5-6} (➲ Figs. 6.10 and ➲ 6.11).

It has been reported that ST segment elevation in lead V_6 occurred in all cases of left circumflex artery occlusion; and ST elevation in lead V_3R was present in 82% of cases with occluded right coronary artery [31]. In one study [32], the presence of ST segment elevation in lead V_6 in patients with acute inferior myocardial infarction was associated with larger infarct size and greater incidence of complications. Also, mortality in patients with inferior MI was increased when maximal ST segment elevation occurred in leads V_{4-6} and not in lead III [33]. ST segment elevation in lead VI may be caused by the presence of right ventricular MI which can be suspected also when in the presence of anterior MI reciprocal ST segment depression in lead VI is absent [34–36].

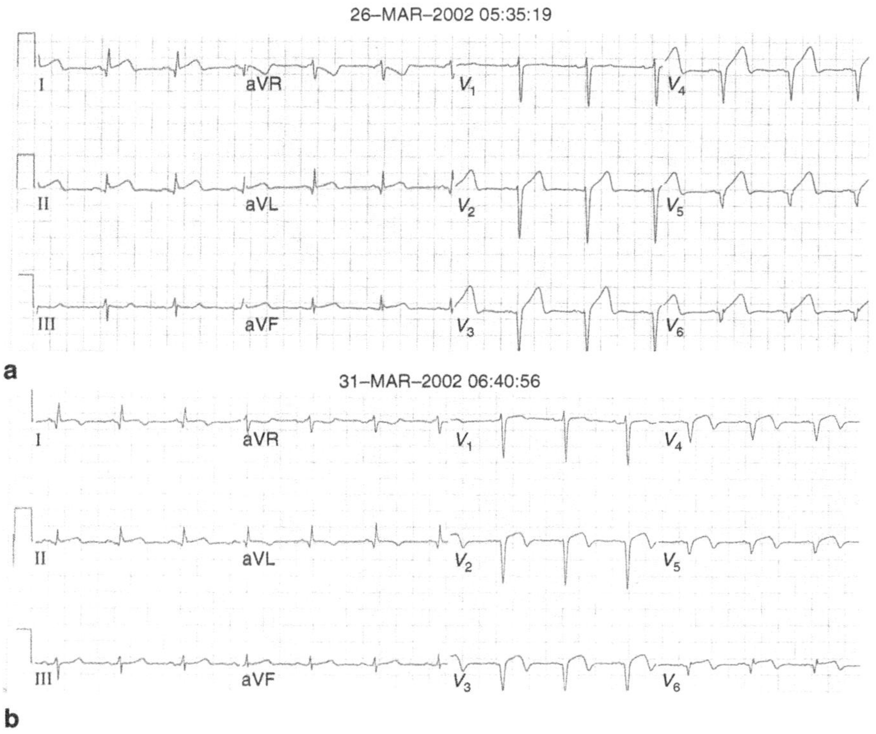

Fig. 6.4
Electrocardiogram of a 47-year-old woman with anterolateral myocardial infarction (MI) caused by total occlusion of left anterior descending coronary artery in midportion associated with 50–70% occlusion of the co-dominant left anterior circumflex artery. Anterior wall and apex were akinetic with an estimated left ventricular ejection fraction of 30%. In (a): Q waves with ST elevation in leads I, aVL, V_{3-6} and reciprocal ST depression in aVR. In (b) 5 days later after an emergent percutaneous intervention evolution of ECG pattern of anterior MI with T wave inversion in leads I, aVL and V_{2-6}. Residual ST elevation is present in the above leads.

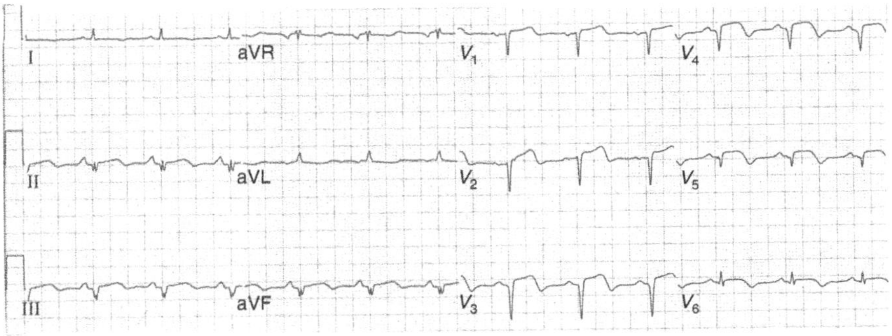

Fig. 6.5
Electrocardiogram of a 70-year-old woman with acute anterior and inferior myocardial infarction caused by complete occlusion of left anterior descending coronary artery proximal to the first septal perforator and to the first diagonal branch without appreciable abnormalities in the remaining large coronary branches. A large portion of anterior wall was akinetic, including apex and an adjoining area of the inferior wall with an estimated left ventricular ejection fraction of 15%. Note Q waves and ST elevation in leads II, III, aVF, V_{1-5} and incipient T wave inversion in leads II, III, V_{3-6}. No reciprocal ST depression in the available leads

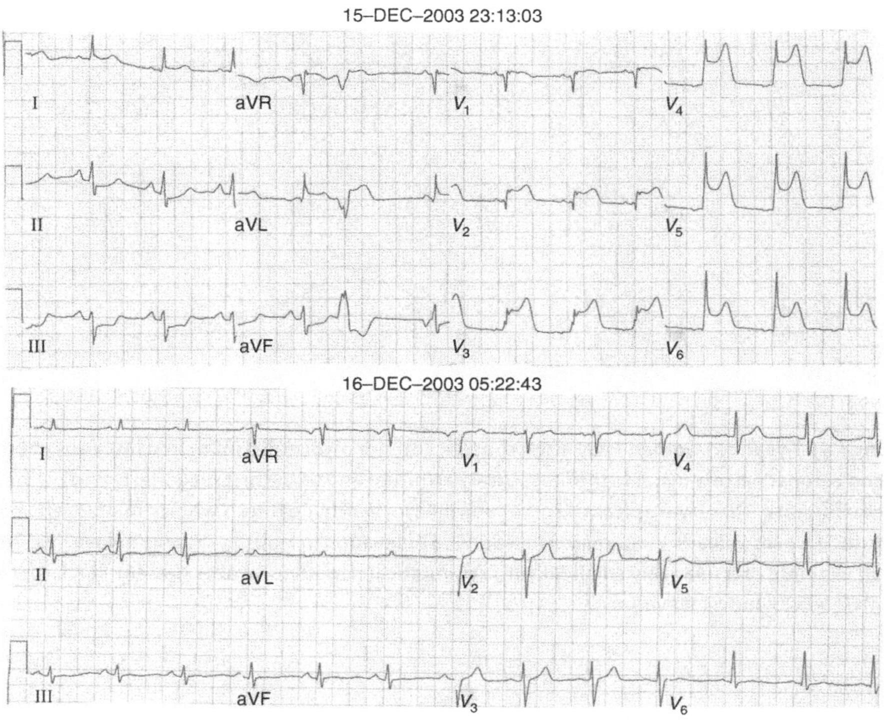

Fig. 6.6
Electrocardiogram of a 51-year-old woman with acute anterior myocardial infarction caused by "very proximal" total occlusion of left anterior descending coronary artery without appreciable obstructions in the remaining large coronary branches. Substantial portion of the anterior wall was akinetic, including the apex, and the estimated left ventricular ejection fraction was 20%. On top: Q wave and ST elevation in leads I, aVL, V_{2-6} and reciprocal ST depression in leads III, aVF and aVR. At the bottom 6 h later ECG is normal after percutaneous intervention

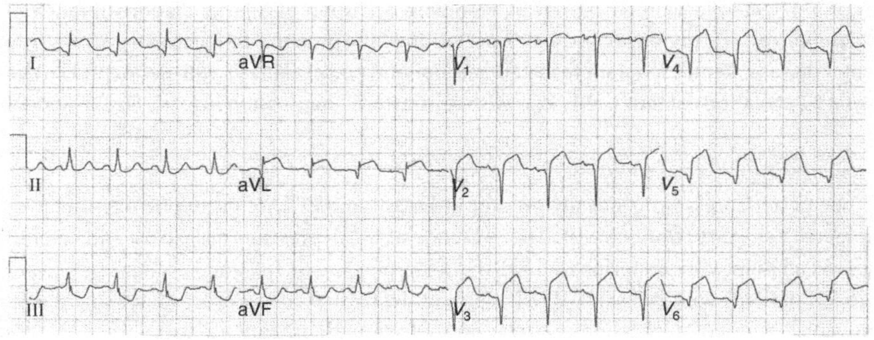

Fig. 6.7
Electrocardiogram of a 56-year-old woman with acute anterior-superior-lateral myocardial infarction caused by occlusion of proximal left anterior descending coronary artery and occlusion of first marginal branch of left circumflex artery. There was severe anteroapical hypokinesis and mild inferior hypokinesis with estimated left ventricular ejection fraction of 20%. In A. before intervention Q wave in lead V_2, ST elevation in I, aVL, V_{2-6} with reciprocal ST depression in leads III, aVF

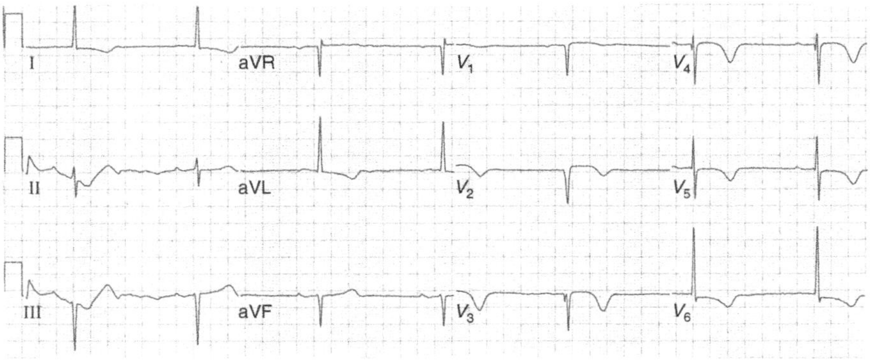

Fig. 6.8
Electrocardiogram of a 94-year-old woman 1 day after an acute anterior myocardial infarction (MI) caused by occlusion of left anterior descending coronary artery distal to the first septal perforator and to the first diagonal branch. Other major coronary branches were free of disease. There was apical and adjoining inferior wall hypokinesis with estimated left ventricular ejection fraction of 40% Note: Q waves in leads V_{1-3}, small Q in lead V_4, ST elevation in leads V_1–V_3 and T wave inversion in leads I, aVL and V_{1-6}. This is an example of a relatively small MI with symmetrical negative T waves present in a larger number of leads than the leads with Q waves and ST elevation

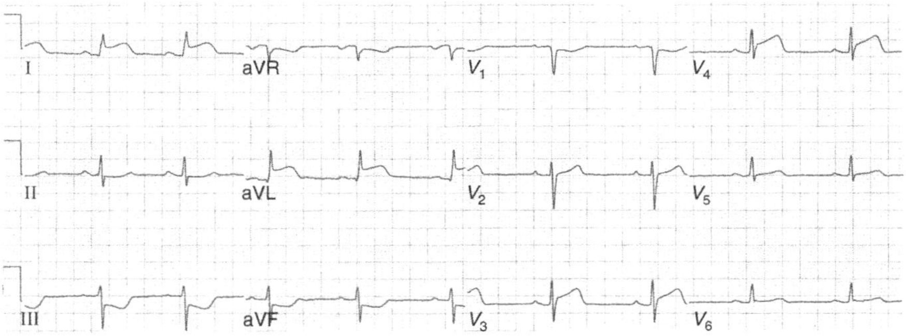

Fig. 6.9
Electrocardiogram of a 47-year-old woman caused by complete occlusion of a large diagonal branch of the left anterior descending (LAD) coronary artery; there was also a 30% occlusion of the proximal LAD coronary artery; other major coronary branches were free of disease. Ventriculogram revealed anterior and apical akinesis with estimated left ventricular ejection fraction of 30%. Note: ST elevation in leads I, aVL, V_{4-5} with reciprocal ST depression in leads III, aVF and aVR

Reciprocal ST segment depression is usually present in leads I and aVL, often in one or more precordial leads, and predominantly in leads V_{2-3} [31] (➋ Fig. 6.10). The presence of ST depression in lead V_1 indicates either a reciprocal change alone or an association with posterior wall MI.

In a study of 16,521 patients with inferior MI, ST segment depression in the precordial leads was present in 61.1% of cases [36]. Reciprocal ST segment depression occurred more frequently in patients with larger MI, greater wall motion abnormalities, and was associated with higher mortality [37, 38]. The magnitude of the sum of ST depression voltage in leads V_{1-6} added significant independent prognostic information with the risk of 30-day mortality increasing by 36% for every 0.5 mV of precordial ST segment depression [34].

In the study of 1,155 patients with inferior MI who took part in the Global Utilization of Streptokinase and TPA for Occluded Arteries Study (GUSTOI-I), subjects with maximum ST segment depression in leads V_{4-6} had more often three-vessel disease than those without precordial ST segment depression or those with ST segment depression in leads

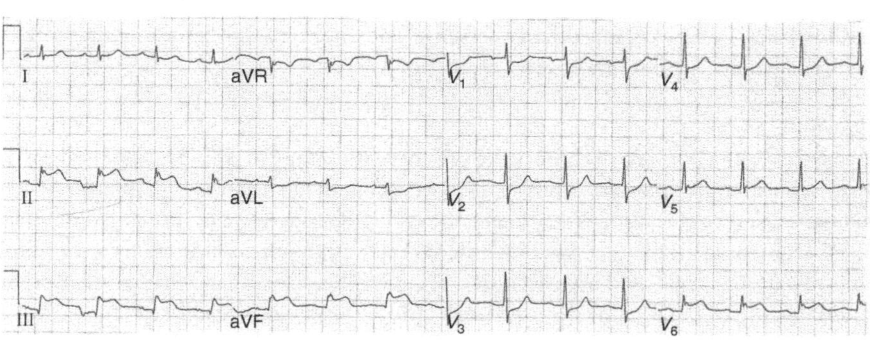

Fig. 6.10
Electrocardiogram of a 69-year-old man with acute inferior and posterior myocardial infarction attributed to occlusion of mid-right coronary artery and mid-left anterior circumflex artery. Left anterior descending coronary artery was free of disease. There was inferior, lateral and posterior hypokinesis with an estimated left ventricular ejection fraction of 50% Electrocardiogram shows Q wave in leads II and III with tall R waves in leads V_{1-2}, ST elevation in leads II, III, aVF and ST depression in leads aVR, V_{1-3}

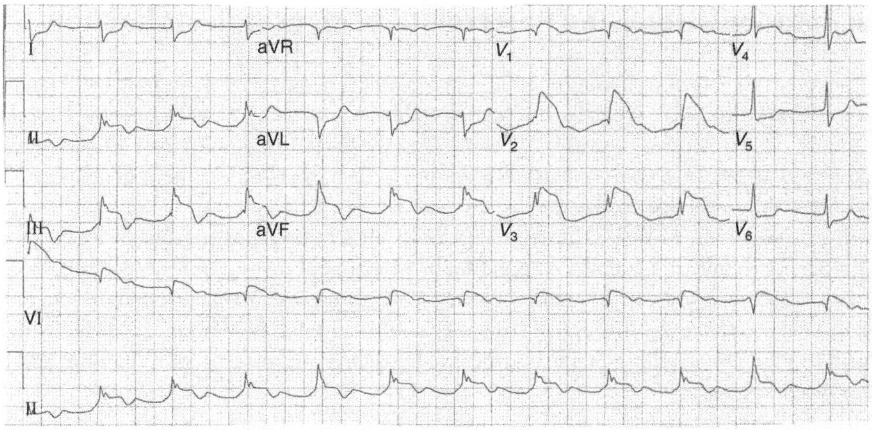

Fig. 6.11
Electrocardiogram of a 58-year-old woman with documented acute myocardial infarction of inferior wall and right ventricle caused by total occlusion of proximal right coronary artery associated with nonobstructive disease of left circumflex and left anterior descending coronary arteries. Note: ST elevation in leads II, III, V_{1-4} with reciprocal ST depression in leads I, aVL and V_{5-6}. The course was complicated by ventricular fibrillation, intraaortic balloon insertion and emergent coronary artery bypass surgery

V_1–V_3 [39]. Patients with maximum depression in leads V_{1-3} had larger infarction as estimated by peak creatine kinase, probably due to posterior or posterobasal extension [40].

6.6 Differences Between Inferior MI Caused by Right and Left Circumflex Occlusion

In patients with inferior myocardial infarction caused by occlusion of the right or the circumflex coronary artery with ST segment elevation in leads II, III, and aVF, the presence of additional elevation of ST segment in the "lateral" precordial leads (V_5, V_6) and/or leads I and aVL was a fairly sensitive and specific marker for left circumflex coronary artery occlusion [40] which accounts for about 18% of cases of inferior MI [41].

In these patients, ST segment in lead I is more likely to be isoelectric or elevated rather than depressed as in most patients with occluded RCA [41].

Huey et al. [42] compared the ECGs of 40 consecutive patients with acute MI caused by left circumflex artery occlusion with those of 107 patients with right coronary artery (RCA) occlusion. In the patients with inferior MI, the presence of ST segment elevation in one or more of leads I, aVL, V_5, and V_6 was highly suggestive of the left circumflex artery occlusion.

Depression of ST segment in leads V_{1-3}, as shown in ➋ Fig. 6.10, tends to indicate large posterolateral perfusion defect [32, 43] and is more often associated with occlusion of circumflex artery (71%) than of RCA occlusion (40%) [30]. Chia et al. [44] found that an ST II/III ratio of 1 or an isoelectric ST segment in lead I represented sensitive and specific markers of left circumflex artery occlusion whereas an ST II/III ratio <1 (ST segment elevation in III greater than in II) and ST depression in lead I were sensitive and specific markers of RCA occlusion. Bairey et al. [40] reported that ST segment elevation in the lateral leads identified circumflex artery occlusion as the cause of inferior MI. In patients with inferior MI, ST segment elevation in lead III exceeding that in lead II, particularly when combined with ST segment elevation in lead V_1 is predictive of occlusion of the RCA proximal to the acute margin of the heart. Herz et al. [45] reported the same results with an added finding that in patients with RCA occlusion reciprocal ST depression in lead aVL was greater than in lead I.

6.7 Lateral, Inferior Lateral and Posterolateral Myocardial Infarction

Localization of ST segment elevation and reciprocal ST segment depression varies in patients with lateral MI, depending on the extent and location of the MI. Typically, ST segment elevation in patients with inferior-lateral MI is present in leads II, III, aVF, and V_6. In many cases, however, ST elevation extends to the right of lead V_6, i.e., leads V_{3-5}. However, the lead with maximal ST segment elevation is usually V_6 or V_5. Reciprocal ST segment depression may be present in leads I, VI, aVL, and V_{1-4} but may also be absent.

In patients with posterolateral MI, ST segment elevation is either absent or present in leads V_{5-6}. Reciprocal ST segment depression occurs usually in leads V_{1-3}. Elevation of ST segment >2 mm in leads V_5 and V_6 correlated with an artery (right or circumflex) supplying a large territory of the myocardium with an expected high ischemic burden [45]. ST segment elevation in posterior leads V_7 through V_9 in patients with an inferior MI was associated with a high incidence of posterolateral wall motion abnormalities, large infarct size, low left ventricular ejection fraction, and high incidence of adverse effects after discharge [46].

In patients with a so-called true posterior MI, i.e., without ECG evidence of inferior and/or lateral MI, ST segment elevation may be present in leads V_{7-9} and reciprocal ST segment depression in leads V_{1-3} [41]. Routine recording of leads V_{7-9} has been recommended in patients with suspected MI but non-diagnostic 12-lead ECG [47–49].

In patients with high lateral MI caused by occlusion of the left circumflex coronary artery, the ST segment is usually elevated in leads I, aVL, and V_{5-6} and is depressed in leads III, aVF, and, occasionally, in lead VI. An abnormally tall R wave in lead V_1-consistent with posterior infarction – also suggests left circumflex artery occlusion.

6.8 Acute Injury Pattern in the Right Precordial Leads and Right Ventricular Infarction and Other Causes

Isolated infarction of the RV free wall seldom occurs [9, 41, 50]. Symptomatic RV MI causing serious hemodynamic complications is usually associated with an acute MI of the inferior or inferoposterior wall. Pathologic studies showed that RV infarction is present in 14–36% of patients with inferior LV Q-wave MI, but no major RV MI is seen in hearts with isolated anterior MI [41, 52–54]. A small portion of the RV, however, was involved with equal frequency in anterior and inferior (posterior) LV infarction.

ST segment elevation in the right precordial leads V_3R and V_4R usually signifies presence of RV MI [51]. In patients with RV MI, ST segment elevation may extend to additional right precordial leads V_5R and V_6R [52–55] and sometimes to precordial leads V_1–V_4 [53] (➋ Fig. 6.11).

In the presence of inferior MI, diagnosis of RV MI is supported by a discordant pattern of ST segment elevation in V_1 and ST segment depression in V_2 [56]. ST segment elevation in leads V_3R–V_4R may be present in patients with acute anterior MI but will seldom extend to lead V_5R [51]. Also, when the ST segment elevation caused by acute anterior MI is present in leads V_3R to V_5R, the magnitude of ST segment elevation diminishes from V_3R to V_5R whereas in the presence of RV MI, ST segment elevation is either the same or increases from V_3R to V_5R [51].

Lead V_4R appears to be most useful among precordial leads in recognition of RV MI. Zehender et al. [57] found ST segment elevation in lead V_4R in 107 (54%) out of 200 consecutive patients with acute inferior infarction. Using autopsy findings, coronary angiography, hemodynamic measurements, and noninvasive imaging, they found that ST segment elevation in lead V_4R had a sensitivity of 88% and diagnostic accuracy of 83% in the diagnosis of the associated acute RV MI.

Braat et al. [58] emphasized the transient nature of the ST elevation in the supplementary leads because this finding was no longer present within 19 h after the onset of chest pain. Saw et al. [59] reported that ST elevation in III > II was more sensitive than ST elevation in lead V_4R in diagnosing RV MI. Menown et al. [60] found that body surface mapping provides improved classification of patients with acute MI of inferior wall, right ventricle, and posterior wall as compared with right ventricular or posterior leads alone.

In patients with RSR' pattern in the right precordial leads and absent anterior infarction, ST segment elevation may be caused by septal ischemia, or by RV MI [52–55]. Other causes of such pattern where the ST segment elevation include the syndrome associated with sudden cardiac death described by Brugada [61] and arrhythmogenic right ventricular dysplasia. The Brugada syndrome [62] consists of RBBB, persistent ST segment elevation in leads V_{1-3} and sudden cardiac death affecting predominantly male gender. Some forms of this syndrome are intermittent and asymptomatic with transient normalization of the ECG. Typically, the ST segment elevation has a saddle back or a coved appearance [63]. The elevation is augmented by selective stimulation of alpha adrenergic or muscarinic receptors or by class 1A antiarrhythmic drugs [64] and vagal activity [65] but reduced by beta adrenergic stimulation or alpha adrenergic block [66]. Many of these patients have no evidence of structural heart disease. Similar ECG pattern was present in young male Southeast Asians who died unexpectedly during sleep [67] and in patients with familial cardiomyopathy (arrhythmogenic RV dysplasia) involving the RV and the conducting system [68–70]. Common to these conditions is QRS widening confined to selected leads with ST segment elevation and normal QRS duration in remote leads such as I and V_6 [71]. Most commonly, ST elevation occurs in leads V_{1-3}, but cases with ST elevation in the inferior leads have been reported [72].

In patients with RV dysplasia, the shape of the terminal QRS portion in the right precordial leads has been likened to the Greek letter epsilon. The pattern of right bundle branch block with ST segment elevation in the right precordial leads is not entirely specific for either right ventricular ischemia or Brugada syndrome because more often it is present in other conditions [73].

6.9 Left Main Coronary Artery Obstruction

In two studies of patients with anterior MI, ST elevation in aVR greater than in lead V_1 was found to be predictive of left main coronary artery obstruction [74, 75]. This requires further confirmation.

6.10 Coronary Spasm, Unstable Angina Pectoris, and Non-Q-Wave Myocardial Infarction*

Acute injury pattern is the diagnostic marker of coronary spasm, and the lead distribution of ST segment deviation during coronary spasm is the same as during myocardial ischemia caused by other types of coronary occlusion. ST segment elevation has been reported also in patients with syndrome x, normal coronary angiograms, and suspected spasm of coronary arterioles [76]. In patients with unstable angina pectoris [77] and non-Q-wave MI [78], acute injury pattern is present in the minority of cases.

*Current nomenclature; non-ST elevation myocardial infarction (NSTEMI)

6.11 ST Segment Changes as a Guide to Thrombolytic and Percutaneous Intervention Therapy

The indication for an emergent thrombolytic therapy of a suspected acute MI is based on the presence of ST segment elevation greater than 0.1 mV in two limb or two or more anatomically contiguous precordial leads. In the cases of pre-existing ST segment elevation such as in LBBB, the same rule applies when the availability of the basic pattern allows the recognition of the ST shift [79] (➋ Fig. 6.12).

Regression of ST segment elevation parallels recanalization [80–82], and incomplete resolution of ST segment elevation is a powerful independent predictor of early mortality [83–86]. Also, in patients with acute MI treated with direct angioplasty, a rapid decrease of ST segment elevation was observed in patients with myocardial reperfusion, but not in those with no-reflow phenomenon [87]. Re-elevation of ST segment is a sign of limited myocardial salvage and suggests extensive myocardial damage [88–92]. In some cases, in the presence of anterior ischemia, transient increase in ST segment elevation (attributed to adenosine release) preceding and following the decrease during the first hour has no adverse consequences [93, 94]. The magnitude of ST segment elevation, measured as a sum of ST-shift voltages, is related to the severity of myocardial ischemia and not to the size of the area at risk [95], but the localization of the ST segment elevation predicts the site of the future loss of QRS voltages.

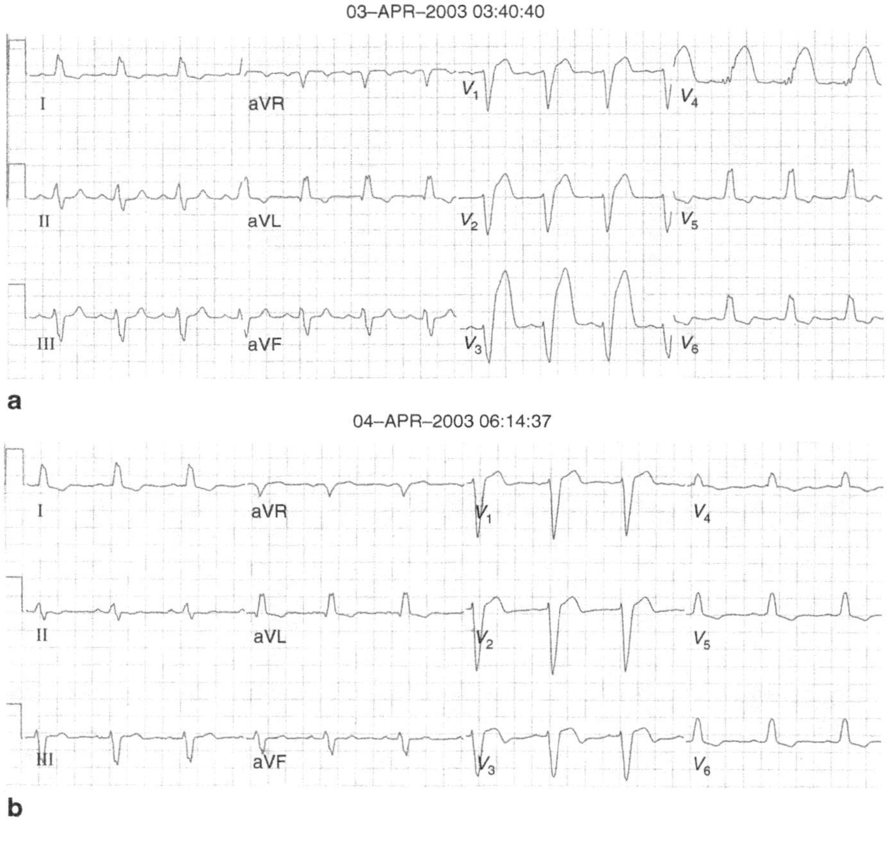

Fig. 6.12
Electrocardiogram of a 58-year-old man with left bundle branch block (LBBB) and acute anterior myocardial infarction (MI). In (a), in addition to secondary ST and T changes of LBBB, there is primary ST elevation in leads V_{2-4}-indicative of acute injury pattern. No reciprocal ST depression is discernible. In (b), after percutaneous intervention, primary ST elevation subsided, but primary T-wave inversion in leads V_{2-3} is compatible with evolution of anterior MI pattern

The depression of the ST segment may be reciprocal or indicative of an additional, presumably subendocardial ischemia. Shah et al. [96] evaluated the prognostic significance of the resolution of ST segment depression in patients with acute MI after thrombolytic treatment. They compared patients with ST segment depression resolving simultaneously with ST segment elevation (simultaneous group) and patients with ST segment depression persisting after ST segment elevation resolution (independent group). In-hospital mortality was significantly higher in the independent group than in the simultaneous group and a control group without ST segment depression. In other studies, early resolution of ST segment elevation was associated with improved wall motion [97] and salvage index [98].

6.12 ST Segment Shift During Percutaneous Coronary Angioplasty

Balloon occlusion of the coronary artery during angioplasty lasts usually from 1 to 3 min. The behavior of ST segment during PTCA is the same as during spontaneous myocardial ischemia but the magnitude of ST segment elevation expressed in percent of QRS amplitude tends to be smaller. Also, the average number of leads with ST segment elevation and those with reciprocal ST segment depression tends to be smaller during PTCA than during acute ischemia. The maximal ST segment elevation during balloon occlusion of LAD coronary artery is located in lead V_2, V_3, or V_4 [99], and during occlusion of RCA in the lead III. During occlusion of diagonal branch of LAD coronary artery maximal ST segment elevation may be located in lead aVL. The results of occlusion of left circumflex coronary artery vary. In about one third of cases, ST segment shift in the standard 12 lead ECG is absent, in another third, ST segment elevation is present in one or more standard leads, and in the remaining one third of cases there is ST segment depression in leads V_{2-3} which is believed to represent a reciprocal change of ST segment elevation localized in the back [99].

In theory, the absence of ST segment displacement at the site of presumed acute injury may be due to cancellation by a contralateral ST segment displacement in an opposite direction but in practice such mechanism is difficult to verify. The nonhomogeneous intensity of ischemia detracts from the accuracy of localizing the site of ischemia. Thus, it has been shown that a balloon occlusion of the partially stenotic left anterior descending coronary artery caused a reversible ST segment elevation in the left precordial leads when the collateral circulation was poor or absent. However, the same procedure in similar patients with good collateral circulation produced ST segment depression in the same leads [100]. Studies during coronary artery angioplasty showed that the site of impaired perfusion could be identified with greater accuracy using a larger array of precordial leads. For instance, ST segment elevation in the left axillary and back leads was specific for occlusions of left circumflex and diagonal branches. The ST segment elevation in lead V_3R was present in 82% of cases with occluded right coronary artery. It has been shown that in patients with acute first anterior myocardial infarction caused by left anterior descending coronary artery lesion, treated with rapid reperfusion by angioplasty, the ST segment behavior has a predictive value. Kobayashi et al. [101] found that the recovery of the left ventricular systolic function was better in patients in whom ST segment elevation resolved than in those in whom it did not. Also, Santoro et al. [102] reported that reduction in ST segment elevation after direct coronary angioplasty was the only independent predictor of left ventricular function recovery. In a more recent collaborative CADILLAC study of 700 patients with prior percutaneous intervention (PCI), ST segment resolution was found to be a strong independent predictor of both survival and freedom from reinfarction [103]. Watanabe et al. [104] found that persistent ST segment elevation present 30 min after primary percutaneous transluminal coronary angioplasty was a highly specific electrocardiographic marker of impaired reperfusion in patients with acute MI. Also in the study by Feldman et al. [105], incomplete (<50%) resolution of ST elevation was a marker of more extensive myocardial damage. It has been suggested to use ST segment resolution as a surrogate end point in reperfusion trials of acute myocardial infarction [106]. Microvascular injury has been suspected to be the cause of persistent ST segment elevation after primary angioplasty for acute myocardial infarction [107, 108].

6.13 Persistent ST Segment Elevation After Myocardial Infarction

Persistent ST segment elevation that lasts more than 1 month after the onset of acute MI is the most helpful sign of nonviable myocardium [109]. The mechanism of such ST segment elevation is poorly understood. A prevailing hypothesis attributes ST displacement to an injury current generated during systole at the junction of the aneurysm with

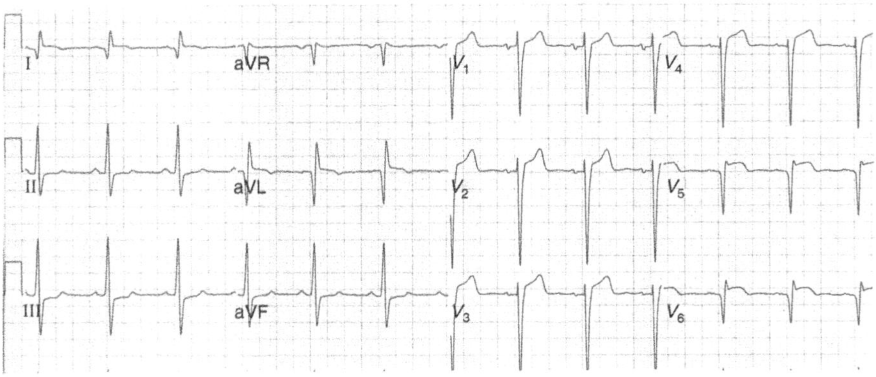

Fig. 6.13

Electrocardiogram of a 61-year-old woman recorded 20 years after anterior myocardial infarction and development of a large calcified ventricular aneurysm with an apical thrombus and an estimated left ventricular election fraction of 15%. The left anterior descending coronary artery was atretic and diffusely diseased whereas the left circumflex and the right coronary artery harbored mild luminal irregularities. Note: Q waves in leads I, aVL, V_{5-6} and ST elevation in the above leads as well as in leads V_{1-4}

the surrounding myocardium. According to this theory, the outward (paradoxical) bulging of the aneurysm produces undue tension at the junction of the aneurysm and normal tissue, resulting in injury (depolarization) of the surviving myocardium next to the border of the aneurysm [110].

After healing of myocardial infarction, ST segment elevation persists in about 60% of patients with anterior infarction (Fig. 6.13) and in about 5% of patients with inferior myocardial infarction [111]. Persistent ST segment elevation correlates with the presence of asynergy. It has been shown that ST segment elevation developed during balloon inflation coincident with the new appearance of hypocontractility in a region of previously normal motion [112] and that there was a close association between the magnitude and extent of ST segment elevation and the extent of asynergy [112]. The most sensitive marker for anterior wall hypocontractility was ST segment elevation in lead V_2 and for inferior wall hypocontractility ST segment elevation in lead III.

The widely held notion that the persistent ST segment elevation is a marker of ventricular aneurysm has not been supported by the recent studies. Radionuclide imaging has shown similar global and regional wall motion abnormalities in patients with and without persistent ST segment elevation after myocardial infarction [113]. If the aneurysm is defined as a "full thickness scar that exhibits a localized convex protrusion during both phases of the cardiac cycle," two-dimensional echocardiography showed that the persistent ST segment elevation correlates with dyskinesia rather than with aneurysm [114]. The well established relation between the persistent ST segment elevation and the paradoxical motion of left ventricular (LV) myocardium [114], suggests that stretch may play role in the process, but the mechanism by which stretch, might cause ST segment displacement has not been elucidated. The study of Toyofuku et al. [115] supports the hypothesis that stretch can cause ST segment elevation in the absence of ischemia. These investigators reported that in patients with arrhythmogenic right ventricular dysplasia (ARVD) who had no coronary artery disease, ST segment elevation was induced by exercise. In their study, significant ST segment elevation in the right precordial leads developed in 11 of 17 (65%) patients with severe right ventricular asynergy; the finding proved to be helpful in diagnosing ARVD noninvasively.

In some patients with dyskinesis, the ST segment becomes elevated after exercise and after cardiac surgery. The phenomenon of ST segment elevation reappearing during exercise-induced ischemia has been reproduced in pigs with a 1-month-old MI [116]. In this model, acute ischemia adjacent to chronic infarction induced ST segment elevation at the surface of the scar despite the virtual absence of viable tissue in the infarction. This suggests a passive ST segment potential transmission from the ischemic peri-infarction area through the infarction.

6.14 Aneurysmectomy

The results of aneurysmectomy have not helped to locate the site of abnormal potential differences [117–119]. In one study of 74 ECGs with ST segment elevation before aneurysmectomy, the pattern remained unchanged in 60.8%, improved in 25.7% and became more pronounced in 13.5% of cases after aneurysmectomy. The average ST segment amplitude after aneurysmectomy in several studies was reduced by only one quarter. Engel et al. [117] found that after encircling endocardial ventriculotomy, ST segment elevation was unchanged. This suggested that the ST segment elevation did not originate in the injured tissue adjacent to the aneurysm. However, the authors admitted the possibility that the encircling procedure could have created new zones of injury.

Anatomic correlations confirm the angiographic findings. In 64 cases of autopsy-proven ventricular aneurysm, the ECG location of the infarction correlated well with the anatomic site of the aneurysm [118]. Among the patients in whom the ECG was recorded more than 30 days after the onset of infarction, 79% of 50 patients with an anterior aneurysm and 50% of 13 patients with a posterior (inferior) aneurysm had persistent ST segment elevation in the appropriate leads. Among 290 patients with an LV pseudoaneurysm, the incidence of ST segment elevation was 20% [119].

Among patients undergoing surgical resection of a ventricular aneurysm [117], the anatomic localization determined at the time of operation was correctly predicted by the ECG changes. Of 26 patients, 21 had abnormal Q waves and 22 had persistent ST segment elevation. Those with wide distribution of the abnormal Q waves had large aneurysms, but the size of the infarction could not be predicted by the magnitude of the ST segment elevation. After aneurysmectomy, there was usually a decrease in QRS duration and an increase in R wave amplitude. The number of leads with abnormal Q waves was reduced, and in some cases Q waves disappeared in all leads. The ST segment elevation also tended to decrease, and in about one third of cases it disappeared after aneurysmectomy. It can be concluded, therefore, that the ECG is a fairly sensitive tool for detecting ventricular aneurysms, particularly at the more common anterior location.

6.15 ECG Findings Predictive of Cardiac Rupture

Oliva et al. [120] retrospectively and prospectively examined ECGs of 70 patients with cardiac rupture after MI. Patients with rupture had a significantly higher incidence of pericarditis, which was detectable on the ECG by progressive or recurrent ST segment elevation in the absence of recurrent ischemia. In patients with anterior infarction, free wall rupture did not occur when the ECG changes of infarction were confined to leads V_1 and V_2. When the anterior wall adjacent to the septum ruptured, the ECG showed changes in leads V_1 through V_4. Of 30 patients with an inferior infarction, 27 had additional involvement of the adjacent lateral wall, or posterior wall, or both. Altogether, 55 patients (79%) had multisegment infarcts, with a mid-lateral or high lateral component in 88%.

Figueras et al. [121] examined clinical and ECG features in patients who died of an acute MI with and without LV free wall rupture. Risk factors of an early rupture included advanced age and first transmural anterior infarction without conduction abnormalities or heart failure. ST segment elevation on admission was higher in patients with early rupture (1 day) than in those with later rupture. On day 2 the ST segment elevation decreased less in patients with the subsequent late rupture (>2 days) than in those without rupture. Among the entire group of 93 patients with rupture, the site of rupture was anterior in 38%, posterior in 33%, and lateral in 29%. Evidence of pericarditis was rarely seen except for extensive pericardial adhesions in ten patients who died late (>4 days). A reported pattern predictive of free cardiac rupture was ST elevation in lead aVL on admission [122] whereas the reported risk factors for the development of ventricular septal defect were: age, female gender, and absence of previous angina. In another study of patients with anterior infarction, less ST segment depression in lead III was a predictor of post-MI ventricular septal defect [123].

6.16 ST Segment Elevation: Normal Variant and Acute Pericarditis (See Chap. 5)

6.16.1 Other Causes of ST Segment Elevation

Persistent multilead ST segment elevation is present in patients with spinal cord injury at C5 to C6 levels, i.e., lesions which completely disrupt cardiac sympathetic influences [124]. These changes were reversed by low doses of infused

Table 6.1
Less Common Causes of ST Segment Elevation

Pulmonary embolism and acute cor pulmonale (usually lead III)
Cardiac tumor
Acute aortic dissection [126]
After mitral valvuloplasty [127]
Pancreatitis, gall bladder disease [128–130] and other catastrophic illnesses [131].
Myocarditis [132]
Septic shock
Anaphylactic reaction [133]
Hyperkalemia ("dialyzable current of injury")
With any marked QRS widening, e.g., antidepressant drug overdose [134] or class IC antiarrhythmic drugs [135, 136]
After transthoracic cardioversion [137, 138]

isoproterenol. Although the mechanism of ST segment elevation in these patients has not been clarified, the findings demonstrate that normal sympathetic tone modulates the course and/or sequence of ventricular repolarization.

Normal "male" pattern with elevated J point and ST segment elevation, mainly in right precordial, is attributed to the effect of testosterone [125] and probably encompasses most cases of a normal variant inappropriately dubbed as "premature repolarization" (see Chap. 5). Less common causes of ST-segment elevation (Table 6.1) which are encountered less frequently than the conditions discussed in the preceding text.

6.16.2 Reciprocal ST Changes in Acute Myocardial Infarction

ST depression in the presence of ST elevation can be a result of either a process which caused the injury current responsible for ST elevation (that is, a true reciprocal change), or the presence of an independent additional area of injury in another location. The magnitude and distribution of ST depression in the baseline ECG of patients with acute coronary syndrome is a strong predictor of cardiac morbidity and mortality [139]. Existence of reciprocal ST depression is supported by experimental studies.

In dogs with anterior myocardial infarction following occlusion of the LAD coronary artery, tachycardia increased ST segment elevation in the anterior precordial leads concomitantly with an increase of reciprocal ST segment depression [140]. It has been shown that a subendocardial lesion associated with ST segment elevation in subendocardial electrograms causes a reciprocal ST segment depression in the epicardial electrograms as long as a layer of nonischemic epicardial muscle is present. However, when ischemia becomes transmural, ST segment elevation occurs in the epicardial electrograms [141].

During acute ischemia, reciprocal ST segment depression is present in all patients with inferior myocardial infarction and in 70% of patients with anterior myocardial infarction. In the cases in which the magnitude of ST segment elevation is small because the overall amplitude of the complex is low, reciprocal ST segment depression may be more conspicuous than the culprit ST segment elevation.

Echocardiographic studies showed that remote-wall changes did not correlate with reciprocal ST segment depression, a finding which is compatible with a true reciprocal change [142]. In other studies, nuclear imaging suggested that reciprocal change indicates an additional region of remote ischemia [143]. Also, angiographic studies performed within 2 weeks of acute myocardial infarction in 84 patients with inferior myocardial infarction showed that patients with anterolateral ST segment depression had larger infarcts and greater incidence of multivessel disease [111]. In the same study, the absence of reciprocal ST segment depression "virtually precluded multivessel disease." Also, in patients with anterior infarction, ST segment depression in inferior leads occurred in 45% of cases and was associated with more extensive infarction, increased morbidity and greater incidence of multivessel coronary disease [144].

During evolution of inferior-wall infarction associated with ST segment elevation in lead III, an absent or disproportionately small reciprocal ST segment elevation in lead V_2 was suggestive of an associated infarction of the right ventricle [145] (Fig. 6.11).

The same principle was shown to be applicable when anterior myocardial infarction caused by occlusion of the left anterior descending coronary artery was accompanied by ischemia of the inferior wall [143]. The latter was caused by either continuation of the occluded left anterior descending coronary artery beyond the apex of the heart onto the inferior wall of the left ventricle, or left anterior descending coronary artery supplying collaterals to the previously infarcted inferior wall. Under such circumstances the ST segment elevation in the anterior precordial leads was associated with either attenuation or reversal of the reciprocal ST segment depression in the "inferior" leads [146].

Boden and Spodick [147] listed the following causes of ST depression in the precordial leads in addition to reciprocal changes in the presence of inferoposterior or inferoseptal or basal (high lateral) acute MI: (1) myocardial ischemia or non-Q-wave infarction; (2) posterior ("transmural") or posteroseptal acute MI, and (3) "benign" reciprocal changes (presumably a normal variant).

6.17 Absence of the Expected Reciprocal ST Segment Deviation

In the presence of the three common types of Q-wave myocardial infarction, i.e., anterior, lateral, and inferior, ST segment elevation is usually associated with reciprocal ST depression in one or more of the standard 12 leads. In the presence of posterior or anterior subendocardial myocardial infarction, the acute injury pattern is manifested by ST segment depression in one or more of the standard leads, and the reciprocal ST segment elevation may be present only in the back in the case of subendocardial infarction, and may be difficult to detect in the anterior leads in the case of posterior infarction because of the low amplitude of ST segment deviation caused by remote location of infarction.

The apparent lack of expected reciprocal ST segment depression in the presence of ST segment elevation in one or more standard precordial leads may be attributed to some of the following factors: (1) Failure to examine leads aVR and V_1 which are probably relatively close to the posterobasal part of the left ventricle; these leads are often less carefully examined than the other ten leads, and therefore the differences between normal and abnormal patterns in these leads may be less recognizable (➋ Fig. 6.4); (2) Difficulty of recognition caused by low amplitude of the ventricular complex in the leads with expected ST segment deviation; (3) Obfuscation by secondary ST segment deviations caused by intraventricular conduction disturbance (➋ Fig. 6.12) or ventricular hypertrophy; common cause is wide terminal QRS deflection in the presence of incomplete or complete RBBB; (4) Co-existence of acute anterior and inferior injury patterns; and (5) Diffuse ST segment elevation in the early stage of anterior infarction with transient extension of ST segment elevation into the territory facing the inferior leads. (➋ Fig. 6.5) Associated pericarditis (➋ Fig. 6.14); It has been suggested [148] that disappearance of reciprocal ST segment depression or appearance of ST segment elevation in the leads with previous ST segment depression may facilitate in some cases the diagnosis of infarction-related pericarditis.

6.18 Hyperacute T Wave Pattern

Pointed tall or deeply negative "coronary" T waves associated with prolonged QT interval may appear either before or after the onset of ST segment shift (➋ Figs. 6.2 and ➋ 6.6). These T wave abnormalities are attributed to prolongation of activity in the ischemic regions of the ventricle [9, 149]. In some cases the increase in T wave amplitude may be modest and not easily recognized [150]. In the presence of posterior infarction tall upright T waves in the precordial leads are similar to "hyperacute" T waves during acute anterior ischemia but usually are less transient.

6.19 Postischemic T Wave Abnormalities

In patients with myocardial infarction or unstable angina pectoris, pointed "coronary" T waves appear when the primary deviation of the ST segment has begun to subside. This is attributed to prolongation of activity in the regions of the ventricle immediately adjoining the area of infarction [151]. The abnormal T wave after myocardial infarction is frequently called the: "ischemic" T wave. However, the same term has been also used to designate the pattern of acute myocardial ischemia which is associated with shortening of the QT interval and deviation of the ST segment from baseline. Since lengthening of the QT interval appears later when the injury becomes subacute or chronic, Lepeschkin [152] proposed

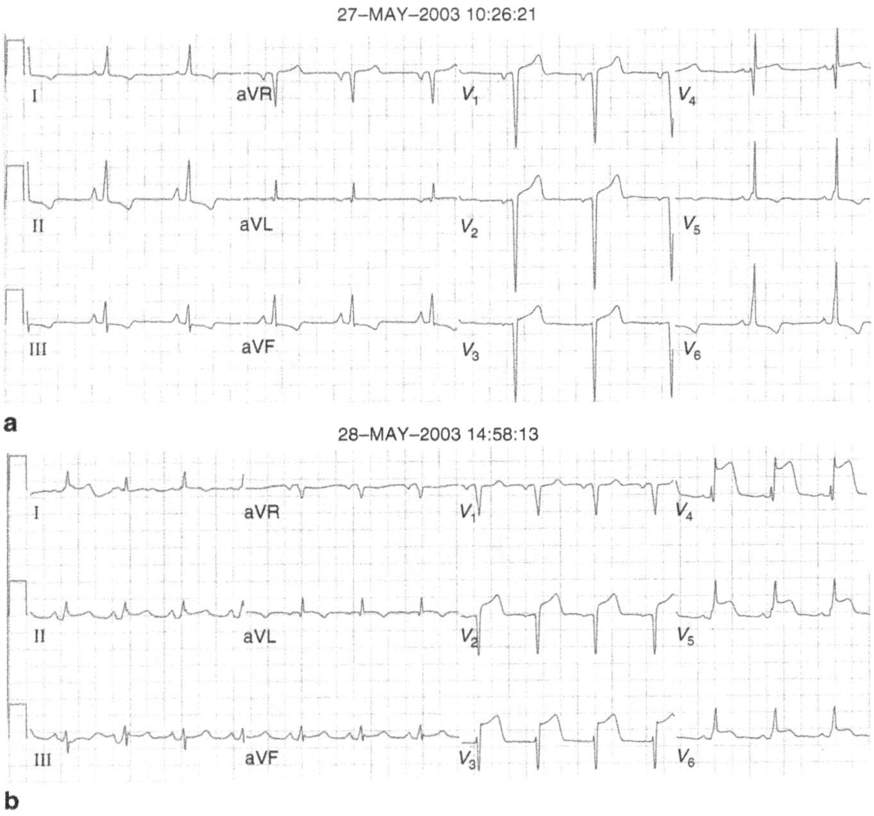

Fig. 6.14

Electrocardiogram of a 40-year-old man with hypertension and three-vessel coronary artery disease. In (a) before coronary artery bypass operation, ECG shows left ventricular hypertrophy pattern with secondary ST and T changes. In (b) on the first post-operative day, ST elevation in II, III, V_{2-6} attributed to postoperative pericarditis. No definite reciprocal ST depression is discernible. The above ST changes regressed 1 day later (not shown)

the term "postischemic T wave pattern". In dogs with myocardial infarction, T wave inversion appears within 2 – 3 days after coronary ligation and is associated with an average 24 ms increase in the functional refractory period at the ischemic site [153]. This suggests lengthening of the ventricular AP in this area, a finding which is supported by experimental data. The possible cause of such a lengthening is not known. The proposed theories include changes in the ionic composition of the partly damaged fibers, a decreased temperature owing to depressed mechanical activity [152], or altered function of repolarizing membrane currents. There is no experimental confirmation of any of these theories. The postischemic T wave abnormalities which appear during exercise-induced or a spontaneous attack of angina pectoris usually regress within minutes, but after myocardial infarction, such changes may persist for several days, weeks, months or years.

The vector of abnormal T waves tends to be directed away from the area of abnormal (prolonged) repolarization; that is negative T waves in leads V_1–V_4 in anterior infarction in V_2–V_5, V_6 in anterolateral infarction in V_1 or V_2–V_4 and I, aVL in antero-superior infarction, in I, aVL, and V_5–V_6 in lateral infarction, in II, III and aVF in inferior infarction and an upright T waves in right precordial leads in posterior infarction. However, the correlation between the distribution of T wave abnormalities and localization of myocardial lesions is not as reliable as the correlation between the distribution of Q waves and the region of myocardial infarction (➋ Fig. 6.8). Therefore, it is not advisable to attempt to localize regions of ischemia or fibrosis based on the T wave vector alone in the absence of QRS abnormalities produced by infarction.

In the differential diagnosis of abnormal T wave following T wave characteristics suggest the presence of myocardial ischemia or non-Q-wave MI: (1) T wave is preceded by a horizontal ST segment; (2) T wave is nearly symmetrical and deep; (3) T wave abnormalities occur in several contiguous leads; (4) QT interval is prolonged. The specificity of diagnosis increases with the increasing number of the above features. In patients with giant negative T waves (see Chap. 5) the presence of coronary artery disease is suggested by the absence of left ventricular hypertrophy and the symmetry of the T wave [154].

In most cases, the T wave abnormalities tend to persist longer than the ST segment deviations. Kloner reported that negative T waves became normal concurrently with the disappearance of wall motion abnormalities within 6 months after coronary angioplasty, presumably owing to the recovery of the stunned (hypoperfused) or hibernating (damaged) but capable of recovery myocardium [155]. The primary "coronary" or postischemic T wave pattern without ST deviation, an abnormal T wave vector, pointed T wave, and prolonged QT interval may appear in patients with various types of pathologic processes discussed in Chap. 5.

6.20 Evolution of ECG Pattern of Acute ST-Elevation Myocardial Infarction (STEMI)**

In a classic sequence of events, during MI the first ECG change is the "hyperacute" T wave followed by ST segment elevation, Q waves (possibly abnormal R waves), decreased ST segment elevation with the beginning of T wave inversion, and return of the ST segment to baseline with symmetric T wave inversion and a prolonged QT interval. During the course of the transition from ST elevation to T wave inversion, a stage of pseudonormalization may occur when the ST segment deviation subsides and the T wave inversion has not yet occurred (see Fig. 6.2). This classic sequence of events is often altered in various ways, particularly in patients undergoing thrombolytic therapy or primary coronary angioplasty (see Figs. 6.3 and 6.6).

The incidence of transient "hyperacute" T wave changes is low even when the ECG is monitored from the time of the onset of symptoms. The patterns of ST segment elevation are described earlier. As a rule, the ST segment elevation is recorded in a larger number of leads than in those with a developing abnormal Q wave. The extent, magnitude, and time course of ST elevation and the associated reciprocal ST segment depression are highly variable. In most cases the initial ST segment elevation decreases markedly during the first 7 to 12 h after the onset of chest pain [90, 156] and subsides within a few days. Mills et al. [157] found that the ST segment elevation resolved within 2 weeks in 90% of patients with inferior infarction and in only 40% of those with anterior infarction. The modern treatment of acute MI has changed the course of ST segment evolution, but the significance of persistent ST segment elevation as a marker of suspected ventricular aneurysm has remained unchanged (see above).

Abnormal T waves are usually more symmetric and more pointed than normal T waves. They are sometimes called "coronary" T waves and are usually associated with lengthening of the QT interval. Pointed "coronary" T waves appear before or after the primary elevation of the ST segment has begun to subside. In the presence of an elevated ST segment the site at which the T wave descent begins to form can be recognizes by the presence of a notch at the summit of repolarization wave (Figs. 6.4 and 6.5). When the notch deepens, the negative deflection is formed. This negative deflection has a characteristic shape known as cove plane T wave [9]. With the increasing descent of the ST segment, the area of the negative T wave increases. When the ST segment becomes horizontal, a symmetric sharply inverted T wave of varying amplitude is inscribed. Such T waves are distinctly different from the secondary T waves of ventricular hypertrophy or intraventricular conduction disturbances but may be indistinguishable from T wave abnormalities caused by other processes (Fig. 6.15; also see Chap. 5).

6.21 Prognostic Implications of Abnormal Repolarization During Acute Myocardial Infarction

The absolute magnitude of the ST segment elevation at hospital admission was found to be of significant prognostic importance [158]. In patients with an inferior infarction, the amplitude of the ST segment elevation was predictive of in-hospital development of a high degree AV block [159]. The degree of reciprocal ST segment depression also was related to infarct size and mortality independent of the ST segment elevation with both anterior and inferior infarctions.

**Previously known as acute Q-wave MI

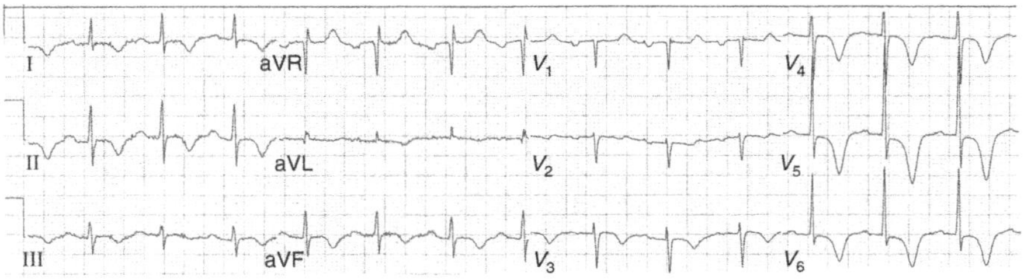

Fig. 6.15
Electrocardiogram of a 70-year-old woman with pulmonary edema and normal coronary arteries shows deeply inverted symmetrical T waves of "coronary" configuration in leads I, II, III, aVF and V_3

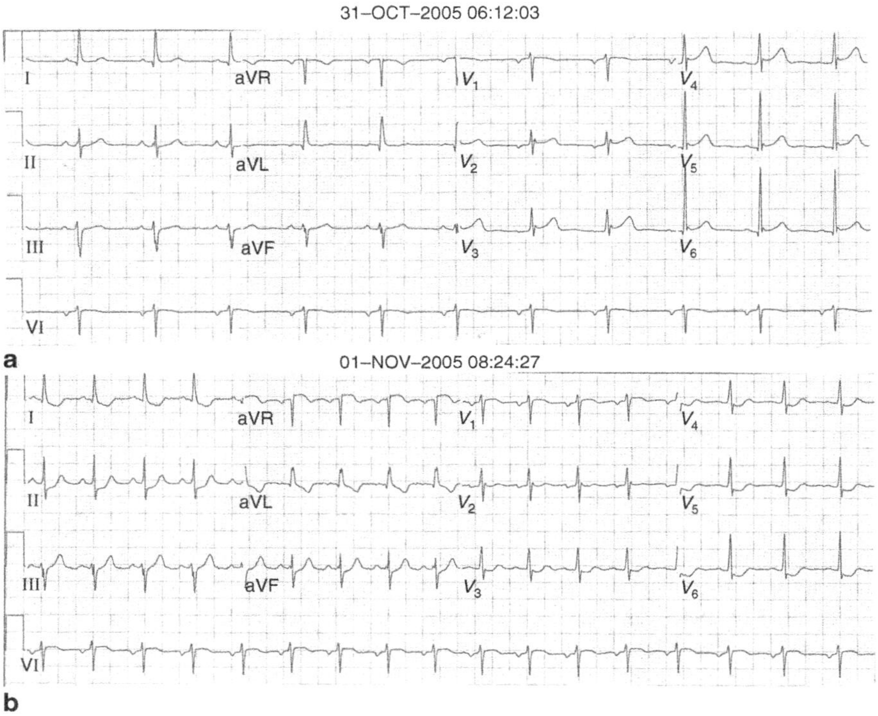

Fig. 6.16
Electrocardiogram of a 72-year-old woman before and after carotid endarterectomy with post-operative chest pain. In (a), normal ECG. In (b), during chest pain ST depression in leads I, II, aVL, $V_{3–6}$ with reciprocal ST-elevation in leads aVR and V_1. See text

T wave abnormalities also have predictive value [160–162]. In one study of patients with acute Q-wave MI, those with ST segment elevation of >2 mm and positive T waves had large infarcts, but a low incidence of recurrent ischemia [162]. In another study [161] persistent negative T waves in leads with Q waves in the chronic stage of MI indicated transmural infarction with a thin fibrotic layer, whereas positive T waves indicated a nontransmural infarct containing viable myocardium within the damaged myocardium. Tamura et al. [163] found that normalization of negative T waves in the infarct-related leads during healing of acute anterior infarction occurred in patients with small infarct and was suggestive of functional recovery of viable myocardium. Lanzelotti et al. [164] reported that persistent negative T waves after first acute MI were independently associated with a worse outcome whereas Q wave regression was of no long-term prognostic importance. Also among patients with non-ST segment elevation acute coronary syndromes, those with abnormal T waves had a significantly greater incidence of adverse effects [165].

6.22 Angina Pectoris

Stress-induced angina is often associated with ST depression in anterior and inferior leads attributed to subendocardial ischemia. ➋ Figure 6.16 shows that these changes are associated with reciprocal ST elevation in leads aVR and V_1. This subject is covered in greater detail in the chapter dealing with stress testing.

6.23 Silent Myocardial Ischemia

Silent myocardial ischemia is observed in patients with asymptomatic coronary artery disease, in patients with symptomatic angina and painless periods and after myocardial infarction [166, 167, 170]. Electrocardiographic manifestations of silent ischemia usually consist of horizontal or downsloping ST segment depression recorded during exercise test or ambulatory monitoring. Silent ST segment elevation may occur but is uncommon.

The review of literature by Rozanski and Berman [170] disclosed that among patients with coronary artery disease, about one third of the episodes of ST segment depression observed during exercise testing occur silently. Ambulatory ECG monitoring in patients with history of angina pectoris and an abnormal exercise test showed that about 75% of the episodes of ST segment depression are silent. The frequency of silent or symptomatic myocardial ischemia follows a typical circadian rhythm, with the highest frequency of the episodes in the morning hours [171, 172].

6.24 QT-Interval

During acute myocardial ischemia QT interval may shorten, lengthen or remain unchanged [31].

6.25 U Wave

During acute myocardial ischemia U wave may become inverted or increase in amplitude. The former occurs more often. In patients with anterior infarction, U wave may become inverted in anterior leads and in those with inferior MI in inferior leads. Transient U wave inversion may be caused, however, not only by regional myocardial ischemia but also by elevation of blood pressure [173, 174] (see ➋ Chap. 5).

References

1. Cascio, W.E., G.X. Yan, and A.G. Kleber, Passive electrical properties, mechanical activity and extracellular potassium in arterially perfused and ischemic rabbit ventricular muscle. *Circ. Res.*, 1990;**66**: 1461–1473.
2. Jennings, R.B., K.A. Reimer, M.L. Hill, and S.E. Mayer, Total ischemia in dog hearts in vitro. 1. Comparison of high energy phosphate production, utilization and depletion and of adenosine nucleotide catabolism in total ischemia in vitro vs severe ischemia in vivo. *Circ. Res.*, 1981: 892–900.
3. Janse, M.J., H. Cinca, J. Morena, et al., The "border zone" in myocardial ischemia. An electrophysiological, metabolic and histochemical correlation in the pig heart. *Circ. Res.*, 1979;**44**: 576–588.
4. Kleber, A.G, Resting membrane potential, extracellular potassium activity and intracellular sodium activity during acute global ischemia in isolated perfused guinea pig hearts. *Circ. Res.*, 1983;**52**: 442–450.
5. Kleber, A.G., C.B. Riegger, and M.J. Janse, Extracellular K+ and H+ in early ischemia: mechanisms and relation to changes in impulse propagation. *J. Moll. Cell. Cardiol.*, 1987;**19**: 35–44.
6. Vleugels, A., J. Vereecke, J. Van der Heyden, and E. Carmeliet, Ionic currents during hypoxia in voltage-clamped ventricular muscle. *Circ. Res.*, 1980;**47**: 501–508.
7. Isenberg, G., J. Vereecke, G. Van der Heyden, and E. Carmeliet, The shortening of the action potential by DNP in guinea pig ventricular myocytes is mediated by an increase of a-time dependent K+ conductance. *Pfluegers Archiv.*, 1983;**397**: 251–259.

8. Van der Heyden, G., J. Vereecke, and R. Carmeliet, The effect of cyanide on the K current in guinea pig ventricular myocytes. *Basic Res. Cardiol.*, 1985;**80**: 93–96.
9. Surawicz, B., *Electrophysiological Basis of ECG and Cardiac Arrhythmias*. Baltimore, MD: Williams and Wilkins, 1995.
10. Samson, W.E. and A.M. Scher, Mechanism of ST segment alteration during acute myocardial injury. *Circ. Res.*, 1960;**8**: 780–787.
11. Downar, E., M.J. Janse, and D. Durrer, The effect of acute coronary artery occlusion on subepicardial transmembrane potential in the intact porcine heart. *Circulation*, 1977;**56**: 217–224.
12. Kleber, A.G., M.J. Janse, P.J. Van Capelle, and D. Durrer, Mechanisms and time course of ST and TQ segment changes during acute regional myocardial ischemia in the pig heart determined by extracellular and intracellular recordings. *Circ. Res.*, 1978;**42**: 603–613.
13. Janse, M.J. and A.L. Wit, Electrophysiological mechanisms of ventricular arrhythmias resulting from myocardial ischemia and infarction. *Physiol. Rev.*, 1989;**69**: 1049–1150.
14. Michelson, E.L., J.F. Spear, and E.N. Moore, Strength-interval relations in a chronic canine model of myocardial infarction. Implications for the interpretation of electrophysiologic studies. *Circulation*, 1981;**63**: 1158–1165.
15. Gardner, P., P.C. Ursell, J.J. Fenoglio, and A.L. Wit, Electrophysiological and anatomical basis for fractionated electrograms recorded from healed myocardial infarcts. *Circulation*, 1985;**72**: 596–611.
16. Taccardi, B., Changes in cardiac electrogenesis following coronary occlusion, in Coronary Circulation and Energetics of the Myocardium, G. Marchetti and B. Taccardi, Editors. Karger, Basel, 1967, pp. 259–267.
17. Cohen, D. and L.A. Kaufman, Magnetic determination of the relationship between the S-T segment shift and the injury current produced by coronary artery occlusion. *Circ. Res.*, 1975;**36**: 414–425.
18. Cohen, D., P. Savard, R.D. Rifkin, E. Lepeschkin, and W.E. Strauss, Magnetic measurement of the S-T and T-Q segment shifts in humans; Part II: Exercise-induced S-T segment depression. *Circ. Res.*, 1983;**53**: 274–279.
19. R. Coronel, F.J. Wilms-Schopman, T. Opthof, F.J. van Cappelle, and M. Janse, Injury current and gradients of diastolic stimulation threshold, TQ potential and extracellular potassium concentration during acute regional ischemia in the isolated perfused pig heart. *Circ. Res.*, 1991;**68**: 1241–1249.
20. Smith, G.T., G. Geary, W. Ruf, T.H. Roelofs, J.J. McNamara, Epicardial mapping and electrocardiographic models of myocardial ischemic injury. *Circulation*, 1979;**60**: 930–938.
21. Cinca, J., J. Figueras, G. Senador, E. Garcia-Moreno, A. Salas, and J. Rius, Transmural DC electrograms after coronary artery occlusion and latex embolization in pigs. *Am. J. Physiol.*, 1984;**246**: H475–H482.
22. Mirvis, D.M., Body surface distribution of repolarization forces during acute myocardial infarction. Isopotential and isoarea mapping. *Circulation*, 1980;**62**: 878–887.
23. Kornreich, F., T.J. Montague, and P.M. Rautaharju, Body surface potential mapping of ST segment changes in acute myocardial infarction. Implications for ECG enrollment criteria for thrombolytic therapy. *Circulation*, 1993;**87**: 773–782.
24. Birnbaum, Y., S. Sclarovsky, A. Solodky, et al., Prediction of the level of left anterior descending coronary artery obstruction during anterior wall acute myocardial infarction by the admission electrocardiogram. *Am. J. Cardiol.*, 1993;**72**: 823–826.
25. Ben-Gal, T., I. Herz, A. Solodky, et al., Acute anterior wall myocardial infarction entailing ST segment elevation in lead V_1; electrocardiographic and angiographic correlations. *Clin. Cardiol.*, 1998;**21**: 399–404.
26. Engelen, D.J.M., A.P.M. Gorgels, E.C. Cheriex, et al., ECG criteria differentiating between proximal versus distal occlusion of the left anterior descending coronary artery. *J. Am. Coll. Cardiol.*, 1997;**30**: 430A (abstr).
27. Assali, A., S. Sclarovsky, I. Herz, et al., Persistent ST segment depression in precordial leads V_5–V_6 after Q-wave anterior wall myocardial infarction is associated with restrictive physiology of the left ventricle. *J. Am. Coll. Cardiol.*, 2000;**35**: 352–357.
28. Lew, A.S., H. Hod, B. Cercek, P.K. Shah, and W. Ganz, Inferior ST segment changes during acute anterior myocardial infarction; a marker of the presence or absence of concomitant inferior wall ischemia. *J. Am. Coll. Cardiol.*, 1987;**30**: 519–526.
29. Iwasaki, K., S. Kusachi, T. Kita, and G. Taniguchi, Prediction of isolated first diagonal branch occlusion by 12-lead electrocardiography; ST segment shift in I and aVL. *J. Am. Coll. Cardiol.*, 1994;**23**: 1557–1561.
30. Surawicz, B., C.M. Orr, J.B. Hermiller, K.D. Bell, R.P. Pinto, QRS changes during percutaneous transluminal coronary angioplasty and their possible mechanisms. *J. Am. Coll. Cardiol.*, 1997;**30**: 452–458.
31. Tsuka, Y., T. Sugiura, A. Yoshiteru, et al., Clinical characteristics of ST segment elevation in lead V_6 in patients with Q-wave acute inferior wall myocardial infarction. *Coron. Art. Dis.*, 1999;**10**: 465–469.
32. Birnbaum, Y., I. Herz, S. Sclarovsky, et al., Prognostic significance of precordial ST segment depression on admission electrocardiogram in patients with inferior wall myocardial infarction. *J. Am. Coll. Cardiol.*, 1996;**28**: 313–318.
33. Wong, C.K., B. Freedman, G. Bautovich, et al., Mechanism and significance of precordial ST segment depression during inferior wall acute myocardial infarction associated with severe narrowing of the dominant right coronary artery. *Am. J. Cardiol.*, 1993;**71**: 1025–1030.
34. Shah, P.K., M. Pichler, D.S. Berman, et al., Non-invasive identification of a high risk subset of patients with acute inferior myocardial infarction. *Am. J. Cardiol.*, 1980;**48**: 915–921.
35. Goldberg, H.L., J.S. Borer, J.S. Jacobstein, et al., Anterior ST depression in inferior myocardial infarction; indicator of posterolateral infarction. *Am. J. Cardiol.*, 1981;**48**: 1009–1015.
36. Peterson, E.D., W.R. Hathaway, K.M. Zabel, et al., Prognostic significance of precordial ST segment depression during inferior myocardial infarction in the thrombolytic era:results in 16,521 patients. *J. Am. Coll. Cardiol.*, 1996;**28**: 305–312.
37. Bates, E.R., P.M. Clemmensen, R.M. Califf, et al., Precordial ST segment depression predicts a worse prognosis in inferior infarction despite reperfusion therapy. *J. Am. Coll. Cardiol.*, 1990;**16**: 1538–1544.
38. Kosuge, M., K. Kimura, T. Ishikawa, et al., New electrocardigraphic criteria predicting the site of coronary artery occlusion in inferior wall acute myocardial infarction. *Am. J. Cardiol.*, 1998;**82**: 1318–1322.

39. Birnbaum, Y., G.S. Wagner, G.I. Barbash, et al., Correlation of angiographic findings and right (V_1 to V_3) versus (V_4 to V_6) precordial ST segment depression in inferior wall acute myocardial infarction. *Am. J. Cardiol.*, 1999;**83**: 143–148.
40. Bairey, C.N., P.K. Shah, A.S. Lew, et al., Electrocardiographic differentiation of occlusion of the left circumflex versus right coronary artery as a cause of inferior acute myocardial infarction. *Am. J. Cardiol.*, 1997;**79**: 182–186.
41. Casas, R.E., H.J.L. Mariott, and D.L. Glancy, Value of leads V_7–V_9 in diagnosing posterior wall acute myocardial infarction and other causes of tall R waves in V_{1-2}. *Am. J. Cardiol.*, 1997;**80**: 508–509.
42. Huey, B.L., G.A. Beller, D.L. Kaiser, and R.S. Gibson, A comprehensive analysis of myocardial infarction due to circumflex artery occlusion; comparison with infarction due to right coronary artery and left anterior descending artery occlusion. *J. Am. Coll. Cardiol.*, 1988;**12**: 1156–1166.
43. Nagahama, Y., T. Sugiura, K. Takehana, et al., PQ segment depression in acute Q wave inferior wall myocardial infarction. *Circulation*, 1995;**91**: 641–645.
44. Chia, B.L., J.W.L. Yip, H.C. Tan, and Y.T. Lim, Usefulness of ST elevation II/III ratio and ST deviation in lead I for identifying the culprit artery in inferior wall acute myocardial infarction. *Am. J. Cardiol.*, 2000;**86**: 341–343.
45. Herz, I., A.R. Assali, Y. Adler, A. Solodky, S.L. Sclarovsky, New electrocardiographic criteria for predicting either the right or left circumflex artery as the culprit coronary artery in inferior wall acute myocardial infarction. *Am. J. Cardiol.*, 1997;**88**: 1343–1345.
46. Assali, A.R., S. Sclarovsky, I. Herz, et al., Comparison of patients with inferior wall acute myocardial infarction with versus without ST segment elevation in leads V_5 and V_6. *Am. J. Cardiol.*, 1998;**81**: 81–83.
47. Dunn, R.F., H.N. Newman, L. Bernstein, et al., The clinical features of isolated circumflex coronary artery disease. *Circulation*, 1984;**69**: 477–484.
48. Agarwal, J.B., K. Khaw, and F. Aurignac, Lo Curto. Importance of posterior chest leads in patients with suspected myocardial infarction, but non-diagnostic routine 12-lead electrocardiogram. *Am. J. Cardiol.*, 1999;**83**: 323–326.
49. Zalenski, R.J., R.J. Rydman, E.P. Sloan, et al., ST segment elevation and the prediction of hospital life-threatening complications. The role of right ventricular and posterior leads. *J. Electrocardiol.*, 1998;**31**(Supplement): 164–171.
50. Matetzky, S., D. Freimark, M.S. Feinberg, et al., Acute myocardial infarction with isolated ST segment elevation in posterior chest leads V 7–9. *J. Am. Coll. Cardiol.*, 1999;**34**: 748–753.
51. Chou, T.C., J. van der Bel-Kahn, J. Allen, et al., Electrocardiographic diagnosis of right ventricular infarction. *Am. J. Med.*, 1981;**70**: 1175–1181.
52. Braat, S.H., A.P.M. Gorgels, F.W. Bar, H.J. Wellens, et al., Value of the ST-T segment in lead V_4 in inferior wall acute myocardial infarction to predict the site of coronary artery occlusion. *Am. J. Cardiol.*, 1988;**62**: 140–142.
53. Kataoka, H., K. Kanzaki, and Y. Mikuriya, An ECG marker of underlying right ventricular conduction delay in the hyperacute phase of right ventricular infarction or ischemia. *J. Electrocardiol.*, 1990;**23**: 369–372.
54. Geft, I.L., P.K. Shah, L. Rodriguez, et al., ST elevations in leads V_1 to V_5 may be caused by right coronary artery occlusion and acute right ventricular infarction. *Am. J. Cardiol.*, 1984;**53**: 991–996.
55. Forman, M.B., J. Goodin, B. Phelan, H. Kopelman, and R. Virmani, Electrocardiographic changes associated with isolater right ventricular infarction. *J. Am. Coll. Cardiol.*, 1984;**4**: 640–643.
56. Mak, K.H., B.L. Chia, A.F. Tan, and T. Johan, Simultaneous ST segment elevation in lead V_1 and depression in lead V_2. A discordant ECG pattern indicating right ventricular infarction. *J. Electrocardiol.*, 1994;**22**: 203–207.
57. Zehender, M., W. Kasper, E. Kauder, et al., Right ventricular infarction as an independent predictor of prognosis after acute inferior myocardial infarction. *N. Engl. J. Med.*, 1993;**328**: 981–988.
58. Braat, S., P. Brugada, C. De Zwaan, J.M. Coenegracht, and H.J. Wellens, Value of electrocardiogram in diagnosing right ventricular infarction in patients with an acute inferior wall myocardial infarction. *Br. Heart J.*, 1983;**49**: 368–372.
59. Saw, J., C. Davies, A. Fung, J.J. Spinelli, and J. Jue, Value of ST elevation in lead III greater than lead II in inferior wall acute myocardial infarction for predicting in-hospital mortality and diagnosing right ventricular infarction. *Am. J. Cardiol.*, 2001;**87**: 448–450.
60. Menown, I.B.A., J. Allen, M.C.C. Anderson, and A.A.J. Adgey, Early diagnosis of right ventricular or posterior infarction associated with inferior wall left ventricular acute myocardial infarction. *Am. J. Cardiol.*, 2000;**85**: 934–938.
61. Brugada, J. and P. Brugada, Further characterization of the syndrome of right bundle branch block, ST segment elevation and sudden death. *J. Cardiovasc. Electrophysiol.*, 1997;**8**: 325–331.
62. Brugada, P. and J. Brugada, Right bundle branch block, persistent ST segment elevation and sudden cardiac death: A distinct clinical and electrocardiographic syndrome. *J. Am. Coll. Cardiol.*, 1992;**20**: 1391–1395.
63. Atarashi, H., S. Ogawa, K. Harumi, et al., Characteristics of patients with right bundle branch block and ST segment elevation in right precordial lead. *Am. J. Cardiol.*, 1996;**78**: 581–585.
64. Ailings, M. and A. Wilde, "Brugada" syndrome. Clinical data and suggested pathophysiological mechanism. *Circulation*, 1999;**99**: 666–671.
65. Wung, S.F. and B. Drew, New electrocardiographic criteria for posterior wall acute myocardial ischemia validated by a percutaneous transluminal coronary angioplasty. Model of acute myocardial infarction. *Am. J. Cardiol.*, 2001;**87**: 970–974.
66. Miayazaki, T., H. Mitamura, H. Miyoshi, et al., Autonomic and antiarrhythmic drug modulation of ST segment elevation in patients with Brugada syndrome. *J. Am. Coll. Cardiol.*, 1996;**27**: 1061–1064.
67. Nademanee, K., G. Veerakul, S. Nimmannit, et al., Arrhythmogenic marker for the sudden unexplained death in Thai men. *Circulation*, 1997;**96**: 2595–2598.
68. Marcus, F.I., G.H. Fontaine, et al., Right ventricular dysplasia; A report of 24 adult cases. *Circulation*, 1982;**65**: 384–389.

69. Corrado, D., A. Nava, G. Guja, et al., Familial cardiomyopathy underlies syndrome of right bundle branch block, ST segment elevation and sudden death. *J. Am. Coll. Cardiol.*, 1996;**27**: 443–448.
70. Tada, H., N. Aihara, T. One, et al., Arrhythmogenic right ventricular cardiomyopathy underlies syndrome of right bundle branch block, ST segment elevation, and sudden death. *Am. J. Cardiol.*, 1998;**81**: 519–523.
71. Marcus, F.I. and G. Fontaine, Arrhythmogenic right ventricular dysplasia/cardiomyopathy: a review Pacing. *Clin. Electrophysiol.*, 1995;**18**: 1298–1314.
72. Takagi, M., N. Aihara, H. Takaki, et al., Clinical characteristics of patients with spontaneous or inducible ventricular fibrillation without apparent heart disease presenting with J wave and ST segment elevation in inferior leads. *J. Cardiovasc. Electrophysiol.*, 2000;**11**: 844–848.
73. Surawicz, B., Brugada syndrome: manifest, concealed, "asymptomatic", suspected and simulated. *J. Am. Coll. Cardiol.*, 2001;**38**: 775–777.
74. Yamaji, H., K. Iwasaki, S. Kusachi, et al., Prediction of acute left main coronary artery obstruction by 12 lead electrocardiography. ST segment elevation in lead aVR with less ST segment elevation in lead V_1. *J. Am. Coll. Cardiol.*, 2001;**38**: 1338–1354.
75. Gaitonde, R., N. Sharma, S. Al-Hasan, J.M. Miller, V. Jayachandran, and V.G. Kalaria, Prediction of significant left main coronary artery stenosis by the 12-lead electrocardiogram in patients with rest angina pectoris and the withholding of clopidogrel therapy. *Am. J. Cardiol.*, 2003;**92**: 846–848.
76. Mukarami, H., K. Urabe, and M. Nishimura, Inappropriate microvascular constriction produced transient ST segment elevation in patients with syndrome X. *J. Am. Coll. Cardiol.*, 1998;**32**: 1287–1292.
77. DeServi, H., E. Arbustini, F. Marsico, et al., Correlation between clinical and morphologic findings in unstable angina. *Am. J. Cardiol.*, 1996;**11**: 128–131.
78. Huey, B., M. Gheorghiade, R.S. Crampton, et al., Acute non-Q wave myocardial infarction with early ST segment elevation: Evidence for spontaneous coronary reperfusion and implications for thrombolytic trials. *J. Am. Coll. Cardiol.*, 1987;**9**: 18–25.
79. Stark, K., M.W. Krucoff, B. Schryver, and K.M. Kent, l: Quantification of ST segment changes during coronary angioplasty in patients with left bundle branch block. *Am. J. Cardiol.*, 1991;**67**: 1219–1222.
80. Blanke, H., H. Scherff, K.R. Karsch, et al., Electrocardiographic changes after streptokinase-induced recanalization in patients with acute left anterior descending artery obstruction. *Circulation*, 1983;**68**: 406–412.
81. Fernandez, A.R., R.F. Sequeira, S. Chakko, et al., ST segment tracking for rapid determination of patency of the infarct-related artery in acute myocardial infarction. *J. Am. Coll. Cardiol.*, 1995;**26**: 675–683.
82. Veldkamp, R.F., S. Sawchak, J.E. Pope, et al., Performance of an automated real-time ST segment analysis program to detect coronary occlusion and reperfusion. *J. Electrocardiol.*, 1996;**29**: 257–263.
83. Schroeder, R., K. Wegscheider, K. Schroder, R. Dissman, and W. Meyer-Sabelle, Extent of early ST segment elevation resolution. A strong predictor of outcome in patients with acute myocardial infarction and a sensitive measure to compare thrombolytic regimens. *J. Am. Coll. Cardiol.*, 1995;**26**: 1657–1664.
84. Pepine, C.J., Prognostic markers in thrombolytic therapy: Looking beyond mortality. *Am. J. Cardiol.*, 1996;**78**: 24.
85. Krucoff, M.W., M.A. Croll, J.E. Pope, et al., Continuous 12-lead ST segment recovery analysis in the TAMI 7 study. *Circulation*, 1993;**88**: 437–446.
86. Mauro, F., P. Maggioni, M.G. Francos, et al., A simple electrocardiographic predictor of outcome of patients with acute myocardial infarction treated with a thrombolytic agent. *J. Am. Coll. Cardiol.*, 1994;**24**: 600–606.
87. Santoro, G.M., R. Valenti, P. Buoanamici, et al., Relation between ST segment changes and myocardial perfusion evaluated by myocardial contrast echocardiography in patients with acute myocardial infarction treated with direct angioplasty. *Am. J. Cardiol.*, 1988;**82**: 932–936.
88. Krucoff, M.W., A.R. Parente, R.K. Bottner, et al., Stability of multilead ST segment "fingerprints" over time after percutaneous transluminal coronary angioplasty and its usefulness in detecting reocclusion. *Am. J. Cardiol.*, 1988;**61**: 1232–1237.
89. Kondo, M., K. Tamura, H. Tania, et al., Is ST segment re-elevation associated with reperfusion an indicator of marked myocardial damage after thrombolysis? *J. Am. Coll. Cardiol.*, 1993;**21**: 62–67.
90. Essen, R., W. Merx, and S. Effert, Spontaneous course of ST segment elevation in acute anterior myocardial infarction. *Circulation*, 1979;**59**: 105–112.
91. Ochiai, M., T. Isshiki, Y. Hirose, et al., Myocardial damage after successful thrombolysis is associated with the duration of ST-re-elevation at reperfusion. *Clin. Cardiol.*, 1995;**18**: 321–327.
92. Kosuge, M., K. Kimura, T. Ishikawa, et al., Relation of absence of ST re-elevation immediately after reperfusion and success of reperfusion with myocardial salvage. *Am. J. Cardiol.*, 1997;**80**: 1080–1083.
93. Schechter, M., B. Rabinowitz, B. Beker, et al., Additional ST segment elevation during the first hour of thrombolytic therapy: an electrocardiographic sign predicting a favorable clinical outcome. *J. Am. Coll. Cardiol.*, 1992;**20**: 1460–1464.
94. Doevendans, P.A., A.P. Gorgels, R. van der Zee, et al., Electrocardiographic diagnosis of reperfusion during thrombolytic therapy in acute myocardial infarction. *Am. J. Cardiol.*, 1995;**75**: 1206–1210.
95. Steg, P.G., M. Faraggi, D. Himbertt, et al., Comparison using dynamic vectorcardiography and MIBI SPECT of ST segment changes and myocardial MIBI uptake during percutaneous transluminal coronary angioplasty of the left anterior descending coronary artery. *Am. J. Cardiol.*, 1995;**75**: 998–1002.
96. Shah, A., G.S. Wagner, R.M. Califf, et al., Comparative prognostic significance of simultaneous versus independent resolution relative to ST segment elevation during acute myocardial infarction. *J. Am. Coll. Cardiol.*, 1997;**30**: 1478–1483.
97. Andrews, J., I.T. Straznicky, J.K. French, et al., for the HERO-1 investigators. ST segment recovery adds to the assessment of TIMI 2 and 3 flow in predicting infarct wall motion after thrombolytic therapy. *Circulation*, 2000;**101**: 2138–2143.
98. Dong, J., G. Ndrepepa, C. Schmitt, et al., Early resolution of ST segment elevation correlates with myocardial salvage assessed by Tc-99m Sestamibi scintigraphy in patients with acute myocardial infarction after mechanical or thrombolytic reperfusion therapy. *Circulation*, 2002;**105**: 2946–2949.

99. Shah, A., G.S. Wagner, C.L. Green, et al., Electrocardiographic differentiation of the ST segment depression of acute myocardial injury due to the left circumflex artery occlusion from that of myocardial ischemia of nonocclusive etiologies. *Am. J. Cardiol.*, 1997;**78**: 512–513.

100. MacDonald, R.G., J.A. Hill, R.L. Feldman, ST segment response to acute coronary occlusion. Coronary hemodynamic and angiographic determinants of direction of ST segment shift. *Circulation*, 1986;**74**: 973–979.

101. Kobayashi, N., N. Ohmura, I. Nakada, et al., Further ST elevation at reperfusion by direct percutaneous transluminal coronary angioplasty predicts poor recovery of left ventricular systolic function in anterior wall AMI. *Am. J. Cardiol.*, 1997;**79**: 862–866.

102. Santoro, G.M., D. Antoniucci, R. Valenti, et al., Rapid reduction of ST segment elevation after successful direct angioplasty in acute myocardial infarction. *Am. J. Cardiol.*, 1997;**80**: 865–869.

103. McLaughlin, M.G., G.W. Stone, E. Aymong, et al., Prognostic utility of comparative methods for assessment of ST segment resolution after primary angioplasty for acute myocardial infarction. The controlled Abciximab and device investigation to lower late angioplasty complications (CADILLAC) Trial. *J. Am. Coll. Cardiol.*, 2004;**44**: 215–223.

104. Watanabe, J., S. Nakamura, T. Sugiura, et al., Early identification of impaired myocardial reperfusion with serial assessment of ST segments after percutaneous transluminal coronary angioplasty during acute myocardial infarction. *Am. J. Cardiol.*, 2001;**88**: 956–959.

105. Feldman, L.J., P. Coste, A. Furber, et al., for the French Optimal STenting (FROST)-2 investigators. Incomplete resolution of ST segment elevation is a marker of transient microcirculatory dysfunction after stenting for acute myocardial infarction. *Circulation*, 2003;**107**: 2684–2689.

106. Brodie, B., T.D. Stuckey, C. Hansen, et al., Relation between electrocardiographic ST segment resolution and early and late outcomes after primary percutaneous coronary intervention for acute myocardial infarction. *Am. J. Cardiol.*, 2005;**95**: 343–348.

107. Claeys, M.J., J. Bosmans, L. Veenstra, et al., Determinants and prognostic implications of persistent ST segment elevation after primary angioplasty for acute myocardial infarction. *Circulation*, 1999;**99**: 1972–1977.

108. Matetzky, S., G. Novikov, L. Gruberg, et al., The significance of persistent ST elevation after primary PTCA. *J. Am. Coll. Cardiol.*, 1999;**34**: 1932–1938.

109. Cokkinos, D.V., G.L. Hallman, D.A. Cooley, O. Zamalloa, and R.D. Leachman, Left ventricular aneurysm: analysis of electrocardiographic features and postresection changes. *Am. Heart J.*, 1971;**82**: 149–157.

110. Chou, T.C., Electrocardiography, in Clinical Practice 1996; 4th ed: Philadelphia, PA: WB Saunders.

111. Roubin, G.S., W.F. Shen, M. Nicholson, et al., Anterolateral ST segment depression in acute inferior myocardial infarction. *Am. Heart J.*, 1984;**107**: 1177–1182.

112. Cohen, M., S.J. Scharpf, and K.P. Rentrop, Prospective analysis of electrocardiographic variables as markers for extent and location of acute wall motion abnormalities observed during coronary angioplasty in human subjects. *J. Am. Coll. Cardiol.*, 1987;**10**: 17–24.

113. Lindsay, J., R.C. Dewey, B.S. Talesnick, and N.G. Nolan, Relation of ST segment elevation after healing of acute myocardial infarction to the presence of ventricular aneurysm. *Am. J. Cardiol.*, 1984;**54**: 84–86.

114. Arvan, S. and M.A. Varat, Persistent ST segment elevation and left ventricular wall abnormalities. A 2 dimensional echocardiographic study. *Am. J. Cardiol.*, 1984;**53**: 1542–1546.

115. Toyofuku, M., H. Takaki, K. Sunagawa, et al., Exercise-induced ST elevation in patients with arrhythmogenic right ventricular dysplasia. *J. Electrocardiol.*, 1999;**32**: 1–8.

116. Cinca, J., A. Bardaji, A. Carreno, et al., ST segment elevation at the surface of a healed myocardial infarction in pigs: conditions for passive transmission from the ischemic peri-infarction zone. *Circulation*, 1995;**91**: 1552–1559.

117. Engel, T.R., R. Caine, P.R. Kowey, and J.O. Finnegan, ST segment elevation with ventricular aneurysm. *J. Electrocardiol.*, 1984;**17**: 75–77.

118. Dubnow, M.H., H.B. Burchell, and J.L. Titus, Post-infarction ventricular aneurysma clinicopathologic and electrocardiographic study of 80 cases. *Am. Heart J.*, 1965;**70**: 753–760.

119. Frances, C., A. Romero, and D. Grady, Left ventricular pseudoaneurysm. *J. Am. Coll. Cardiol.*, 1998;**32**: 537–541.

120. Oliva, P.B., S.C. Hammill, and W.D. Edwards, Cardiac rupture, a clinically predictable complication of acute myocardial infarction: report of 70 cases with clinico-pathologic correlations. *J. Am. Coll. Cardiol.*, 1993;**22**: 720–726.

121. Figueras, J., A. Curos, J.M. Cortodellas, and J. Soler-Soler, Relevance of electrocardiographic findings, heart failure and infarct site in assessing and timing of left ventricular free wall rupture during acute myocardial infarction. *Am. J. Cardiol.*, 1995;**76**: 543–547.

122. Yoshino, H., M. Yotsukara, K. Yano, et al., Cardiac rupture and admission electrocardiography in acute anterior myocardial infarction: Implication of ST elevation in aVL. *J. Electrocardiol.*, 2000;**33**: 49–53.

123. Birnbaum, Y., G.S. Wagner, K.B. Gates, et al., Clinical and electrocardiographic variables associated with increased risk of ventricular septal defect in acute anterior myocardial infarction. *Am. J. Cardiol.*, 2000;**86**: 830–834.

124. Lehmann, K.G., A.H. Shandling, A. Yusi, and V.F. Froelicher, Altered ventricular repolarization in central sympathetic dysfunction associated with spinal cord injury. *J. Am. J. Cardiol.*, 1989;**63**: 1498–1504.

125. Surawicz, B. and S.R. Parikh, Prevalence of male and female patterns of early ventricular repolarization in the normal ECG of males and females from childhood to old age. *J. Am. Coll. Cardiol.*, 2002;**40**: 1870–1876.

126. Hirata, K., M. Kyushima, and H. Asato, Electrocardiographic abnormalities in patients with acute dissection. *Am. J. Cardiol.*, 1995;**76**: 1207–1212.

127. Ludman, P.F., D. Hildick-Smith, A. Harcombe, and L.M. Shapiro, Transient ST segment changes associated with mitral valvuloplasty using the Inoue balloon. *Am. J. Cardiol.*, 1997;**79**: 1704–1705.

128. Patel, J., A. Mohaved, and W.C. Reeves, Electrocardiographic and segmental wall motion abnormalities in pancreatitis mimicking myocardial infarction. *Clin. Cardiol.*, 1994;**17**: 505–509.

129. Chandraratna, P.A.M., A. Nimalasurya, C.L. Reid, S. Cohn, and S.H. Rahimtoola, Left ventricular asynergy in acute myocarditis. Simulation of acute myocardial infarction. *JAMA*, 1983;**250**: 1428–1430.
130. Dec, G.W., H. Waldman, J. Southern, et al., Viral myocarditis mimicking acute myocardial infarction. *J. Am. Coll. Cardiol.*, 1992;**20**: 85–89.
131. Thomas, I., J. Mathew, V.P. Kumar, R. Cooper, and J. Ferlinz, Electrocardiographic changes in catastrophic abdominal illness mimicking acute myocardial infarction. *Am. J. Cardiol.*, 1987;**59**: 1224–1225.
132. Chida, K., S.I. Ohkawa, and Y. Esaki, Clinicopathologic characteristics of elderly patients with persistent ST segment elevation and inverted T waves: Evidence of insidious or healed myocarditis? *J. Am. Coll. Cardiol.*, 1995;**25**: 1641–1649.
133. Rich, M.W., Myocardial injury caused by an anaphylactic reaction to ampicillin/sulbactam in a patient with normal coronary arteries. *Tex. Heart Inst. J.*, 1998;**25**: 194–197.
134. Bolognesi, R., D. Tsialtas, P.E. Vasini, M. Conti, and C. Manca, Abnormal ventricular repolarization mimicking myocardial infarction after heterocycling antidepressant overdose. *Am. J. Cardiol.*, 1997;**79**: 242–245.
135. Nakamura, W., K. Segawa, H. Ito, and N. Yoshimoto, Class IC antiarrhythmic drugs, flecainide and pilsicainide, produce ST segment elevation simulating inferior myocardial ischemia. *J. Cardiovasc. Electrophysiol.*, 1998;**9**: 585–558.
136. Krishanan, S. and M.E. Josephson, ST segment elevation induced by class IC antiarrhythmic agents: underlying electrophysiologic mechanisms and insight into drug-induced proarrhythmia. *J. Cardiovasc. Electrophysiol.*, 1998;**9**: 1167–1174.
137. Kok, L.C., M.A. Mitchell, D.E. Haines, J.P. Mounsey, and J.P. Di Marco, Transient ST elevation after transthoracic cardioversionn in patients with hemodynamically unstable ventricular tachyarrhythmia. *Am. J. Cardiol.*, 2000;**85**: 877–881.
138. Wang, K., R.W. Asinger, and H.J.L. Marriott, ST segment elevation in conditions other than acute myocardial infarction. *N. Engl. J. Med.*, 2003;**349**: 2128–2135.
139. Kaul O, We-Ching C, Harrington RA, Wagner GS, et al. for the PARAGON-A and GUSTO-IIb Investigators. Prognostic value of ST segment depression in acute coronary syndromes: Insights from PARAGON-A applied to GUSTO-IIb. *J. Am. Coll. Cardiol.*, 2001;**38**: 64–71.
140. Mirvis, D.M., J.L. Wilson, and K.B. Ramanathan, Effects of experimental myocardial infarction on the ST segment response to tachycardia. *J. Am. Coll. Cardiol.*, 1985;**6**: 665–673.
141. Guyton, R.A., J.H. McClenathan, G.E. Newman, and L.L. Michaelis, Significance of subendocardial S-T segment elevation caused by coronary stenosis in the dog. *Am. J. Cardiol.*, 1977;**40**: 373–380.
142. Camara, E.J.N., N. Chandra, P. Ouyang, S.H. Gottlieb, and E.P. Shapiro, Reciprocal ST change in acute myocardial infarction. Assessment by electrocardiography and echocardiography. *J. Am. Coll. Cardiol.*, 1983;**2**: 251–257.
143. Pichler, M., P.K. Shah, T. Peter, et al., Wall motion abnormalities and electrocardiographic changes in acute transmural myocardial infarction: Implications of reciprocal ST segment depression. *Am. Heart J.*, 1983;**106**: 1003–1009.
144. Haraphongse, M., S. Tanomsup, and B.I. Jugdutt, Inferior ST segment depression during acute anterior myocardial infarction: Clinical and angiographic correlations. *J. Am. Coll. Cardiol.*, 1984;**4**: 467–476.
145. Lew, A.S., P. Laramee, P.K. Shah, J. Maddahi, T. Peter, and W. Ganz, Ratio of ST segment depression in lead V_2 to ST segment elevation in lead aVF in evolving inferior acute myocardial infarction; an aid to recognition of right ventricular ischemia. *Am. J. Cardiol.*, 1986;**57**: 1047–1051.
146. Lew, A.S., H. Hod, B. Cercek, P.K. Shah, and W. Ganz, Inferior ST segment changes during acute anterior myocardial infarction. A marker of the presence or absence of concomitant inferior wall ischemia. *J. Am. Coll. Cardiol.*, 1987;**10**: 519–526.
147. Boden, W.E. and D.H. Spodick, Diagnostic significance of precordial ST segment depression. *Am. J. Cardiol.*, 1989;**63**: 358–361.
148. Oliva, P.B., S.C. Hammill, and W.D. Edwards, Electrocardiographic diagnosis of postinfarction regional pericarditis. *Circulation*, 1993;**88**: 896–904.
149. Wilson, F.N., A.G. Macleod, and P.S. Barker, The T deflection of the electrocardiogram. *Trans. Assoc. Am. Phys.*, 1931;**46**: 29–38.
150. Goldberger, A.L., Hyperacute T waves revisited. *Am. Heart J.*, 1982;**104**: 888–890.
151. Wilson, F.N., F.F. Rosenbaum, and F.D. Johnston, Interpretation of the ventricular complex of the electrocardiogram. *Adv. Intern. Med.*, 1947;**2**: 1–63.
152. Lepeschkin, E., *Modern Electrocardiography*. Baltimore, MD: Williams and Wilkins, 1951, pp. 307, 420.
153. Kleber, A.G., M.F. Janse, F.J.L. van Capelle, and D. Durrer, Mechanism and time course of S-T and T-Q segment changes during acute regional myocardial ischemia in pig heart determined by extracellular and intracellular recordings. *Circ. Res.*, 1978;**42**: 603–613.
154. Otrusinik, R., M.A. Alpert, C.R. Hamm, et al., Factors predicting coronary artery disease in patients with giant negative T waves. *Am. J. Cardiol.*, 2000;**85**: 873–875.
155. Kloner, R.A., Inverted T waves. An electrocardiographic marker of stunned or hibernating myocardium in man? *Circulation*, 1990;**82**: 1060–1061.
156. Zmyslinski, R.W., T. Akiyama, T.L. Biddle, et al., Natural course of S-T segment and QRS complex in patients with acute anterior myocardial infarction. *Am. J. Cardiol.*, 1979;43: 29–34.
157. Mills, R.M., E. Young, R. Gordon, et al., Natural history of S-T segment elevation in acute myocardial infarction. *Am. J. Cardiol.*, 1975;**35**: 609–614.
158. Willems, J.L., R.J. Willems, G.M. Willems, et al., Significance of initial ST segment elevation and depression for the management of thrombolytic therapy in acute myocardial infarction. *Circulation*, 1990;**82**: 1147–1158.
159. Birnbaum, Y., S. Sclarovsky, and I. Herz, Admission clinical and electrocardiographic characteristics predicting in-hospital development of high-degree atrioventricular block in inferior acute myocardial infarction. *Am. J. Cardiol.*, 1997;**80**: 1134–1138.
160. Hochrein, J., F. Sun, K.S. Pieper, et al., Higher T wave amplitude associated with better prognosis in patients receiving thrombolytic therapy for acute myocardial infarction (a GUSTO-I-substudy). *Am. J. Cardiol.*, 1998;**81**: 1078–1084.
161. Sclarovsky-Benjaminov, F., S. Sclarovsky, and Y. Birnbaum, The predictive value of the electrocardiographic pattern of acute Q-wave myocardial infarction for recurrent ischemia. *Clin. Cardiol.*, 1995;**18**: 710–715.
162. Maeda, S., T. Imai, K. Kuboki, et al., Pathologic implications of restored positive T waves and persistent negative T waves after Q wave myocardial infarction. *J. Am. Coll. Cardiol.*, 1996;**28**: 1514–1518.

163. Tamura, A., K. Nagase, Y. Mikurya, et al., Significance of spontaneous normalization of negative T waves in infarct-related leads during healing of anterior wall acute myocardial infarction. *Am. J. Cardiol.*, 1999;**84**: 1341–1344.
164. Lanzellotti, P., P.L. Gerard, H.E. Kulbertus, and L.A. Pierard, Persistent negative T waves in the infarct-related leads as an independent predictor of poor long-term prognosis after acute myocardial infarction. *Am. J. Cardiol.*, 2002;**90**: 833–837.
165. Jacobsen, M.D., G.S. Wagner, L. Holmvang, P.W. Macfarlane, U. Nasllund, P. Grande, and P. Clemmensen, on behalf of the TRIM investigators. Clinical significance of abnormal T waves in patients with non-ST segment elevation acute coronary syndromes. *Am. J. Cardiol.*, 2001;**88**: 1225–1229.
166. Chierchia, S., M. Lazzari, B. Friedman, C. Brunelli, and A. Maseri, Impairment of myocardial perfusion and function during painless myocardial ischemia. *J. Am. Coll. Cardiol.*, 1983;**1**: 294–330.
167. Deanfield, J.E., M. Shea, P. Ribiero, et al., Transient ST segment depression as a marker of myocardial ischemia during daily life. *Am. J. Cardiol.*, 1984;**54**: 1195–1200.
168. Maseri, A., Role of coronary artery spasm in symptomatic and silent myocardial ischemia. *J. Am. Coll. Cardiol.*, 1987;**9**: 249–262.
169. von Arnim, T., B. Hoffling, M. Schreiber, et al., Characteristics of episodes of ST elevation or ST depression during ambulatory monitoring in patients subsequently undergoing coronary angiography. *Br. Heart J.*, 1985;**54**: 484–488.
170. Rozanski, A. and D.S. Berman, Silent myocardial ischemia: I. Pathophysiology, frequency of occurrence and approaches toward detection. *Am. Heart J.*, 1987;**114**: 615–626.
171. Quyumi, A., C.M. Wright, L.J. Mockus, and K.M. Fox, How important is history of chest pain in determining the degree of ischemia in patients with angina pectoris? *Br. Heart J.*, 1985;**54**: 22–26.
172. Rocco, M.B., J. Barry, S. Campbell, et al., Circadian variation of transient myocardial ischemia in patients with coronary artery disease. *Circulation*, 1987;**75**: 395–400.
173. Gerson, M.C., J.F. Phillips, S.N. Morris, and P.L. McHenry, Exercise-induced U wave inversion as a marker of stenosis of the left anterior descending coronary artery. *Circulation*, 1979;**60**: 1014–1020.
174. Kishida, H., J.S. Cole, and B. Surawicz, Negative U wave: A highly specific but poorly understood sign of heart disease. *Am. J. Cardiol.*, 1982;**49**: 2030–2036.

7 The QT Interval

Wojciech Zareba · Iwona Cygankiewicz

P. W. Macfarlane et al. (eds.), *Electrocardiology*, DOI 10.1007/978-0-85729-874-4_7,

7.1 Introduction

The QT interval in an electrocardiogram is a global reflection of complex processes governing the repolarization of ventricular myocardium. Most frequent concerns regarding the QT interval relate to its prolongation whereas QT shortening is relatively rare. QT interval prolongation may result from inherited long QT syndrome (LQTS), but more frequently is observed in the course of ischemic and nonischemic cardiomyopathies, or can be induced by drugs or abnormal electrolyte/metabolic disorders [1–10]. The LQTS is characterized by prolongation of the QT interval on the electrocardiogram and is associated with an increased propensity to ventricular tachyarrhythmias that can lead to cardiac events such as syncope, cardiac arrest, or sudden death [1–6]. The LQTS is a pure electrical disorder, which became a paradigm to understand QT interval and repolarization in general, and its role in cardiac electrophysiology. In particular, clinical observations in LQTS patients and related basic science research have led to a better understanding of the role of repolarization in cardiac arrhythmias and cardiac electrophysiology. Recognition of the association between QT prolongation and risk of torsades de pointes (TdP) ventricular tachycardia (VT) has lead to increasing interest in evaluating QT prolongation as a surrogate marker of cardiac arrhythmias, first in congenital LQTS, second, in drug-induced abnormalities of repolarization, and in more common conditions as well as in healthy subjects [1–6, 10].

In this chapter, we aim to provide an overview of current concepts on ventricular repolarization and its pathophysiology, describe clinical and electrocardiographic aspects of QT interval analysis, explore prognostic significance of repolarization abnormalities, describe clinical aspects of drug-induced repolarization abnormalities, and describe dynamic features of the QT interval.

7.2 QT Interval and Ventricular Repolarization

7.2.1 Long QT Syndrome (LQTS) as a Paradigm for Understanding Ventricular Repolarization

During the last decades, several mutations in specific genes encoding cardiac ion channels have been identified in patients with the congenital form of LQTS [11–22]. These mutations cause alterations in the ion-channel proteins leading to abnormalities in ion-channel function that prolong ventricular repolarization (Fig. 7.1). The KVLQT1 (LQT1) gene [11, 14] encodes a potassium channel protein (α-subunit) that when coexpressed with a protein (β-subunit) from the minK (KCNE1; LQT5) gene produces a reduction in the slowly activating, delayed rectifier (repolarizing) potassium current (I_{Ks}). The reduction in I_{Kr} (rapidly activating delayed rectifier) current is caused by mutations in the HERG (LQT2) gene [11, 12] regulating the major pore-forming subunit or by mutations in the MiRP1 (LQT6) gene coding the putative regulatory subunit of the I_{Kr} channel. The SCN5A (LQT3) sodium channel gene [13] mutations cause abnormal inactivation of sodium channel with an inward leakage of sodium ions during the repolarization phase contributing to QT prolongation. There are currently 12 different genes recognized as causing QT prolongation (Table 7.1). About 60–70%

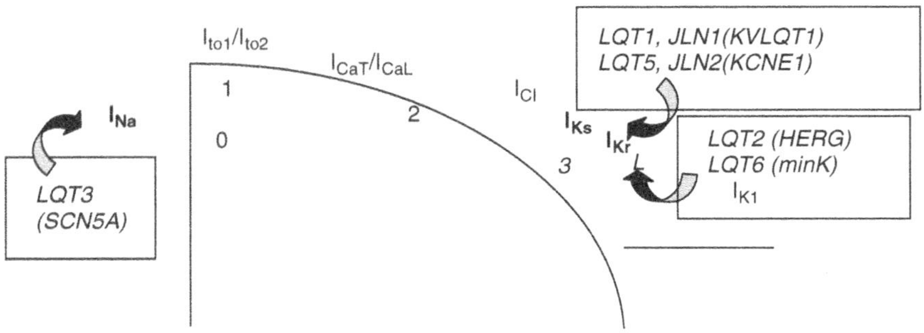

Fig. 7.1
Schematic presentation of action potential with key ion currents and related long QT syndrome (LQTS) genes

Table 7.1
Genetic types of the Long QT Syndrome (LQTS)

Genotype	Chromosome	Affected gene	Channel protein	Ion-channel current
LQT1	11	KCNQ1	Four α-subunits each with six membrane spanning segments	$\downarrow I_{Ks}$
LQT2	7	KCNH2	Four α-subunits each with six membrane spanning segments	$\downarrow I_{Kr}$
LQT3	3	SCN5A	One α-subunit with 24 membrane spanning segments	$\uparrow I_{Na}$
LQT4	4	Ankyrin-B (ANK2)	Sodium pump and Na/Ca exchanger	I_{Na}[a]
LQT5	21	KCNE1	β-subunit of KCNQ1 with one membrane spanning segment	$\downarrow I_{Ks}$
LQT6	21	KCNE2	β-subunit of KCNH2 with one membrane spanning segment	$\downarrow I_{Kr}$
LQT7	17	KCNJ2	Two membrane spanning segments	$\downarrow I_{K1}$
LQT8	6	CACNA1C	One α_1-subunit with 24 membrane spanning segments	$\uparrow I_{Ca}$
LQT9	3	CAV3 (Caveolin)	Altered gating kinetics of $Na_V1.5$	I_{Na}[a]
LQT10	11	SCN4B	β-subunit of SCN5A with one membrane spanning segment	$\uparrow I_{Na}$
LQT11	7	AKAP9	A-kinaze anchor protein	$\downarrow I_{Ks}$[a]
LQT12	20	SNTA1	Sodium current (SCN5A) regulator	$\uparrow I_{Na}$[a]

[a]Channel-related proteins, these are not proteins forming channels

of genetically tested patients have mutations found in one of the recognized causative genes [22]. It is estimated that among patients with known genotype, LQT1 and LQT2 account for the majority (87%) of cases of congenital LQTS, LQT3 accounts for 8%, whereas LQT5 and LQT6 are extremely rare accounting for less than 5% of LQTS cases [11]. The remaining types of LQTS: LQT4 [15], LQT7 [16], LQT8 [17], LQT9 [18], LQT10 [19], LQT11 [20], and LQT12 [21] are extremely rare conditions accounting when combined for less than 1% of clinical LQTS cases, but their importance should not be underappreciated since they provide crucial insight into mechanisms of cardiac repolarization. Identification of some of these rare forms has led to recognizing the role of not only ion-channel proteins but also proteins associated with and regulating ion-channel function in repolarization.

7.2.2 Ion-Channel Function and Arrhythmogenesis

There are significant differences in repolarization in the various layers of the myocardium, with the epicardial cells having the shortest action potential duration, endocardial cells having an intermediate duration, and M cells having the longest action potential duration [23–25]. QT duration on ECG represents the longest repolarization in the M cell zone. This physiologic transmural dispersion of repolarization usually does not lead to TdP. However, proarrhythmic states may arise as a result of specific gene mutations or actions of medications causing selective action potential prolongation in certain areas of the heart (usually M cells) that lead to increased transmural repolarization gradients (Fig. 7.2) [25]. This increased transmural gradient may contribute to reentrant arrhythmias leading to TdP. It is worth stressing that not all drugs prolonging repolarization cause TdP. For example, amiodarone is known to prolong QT duration, but since this drug is not increasing transmural heterogeneity of repolarization (or it might decrease it), TdP is not observed in patients taking this drug. Similarly, the novel compound ranolazine may increase QT duration but simultaneously decreases heterogeneity of repolarization. Interestingly, both of these drugs are mild calcium and sodium channel blockers, which might contribute to a decreased propensity to proarrhythmias [26].

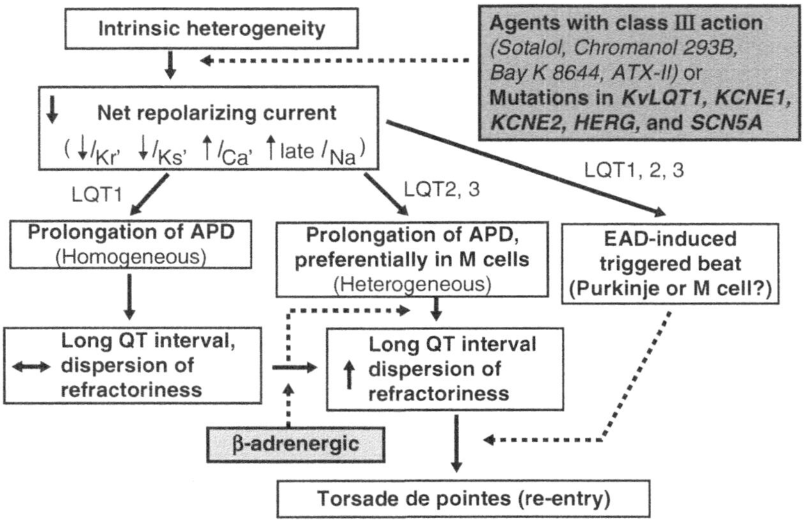

Fig. 7.2
Proposed cellular and ionic mechanisms for the long QT syndrome. ***APD*** **action potential duration,** ***EAD*** **early after depolarization (Antzelevitch et al. [25]. © Elsevier Limited. Reproduced with permission)**

Recent progress in the understanding of ion-channel structure and function has provided evidence for the mechanisms associated with HERG channel and I_{Kr} current abnormalities [27–29]. Numerous medications cause QT prolongation by blocking I_{Kr} due to their binding affinity to sites within the HERG channel cavity, while others may cause abnormal trafficking of proteins forming the channel from inside the cell toward the cellular membrane. Abnormal trafficking of channel proteins may result in a decreased number of channels in the cellular membrane or expression of dysfunctional channels [29]. Some of the proteins do not reach the membrane at all, and some reach it as imperfect, defective proteins that are not fully functional, therefore unable to pass the expected number of potassium ions through the pore of the channel. LQT2 patients as well as patients who never had an LQTS diagnosed but might have genetic polymorphism of HERG protein are particularly prone to developing QT prolongation due to drugs blocking this channel. Other individuals with normal function and structure of the channel who develop drug-induced QT prolongation might have an affinity to experience an entrapment of the drug molecule within the pore of the channel causing decreased outward potassium current.

Although dysfunction of different ion channels has been found to cause inherited forms of LQTS, the HERG channel conducting I_{Kr}, the rapid delayed rectifier current, seems to play a critical role in drug-induced QT prolongation and TdP [10, 30–32]. Numerous medications including some antiarrhythmics, antihistamine, antibiotics, psychotropic, and gastrointestinal prokinetic drugs have been found to block I_{Kr}. The reason for so many different drugs blocking the same channel is found in a different molecular structure and dysfunction of the channel caused by prolonged entrapment of drug molecules in the channel cavity leading to enhanced binding affinity of the drug to the sites in the channel [27–29]. The other potassium channels have a protective mechanism (a proline-X- proline sequence in S6 domain) that reduces the volume of the channel cavity precluding drug molecules to be trapped there. The HERG channel does not have proline residues in the S6 location and, therefore, this channel is more prone to bind drug molecules inside the channel with subsequent blocking of the channel and reduction in I_{Kr} current. Since not all drugs that block I_{Kr} produce TdP, other mechanisms might be involved in the proarrhythmic response including other actions of the drugs. Amiodarone and verapamil are examples of I_{Kr} blockers that are not associated with increased risk of TdP possibly due to concomitant blocking of calcium channels or homogenous prolongation of repolarization in various layers of the myocardium.

Transmural dispersion of repolarization seems to play the most important role in arrhythmogenesis in both drug-mediated and congenital forms of LQTS [24, 25]. There is a physiologic transmural dispersion of repolarization with M cells showing the longest action potential duration, epicardial cells the shortest, and endocardial cells intermediate

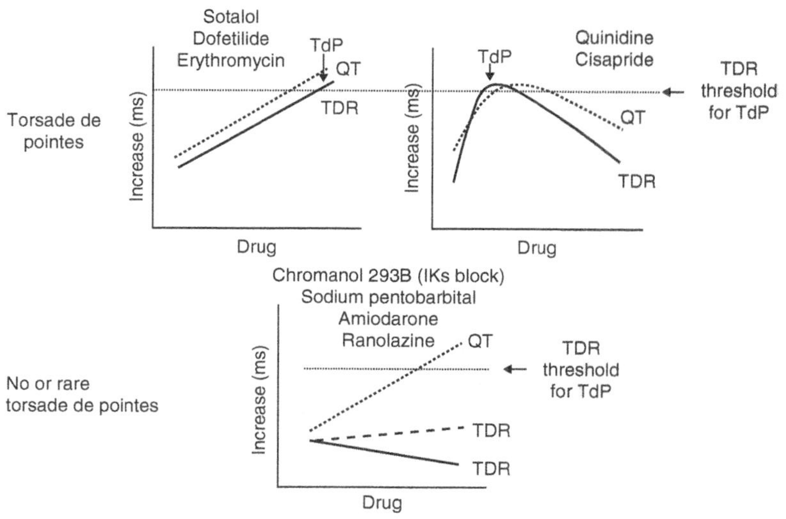

Fig. 7.3
Correspondence between changes in QT interval and transmural dispersion of repolarization, and propensity for development of torsade de pointes (Antzelevitch et al. [25]. © Elsevier Limited. Reproduced with permission)

action potential duration. The magnitude of this physiologic transmural dispersion of repolarization is not sufficient to cause conditions leading to TdP, unless there is selective prolongation of the action potential in one of the layers (M cells) due to action of drugs or due to a specific genetic mutation (➋ Fig. 7.3). This excessive prolongation increases the magnitude of transmural gradient of repolarization, which may cause functional block and reentry in response to a premature beat [24, 25].

7.3 QT Interval

7.3.1 QT Interval Measurement

The routine QT interval measurements in ECGs are used to assess global repolarization duration. The QT interval includes the QRS complex, nevertheless, the entire QT interval is considered as a measure of repolarization since the repolarization process already takes place during the QRS complex for early activated regions of myocardium. The QT interval should be measured from the onset of the QRS complex to the offset of the T wave, defined as a deflection point terminating the descending arm of the T wave usually at the level of isoelectric line or as the nadir between the T and U waves [33, 34]. When T and U waves are merged or when the T wave has a bifid appearance with two components of the T wave, clinicians might have difficulties where to identify the end of the repolarization segment. In such a case, careful inspection of repolarization duration in all 12 leads might be helpful in determining proper approach to quantify QT interval in such situation, or a QTU duration is sometimes reported with proper acknowledgment that the measurement includes a second component that might be part of the T wave or superimposed U wave (➋ Fig. 7.4). In case of repolarization morphologies with the presence of a second component of T wave or U wave, some investigators suggest using the rule that U wave usually should be at least 150 ms behind the peak of the T wave, whereas closer deflections might be considered as the second component of the T wave [35, 36]. However, there are no systematic data validating this rule. There is no doubt that complex patterns of repolarization usually reflect more heterogeneous repolarization patterns which are likely to contribute to arrhythmogenic conditions. Identifying the end of theT wave and measurement of QT may lead to quite

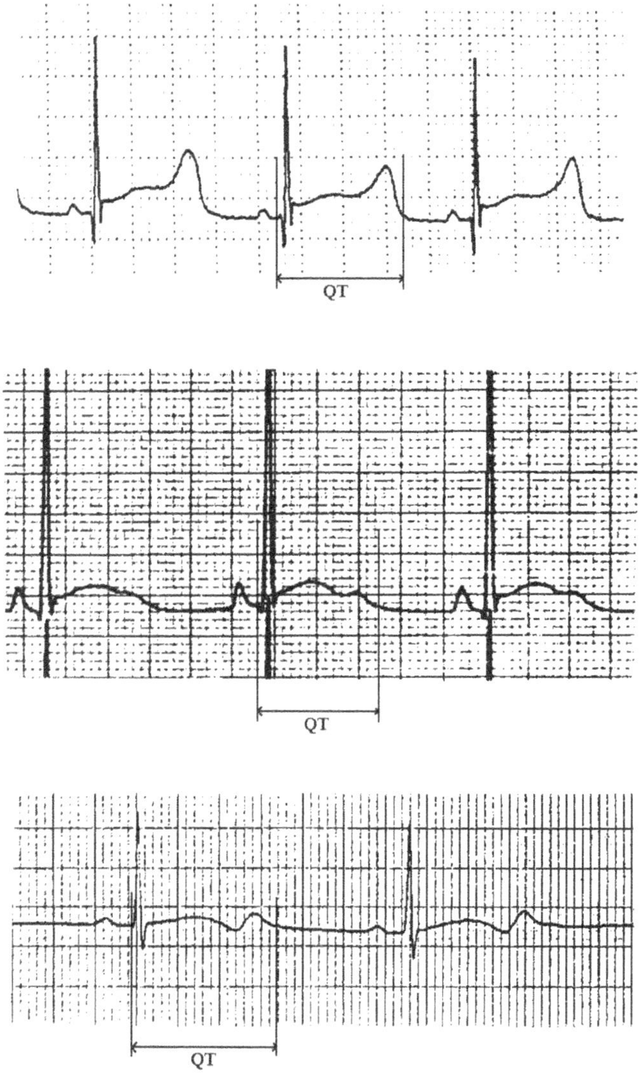

Fig. 7.4
QT interval measurement in different T wave morphologies

significant differences based on the experience of the reader, as it was shown by Viskin et al. [37] who demonstrated that only about 40% of internists and 70% of cardiologists were able to measure it properly in comparison to measurements done by a group of experts.

7.3.2 Lead Selection for QT Duration

Physiologically, the optimal method of measuring the QT in ECG is to take the earliest onset of the QRS complex in any of 12 leads and the latest offset of the T wave in any of the 12 leads, reflecting global duration of the repolarization process [38]. This approach is rarely exercised in manual measurements since it is time consuming and in most cases does not provide major benefit on top of routine measurements done in lead II. In some cases with borderline QT prolongation, careful investigation of repolarization duration and morphology in all leads might help identify QT prolongation and repolarization abnormalities.

Automatic algorithms evaluating repolarization duration might also utilize the concept of a so-called global lead represented as a superimposition of all 12 leads in the ECG [38]. The QT interval in such presentation is measured from the earliest onset of the QRS complex in any lead to the latest offset in any lead verified visually with all T wave ends superimposed.

The QT duration varies among standard 12 leads, and QT dispersion has been measured in numerous studies as a possible marker of arrhythmogenic conditions [39, 40]. However, due to conceptual and methodological limitations of QT dispersion, this method has not been approved as a standard tool in clinical practice or in drug studies. Interlead differences in repolarization morphology rather than just QT duration seem to better reflect the complexity of repolarization process [40–44]. Interlead differences in repolarization morphology could be quantified utilizing various methods including principal component analysis, area-based analysis of repolarization segment, and other methods [41–44]. Principal component analysis of the repolarization segment allows quantifying the length ($\lambda 1$) and width ($\lambda 2$) of the T wave loop [41, 43]. The roundness of the T-loop in its preferential plane ($\lambda 2/\lambda 1$) has been considered as an index of increased T wave complexity.

7.3.3 Adaptation of QT Duration to Heart Rate

In 1920, Bazett described a curvilinear association between the QT and RR intervals and the formula based on his observation ($QTc = QT/(RR^{1/2})$) is most frequently used [45]. The Fridericia's [46] formula ($QTc = QT/(RR^{1/3})$) is increasingly used especially in studies evaluating the effects of medications on the QT interval. Both these formulae adjust the QT interval to the conditions seen for a heart rate of 60 bpm. Bazett's QTc formula has limitations of overestimating repolarization duration at fast heart rates and underestimating it at slow heart rates. Fridericia's formula causes less misjudgment, however, clinicians are not comfortable in using this formula on a daily basis due to a need of cubic root equation and more importantly due to limited clinical data on normal values and the diagnostic and prognostic significance of this measurement. Few other QTc formulae were proposed including (1) Framingham [47] – a more linear formula ($QTc = QT + 0.154(1 - RR)$); (2) Hodges et al. [48] – utilizing the heart rate ($QTc = QT + 1.75(\text{heart rate}-60)$); (3) Rautaharju et al. [49] – where QT is entered in milliseconds and where the formula is different for males and females depending on age: for all females and males <15 and >50 years $QTI = QT(HR + 100)/656$ ms and for males 15–50 years: $QTI = (100 \times QT)/((656/(1 + 0.01HR)) + 0.4\,\text{age} - 25)$; and Karjalainen et al. [50] – where both QT and RR are entered in milliseconds, and it varies by heart rate: for heart rate <60 bpm, $QT_{Nc} = (QT \times 392)/(0.116\,RR + 277)$; for heart rate 60–99 bpm $QT_{Nc} = (QT \times 392)/(0.156\,RR + 236)$; and for heart rate ≥ 100 bpm, $QT_{Nc} = (QT \times 392)/(0.384\,RR + 99)$. All of these formulas tend to adjust well for the QT/RR association; however, each has some limitations. The QTc formulae provide good estimation of QT duration at heart rates close to the normal resting range of 55–75 bpm as observed in the vast majority of ECGs. However, below and above those limits there could be room for misclassification of the QTc value. Heart rates below 55 bpm or above 75–80 bpm are usually recorded using Holter recordings and exercise testing and for these ranges of heart rates, the Fridericia's (cubic) formula is of preference due to its simplicity of application, although other more complex formulae including Rautaharju's or Karjalainen's could be used.

For evaluation of ECGs recorded off and on a drug, the analysis of QT/RR regression with the subject-specific QT/RR relationship plots is of increasing use [51, 52]. One could also use the so-called RR-bin method that relies on measurement of QT intervals in absolute value for matched RR intervals for recordings off and on drugs without a need of using correction formulas [53]. The QT/RR subject-specific method and the RR-bin approach are particularly valuable when evaluating drugs affecting heart rates.

7.3.4 Normal QTc Values for Age and Gender

QT interval duration is different according to age and gender. ➋ Table 7.1 shows proposed normal and abnormal QTc values (using Bazett heart rate correction) by age and gender [54]. Women and children have longer duration of repolarization than men (➋ Table 7.2).

Table 7.2
QTc values by age and gender

QTc value (s)	Children 1–15 years	Men	Women
Normal	< 0.44	< 0.43	< 0.45
Borderline	0.44–0.46	0.43–0.45	0.45–0.46
Prolonged	> 0.46	> 0.45	> 0.46

Adapted with permission from Ref [54].

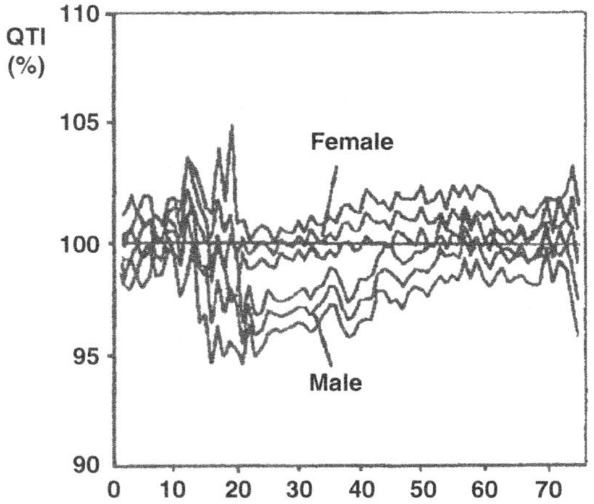

Fig. 7.5
Age and sex-related pattern of QTI (QT index by Rautaharju) (Rautaharju et al. [49]. © Pulsus Group Inc. Reproduced with permission)

Rautaharju et al. [49] demonstrated that a sex-related difference in QT is due to a shorter QT duration in men than women at age 15–55 years, not because of QT prolongation in women (Fig. 7.5). Slower heart rate in men is one of the important factors contributing to this difference, but it is postulated that other important modulators include different density of potassium ion channels in male versus female myocardium, effects of female hormones contributing to longer QT duration in women, or possibly the effect of male hormones contributing to their shorter QT duration. Sex-related differences in repolarization are also observed for parameters describing T wave morphology with men having a steeper ascending arm of the T wave than women [55]. Women dominate cases of drug-induced torsade de pointes and long QT cases in adulthood which is explained by a longer QTc in women than men.

7.3.5 QT Prolongation and Risk of Cardiac Arrhythmias and Mortality

The risk of arrhythmic events is significantly associated with QT prolongation in LQTS [1–6]. For every 10 ms increase of QTc duration, there is 5% exponential increase of the risk of cardiac events [1]. Therefore, a patient showing an increase in QTc duration from 440 to 500 ms has a 34% increase in the risk of cardiac events (60 ms difference indicates $1.05^6 = 1.34$). Figure 7.6 shows the association between QTc interval and risk of aborted cardiac arrest or death in LQTS patients evaluated during adulthood from age 18 to 40 years [56]. Subjects with QTc > 500 ms are particularly prone to developing cardiac events. Genotype–phenotype correlations indicate that about a third of LQTS carriers have normal or borderline QTc values [2–4]. These observations indicate that the magnitude of QTc duration is not the sole factor when evaluating the risk of arrhythmic events. In the case of drug-induced QTc prolongation, the QTc duration above 500 ms or prolongation by more than 60 ms in response to a drug indicates an increased risk of TdP [57].

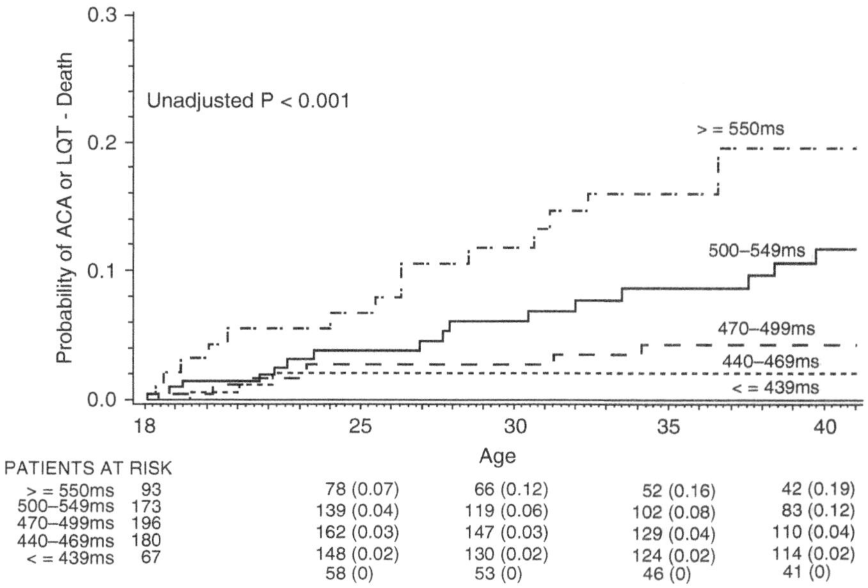

Fig. 7.6
Cumulative probability of cardiac events by QTc duration in adult LQTS patients (Sauer et al. [56]. © Elsevier Limited. Reproduced with permission)

QT prolongation is also considered as a risk factor in non-LQTS subjects. The Rotterdam Study [58], a prospective population-based cohort study of 3,105 men and 4,878 women aged 55 years and older, demonstrated that an abnormally prolonged QTc interval (>450 ms in men, >470 ms in women) was associated with a threefold increased risk of sudden cardiac death after adjustment for age, gender, body mass index, hypertension, cholesterol/high-density lipoprotein ratio, diabetes mellitus, myocardial infarction, heart failure, and heart rate (➲ Figure 7.9). The Framingham study did not show an association of baseline QTc prolongation with total mortality, sudden death, or coronary mortality [59]. The Cardiovascular Health Study [60], on the other hand, showed an association between a QTc interval of >450 ms and total mortality, and in the Strong Heart Study [61], a QTc interval of ≥ 460 ms was associated with a twofold increased risk of cardiac and total mortality.

Data regarding the predictive value of QT interval prolongation in patients with coronary disease and heart failure are controversial [62–68]. In a recent study of Attar et al. [63], 682 individuals underwent diagnostic coronary angiography of whom 17 (2.5%) died or had a nonfatal myocardial infarction during 1-year follow-up. In multivariate analysis, QRS duration, extent of coronary disease, and prolonged corrected QT peak interval were independently associated with events. However, most of the studies are not able to confirm practical usefulness of QT prolongation for predicting cardiac events in patients with underlying coronary disease and cardiomyopathy since these conditions alter repolarization and QT prolongation is reflecting more a severity of the disease than the risk of cardiac events [64–68].

7.3.6 Changes in T wave Morphology

The T wave morphology varies among LQTS patients and this variation could be related to the type of affected ion channel, the magnitude of ion-channel dysfunction, as well as other factors including age, heart rate, and the status of the autonomic nervous system. It has been recognized that specific genetic types of LQTS could be associated with distinct ECG patterns of repolarization [69]. ➲ Figure 7.7 shows specific patterns associated with distinct genetic types of the disorder: LQT1 characterized by wide, broad-based T waves, LQT2 usually showing low-amplitude and frequently notched

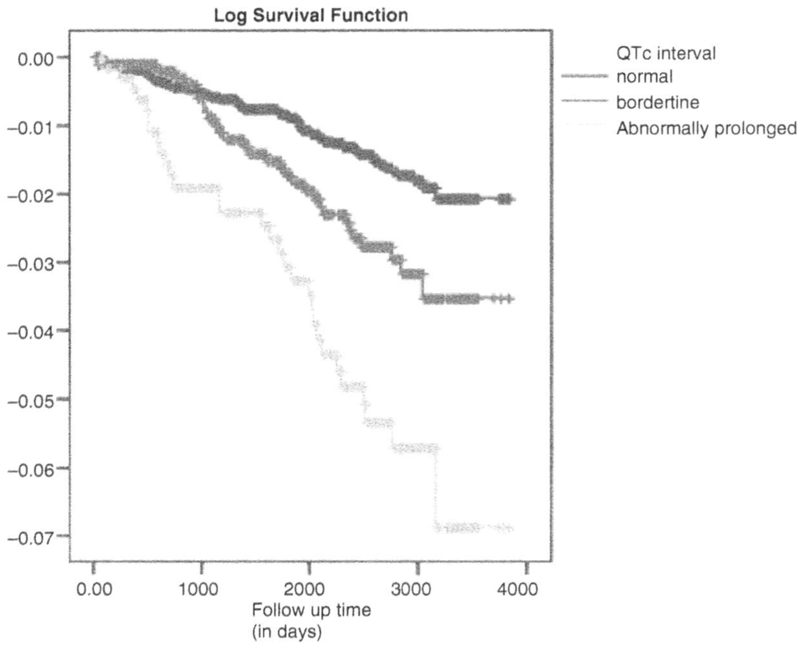

Fig. 7.7
Risk of sudden death and QTc in elderly subjects enrolled in the Rotterdam study (Straus et al. [58]. © Elsevier Limited, Oxford, UK. Reproduced with permission)

T waves, and LQT3 characterized by a relatively long ST segment followed by a peaked, frequently tall, T wave. The abnormal T wave morphology might be particularly useful in diagnosing patients with borderline QTc duration (420–470 ms). In such patients, presence of an abnormal (notched, flat) T wave may indicate the possibility of LQTS.

The HERG gene mutation encodes the I_{Kr} current (the current most frequently affected by drugs) and is associated with decreased T wave amplitude with increased presence of notches [69, 70]. Similar observations could be made when evaluating drug-induced changes in repolarization. Drug-induced changes in T wave morphology reflect changes in the transmural gradient of repolarization with propensity to arrhythmogenesis (Fig. 7.8) [71, 72]. Therefore, identification of drug-induced changes in repolarization morphology in clinical studies should always trigger attention since those changes may indicate a propensity to proarrhythmia.

7.4 Drug-Induced QT Prolongation

Numerous cardiac and noncardiac drugs have been found to prolong the QTc interval duration and cause TdP (Table 7.3). Most of them directly block the I_{Kr} current, while others exert such action if administered together with a drug affecting the function of the cytochrome P-450 enzymatic system. The quinidine-induced sudden deaths and subsequently the results of the CAST trial brought further attention to the proarrhythmic effects of antiarrhythmic drugs [73]. In the early 1990s, the adverse effects of terfenadine (an antihistamine drug) brought much attention to the possibility of noncardiac drugs being associated with torsade de pointes and sudden cardiac death [74]. Terfenadine, an anithistamine agent, blocks the I_{Kr} current (also blocking sodium current and the L-type calcium channel) causing a mean 6 ms QTc prolongation, which should not have clinical implications. Cardiac events were reported in patients taking terfenadine, almost exclusively when used in combination with other medications (ketoconazole, antibiotics) also metabolized by the same enzymatic system of the cytochrome P-450 3A4. Such a combination causes increase in plasma concentration of terfenadine due to inhibition of its metabolism by a concomitantly administered drug with subsequent substantial QTc

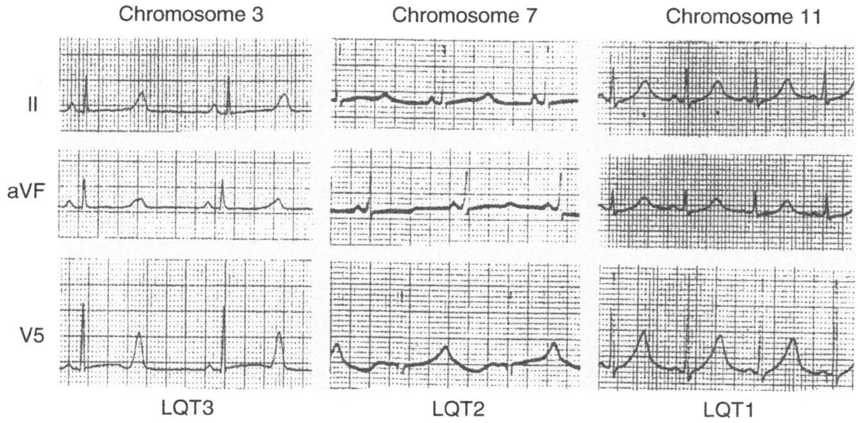

Fig. 7.8
T wave morphology in ECG recordings from leads II, aVF, and V5 from patients with LQT1, LQT2, and LQT 3 (Moss et al. [69], © American Heart Association, Dallas, Texas, Reproduced with permission)

Table 7.3
Drugs that prolong the QT interval

Category	Drugs
Antihistamines	Astemizole, terfenadine
Anti-infectives	Amantadine, clarithromycin, chloroquine, erythromycin, grepafloxacin, moxifloxacin, pentamidine, sparfloxacin, trimethoprim-sulfamethoxazole
Antineoplastics	Tamoxifen
Antiarrhythmics	Quinidine, sotalol, procainamide, amiodarone, bretylium, disopyramide, flecainide, ibutilide, moricizine, tocainide, dofetilide
Antilipemic agents	Probucol
Calcium channel blockers	Bepridil
Diuretics	Indapamide
Gastrointestinal agents	Cisapride
Hormones	Fludrocortisone, vasopressin
Antidepressants	Amitriptyline, amoxapine, clomipramine, imipramine, nortriptyline, protriptyline
Antipsychotic	Chlorpromazine, haloperidol, perphenazine, quetiapine, risperidone, sertindole, thioridazine, ziprasidone, doxepin, methadone

prolongation (>60 ms in majority of reported cases) and TdP. Among noncardiac drugs, several antipsychotic drugs block I_{Kr} current and cause QTc prolongation and some of them were reported to be associated with sudden death [75].

Based on transmural recordings from perfused wedge preparations [71, 72] it was postulated that the peak of the recorded T wave coincides with the end of repolarization in the epicardium and the end of the T wave with the end of repolarization in the M cell zone, thus measurement of the T peak – T end duration and its ratio to the QT interval was proposed to reflect transmural dispersion, at least in the experimental setting. Liu et al. [76] applied this approach effectively in laboratory conditions identifying drugs prone to induce TdP ➲ Figure 7.9. ➲ Figure 7.10 shows drug-induced changes in the TpTe/QT ratio for drugs known to cause QT prolongation and TdP in comparison to drugs with no such effect. These findings provide the foundation for applying T wave morphology for identifying patients prone to developing TdP.

Drug-induced QT prolongation and TdP usually occur in susceptible individuals; ➲ Table 7.4 lists common factors predisposing to QT prolongation and TdP [77]. Females have faster resting heart rates and longer QTc intervals than men,

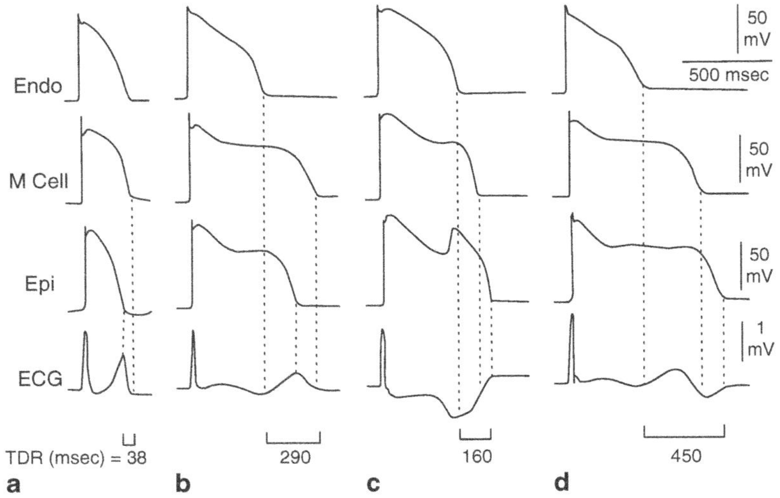

Fig. 7.9
Transmural dispersion of action potentials and changes in T wave morphology on ECG. (a) Normal T wave with normal transmural gradient of repolarization. (b) Biphasic T wave: increase in transmural gradient with end of endocardial action potential coinciding with negative phase of T wave. (c) Inverted T wave: epicardial layer shows longest repolarization duration contributing to increased and inverted transmural gradient. (d) Polyphasic T wave with markedly increased transmural gradient: negative phases of T wave coincide with end of action potential in endocardial and M cell layers (Emori et al. [72]. © Wiley–Blackwell. Reproduced with permission)

and not surprisingly about 70% of cases of drug-induced TdP are found in women [77]. The elderly and patients with underlying heart diseases (cardiomyopathies), those with electrolyte abnormalities, especially hypokalemia and bradycardia, are at particularly increased risk for drug-induced QT prolongation and TdP. In some patients, there is evidence for a genetic predisposition to drug-induced QT prolongation although there are not yet data supporting that all cases are genetically predetermined [78].

The Food and Drug Administration (FDA) in the United States and the Committee for Proprietary Medicinal Products (CPMP) of the European Agency for the Evaluation of Medicinal Products mandate evaluating the potential QT prolonging effects of all new drugs undergoing regulatory approval [79, 80]. Each drug has to be evaluated individually after full considerations of risks associated with the drug in relationship to benefit of the drug for the population at risk. A number of drugs which show some QT prolonging effects in Phase I or Phase II studies might require further testing in a so-called Thorough QT Study. The Thorough QT Study consists of repeated monitoring of QT and RR parameters as well as T wave morphology during administration of a tested drug and during administration of moxifloxacin, an antibiotic with known QT prolonging effect considered as a positive control (to validate the ability of the ECG core lab to detect the expected repolarization changes). Drugs with QT prolongation showing upper confidence intervals exceeding 10 ms might require additional safety measures during the next phases of development, possibly requiring specific labeling about the QT prolonging effect, or may not be recommended for entering the market.

7.5 Dynamics of QT Interval

The QT interval may be influenced by several factors including heart rate, sympathovagal balance, metabolic and electrolyte changes, disease entities, or drugs. Heart rate dependency of the repolarization process represents a form of repolarization dynamics appreciated already in the 1920s by several researchers including Bazett and Fridericia who described the QT/RR relationship and established the first heart rate correction formulae [45, 46]. It is well accepted

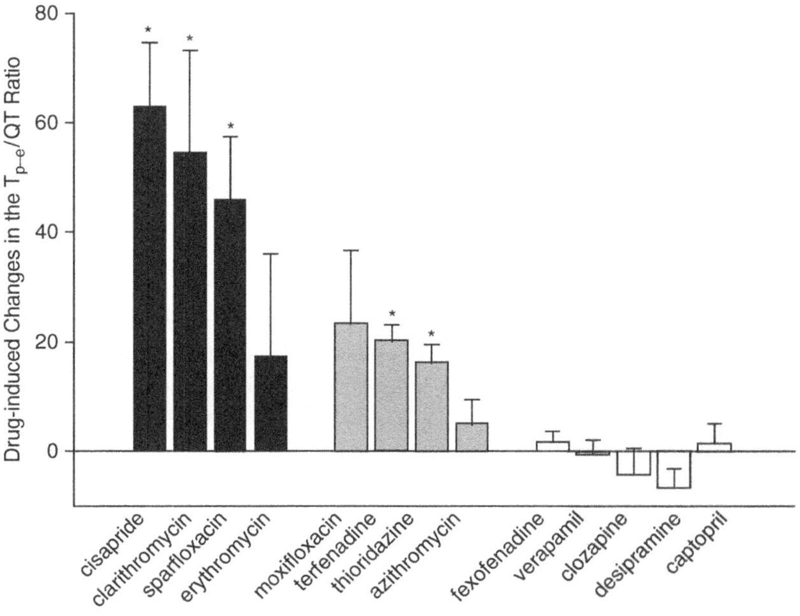

Fig. 7.10

Maximal drug-induced change in TpTe/QT ratio at concentrations <100-fold of their free therapeutic plasma concentration. The black bars represent the compounds that resulted in significant QT prolongation accompanied by the development of EAD, R-on-T extrasystoles, and torsades de pointes (TdP); the gray bars represent the compounds that led to a significant increase in the QT interval but without EAD and EAD-dependent phenomena; and the blank bars represent the negative compounds. * indicates $p < 0.05$ when compared with the control value of the compound (Liu et al. [76]. © Elsevier Limited. Reproduced with permission)

Table 7.4

Factors associated with increased risk of QT prolongation and torsades de pointes (TdP)

Prolonged QTc
Female sex
Advanced age
Bradycardia
Hypokalemia
Hypomagnesemia
Congestive heart failure (low EF)
Cardiac arrhythmias
Combinations of drugs (cytochrome P450 enzymes inhibitors)
Genetic polymorphisms of gene coding cardiac ion channels or enzymes in liver metabolising drugs

that during controlled exercise the uncorrected QT interval shortens with decreasing RR intervals. In case of progressively increasing or decreasing heart rate, the QT interval shows a linear correlation with heart rate within physiological limits. However, in cases of abrupt RR changes, the QT interval does not change adequately, and a lag of QT adaptation to changing heart rate is frequently observed. It is also recognized that RR interval changes in the form of a "short–long cycle" may precede the onset of VT. The presence of this sequence might prolong action potential duration (reflected as QT prolongation on surface ECG), facilitating early after depolarizations and triggering TdP VT.

Advances in Holter technology in recent years have allowed for continuous tracking of RR intervals and corresponding QT intervals and brought an increased interest in the analysis of the dynamic behavior of repolarization. Changes in not only duration but also in morphology of the QT interval have been explored within the last decade. This dynamic behavior of repolarization could be evaluated by identifying specific patterns of the QT and RR intervals' relationship in long-term recordings, by measuring beat-to-beat QT or T wave variability, and by measuring 2:1 pattern of variability defined as T wave alternans (TWA) [81].

7.5.1 Methods to Assess QT/RR Dynamics

Adjustment of the QT to changing heart rate is a dynamic phenomenon consisting of fast adaptation and slow adaptation phases. Franz et al. [82] showed that after a rapid change in heart rate, the fast adaptation phase of repolarization usually lasts 30–60 s followed by a 2-min slow adaptation. This adjustment also seems highly individual and among other factors is dependent on the nature of heart rate changes. Repolarization adapts faster to increasing heart rate than it does to decreasing heart rate. This differential response is known as repolarization hysteresis [83]. Measures of repolarization hysteresis are proposed for diagnosing LQTS patients who usually show a larger difference in QT duration between exercise and recovery than control subjects [84].

Several methods have been developed to describe the dynamicity of repolarization [85–87], however, QT/RR slope is increasingly used, mainly due to incorporation of the algorithm into commercial Holter software. Repolarization dynamics are then measured by the slope of the linear regression between QT and RR intervals (➲ Fig. 7.11). To compute the QT/RR slope, RR and QT intervals included in 30- or 60-s epoch of ECG are calculated and averaged to diminish possible influence of erroneous measurements and to decrease the effect of sudden and short-acting changes in RR on QT interval duration [88]. These averaged QT and RR intervals may be then linearly fitted from the period of prolonged recording, typically 24 h of Holter. Measurement of slope is usually performed separately for both the QT apex (QTa) and QT end (QTe). In contrast to the short beat-to-beat QT interval adaptation and hysteresis, the QT/RR slope refers to overall behavior of QT in response to changes in RR. Steeper slope indicates excessive prolongation of QT at longer RR cycle lengths and adequate or excessive shortening of QT at shorter RR cardiac cycles (➲ Fig. 7.11). Flat slope indicates that QT interval is less dependent on the RR cycle and fails to adequately shorten at faster heart rates (shorter cycle). Both of these features

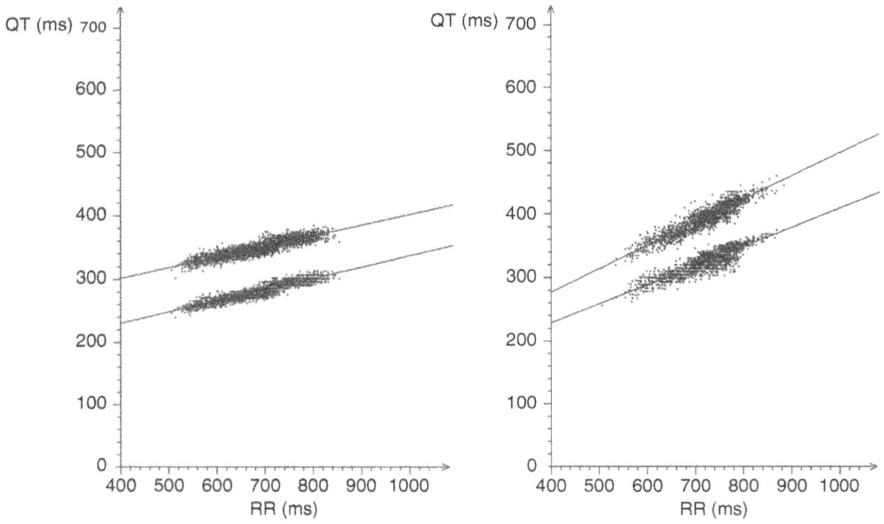

Fig. 7.11
Example of repolarization dynamics measured by QT/RR slopes

might contribute to an increased risk of arrhythmias. Steeper QT/RR indicates decreased vagal tone and increased sympathetic activity, which might contribute to a higher vulnerability of myocardium to arrhythmias. At the cellular level, sympathetic stimulation prolongs ventricular refractoriness. Therefore, abnormal QT slope represents increased vulnerability of myocardial substrate to its modulation by the autonomic nervous system. Lengthening of the QT at slower rates might be associated with arrhythmogenic increase in dispersion of refractoriness in the myocardium while excessive shortening of QT at fast heart rates might facilitate arrhythmia by diminished heterogeneity of refractoriness. QT dynamics reflects both the rate dependence of ventricular repolarization as well as the modulation of this dependence by a variety of factors such as autonomic nervous system, hormones, metabolic equilibrium, disease entities, and drugs. As significant diurnal variation of QT/RR was reported, QT/RR is usually evaluated separately for day and night time [89].

7.5.2 Clinical Factors Influencing QT/RR Slope

QT dynamicity is known to be influenced by a variety of clinical covariates. Advanced age was related to abnormal QT/RR dynamicity in healthy subjects [89], however, in patients with cardiac diseases, as shown in other studies, this relationship was absent or weak [90, 91]. It is most likely that advanced age and underlying heart disease influence repolarization parameters to a higher degree than age itself. Gender-related changes in repolarization parameters have been reported for several decades showing that women have longer QTc interval duration, and that women are more prone to develop torsade de pointes arrhythmias. Consequently, women tend to present higher QT/RR slopes than men, suggesting that QT dynamicity (both QT and RR duration) is influenced not only by autonomic nervous tone but also by other factors like hormones, and gender-specific differences in repolarizing currents [87, 89, 92, 93]. Hormone-related changes in QT/RR behavior were observed in subsequent phases of menstrual cycle [94] as well as during estrogen replacement therapy [95].

The QT/RR slope was found to be a strong marker of existing cardiac pathology. Abnormal QT dynamicity was observed in different populations including patients with long QT syndrome, ischemic heart disease, dilated and hypertrophic cardiomyopathy, congestive heart failure, mitral valve prolapse, hypertension, TakoTsubo syndrome, obstructive sleep apnea, or diabetes – all of the settings known to present some degree of impaired autonomic nervous system control [96–107].

Merri et al. [96] were the first to develop a Holter-based algorithm to assess the QT/RR relationship, and to report that patients with LQTS have a significantly increased relationship between repolarization duration and preceding sinus cycle length with an exaggerated prolongation of QT interval at slower heart rates. In this relatively small study, 16 subjects with LQTS were compared with ten matched healthy volunteers. Each RTm interval (the interval from R peak to the maximum amplitude of a T wave) was coupled to the RR interval of the preceding beat to avoid problems related with identification of Q wave onset and T wave end. The mean value for RTm/RR slope was significantly ($p = 0.003$) higher in LQTS patients (0.21 ± 0.08) than in normal subjects (0.14 ± 0.03) (➋ Fig. 7.12).

An abnormal QT/RR relationship indicates an exaggerated delay in repolarization with prolonged cycle length. In these cases, the T wave of the beat immediately following a long pause may have a bizarre configuration and prolongation of the QT interval, and reflect the presence of afterdepolarizations contributing to triggered ventricular arrhythmias. This pattern may explain bradycardia-related occurrence of TdP in LQTS patients. In patients with LQTS heterogeneous channel, abnormalities may contribute to differences in the QT/RR relationship. Some reports indicate that patients with LQTS may be characterized by flatter than normal QT/RR slopes [108].

Lower values of QTa/RR (QTa – QTapex duration) slopes were observed in patients with idiopathic ventricular fibrillation (VF) [109, 110]. The decrease in QT/RR slopes was particularly prominent at night time, which may contribute to the nocturnal occurrence of VF in this subset of patients. On the other hand, inappropriate QT shortening at higher rates may also result in a lower slope. A similar pattern with significantly reduced QT/RR slopes at night time was observed also in patients with Brugada syndrome. Of note, QT/RR slopes were significantly decreased in patients with spontaneous Brugada syndrome as compared to those with induced Brugada ECG pattern [111].

Coronary artery disease may influence repolarization dynamics by alteration of the autonomic nervous system as well as by structural changes in myocardium. Among patients with coronary artery disease, higher slopes are observed in patients with multi-vessel as compared to single-vessel coronary patients [112]. In patients with diseased hearts, impaired dynamicity of repolarization may be related to the degree of left ventricular dysfunction and may progress with severity of symptoms in patients with heart failure [90, 100, 102]. In general, patients with congestive heart failure present steeper

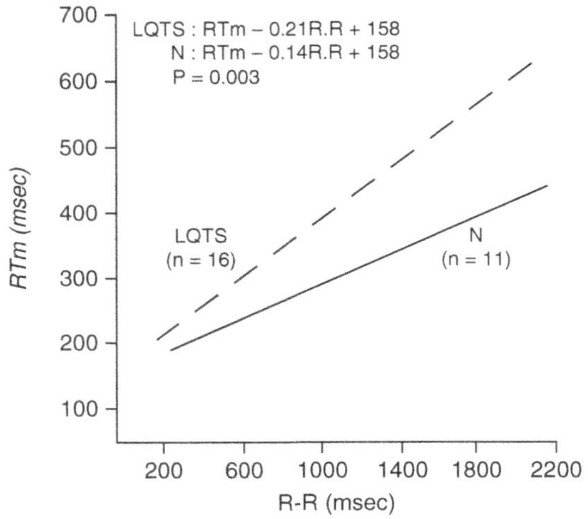

Fig. 7.12

Mean regression RTm/RR lines for one normal subject (N) and 16 patients with LQTS. The RTm/RR slope is significantly larger in the LQTS patients than in the normal subjects (Merri et al. [96]. © American Heart Association, Dallas, Texas. Reproduced with permission)

slopes not only than healthy subjects but also than those with coronary disease [100]. This finding may be related to both more advanced structural changes expressed by low ejection fraction and also by coexisting impairment of the autonomic nervous system. Alteration in autonomic nervous system functioning may also explain the loss of the typical night–day variation in QT/RR slope reported in healthy subjects (➋ Fig. 7.13).

Studies on the influence of reperfusion treatment on repolarization dynamics provide further insight into the potential mechanism underlying the observation about the relationship between steeper QT slopes and arrhythmic events in postinfarction patients. Bonnemeier et al. [113] found that in patients with first acute myocardial infarction undergoing PCI procedures, the QT/RR slopes were significantly increased in patients with TIMI 2 flow subgroup whereas they remained constant in those with complete reperfusion. Patients with increased QT/RR slopes after PCI more frequently presented with major arrhythmic events during a 1-year follow-up. Therefore, the authors concluded that impaired QT dynamicity reflects an altered electrical restitution after incomplete reperfusion PCI, potentially providing a substrate for life-threatening arrhythmias. Such an incomplete reperfusion might affect ventricular repolarization by directly influencing electrophysiological properties or interplaying with autonomic nervous tone (➋ Fig. 7.14).

7.5.3 Prognostic Value of QT/RR Slopes

Evaluation of the repolarization process limited to QT interval duration in a surface ECG only may not correspond to what happens in the period directly preceding malignant arrhythmias. Abrupt changes in QT behavior were observed in patients with life-threatening arrhythmias on Holter monitoring. Singh et al. [114] reported an abrupt increase in the QT/RR slope associated with a prolonged QTc and reduced heart rate variability in the interval immediately preceding the onset of VF that led to cardiac arrest in a 71-year-old man with hypertension and chronic renal failure. QT/RR slope increased from 0.032 at 60 min before VF to 0.293 as observed 10 min before cardiac arrest (➋ Fig. 7.15). Similarly, Sredniawa et al. [115] described an abrupt increase in QT/RR slope (from 0.223 to 0.483) in the period preceding a burst of frequent ventricular ectopic beats on Holter monitoring in coronary patients with documented cardiac arrest due to sustained VT. Transitory QT lengthening may express a temporal imbalance of the autonomic nervous system that may lead to heterogeneity of the ventricular refractory periods and may predispose to the development of reentry phenomena.

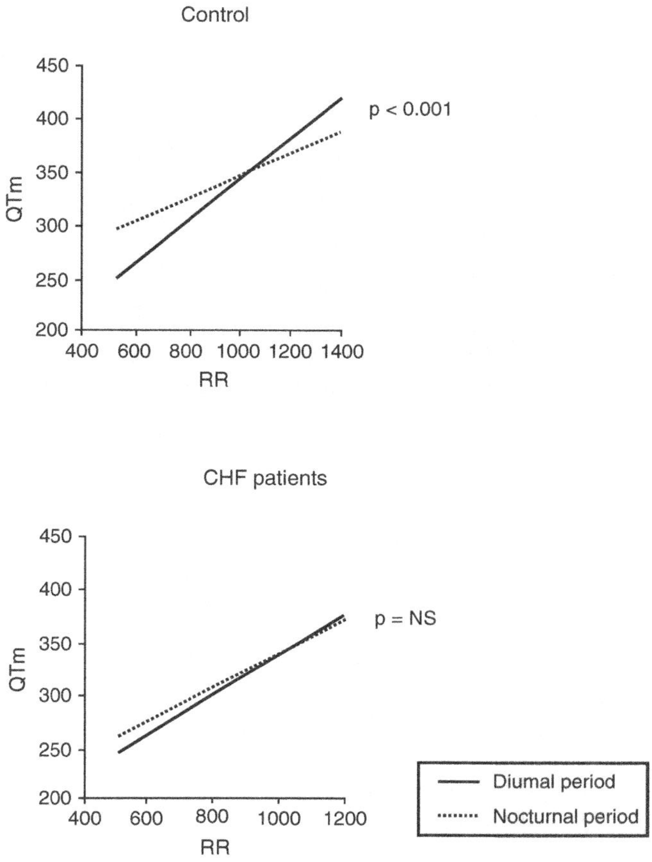

Fig. 7.13

Circadian modulation of QTm rate dependence in control patients (top panel) and in CHF patients (bottom panel). In the CHF group, the physiological circadian modulation of QTm rate dependence is lacking. CHF: congestive heart failure; solid lines: diurnal period; dotted lines: nocturnal period (Faber et al. [100]. © Wiley–Blackwell. Reproduced with permission from reference)

Several investigators evaluated the prognostic value of QT dynamics in predicting cardiac and arrhythmic events. In 1999, Extramiana et al. [98] compared postinfarction patients with a history of VT and positive programmed electrical stimulation with a control group without VT history, negative electrophysiologic study and arrhythmia-free 3-year survival after myocardial infarction. The analysis showed significantly enhanced QT dynamicity in postinfarction patients with a history of VT. In this group, QT/RR slopes were much higher than in control subjects within the three assessed circadian periods (awake, sleep, morning awakening). Furthermore, the difference was even more pronounced during awaking hours – a period considered as the high-risk time for sudden death occurrence (0.251 vs. 0.179 in VT and control groups, respectively). Of note, neither static QT parameters nor HRV parameters, potentially indicating abnormal autonomic nervous system modulation, could differentiate the VT group from controls.

Strong evidence of the prognostic value of QT/RR slopes in prediction of sudden death was provided by the GREPI study (Groupe d'Etude du Pronostic de l'Infarctus du myocarde) published in 2002 [116]. This multicenter, prospective study including 256 patients with acute myocardial infarction demonstrated that abnormal QT/RR evaluated nine to 14 days after infarction is an independent risk marker for sudden death during an average 7-year follow-up. As no normal limits of QT/RR exist, patients with QT/RR values corresponding to upper quartile were arbitrary defined as a high-risk subgroup. Steeper QT/RR slope (>0.18 during daytime) was associated with total mortality as well as with sudden death,

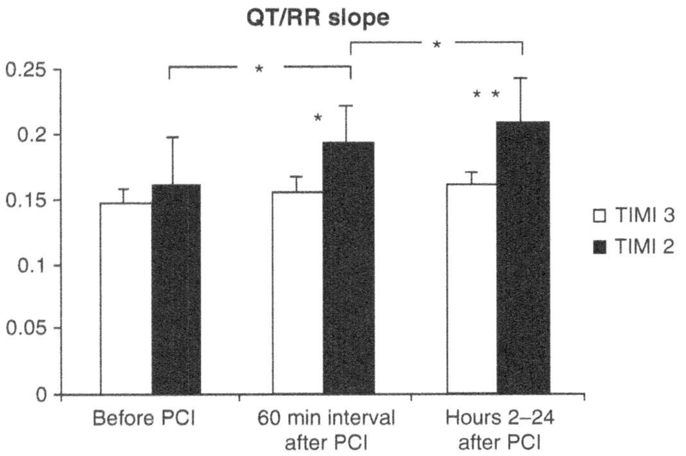

Fig. 7.14
QT/RR slope, in the first hour after PCI, and in interval from hour 2 to 24 after PCI in patients with TIMI 2 and 3 flow (Bonnemeier et al. [113], © American Heart Association, Dallas, Texas. Reproduced with permission)

indicating that excessive shortening at fast rates and/or excessive lengthening at slow rates may contribute to arrhythmic events (Fig. 7.16). The increased QT/RR slope was the most powerful predictor when tested simultaneously with clinical variables in the Cox multivariate model. It is worth emphasizing that the hazard ratio for sudden death was three times higher than for mortality of all causes (hazard ratio: 6.07 vs. 2.25, respectively). At the same time, other ECG stratifiers like SDNN and late potentials did not provide any prognostic information. Interestingly, only daytime, but not nighttime, QT slopes were predictive for events during follow-up.

In the EMIAT (European Myocardial Infarct Amiodarone Trial) study, QT dynamicity was assessed in postinfarction patients with LVEF $\leq$ 40% and was compared between patients with arrhythmic cardiac death (ACD) and non-ACD during a mean of 21 months follow-up [117]. The QT slopes were significantly higher in the cardiac death group, but only increased morning QT/RR slope differentiated patients with arrhythmic versus non- ACD (QT/RR slope: 0.272 vs. 0.239, respectively). Therefore, QT dynamicity not only discriminated postinfarction patients who died of cardiac death from survivors but also predicted the type of death. Other data from the EMIAT trial indicated that chronic amiodarone treatment affects the QT/RR relationship and the lack of treatment-related QT/RR changes predicts arrhythmic death [118].

Another study in postinfarction patients [87] documented higher QT/RR slopes in patients who died versus survived during a 3-year follow-up (0.187 vs. 0.139, $p < 0.001$). As in this case, increased QT/RR slope was associated with high risk of mortality and sudden death only in univariate analysis, the authors developed an additional novel parameter: QT/RR variability ratio, defined as SDQT/SDNN remained the only significant multivariate risk stratifier among all studied repolarization measures.

Several noninvasive Holter-based parameters were documented as strong risk markers in postinfarction patients, but arrhythmic risk stratification in patients with dilated cardiomyopathy and/or heart failure is still an open, unanswered issue. Even though the majority of noninvasive parameters predicts arrhythmic events in post-MI patients, these parameters fail to be independent markers in patients with DCM, and data in patients with heart failure are scarce and conflicting.

Pathak et al. [119] demonstrated that increased QT/RR slope (>0.28) assessed over 24 h was predictive for sudden death in patients with chronic heart failure class II–III due to ischemic (43%) or idiopathic (57%) cardiomyopathy with mean LVEF 28%. It is worth emphasizing that similar to studies in postinfarction patients, abnormal QT dynamicity was more related with sudden death than with total mortality. The hazard ratio of 24-h QT dynamicity (QTe) was over 50% higher for sudden death than for total mortality (HR = 3.4 vs. 2.2 in univariate analysis). A study by Watanabe et al. [120] confirmed that impaired QT dynamics is an independent risk marker in patients with heart failure followed for an average

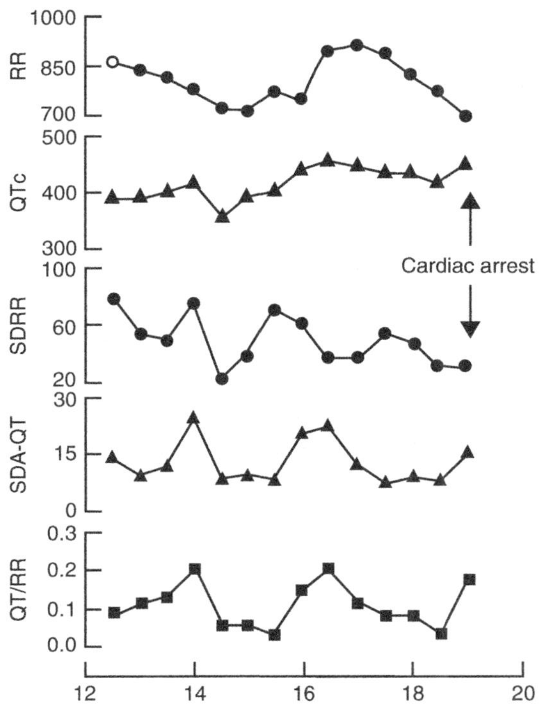

QT/RR slope and SDRR in the hour preceding the terminal rhythm

Time(min)	*QT/RR slope*	*SDRR (ms)*
−60	0.032	43.2
−50	0.043	37.3
−40	0.068	56.8
−30	0.026	40.5
−20	0.018	25.3
−10	0.293	33.1

SDRR, standard deviation of consecutive RR intervals over 5 min intervals.

Fig. 7.15

Half-hourly distribution of electrophysiological parameters assessed preceding cardiac arrest. SDRR: standard deviation of the consecutive RR intervals over 5-min segments; SDA-QT: standard deviation of the average of consecutive uncorrected QT intervals over 5-min segments; QTc: corrected QT interval; QT/RR: the slope of the regression line between the QT and RR intervals (Singh et al. [114]. © BMJ Publishing Group Ltd. Reproduced with permission)

of 34 months. Similar to other studies increased QT/RR slope (>0.17 over the day) was a stronger predictor of sudden death than cardiac death (HR 11.2 vs. 4.73, respectively).

Analysis of repolarization dynamics was performed in the MUSIC study [121], which analyzed 542 patients with mild to moderate heart failure (49% with ischemic cardiomyopathy; mean LVEF 37%). The mean value of QTa/RR slope was 0.172 and QT/RR was 0.193. During the 44-month follow-up there were 119 deaths including 47 sudden deaths. Non-survivors were characterized by steeper QT/RR slopes. In this study, increased QT/RR slopes during the daytime (>0.20 for QTa and >0.22 for QTe) were independently associated with increased total mortality during an average 44-month follow-up (hazard ratio = 1.57 and 1.58 for QTa and QT, respectively) (➋ Fig. 7.17). None of the dynamic repolarization parameters was associated with increased risk of sudden death.

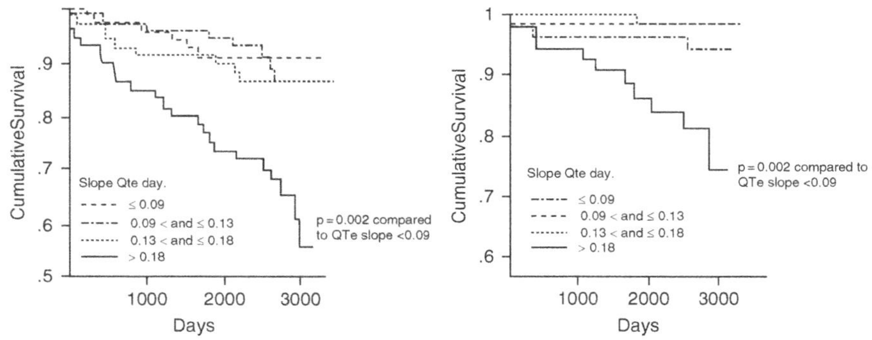

Fig. 7.16
Event-free curves of total mortality (left) and sudden death (right) according to daytime slope of QTe/RR using the Kaplan Meier method (Chevalier et al. [116]. © Wiley–Blackwell. Reproduced with permission)

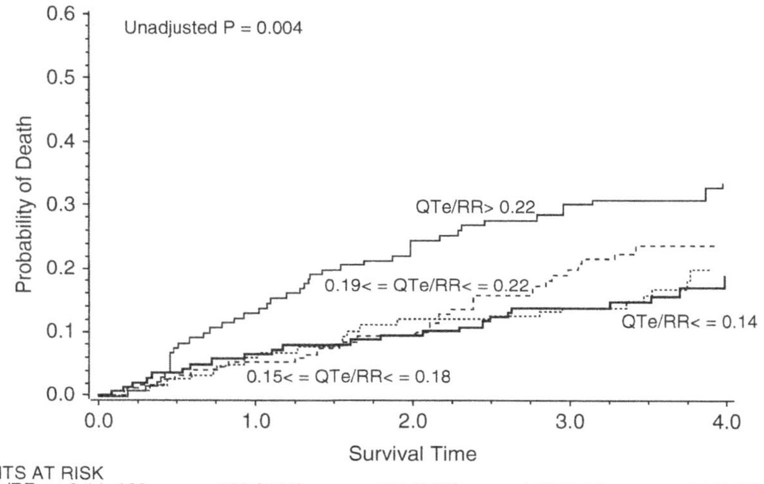

PATIENTS AT RISK					
QTe/RR< = 0.14	139	129 (0.06)	125 (0.09)	118 (0.14)	23 (0.20)
0.15< = QTe/RR< = 0.18	152	143 (0.05)	137 (0.09)	128 (0.14)	25 (0.20)
0.19< = QTe/RR< = 0.22	118	109 (0.06)	102 (0.12)	91 (0.20)	17 (0.24)
QTe/RR> 0.22	133	114 (0.13)	97 (0.25)	90 (0.30)	20 (0.36)

Fig. 7.17
Probability of death according to the QTe/RR slope value in patients with congestive heart failure (Cygankiewicz et al. [121]. © Wiley–Blackwell. Reproduced with permission)

Independent prognostic value of QT dynamicity in patients with idiopathic dilated cardiomyopathy was reported by Iacoviello et al. [90] who found that abnormal QT dynamicity was significantly associated with arrhythmic events (VT/VF or SCD) during a mean 39-month follow-up. At multivariate analysis only the QT slope (>0.19) decreased LVEF (Left Ventricular Ejection Fraction) and nsVT (non-sustained Ventricular Tachycardia) were independent predictors of poor outcome.

In summary for the section on QT/RR dynamics, there is increasing evidence that abnormal QT/RR slope is a powerful predictor of cardiac events, mainly mortality in various groups of patients with ischemic heart disease and nonischemic cardiomyopathies. Modern Holter technology provides algorithms for computing QT/RR slope automatically with very much needed preprocessing and filtering that aims to decrease the effects of outliers and effects of instantaneous changes of QT and RR behavior. However, it is worth pointing out that apart from the overall pattern of QT/RR behavior, there is

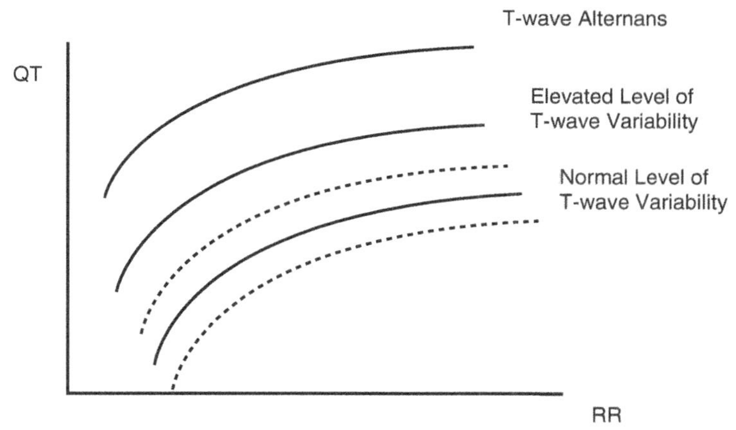

Fig. 7.18
Conceptual link between ECG measures of myocardial vulnerability: QT/RR relationship, T wave (or QT) variability and T wave alternans (TWA) (Zareba [122]. © Wiley–Blackwell. Reproduced with permission)

an increased interest in exploring beat-to-beat changes in the QT interval (QT variability), especially since such instantaneous changes might lead to development of life-threatening ventricular tachyarrhythmias. QT dynamics expressed as overall QT/RR slope representing overall underlying substrate for arrhythmia might be complemented by analysis of QT variability reflecting transient changes in vulnerability of myocardium to arrhythmias.

7.6 QT Variability

The QT interval being influenced by a variety of factors may change not only in terms of its duration but also morphology. QT variability is an ECG phenomenon consisting of beat-to-beat changes in repolarization duration and morphology appearing without the 2:1 pattern typical for TWA. These beat-to-beat changes in the T wave amplitude and shape as well as in QT duration, similar to what was observed in the case of QT dynamics, can be analyzed by several novel computerized ECG methods enabling for detection and quantification of subtle, microvolt-level changes, which otherwise remain undetected by the naked eye.

In a healthy heart, there is some small level of beat-to-beat variation of action potential duration which could be elevated by autonomic stimuli, a disease process, or effects of drugs [122]. The QT variability is dependent on both QT and RR duration and either QT prolongation, RR shortening, or both occurring simultaneously might contribute to excessive QT variability and in the case of further challenges to TWA (➋ Fig. 7.18). Along the line of this concept, TWA occur in most of the healthy subjects if heart rate exceeds 120–140 bpm, and this is why exercise-induced TWA are evaluated in a range of heart rates not exceeding 110 bpm.

7.6.1 Methods of QT Variability Assessment

In 1997, Berger and coworkers published a new method to assess the QT variability which they named QT lability [123]. A time-stretching algorithm was developed to quantify changes in repolarization duration and morphology. Beat-to-beat QT interval variability was measured on the basis of 256-s records of surface ECGs. A QT variability index was calculated as the logarithm of the ratio of normalized QT variance to heart rate variance. Using this algorithm, the authors documented that patients with dilated cardiomyopathy had higher QT variability as compared to control subjects (➋ Fig. 7.19).

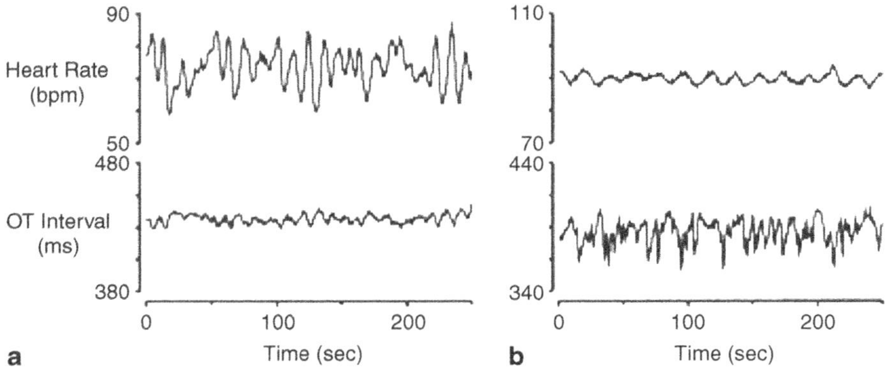

Fig. 7.19
Left part of the figure (a) shows normal subject [with high HRV and low QTV], while (b) is the patient with dilated cardiomyopathy [low HRV and high QTV]

Changes in heart rate and heart rate variability influence changes in the QT interval; however, QT variability cannot be entirely explained by changes in the autonomic nervous system. It is likely that beat-to-beat changes in action potential duration are dependent on instantaneous changes in ion-channel activity or the number of channels involved in the repolarization process. Even with a stable RR interval, there is a possibility of repolarization changes due to variations in the number of channels involved [124]. Myocardial conditions might alter the number of channels involved and changes in cycle length might further potentiate beat-to-beat variability of repolarization.

Exact detection of the end of the T wave is one of the main limitations of a proper assessment of QT-related parameters. Random noise, baseline wandering, and respiration modulation of T wave shape may influence the beat-to-beat QTe evaluation. Our group developed a T wave endpoint-independent method to quantify repolarization variability based on a wavelet transformation. The wavelet-based method showed that LQTS patients (SCN5A carriers) have significantly increased repolarization variability both in time and amplitude as compared to noncarriers [125]. Recently, we focused on a time-domain technique quantifying T wave variability (TWV) based on a beat-to-beat change in T wave amplitude without a need to identify the end of the T wave. As shown in ➋ Fig. 7.20, the variation of mean amplitude inside each of the four windows encompassing the repolarization segment (T1–T4) is analyzed across beats, and the level of variability is computed in each window based on the estimated variance of the average amplitude across beats in the selected window. The square-root value is reported and expressed in microvolt. The prognostic significance of this method was validated in the MADIT II cohort [126].

7.6.2 Clinical Factors Influencing QT Variability

Increased QT variability has been demonstrated in patients with heart failure, dilated cardiomyopathy, hypertrophic cardiomyopathy, coronary disease, LQTS as well as in patients with anxiety, depression, and panic disorders [127–133]. There are also data indicating that cocaine use may increase QT variability in a dose-dependent manner [134]. QT variability increases prior to drug-induced torsade de pointes in experimental conditions [135, 136]. QT variability was also reported to be influenced by external factors such as air pollution [137].

Little is known about the clinical covariates influencing QT variability. In the original paper by Berger et al. [123], no differences were found in QT variability between patients with ischemic and nonischemic dilated cardiomyopathy. Several reports indicate that QTVI (QT variability index) depends more on NYHA functional class than on LVEF, indicating that QT variability might be more related to disintegration of the autonomic nervous system than to structural changes in myocardium [98, 99]. Long-term treatment with beta-blockers (metoprolol or carvedilol) in patients with congestive heart failure in NYHA class II–III was documented to significantly reduce QTVI as compared to placebo [138]. Not only pharmacotherapy but also reperfusion may influence QT variability. As documented by Bonnemeier et al. [139], successful

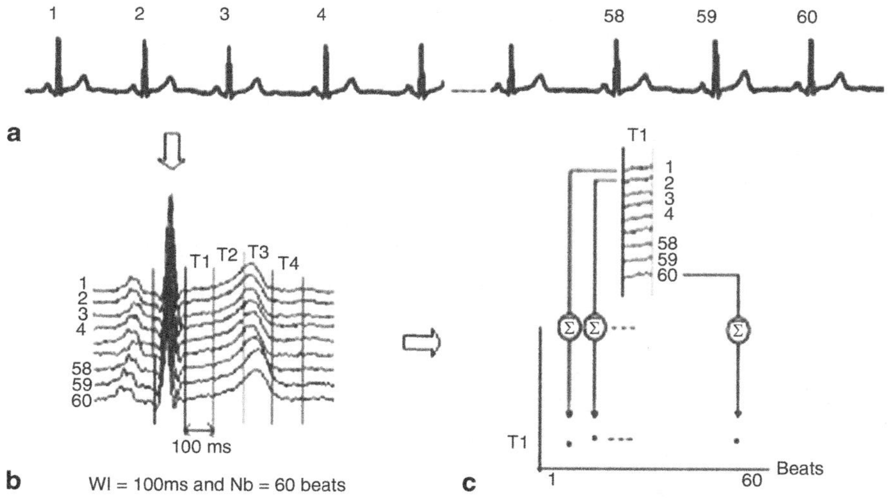

Fig. 7.20
Schematic presentation of the ECG processing for the measurements of T wave amplitude variability. (a) A set of 60 continuous cardiac beats are identified; (b) the beats are aligned based on the QRS beginning and the repolarization segment is windowed using 100 ms duration interval (T1–T4), (c) mean amplitude of each beat inside each window (T1–T4) are computed and plotted across beats, this panel represents the computation for T1 only (Couderc et al. [126]. © Oxford University Press. Reproduced with permission)

reperfusion resulted in a significant decrease in QT variability in patients with TIMI 2 and 3 flow grade. Interestingly, patients who experienced major arrhythmic events (sudden death, survived sudden death due to VF or sustained VT) during a 1-year follow-up were characterized by significantly higher mean 24-h QT variability (QTcSD 26.7 ± 2.9 vs. 25.4 ± 2.9, $p < 0.05$). This observation indicates that despite the opening of the infarct-related artery, impaired microcirculation may lead to persistent repolarization liability being an electrophysiological substrate for arrhythmic events.

7.6.3 Prognostic Value of QT Variability

The first study to demonstrate the usefulness of QT variability (assessed according to Berger' algorithm) in recognition of elevated arrhythmic risk was published in 1998 by Atiga et al. [140]. This study analyzed QTVI in 95 patients undergoing electrophysiological study. The QTVI was higher in patients with structural heart disease than in controls (−0.7 ± 0.7 vs. −1.1 ± 0.5, $p < 0.05$), and higher in patients who died suddenly during a 2-year follow-up than in other patients with heart disease (0.0 ± 0.6 vs. −0.8 ± 0.5, $p < 0.05$). After adjustment for significant clinical covariates, increased QTVI (≥0.1) was the only parameter identifying patients at risk of arrhythmic events (OR = 12.5, $p = 0.004$). The event-free survival rate was 67% for patients with QTVI ≥ 0.1 as compared to 85% with those with QTVI <0.1. It is important to emphasize that QTVI outperformed the following parameters tested simultaneously in studied patients as a predictor: QT dispersion, TWA during atrial pacing, VT inducibility, SAECG, HRV, and ejection fraction.

Berger's algorithm was applied by our group to the MADIT II population to investigate whether abnormal QT repolarization is related to spontaneous VT/VF detected by ICD (141). In this study, QT variability was assessed in a 10-min resting ECG recording. A high-risk QT variability subgroup was defined by identifying patients from the highest (>75th percentile) QTVI distribution. The beat-to-beat QT variability algorithm applied to MADIT II patients showed an independent prognostic value of QTVI (> −0.52 log units) to predict an increased risk of arrhythmic events in postinfarction patients with severe left ventricular dysfunction (EF <30%). The mean QTVI and QTVN (QT variability numerator) were significantly higher in subjects requiring an appropriate therapy for VF/VT during a mean of 21 ± 12 months of follow-up (−0.80± vs. −0.94 ± 0.60, $p = 0.037$; and 0.39 ± 0.59 vs. 0.25 ± 0.56, $p = 0.001$ for QTVI and QTVN, respectively).

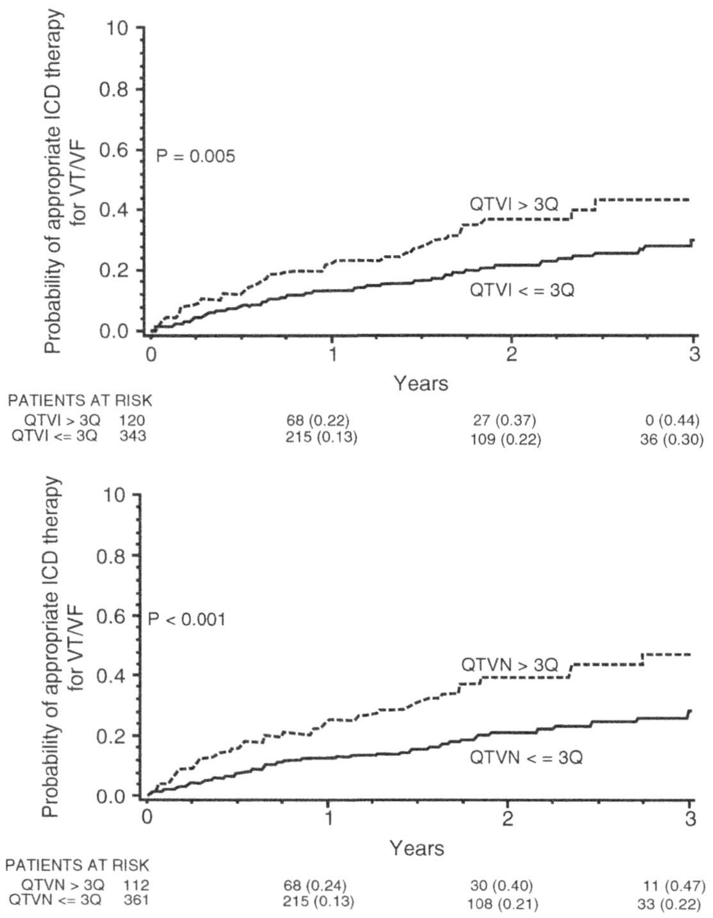

Fig. 7.21

Cumulative probability of first appropriate defibrillator therapy for ventricular tachycardia (VT) or ventricular fibrillation (VF) in patients with QT variability numerator (QTVN) in the highest quartile versus lower three quartiles for QT variability index (QTVI) (*top panel*) and QTVN (*bottom panel*) (Haigney et al. [141]. © Elsevier Limited. Reproduced with permission)

Of the subjects in the highest quartile for QTVI, 37% experienced an episode of VT/VF as compared to 22% in the lower three quartiles. An even stronger difference was observed in respect to QTVN (40 vs. 22%, $p < 0.001$) (Fig. 7.21). Multivariate Cox analysis showed that both QTVI and QTVN were independent risk factors for VT/VF (HR = 1.80 and 2.18, respectively), after adjustment for significant clinical covariates. It is worth emphasizing that neither low ejection fraction nor inducibility of VT/VF during programmed ventricular stimulation was a significant predictor of spontaneous VT/VF. Additional analysis focusing on survival showed that increased QTVI was related to a higher incidence of death within the defibrillator arm.

Recently, we developed a new method to quantify repolarization variability focusing on the variability of T wave amplitude in scalar ECGs instead of analyzing the variability of QT interval duration. Our newly developed method to estimate TWV was tested in a group of 275 ICD patients from the MADITII trial. TWV >0.59 μV was an independent risk predictor of ICD therapy for VT or fibrillation. Patients with increased TWC had 47% probability of appropriate ICD therapy as compared to 29% in those with TWV <= 59 μV during a mean 3-year follow-up (Fig. 7.22). Concordance of the findings by two different methods (Berger's and ours) support the observation that the phenomenon of QT variability exists and might be considered as a risk stratifier [126].

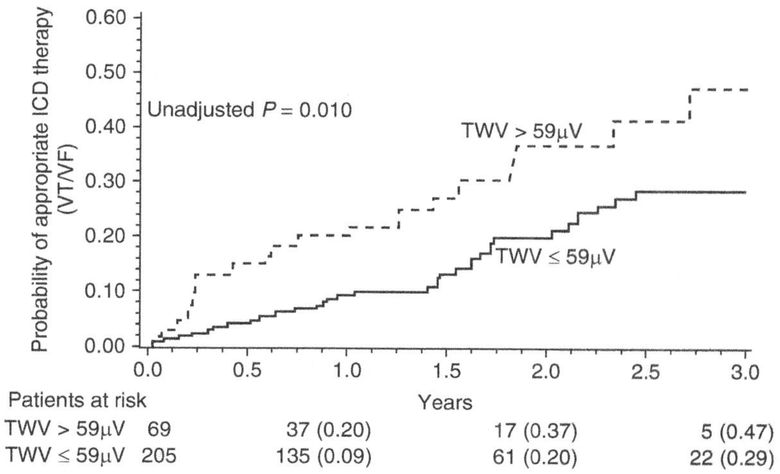

Fig. 7.22
Cumulative probability of VT/VF requiring ICD therapy in MADIT II patients (Couderc et al. © Oxford University Press. Reproduced with permission)

More and more attention is recently paid to patients with relatively preserved LVEF. Due to advancement in modern treatment, this population of patients is growing, and despite a lower incidence of sudden death in patients with significantly depressed LVEF, the absolute number of patients experiencing sudden death in absolute values is very high. As recently documented by Piccirillo et al. [142], abnormal QT variability can identify the sudden cardiac death high-risk group among asymptomatic patients with only mild to moderate left ventricular dysfunction. In a group of 396 patients with congestive heart failure due to ischemic cardiomyopathy with LVEF between 35 and 40% and NYHA class I, QTVI greater or equal to the 80th percentile (−0.47) indicated an independent high risk for SCD with HR of 4.6 (1.5–13.4, $p = 0.006$). This finding might suggest that abnormal QT variability may serve as a marker to identify possible candidates for ICD therapy among patients with a moderately depressed LVEF. However, this requires further prospective studies.

In comparison to the QT/RR slope analyses where computer algorithms take advantage of averaging a series of beats, the methodology of quantifying beat-to-beat QT or TWV requires very robust identification of repolarization in consecutive beats. Although QT measurement on a beat-to-beat basis is of primary interest, it is frequently difficult to accomplish in ambulatory recordings due to challenges in identifying the end of the T waves. Both the above mentioned methods, QT variability/lability developed by Berger et al. [123] and TWV developed by Couderc et al. [126], do not require precise identification of the T wave end since they both rely on quantifying QT and T wave morphology on a beat-to-beat basis. Despite these advances in signal processing, it has to be recognized that there are limitations of quantifying beat-to-beat QT or TWV in recordings with flat T waves, in recordings with non-sinus rhythms, frequent arrhythmias, or excessive noise.

TWA is yet another parameter reflecting beat-to-beat changes in T wave morphology and there is a large body of literature describing the electrophysiologic understanding of this electrical phenomenon and clinical applications in the risk stratification of ventricular arrhythmias and sudden death. This broad topic was purposefully not covered by this chapter, which specifically focused on the QT interval and its dynamics.

7.7 Summary

During the last decade, we have observed increasing interest in analysis of the QT interval, which is considered an important ECG parameter reflecting the complexity of ventricular repolarization driven by an interplay of ion-channel activity, myocardial cell connectivity, disease processes (ischemia, hypertrophy), and external factors including drugs. Despite the 100 years of science and clinical practice in electrocardiography, there is still room for improvement in developing reproducible methods of manual and automatic measurements of the QT interval. Computerized method quantifying QT duration and T wave morphology are increasingly used in everyday practice and in drug safety studies. There also is an increasing appreciation for T wave morphology that offers additional clinically relevant information in addition to QT duration, particularly in electrical disorders of the heart and drug safety concerns. Evaluation of static measures of QT interval duration and T wave morphology is increasingly accompanied by analyses of dynamic features of the QT interval behavior that could be quantified by measuring QT adaptation to changing heart rate, QT or T wave variability, as well as TWA. These dynamic measures of repolarization seem particularly promising in the risk stratification of mortality in patients with ischemic heart diseases and patients with cardiomyopathies.

References

1. Moss, A.J., P.J. Schwartz, R.S. Crampton, et al., The long QT syndrome. Prospective longitudinal study of 328 families. *Circulation*, 1991;**84**: 1136–1144.
2. Vincent, G.M., K.W. Timothy, M. Leppert, et al., The spectrum of symptoms and QT intervals in carriers of the gene for the long-QT syndrome. *N. Engl. J. Med.*, 1992;**327**: 846–852.
3. Zareba, W., A.J. Moss, S. le Cessie, et al., Risk of cardiac events in family members of patients with long QT syndrome. *J. Am. Coll. Cardiol.*, 1995;**26**: 1685–1691.
4. Zareba, W., A.J. Moss, P.J. Schwartz, et al., Influence of genotype on the clinical course of the long-QT syndrome. International Long-QT Syndrome Registry Research Group. *N. Engl. J. Med.*, 1998;**339**: 960–965.
5. Priori, S.G., P.J. Schwartz, C. Napolitano, et al., Risk stratification in the long-QT syndrome. *N. Engl. J. Med.*, 2003;**348**: 1866–1874.
6. Zareba, W. and I. Cygankiewicz, Long QT syndrome and short QT syndrome. *Prog. Cardiovasc. Dis.*, 2008;**51**: 264–278.
7. Schouten, E.G., J.M. Dekker, P. Meppelink, et al., QT interval prolongation predicts cardiovascular mortality in an apparently healthy population. *Circulation*, 1991;**84**: 1516–1523.
8. Sohaib, S.M., O. Papacosta, R.W. Morris, et al., Length of the QT interval: determinants and prognostic implications in a population-based prospective study of older men. *J Electrocardiol.*, 2008;**41**: 704–710.
9. Piotrowicz, K., W. Zareba, S. McNitt, and A.J. Moss, Repolarization duration in patients with conduction disturbances after myocardial infarction. *Am. J. Cardiol.*, 2007;**99**: 163–168.
10. Zareba, W., Drug induced QT prolongation. *Cardiol. J.*, 2007;**14**: 523–533.
11. Splawski, I., J. Shen, K.W. Timothy, et al., Spectrum of mutations in long-QT syndrome genes: KVLQT1, HERG, SCN5A, KCNE1, and KCNE2. *Circulation*, 2000;**102**: 1178–1185.
12. Curran, M.E., I. Splawski, K. Timothy, et al., A molecular basis for cardiac arrhythmia: HERG mutations cause long QT syndrome. *Cell*, 1995;**80**: 795–803.
13. Wang, Q., J. Shen, I. Splawski, et al., SCN5A mutations cause an inherited cardiac arrhythmia, long QT syndrome. *Cell*, 1995;**80**:805–811.
14. Wang, Q., M.E. Curran, I. Splawski, et al., Positional cloning of a novel potassium channel gene: KVLQT1 mutations cause cardiac arrhythmias. *Nat. Genet.*, 1996;**12**:17–23.
15. Mohler, P.J., J.J. Schott, A.O. Gramolini, et al., Ankyrin-B mutation causes type 4 long-QT cardiac arrhythmia and sudden cardiac death. *Nature*, 2003;**421**:634–639.
16. Plaster, N.M., R. Tawil, M. Tristani-Firouzi, et al., Mutations in Kir2.1 cause the developmental and episodic electrical phenotypes of Andersen's syndrome. *Cell*, 2001;**105**:511–519.
17. Splawski, I., K.W. Timothy, L.M. Sharpe, et al., Ca(V)1.2 calcium channel dysfunction causes a multisystem disorder including arrhythmia and autism. *Cell*, 2004;**119**:19–31.
18. Medeiros-Domingo, A., T. Kaku, D.J. Tester, et al., SCN4B-encoded sodium channel beta4 subunit in congenital long-QT syndrome. *Circulation*, 2007;**116**: 134–142.
19. Vatta, M., M.J. Ackerman, B. Ye, et al., Mutant caveolin-3 induces persistent late sodium current and is associated with long-QT syndrome. *Circulation*, 2006;**114**:2104–2112.
20. Chen, L., M.L. Marquardt, D.J. Tester, et al., Mutation of an A-kinase-anchoring protein causes long-QT syndrome. *Proc. Nat. Acad. Sci. USA*, 2007;**104**:20990–20995.
21. Ueda, K., C. Valdivia, A. Medeiros-Domingo, et al., Syntrophin mutation associated with long QT syndrome through activation of the nNOS-SCN5A macromolecular complex. *Proc. Natl. Acad. Sci. USA*, 2008;**105**: 9355–9360.
22. Napolitano, C., S.G. Priori, P.J. Schwartz, et al., Genetic testing in the long QT syndrome: development and validation of an efficient approach to genotyping in clinical practice. *JAMA*, 2005;**294**: 2975–2980.
23. Fadi, A.G., G.X. Yan, C. Antzelevitch, and D.S. Rosenbaum, Unique topographical distribution of M cells underlies reentrant mechanism of torsades de pointes in the long-QT syndrome. *Circulation*, 2002;**105**: 1247–1253.
24. Antzelevitch, C., and W. Shimizu, Cellular mechanisms underlying the long QT syndrome. *Curr. Opin. Cardiol.*, 2002;**17**: 43–51.
25. Antzelevitch, C. Role of transmural dispersion of repolarization in the genesis of drug-induced torsades de pointes. *Heart Rhythm*, 2005;**2**: S9–S15.
26. Antzelevitch, C., L. Belardinelli, A.C. Zygmunt, et al., Electrophysiologic effects of ranolazine: a novel anti-anginal agent with antiarrhythmic properties. *Circulation*, 2004;**110**: 904–910.
27. Moss, A.J. and R.S. Kass, Long QT syndrome: from channels to cardiac arrhythmias. *J. Clin. Invest.*, 2005;**115**: 2018–2024.
28. Keating, M.T. and M.C. Sanguinetti, Molecular and cellular mechanisms of cardiac arrhythmias. *Cell*, 2001;**104**: 569–580.
29. Sanguinetti, M.C., C. Jiang, M.E. Curran, and M.T. Keating, A mechanistic link between an inherited and an acquired cardiac arrhythmia: *HERG* encodes the IKr potassium channel. *Cell*, 1995;**81**: 299–307.

30. Roden, D.M., R.L. Woosley, and R.K. Primm, Incidence and clinical features of the quinidine-associated long QT syndrome: implications for patient care. *Am. Heart. J.*, 1986;**111**: 1088–1093.
31. Kay, G.N., V.J. Plumb, J.G. Arciniegas, et al., Torsades de pointes: the long-short initiating sequence and other clinical features: observations in 32 patients. *J. Am. Coll. Cardiol.*, 1983;**2**: 806–817.
32. Makkar, R.R., B.S. Fromm, R.T. Steinman, et al., Female gender as a risk factor for torsades de pointes associated with cardiovascular drugs. *JAMA*, 1993;**270**: 2590–2597.
33. Moss, A, Measurement of the QT interval and the risk associated with QTc interval prolongation: a review. *Am. J. Cardiol.*, 1993;**72**: 23B–25B.
34. Goldenberg, I, A.J. Moss, and W. Zareba, QT interval: how to measure it and what is "normal". *J. Cardiovasc. Electrophysiol.*, 2006;**17**: 333–336.
35. Lepeschkin, E., The U wave of the electrocardiogram. *Mod. Concepts Cardiovasc. Dis.*, 1969;**38**: 39–45.
36. Pérez Riera, A.R., C. Ferreira, C.F. Filho, et al., The enigmatic sixth wave of the electrocardiogram: the U wave. *Cardiol. J.*, 2008;**15**: 408–421.
37. Viskin, S., U. Rosovski, A.J. Sands, et al., Inaccurate electrocardiographic interpretation of long QT: the majority of physicians cannot recognize a long QT when they see one. *Heart Rhythm*, 2005;**2**: 569–574.
38. Kligfield, P., L.S. Gettes, J.J. Bailey, et al., Recommendations for the standardization and interpretation of the electrocardiogram: part I: the electrocardiogram and its technology a scientific statement from the American Heart Association Electrocardiography and Arrhythmias Committee, Council on Clinical Cardiology; the American College of Cardiology Foundation; and the Heart Rhythm Society endorsed by the International Society for Computerized Electrocardiology. *J. Am. Coll. Cardiol.*, 2007;**49**: 1109–1127.
39. Zareba, W., A.J. Moss, S. le Cessie, Dispersion of ventricular repolarization and arrhythmic cardiac death in coronary artery disease. *Am. J. Cardiol.*, 1994;**74**: 550–553.
40. Zareba, W., Dispersion of repolarization: time to move beyond QT dispersion. *Annals of Noninvasive Electrocardiol.*, 2000;**5**: 373–381.
41. Priori, S.G., D.W. Mortara, C. Napolitano, et al., Evaluation of the spatial aspects of T-wave complexity in the long-QT syndrome. *Circulation*, 1997;**96**: 3006–3012.
42. Zareba, W., A.J. Moss, and J. Konecki. TU wave area-derived measures of repolarization dispersion in the long QT syndrome. *J. Electrocardiol.*, 1998;**30**(Suppl.): 191–195.
43. Okin, P.M., R.B. Devereux, R.R. Fabsitz, et al., Principal component analysis of the T wave and prediction of cardiovascular mortality in American Indians: the Strong Heart Study. *Circulation*, 2002;**105**: 714–719.
44. Couderc, J.P., S. McNitt, J. Xia, et al., Repolarization morphology in adult LQT2 carriers with borderline prolonged QTc interval. *Heart Rhythm*, 2006;**3**: 1460–1466.
45. Bazett, H.C., An analysis of time relations of electrocardiograms. *Heart*, 1920;**7**: 353–367.
46. Fridericia, L.S., Duration of systole in electrocardiogram. *Acta. Med. Scandinav.*, 1920;**53**: 469–475.
47. Sagie, A., M.G. Larson, R.J. Goldberg, et al., An improved method for adjusting the QT interval for heart rate (the Framingham Heart Study). *Am. J. Cardiol.*, 1992;**70**: 797–801.
48. Hodges, M., D. Salerno, and D. Erlien, Bazett's QT correction reviewed: evidence that a linear QT correction for heart rate is better. *J. Am. Coll. Cardiol.*, 1983;**1**: 694.
49. Rautaharju, P.M., S.H. Zhou, S.Wong, et al., Sex differences in the evolution of electrocardiographic QT interval with age. *Can. J. Cardiol.*, 1992;**8**: 690–695.
50. Karjalainen, J., M. Viitasalo, M. Manttari, et al., Relation between QT intervals and heart rates from 40-to 120 beats/min in rest electrocardiogram of men and a simple method to adjust QT interval values. *J. Am. Coll. Cardiol.*, 1994;**23**: 1547–1553.
51. Batchvarov, V.N., A. Ghuran, P. Smetana, et al., QT-RR relationship in healthy subjects exhibits substantial intersubject variability and high intrasubject stability. *Am. J. Physiol. Heart Circ. Physiol.*, 2002;**282**: H2356–H2363.
52. Malik, M., K. Hnatkova, and V. Batchvarov, Differences between study-specific and subject-specific heart rate corrections of the QT interval in investigations of drug induced QTc prolongation. *Pacing Clin. Electrophysiol.*, 2004;**27**: 791–800.
53. Extramiana, F., P. Maison-Blanche, A. Haggui, et al. Control of rapid heart rate changes for electrocardiographic analysis: implications for thorough QT studies. *Clin. Cardiol.*, 2006;**29**: 534–539.
54. Moss, A.J. and J. Robinson. Clinical features of the idiopathic long QT syndrome. *Circulation*, 1992;**85**(Suppl. 1): I140–I144.
55. Lehmann, M.H. and H.Yang, Sexual dimorphism in the electrocardiographic dynamics of human ventricular repolarization: characterization in true time domain. *Circulation*, 2001;**104**: 32–38.
56. Sauer, A.J., A.J. Moss, S. McNitt, et al., Long QT syndrome in adults. *J. Am. Coll. Cardiol.*, 2007;**49**: 329–337.
57. Fenichel, R.R., M. Malik, C. Antzelevitch, et al., Drug-induced Torsade de Pointes and implications for drug development. *J. Cardiovasc. Electrophysiol.*, 2004;**15**: 475–495.
58. Straus, S.M., J.A. Kors, M.L. De Bruin, et al., Prolonged QTc interval and risk of sudden cardiac death in a population of older adults. *J. Am. Coll. Cardiol.*, 2006;**47**: 362–367.
59. Goldberg, R.J., J. Bengtson, Z.Y. Chen, et al., Duration of the QT interval and total and cardiovascular mortality in healthy persons (the Framingham Heart Study experience). *Am. J. Cardiol.*, 1991;**67**: 55–58.
60. Robbins, J., J.C. Nelson, P.M. Rautaharju, and J.S. Gottdiener, The association between the length of the QT interval and mortality in the cardiovascular health study. *Am. J. Med.*, 2003;**115**: 689–694.
61. Okin, P.M., R.B. Devereux, B.V. Howard, et al., Assessment of QT interval and QT dispersion for prediction of all-cause and cardiovascular mortality in American Indians: the Strong Heart Study. *Circulation*, 2000;**101**: 61–66.
62. Algra, A., J.G. Tijssen, J.R. Roelandt, et al., QTc prolongation measured by standard 12-lead electrocardiography is an independent risk factor for sudden death due to cardiac arrest. *Circulation*, 1991;**83**: 1888–1894.
63. Attar, M.N., K. Wong, D.G. Groves, et al., Clinical implications of QRS duration and QT peak prolongation in patients with suspected coronary disease referred for elective cardiac catheterization. *Ann. Noninvasive Electrocardiol.*, 2008;**13**: 106–112.
64. Davey, P., QT interval and mortality from coronary artery disease. *Prog. Cardiovasc. Dis.*, 2000;**42**: 359–384.

65. Davey, P., QT interval lengthening in cardiac disease relates more to left ventricular systolic dysfunction than to autonomic function. *Eur. J. Heart Fail.*, 2000;**2**: 265–271.
66. Montanez, A., J.N. Ruskin, P.R. Hebert, et al., Prolonged QTc interval and risks of total and cardiovascular mortality and sudden death in the general population: a review and qualitative overview of the prospective cohort studies. *Arch. Intern. Med.*, 2004;**164**: 943–948.
67. Breidthardt, T., M. Christ, M. Matti, et al., QRS and QTc interval prolongation in the prediction of long-term mortality of patients with acute destabilised heart failure. *Heart*, 2007;**93**: 1093–1097.
68. Zareba, K.M., H.J. Shenkman, and J.D. Bisognano, Predictive value of admission electrocardiography in patients with heart failure. *Congest. Heart Fail.*, 2008;**14**: 173–179.
69. Moss, A.J., W. Zareba, J. Benhorin, et al., ECG T-wave patterns in genetically distinct forms of the hereditary long QT syndrome. *Circulation*, 1995;**92**: 2929–2934.
70. Zhang, L., K.W. Timothy, G.M. Vincent, et al., Spectrum of ST-T-wave patterns and repolarization parameters in congenital long-QT syndrome: ECG findings identify genotypes. *Circulation*, 2000;**102**: 2849–2855.
71. Yan, G.X. and Antzelevitch C., Cellular basis for the normal T wave and the electrocardiographic manifestations of the long-QT syndrome. *Circulation*, 1998;**98**: 1928–1936.
72. Emori, T. and C. Antzelevitch Cellular basis for complex T waves and arrhythmic activity following combined I_{Kr} and I_{Ks} block. *J. Cardiovasc. Electrophysiol.*, 2001;**12**: 1369–1378.
73. The CAST Investigators. Increased mortality due to encainide or flecainide in a randomized trial of arrhythmia suppression after myocardial infarction. *N. Engl. J. Med.*, 1989;**321**: 406–412.
74. Woosley, R.L., Y. Chen, J.P. Freiman, and R.A. Gillis. Mechanism of the cardiotoxic actions of terfenadine. *JAMA*, 1993;**269**: 1532–1536.
75. Glasman, A.H. and T.J. Biggert. Antipsychotic drugs: prolonged QTc interval, torsade de point sudden death. Am. J. Psychiatry, 2001;**158**(1): 774–782.
76. Liu, T, B.S. Brown, Y. Wu, et al., Blinded validation of the isolated arterially perfused rabbit ventricular wedge in preclinical assessment of drug-induced proarrhythmias. *Heart Rhythm*, 2006;**3**: 948–956.
77. Makkar, R.R., B.S. Fromm, R.T. Steinman, et al., Female gender as a risk factor for torsades de pointes associated with cardiovascular drugs. *JAMA*, 1993;**270**: 2590–2597.
78. Roden, D.M. and P.C. Viswanathan. Genetics of acquired long QT syndrome. *J. Clin. Invest.*, 2005;**115**: 2025–2032.
79. Haverkamp, W., G. Breithardt, A.J. Camm, et al., The potential for QT prolongation and proarrhythmia by non-antiarrhythmic drugs: clinical and regulatory implications: report on a policy conference of the European Society of Cardiology. *Eur. Heart J.*, 2000;**21**: 1216–1231.
80. International Conference on Harmonisation; guidance on E14 clinical evaluation of QT/QTc interval prolongation and proarrhythmic potential for non-antiarrhythmic drugs; availability. *Fed. Regist.*, 2005;**70**: 61134–61135.
81. Zareba, W. and A. Bayes de Luna, QT dynamics and variability. *Ann. Noninvasive Electrocardiol.*, 2005;**10**: 256–262.
82. Franz, M.R., C.D. Swerdlow, L.B. Liem, et al., Cycle length dependence of human action potential in vivo. Effects of single extrastimuli, sudden sustained rate acceleration and deceleration, and different steady-state frequencies. *J. Clin. Invest.* 1988;**82**: 972–979.
83. Lau, C.P., A.R. Freedman, S. Fleming et al., Hysteresis of the ventricular paced QT interval in response to abrupt changes in pacing rate. *Cardiovasc. Res.*, 1988;**22**: 67–72.
84. Krahn, A.D., G.J. Klein, and R.Yee, Hysteresis of the RT interval with exercise. A new marker for the long QT syndrome? *Circulation*, 1997;**96**: 1551–1556.
85. Merri, M., M. Alberti, and A.J. Moss, Dynamic analysis of ventricular repolarization duration from 24 hour Holter recordings. *IEEE Trans. Biomed. Eng.*, 1993;**40**: 1219–1225.
86. Homs, E., V. Marti, J. Offndo, et al., Automatic measurement of corrected QT interval in Holter recordings: comparison of its dynamic behavior in patients after myocardial infarction with and without life-threatening arrhythmias. *Am. Heart. J.*, 1997;**134**(2 Pt 1): 181–187.
87. Jensen, B.T., C.E. Larroude, L.P. Rasmussen, et al., Beat-to-beat QT dynamics in healthy subjects. *Ann. Noninvasive Electrocardiol.*, 2004;**9**: 3–11.
88. Badilini, F., P. Maison-Blanche, R. Childers et al., QT interval analysis on ambulatory electrocardiogram recordings. A selective beat averaging approach. *Med. Biol. Eng. Comput.*, 1999;**37**: 71–79.
89. Extramiana, F., P. Maison-Blanche, F. Badilini et al., Circadian modulation of QT-rate dependence in healthy volunteers: gender and age differences. *J. Electrocardiol.*, 1999;**32**: 33–43.
90. Iacoviello, M., C. Forleo, P. Guida, et al., Ventricular repolarization dynamicity provides independent prognostic information toward major arrhythmic events in patients with idiopathic dilated cardiomyopathy. *J. Am. Coll. Cardioi.*, 2007;**50**: 225–231.
91. Jensen, B.T., S.Z. Abildstrom, C.E. Larroude, et al., QT dynamics in risk stratification after myocardial infarction. *Heart Rhythm*, 2005;**2**: 357–364.
92. Stramba-Badiale, M., E. Locati, A. Martinelli, et al., Gender and the relationship between ventricular repolarization and cardiac cycle length during 24-hour Holter recordings. *Eur. Heart. J.*, 1997;**18**: 1000–1006.
93. Sredniawa, B., A. Musialik-Lydka, P. Jarski, et al., Circadian and sex-dependent QT dynamics. *Pacing Clin. Electrophysiol.*, 2005;**28**(Suppl. 1): S211–S216.
94. Nakagawa, M., T. Ooie, N. Takahashi, et al., Influence of menstrual cycle on QT dynamics. *Pacing Clin. Electrophysiol.*, 2006;**29**: 607–613.
95. Vrtovec, B., V. Starc, and H. Meden-Vrtovec, The effect of estrogen replacement therapy on ventricular repolarization dynamics in healthy postmenopausal women. *J. Electrocardiol.*, 2001;**34**: 227–283.
96. Merri, M., A.J. Moss, J. Benhorin, et al., Relation between ventricular repolarization duration and cardiac cycle length during 24 hour Holter recordings. Findings in normal patients and patients with long QT syndrome. *Circulation*, 1992;**85**: 1816–1821.
97. Perkiomaki, J.S., W. Zareba, A. Nomura, et al., Repolarization dynamics in patients with long QT syndrome. *J. Cardiovasc. Electrophysiol.*, 2002;**13**: 651–656.

98. Extramiana, F., N. Neyroud, H. Huikuri, et al., QT interval and arrhythmic assessment after myocardial infarction. *Am. J. Cardiol.*, 1999;**83**: 266–269.
99. Savelieva, I., Y.G. Yap, G.Yi, et al., Relation of ventricular repolarization to cardiac cycle length in normal subjects, hypertrophic cardiomyopathy and patients with myocardial infarction. *Clin. Cardiol.*, 1999;**22**: 649–654.
100. Faber, T.S., A. Grom, M. Schopflin, et al., Beat-to-beat assessment of QT/RR ratio in severe heart failure and overt myocardia ischemia: a measure of electrical integrity in diseased hearts. *Pacing Clin. Electrophysiol.*, 2003;**26**: 836–842.
101. Roche, F., J.M. Gaspoz, I. Court-Fortune, et al., Alteration of QT rate dependence reflects cardiac autonomic imbalance in patients with obstructive sleep apnea syndrome. *Pacing Clin. Electrophysiol.*, 2003;**26**: 1446–1453.
102. Pellerin, D., P. Maison Blanche, F. Extramiana, et al., Autonomic influences on ventricular repolarization in congestive heart failure. *J. Electrocadiol.*, 2001;**34**: 35–40.
103. Lang, C.C., J.M. Neilson, and A.D. Flapan. Abnormalities of the repolarization characteristics of patients with heart failure progress with symptom severity. *Ann. Noninvasive Electrocardiol.*, 2004;**9**: 257–264.
104. Digeos-Hasnier, S., X. Copie, O. Paziaud, et al., Abnormalities of ventricular repolarization in mitral valve prolapse. *Ann. Noninvasive Electrocardiol.*, 2005;**10**: 297–304.
105. Bonnemeier, H., J. Ortak, F. Bode, et al., Modulation of ventricular repolarization in patients with transient left ventricular apical ballooning: a case control study. *J. Cardiovasc. Electrophysiol.*, 2006;**17**: 1340–1347.
106. Lieb, W., C. Voss, J. Ortak, et al., Impact of diabetes on QT dynamicity in patients with and without myocardial infarction: the KORA Family Heart Study. *Pacing Clin. Electrophysiol.*, 2007;**30**: S183–S187.
107. Valensi, P.E., N.B. Johnson, P. Maison-Blanche, et al., Influence of autonomic neuropathy on heart rate dependence of ventricular repolarization in diabetic patients. *Diabetes Care*, 2002;**25**: 918–923.
108. Nakagawa, M., T. Iwao, S. Ishida, et al., Dynamics of QT interval in a patient with long QT syndrome and a normal QT interval. *Jpn. Circ. J.*, 1998;**62**: 215–218.
109. Fujiki, A., M. Suago, K. Nishida, et al., Repolarization abnormality in idiopathic ventricular fibrillation: assessment using 24-hour QT-RR and QTa-RR relationship. *J. Cardiovasc. Electrophysiol.* 2004;**15**: 59–63.
110. Tavernier, R., L. Jordaens, F. Haerynck, et al., Changes in the QT interval and its adaptation to rate, assessed with continuous electrocardiographic recordings in patients with ventricular fibrillation, as compared to normal individuals without arrhythmias. *Eur. Heart J.*, 1997;**18**: 994–999.
111. Pierre, B., D. Babuty, P. Paret, et al., Abnormal nocturnal heart rate variability and QT dynamics in patients with Brugada syndrome. *Pacing Clin. Electrophysiol.*, 2007; **30**(Suppl. 1): 188–191.
112. Yavuz, B., A. Deniz, G. Abali, et al., Impaired ventricular electrical stability and sympathetic hyperactivity in patients with multivessel coronary artery disease. *Coron. Artery Dis.*, 2007;**18**: 241–245.
113. Bonnemeier, H., U.K.W. Wiegand, F. Bode, et al., Impact of infarct-related artery flow on QT dynamicity in patients undergoing direct percutaneous coronary intervention for acute myocardial infarction. *Circulation*, 2003;**108**: 2979–2986.
114. Singh, J.P., P. Sleight, A. Kardos, and G. Hart, QT interval dynamics and heart rate variability preceding a case of cardiac arrest. *Heart*, 1997;**77**: 375–377.
115. Sredniawa, B., P. Jarski, A. Musialik-Lydka, et al., QT dynamics and the risk of sudden arrhythmic cardiac death In ischemic heart disease. *Pacing Clin. Electrophysiol.*, 2004;**27** (Pt 1): 827–828.
116. Chevalier, P., H. Burri, P. Adeleine, et al., QT dynamicity and sudden death after myocardial infarction: results of long term follow up study. *J. Cardiovasc. Electrophysiol.*, 2002;**14**: 227–233.
117. Milliez, P., A. Leenhardt, P. Maison Blanche, et al., Usefulness of ventricular repolarization dynamicity in patients with ischemic cardiomyopathy (from the European Myocardial Infarct Amiodarone Trial). *Am. J. Cardiol.*, 2005;**95**: 821–826.
118. Smetana, P., E. Pueyo, K. Hnatkowa, et al., Individual pattern of dynamic QT/RR relationship in survivors of acute myocardial infarction and their relationship to antiarrhythmic efficacy of amiodarone. *J. Cardiovasc. Electrophysiol.*, 2004;**15**: 1147–1154.
119. Pathak, A., D. Curnier, J. Fourcade, et al., QT dynamicity: a prognostic factor for sudden death in chronic heart failure. *Eur. J. Heart Fail.*, 2005;**7**: 269–275.
120. Watanabe, E., T. Arakawa, T. Uchiyama, et al., Prognostic significance of circadian variability of RR and QT intervals and QT dynamicity in patients with chronic heart failure. *Heart Rhythm*, 2007;**4**: 999–1005.
121. Cygankiewicz, I., W. Zareba, R. Vazquez, et al., Prognostic value of QT/RR slope in predicting mortality in patients with congestive heart failure. *J. Cardiovasc. Electrophysiol.*, 2008;**19**: 1066–1072.
122. Zareba, W., QT-RR slope: dynamics of repolarization in the risk stratification. *J. Cardiovasc. Electrophysiol.*, 2003;**14**: 234–235.
123. Berger, R.D., E.K. Kasper, K.L. Baughman, et al., Beat-to-beat QT interval variability. Novel evidence for repolarization lability in ischemic and nonischemic dilated cardiomyopathy. *Circulation*, 1997;**96**: 1557–1565.
124. Zareba, W., F. Badilini, and A.J. Moss, Automatic detection of spatial and dynamic heterogeneity of repolarization. *J. Electrocardiol.*, 1994;**27**(Suppl.): 66–72.
125. Couderc, J.P., W. Zareba, L. Burattini, and A.J. Moss, Beat-to-beat repolarization variability in LQTS patients with SCN5A sodium channel gene mutation. *Pacing Clin. Electrophysiol.*, 1999;**22**: 1581–1592.
126. Couderc, J.P., W. Zareba, S. McNitt, et al., Repolarization variability in the risk stratification of MADIT II patients. *Europace*, 2007;**9**: 717–723.
127. Goldenberg, I., J. Mathew, A.J. Moss, et al., Corrected QT variability in serial electrocardiograms in long QT syndrome: the importance of the maximum corrected QT for risk stratification. *J. Am. Coll. Cardiol.*, 2006;**48**: 1047–1052.
128. Vrtovec, B., V. Starc, and R. Starc, Beat-to-beat QT interval variability in coronary patients. *J. Electrocardiol.*, 2000;**33**: 119–25.
129. Cuomo, S., F. Marciano, M.L. Migaux, et al., Abnormal QT interval variability in patients with hypertrophic cardiomyopathy: can syncope be predicted? *J. Electrocardiol.*, 2004;**37**: 113–119.
130. Hiromoto, K., H. Shimizu, T. Mine, et al., Correlation between beat-to-beat QT interval variability and impaired left ventricular function in patients with previous myocardial infarction. *Ann. Noninvasive Electrocardiol.*, 2006;**11**: 299–305.
131. Desai, N., D.S. Raghunandan, M. Mallavarapu, et al., Beat-to-beat heart rate and QT variability in patients with congestive

cardiac failure: blunted response to orthostatic challenge. *Ann. Noninvasive Electrocardiol.* 2004;**9**: 323–329.
132. Yeragani, V.K., M. Tancer, and T. Uhde, Heart rate and QT interval variability: abnormal alpha-2 adrenergic function in patients with panic disorder. *Psychiatry*, 2003;**121**: 185–196.
133. Carney, R.M., K.F. Freedland, P. Stein, et al., Effects of depression on QT interval variability after myocardial infarction. *Psychosomatic Medicine*, 2003;**65**: 177–180.
134. Haigney, M.C., S. Alam, S. Tebo, et al., Intravenous cocaine and QT variability. *J. Cardiovasc. Electrophysiol.*, 2006;**17**: 610–616.
135. Thomsen, M.B., P.G. Volders, J.D. Beekman, et al., Beat-to-beat variability of repolarization determines proarrhythmic outcome in dogs susceptible to drug-induced Torsades de Pointes. *J. Am. Coll. Cardiol.*, 2006;**48**: 1268–1276.
136. Thomsen, M., A. Oros, M. Schoenmakers, et al., Proarrhythmic electrical remodeling is associated with increased beat-to-beat variability of repolarization. *Cardiovasc. Res.*, 2007;**73**: 521–530.
137. Henneberger, A., W. Zareba, A. Ibald-Mulli, et al., Repolarization changes induced by air pollution in ischemic heart disease patients. *Environ. Health. Perspect.*, 2005;**113**: 440–446.
138. Piccirillo, G., R. Quaglione, M. Nocco et al., Effects of long-term beta-blocker (metoprolol or carvedilol) therapy on QT variability in subjects with chronic heart failure secondary to ischemic cardiomyopathy. *Am. J. Cardiol.* 2002;**90**: 1113–1117.
139. Bonnemeier, H., F. Hartmann, U.K. Wiegand, et al., Course and prognostic implications of QT interval and QT variability after primary coronary angioplasty in acute myocardial infarction. *J. Am. Coll. Cardiol.*, 2001;**37**: 44–50.
140. Atiga, W.L., Calkins, H., Lawrence, J.H., et al., Beat-to-beat repolarization lability identifies patients at risk for sudden cardiac death. *J. Cardiovasc. Electrophysiol.*, 1998;**9**: 899–908.
141. Haigney, M.C., W. Zareba, P.J. Gentlesk, et al., and the MADIT II Investigators. QT interval variability and spontaneous ventricular tachycardia or fibrillation in the Multicenter Automatic Defibrillator Implantation Trial (MADIT) II patients. *J. Am. Coll. Cardiol.*, 2004;**44**: 1481–1487.
142. Piccirillo, G., D. Magri, S. Matera, et al. QT variability strongly predicts sudden cardiac death in asymptomatic subjects with mild or moderate left ventricular dysfunction: a prospective study. *Eur. Heart. J.* 2007;**28**: 1344–1350.

8 Miscellaneous Electrocardiographic Topics

J.E. Madias

P. W. Macfarlane et al. (eds.), *Electrocardiology*, DOI 10.1007/978-0-85729-874-4_8,

8.1 Introduction

A chapter, entitled as this one is, aims at providing a systematic presentation on a number of topics, which are either not included elsewhere in this book, or they receive a cursory treatment as mere components of an overall exposition. In the first category, one could consider the attenuation of ECG voltage resulting from the development of peripheral edema of varying etiology [1], while in the second the giant T waves could represent an example of a topic included here, but also mentioned under ST-T changes found in chapters about myocardial infarction, ischemia, intraventricular conduction abnormalities or ventricular hypertrophy. In such a venture some redundancy is inevitable, but overall it proves to be beneficial. Some ECG abnormalities, which were included in this chapter in the first Edition, became so pervasive as to deserve their separate handling (e.g., QT interval, ➋ Chap. 7). Many ECG topics, not considered previously, had to be included in this Edition because of their expanding role in the practice of medicine. Finally, one should envisage that undescribed ECG changes and associations are still awaiting detection, and thus a chapter like this is open-ended in terms of its contents, and serves as a "gate" or "filter" for what eventually becomes established. The author is much indebted to Professor C.Y. Chen and the late Professor K. Harumi, authors of this chapter in the first Edition, for the aid received from their original text and associated references, and for the marvelous panel of their figures, most of which have been retained.

8.2 Electrolyte, Acid Base, and Blood Abnormalities

Imbalances of the various cations, and disturbances in the acid-base, blood gas, and hemoglobin concentration affect the ECG most often in a nonspecific fashion, although occasionally may produce characteristic changes, as in the alterations of K^+ and Ca^{2+}.

Electrophysiologic properties of myocardial cells depend on the movement of electrolytes across their membranes, setting up ionic currents [2, 3]. ➋ Table 8.1 summarizes the effects of various types of electrolyte imbalance on the transmembrane action potential, which result in ECG changes of depolarization (P wave and QRS complex), repolarization (ST segment and T wave), and impulse generation and conduction.

In the clinical domain, the characteristic ECGs resulting from electrolyte imbalance are encountered in patients with malabsorption, starvation, various endocrinopathies and sizeable loss of electrolytes due to severe vomiting, diarrhea, burns, diabetic ketoacidosis, and diuretic therapy. Patients with renal failure are the ones most frequently troubled by electrolyte imbalance. Among all the electrolyte disorders, changes in serum K^+ are the most prevalent, leading to alterations in the ECG and occasionally serious cardiac rhythm and conduction disturbances.

8.2.1 Hyperkalemia

8.2.1.1 P Wave, QRS Complex, and Conduction Disturbance

Normally the extracellular concentration of K^+ (3.5–5.0 $mEq\,L^{-1}$) is much lower than the intracellular K^+ (140 $mEq\,L^{-1}$), and thus the intracellular to extracellular concentration gradient of this cation can be easily increased or decreased by small changes in the serum K^+ [2, 3]. An increase in the extracellular K^+ concentration and the consequent decrease of this gradient will rapidly decrease the resting membrane potential, the magnitude of the action potential, and the maximum rate of rise of phase 0 $(dV/dt)_{max}$, the last resulting from its dependence on the resting membrane potential (➋ Fig. 8.1). Also, since the conduction velocity in the Purkinje fibers and cardiac muscle is determined primarily by $(dV/dt)_{max}$, and this is reduced in hyperkalemia (↑K), conduction through the heart will be depressed [4]. During phase 4, the membrane potential is approximately compatible with the equilibrium potential of K^+. If there is an excess of extracellular K^+, as in ↑K, the membrane potential is reduced according to the Nernst equation [2]. ↑K, however, produces a biphasic effect on the atrioventricular (AV) conduction system, with mild degrees accelerating the AV conduction, and severe ↑K (≥7.5 $mEq\,L^{-1}$) depressing it. In experimental studies, conduction is most rapid at a K^+ level of ~6.0–6.5 $mEq\,L^{-1}$. This enhancing effect of mild ↑K may improve conduction in patients with sinus rhythm and AV block, or accelerate the ventricular response in atrial fibrillation [4–6]. Severe ↑K may produce all kinds of AV blocks, although high-degree AV

Table 8.1
Effects of K^+ and Ca^{2+} on electrophysiological properties

	Hyperkalemia	Hypokalemia	Hypercalcemia	Hypocalcemia
Phase 0				
Upstroke rate of rise (dV/dt)	Decreased	Unchanged or increased	Decreased	Increased
Action potential Amplitude	Decreased	Increased		
Phase 2				
Plateau of action Potential	Shortened	Prolonged	Shortened	Prolonged
Phase 3				
Action potential Duration	Shortened	Prolonged	Shortened	Prolonged
Phase 4				
Resting membrane Potential	Decreased	Increased Decreased (≤2 mEq)	Unchanged	Unchanged
Pacemaker activity	Enhanced (5.5–6 mEq) Depressed (≥7 mEq)	Enhanced	Increased	Increased
Conductivity	Enhanced (5.5–6 mEq) Depressed (≥7 mEq)	Depressed	Decreased	Increased

block is infrequent. Electrophysiological studies show that the sites of AV block in ↑K are at the atrionodal, nodal-His or His-Purkinje regions, and that the N (true nodal) regions are relatively insensitive to it [7].

The action of increased serum K^+ on the various types of cardiac fibers may be nonuniform [5], with the atrial fibers being more sensitive than the ventricular myocardium. Intra-atrial conduction is depressed in ↑K (7.0–7.5 $mEq\,L^{-1}$), resulting in wide and flattened P waves (➋ Table 8.2), and in severe ↑K (≥9 $mEq\,L^{-1}$), intra-atrial conduction is markedly slowed and the P waves often disappear (➋ Fig. 8.2), leading to the so-called sinoventricular rhythm. In this condition, where absence of P waves hinders its differentiation from complete AV block, there is no influence of ↑K on the sinus pacemaker properties, and conduction from the sinus node to the ventricular fibers is maintained.

Intraventricular conduction is also affected by ↑K, and its mild to severe forms lead to diffuse widening of the QRS complexes, often simulating all kinds of bundle branch blocks (➋ Fig. 8.2). Left anterior or posterior fascicular blocks may be observed transiently [8], and might be caused by the nonuniform effects of ↑K on the intraventricular conduction [9]. The same mechanism may be responsible for the pseudoinfarctional QRS patterns occasionally noted and mistaken for real myocardial infarcts (MI). Also a reduction of cardiac excitability manifest as an increase in the threshold or failure to capture by an electronic pacemaker has been noted with ↑K, involving the atrium or the ventricle [10–12]. Indeed, failure to capture the atrium with preservation of capture of the ventricle in DDD pacemaking attests to the greater sensitivity of the former to ↑K [11]. With levels of serum $K^+ \geq 8\,mEq\,L^{-1}$ a sine-wave pattern may appear [13], consisting of a wide QRS complex with an inverted T wave leading to ventricular fibrillation and cardiac standstill.

8.2.1.2 ST Segment and T Wave

Increase in the extracellular K^+ concentration (≥6.0 $mEq\,L^{-1}$) shortens the duration of the action potential, mainly by increasing the steepness of phase 2 [9] (➋ Fig. 8.1). This action of K^+ may depend on an increase of K^+

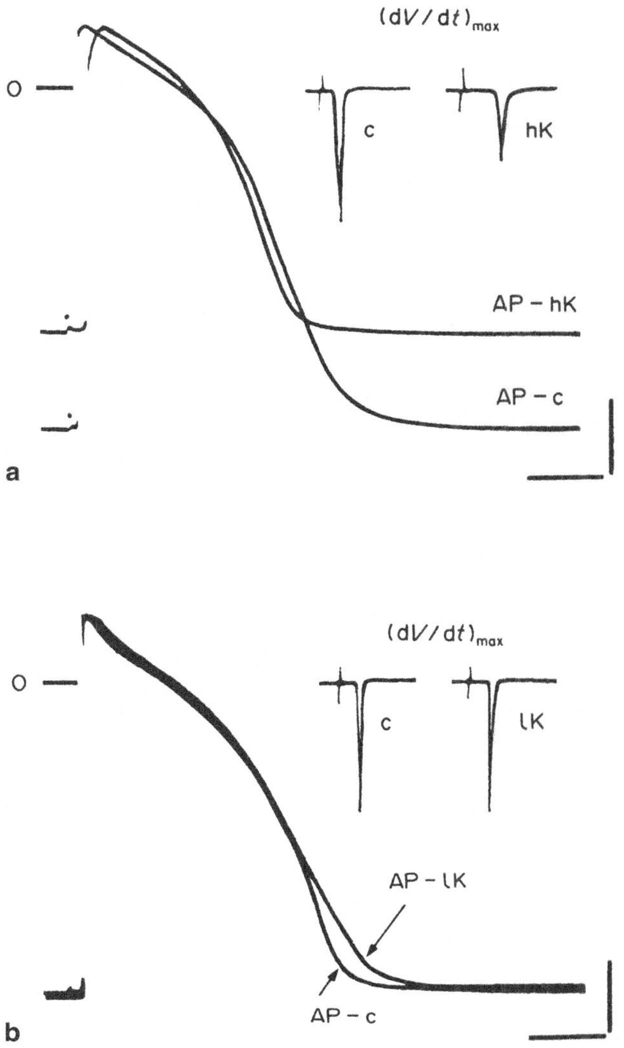

Fig. 8.1
Action potentials from the guinea pig's heart: (a) action potentials in normal (2.7 mM) and altered Tyrode's solution (K^+; 8.0 mM) are depicted. In a higher concentration of K^+, the resting membrane potential and the maximum upstroke velocity of phase 0 are reduced, and the duration of repolarization is shortened (c, control; hK, higher concentration of K^+; AP, action potential); (b) action potentials in normal (K^+; 2.7 mM) and altered Tyrode's solution (K^+; 1.0 mM) are depicted. In a lower concentration of K^+ (lK), the resting membrane potential and the maximum upstroke velocity are unchanged, while the duration of repolarization is slightly prolonged

conductance (gK) [3]. These changes in the shape of the action potential are probably the reason for the shortening of the QT interval and the peaked tent-shaped T wave, which is the most common and the sole ECG sign of serum K^+ concentrations between 5.5 and 6.5 mEq L^{-1}. The corresponding change in the vectorcardiogram is a linear T wave loop. The T wave changes are more frequently seen in leads II, III and in the precordial leads, and are nonspecific for ↑K, since they are also seen in many other conditions, i.e., myocardial ischemia, bradycardia, and subjects with early repolarization (➋ Fig. 8.3). In differentiating acute ischemic syndromes from ↑K, the regional presence in the former with normal or prolonged QTc, in contrast to the diffuse occurrence in the latter of similarly appearing T waves with shortened

Table 8.2
ECG abnormalities in hyperkalemia

	Abnormalities
P and QRS waves	Flat and broad P wave (7–7.5 mEq L^{-1}) Disappearing P wave (8–9 mEq L^{-1}) Widening of QRS wave (≥6.5 mEq L^{-1}) Sine-wave patterns of QRS wave (≥8–9 mEq L^{-1}) Cardiac arrest (8 mEq L^{-1} or higher)
ST segment and T waves	Tent-shaped T wave (≥5.5 mEq L^{-1}) Shortening QT_c interval (≥5.5 mEq L^{-1}) Opposing T wave (8–9 mEq L^{-1}) Depression or elevation of ST segment (6.5–7.5 mEq L^{-1})
Conduction and impulse formation	Accelerated AV conduction (5.5–6 mEq L^{-1}) Slow AV conduction (≥7–7.5 mEq L^{-1}) Failure of cardiac capture by artificial pacemaker (6–7.5 mEq L^{-1}) Reversible fascicular block (6.5–7.5 mEq L^{-1}) Reentrant ectopic beats (7.5–8.5 mEq L^{-1}) Ventricular fibrillation (8–9 mEq L^{-1})

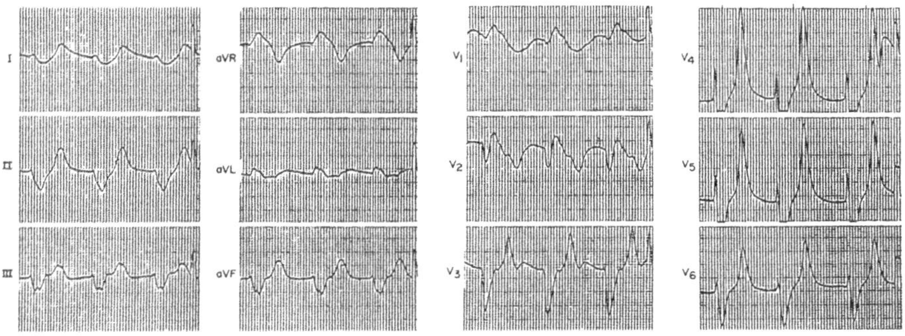

Fig. 8.2
The ECG was recorded from a patient suffering from severe chronic renal failure, and advanced hyperkalemia (serum K^+ level was 8.3 mEq L^{-1}). The characteristic sinoventricular rhythm (no discernible P waves), and the intraventricular conduction disturbance, simulating right bundle branch block, are shown

QTc, is helpful [2]. Occasionally, the tent-shaped T waves may be of normal amplitude, [14], and this should be kept in mind so that ↑K is not overlooked. In severe ↑K (7.5 mEq L^{-1}), the T wave changes may be associated with widening of the QRS and a decrease in the amplitude of the R waves. The T wave changes in advanced ↑K may be secondary to intraventricular conduction disturbances [13, 15], rather than due to the alteration of the action potential. In very severe ↑K, an inverted T wave with a wide QRS complex may be observed and may be followed by the development of ventricular tachycardia, fibrillation, and asystole [16].

ST segment depression, and even rarely ST segment elevation, may be observed in ↑K, probably as a result of the shortening of the plateau of the action potential and the decrease of diastolic potential (➋ Fig. 8.1). ST segment elevation indistinguishable from a current of injury has been recognized for a long time, and has led to numerous reports in the literature of ↑K, simulating acute MI [17]; in such cases correction of ↑K has abolished the pseudoinfarctional ECG pattern, hence the expression "dialyzable currents of injury" has been coined to characterize these transient ECG alterations [18]. The ST segment elevation probably is due to inhomogeneous depolarization of different myocardial territories, resulting

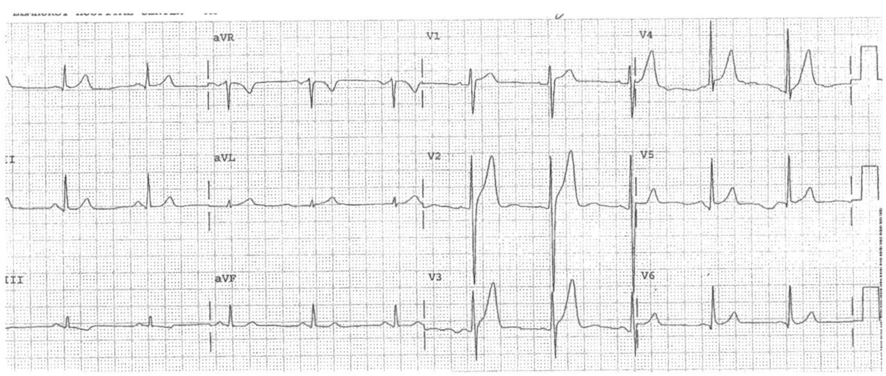

Fig. 8.3
ECG changes simulating hyperkalemia in a 27-year old healthy male subject, due to early repolarization; automated systems often interpret these changes as due to "metabolic or ischemic abnormalities". A QTc of 358 ms was present, in the absence of hypercalcemia, or hyperkalemia

in voltage gradients and current flow between these regions. A pseudoinfarctional ST segment elevation has been noted in a hypokalemic patient undergoing rapid K^+ replenishment, and while she was still hypokalemic (K^+: 3.0 mEq L^{-1}) (➋ Fig. 8.4), and it was attributed to the reduction of the intracellular to extracellular gradient, not unlike what occurs with true serum ↑K [19]. Finally, it should be always kept in mind that profound ↑K may be encountered without ECG manifestations [20].

8.2.2 Hypokalemia

8.2.2.1 P Wave and QRS Complex

Increase in the resting membrane potential and the amplitude of the action potential are mediated by a progressive decrease of serum K^+ at a level ~2.7 mEq L^{-1}, although with even lower concentrations, the conduction velocity might be reduced, indicating a decrease in resting membrane potential and prolongation of repolarization [2]. Thus, with severe hypokalemia (↓K), the amplitude and the duration of the QRS increase (➋ Table 8.3). The widened QRS complexes indicate that the intraventricular conduction disturbance is due to a generalized slowing of conduction in the peripheral conduction system and/or myocardium. The amplitude and duration of the P waves also are usually increased in ↓K, as seen in leads II, III and aVF, with such changes resembling P-pulmonale, or "pseudo P-pulmonale" found in left atrial abnormality.

8.2.2.2 ST Segment and T and U Waves

The earliest abnormalities consequent to a modest reduction of the serum K^+ are those of repolarization, and are commonly appreciated in the ECG. Electrophysiologically, there is an increase in the action potential duration. Further lowering of K^+ leads to shortening of the plateau phase of the action potential, and a progressively steeper slope of phase 2. This change in the slope of the action potential, mediated by decreased conductance, can occur with milder ↓K (2.7–2.4 mEq L^{-1}), but it is associated with insignificant effect on the resting potential.

The ECG (usually leads II, III and V_2–V_4) reveals abnormalities of the ST segment, T and U waves, which constitute the most common and helpful changes for the detection of ↓K (➋ Table 8.3). The amplitude of the T and U wave reflect relatively accurately the levels of the deficit in the serum concentration of K^+ (➋ Fig. 8.5). The diagnosis of ↓K in patients

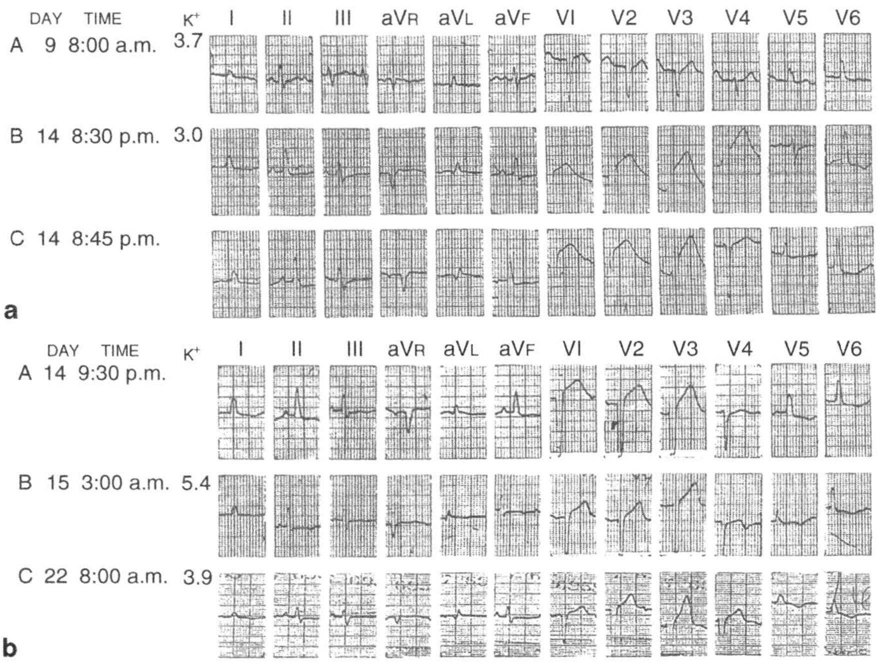

Fig. 8.4

(a) ST segment elevation, simulating an acute myocardial infarction in a 65-year-old woman, which persisted for a few hours while she was receiving K^+ supplementation for hypokalemia resulting from intravenous hyperalimentation. (b) The highest serum K^+ recorded in this patient was 5.4 mEq L^{-1}, at which time the ST segment elevation had resolved (Reproduced from Ref. [19]. With permission of the *Journal of Electrocardiology*)

Table 8.3

ECG abnormalities in hypokalemia

	Abnormalities
P and QRS waves	Increased QRS wave amplitude Increased QRS wave duration Increased P wave amplitude Increased P wave duration
ST segment, T and U waves	Prominent U wave Flat or inverted T wave ST segment depression
Conduction and impulse formation	Atrial premature contractions Atrial tachycardia Supraventricular tachycardia AV junctional rhythm AV dissociation First degree AV block Ventricular premature contractions Bidirectional ventricular tachycardia Ventricular fibrillation

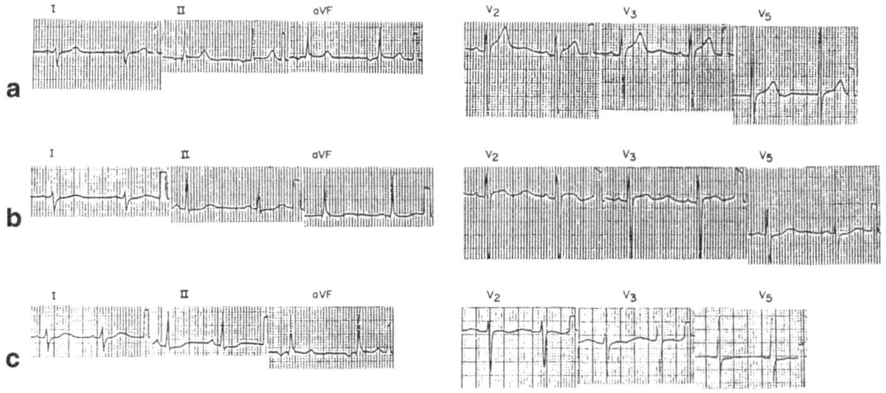

Fig. 8.5
ECG changes at different degrees of hypokalemia, in a patient with primary aldosteronism: (a) Na 147 mEq L^{-1}, K 4.3 mEq L^{-1}, Cl 106 mEq L^{-1}; (b) Na 146 mEq L^{-1}, K 2.8 mEq L^{-1}, Cl 98 mEq L^{-1}; (c) Na 147 mEq L^{-1}, K 1.7 mEq L^{-1}, Cl 97 mEq L^{-1}. With increasing ↓K the T wave becomes lower and the U wave taller

can be facilitated by employing ST segment depression ≥0.05 mV, U wave amplitude >0.1 mV, and U wave amplitude >T wave amplitude in the same lead as the other criteria, with the frequency of a positive diagnosis paralleling the severity of ↓K [21]. The depressed ST segment and the low or inverted T wave may fuse with the prominent U wave in ↓K without significant changes of QT or QU intervals. In severe ↓K, the ST segment depression is accompanied by a prominent U wave and a dwarfed T wave.

The effects of ↓K on the Purkinje fibers differ from those on the ventricular fibers, prolonging the plateau phase in the former and shortening it in the latter, thus increasing the difference between the action potential durations [22]; this difference in the sensitivity of Purkinje and myocardial fibers to ↓K might underlie the development of the U wave.

8.2.2.3 Conduction and Impulse Generation

A clinically relevant effect of ↓K is the enhancement of automaticity of latent pacemakers, which is probably mediated by the acceleration of the decay of pacemaker current (i_{K2}) in the Purkinje fibers resulting from a decreased K^+ conductance [3]. Accordingly, unifocal or multifocal ectopic beats have been found in experimental and clinical studies. Common cardiac arrhythmias at serum K^+ levels ≤3.0 mEq L^{-1} are atrial premature beats, atrial tachycardia with or without AV block, supraventricular tachycardia, AV junctional rhythm and AV junctional parasystole. However, in a study employing ambulatory ECG monitoring of hypertensive patients without coronary artery disease treated with diuretics, K^+ levels of 2.5 to 3.4 mEq L^{-1} were not associated with arrhythmias [23]. The important issue of whether mild to moderate ↓K *per se* is arrhythmogenic has not been resolved thus far conclusively, but even resolution of this matter may not be clinically relevant most of the time, in terms of the need for correction of ↓K; patients usually present with clusters of conditions and abnormal tests, and in that setting management should be individualized and mostly in favor of K^+ replenishment [24]. The duration of the action potential is prolonged in severe ↓K (➋ Fig. 8.1), making it more likely for a propagated simple ectopic ventricular impulse to fall into the vulnerable period of the fused TU complex, and easily initiate reentrant arrhythmias by a complex interplay of ectopy and depressed conduction. In such a setting, "torsade de pointes" (TdP), the unusual multidirectional ventricular tachycardia characteristic of ↓K [25], may emerge; in fact ↓K is an important cause of acquired long QT syndrome, and associated TdP. ↓K also causes arrhythmias due to enhanced automaticity. The enhancement of digitalis-induced arrhythmias by ↓K has been known for a long time and thus it is recommended that serum K^+ be kept between 4.5 and 5.0 mEq L^{-1} [26]. Also, arrhythmias occur in the interplay of ↓K and myocardial ischemia [27]. Significant AV and intraventricular conduction disturbances secondary to ↓K have been noted in patients, with 1° AV block appearing at serum K^+ levels ≤2.7 mEq L^{-1}, and variable degrees of AV block at levels ≤1.01 mEq L^{-1} [2, 28].

8.2.3 Hypercalcemia and Hypocalcemia

8.2.3.1 P Wave and QRS Complex

The resting potential, the amplitude of the action potential, or the shape of phase 3 are not significantly affected even with extremes of serum Ca^{2+} concentrations (1.2–20.8 mEq L^{-1}) [29]. Primarily, an abnormal Ca^{2+} level impacts the ventricular repolarization. However, severe hypercalcemia (↑Ca) reduces the upstroke and conduction velocities in ventricular muscle fibers, and increases the QRS duration, in contrast to hypocalcemia (↓Ca), which decreases the QRS duration [2, 30]. An increased amplitude of the QRS complex, suggesting an increase in the ventricular muscle mass, has been observed with ↑Ca [31]. Furthermore, the duration of the T wave was significantly prolonged in patients with hyperparathyroidism. Abnormal serum Ca^{2+} concentrations have no discernible effect on the P wave. All degrees of AV block can be seen with ↑Ca [2]. Also sinus node dysfunction and tachy-brady syndrome have been described with ↑Ca [32, 33].

8.2.3.2 ST Segment and T Wave

↑Ca shortens the duration of phase 2 of the action potential in all cardiac fibers (➋ Table 8.1) and increases the amplitude of the plateau, a feature enhanced by increased catecholamines [2, 34]. Consequently, the duration of the action potential and the effective refractory period are decreased. Phase 2 of the action potential should be prolonged since, as per the Nernst equation, ↑Ca increases the inward calcium current. However, ↑Ca actually produces a rapid repolarization, probably resulting from the simultaneous enhancement of the K^+ outward current [3]. As the slope of phase 2 and its duration are reflected in the shape of the ST segment of the ECG, the shortening of Q-oT (onset of QRS complex to onset of T wave) and Q-aT (onset of the QRS complex to the apex of the T wave) are the most common early ECG abnormalities in ↑Ca [35] (➋ Fig. 8.6); the total duration of ventricular repolarization does not decrease though, and thus ↑Ca has less effect on the QTc or QU intervals [36, 37]. Occasionally in ↑Ca, the onset of the T wave appears to be at the J-point [38]. An Osborn-like wave has been described with ↑Ca [39]. Short QTc is frequently encountered, particularly in young subjects without ↑Ca (➋ Fig. 8.3) [38], sometimes bordering the measurements seen in patients with the short QT interval syndrome [40]. However, an increased T wave duration has been documented with ↑Ca [31]. By contrast, ↓Ca increases the duration of plateau phase (➋ Table 8.1), leading to prolongation of the ST segment and QT interval, which are both early ECG signs of ↓Ca [2]. In both ↑Ca and ↓Ca, the effect on the QT interval is primarily exerted on the ST segment [2]. The T wave morphology can be affected in both ↑Ca and ↓Ca [2]. Barring the confounding influence of other electrolyte abnormalities, the change of the Q-oTc interval duration may significantly correlate with the serum Ca^{2+} level [41]. The duration of the T wave is not usually affected by ↓Ca, but its amplitude is decreased or sometimes it becomes flattened (➋ Fig. 8.6). The combined ↓Ca and hyperkalemia of renal failure produces ST segment prolongation with narrow-based tall T waves [2]. ↓Ca may mimic acute MI with ST elevation, reciprocal ST segment depression, and regional contraction abnormalities; all these abate with calcium and vitamin D_3 therapy [42]; coronary spasm is implicated in this condition.

8.2.3.3 Conduction and Impulse Generation

Although cardiac arrhythmias and 1° AV block are infrequent in ↓Ca and ↑Ca [5], extreme ↓Ca can produce sinus bradycardia with intermittent sinoatrial block, 2:1 AV block and complete AV block [43, 44], especially in children, and ventricular fibrillation (VF) [45], while ventricular tachycardia and VF have also occurred with ↑Ca [46, 47]. Moreover, torsade de pointes has occurred with both ↓Ca and ↑Ca [48, 49].

The hereditary prolonged QT syndrome and the prolonged QT interval seen with ischemic heart disease are predisposing factors for VF. A possible explanation for the absence of cardiac arrhythmias in sodium EDTA induced ↓Ca with prolonged QT interval [50] is that ↓Ca produces a uniform prolongation of repolarization, thus preventing reentry. Continuous injection of calcium chloride until death in animal experiments led to a change in AV conduction, followed by VF [51].

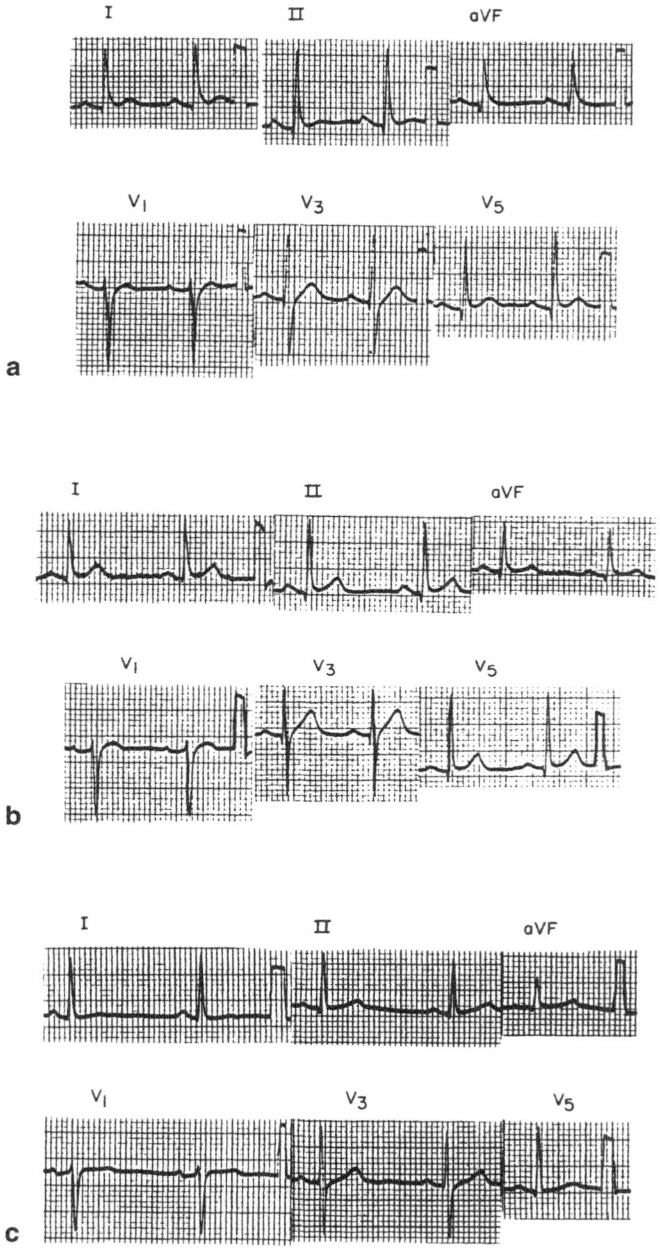

Fig. 8.6
ECG changes at different serum Ca^{2+} levels. (a) 7.2 mEq L^{-1}; (b) 4.2 mEq L^{-1}; (c) 2.6 mEq L^{-1}

In hyperparathyroidism with severe ↑Ca, sinus arrest, Wenckebach 2° AV block and atrial fibrillation have been reported [52, 53]. ↑Ca also may accentuate digitalis-induced ectopy. Finally, the interaction between K^+ and Ca^{2+}, in which ↑Ca reverses the conduction abnormality and cardiac arrhythmias induced by ↑K, has been put to therapeutic use.

8.2.4 Hypomagnesemia and Hypermagnesemia

Clinically encountered abnormalities of serum Mg^{2+} do not affect the action potential significantly. However, the combination of hypomagnesemia (↓Mg), ↓K and digitalis intoxication can lead to cardiac arrhythmias [2, 26]. The influence of ↓Mg in digitalis-induced arrhythmias may be related to the role of Mg^{2+} as a cofactor for membrane sodium and potassium (Na^+–K^+) adenosine triphosphatase, which maintains mitochondrial integrity [54]. Nevertheless, hypomagnesemic patients have suffered paroxysmal VF in the absence of digitalis therapy [55]. ↓Mg in patients with alcoholic heart disease leads to ECG changes similar to the ones noted with ↑K (slightly widened QRS complexes, mild ST depression, peaked T waves and prolonged QT intervals) [56]. Simultaneous correction of ↓Mg and ↓K, in cases of ↓K resistant to adequate replenishment of K^+, is required [24, 26]. Depressed AV conduction with severe hypermagnesemia (↑Mg) may be due to slowing of the velocity of the upstroke of the action potential. In attributing changes in the ECG to ↑Mg, attention should be paid to the associated electrolyte and metabolic disorders [2]. Whether ↓Mg and ↑Mg are arrhythmogenic has not as yet been determined [57].

8.2.5 Sodium

The amplitude of the action potential, and the upstroke velocity, increase with hypernatremia (↑Na) and decrease with hyponatremia (↓Na) [2]. However, since the concentrations of Na^+ required to change the ECG are usually incompatible with life, no ECG abnormalities are encountered with the range of changes seen in the clinical setting [2]. Widened QRS due to intraventricular conduction disturbances resulting from ↑K is shortened by ↑Na, and further prolonged by ↓Na [2].

8.2.6 Lithium

Li^+ readily replaces intracellular K^+, and in patients treated for bipolar depression, may cause minor T wave abnormalities, sinus bradycardia and sinus node dysfunction, with stimulation testing revealing that only the sinus node is reversibly affected by this cation [58]. High Li^+ levels (>1.2 mEq L^{-1}) are also associated with prolongation of PR interval and other AV blocks, ventricular arrhythmias, reversible diffuse T wave inversions, and QTc interval prolongation [59]. The T wave inversions may be due to intracellular displacement of K^+ by Li^+, and respond to K^+ administration. The SA and AV node dysfunction are attributed to alterations of Ca^{2+} flux caused by Li^+. Frequent recording of the ECG, particularly in patients with renal failure or concomitant therapy with β-blockers and Ca^{2+} channel inhibitors, could detect treated patients with over-range Li^+ levels [59].

8.2.7 Hypertonicity and Hypotonicity

Cardiac cells become hyperpolarized and reveal a decrease in action potential upstroke by hypertonic sucrose and other type of solutions [60, 61], and this slows conduction probably because of the widened resting-threshold membrane potential gradient. In canine cardiac Purkinje fibers, hypertonicity increases the action potential duration [61], and in ventricular fibers from guinea pigs and cats, it leads to disappearance of phase 3 of the action potential [60]. Information on hypotonicity is lacking. An anisotonic solution application on the heart causes T wave changes. However, in the clinical setting changes in osmolarity occur in various combinations with alterations in electrolytes, pH, and oxygenation, and thus the impact on electrophysiology and the ECG is variable.

8.2.8 pH

It is difficult to evaluate the effects of pH changes on the ECG, since acidosis and alkalosis are closely linked to alterations in the serum concentration of K^+ and Ca^{2+}. Resting membrane potential and repolarization of canine Purkinje fibers were little affected by a pH of 6.8, while decreasing the bicarbonate concentration to 12 mM independent of acidosis led to an increase in the action potential duration [62]. In diseases leading to metabolic and respiratory acidosis, an increase in the amplitude of the T wave would be expected, while alkalosis would lead to flattening or even inversion of T waves [63]. The above are stated by extrapolation from results of human experimentation with voluntary hyperventilation, exercise, and ingestion of Na bicarbonate and ammonium chloride. Alkalosis and acidosis increase the pacing threshold [12].

8.2.9 Oxygen and Carbon Dioxide

Hypoxemia (↓PaO_2), rise of PaO_2 through breathing of high oxygen concentrations, hypercapnia (↑$PaCO_2$), and hypocapnia (↓$PaCO_2$) are encountered in patients with respiratory and metabolic conditions; thus inevitably alterations in pH and concentrations of serum electrolytes also occur. ↓PaO_2 in canine experiments leads to sinus tachycardia [64], while normal human subjects develop reduction of the T wave amplitude and in patients with coronary artery disease, similar T wave changes develop and are associated with ST segment depression [65]. Atrial and ventricular extrasystoles are rare in the absence of cardiac pathology. There is no literature on breathing high oxygen concentrations under normobaric conditions and the ECG, although data on ECG with hyperventilation may be only tangentially relevant, due to the associated ↓$PaCO_2$. ↑$PaCO_2$ increased QTc interval and QT dispersion in normal subjects [66], and in dogs caused an increase in respiratory sinus arrhythmia, in contrast to the decrease produced by ↓PaO_2 [67]. ↓$PaCO_2$ induced by voluntary hyperventilation led to mild increase in heart rate, and a decrease in the mean amplitude of the T waves [68]. Up to 15% of apparently healthy subjects had nonspecific ST-T changes with hyperventilation [69].

8.2.10 Anemia and Polycythemia

ECG changes in anemia (↓Hb) and polycythemia (↑Hb) are partially modulated by underlying cardiac pathology. Thus, chronic ↓Hb results in high output failure, cardiac dilatation, and resultant increase in the amplitude of QRS complexes. ↓Hb may also lead to left ventricular hypertrophy on the ECG in renal transplant recipients [70], and low heart rate variability in patients with stable coronary heart disease [71]. ↑Hb with its prothrombotic effects may lead to MI or pulmonary embolism, with corresponding ECG changes. ↓Hb and ↑Hb lead to increase and decrease in the amplitude of QRS complexes correspondingly, both in animal experiments and human subjects [72, 73].

8.3 Atmospheric Pressure Changes

Exposure to high altitude (hypoxemic stress) impacts normal subjects and patients, producing pulmonary hypertension, which is reversible on return to low altitudes. At 4,700 m altitude, normal subjects showed striking low frequency (0.04–0.06 Hz) heart rate oscillations during sleep, which correlated with low frequency (0.05 Hz) respiratory oscillations consistent with an unstable cardiopulmonary control system, not merely attributable to increased sympathetic modulation of heart rate [74]. The same high altitude, as simulated in a hypobaric chamber, had no impact on ventricular stimulation thresholds, thus ensuring the safety of pacing in pacemaker patients exposed to high altitude [75]. At a simulated altitude of 4,500 m, an increase in myocardial blood flow by 62% was documented in normal subjects inhaling a hypoxic gas mixture, expected to induce myocardial ischemia in patients with coronary artery disease (CAD); however, airplane travel corresponds to exposure to an altitude of ~2,000 m (cabin pressure in most airplanes during flight), does not lead to changes in myocardial blood flow, and thus it is tolerated even by patients with CAD [76]. However, all the above reflect changes imparted by associated hypoxemia. Apnea due to underwater diving results in bradycardia and increase in R wave amplitude [77], and scuba diving may lead to ECG signs of right ventricular hypertrophy, sinus bradycardia, and sinus arrhythmia [78]. Premature atrial and ventricular beats may occur even in normal subjects during deep breath-hold dive [79]. Two other influences are included herein, although they are not experienced necessarily in association with changes in increases in atmospheric pressure: (1) The Bezold-Jarisch reflex involves a marked increase in vagal efferent discharge to the heart with profound bradycardia-hypotension responses, and can occur with many ordinary activities [80], various pathologies, and medical procedures; and (2) face immersion increases heart rate variability via an increase in vagal activity [81], and total body immersion in cold water increases QT dispersion in normal subjects, particularly older persons[82].

8.4 Gravity Changes

Aerial combat and space travel entails changes in gravity exerted on the body. In experiments with normal subjects, employing a special aircraft, increase in gravity (1.7–1.8 G) led to increase in the R wave of Z lead, while decrease in gravity resulted in the opposite effect. The mechanism by which gravity changes the amplitude of QRS complexes appears to be dependent on alterations in thoracic and heart geometry, thoracic conductivity, and the heart-electrode distance [83]. Sustained high gravity acceleration led to tall narrow-based T waves 1 min after the stress period; since hyperkalemia was found immediately after stress, its role in the T wave changes is implicated, although adrenergic stimulation is also a possible alternative cause [84].

8.5 Temperature Changes

8.5.1 Hypothermia

Low body temperature imparts characteristic changes to the ECG. These include sinus bradycardia, prolonged PR, QRS, and QTc intervals, and the "Osborn waves", i.e., slowly inscribed camel-hump like deflections of the J point in the same direction as the QRS complexes, bridging the end of the QRS and the beginning of the ST segment, seen most prominently in leads facing the left ventricle and in the inferior limb leads [85–89] (➋ Fig. 8.7). The amplitude and duration of the J waves bear some relationship to the fall of the body temperature. Flat or even inverted T waves appear when the J waves become very prominent. The resultant QRS complex widening is occasionally misinterpreted as an intraventricular conduction delay or right bundle branch block. The prolongation of the PR interval suggests a slowed conduction in the atria and the AV junction. Atrial arrhythmias encountered include junctional rhythm, atrial flutter, and atrial fibrillation [90], with the latter being the most common, particularly with temperatures below 32°C; ventricular extrasystoles and ventricular fibrillation also occur with temperatures below 28°C [91]. Body shivering, even when not visually noticeable, results in intermittent or continuous baseline oscillation (➋ Fig. 8.7). Rewarming abolishes both the arrhythmias and the "Osborn waves", although the latter may persist in an attenuated form for 12–24 h [87].

It has been thought that the "Osborn waves" may represent a current of injury, or early repolarization in a ventricular territory while delayed depolarization is under way in some other territory, or due to delayed ventricular depolarization [86, 92]. These waves are not pathognomonic of hypothermia, and may also be seen in patients with cerebral injuries, e.g., subarachnoid hemorrhage [93, 94], hypothalamic lesions, Prinzmetal's angina or other types of myocardial ischemia, infarction, coronary angioplasty [95] (➋ Fig. 8.8), hypercalcemia [35], and as a normal variant [89]. These waves often simulate ischemic injury [16], resulting in problems in the differential diagnosis. Also, regional epicardial cooling of the heart in canine experiments led to "Osborn waves" indistinguishable from the ECG changes of Brugada pattern [96], suggesting a pathophysiological similarity of the two conditions, due to activation of transient outward current (Ito) [97]. A J wave is caused by the transmural (epicardial–endocardial) voltage gradient resulting from a prominent action potential notch in the epicardial, but not in the endocardial, cells. Hypothermia-related delayed conduction of action potential from the endocardial cells to epicardium also moves a latent J wave out of the QRS complex, making it even more prominent [98]. Experimental cooling of the ventricle causes T wave inversion [96], also seen in clinical hypothermia (➋ Fig. 8.7).

8.5.2 Hyperthermia

Warming of the inside of the heart causes T wave changes [86]; this may have relevance in therapeutic ablations, where an increased temperature is produced in different heart chambers. Fever causes sinus tachycardia with or without nonspecific ST-T changes. Since fever accompanies many underlying pathologies, it is difficult to evaluate the effect of fever per

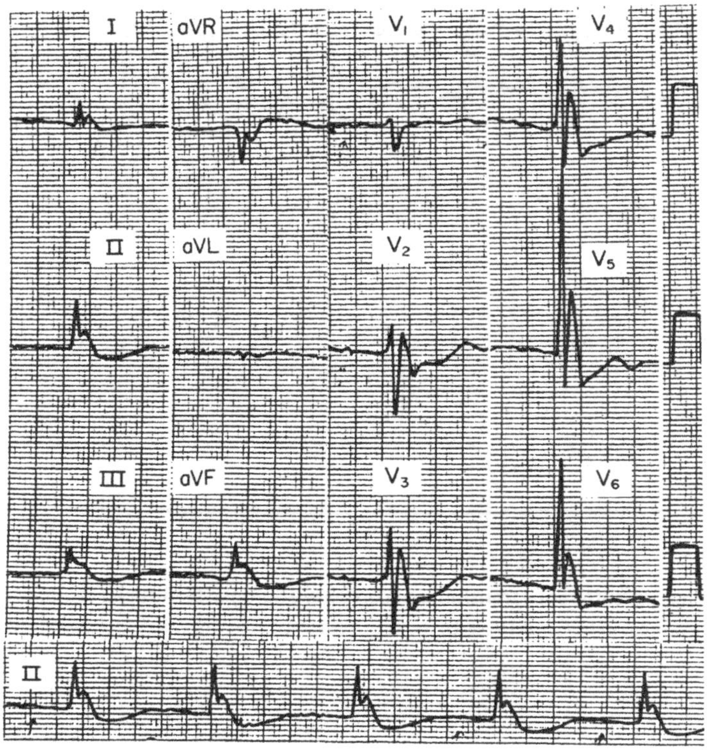

Fig. 8.7
An ECG recorded from a patient with hypothermia, whose body temperature was below 32° C. "Osborn waves" in all leads, sinus bradycardia and 1° AV block (rhythm strip, lead II), low T waves, prolonged QT interval, and intermittent baseline oscillation from somatic muscle tremor are evident

se on the ECG. All types of arrhythmias, from trivial to life threatening, have been described with febrile illnesses. The ECG phenotype in Brugada syndrome is temperature-dependent, and thus it may emerge with fever, in association with arrhythmias and T wave alternans [99–101]. Paroxysmal atrial fibrillation with fever most probably is due to an intercurrent illness. Malignant hyperthermia may lead to sudden death [102], and since anesthesia is a frequent precipitant, close ECG monitoring is emphasized [103].

8.6 Endocrine Disorders

Frequently, it is the ECG that alerts the physician to the fact that what is perceived initially as a primary cardiac disorder is indeed a secondary cardiac involvement of a systemic affliction [16]. Endocrine disorders impact the heart by direct and indirect ways producing occasionally pathognomonic ECG appearances.

8.6.1 Thyroid Heart Diseases

Deficiency or excess of thyroid hormones exert direct effects on the cardiac electrical activity, leading to changes in the ECG; in addition, the secondary activation of the sympathetic nervous system (SNS) influences indirectly the heart's electrical activity [104, 105]. Direct effects of hyperthyroidism (↑TH) on the sinoatrial node fibers of the rabbit included shortening of the action potential duration (APD) and increase in the diastolic rate of depolarization, while the opposite

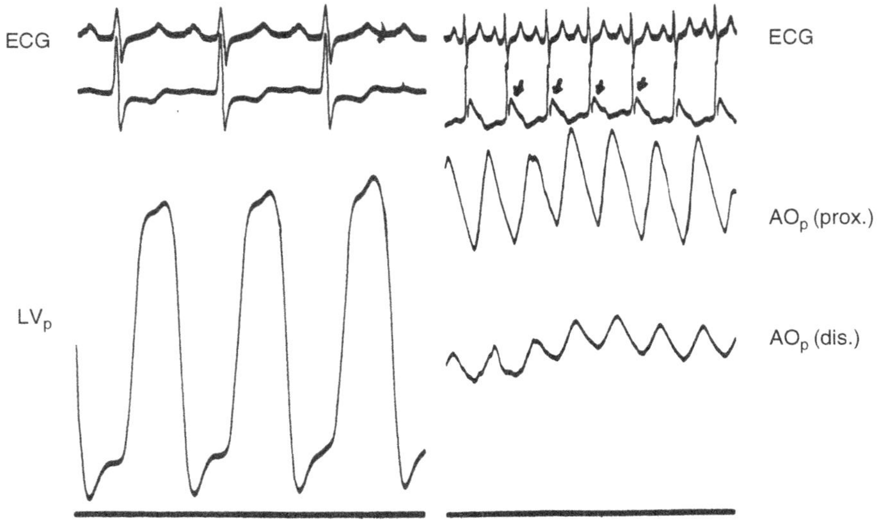

Fig. 8.8
Inflation of the balloon during percutaneous transluminal coronary angioplasty induced regional myocardial ischemia; note *arrows* pointing to "Osborn waves" in ECG lead V_5 (*AOp* aortic pressure, *prox.* proximal, *dis.* distal, *LVp* left ventricular pressure)

was observed in hypothyroid animals [106]. ↑TH also induced shortening of the APD of atrial fibers [106, 107], AV conduction and functional refractory period, with opposite effects in hypothyroidism (↓TH). ↑TH prolonged APD in canine Purkinje fibers [108], and shortened it in guinea pigs [109], while in ventricular papillary muscle from rabbits, ↑TH prolonged APD at slow rates and shortened it at rapid stimulation [110]. It can be speculated that the lowered stimulation threshold for repetitive atrial activity in the hyperthyroid rabbit [107] and the shortened refractory period of atrial cells [105] are etiologically linked to the frequent association of atrial fibrillation (AF) and clinical ↑TH. The effect of thyroid hormone on sinoatrial, atrial and AV nodal fibers appears to be direct, and independent of the influence of the SNS.

8.6.2 Hyperthyroidism

8.6.2.1 Arrhythmias

Atrial arrhythmias encountered in ↑TH include sinus tachycardia, AF, and atrial flutter in descending order of frequency [111]. Sinus tachycardia is persistent throughout the 24 h, and its rate reflects the severity of ↑TH [105, 112, 113]. AF reversed to normal sinus rhythm in 62% of patients, but this occurs with some delay, or follows establishment of euthyroidism by several months [114]. Persisting AF in patients rendered euthyroid may require cardioversion [114], and may reflect the presence of comorbidity. A role for subclinical ↑TH in facilitating emergence of AF has been identified [115]. Young thyrotoxic patients rarely have AF [116]. Prospective data on the above are lacking. Paroxysmal atrial tachycardia, and premature atrial and ventricular beats are rare [111]. The Wolff-Parkinson-White ECG pattern is more frequent in hyperthyroid subjects than in the general population [2, 117]. Paradoxical intraatrial conduction disturbances, manifesting as prolongation and notching of P waves, and 1°, 2° and 3° AV block are also found [105, 112, 113]. The AV block, which often precedes the emergence of atrial fibrillation, is also paradoxical since canine experiments have documented enhanced AV conduction (see ➋ Sect. 8.6.1) [111]. Even intraventricular conduction blocks can occur, most commonly left anterior fascicular block and right bundle branch block (RBBB) [111, 113]. These changes are reversible with management of ↑TH [111, 113].

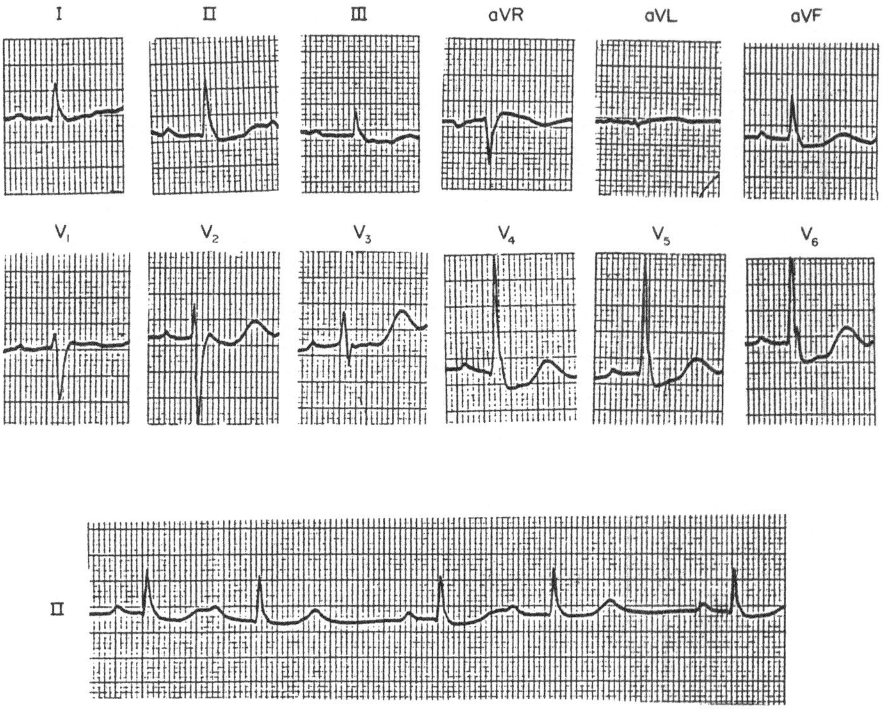

Fig. 8.9
ECG recorded in a patient during an episode of thyrotoxic periodic paralysis, showing marked ST-T changes and QT interval prolongation (*upper* panel), and periods of Mobitz II 2° AV block (*lower* panel)

8.6.2.2 P Wave, QRS Complex, ST Segment, T Wave

Increased amplitude of QRS complexes and P waves, simulating left ventricular hypertrophy and P-pulmonale may be seen with ↑TH, and can lead to such erroneous diagnoses. Perhaps these increased amplitudes are due to the influence of the thyroid hormone, or the aroused SNS [104], or the rapid heart rates per se [118]. Nonspecific ST-T abnormalities were observed in 25% of patients with hyperthyroidism, particularly in women 20–30 years old [112, 113].

While a shortened QT interval was detected in hyperthyroid patients by some [112], others have observed prolonged QTc in patients with ↑TH, with a good positive relationship between the QTc interval and serum levels of tri-iodothyronine, thyroxine, and tri-iodothyronine uptake, but not heart rate, suggesting that a direct effect of elevated thyroid hormones on the myocardium must be at play [119].

Thyrotoxic periodic paralysis is characterized by episodic weakness and paralysis of skeletal muscles. In a study of this syndrome, serum K^+ was ≤ 2.8 mEq L^{-1} in all patients during paralysis and the ECGs showed sinus arrest and 2° AV block in a few patients (Fig. 8.9), while none had extrasystoles [120]; nevertheless, ventricular fibrillation has been reported during periodic paralysis [121]. Other typical ECG features are sinus tachycardia, high QRS voltage, and prominent U waves [122–124].

8.6.3 Hypothyroidism

A combination of sinus bradycardia and low-voltage P, QRS and T waves (Fig. 8.10) is seen in the ECG of patients with ↓TH [105]. These changes may be related to the direct effects of low levels of circulating thyroid hormones on the

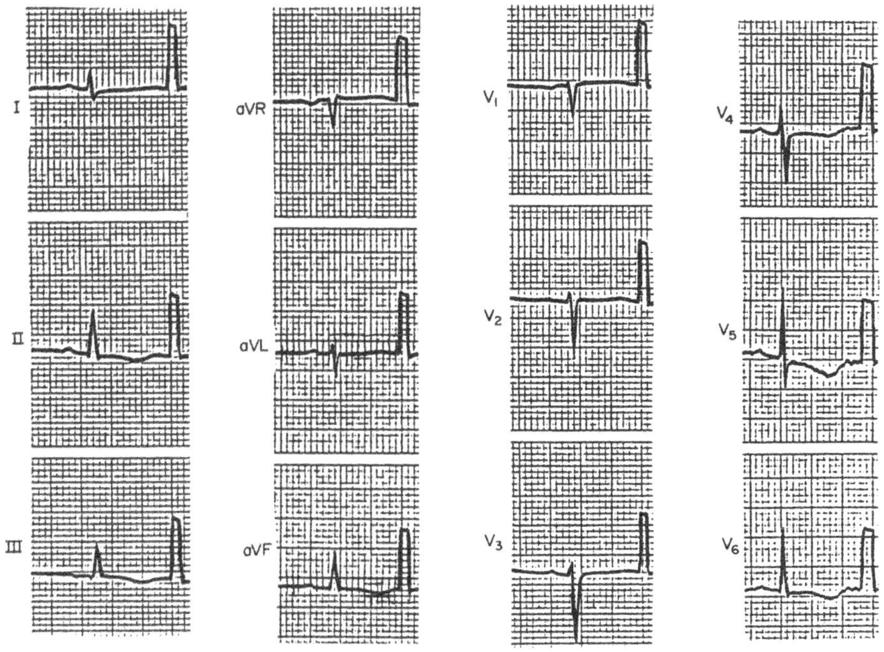

Fig. 8.10
ECG of a 40-year-old woman with hypothyroidism

myocardium, associated pericarditis or pericardial effusion, intracardiac and extracardiac deposits of myxomatous material. The frequently prolonged QT interval associated with low T wave amplitude may render the accurate measurement of the QT interval problematic [111]. The low-voltage ECG does not correlate with pericardial effusion [125], suggesting that other causes for this may be implicated.

The incidence of AV and intraventricular conduction blocks (particularly incomplete and complete RBBB) is greater by a factor of 3 in patients with myxedema than in the general population [105, 126], but complete AV block associated with syncope is less common [127]. Both sinus bradycardia and 1° AV block improve with the administration of thyroid hormone. Atrial flutter, AF, and nodal tachycardia, are rarely seen. Ventricular tachycardia in association with syncope in patients with myxedema coma has been reported [128, 129]. An increased rate of reentrant ventricular tachycardias may be due to the prolonged action potential duration [130].

8.6.4 Parathyroid Diseases

Hyperparathyroidism and hypoparathyroidism, along with many other mechanisms, lead to hypercalcemia and hypocalcemia respectively with ECG changes caused by these biochemical abnormalities (see Sect. 8.2.3).

8.6.5 Hypothalamus and Pituitary Gland

The hypothalamus is the center of autonomic sympathetic and vagal control of the heart. Animal experiments with stimulation of the hypothalamus led to arrhythmias and repolarization abnormalities, and its injury may be the reason for the characteristic T wave changes in subarachnoid hemorrhage (see Sect. 8.7) [111]. Pituitary insufficiency is associated with T wave abnormalities and prolonged QTc, but no changes in the QRS complex or ST segment; these T wave changes, which are similar to those seen in adrenal insufficiency and myxedema, are abolished transiently with isoproterenol, and usually disappear with hormonal therapy [131]. There are no specific electrophysiologic or ECG abnormalities noted with acromegaly, but the 50–80% incidence of ECG changes, arrhythmias and conduction disturbances encountered with this disease are secondary to the associated cardiac hypertrophy and cardiomyopathy. Changes noted include ST segment depression and T wave inversion, septal Q waves, left axis deviation, increased QT dispersion, conduction abnormalities, atrial and ventricular ectopic beats, sick sinus syndrome, supraventricular and ventricular tachycardias, and late potentials in signal averaged ECG [132–134]. AF or sinus tachycardia in acromegaly should prompt evaluation of associated hyperthyroidism.

8.6.6 Cushing's Disease and Cushing's Syndrome

High levels of cortisol secretion are associated with hypertension and accelerated atherosclosis with resultant changes in the ECG; left ventricular hypertrophy with inverted T waves has also been described in Cushing's syndrome [135]. An increase in the PR and QTc intervals has been observed with cortisol hypersecretion [104].

8.6.7 Hyperaldosteronism and Hypoaldosteronism

Aldosterone hypersecretion (Crohn's disease) leads to hypertension and hypervolemia associated with increased QRS complexes, and ECG signs of hypokalemia (see ➲ Sect. 8.2.2). In cases of hypoaldosteronism (Addison's disease), the ensuing hyperkalemia leads to all the expected ECG changes (see ➲ Sect. 8.2.1) [136]. Sinus bradycardia, low ECG voltage, low or inverted T waves, and prolonged QTc are also seen with Addison's disease. Adrenal insufficiency in rats and cats did not alter the resting or action potentials [137].

8.6.8 Pheochromocytoma

A large variety of ECG abnormalities has been noted in patients with pheochromocytoma. Sinus tachycardia, left ventricular hypertrophy, sinus node dysfunction with intermittent sinus arrest and AV-nodal escape rhythm, are found; also ST segment depression, elevation, and inverted, upright, and sometimes positive "giant T waves" diagnostic of acute myocardial infarction (MI) have been documented. The postulated mechanisms for these changes include "catecholamine myocarditis", myocardial infarction, hypertrophic, apical (Japanese), dilated and "tako-tsubo" cardiomyopathies, and coronary vasospasm [138–140]. Other findings include a decreased low frequency component of heart rate variability, "pseudo-P-pulmonale" due to high circulating catecholamines, frequent premature ventricular beats, monomorphic ventricular tachycardia, torsade de pointes, and long QT interval [38, 141–147].

8.6.9 Diabetes Mellitus

In experimental diabetic animals, sinus bradycardia, prolongation of the sinus node recovery time, inhomogeneity of atrial conduction and AV nodal block, have been found [148]. In diabetic patients without hypertension and coronary artery disease (CAD), diffuse T wave abnormalities are frequently noted. Also the expected ECG changes due to hyperkalemia with diabetic ketoacidosis are seen, while hypokalemia, and its attendant ECG changes may ensue with intracellular influx of K^+ following therapy of acidosis (alkali, fluids, and insulin). Transient deep T wave inversions with prolonged QT interval may be present during therapy of diabetic acidosis while serum K^+ is normal. These are attributed to a central nervous system abnormality coinciding with sensorial disturbances [149]. Sulfonylurea attenuates the magnitude of ST segment elevation during an acute myocardial infarction, leading to inappropriate withholding of thrombolytic therapy [150]. Diabetic patients with CAD have a higher risk of developing silent myocardial ischemia (ST segment depression) during exercise than non-diabetic patients [151]. Autonomic neuropathy in diabetic individuals results in a decrease in heart rate variability and a disappearance of the heart rate dependency of the QT interval, a plausible mechanism for the increased risk of ventricular arrhythmias and sudden death in such patients [152].

The most frequent conduction disorders in type 2 diabetes are RBBB and left anterior fascicular block [153]. Hypoglycemia can induce angina and silent myocardial ischemia with classic ST-T changes, in diabetic patients with and without CAD, which are abolished with glucose administration [154, 155]. Hyperglycemia increases the pacing threshold [12].

8.7 Neurological and Neuromuscular Diseases

8.7.1 Cerebrovasular Accidents

An increased incidence mainly of repolarization ECG abnormalities, e.g., flat, large broad inverted, and rarely positive "giant T waves", depressed or elevated ST segments, prominent U waves, and prolonged QT intervals are noted in patients with cerebrovascular accidents (CVA) [156, 157], particularly in those with subarachnoid or intracerebral hemorrhage, who show more severe such changes [158, 159]. Similar ECG abnormalities are seen with ischemic strokes, neurosurgical procedures, head injuries, meningitis, epilepsy, and intracranial tumors. Prolonged QT intervals are associated with the risk of torsade de pointes [160, 161]. The prevalence of ECG abnormalities with subarachnoid hemorrhage has been reported to be 50–90% [159–166]. The ECG changes resemble those of myocardial ischemia (➲ Fig. 8.11), with wide and deeply inverted T waves noted usually in leads I, aVL, and left precordial leads, although the QRS complexes are not usually altered [164, 167]. Q waves may occasionally develop and in combination with ST segment elevation (➲ Fig. 8.11) simulate the ECG of patients with acute MI [168, 169]. In the latter, usually the duration of the T wave and QT interval is shorter, and the amplitude smaller. These ECG abnormalities may be either short-lived or persist for several weeks [169, 170]. Arrhythmias are noted in >75% of patients, and include sinus bradycardia and tachycardia, atrial and ventricular extrasystoles and atrial fibrillation (AF) [168, 171, 172]. Often it is not clear whether the last is the consequence or the cause of a CVA [173]. After acute CVA ambulatory 7-day ECG monitoring surpassed the standard ECG and 24-h Holter

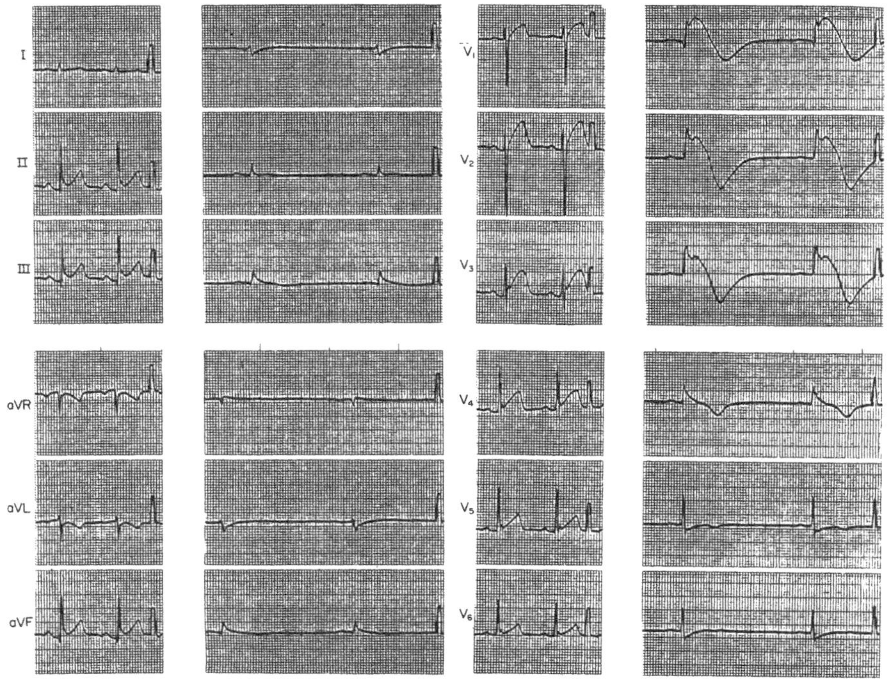

Fig. 8.11
Marked bradycardia with precordial ST segment elevation and giant T wave inversions resembling changes seen in the acute phase of myocardial infarction, in serial ECGs recorded in the acute stage of subarachnoid hemorrhage

monitoring, in the detection of AF [174]. All varieties of AV blocks have been encountered with CVAs [175]. Heart rate variability decreases and heart rate increases after the acute phase of CVA [176].

The exact cause of these ECG changes has not been delineated, but it appears that cerebrovascular pathology leads to myocardial injury [177]. Moreover it appears that specific brain lesions lead to specific ECG abnormalities; e.g., insular lesions were related to sinus tachycardia, ectopic beats, and ST elevation, with right insular lesions related to AF, atrioventricular block, ectopic beats, and inverted T waves, and right insular lesions, compared with left or no insular lesions, increased the odds of death within 3 months independent of stroke severity and age [178]. Postmortem study of hearts revealed interruption of myocyte bundles and disarray of myocyte architecture with more severe such changes in patients who had tall inverted or peaked T waves [157]. Also focal subendocardial hemorrhagic lesions were found in some patients who died of subarachnoid hemorrhage [179], and prospective studies with a variety of intracranial lesions documented subendocardial hemorrhage in 40% and epicardial hemorrhage or myocytolysis in 8% of patients [180]. The rise of the myocardial biomarker troponin I, noted in patients with neurological syndromes, further supports the occurrence of cardiac damage [181]. This direct proof of heart injury is also corroborated by evidence for regional wall motion abnormalities in ventriculographic and echocardiographic studies [182–184]. The arrhythmias and ECG changes, observed after manipulation of the circle of Willis during surgical procedures in humans and experimental animals, provide evidence that a pathophysiologic link between the central nervous system and the heart is at play [185].

Mechanistically the T wave changes have been attributed to functional repolarization abnormalities [186, 187], structural heart disturbances [188], parasympathetic nerve stimulation [189], and surge of sympathetic tone and catecholamine release [190]. Animal studies have demonstrated that infusions of catecholamines and stimulation of hypothalamus and insula produce the same hemodynamic alterations and necrotic myocardial lesions seen in subarachnoid hemorrhage [168, 191]; these lesions appear similar to those seen in patients with pheochromocytoma (see ➋ Sect. 8.6.8) or cocaine abuse, conditions previously linked to sympathetic stimulation [192]. Of course it is possible that this sympathetic arousal leads to myocardial damage mediated by increase in the myocardial oxygen demands in patients with neurologic syndromes and coronary artery disease. Nevertheless, autopsies in patients with head trauma or subarachnoid hemorrhage have identified myocardial injury in the presence of normal coronary arteries [190, 193]. It is also hypothesized that the myocardial lesions found at autopsy are caused by disturbances in the cardiac contraction pattern resulting from abnormal excitation of the origins of the autonomic nerves at the central nervous system mediated by the extravasation of blood [157]. The bulk of evidence indicates that sympathetic arousal is the pathophysiologic mechanism for myocardial damage, via a direct effect or an intense coronary vasoconstrictive influence [192]. This is further corroborated by animal studies showing that adrenergic blockade, reserpine, and occasionally, atropine prevented the ECG abnormalities [180].

8.7.2 Seizures

At least a dozen electrophysiological disorders (torsade de pointes, Brugada syndrome, long-, and short-QT syndromes and arrhythmogenic right ventricular dysplasia) as well as cardiogenic syncope, often masquerade as "epilepsy" or "seizures" in both the adult and pediatric population, emphasizing the importance of the ECG and continuous ECG monitoring in unraveling many of the above diagnostic conundrums [194]. On the other hand, the higher incidence of sudden death in epilepsy than in the normal population points to ventricular tachyarrhythmias as the possible culprit. The reduction of high frequency and increase of low frequency values in heart rate variability in the frequency domain analysis in such patients suggests that increased sympathetic activity may be the incriminating factor [195].

8.7.3 Neuromuscular Diseases

Friedreich's ataxia, progressive muscular dystrophy and myotonic muscular dystrophy (MD) are hereditary neuropathic diseases associated with cardiomyopathy. MD is associated with very slow pulse, high incidence of all types of AV block, Q waves and slurring of the QRS complexes resulting from changes in the intraventricular conduction, left axis deviation,

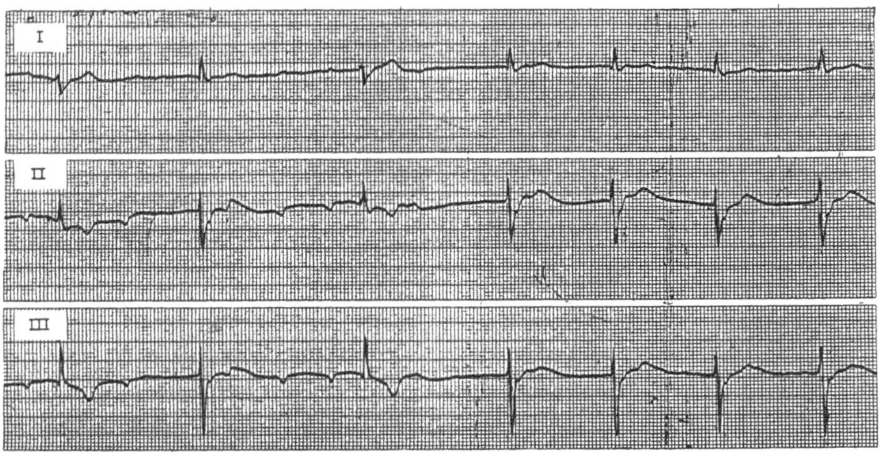

Fig. 8.12
An ECG from a patient with myotonic dystrophy during syncopal seizure, showing complete AV block and AV junctional escape rhythm

P waves of low amplitude, ST segment abnormalities, and flat or inverted T waves [196–199]. Most frequent cardiac manifestations of this disease are conduction abnormalities (Fig. 8.12) for which electronic pacing is often required (Fig. 8.13).

Atrial arrhythmias also occur more frequently (flutter and fibrillation) than ventricular arrhythmias. An association of the frequency of arrhythmias and conduction disturbances with the severity of the disease has been documented [199]. In spite of the high prevalence of conduction abnormalities in MD, the incidence of complete heart block is lower than expected [200, 201]. A tall R wave in V_1 is seen in Duchenne muscular dystrophy. Cardiac involvement in facioscapulohumeral MD was characterized by myocardial thickening in the echocardiogram and incomplete right bundle branch block, ST elevation in V_2–V_4, and tall T waves in V_3–V_5 [202, 203]. Short and prolonged QTs are seen in different forms of MD [204].

8.8 Thoracic Diseases

8.8.1 Thoracic Skeletal Abnormalities

Posterior depression of the sternum and costal cartilages (pectus excavatum) (PEX) may be associated with ECG changes, which are not specific for the condition and are attributed to the compression and leftward displacement of the heart between the sternum and the spine. These ECG changes, which may not necessarily signify any cardiac abnormality, include non-ischemic and ischemic type T wave inversions (Fig. 8.14), late transition of the precordial QRS complexes with the Q waves in V_1–V_4 simulating an anterior myocardial infarction (MI), complete right bundle branch block (RBBB), an rSr' pattern in lead V_1, and a negative P wave in lead V_1, similar to that of lead aVR; this last finding may be due to the direction of the atrial depolarization vector away from the V_1 position, because of the leftward displacement of the heart [205–208]. PEX was associated with incomplete blockade of the bundle of His, ventricular extrasystoles, Wolff-Parkinson-White syndrome, and mitral valve prolapse (MVP) (97% of cases) [209]. With thoracic deformities, the distance of the heart from certain precordial electrodes may increase or decrease, resulting in low or high QRS complexes. Paroxysmal tachycardias have been described in association with PEX [206], but as in patients with MVP, it is uncertain whether they are truly related to the condition. In patients

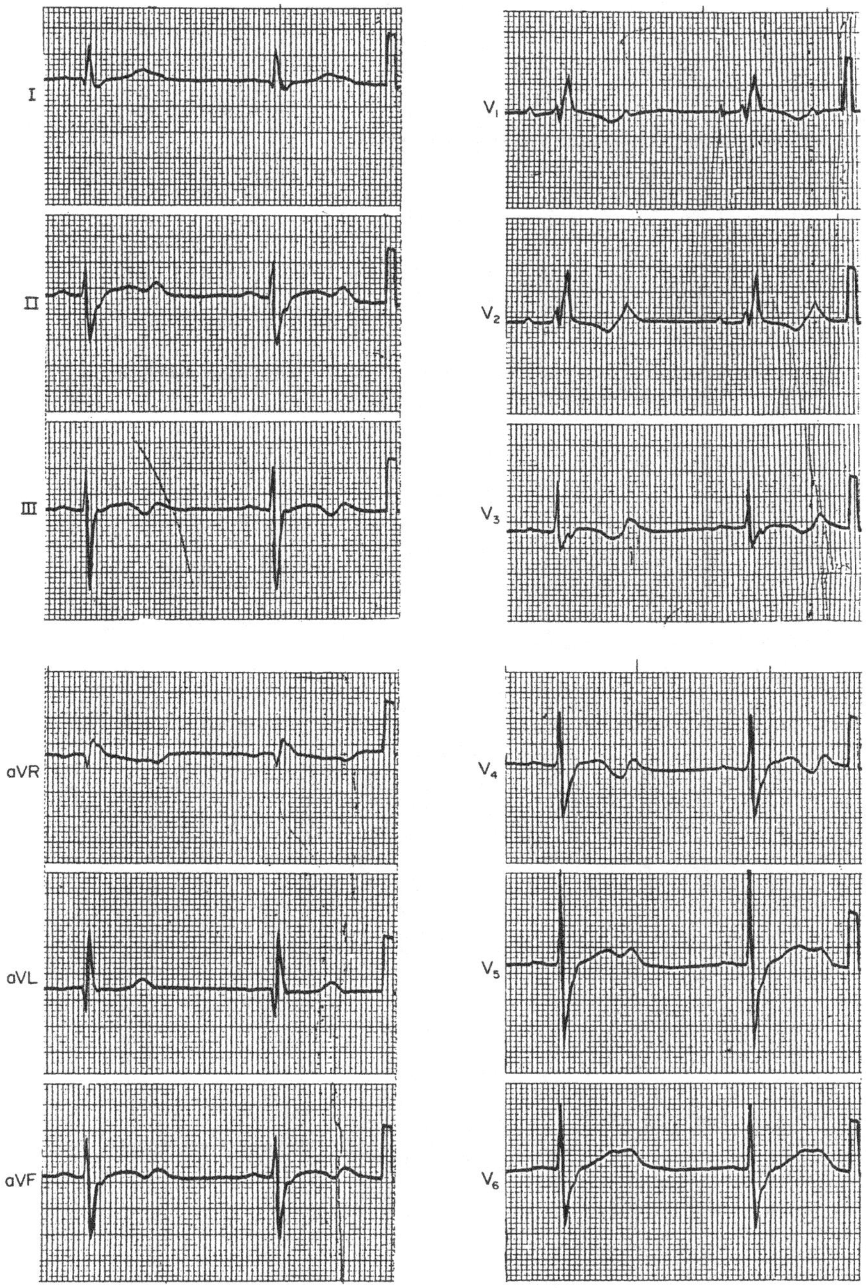

Fig. 8.13
The ECG obtained after recovery from syncopal seizure of the same patient as in Fig. 8.12, shows marked sinus bradycardia, prolonged QT interval, prominent U wave, 1° AV block, and complete right bundle branch block with left anterior fascicular block (frontal QRS axis of −60°). This patient underwent implantation of an artificial pacemaker

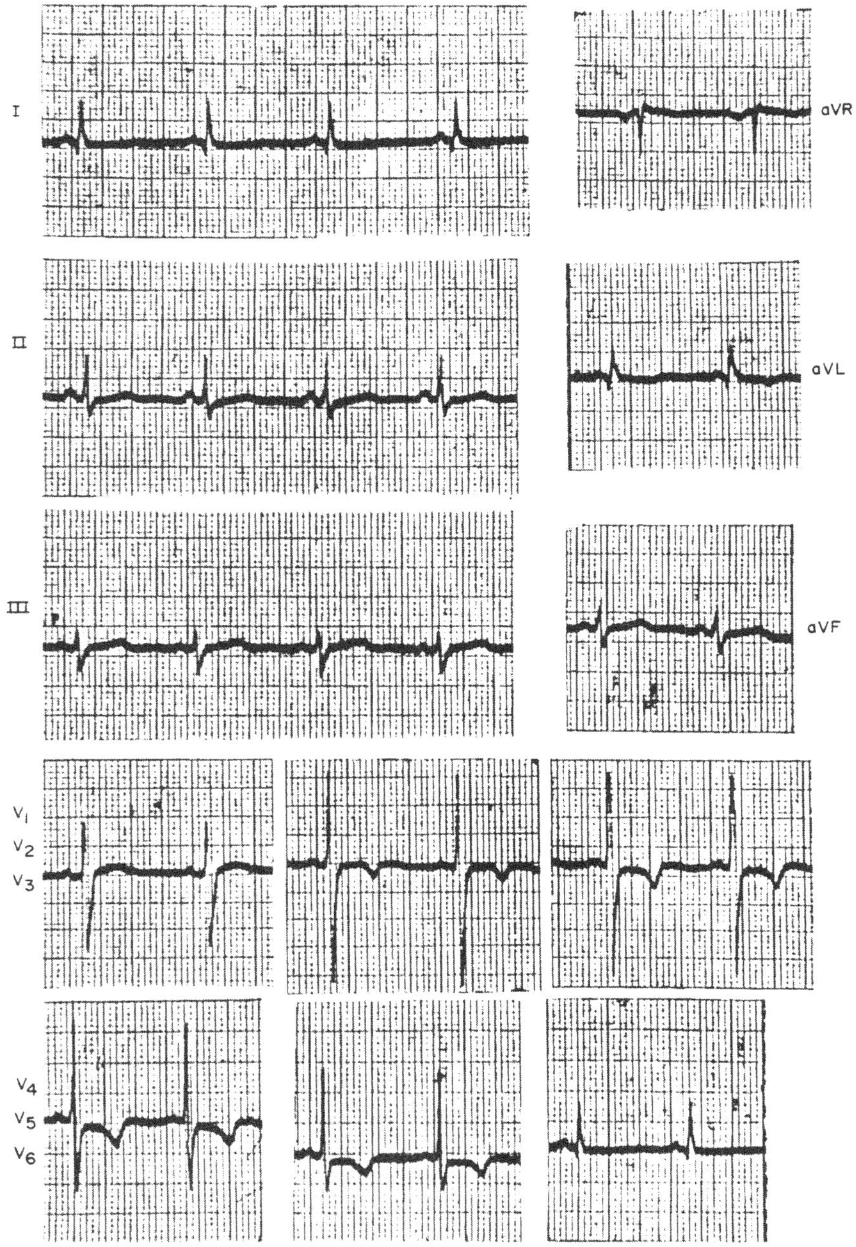

Fig. 8.14

ECG of a patient with pectus excavatum showing ischemic-appearing T waves in the precordial leads

with the "straight back syndrome", in which the heart is compressed and leftwardly displaced between a "straightened" dorsal spine and the unaffected sternum, ECG changes similar to those described in patients with PEX have been noted. Noninfarctional Q waves in the inferior leads or severe frontal QRS left axis deviation has been observed [86]. Severe degrees of kyphosis, scoliosis or kyphoscoliosis are accompanied by deranged lung function, hypoxemia, and pulmonary hypertension. In such situations, the ECG changes may be related to chronic cor pulmonale (see

Sect. 8.9.1). An association of thoracic skeletal abnormalities and MVP has been documented [210]; also it has been postulated that MVP may be an acquired condition caused by a growth disproportion between the heart and the chest cavity [211].

8.8.2 Parenchymal Lung Diseases

Chronic obstructive lung disease (COPD) and its clinical expressions of bronchitis and emphysema may lead to a decrease in the ECG voltage, particularly in the limb leads; also the precordial leads may show an attenuated ECG voltage, especially in the left precordial leads, which partially may be due to the increase of the distance of the heart from the recording electrodes. Of course this occurs when there is a lung-inflated consequence of the underlying pathology, as in emphysema. Theoretically, in asthma, lung hyperinflation also may be present episodically. In severe asthma, transient sinus tachycardia, right axis deviation, right atrial enlargement, right ventricular hypertrophy, ventricular premature complexes, and RBBB were noted, and correlated with the degree of airway obstruction [212]. Asthmatics show reversible inferior T wave inversions [213], and increase in heart rate and decrease in heart rate variability, when exposed to ambient coarse particles [214]. The presence of hypoxia ($\downarrow O_2$), hypercapnea ($\uparrow CO_2$), respiratory acidosis, alkalosis or exacerbations of COPD may set the stage for more ECG abnormalities to appear (see Sects. 8.2.8 and 8.2.9). The frontal QRS axis is vertical or rightward, and poor R wave progression in the precordial leads is noted simulating an anterior MI. Both are due to the downward displacement of the diaphragm resulting in an anatomical, and thus an electrical, vertical heart position and a high placement of the precordial leads relative to the heart [38, 86]. In addition, right ventricular dilatation contributes to the leftward shift of the transition zone. P waves are tall in leads II, III, and aVF with a vertical or rightward frontal axis, due to the heart's vertical position; P-R segment and ST segment depressions in the same leads are due to exaggerated atrial repolarization [38]. Some of the above changes are stable in established COPD, or transient, as in patients with asthmatic attacks. Exercise, even when associated with $\downarrow O_2$, does not cause myocardial repolarization abnormalities (altered QTc dispersion) in patients with COPD [215]; others, however, have documented increase in QTc dispersion with $\downarrow O_2$ and $\uparrow CO_2$, and decrease of QTc dispersion with partial correction of $\downarrow O_2$ [216].

Theoretically lung tissue, particularly in its hyperinflated state, is a poor electrical conductor and should produce an increase in ECG potentials based on its increased impedance [217]. However, this may be offset by the increase in the heart surface-electrode distance due to hyperinflation. When acute or chronic cor pulmonale ensues, the expected ECG pictures emerge (see Sects. 8.9.1 and 8.9.2). Extensive atelectasis and infiltration due to pneumonia, pleural effusions, and other complications are expected to influence the ECG further. The ECG voltage is routinely attenuated in patients cared for in respiratory critical care units (Fig. 8.15).

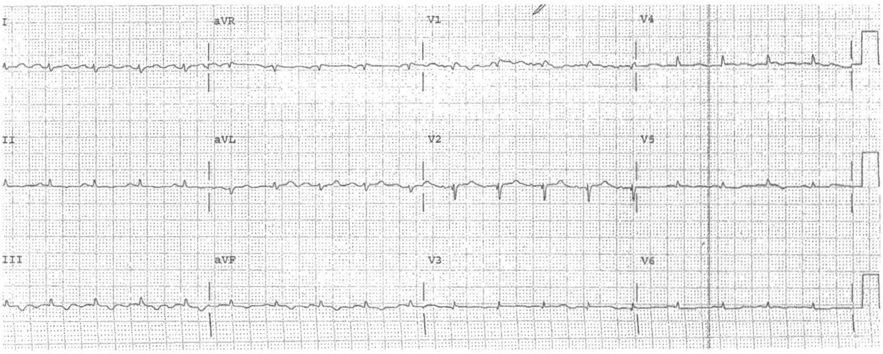

Fig. 8.15
ECG of a 74-year-old woman hospitalized in the Respiratory Intensive Care Unit. The chest X-ray showed infiltrates and atelectases, an endotracheal tube in place, bilateral pleural effusions and cardiomegaly. The echocardiogram showed normal size and function of the left ventricle, and enlarged hypocontractile right ventricle with pulmonary hypertension. Note the low ECG voltage, tachycardia, and a frontal QRS axis of 95°

COPD is associated with atrial and ventricular arrhythmias, particularly multifocal atrial tachycardia, which typically is seen in elderly patients with severe decompensation [218]. Although not firmly established, the mechanism of this arrhythmia may be delayed afterdepolarizations leading to triggered activity [218]. Several factors may be potentially arrhythmogenic in patients with COPD, including $\downarrow O_2$, $\uparrow CO_2$, acid-base disturbances, cor pulmonale and the use of sympathomimetic drugs, methylxanthines, digitalis, preexisting cardiopulmonary pathology, conscious sedation, endotracheal intubation, anesthesia, invasive procedure and surgery. Cough related syncope has been traced to inappropriate chronotropic response to hypotension [219].

8.8.3 Sleep Apnea/Hypopnea Syndrome

Marked obesity and COPD, with associated $\downarrow O_2$, $\uparrow CO_2$, and oropharyngeal obstruction, result in the sleep apnea/hypopnea syndrome (SAS), which is associated with autonomic nervous system dysfunction and culminates in pulmonary hypertension, and heart disease. ECG changes noted in SAS include sinus tachycardia, bradycardia, arrhythmia and arrest, supraventricular and ventricular couplets and tachycardia, nocturnal ST segment depression, 2° AV block Mobitz II, high ULF, VLF, LF components and high LF/HF, but low HF values in spectral analysis of heart rate variability, and increased QTc dispersion [220–222]. Continuous positive airway pressure therapy and bariatric surgery ameliorates or eradicates all or many of the above [222, 223]. Heart rate tachograms derived from Holter ECG monitoring can be used, in lieu of polysomnography, to detect SAS [224].

8.8.4 Lung Congestion and Lavage

In pulmonary edema, reduced ECG voltage is noted, due to the short-circuiting effect on the cardiac potentials from the congested lungs surrounding the heart; this phenomenon can be exploited in monitoring patients for congestive heart failure; however, the interplay of cardiac volume changes during episodes of acute pulmonary edema may offset the attenuation of ECG complexes, leading to unchanged ECG potentials [225]. Lung lavage, particularly of the left lung, used in the therapy of pulmonary proteinosis, results in attenuated ECG potentials [226].

8.8.5 Pneumothorax and Pneumopericardium

The ECG of pneumothorax and pneumomediastinum simulates appearances found in cardiac pathology [227–231], with the left pneumothorax producing a decrease in QRS and T wave voltage, inverted T waves in the precordial leads, and right frontal QRS axis deviation [231], which leads to an increase in the voltage of the R wave in lead III (➔ Fig. 8.16). Occasionally right pneumothorax may not produce discernible ECG changes but when it does, the transitional zone moves to the left, T waves decrease in the right precordial leads, R and T waves increase in the left precordial leads, and can simulate anterior MI [232]. In left pneumothorax, the transitional zone is unchanged, but the voltages of QRS and T waves in the precordial leads and the R waves in V_4–V_6 decrease. Tension pneumothorax may alter the ECG in unexpected ways and may imitate other pathologies, particularly pulmonary embolism, and MI. The underlying mechanisms for these ECG findings are probably the drastic positional changes of the heart, and the resultant change in its distance from the recording electrodes due to alterations (particularly with left pneumothorax) in the intrathoracic volume conductor properties, overloading of the right ventricle, and a rotation of the heart. Pneumomediastinum can cause T wave inversions [233].

8.8.6 Pleural and Mediastinal Effusions

Pleural effusion, depending on its size and location, results in lung and heart displacement, influencing the ECG appearance. When it is left-sided and large, attenuation of QRS complexes and R waves and pseudo-infarctional Q waves are

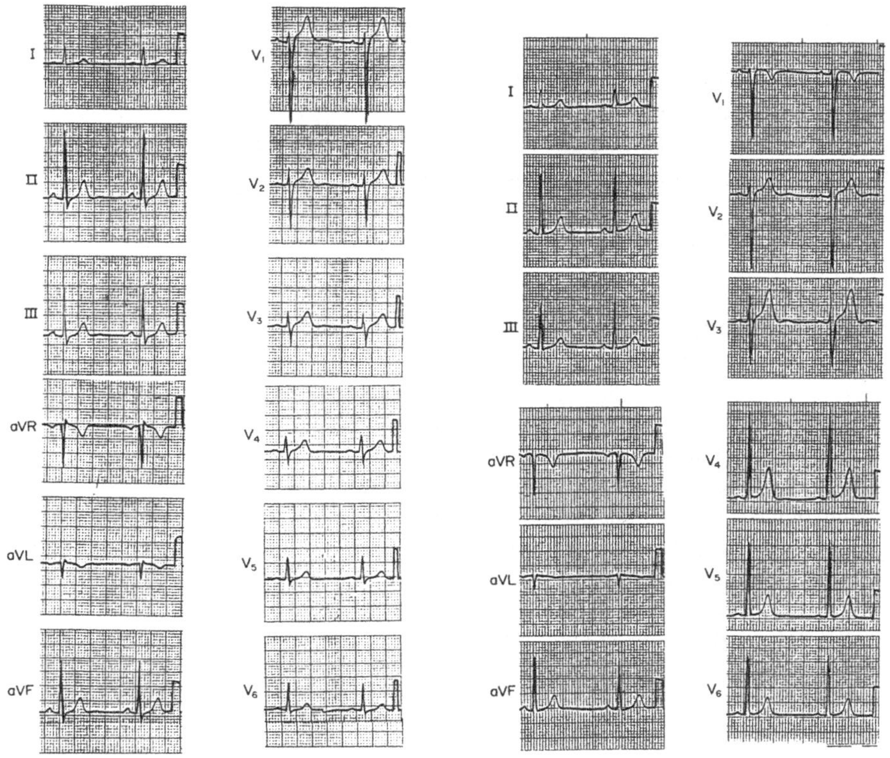

Fig. 8.16
ECG in spontaneous left pneumothorax showing reduced QRS voltage in V_3–V_6 (*left* panel), with increased voltage after recovery (*right* panel)

observed, mediated by an increase in the heart-electrode distance and the short-circuiting of heart's potentials due to the intervening fluid [217, 234]. In addition to pathological causes, pleural effusion may follow intrathoracic procedures [234] and insertion of central venous catheters (CVC), the latter employed for hemodynamic monitoring, hemodialysis, or facilitation of monitoring the intracardiac P wave via the CVC [235]. ECG changes are further affected when pleural effusion is combined with pericardial effusion.

8.8.7 Pleural Disease

Thickening of pleura due to inflammatory, infectious (tuberculosis) and neoplastic diseases, or radiation therapy, particularly involving the left side of the thorax is associated with attenuation of the ECG voltage. Often these pleural changes are coupled with pleural effusion, resulting in further loss in ECG voltage.

8.8.8 Aortic Dissection

Acute or chronic aortic dissection can lead to a spectrum of complications (outflow tract stenosis, aortic valve and coronary insufficiency, and myocardial infarction [MI], with suggestive ECG abnormalities). The ECG may be normal or indicative of prior pathologies. Typical of the ECG in acute aortic dissection is its fluidity in time as the clinical picture evolves. Differentiation of aortic dissection from acute MI is imperative, to avoid administration of thrombolytic therapy [236].

8.9 Pulmonary Hypertension

Pulmonary hypertension may arise acutely or gradually, be transient or progressive, and be primary, or secondary to lung or heart disease. Paralleling this variability in pathology, a spectrum of ECG changes is observed reflecting functional or structural alterations of the right ventricle and atrium. ECG changes observed in pulmonary hypertension are also modulated by other intercurrent conditions and left ventricular and atrial pathology.

8.9.1 Chronic Cor Pulmonale

Chronic conditions including COPD, other pulmonary diseases, congenital heart disease, recurrent pulmonary embolism, left ventricular systolic and diastolic dysfunction, obstructive sleep apnea syndrome, and primary pulmonary hypertension lead to chronic cor pulmonale. The ECG of chronic cor pulmonale includes frontal right axis QRS deviation, tall R waves in V_1–V_3, early R wave progression (counterclockwise rotation), R/S ≥ 1 in V_1, R amplitude in $V_1 \geq 5$ mm, R/S $V_5 \leq 1$, incomplete or complete right bundle branch block (RBBB), T wave inversion in V_1–V_3, and P pulmonale [237]; rarely ST segment depression or elevation in inferior leads is seen [238]. Chronic cor pulmonale with evidence of right ventricular hypertrophy and/or dilatation is occasionally presenting as reversed R wave progression, where the R waves decrease progressively from V_1 or V_2 to V_3–V_6. Arrhythmias encountered include sinus tachycardia, supraventricular and ventricular extrasystoles, atrial flutter and fibrillation, and multifocal atrial tachycardia.

8.9.2 Acute Cor Pulmonale and Pulmonary Embolism

All the above conditions culminating in chronic cor pulmonale may also cause acute cor pulmonale, which by definition is transient, although it can evolve to the chronic type. Pulmonary embolism, transient heart failure, or rise of left ventricular afterload, can lead to acute cor pulmonale. The ECG is not sensitive or specific for the recognition of pulmonary embolism, and changes and their severity depend on time and the frequency of recording, the size and location of the embolus and its hemodynamic consequences, and preexisting pulmonary and/or heart diseases [16]. The latter may complicate the diagnosis by either accentuating or masking the ECG abnormalities. The most frequent ECG abnormalities in patients with pulmonary embolism reported in three series were clockwise cardiac rotation and sinus tachycardia [239], RBBB and sinus tachycardia [240], and T wave inversion in the right precordial leads [241]. Also, the ECG was found to be normal in 72% and 27% of the patients with PEM [242, 243]. Other ECG findings include P-pulmonale, right axis deviation (RAD) and left axis deviation (LAD), an S_1Q_3 pattern, Q waves in leads III and aVF (but not II), S waves in leads I and aVL, R > 0.5 mV or R/S ratio >1 in lead V_1, QR pattern in lead V_1, nonspecific ST-T changes, 1° AV block, atrial and ventricular premature beats, and atrial flutter and fibrillation [86, 244–247]. The ST-T changes include T wave inversion in leads III and aVF, in addition to those in precordial leads, and ST segment elevation in leads III, aVR and V_1. ST-T changes in limb and precordial leads may be due to the right ventricular conduction disturbances, myocardial ischemia resulting from low cardiac output and/or pulmonary hypertension, and in some patients underlying coronary artery disease. In pulmonary embolism, ECG changes are transient, as compared to myocardial infarction (MI); also T wave inversions constitute an early feature, while they appear later in MI. An otherwise unexplainable episode of atrial fibrillation occasionally may be due to acute pulmonary embolism. The SIQ3T3 pattern, thought in the past, and even by some today, to be pathognomonic of pulmonary embolism [244] (➋ Fig. 8.17), has been found to be equally prevalent in patients with and without this condition [246]. It is postulated that the SIQ3T3 pattern is due to left posterior fascicular block, mediated by selective stretch of the posterior part of the septum due to the high right ventricular pressure, leading to conduction delay in the posteroinferior fibers of the left bundle. Accordingly, LAD, which is twice as frequent as RAD, may be due to selective stretching of the anterosuperior branch of the left bundle [248]. Also the SIQ3T3 pattern may be due to mere right ventricular dilatation and change in this chamber's position relevant to the left ventricle and/or thorax.

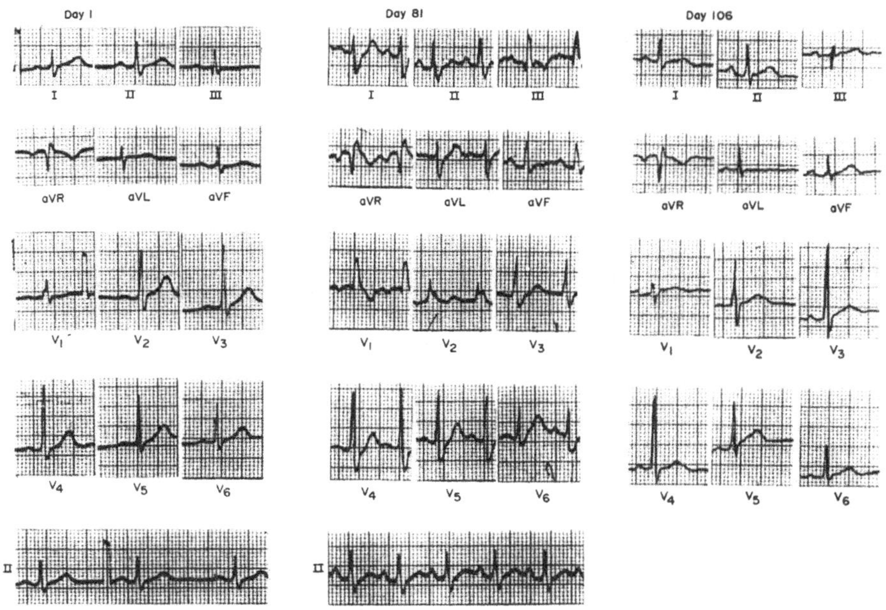

Fig. 8.17
The ECG on day 1 before the occurrence of acute pulmonary embolism, showed normal axis and incomplete right bundle branch block (RBBB). The ECG on day 81, the day of the event, showed sinus tachycardia, marked right axis deviation, $S_1Q_3T_3$ pattern, complete RBBB, and T inversion in leads V_1 and V_2. The ECG on day 106, 1 month after successful thrombolytic treatment, showed a normal axis and no sign of right heart overload

Right ventricular pressure overload may direct the initial left septal force superiorly and the terminal QRS vector rightwardly, resulting in a Q wave in lead III and an S wave in lead I, respectively; the same mechanism may also lead to a clockwise rotation of the heart along its longitudinal axis, i.e., a leftward displacement in the transitional zone of the precordial leads. The occasional appearance of Q waves is due to marked changes in the position of the left and right ventricle due to the latter's dilatation. Incomplete or complete RBBB with RAD is also attributed to the acute right ventricular dilatation.

Since the above ECG changes are nonspecific for acute right ventricular strain due to pulmonary embolism, they should be differentiated from those of normals, inferior or anterior MI or ischemia, extensive pneumonia, massive atelectasis, chronic cor pulmonale, pneumothorax, and large pleural effusion. A previous ECG available for comparison [86], and the repetition of the ECG, has enhanced its sensitivity in diagnosing pulmonary embolism [249]. Accordingly, a shift in the axis even if it remains within the normal limits may be indicative of pathology. Pulmonary embolism with severe hemodynamic consequences has been linked to precordial T wave inversions [250], and high ECG scores consisting of a number of weighted ECG findings described above [251].

8.10 Mitral Valve Prolapse Syndrome

Degeneration or myxomatous infiltration of the mitral leaflets leads to their characteristic abnormal systolic sagging, known as mitral valve prolapse [104]. The ECG in patients with MVP can be normal, but various arrhythmias and nonspecific ST-T changes, involving mostly the inferior leads, may be present in 15–42% of patients [86, 252], often misinterpreted as ischemic in origin. The T wave abnormalities may be confined only to the precordial leads (➲ Fig. 8.18), or may be diffuse. While the T wave inversions may vary spontaneously, exercise may normalize them, and inhalation of amyl nitrate

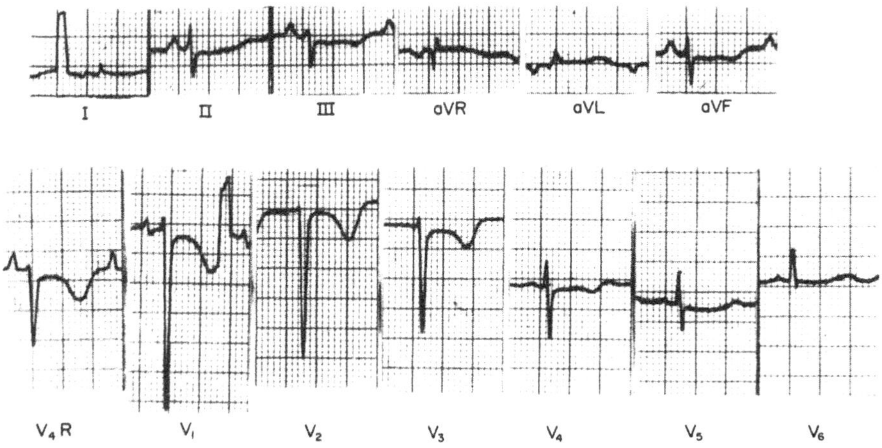

Fig. 8.18
ECG of a patient with mitral valve prolapse (MVP) showing ischemic-appearing T wave inversion in precordial leads V_1–V_4, with a prolonged QT interval

will accentuate them or convert flat to inverted T waves. An ECG false-positive exercise response, with marked ST segment depression during exercise or on recovery, is not at all uncommon, with a 53% incidence reported in one series [253]. Other ECG abnormalities occasionally noted are prolongation of the QT interval (Fig. 8.18), prominent U waves and abnormal Q waves without evidence of infarction [86]. Heart rate variability in patients with MVP was not different than in control subjects, but the QT duration was increased; also the QT/RR slope revealed an increased nocturnal rate dependence, which might explain the risk of arrhythmic events in these patients [254].

The pathogenesis of flattened or inverted T waves is still elusive, although ischemia or even infarction of the papillary muscle and the adjacent myocardium is implicated [255]. It has been postulated that the underlying mechanism might be the increased traction to the papillary muscle(s) exerted by the billowing leaflet(s) via the attached chordae, which thus interferes with the rather tenuous vascular supply of the region.

Studies with Holter monitoring show that patients with MVP have a higher incidence of supraventricular and ventricular arrhythmias than normal subjects [255–259]. Arrhythmias noted run the gamut from atrial, junctional, or ventricular extrasystoles to paroxysmal supraventricular tachycardia, premature ventricular extrasystoles in a bigeminal, trigeminal, or R-on-T patterns, or even ventricular tachycardia and fibrillation [86, 104]. It is believed that the latter is the cause of syncope or sudden death in some patients with MVP [86, 104, 260]. Possible predisposing mechanisms for arrhythmias in patients with MVP could be the mechanical stress to which the left atrium and ventricle are subjected, an underlying myocardial ischemia, as evidenced by the nonspecific ST-T abnormalities, possible coexisting bypass tracts, usually left-sided which would precipitate reentrant tachycardias, and a QT-interval prolongation [86]. Although it cannot be denied that arrhythmias in patients with MVP may be associated with an increased risk of sudden death, the previously reported increased incidence probably had been due to a selection bias (study of patients with the most severe form of the syndrome) [261]. In the same vein, the occurrence of complex ventricular arrhythmias in some patients with MVP may be a reflection of their underlying consequent mitral regurgitation, and not due to the syndrome per se, since such arrhythmias are common in patients with nonischemic hemodynamically significant mitral regurgitation, regardless of the specific etiology [262].

8.11 Infectious Heart Diseases

The heart can be affected by any of the entire range of infectious agents. Depending on the topography of physiological and structural derangements and the subsequent pathophysiological consequences, as for example in endocarditis, viral

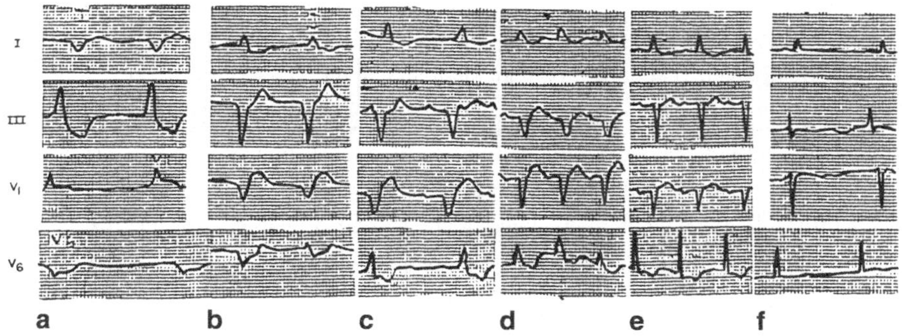

Fig. 8.19
Serial ECG changes in acute viral myocarditis: (a) junctional escape rhythm with RBBB-type intraventricular conduction defect (IVCD) and ST abnormality; (b) junctional escape rhythm with LBBB-type IVCD; (c) normal sinus rhythm with LBBB-type IVCD; (d) sinus tachycardia with LBBB; (e) sinus tachycardia with normal QRS morphology; (f) atrial fibrillation with normal QRS morphology

myocarditis, echinococcosis, syphilis, Chagas disease, and others, the gamut of arrhythmias, conduction abnormalities, and evidence of chamber hypertrophy/dilatation may be seen in the ECG.

8.11.1 Myocarditis

While most cases of acute "idiopathic" myocarditis are probably due to viruses [263], any infectious organism or toxic agent can cause this condition. ECG changes of acute viral myocarditis are frequent but nonspecific, and consist of diffuse low voltage, ST-T abnormalities, QT interval prolongation, sinus tachycardia, atrial and ventricular arrhythmias, and AV and intraventricular conduction defects (Fig. 8.19) [86]. The ST segment and T wave changes may be related to the associated pericarditis. A "fulminant" form of myocarditis is seen in association with Q waves plus ST segment elevation, and heralds a rapidly fatal course; in general, abnormal QRS complexes and left bundle branch block are markers of poor survival and sudden cardiac death [264]. Frequently "idiopathic" ventricular tachycardia is linked to macroscopic and/or microscopic ventricular abnormalities of myocarditis [265].

Acute rheumatic fever, still of major prevalence in developing countries, may lead to "rheumatic carditis", a form of "pan-carditis" with involvement of endocardium, and pericardium, but also with a "myocarditis" component. The most frequent encounter in such patients is 1° AV block (Fig. 8.20), with 2° AV block of the Wenckebach type or complete AV block occurring rarely. The length of P-R interval does not bare any relationship with the severity of the carditis, or the eventual occurrence of valvular sequelae [266].

Rarely a patient with acute MC may show changes suggestive of myocardial infarction (ST segment elevation, reciprocal ST segment depression, or even Q waves). A possible myocarditis should be suspected when a previously healthy young adult presents with serious atrial or ventricular arrhythmias, high-degree AV block, intraventricular conduction disturbances, or cardiac arrest (Figs. 8.19, 8.21 and 8.22).

8.11.2 Chagas Disease

Chagas disease, a progressive disease leading to congestive heart failure and a variety of ECG abnormalities is essentially endemic in Central and South America. A study of symptomatic seropositive patients revealed an incidence of arrhythmias, including extrasystoles, of 100%. 1° or 2° AV block occurred in 14.3%, 3° AV block in 2.5%, atrial fibrillation in 18.6%, ventricular extrasystoles in 75.2%, right bundle branch block (RBBB) in 39.8% and left anterior fascicular block (LAFB) in 38.6% of patients, with the last two being the most commonly occurring conduction defects [267]. Another study of

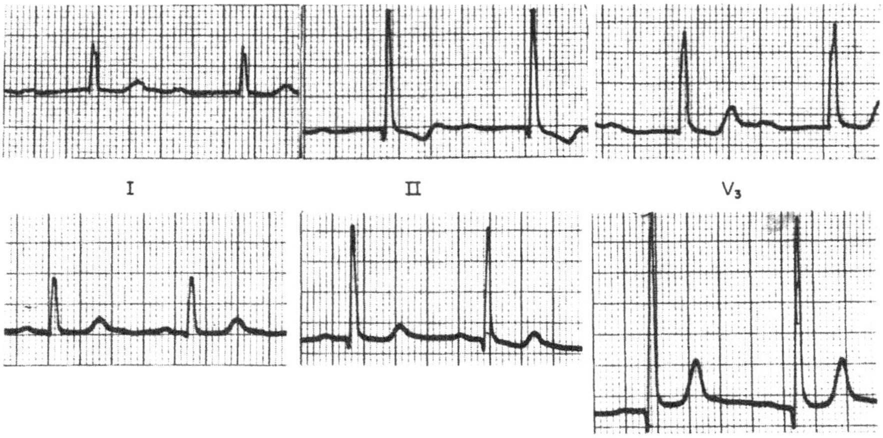

■ Fig. 8.20
Marked PR prolongation (0.46 s) during the acute phase of rheumatic fever (*upper* trace) has returned to normal AV conduction 4 days later (*lower* trace)

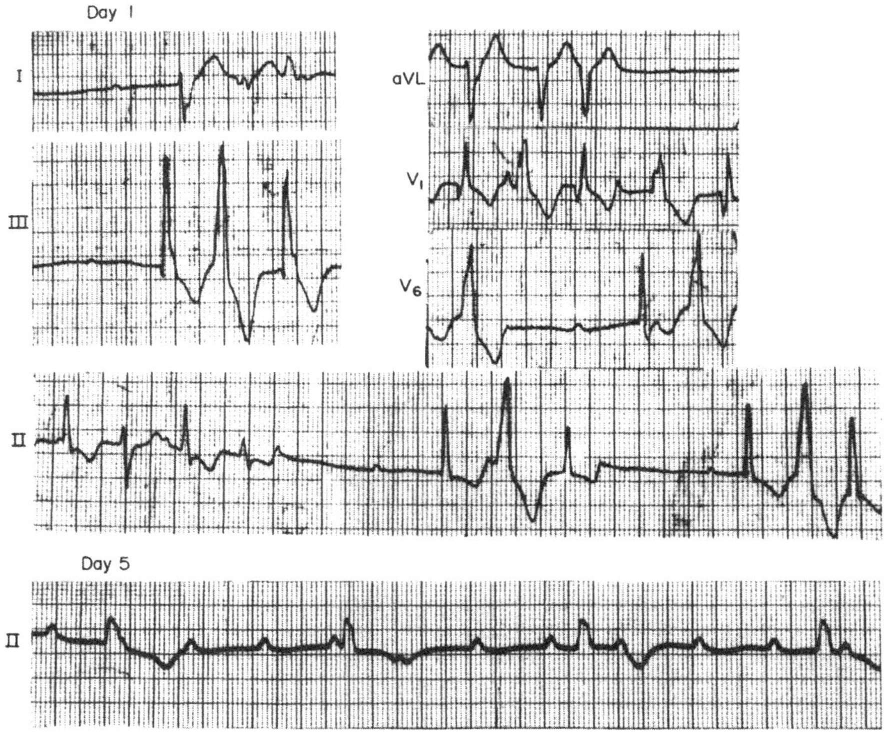

■ Fig. 8.21
ECG showing AV dissociation and frequent VPCs during the acute phase of viral myocarditis. Four days later, the ECG rhythm has changed to complete AV block with a normal atrial rate

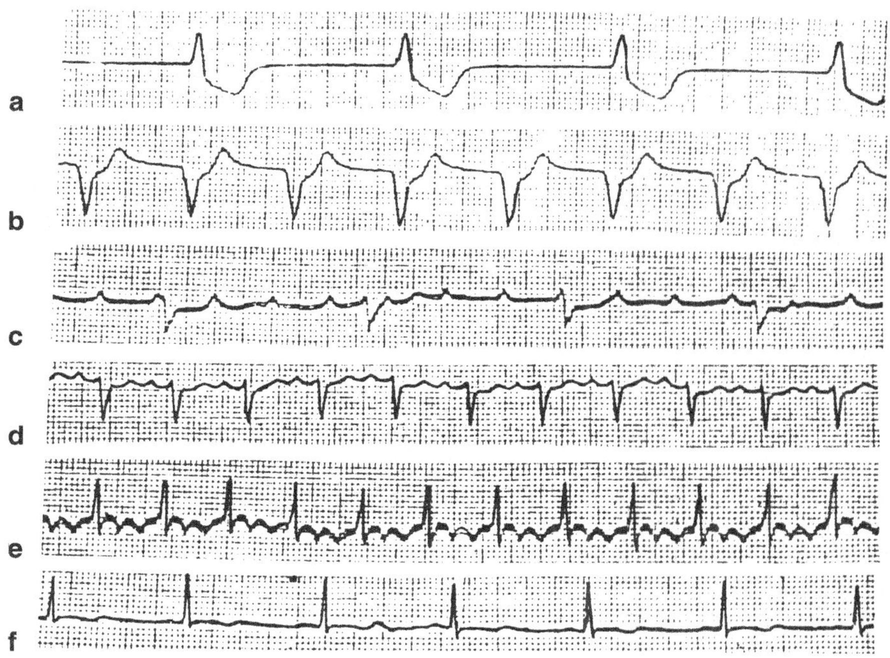

Fig. 8.22
Serial ECG changes in acute viral myocarditis: (a) idioventricular rhythm; (b) accelerated idioventricular rhythm; (c) complete AV block; (d) sinus tachycardia with left axis deviation; (e) atrial flutter with right axis deviation; (f) atrial fibrillation

seropositive subjects showed that RBBB was also the most commonly found ECG abnormality [268]. An incidence of RBBB of 9.3% versus 1.3%, and of LAFB of 9.3% versus 3.9% were the only significant differences between asymptomatic Chagas seropositive and seronegative subjects, while the most frequently occurring ECG finding in these two groups was a T wave change (11.2% vs. 9.1%, respectively) [267]. An early cardio-vagal dysfunction was documented in asymptomatic seropositive subjects regardless of ECG appearance, based on a large panel of tests, suggesting that such change may be useful for identification of subclinical disease [269]. Abnormal values for heart rate turbulence have been noted in patients with Chagas disease [270].

8.12 Connective Tissue Diseases

Connective tissue diseases, e.g., lupus erythematosus, scleroderma, rheumatoid arthritis, etc., frequently impact the cardiovascular system, leading to a variety of cardiac sequelae, and ECG abnormalities. Thus, patients with rheumatoid arthritis were found to have increased sympathetic activity [271]; the signal averaged ECG in patients with scleroderma revealed late potentials in the absence of overt cardiac disease [272], which could be related to the high incidence of ventricular arrhythmias and sudden death in this disorder. In Marfan's syndrome, atrial and ventricular extrasystoles and T wave changes were detected [273]; in patients with systemic lupus erythematosus, atrial and ventricular arrhythmias, 1° AV block, and acquired complete heart block, along with a myriad of ECG abnormalities depending on the associated cardiac complications have been found [274]. Q waves, ST segment changes, increased P wave terminal force, conduction defects, and features of cor pulmonale (see Sect. 8.9.1) were found in patients with connective tissue diseases [275, 276].

8.13 Cardiomyopathy

8.13.1 Hypertrophic Cardiomyopathy

The ECG is abnormal in 93% of patients with hypertrophic cardiomyopathy showing left ventricular hypertrophy (LVH), pseudoinfarctional Q waves, abnormalities of the P waves, ST segments, or T waves, QTc prolongation, and atrial and ventricular arrhythmias, irrespective of the presence of left ventricular outflow obstruction; however, none of these findings is diagnostic of the disease [277, 278]. Left atrial enlargement (LAE), secondary to either poor left ventricular compliance or mitral regurgitation was more common than right atrial enlargement [278]; P-pulmonale noted in patients with HCM may be of the "pseudo-P pulmonale" type, occasionally seen with LAE [86]. LVH, mostly associated with secondary T wave inversion, was present in 81% of patients [278]. ECG LVH may reflect primary involvement of the left ventricular myocardium or hypertrophy in response to the outflow tract obstruction [279]. A frontal axis superior to 0° noted in 52% of patients might have been related to LVH. [278]. The most common ECG findings in hypertrophic cardiomyopathy are the ST segment and T wave abnormalities [86, 277], which may be of the nonspecific type, or those secondary to LVH and conduction defects. Sinoatrial or AV blocks are uncommon [86, 280, 281], with a 4% incidence of complete AV block, requiring permanent pacemaking [278]. T wave alternans (TWA) was more frequent in patients with hypertrophic cardiomyopathy than in hypertensive LVH, and there was a correlation of TWA with myocardial disarray and/or fibrosis, the maximal numbers of successive ventricular ectopic beats and episodes of nonsustained ventricular tachycardia (VT), reflecting myocardial electrical instability [282, 283]. Longer QRS and QT intervals are consequences of increased left ventricular mass in patients with hypertrophic cardiomyopathy, while abnormalities in the T wave complexity index, QT dispersion, activation-recovery interval and its dispersion, and duration of the signal in the terminal portion of the QRS predicted cardiogenic syncope [284].

Pseudoinfarctional Q waves, the most distinctive ECG abnormality in hypertrophic cardiomyopathy (➔ Figs. 8.23–➔ 8.25), are more commonly seen in the anterolateral than the inferior leads [278], and may be due to ventricular septal hypertrophy, septal fibrosis, or abnormal septal activation caused by disarray of the myofibrils [86, 285]. These abnormal Q waves, seen in both the obstructive and non obstructive types of hypertrophic cardiomyopathy have no apparent relationship to the severity of the outflow tract obstruction [86], and they may change in amplitude, or even disappear during the course of the disease [285]. It is intriguing that the segmental muscle hypertrophy of hypertrophic cardiomyopathy produces Q waves similar to those resulting from muscle necrosis. A study employing intracoronary electrograms identified the mechanisms of Q wave generation in hypertrophic cardiomyopathy to be both transmural myocardial fibrosis and altered direction of resultant initial vectors due to disproportionate hypertrophy of septal and/or free wall, unopposed by apical forces; areas of fibrosis were associated with regional contraction abnormalities while hypertrophic territories were not [286]. The above were corroborated by newly appearing and disappearing Q waves after alcohol septal ablations in patients with hypertrophic cardiomyopathy [287]. Occasionally patients with hypertrophic cardiomyopathy can suffer a true myocardial infarction (➔ Fig. 8.26).

Atrial fibrillation (AF) has been reported to occur in 7–45% of the patients, while atrial and ventricular premature beats were found in 9–27% when employing 24 h ambulatory ECG monitoring [86, 278, 280]. VT was observed in 4% of patients (➔ Fig. 8.27a) during Holter monitoring [278], with a higher incidence reported in other literature [86, 280, 281]. AF and the Wolff-Parkinson-White syndrome are more commonly associated with certain genetic mutations in patients with hypertrophic cardiomyopathy. Nonsustained VT particularly in the young has a poor prognosis, and sustained VT and ventricular fibrillation are rarely documented [288]. Invasive electrophysiology studies have little advantage over non-invasive risk stratification [289], and along with a host of risk factors, both need to be considered for prophylactic implantation of an automatic defibrillator [288, 289].

8.13.2 Dilated Cardiomyopathy

The most common ECG findings in patients with dilated cardiomyopathy are left ventricular hypertrophy (LVH) and left atrial enlargement (LAE) [86]. The pathophysiologic pathways leading to dilated cardiomyopathy are ever expanding.

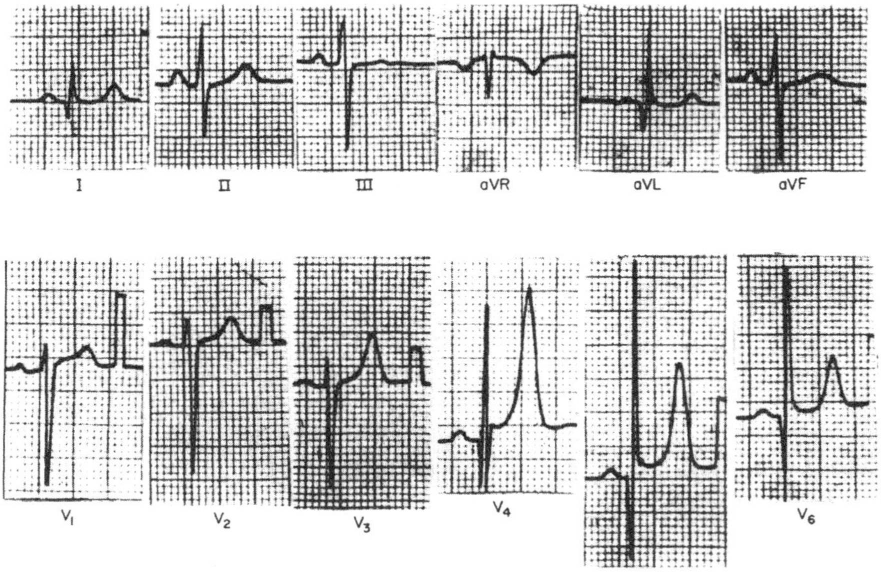

Fig. 8.23
Pseudoinfarctional Q waves in leads I, aVL, and V_4–V_6, with evidence of left ventricular hypertrophy in a patient with HCM

A newly described form of apical dilated cardiomyopathy ("takotsubo") induced by acute physical and psychological stress leads to ST segment elevation, diffuse T wave inversion, and prolonged QT interval indistinguishable from acute myocardial infarction syndrome [290–292]. A reversible arrhythmogenic dilated cardiomyopathy due to tachyarrhythmias, mainly atrial fibrillation (AF) [293], but rarely even due to "chronic" sustained ventricular tachycardia [294] should be kept in mind. Arrhythmogenic right ventricular dysplasia may lead to right and rarely left ventricular dilated cardiomyopathy [295]. Right ventricular hypertrophy (RVH) and biventricular hypertrophy/dilatation (BVH) are commonly documented by echocardiography or autopsy, although are not always paired with suggestive ECG findings. The ECG cannot distinguish hypertrophy from dilatation [296]. Although BVH due to congenital heart disease is occasionally associated with the Katz–Wachtel pattern [297] characterized by large diphasic QRS complexes in the standard bipolar leads, BVH may lead to a reduction of QRS voltage or an almost normal ECG due to cancellation [2]. The author has observed large diphasic QRS complexes in the precordial leads in patients with BVH, while a normal-sized diphasic QRS complex in these leads is a normal finding [297]. An R/S ratio ≥1 in V_1 is the most sensitive among the conventional ECG criteria of RVH [298]. Diastolic overload is associated with LVH in the ECG, and tall symmetrical T waves with some ST segment elevation (not commented upon by the author) of upward concave type, in contrast to ST segment depression and inverted T waves, found with systolic overload [299]. Diffuse myocardial fibrosis may be the mechanism of the reduced QRS voltage in dilated cardiomyopathy. This attenuation of QRS complexes may involve only the limb leads, while the precordial leads may be normal or prominent in amplitude and show poor R wave progression in patients with dilated cardiomyopathy, or congestive heart failure (➋ Fig. 8.27b) [300, 301]. Low voltage ECG in patients with peripheral edema is seen in spite of the cardiac dilatation (see ➋ Sect. 8.25.6). Also the amplitude of cardiac signals, acquired by body surface potential mapping, decreased by approximately 30% after partial left ventriculotomy [302].

Pseudoinfarctional Q waves in patients with dilated cardiomyopathy may be seen, although with lower frequency than in dilated cardiomyopathy; such Q waves are mostly present in the right and mid-precordial leads (➋ Fig. 8.27b), and are probably due to LVH and/or intraventricular conduction defects (IVCD) [86, 303, 304]. IV conduction defects, particularly left bundle branch block (LBBB) (➋ Fig. 8.28), are common in dilated cardiomyopathy, with incidences varying between 9% [305] and 44% [86, 300, 303, 306]. LBBB is so prevalent that its presence, particularly in patients

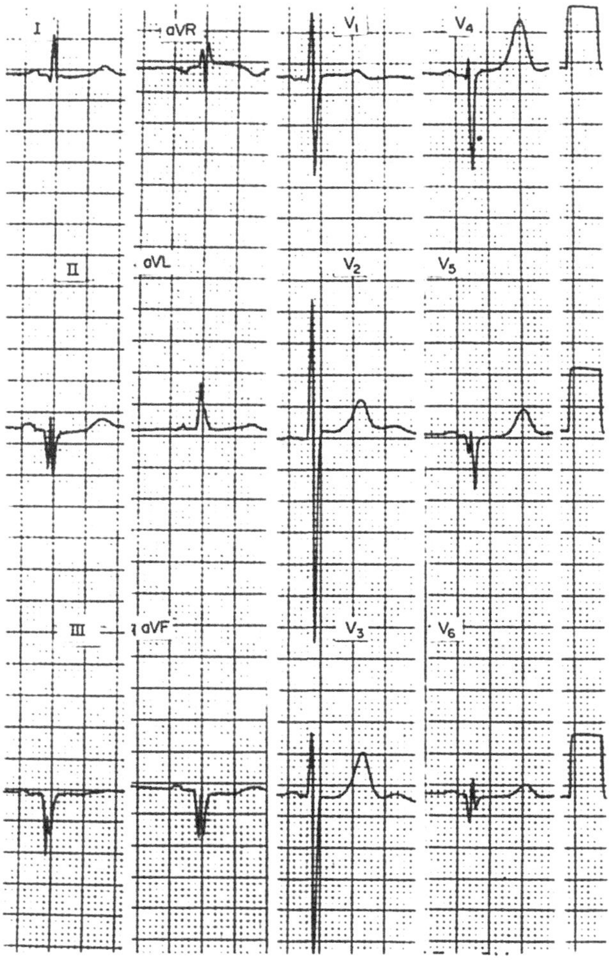

Fig. 8.24

Pseudoinfarctional Q waves in leads II, III, aVF, V_5 and V_6, and reversed R wave progression in V_1–V_4 in a patient with documented HCM

younger than 40 years of age, would support the diagnosis of the disease. An association of extreme frontal right axis deviation with the LBBB has been noted in some patients, and may indicate extreme severity of dilated cardiomyopathy [307]. QRS duration and its perturbations are employed as a predictor, in the monitoring of patients with dilated cardiomyopathy, and their response to resynchronization therapy [308–310]. Heart rate turbulence (onset and slope), microvolt-level T-wave alternans, abnormal baroreflex sensitivity and heart rate variability are powerful independent predictors of ventricular tachyarrhythmic events in patients with dilated cardiomyopathy [311, 312]. Commonly, the prolongation of the QRS complexes, in the absence of typical features of either LBBB or right bundle branch block, qualifies for the diagnosis of IVCD (➋ Fig. 8.29). Most of the ST segment and T wave changes seen in the left precordial leads in dilated cardiomyopathy are nonspecific or secondary to LVH, IVCD, or digitalis effect. Atrial arrhythmias, particularly AF (➋ Fig. 8.29), and ventricular arrhythmias are common in this disease. ECGs pertaining to employment of pacing, implantable cardioverter/defibrillators, and resynchronization therapy, with changes associated with their advanced operational features and occasional malfunction, are frequently encountered in patients with dilated cardiomyopathy [313].

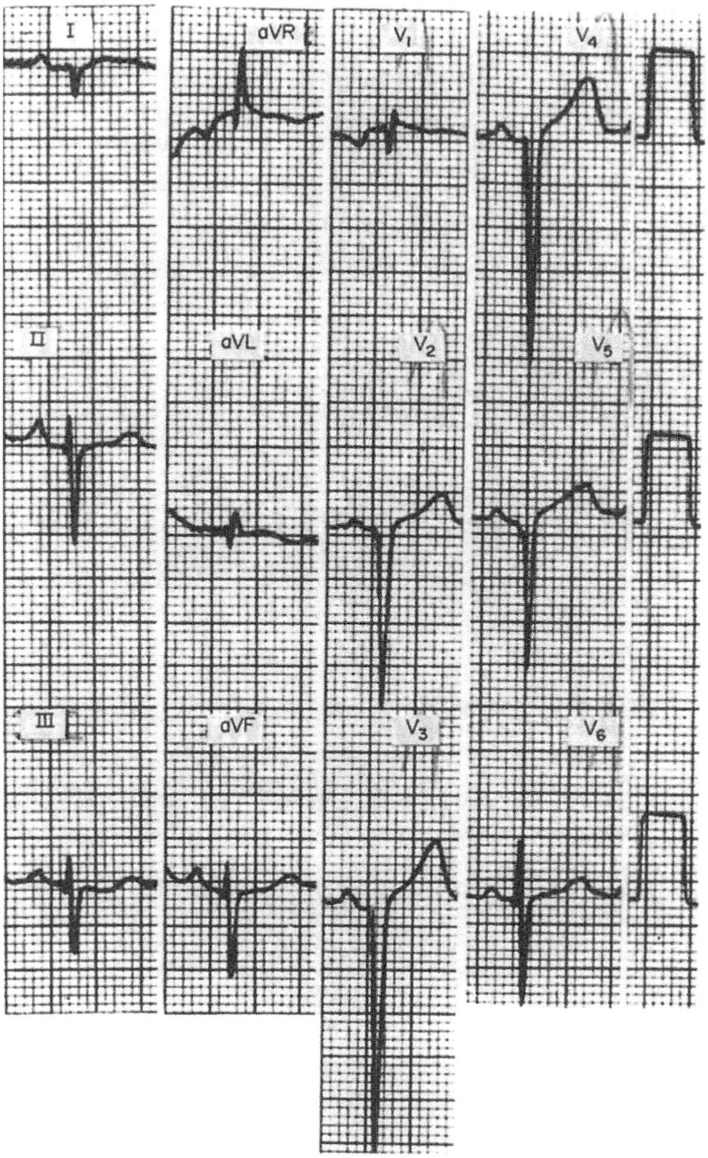

Fig. 8.25
Pseudoinfarctional Q waves in V_1–V_5 in a patient with documented HCM

8.13.3 Restrictive Cardiomyopathy

Restrictive cardiomyopathy is characterized by low-voltage QRS complexes, left and right atrial enlargement, LVH, nonspecific ST-T changes, AV conduction defects, IVCD, and arrhythmias, particularly AF [2]. Pseudoinfarctional Q waves and low voltage ECG complexes are noted in amyloid heart disease [2, 314], while body surface potential maps revealed correlation of the amplitude of positive potentials on the anterior and lateral chest wall with disease severity, and prolongation of ventricular activation time [315]. It is possible that the low voltage in advanced stages of restrictive cardiomyopathy

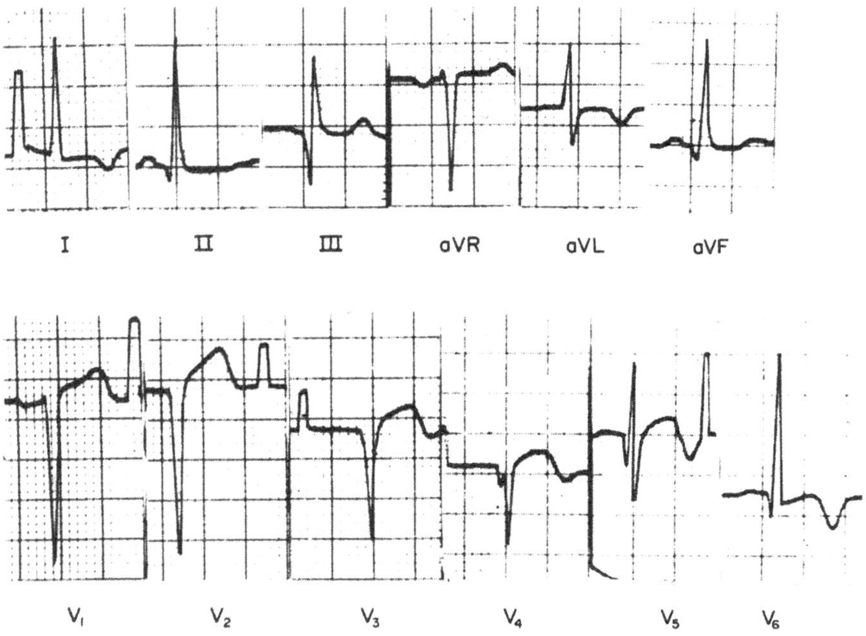

Fig. 8.26
ECG of a patient with documented HCM complicated by acute anterior myocardial infarction

may be in part related to the associated peripheral edema (see Sect. 8.25.6). Other infiltrative diseases causing restrictive cardiomyopathy are Fabry disease [316], hemochromatosis, in which chelation therapy restores the amplitude of QRS complexes [317], hypereosinophilia [318], mucopolysaccharide (Hurler's) and glycogen storage (Pompe's) diseases [319]. The last is associated with very high QRS complexes, possibly related to high extracellular resistance [2].

8.14 Cardiac Transplantation

ECG changes at some point after cardiac transplantation (CT) are seen in approximately 75% of patients, consisting of bundle branch block, atrial flutter or fibrillation, and ventricular arrhythmias with coronary vasculopathy [320]. A direct association of increase in QTc duration over time with mortality has been identified [321]. However, with contemporary treatment, ECG changes develop only in severe forms of rejection. Diffuse low QRS voltage, loss of precordial R wave amplitude, right axis deviation, 1° AV block progressing to nodal rhythm, atrial arrhythmias, and occasionally ischemic ST segment changes are looked for in the monitoring of patients following CT [322, 323]. However, these changes are nonspecific, and particularly in reference to the QRS voltage, attenuation has not correlated with acute rejection [324]; pericardial and pleural effusions, or other complications in the post cardiac transplantation course could also be the cause of low QRS voltage [325]. Linear or nonlinear analyses of heart rate variability provide detection of acute rejection following allograft CT [326]. Increased QTc dispersion, independent of the reduction of the ejection fraction, has been found in patients with post CT coronary vasculopathy [327]. However, increase in QTc dispersion and right bundle branch block have not been found to discriminate between patients with and without biopsy-proven cellular rejection [328–330], although a trend has been noted linking increased QTc dispersion and rejection, calling for a change of management [330]. The study of the frequency content of the ECG has been found useful for the detection of rejection, and its management, while changes in QRS or signal averaged ECG were noncontributory [331, 332]. Analysis of the ventricular evoked response obtained by programmed electrical stimulation may be suitable for detection and monitoring of cardiac allograft rejection [333].

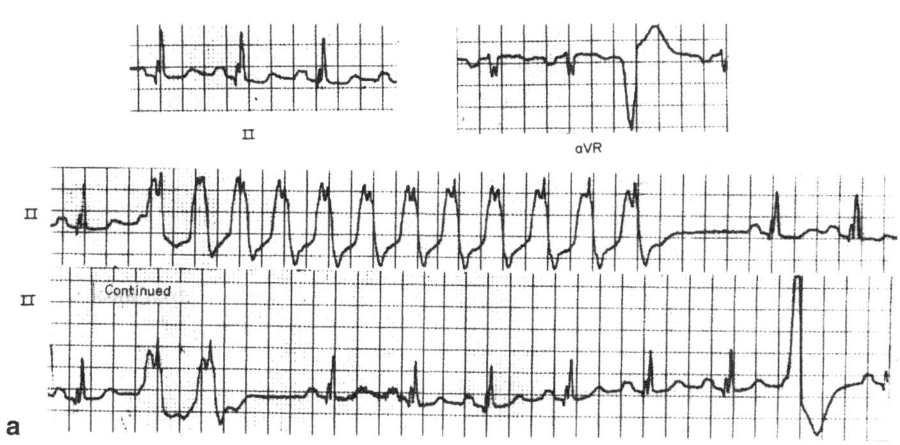

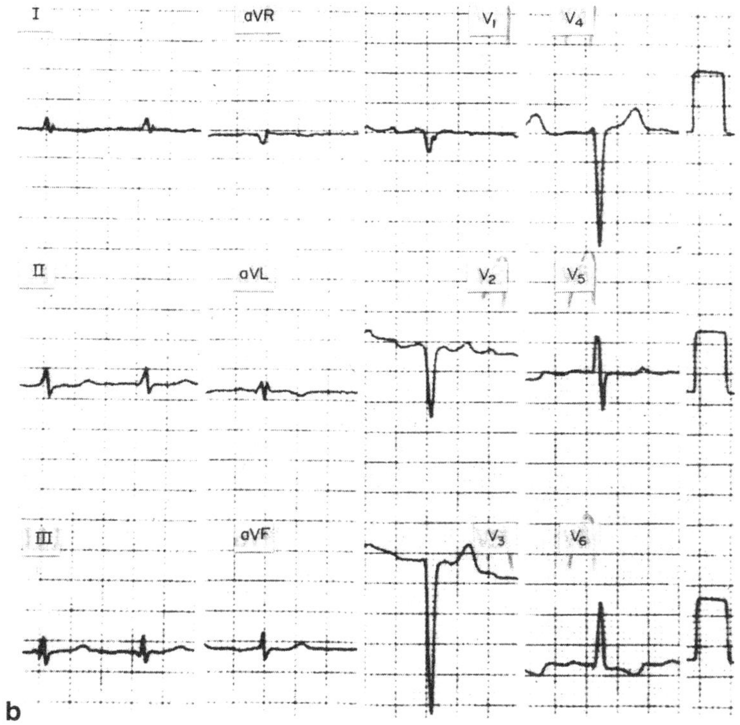

Fig. 8.27

(a) Ventricular tachycardia in a patient with documented hypertrophic cardiomyopathy. (b) ECG of a patient with autopsy-proven idiopathic congestive cardiomyopathy, simulating an old anteroseptal myocardial infarction. The low voltage in standard leads is the result of pericardial effusion, which often appears not to have involved the precordial leads in patients with enormous QRS complexes prior to the development of the effusion

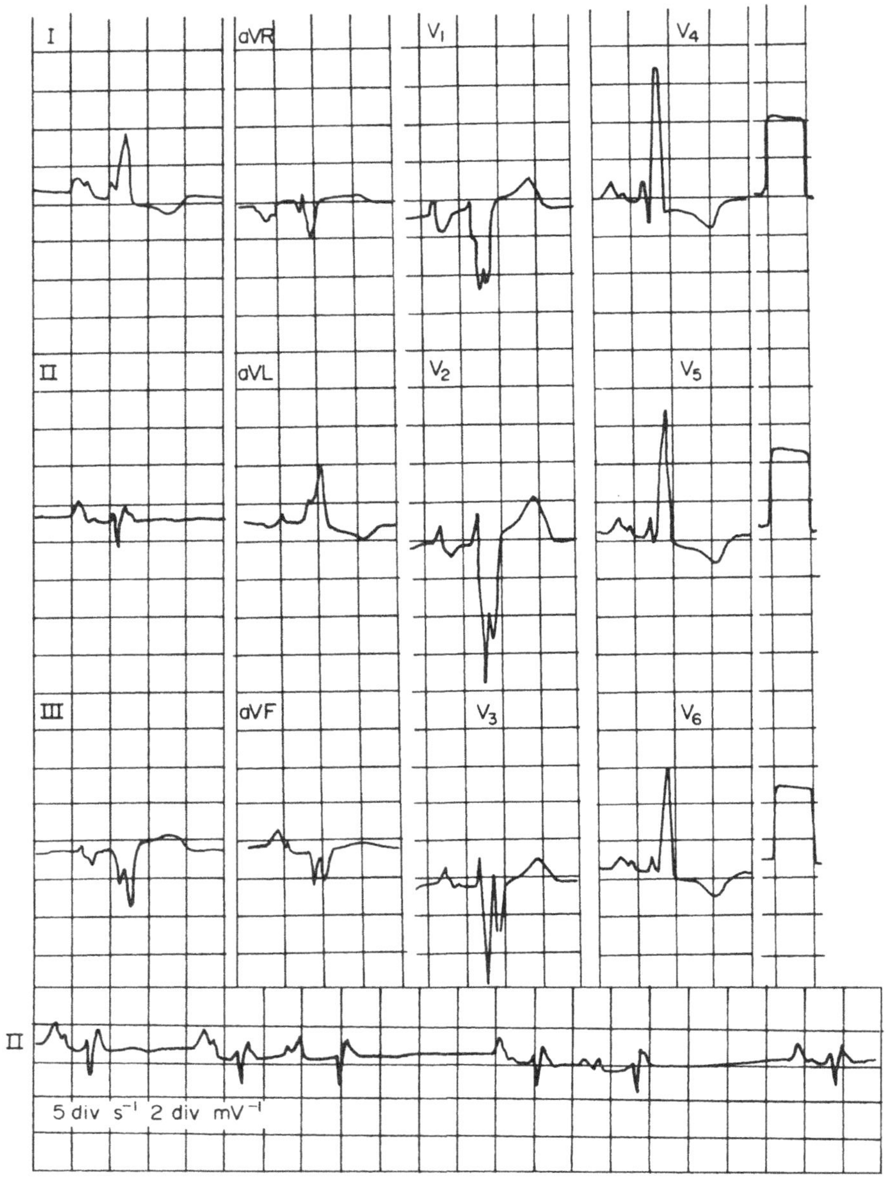

Fig. 8.28
ECG showing left atrial enlargement and LBBB in a patient with dilated cardiomyopathy

8.15 Heart Injury

Trauma to the heart and large vessels may lead to ECG changes, which depend on the nature of injury and the particular anatomic site of cardiac involvement. Blunt trauma to the chest wall can involve the underlying heart in "commotio cordis", "contusio cordis", and "steering wheel injury" where experimental work and clinical experience has shown the gamut of ECG abnormalities occurring, with various outcomes from sudden death due to ventricular fibrillation (VF), to quick, but sometimes more protracted, recovery [334]. Atrial and ventricular arrhythmias, AV and intraventricular

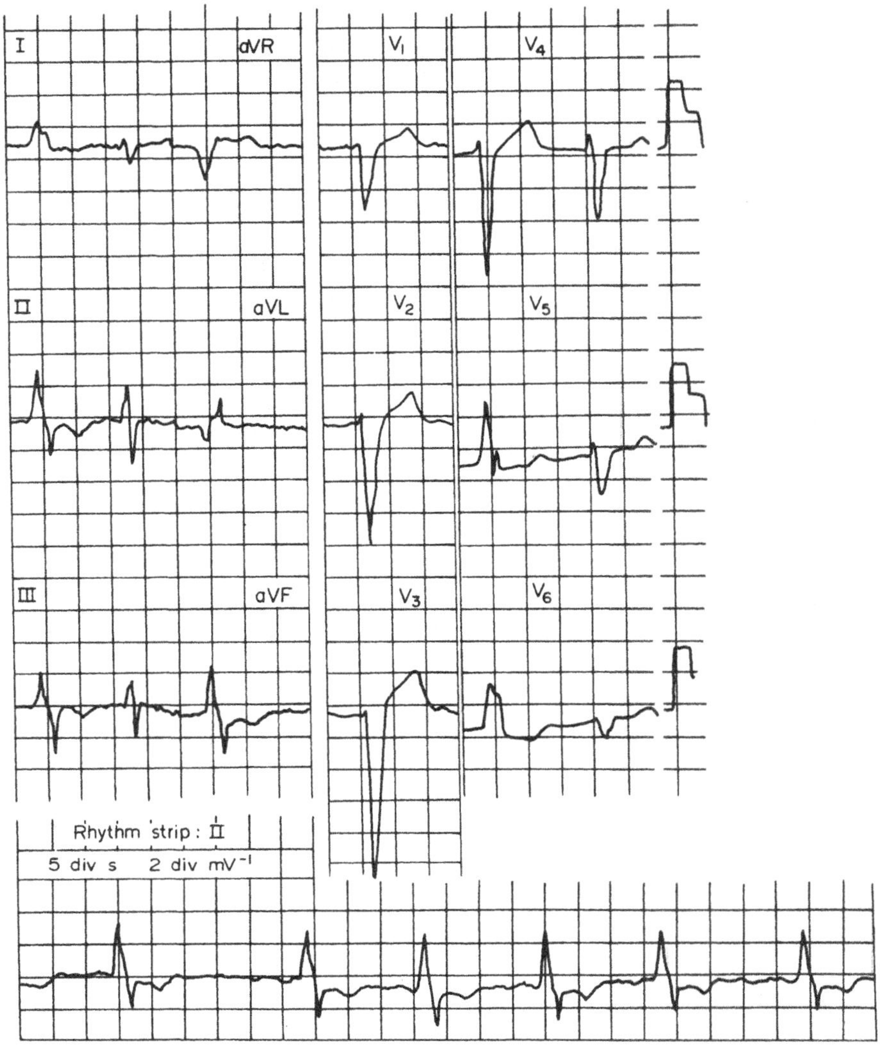

Fig. 8.29
Atrial fibrillation and LBBB-like IVCD in a patient with dilated cardiomyopathy

conduction disturbances, evidence of pericarditis, pericardial effusion and frank myocardial infarction (MI) (resulting from damage to the myocardium itself or the perfusing coronary artery) are found. Some of the above may be noted only transiently, while others may leave a permanent change on the ECG. Attenuated ECG complexes or such changes becoming more pronounced in serial ECGs indicate hemopericardium, which is often expanding rapidly. Minor repolarization ECG changes may be seen in "contusio cordis", which can be followed by ventricular pseudoaneurysm and sudden cardiac death. Similar changes lasting for a few hours can be seen in boxers [335]. Involvement of valves leads to atrial and myocardial after effects, which manifest as progressive ECG changes as the pathophysiology of cavity enlargements evolves.

A variety of arrhythmias result from electrical injuries including the effect of lightning to the heart, with the alternating current being worse than the direct current at the same voltage. Current of high frequencies is not damaging, and the vulnerability of patients varies with the degree of skin resistance. Levels of current intensity (approximately 80 mA is fatal), duration of exposure, and its trajectory passing through the heart, determine the seriousness of the outcome.

Sinus tachycardia, ST segment elevation, nonspecific ST-T changes, prolonged QTc interval, atrial and ventricular tachycardia, VF, conduction abnormalities, and MI can occur with low and high voltage electrical injuries; QTc prolongation results only from direct lightning hits, and for MI coronary vasospasm is implicated [336, 337]. The transient collapse, noted in some victims, implies that VF may be occasionally reversible. After exposure in survivors, sinus tachycardia and non-specific ST-T changes can be seen in the ECG, which partially may be due to underlying myocardial injury [337].

After electroconvulsive therapy, no new persisting ECG changes were found even in patients with prior cardiac disease [338]. Internal cardioversion of atrial fibrillation may lead to prolongation of QTc [339]. Brief ST segment elevation may follow external DC cardioversion [340]. Internal and external cardioversion of ventricular arrhythmias resulted in brief sinus bradycardia, supraventricular and rare ventricular tachycardias [341]. The external and internal defibrillation during procedures or after implantation of automatic defibrillators, has the potential rarely to cause epicardial injury, or biochemical evidence of necrosis [342–344].

8.16 Pericardial Diseases

Acute and chronic diseases of the pericardium produce various ECG abnormalities, some of which are nonspecific, while others are very distinctive of the underlying pathology.

8.16.1 Pericarditis

Acute pericarditis causes diffuse ST segment elevation and T wave inversion, attributed to subepicardial myocarditis or myocardial damage along with the type involving the pericardium per se (➲ Fig. 8.30). Although the condition is usually generalized, local or loculated pericarditis occasionally occurs and results in regional ST-T changes. Four stages of evolutionary ST segment and T wave changes have been described in association with acute pericarditis [120, 345]: (a) stage 1: diffuse ST elevation in almost all leads except aVR and possibly V_1, i.e., absence of reciprocal changes; (b) stage 2: return of ST junction to the baseline, with diminishing amplitude of the T wave; (c) stage 3: inversion of

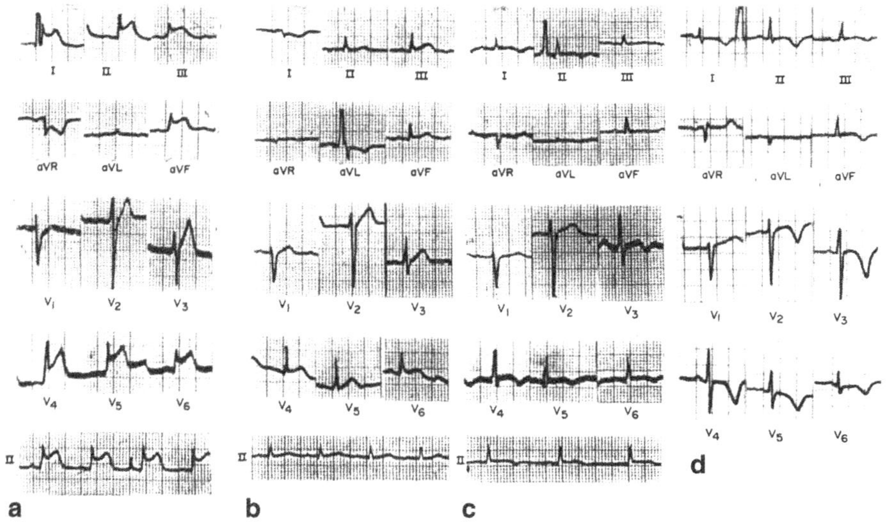

Fig. 8.30
Serial ECG changes in a patient with acute viral pericarditis: (a) Diffuse ST elevation seen on day 1; (b) Normal ST segment and T wave seen on day 2; (c) Normal ST segment, but the T wave begins to be inverted on day 3; (d) Marked T wave inversion seen on day 16

the T wave with an isoelectric ST segment; and (d) stage 4: return of the T wave to its normal pattern. One or more stages may be absent, or features of one stage may be intermingled with features of another, depending on the frequency of observation, severity of the disease, and time interval between the recording and the onset of illness. Although characteristic ST segment displacement has been reported in ≥90% of the cases of the disease, the sensitivity and specificity of ECG changes in the diagnosis of acute pericarditis are very difficult to evaluate [345]. The typical ST segment and T wave abnormalities are more often seen in acute purulent pericarditis than in the type resulting from tuberculosis, uremia, or as a complication of acute myocardial infarction (MI) either shortly after inception, or later (Dressler's syndrome). Perhaps the associated QRST alterations of the subacute or chronic MI explain the apparent paucity of characteristic ST-T changes of pericarditis in Dressler's syndrome, although others feel that the latter has truly decreased in incidence in the thrombolytic era [346]. Etiology of pericarditis and the extent of the associated myocardial damage determine the duration of the ECG changes [86]. Thus, while purulent pericarditis is likely to be associated with persistent ECG abnormalities, the ST segment displacement in acute viral or idiopathic pericarditis may return usually to normal within a week. However the succeeding T wave inversion may last longer, perhaps for weeks or months, even in patients who have fully recovered.

Other less frequent and specific ECG findings in acute pericarditis include a depressed PR segment, and atrial arrhythmias, both of which are probably responses to atrial injury. Some PR segment depression (occasionally up to 200 μV) is the normal expression of atrial repolarization (secondary) and may extend into the ST segment and T wave [347]; consequently, the exaggerated PR segment should be viewed as a primary alteration of the atrial repolarization, and is encountered in 23% of patients with clinically silent pericarditis, particularly with inflammatory pericardial involvement [348].

The ST segment displacement observed in acute pericarditis should be differentiated from those occurring in acute MI, ST elevation in healthy young people caused by vagotonia, and early repolarization. In reference to the differentiation from acute MI [349], the following are helpful: (a) There is no reciprocal ST segment depression in acute pericarditis – ST depression is only seen in lead aVR (➲ Figs. 6.25 and ➲ 8.30), and rarely in leads V_1, III and aVL; (b) Less severe ST segment elevation (usually <0.4 mV) occurs in pericarditis, but more leads are involved; (c) Upward concave ST segment elevation, rather than upward convex ST segment elevation, is observed in pericarditis; (d) During the period of ST segment elevation, the T wave remains upright in pericarditis, until the ST segment returns to the isoelectric line; (e) More diffuse but less deep T wave inversion occurs in pericarditis; and (f) The QT interval in pericarditis is normal. Regarding the differentiation of pericarditis from early repolarization, it has been reported that the ratio of ST segment elevation to the corresponding upright T wave is higher in the former than in the latter [350] (➲ Fig. 8.30).

8.16.2 Pericardial Effusion

Low QRS voltage is traditionally thought to be due to the "insulating" effect of fluid or fibrin deposits [86], or changes in the electrical properties of the pericardium, although an alternative explanation is that of a short-circuiting effect of the fluid enveloping the heart [351]. There is continuing debate about the correlation of the presence of low voltage ECG or the degree of QRS attenuation and the magnitude of pericardial effusion and it appears that the interplay of the above is complex [352]. Generalized low QRS voltage with electrical alternans is seen with large pericardial effusions, and is attributed to a swinging motion of the heart maintaining a two-beat periodicity [86, 353].

8.16.3 Pericardial Tamponade

There are no specific ECG changes of pericardial tamponade; however the low voltage ECG in tamponade may be due to the associated (usually large) PE although a possible compressive effect of the increased pericardial pressure reducing the ventricular volume has also been implicated [354].

8.16.4 Pericardial Constriction

ECG changes with chronic pericardial constriction include all the above findings seen in pericarditis, particularly the T wave inversion seen in its third stage, and the low QRS voltage found with pulmonary embolism [355]; the depth of T waves has been felt to correlate with the degree of myocardial-pericardial adherence [356], and may have implications on the feasibility of surgical pericardial "stripping".

8.17 Heart Tumors

A variety of benign and malignant primary and metastatic heart tumors are associated with Q waves, ST segment deviations, T wave inversions, conduction abnormalities, and atrial and ventricular arrhythmias. ECG changes may simulate all appearances of myocardial ischemia and infarction [357, 358]. The entire range of ECG changes of pericarditis (see ➋ Sect. 8.16) may be seen with tumor invasion of the pericardium [359]. Cardiac rhabdomyomas associated with tuberous sclerosis may show ECG evidence of right or left ventricular hypertrophy depending on the ventricular cavity involved, in the absence of pressure overload or cardiac enlargement, with such changes disappearing with regression of the tumors [360]. Atrial myxomas lead mainly to P-mitrale (broad P waves in lead II and enhanced terminal force of P waves in lead V_1) [361].

8.18 Electrical Alternans

Electrical alternans, i.e. a regular alternating change in the configuration or magnitude and axis of the ECG complexes, arising from the same pacemaker, and associated with a stable R-R interval, is an extracardiac phenomenon [86]. It may involve the P, QRS or T waves, and when all these three occur together, "total electrical alternans" is said to be present. ST segment alternans occasionally occurs in the setting of variant angina [362], myocardial infarction [363], exercise testing [364], or during coronary angioplasty [365], and even alternans in conduction can occur. P, T, and U wave, and ST segment alternans is rare, while QRS alternans, with or without T wave change, is the most common pattern.

Pericardial effusion, with or without cardiac tamponade, is the most common clinical cause of electrical alternans (see ➋ Sect. 8.16.2) (➋ Fig. 8.31), and is often associated with low ECG voltage and tachycardia. QRS alternans may also occur in hypertensive heart disease with left ventricular hypertrophy, coronary artery disease (CAD), and supraventricular tachycardia associated with the Wolff-Parkinson-White syndrome (WPW). Alternating WPW pattern might be misinterpreted as QRS alternans (➋ Fig. 8.32), although the mechanism obviously is different (pseudo-alternans). In pericardial effusion or cardiac tamponade, electrical alternans most likely results from cardiac displacement in the pericardial sac as well as the reduction of the restraining interference of the lungs on the heart [366]. In the absence of pericardial effusion or cardiac tamponade, the possible mechanism of electrical alternans is an alternation in the pattern of depolarization,

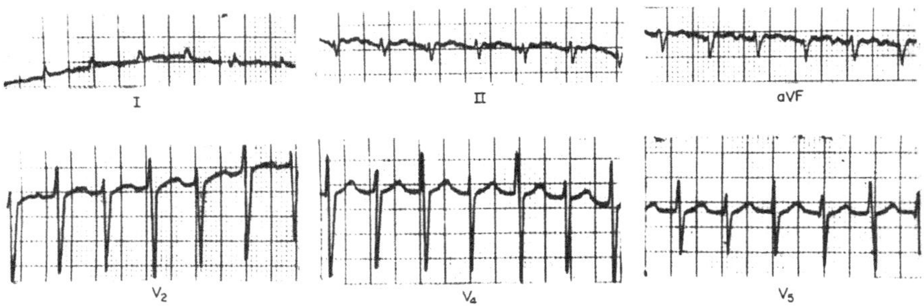

Fig. 8.31
QRS alternans in a patient with complicated large pericardial effusion due to a hepatoma

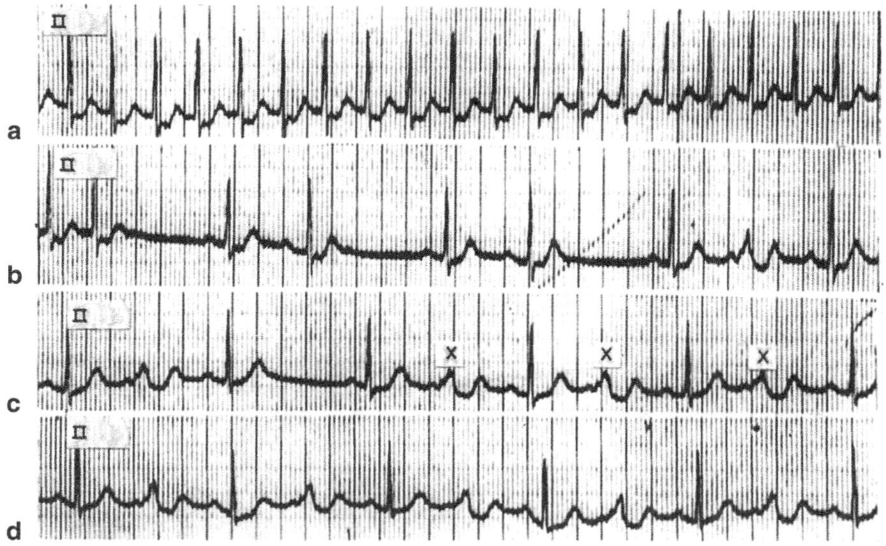

Fig. 8.32
QRS alternans in a patient with alternating WPW ECG pattern (lead II (b, c, d). Note the regularity of the P–P interval, and the xs indicating the QRSs with preexcitation)

which is the consequence of the inhomogeneous refractory phase of the myocardium [367]. However, this should be termed "depolarization alternans" and the implication is that this is a cardiac rather than extracardiac phenomenon. Currently T wave alternans, expressed in μV, has been employed in research and practice [368]; particularly its application during exercise testing is touted as useful for evaluation of patients with CAD, or for selection of patients for implantation of cardioverter/defibrillators [369].

8.19 Cardiac Memory

T wave changes can be thought of as primary, implying a change in ventricular gradient, like the ones caused by electrolytic or ischemic disturbances, or secondary, due to changes in the ventricular depolarization sequence, as in bundle branch block (BBB) or sequence of repolarization as in some forms of left ventricular hypertrophy. Experimental work [370–372] and the repolarization changes noted in left bundle branch block (LBBB) and right ventricular pacing led to the proposition that a change in the sequence of ventricular activation may also induce variation in the duration of the excited state resulting in a change in the ventricular gradient, i.e. emergence of "primary" or "pseudoprimary" T wave abnormalities [373–375]. Such T wave changes are unlike the secondary changes that are seen as "obligatory" components of LBBB or right ventricular pacing, and have the following characteristics: they develop gradually; a long time may be needed for maximal effect to appear and subsequently to dissipate, and a shorter time for these to take place when the heart has been previously exposed to BBB or pacing. They are manifest during return to normal activation; and their direction is the same as that of the inciting abnormal QRS complexes (➋ Fig. 8.33). These "pseudoprimary" T wave changes may also be seen in some cases of transient complete AV block with wide QRS complexes, single or combined fascicular blocks, preexcitation, after tachycardias especially ventricular, following premature ventricular beats (VPBs) (➋ Fig. 8.34a) and premature atrial beats (➋ Fig. 8.35) and even after myocardial infarction [375]. It has been stated that with single VPBs, cardiac memory can be detected when the VPBs are interpolated (➋ Fig. 8.34a) or they are followed by a non-fully compensatory period (➋ Fig. 8.34b), while it does not occur or is barely detected with fully compensatory periods; however, occasionally evidence of memory is seen in association with a fully compensatory period (➋ Fig. 8.36). Also the change in the T wave may require a few beats for full return to the appearance present prior to the VPCs.

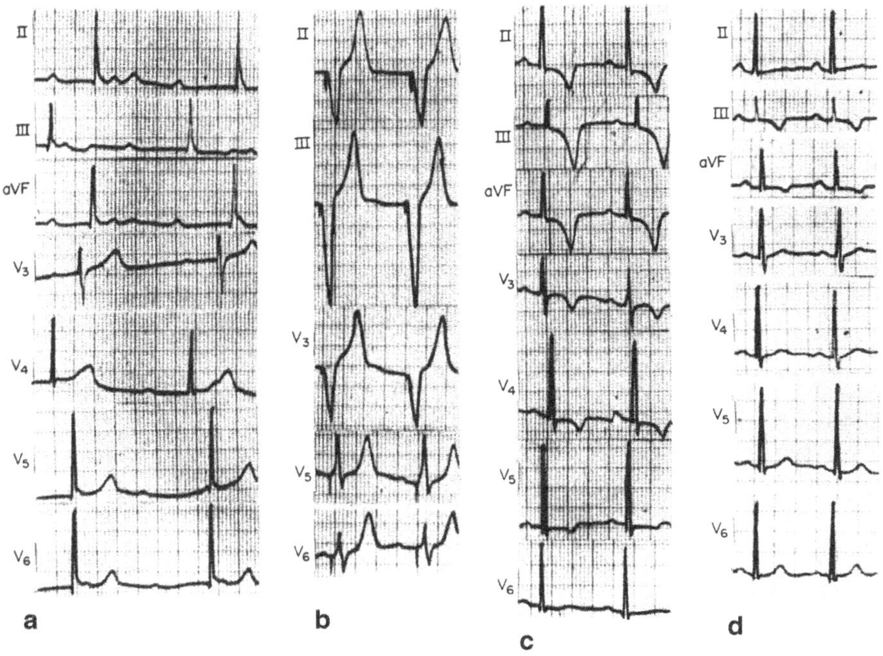

Fig. 8.33
(a) ECG of a patient with acute myocarditis shows complete AV block. (b) ECG shows RV pacing rhythm. (c) ECG 6 days later, after discontinuation of the pacemaker, shows remarkable T wave inversion in leads II, III, aVF, V_3–V_6, with the T waves in the same direction as the wide QRSs during RV pacing. (d) ECG further 4 days later has returned to normal

Multiple single VPBs may gradually enhance the observed post-VPB T wave changes. Evidence for cardiac memory is ubiquitous in both standard ECGs, exercise stress ECGs, and Holter monitoring tracings (➋ Figs. 8.34 and ➋ 8.35).

The mechanism, by which the ventricular gradient is affected when the sequence of ventricular activation changes as in LBBB, has been thought to be an electrotonic modulation occurring during cardiac activation, accelerating repolarization at sites where depolarization starts, and delaying it at sites where it terminates [375]. A cumulative modulation of the T wave change ensues, which can be appreciated in serial ECGs, and suggests some form of "storage", simulating "memory". Such change may persist for days or weeks after the discontinuation of the inciting stimulus. Although the mechanism of these T wave changes has been debated for a long time, the existence of cardiac memory is not any more disputed, and is currently viewed as a form of remodeling via similar processes determining memory in the central nervous system [374, 376–378]. Cardiac memory consequent to pacing has been shown to depend on changes in ionic currents, and the distinction between secondary and "pseudoprimary" T wave changes is becoming less clear, since pacing for example alters slightly the post-pacing QRS complexes, which are not exactly as they appeared prior to the initiation of artificial cardiac stimulation [378].

The clinical significance of these T wave changes was and still is the object of controversy [377–379]. The post PVB T wave abnormality is a case in point, where arguments persist as to whether it reflects latent pathology, or merely it is a consequence of cardiac memory [377–379]. The same applies to T wave changes in the intrinsic ventricular capture beats in patients with intermittent pacing (➋ Fig. 8.37), and whether this signifies underlying pathology, injury to the myocardium, or merely "an ECG curiosity" [378, 379]. In terms of the causative mechanism, T wave change after a VPB could also be due to myocardial ischemia resulting from post-ectopic potentiation of ventricular contraction, transiently increasing regional myocardial oxygen demands [380, 381]. A way to discriminate between the T wave changes due to cardiac memory and those reflecting ischemic alterations regardless of the coronary artery involved has been reported, and relies on the polarity and amplitude of the T waves in particular ECG leads [382].

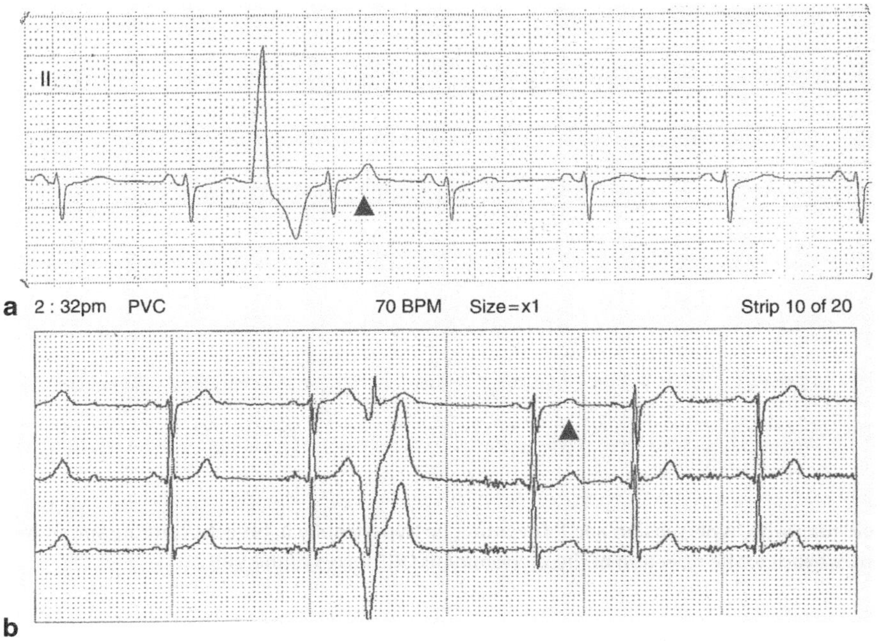

Fig. 8.34
(a) ECG of a 66-year-old man with hypertension, and normal coronary arteries and left ventricular function shows T wave changes after an interpolated VPB (*arrowhead*) (b) A Holter ECG recording of a 53-year-old man with normal coronary arteries and left ventricular function complaining of palpitations reveals post VPB T wave changes (*arrowhead*)

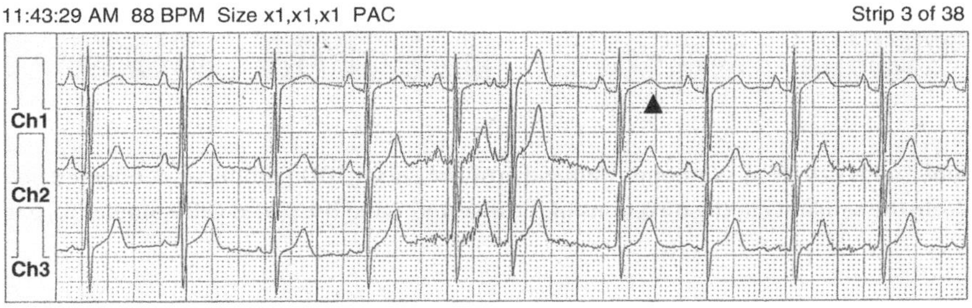

Fig. 8.35
Holter ECG of a 54-year-old man with complaints of dizziness and a normal exercise treadmill/thallium-201 test shows post premature atrial beat (PAB) lowering of the T wave (arrowhead) to the direction of the predominant QRS forces of the PAB

8.20 Gastrointestinal Disease

A number of diseases of abdominal organs (pancreatitis, cholecystitis, duodenal ulcer disease) are associated with ECG changes, mainly nonspecific ST-T changes; however, occasionally the ECG changes are more impressive, i.e., deep T wave inversion and ST segment elevation of ≥ 1.0 mm, and rarely Q waves simulating myocardial ischemia or infarction [383, 384]. ST-T changes in patients with gastrointestinal diseases may occasionally represent a normal variant. In esophageal disorders in particular, due to the frequent presentation with chest pain indistinguishable from the one due

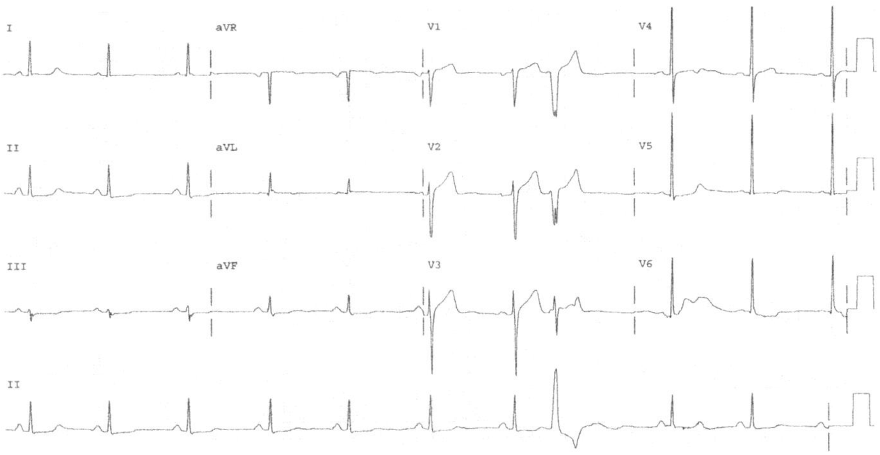

Fig. 8.36
ECG of a 65-year-old man with hypertension and left ventricular hypertrophy in his echocardiogram, shows T wave enhancement post VPB (arrowhead) to the direction of the predominant QRS forces of the VPB

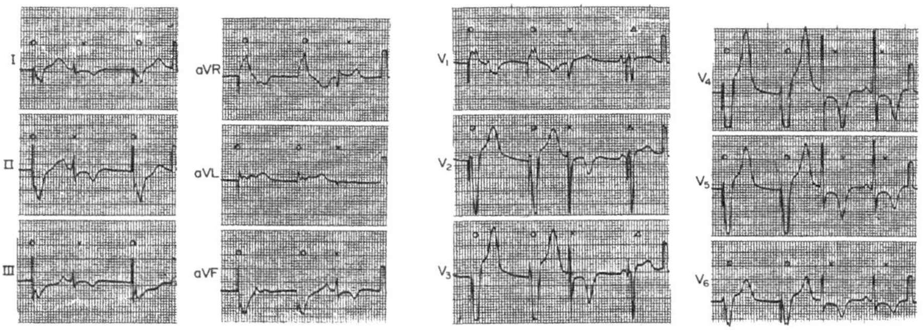

Fig. 8.37
In a 72-year-old woman with sick sinus syndrome, demand artificial pacing (DDI) produced conducted beats (x), with deeply inverted T waves. Note the similarity in the directions of the inverted T and the paced QRS complex (o, paced beat; Δ, fusion beat)

to myocardial ischemia, evaluation of ECG changes is problematic [16]. Although real myocardial ischemia has been occasionally attributed to esophageal reflux, ECG changes did not occur with decrease in the esophageal pH [385]. Upper gastrointestinal endoscopy is associated with sinus tachycardia, ST segment depression, and in some patients, evidence of myocardial ischemia by cardiac scintigraphy [386]; no protective effect was documented by sedation or supplemental oxygen, and the tachycardia rather than hypoxemia was found to be the mediator of ST segment depression [387, 388]. Myocardial ischemia with ST segment depression or elevation during colonoscopy (under conscious sedation and without supplementary oxygen) may be associated with tachycardia and/or hypoxemia, while probably viscerocardiac reflexes may be contributing to the pathogenesis of myocardial ischemia [389]. In general, arousal of the sympathetic nervous system, sinus tachycardia, atrial and ventricular ectopy, and ST segment deviations are noted, particularly in elderly patients and/or those with cardiac disease, and supplemental oxygen, sedation, and monitoring during and after endoscopic procedures is recommended. A frequent affliction, the "irritable bowel syndrome" is associated with palpitations [390], and functional gastric dilatation may present with atypical chest pain and dramatic T wave inversions, resolving with gastric decompression [391].

8.21 Renal Disease and Hemodialysis

Renal diseases, with the culminating coronary artery disease and hypertension, may lead to all the commonly encountered ECG abnormalities of these complications. Patients with renal failure and pericarditis/pericardial effusion may have the expected ECG changes (see ➋ Sect. 8.16), and those with end stage disease show increase in ECG voltage after hemodialysis, most probably due to alleviation of fluid overload [392–394]. Patients with renal failure suffer an excessive mortality, particularly cardiovascular in nature and due to sudden death [395], and their ECGs reveal abnormal late potentials [396], decreased heart rate variability [397], and prolongation of the P wave and QTc intervals [398, 399]. Some of these changes may become accentuated with hemodialysis but a confounding influence contributing to these abnormalities may be the fluid shifts which such patients experience [400].

8.22 Psychiatric Disease

Psychiatric disease aggravates the condition of patients with coronary artery disease or heart failure. In addition, psychiatric disease, in the absence of cardiac disease, increases mortality. Psychiatric disorders are linked to autonomic dysregulations, and heart rate variability (HRV) is reduced in patients with major depression, panic disorders, Alzheimer's disease, and schizophrenia [401]. The magnitude of HRV reduction correlates with the severity of the depression and there is suspicion that these dysregulations are partly responsible for the increased mortality in patients with psychiatric disease. Mostly reduced parasympathetic activity, but also elevated sympathetic activities have been found in psychiatric patients. Antidepressive therapy with serotonin reuptake inhibitors has failed to improve the prognosis of these patients. Anorexia nervosa, bulimia, depression, anxiety, and panic attacks prolong QTc, while weight recovery in patients with anorexia nervosa reduces the increased QT duration and QT dispersion [402]. Such patients with psychiatric disease and QT abnormalities should be evaluated for underlying hypokalemia [403]. Certain antipsychotic drugs cause T wave changes and QTc prolongation and confer an arrhythmic risk to patients with psychiatric disease [404]. Although ECG screening of all patients with psychiatric disease is felt not to be cost-effective, the high prevalence of electrophysiologic abnormalities in such patients and the importance of monitoring such prognostic parameters, as the above, and their response to drug therapy, emphasizes the importance of routine use of the ECG [405].

8.23 Non-Specific ST-T Changes

The "non-specific ST-T changes" designation is employed widely by electrocardiographers, mostly without adherence to specific criteria. Implicitly this diagnosis encompasses "mild" ST-T alterations for some, while others refer to criteria (<0.1 mV ST segment elevation or depression with or without flattened or inverted T waves <0.5 mV) [406]. Although such changes can be found as a normal variant, or as a response to many drugs, other environmental influences or substances, and in a large array of pathological conditions, most often there is no explanation for their presence. Since many causes lead to similar ECG appearances, the designation "non-specific ST-T changes" in describing these changes is appropriate. The term "non specific" is employed in contrast to "specific", e.g. the tall T waves of hyperkalemia; however, even "specific" changes can occasionally occur without a specific inciting pathology. Interpretation of ST-T changes should always take into consideration the clinical context. A partial list of conditions causing non specific ST-T changes, contained in a book, includes 90 items [406].

Non specific ST-T changes are frequently the reason for cardiology consultation (e.g. in healthy pregnant women) (➋ Fig. 8.38) (see ➋ Sect. 8.27), and the cause for anxiety or iatrogenic disease, in normal subjects [407]. Only up to 8% of patients presenting to an emergency department with chest pain and normal ECG or non specific ST-T changes were diagnosed with an acute myocardial infarction [408]. Also, transient ST segment changes were found in up to 8% of patients' ambulatory ECG recordings in the absence of coronary artery disease [409]. Non specific ST-T changes were detected in ambulatory ECG monitoring after meals, with the Valsalva maneuver, and with a change in body position [410].

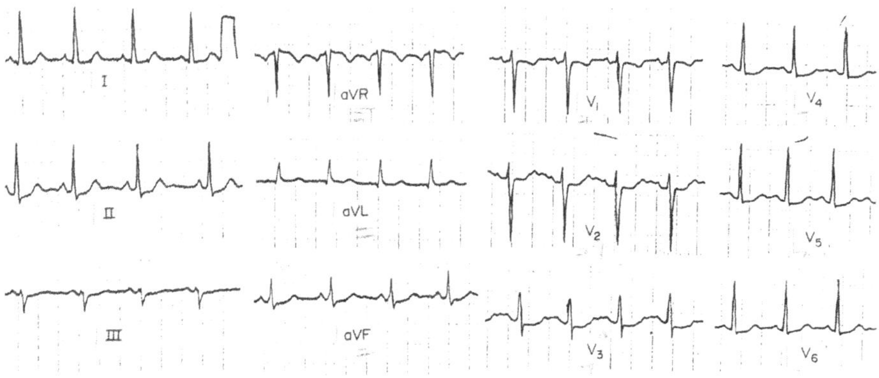

Fig. 8.38
ECG of a young woman 24 weeks pregnant who was referred for evaluation after a heart murmur was detected; this turned out to be a functional murmur, and echocardiography showed a hyperdynamic normal-sized heart

Variation in anatomical position of the heart and the spread of excitation and repolarization may generate a wide range of normalcy. Multiple gradients of repolarization are generated, with cancellation from simultaneously recovering territories, resulting in the appearance of what is called normal ST-T waves. When cardiac activation is abnormal, such gradients are altered, their cancellation patterns are different, and the associated changes in the shape of action potentials (particularly the slope and duration of phases 2 and 3) conspire to produce ST-T wave abnormalities. These types of changes, called "secondary" changes, are due to abnormal activation seen with bundle branch blocks or ventricular hypertrophies, in distinction from "primary" ST-T wave abnormalities resulting from alterations of the recovery process per se. [131]. Examples of the latter are changes imparted by various cardiac and non-cardiac conditions, and drugs. Non specific ST-T changes may be similar in morphology and amplitude to the above "primary" and "secondary" changes.

8.24 Giant and Low Voltage ECG Complexes and Waves

The "giant" ECG voltage characterization is often employed without criteria, although it is occasionally used for high amplitude T waves, e.g., T amplitude >1.0 mV is considered a diagnostic demarcation [406]. Conventionally, low voltage ECG is diagnosed when the QRS peak to peak voltage is ≤0.5 mV in the limb leads and ≤1 mV in the precordial leads.

8.24.1 Giant R Waves

Giant R waves are noted transiently with myocardial infarction (MI) (➊ Fig. 8.39) [411], Prinzmetal's angina (➊ Fig. 8.40) [412], and during exercise stress testing (➊ Fig. 8.41) [413]. Often they appear as monophasic QRS complexes with merging of the QRS and ST segment, some widening of QRS, and in the presence of tachycardia may simulate ventricular tachycardia [414]. Mechanistically, giant R waves may represent intraventricular (unopposed) ventricular conduction delay [415].

8.24.2 Positive Giant T Waves

If positive or negative T waves >1.0 mV are considered as "giant", their incidence is frequent. Positive "giant T waves" are seen with electrolytic abnormalities, Prinzmetal's angina, hyperacute phase of MI, hyperkalemia, and rarely cerebrovascular accidents [406]. Transient positive giant T waves are seen in leads V_1–V_3 in posterior MI, left ventricular hypertrophy

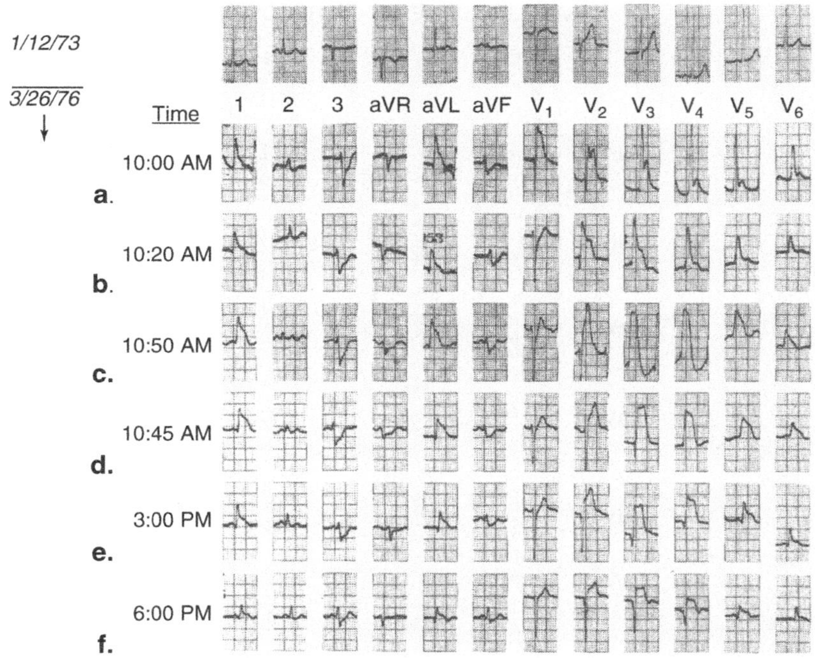

Fig. 8.39
ECG of a 43-year-old man who presented minutes after onset of chest pain; an acute myocardial infarction (MI) was associated with early changes in the amplitude and duration of the QRS complexes before the emergence of the classic ECG changes of MI (Reproduced from Ref. [411]. With permission of the *Journal of Electrocardiology*)

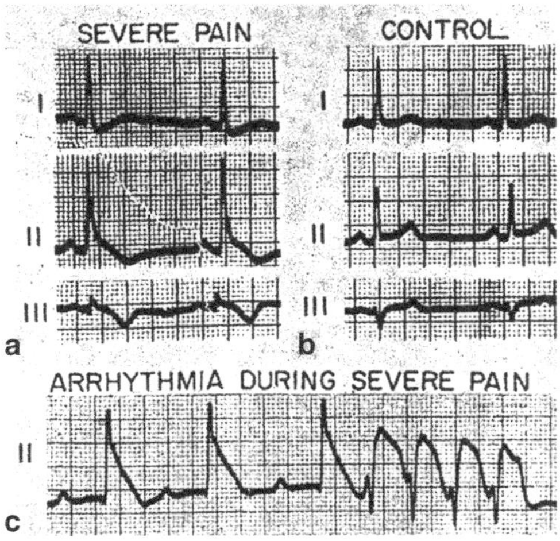

Fig. 8.40
ECG of a 42-year-old man, subjected to anginal attacks of Prinzmetal's angina; increase in the amplitude of the R wave particularly in lead II (a) in comparison with the resting ECG (b) occurred and was followed by ST segment elevation. A burst of ventricular tachycatrdia occurred at the peak of the attack (c) (Reproduced from Ref. [412]. With permission of the *Journal of the American Medical Association*)

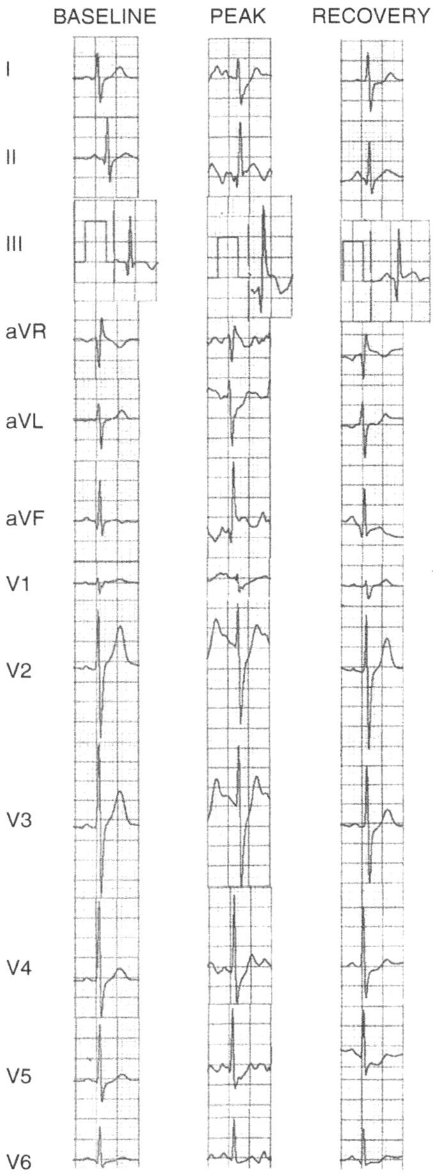

Fig. 8.41
Exercise stress ECG from a 39-year-old man who showed transient increase in the amplitude of R-wave in leads II, III, and aVF; cardiac enzymes did not rise after the stress test, coronary arteriography revealed three-vessel coronary artery disease with an occluded right coronary artery, and a left ventricular ejection fraction of 75% with mild hypokinesis of the inferior ventricular wall (Reproduced from Ref. [413]. With permission of the *Journal of Electrocardiology*)

and left bundle branch block, and in left precordial leads in association with aortic and mitral regurgitation and other left ventricular volume overload states [299]. Positive giant T waves are very occasionally encountered in the early phase of acute pericarditis, or as a normal variant in early repolarization with occasionally marked (➋ Fig. 8.3), but most often modest, ST segment elevation. Automated ECG interpretation often ascribes the positive giant T waves to "metabolic abnormalities".

8.24.3 Negative Giant T Waves

Many clinical entities are associated with negative "giant T waves", pointing to a common underlying ventricular repolarization disturbance [416–421], but with diverse pathophysiological underpinnings, or rarely as a normal variant in young subjects [406], particularly of the black race. A variety of morphologies of the negative giant T waves are encountered in different leads and in different patients associated with abnormalities in the ST segment and prolongation of the QT interval. Deeply inverted T waves and QT prolongation, both being abnormalities of ventricular repolarization, often coexist in many conditions. T wave morphology is not expected to change from a diffuse increase of the action-potential duration, which results however in a QT prolongation, as in hypocalcemia. On the other hand, T wave changes imply underlying regional differences in the repolarization duration. However, minor local dispersion of the action potential is often accompanied by QT prolongation. Theoretically the negative giant T waves could be due to shortening of the action potentials somewhere in the ventricles. In general, negative giant T waves are almost always associated with some QT prolongation, but the separation of the ECG entities of negative giant T waves with and without QT interval prolongation may be useful. Furthermore, mild QT interval prolongation may not have the same diagnostic and prognostic significance as marked QT prolongation. The particulars of prolonged congenital and acquired long QT interval are dealt with in ➋ Chap. 7, while here the focus is mainly on the negative giant T waves.

8.24.3.1 Myocardial Infarction and Ischemic Heart Disease

Symmetrical negative giant T waves are frequently found in patients with MI in the subacute phase and beyond, and in leads overlying the infarcted territory. Also, they are seen in non-ST segment elevation or non-Q wave MIs (➋ Fig. 8.42), angina pectoris, and variant angina [422–425]. Some prolongation of the QT interval is seen in the above conditions, suggesting a repolarization delay of the ischemic territory, and explains the interest in employing the QT interval as a prognostic index [426–428].

8.24.3.2 Ventricular Hypertrophy and Hypertrophic Cardiomyopathy

Occasionally, secondary negative giant T waves are seen in leads V_1–V_4 with right ventricular hypertrophy (RVH) [416], particularly in association with the acute right ventricular pressure overload of pulmonary embolism. Similar T waves in leads V_4–V_6, with less impressive changes in the limb leads, and tall R waves in V_2 and V_3 resembling the pattern of RVH are noted in the "Japanese" hypertrophic cardiomyopathy with confinement of hypertrophy to the apical region (➋ Figs. 8.43 and ➋ 8.44) [429–431]. The above ECG picture evolves gradually over the course of many years and then

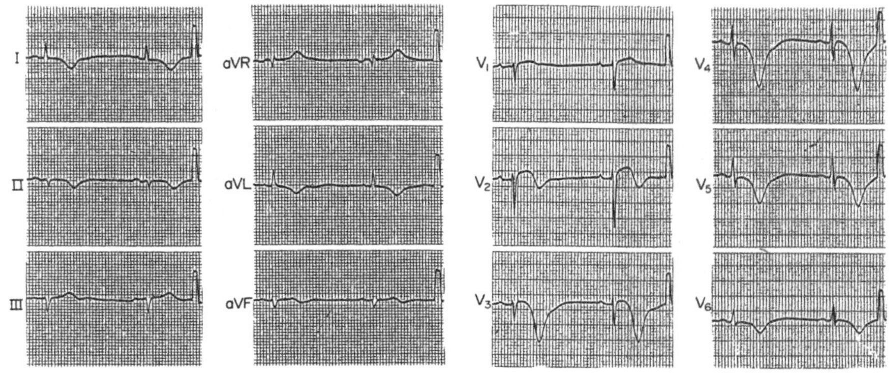

Fig. 8.42
Negative "giant T waves" in the ECG recorded from a 70-year-old woman with anterior and inferior myocardial infarction

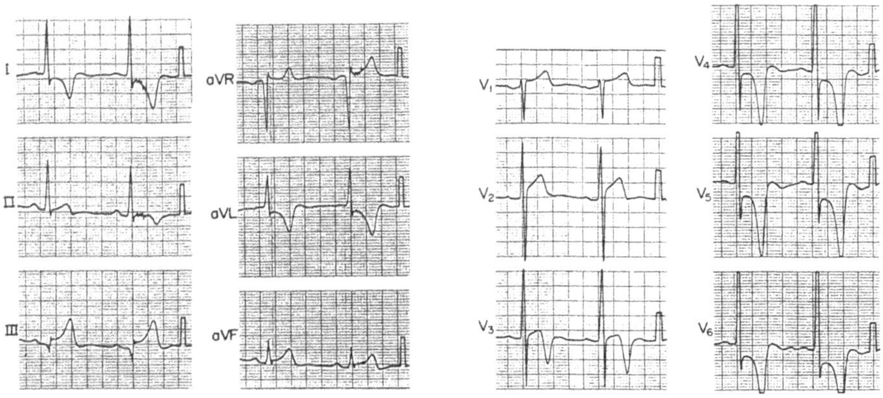

Fig. 8.43
ECG showing negative "giant T-waves" in a 55-year-old man with apical hypertrophic cardiomyopathy

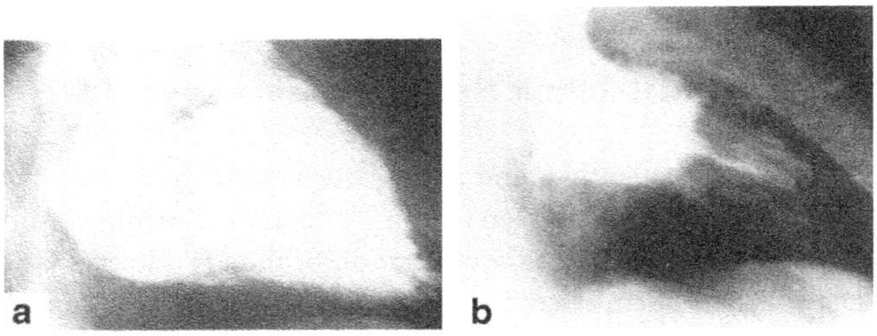

Fig. 8.44
Ventriculogram at end diastole (a) and end systole (b) of the patient whose ECG is shown in Figs. 8.43 and 6.44

may persist for a long time. Some QT interval prolongation, attributed to a recovery delay of the abnormal hypertrophic myocardium, is usually seen in these patients. Similar T wave abnormalities may be found in other cardiomyopathies [277, 432].

8.24.3.3 Central Nervous System

Negative giant T waves resembling changes found in MI may be seen in patients with cerebral pathology, e.g. brain tumors, or subarachnoid hemorrhage (Fig. 8.45), [418, 433–441]. Frequently, pronounced QT interval prolongation and occasionally abnormal Q waves are also noted. Similar ECG changes have been reported in brain surgery and cranial injuries [442, 443]. Subarachnoid hemorrhage and lesions in the frontal cortex and basal portion of the brain are frequent correlates of these ECG abnormalities, and are probably due to abnormal autonomic nervous system discharges and electrolyte or other metabolic problems (see Sect. 8.7.1).

8.24.3.4 Electrolyte Abnormalities

Myocardial repolarization disturbances are frequently linked to abnormal serum electrolyte concentration [13, 419]; prominent U waves with hypokalemia and QT prolongation with hypocalcemia are prime examples. Such conditions are rarely associated with significant T wave abnormalities, since they exert a diffuse influence on the myocardium. Nevertheless in severe or chronic K^+ or Ca^{2+} deficiencies, deeply inverted T waves, marked ST segment changes, and ventricular arrhythmias have been noted [25, 416, 444]. The underlying mechanism appears to be the changes in the membrane or

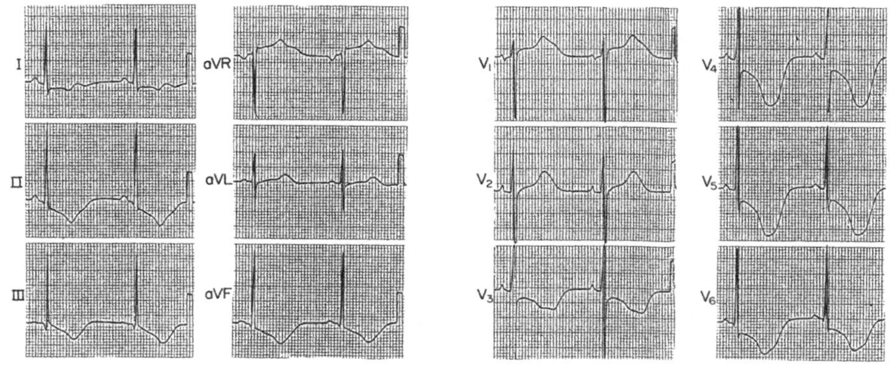

Fig. 8.45
Giant negative T-waves with prolonged QTU-interval in a 55-year-old woman with subarachnoid hemorrhage, resembling myocardial ischemia (compare with Figs. 8.42 and 6.43)

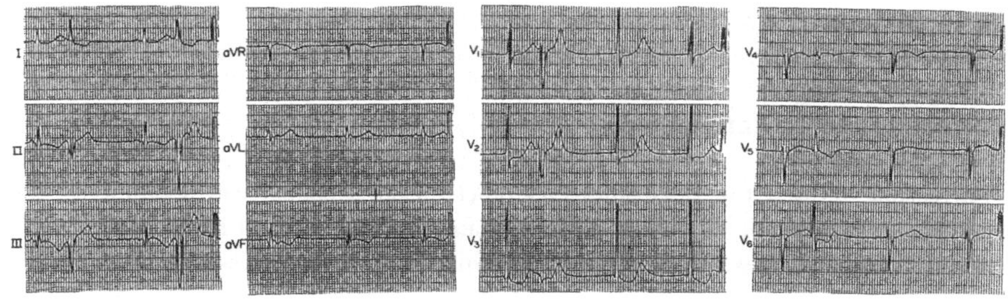

Fig. 8.46
Markedly prolonged QT interval, ST-T abnormalities, and negative T waves in leads II, III and aVF. T-waves seen in a 62-year-old woman with an inferior myocardial infarction, potassium of 2.5 mEq L^{-1}, and digoxin level of 1.8 ng mL^{-1}. The T wave was normalized after these values became normal

intracellular distribution of ions and an enhanced sensitivity to sympathetic activity. Myocardial ischemia, infarction and high serum digoxin level may complicate the picture further (Fig. 8.46).

8.24.3.5 Sympathetic Nerves and Catecholamines

Clinical doses of catecholamines administered to normal subjects lead to sinus tachycardia, minor changes in the morphology of QRS complex, and flattening of the T waves [445, 446]; these are partly caused by the β_2-mediated lowering of the serum potassium level [446, 447]. Slight shortening in the action potential duration of normal ventricular muscle has been observed with isoproterenol [448–450], but such changes could alter the ECG drastically. Negative giant T waves can be generated with unilateral stimulation of the stellate ganglion or local application of catecholamines [451–454]. Right and left sympathetic nerves innervate the anterior and posterior aspects of the ventricles, respectively [455], and thus when either of the right and left sides is stimulated, a small local difference in repolarization leads to T wave changes.

In contrast, high doses of catecholamines superimposed on myocardial pathology or electrolyte abnormalities could influence the ECG markedly [456, 457]. Accordingly, negative giant T waves can be produced by experimental isoproterenol infusions combined with a high calcium environment [458]. Repeated or chronic catecholamine exposure may have somewhat different outcomes from that of acute single dose administration. Negative giant T waves have been

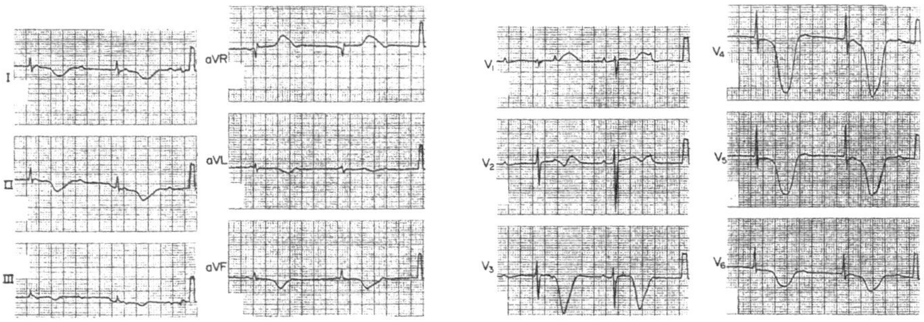

Fig. 8.47
ECG of a 76-year-old woman with complete AV block and giant negative T-waves

reported with pheochromocytoma [459, 460], and it is probable that the effect of catecholamines is modified by underlying myocardial ischemia, abnormalities in electrolyte distribution, or other reasons. Also catecholamines could induce focal toxic "myocarditis" and cardiomyopathy [461, 462].

8.24.3.6 AV Block and Heart-Rate Change

Occasionally in bradycardia, in the setting of advanced AV block, negative giant T waves with marked QT prolongation have been observed (➋ Fig. 8.47) [416, 417]. Bizarre repolarization waves are most likely to occur after Adams-Stokes attacks resulting from tachyarrhythmias, where abnormalities in the recovery process are, in turn, considered to predispose to ventricular arrhythmias (VT) and initiate repeated attacks over a period of time. Hence, it is often difficult to determine which is the primary event. Similar repolarization abnormalities have been seen in association with torsades de pointes [463, 464], suggesting a common underlying mechanism; this atypical VT is caused by certain antiarrhythmic drugs and other agents (see ➋ Chap. 7).

Post-tachycardia inverted T waves, not necessarily with marked QT prolongation, have been observed after the termination of supraventricular or ventricular tachycardia [465, 466]. Inverted T waves, not always of the "giant" variety, have been observed also after artificial ventricular pacing [467, 468], but since the pacing rate inducing them is not high (as in the post-tachycardia states) the mechanism is different (see ➋ Sect. 8.19). Of similar mechanism are the changes noted after transient or intermittent LBBB [469], and radiofrequency catheter ablation of accessory bypass tracts [470]; in the latter case the T wave changes secondary to such tracts are replaced after ablation by the "memory" primary T wave changes [471].

8.24.3.7 Antiarrhythmic Drugs and Miscellaneous Conditions

The list of drugs leading to ST-T changes, with QT prolongation and ventricular arrhythmias, is perpetually expanding. Association with negative giant T waves is not reported with all such drugs, but since they cause long QTc or ventricular arrhythmias, they are considered as potential causes of giant T waves. Since these agents primarily prolong the QT interval, they are dealt with in ➋ Chap. 7. During angiography (see ➋ Sect. 8.29.6) and surgical procedures [472–476], low temperature and tissue injuries may also be responsible for pronounced ST-T abnormalities.

8.24.4 Low Voltage ECG

The "low voltage ECG" is characterized by a decrease in amplitude of all components of the ECG curve; thus the P waves, the QRS complex and the T waves are of low amplitude, although diagnostic criteria conventionally refer only to the

QRS complexes. Traditionally the list of conditions associated with the low voltage ECG includes among others, obesity, emphysema, pneumothorax, pericardial and pleural effusions, infiltrative heart disease, multiple MIs, and myocarditis [477]; also other factors can induce such ECG changes (see Sect. 8.25.6).

8.25 Extracardiac Factors

Amplitude, morphology, and orientation of the various components of the ECG curve are influenced by a number of factors exerting an effect beyond the heart's surface. What is recorded at the body surface are "residual currents" after the extracardiac influences (pericardial, and body volume conductor) have exerted their effects on the currents emanating from the heart [217]. Additionally, the intracavitary blood volume influences the potentials recorded at the body surface [478].

8.25.1 Heart-Electrode Distance

Distance of the heart from the chest wall (and therefore from the recording electrode), irrespective of the intervening tissues and organs, affects the surface ECG voltage [479]. The prime example of such influence is the large voltages recorded in the precordial leads in comparison with the unipolar limb leads [480]. The drop of ECG voltage is precipitous, as the "exploring" electrode is positioned at gradually increasing distances from the heart, and this relationship follows the inverse square law. The increase in the V_4–V_6 QRS voltage in tachycardia may be due to the enhanced closeness of the heart's "centroid" to the chest wall precipitated by a reduction of its volume due to tachycardia [118]; hypovolemia leading to an underfilling of the heart may exert a similar influence. These associations are discordant to what is expected as a result of "Brody effect" [478].

8.25.2 Body Habitus

Anthropometric designations of ectomorphic, mesomorphic, or endomorphic with their attendant different amount and proportion and distribution of muscle and fat, have an effect on the appearance of ECG, which is exerted via the variation in the heart-electrode distance (see Sect. 8.25.1), and heart position (see Sect. 8.25.3). The chest configuration also influences potentials. The ECG of emaciated patients may show enormous deflections in all leads [481], while thin-chested individuals have such changes only in precordial leads [482]. Both factors prevent great losses in potentials on the way to the body surface (Wilson's "proximity effect") [480]. Muscular or obese (see Sect. 8.26) individuals, or those with large cylindrical chests have attenuated potentials. Consequently knowledge of the patient's height, weight, and body build is useful in accurately interpreting the ECG.

8.25.3 Heart Position

The anatomical versus "electrical" heart positions should be viewed as distinct, with the former however influencing the latter. There is a relation between the ECG and the anatomical position of the heart in the thorax [479]; thus a vertical position of the QRS loop is found with a vertical anatomical axis of the heart, as seen in lean subjects and/or with a low-positioned diaphragm, while a leftward rotation of the loop is seen with transversely placed heart in association with a raised diaphragm in a stocky individual and/or with a prominent abdomen. In a person with average body build the anatomic and electrical orientation of the heart is from upper right to lower left. In slender tall individuals the heart is anatomically more vertical and shows a vertical axis [482], while it is more horizontal in heavy-set corpulent subjects who have more squat hearts [481]. Occasionally, there is a discordance of the anatomical and electrical axes of the heart.

Rotations of the body and heart can be about the sagittal body axis (e.g. dextrocardia), the anatomical longitudinal axis of the heart or the long axis of the body, or the transverse axis (anterior or posterior position of the apex).

The last is associated with low QRS voltage in the frontal plane, as with emphysema. Similar changes are seen in congestive heart failure (CHF), and can be attributed to the left ventricular posterior displacement due to right ventricular dilatation in patients with CHF [301]. Even Q waves can be found in some ECG leads as a result of an unusual position of the heart. The P waves and T waves are also affected, and the R/S ratios may be changed markedly. Physiological and pathological changes in the position of the diaphragm, i.e. pregnancy (see ❯ Sect. 8.27), obesity (see ❯ Sect. 8.26), ascites, and tumors may resemble the ECG appearances of deep expiration, while emphysema, asthma, and wasting mimic the state of deep inspiration. All these changes can be compounded by pathological alterations, thus becoming atypical. The "electrical centers" or "centers of gravity" of the atrial and ventricular depolarization and their relationship to various positions of surface electrodes determine the ECG appearance [481].

8.25.4 Body Posture

Different body positions influence the ECG, since they change the relationship of the heart with the recording electrodes; this may apply particularly for lateral decubitus and for prone, in contrast to supine, body positions. Both stable ECGs in the supine, sitting, and standing positions, using the standard and the Mason-Likar exercise testing electrode "hook-up" [483, 484] (❯ Fig. 8.48), and decrease in the R wave amplitude in the standing position has been reported [485]. A heart rate increase is expected by assuming the sitting and standing positions [484, 485]. Nevertheless, mild T wave changes and alterations of repolarization occur with change in position [486]. Also, non-specific ST-T changes, tall P waves in leads II and III, and right QRS frontal axis deviation have been recorded in young patients with a labile autonomic nervous system on assuming the upright position [481]. Since the ECG is routinely recorded in a supine body posture, changes are expected mostly in ambulatory ECG recordings, where drastic variation of the entire PQRST curve has been noted with

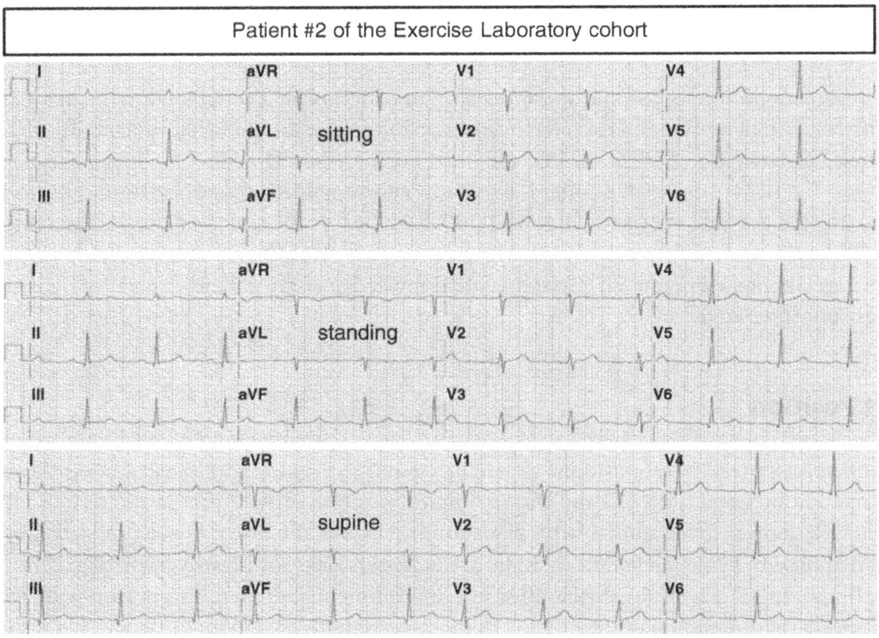

Fig. 8.48
ECGs in the sitting, standing and supine positions, employing the Mason-Likar electrode "hook-up", from a patient undergoing a Bruce treadmill exercise stress test, were similar in appearance (Reproduced from Ref. [484]. With permission of the *Journal of Electrocardiology*)

different body postures [487]. Lying on the right or left side, or the prone position produces expected ECG alterations (shift of the entire PQRST three dimensional vector loop toward the lowest body point). The R wave in V_5 increases in amplitude in the left decubitus position [479]. Absence of changes in the amplitude and frontal axis of QRS complexes in the standard bipolar ECG leads with lying on the right and left sides is indicative of pathology causing fixation of the heart in the thorax (adhesive pericardiomediastinitis) [488]. Also, the inelastic dilated lungs of an emphysematous patient can lead to a "fixation" of the heart in the thorax, leading to a stable ECG, unaffected by changes in the body position [481]. Perhaps recording of the ECG in the standing position, in a patient who complains of orthostatic symptoms, may be more informative of his/her condition than the traditional recording in the supine position; ECGs recorded during "tilt table" testing may not be equivalent to those recorded in self-supported standing patients, and thus the latter should also be employed [484].

8.25.5 Respiration

The frontal QRS axis is deflected to the right in inspiration and to the left in expiration [489] (➋ Fig. 8.49). Lead III is particularly affected, and its positivity of P, R, and T waves may be increased, or be reversed especially in deep inspiration and expiration respectively [482]. Of diagnostic significance for non existing inferior myocardial infarction is the conversion of a considerable Q wave to a nonpathological q wave or even to an R wave in lead III, during deep inspiration. Also morphological changes are seen in the QRS complex related to the projection of a changed loop in its 3D space orientation, on the recording thoracic electrode lattice. Of course, the outcome of deep inspiration depends on the amplitude and polarity of waves and complexes at expiration. ECG changes due to respiration reflect a special and reproducible change in the heart's position (see ➋ Sect. 8.25.3), [489] along with other electrophysiological influences not examined herein.

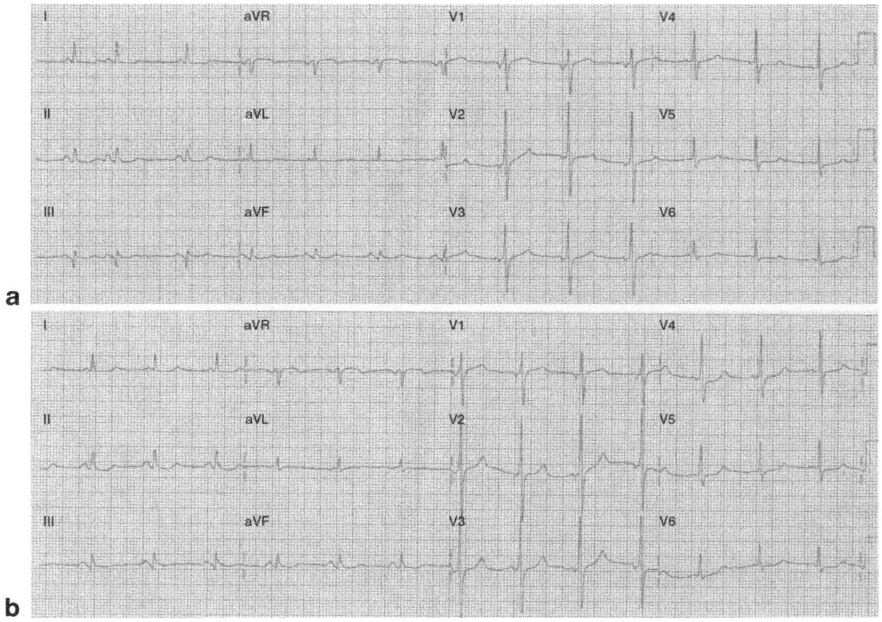

➋ Fig. 8.49
ECGs of a 63-year-old patient with history of coronary artery disease and chronic obstructive lung disease, obtained in the supine position at the points of modest expiration (a) and inspiration (b) showing a corresponding shift of the frontal QRS axis from 20° to 52°

8.25.6 Peripheral Edema

Peripheral edema of varying etiology (sepsis, pneumonia, chronic obstructive lung disease, congestive heart failure [CHF], end stage-renal failure) leads to attenuation of all parts of the ECG curve [1, 490], which is more prominent in the limb and lateral precordial leads. Some of these changes do not necessarily reach the point of "low voltage" ECG. Peripheral edema in supine patients involves more the dorsal torso due to gravity. Also, due to the eccentric anterior/lateral position of the heart in the chest, V_5 and V_6 are much more affected than V_1 and V_2 (➋ Fig. 8.50). Weight gain due to peripheral edema correlates well with the reduction of the amplitude of QRS complexes [1]. Augmentation of the ECG voltage (the inverse phenomenon) has also been observed with treatment of peripheral edema due to CHF [491, 492] (➋ Fig. 8.51), or after hemodialysis [493, 494]. The attenuation of the QRS complexes in the limb leads reflect the overall (peripheral/distal changes) while the changes in the precordial leads reflect also the influence of peripheral edema on local thoracic ECG expression [1]. Clinical consequence of this phenomenon is the false negative ECG diagnosis of left ventricular hypertrophy [495], as well as atrial abnormalities [496].

The attenuation of the ECG voltage with peripheral edema appears to be due to a decreased electrical impedance of the passive volume conductor influencing the transfer of cardiac potentials from the surface of the heart to the recording sites [1, 217]. Other consequences of peripheral edema are shortening of the QRS and the QT intervals, which are attributed to a measurement failure in detection of early onset and late offset of these intervals resulting from the overall attenuation of the ECG curves [497, 498]. There may be clinical implications of these shortenings of the QRS and QT durations for patients with heart failure and peripheral edema who are being considered for cardioverter/defibrillator implantation, or biventricular resynchronization pacing [490]. Continuous impedance monitoring incorporated in the permanent pacemakers can be employed to monitor the intrathoracic edema in patients with heart failure [499]; the principle involved is similar to the one discussed above to explain the changes in the ECG amplitude with peripheral edema, although applied locally.

8.26 Obesity

Traditionally low voltage ECG comes to mind in association with obesity, resulting from increase in the distance of the heart from the recording electrodes due to the excess of adipose tissue. In addition, some influence must be exerted by the resistivity characteristics of the fat, which may increase the amplitude of body surface potentials [217]. The condition also tends to shift the frontal axis to the left, due to elevation of the diaphragm (see ➋ Sect. 8.25.3); such a shift may lead to a false diagnosis of an inferior myocardial infarction [500]. Increases in the QRS amplitude, QRS duration, QTc and PR intervals, and heart rate have also been reported in obesity [501]; increase in the cardiac workload leading to left ventricular hypertrophy may be the reasons for this. ECG abnormalities change after bariatric surgery for obesity but are not eliminated [502]. Liquid protein diets result in QTc or QTUc prolongation, ST-T abnormalities, left axis deviation, torsade de pointes, and ventricular fibrillation [503, 504].

8.27 Pregnancy

Although pregnancy is associated with augmented blood volume and cardiac output, the ECG of most pregnant women is normal. In the late stages of pregnancy, sinus tachycardia is frequently present, and the frontal QRS axis gradually shifts leftward or towards horizontal, or rarely even rightward due to elevation of the left hemidiaphragm, consequent to uterine enlargement [505]. Also with advancing pregnancy, atrial and ventricular premature beats are common. In young women during pregnancy, first onset of reentrant supraventricular tachycardias (RSVT) is rare, but symptoms of recurrent RSVT are exacerbated [506]. AV conduction defects are extremely rare, and they are of the 2° AV block

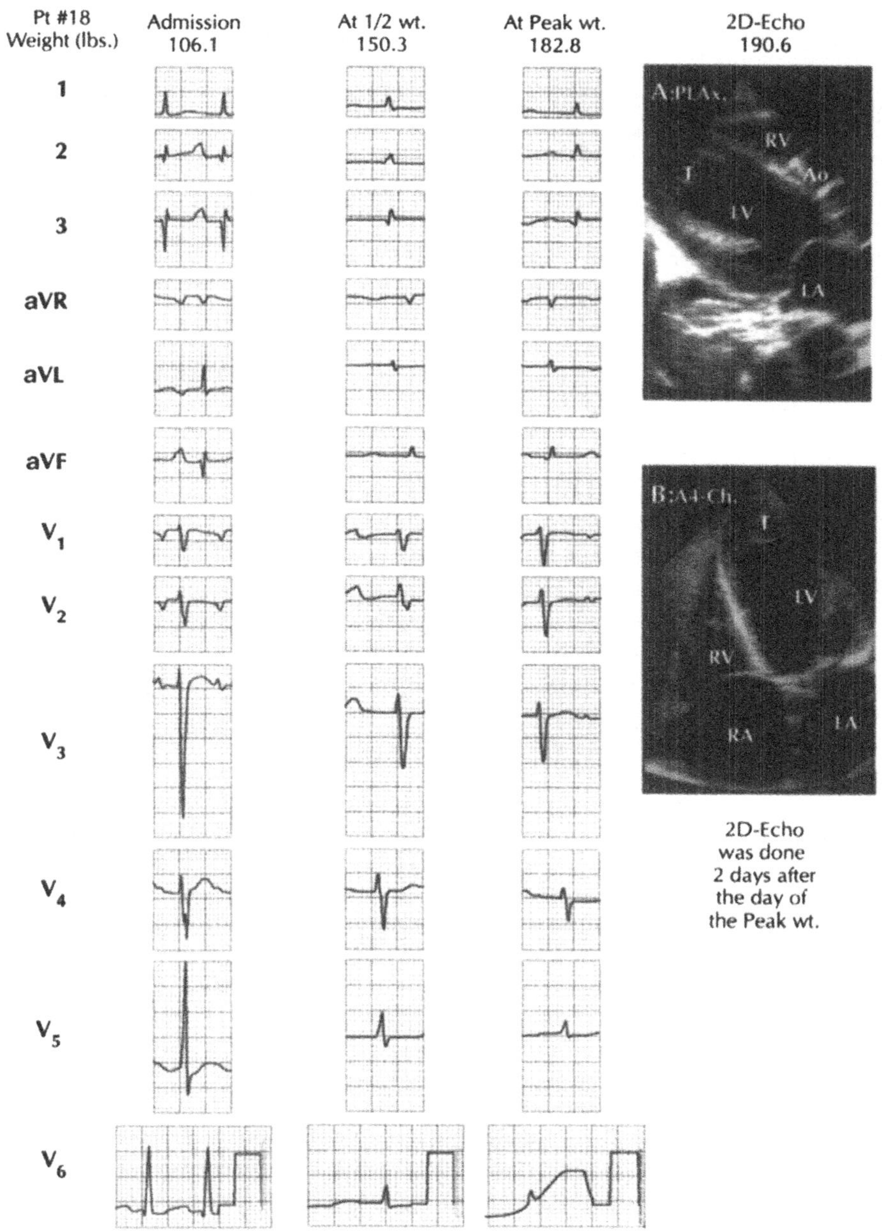

Fig. 8.50
ECGs of a 53-year-old man who had suffered pneumonia and sepsis and in the process had fluid overload gaining 84.5 lbs showed gradual attenuation of the voltage of his ECGs; an echocardiogram obtained close to the date of the peak fluid accumulation showed that there was no pericardial effusion to account for the attenuated ECG voltage (Reproduced from Ref. [1]. With permission of the *Journal of the American College of Cardiology*)

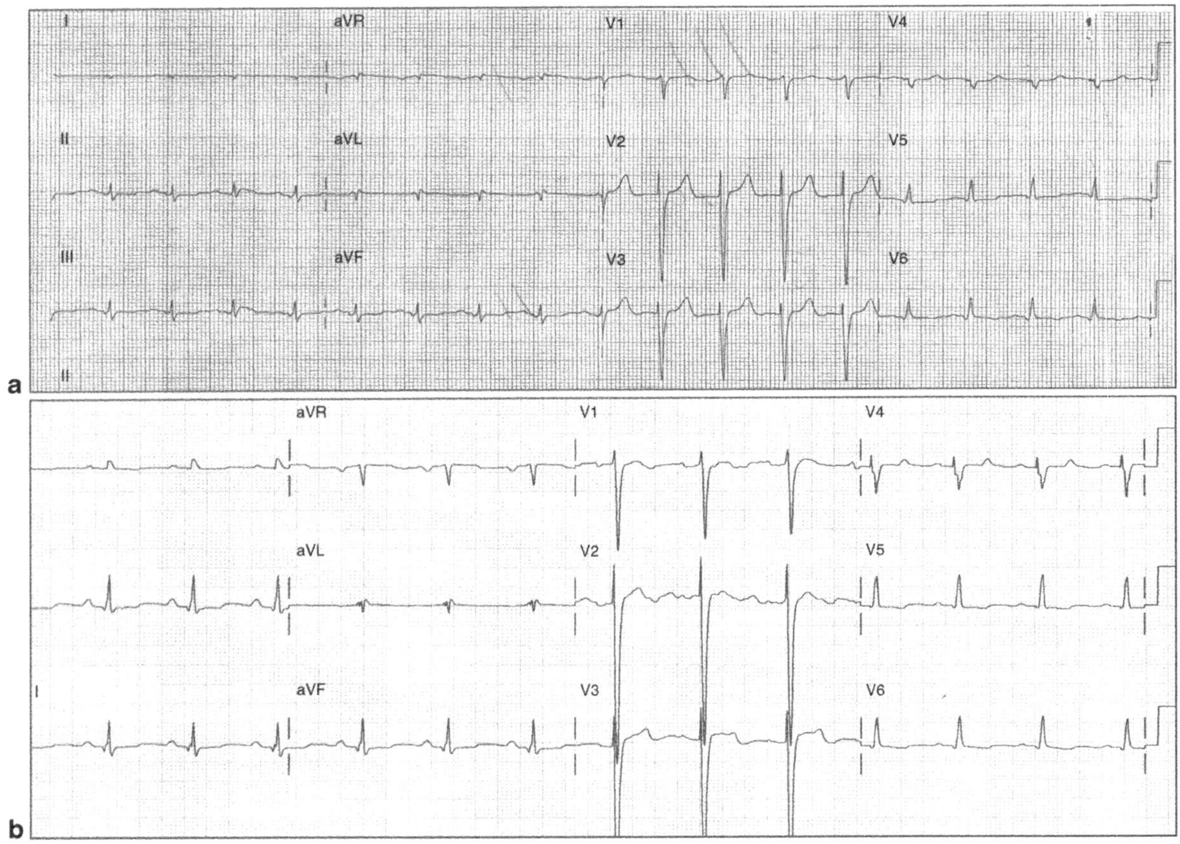

Fig. 8.51

ECGs of a 54-year-old man with congestive heart failure who lost 48 lbs in the course of 2 weeks in response to diuresis, showed augmentation of the voltage of his discharge ECG (b) in comparison with the one from his admission (a) (Reproduced from Ref. [492]. With permission of the *Congestive Heart Failure*)

of Wenckebach type [507]. Increase in size and mass of the left ventricle, as assessed by echocardiography, is occasionally associated with QRS voltage compatible with left ventricular hypertrophy.

Transient ST segment depression with flat or inverted T waves may be registered in both the limb and precordial leads (➋ Fig. 8.38) [508], and such changes are abolished after delivery but may recur with succeeding pregnancies [509]. Follow-up for 20–30 years of women with such changes has not disclosed any pathology. A cause for these ST-T changes has not been found, and myocardial ischemia does not appear to be contributory. Occasionally Q waves with inverted T waves may occur in the limb leads in older patients, suggestive of an inferior myocardial infarction [500] (see ➋ Sect. 8.25.3), but such changes are not registered in aVF and are abolished by deep breathing.

Peripartum cardiomyopathy, a form of an idiopathic congestive cardiomyopathy characteristic of pregnancy, is manifest in a few women during the last month of gestation or the first few months after delivery. It is associated with cardiomegaly and all the hallmarks of heart failure (see ➋ Sect. 8.13.2). Nonspecific ST segment depression and T wave inversions are seen in the ECG of patients afflicted with this condition.

Cardiovascular abnormalities in pregnant women such as hypertension, rheumatic heart disease, congenital heart disease, and obstructive cardiomyopathy may become aggravated, by the increased circulatory load. The ECG tends to show changes in keeping with these associated diseases, occasionally expressing right and/or left ventricular hypertrophy.

8.28 Fetal Electrocardiography

The fetal ECG (FECG), albeit initially of low signal-to-noise ratio and poor quality of tracings, has permitted the detection of the fetal heart rate [510]; the fetal and maternal heart rates are independent of each other in the absence of pathology [511]. To obtain analyzable tracings, amplification of the fetal heart currents is necessary [512], since such currents are expected to be miniscule at the maternal abdominal surface due to the large distance between their source and the recording electrodes, and the short-circuiting effect of the amniotic fluid. The fetal ECG has important clinical applications [513]. Directly applied fetal electrodes and computerized signal-enhancement techniques [514] have led to improvement in the quality of tracings [515]. This, in turn, has provided the basis for correlative studies of ECG parameters (P, QRS, ST amplitudes, heart rate variability) with the condition of the fetus as assessed by laboratory data such as blood gas analysis, blood pH, or hemoglobin content [516]. As a minimum, digital signal processing techniques applied to maternal abdominal fetal ECGs (➋ Fig. 8.52) can improve monitoring and analysis of fetal heart rate [517, 518]. A study of the PR–RR relationship during normal labor found both positive and negative relationship between P-R and R-R intervals, but the latter did not discriminate between bradycardia with or without hypoxemia [519]. The problem of fetal ECG extraction is being addressed by a multitude of innovative techniques [520, 521]. In some of these studies, the intrapartum fetal ECG is obtained by fetal scalp electrodes [522]. Modern fetal electrocardiography has extended its scope to monitoring and analysis of the fetal ST waveforms [519].

8.29 Food, Drink and Other Compounds

8.29.1 Prandial and Postprandial Changes

The effect of eating solid food and drinking fluids, both cold and hot, on the ECG has been reported; changes occur in the T waves with cold [523] and hot drinks, and supraventricular tachyarrhythmias, focal atrial tachycardia, atrial fibrillation, and ischemic ST segment changes have been elicited [524–527]. The arrhythmogenic influences may be due to neural or local sensitivity of the atria or pulmonary veins, while the ST segment changes may partially reflect coronary vasospasm. Water ingestion in normals increased cardiac vagal control, but this is not seen in the elderly, transplant recipients, or subjects with autonomic failure [528]. Tachyarrhythmias, syncope, and silent myocardial ischemia have been observed with swallowing, belching and mastication [529–531]. Post-prandially, exertional angina indicates obstructive coronary artery disease, rest angina reflects an unexplained myocardial oxygen supply deficit [532], and heart rate variability assessment suggests diminished vagal activity [533]. Starvation in ex-prisoners of wars increased QTc duration and dispersion [534], and in patients with anorexia nervosa, enhanced heart rate variability due to increased vagal control was detected [535]; QTc abnormalities in the latter were abolished with oral potassium administration and refeeding [536, 537].

8.29.2 Alcohol

Alcohol drinking induces, in healthy subjects, sinus tachycardia, atrial and ventricular ectopic beats, and prolongation of the P-R, QRS and QTc intervals [538]. The interplay of pathology and alcohol drinking in patients may exacerbate the above, and can cause more abnormalities. Rarely, heavy alcohol drinking leads to myocardial infarction [539]. Sinus

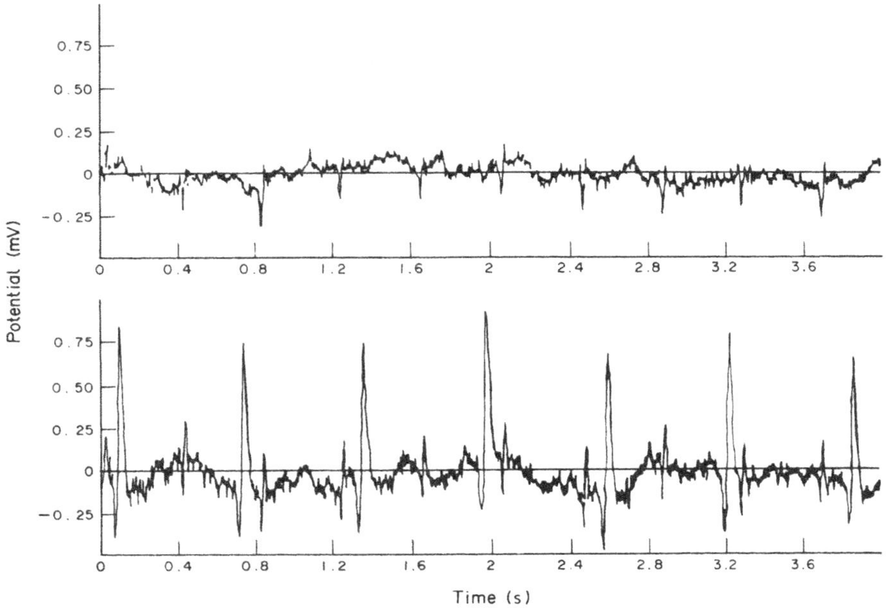

Fig. 8.52
The lower tracing shows the abdominal ECG containing maternal and fetal ECG signals. The upper tracing shows the fetal ECG obtained after mathematical treatment to remove the maternal signal (After van Oosterom. In: Ruttkay I, Macfarlane P, eds. *Electrocardiology* 83, 1984, 175. © Excerpta Medica, Amsterdam. Reproduced with permission)

tachycardia and decrease in heart rate variability is determined by the aldehyde dehydrogenase-2 genotype and is probably mediated by catecholamine secretion [540]. Heavy alcohol drinking may render an implantable cardioverter defibrillator transiently ineffective [541]. Signal averaging of the P waves identifies patients who are prone to alcohol-induced paroxysmal atrial fibrillation [542]. Alcohol withdrawal may culminate in a catecholamine-driven state characterized by ST segment depressions and release of myocardial enzymes [543].

8.29.3 Caffeine

The effective and functional antegrade and retrograde refractory periods of the atrioventricular node decrease after coffee ingestion, most probably due to a rise in catecholamines [544]. In normal adults, even high dose caffeine does not affect the heart rate or cause atrial or ventricular ectopy [545]. Caffeine did not increase the rate of PVCs, ventricular couplets, and ventricular tachycardia in patients with a recent myocardial infarction [546], or even among patients with known life-threatening arrhythmias [547]; also coffee was not associated with risk of atrial fibrillation or flutter [548]. In patients referred with symptomatic idiopathic ventricular premature beats (VPBs), caffeine restriction did not result in significant change in the frequency of VPBs [549].

8.29.4 Tobacco

Smokers have elevated mean heart rates, mediated by sympathetic stimulation, while the vagal cardiac control is not altered. Thus, no change in respiratory sinus arrhythmia is detected [550]. However, environmental tobacco exposure in nonsmokers led to a decrement in the heart rate variability [551]. In ambulatory ECG studies, smokers had a higher heart rate and prevalence of supraventricular and ventricular extrasystoles than non-smokers, and smoking cessation led to reversion of these differences [552]. Electrophysiologic studies at baseline and after smoking showed an increase in heart rate and improved atrioventricular conduction both in patients on and off beta-blockers, suggesting a direct effect of sympathomimetic action of smoking; also atrial and ventricular arrhythmias were not increased by smoking [553]. In the absence of an arrhythmogenic substrate, smoking does not induce late potentials in smokers [554].

8.29.5 Drugs

The tricyclic anti-depressants, not favored any more for treatment of depression, mediate their cardiovascular side effects via a quinidine-like influence and anticholinergic action, leading to sinus bradycardia, prolongation of P-R, QRS and QTc intervals, 2° and 3° AV blocks, and torsade de pointes [555, 556]. Premonitory ECG features of cardiac toxicity include QRS duration >100 ms, and a rightward shift of the terminal 40 ms frontal axis of the QRS vector [556]. Arrhythmias, nonspecific ST-T changes, QTc prolongation and decrease in the amplitude of the QRS complexes have been described with some chemotherapeutic drugs [557]. Although cardiomyopathy due to anthracycline-related toxicity and lethal arrhythmias is well recognized, many other chemotherapeutic drugs are associated with bradycardia, ischemic ST-T changes, myocardial infarction, and serious arrhythmias [16]. The electrophysiologic and ECG effects of drugs are beyond the scope of this chapter; also drug-induced prolongation of QTc is dealt with in ➋ Chap. 7.

8.29.6 Contrast Agents

Employment of contrast agents in cardiac catheterization is associated with frequent ECG changes, like inversion or peaking of the T waves in the inferior leads, prolongation of the QTc and QRS complexes, and significant ST segment shifts [558]. Transient bradycardia, sinus arrest, and various degrees, including complete AV blocks, are encountered. Ventricular fibrillation is reported in 0.6% to 1.3% of patients [559]. Hyperosmolarity mediates partly the toxicity of contrast agents, while transiently induced hypocalcemia may contribute to ventricular fibrillation [560]. Newer contrast agents are lower in osmolarity, and have a lower calcium-binding potential, thus resulting in fewer ECG changes and arrhythmias, including ventricular fibrillation [561].

8.29.7 Illicit Drugs

Amphetamines and cocaine may be associated with ECG changes suggestive of ischemia most probably mediated by a strong sympathomimetic influence, although coronary vasospasm may also be contributing particularly with cocaine [562]. An abundance of literature, mainly case reports, documents occurrence of ST segment deviations, atrial and ventricular arrhythmias, myocardial infarction, QTc prolongation, and decrease in heart rate variability with the use of cocaine.

8.29.8 Poisons

CO poisoning results in ST-T changes reflective of myocardial ischemia, which could culminate in myocardial infarction [563, 564], and may require hyperbaric oxygen administration [565]. CO, in contrast to cyanide, which commonly coexist in exhaust fumes and smoke, led to slowing of AV conduction and ventricular repolarization in animal experiments [566]. Organophosphates lead to acetylcholine accumulation with resultant sinus tachycardia, bradycardia, ST-T changes, prolonged QTc, atrial fibrillation, monomorphic ventricular tachycardia (VT), torsade de pointes, and ventricular fibrillation (VF) [567, 568]. The commonest heavy metal poisoning is with arsenic, and is associated with T wave inversion,

QTc prolongation, torsade de pointes, and VF [569]. Emetine results in a host of ECG changes including T wave alterations, and prolongation of PR, QRS and QT intervals [570]. Antimony poisoning produces flattening and/or inversion of T waves and prolongation of the QTc, particularly in large doses and with prolonged exposure [571]. Poisoning can result from herbal agents used singly in the context of alternative medicine, or by interacting with conventional medications. Bradycardia, heart blocks and VT result from oleander, a cardiac glycoside containing plant [572]. Many toxins from scorpion venoms activate sodium channels and the sympathetic nervous system; scorpion envenomation resulted in 1° atrioventricular block, intraventricular conduction disturbances, predominantly right bundle branch block, reversible ventricular repolarization changes, and arrhythmias [573].

8.30 Physical Activities

8.30.1 Exercise

Exercise and its lack impart certain changes in the ECG. The rapid increase in the heart rate early during exercise is typical of underconditioning, with a much slower heart rate rise encountered in fit individuals. In a study of monozygotic twin pairs discordant for physical fitness, the ones who engaged in more physical activities had ECG evidence of left ventricular hypertrophy (LVH), not corroborated by echocardiography [574]; this suggests a different role of ECG in the assessment of effects of exercise beyond that of the anatomic LVH. Heart rate at 1 or 2 min of recovery after exercise is a prognostic index of mortality [575] and morbidity and should be employed unfailingly. Heart rate variability increases with exercise, even after a single such session or mild exercise in sedentary individuals [576]. T wave alternans during exercise is rarely found in normal subjects [577]. In view of the prognostic importance of the long QTc interval, physicians should look for it when evaluating normal subjects embarking in an exercise program. Swimming, jogging, running, mild, moderate, or heavy exercise, the isotonic or isometric nature of exercise, and the age, sex, weight, and sedentary status of healthy subjects and patients, all are factors influencing the ECG derived diagnostic and prognostic parameters.

8.30.2 Bathing

Bathing and showering is associated with tachycardia, atrial and ventricular extrasystoles and even ventricular tachycardia, particularly in the elderly and during winter [578]; the ambient temperature, the temperature of the bathing water and underlying pathology are influential. Heart rate variability showed changes in the elderly during hot bathing with the LF/HF ratio in the frequency domain analysis decreasing, which suggests a decrease in sympathetic tone predisposing to syncope. The high ambient temperatures of sauna bathing with its resultant reduction in the intraventricular volume is associated with increases in the magnitudes of the R and Q waves in lead Z, and of the S wave in lead X, which contradict the Brody effect [478, 579]. Showering or bathing lead to changes in the autonomic nervous tone, while addition of light exercise in predisposed individuals may lead to myocardial ischemia [580]. Cold packs on the chest wall cause nonspecific ST-T changes [406].

8.30.3 Athlete's Heart

The range of athletic activities is wide, encompassing increase of strength or endurance objectives, length of involvement, status (amateur to elite) and intensity. ECG changes are seen in athletes, in subjects with "athlete's heart", and in athletes with heart disease. These distinctions should be kept in mind. Vagally mediated sinus bradycardia, sinus arrhythmia, escape rhythms (both atrial and ventricular), incomplete right bundle branch block, various atrial and ventricular arrhythmias, all degrees of AV blocks are noted, with the disappearance of many of the above under stress, attesting to the non pathological nature of these findings [581, 582]. Other ECG features often seen in athletes include increased amplitude of Q, R, and S waves, ST segment changes, and T wave flattening or inversion, often mimicking LVH or cardiomyopathy [583]. The ECG is more sensitive in diagnosing athlete's heart than the imaging modalities focusing on change in left ventricular dimensions and myocardial wall thickness. Reversibility of LVH is seen in the ECG of athletes undergoing detraining, who also experience resolution of ventricular extrasystoles and episodes of ventricular tachycardia, and absence of cardiac events at follow-up; all these support the notion that LVH and these rhythm disturbances are of benign nature, or they represent another expression of AH [584]. QT duration and QT dispersion do not increase in athletes, as they do in patients with LVH due to hypertension, even in the presence of LVH [585, 586]. Heart rate variability is increased in athletes [582]. The ECG is used in screening individuals who potentially could be "athletes" – see ➋ Chap. 1.

8.31 Bodily Functions

8.31.1 Sleep

ECGs during sleep may normally show isorhythmic AV dissociation, marked bradycardia, sinus arrhythmia, sinus nodal blocks, 1° and 2° Mobitz AV blocks, and supraventricular and ventricular beats; atrial extrasystoles are less frequent, and ventricular extrasystoles are more frequent, than during wakefulness, while both increase with age [587]. In Holter ECG recordings, long asymptomatic pauses are occasionally seen during sleep, but these should not lead to interventions. Recumbent episodes at night, while awake, cannot be distinguished from sleep in the evaluation of such recordings. Heart rate variability changes during sleep, and is related to changes in the encephalogram and cycles of rapid, and non-rapid, eye movement sleep [588], while QT interval duration increases [589]. Sleep deprivation results in increased sympathetic and decreased parasympathetic cardiovascular modulation [590].

8.31.2 Diurnal Changes

The ECG is subject to diurnal changes; thus the heart rate, cardiac refractoriness and conduction, pacing and defibrillation thresholds, heart rate variability indices, QT duration, QT dispersion and T wave alternans show diurnal variability [591]. Autonomic tone mediated physiologic variations, during eating, sleeping, and exercise result in day-to-day fluctuations in pacing threshold [12], while some have not found a role of the autonomic tone for such variation [592]. Studies of the reproducibility of ECGs over time have disclosed diurnal changes, e.g., the P wave duration and PR interval show a significant circadian variation in healthy subjects [593]. These variations require that the "time" factor is considered in the analysis of electrophysiological and ECG test results, and may provide an explanation for the clustering of clinical "events" at particular time windows. These diurnal changes of electrophysiological/ECG variables are influenced by a large number of factors, e.g. age effect on QT intervals [594], and cardiac pathology.

8.31.3 Sexual Activity

Sexual activity may precipitate ischemic ST segment changes [595] and ventricular arrhythmias [596] in patients with coronary artery disease. In normal subjects, sexual activity leads to sinus tachycardia, equal to 60–70% of maximum predictive value, persisting longer in women [597], and affecting the post exercise heart rate recovery for at least 2 h after sexual activity [598]. All the above changes are modulated by the arousal of the sympathetic nervous system, which exerts an effect on all electrophysiologic and ECG parameters.

8.31.4 Belching, Nausea, Vomiting

Atrial arrhythmias, including atrial fibrillation, can be precipitated by esophageal stimulation during swallowing and belching [599]. Ischemic like ST depression and T wave inversion can be found in patients experiencing nausea [600]. Spontaneous or self-induced vomiting is associated with prolonged QTc, although inter-current pathology or electrolyte abnormalities are confounding factors [601].

8.31.5 Urination and Defecation

Situational syncope is diagnosed with bradycardia immediately after urination or defecation [602]. Profound sinus bradycardia due to increased vagal tone, while straining during a bowel movement, could result in severe cerebral and myocardial hypoperfusion with cardiac arrest, particularly in elderly patients. Syncope during straining is rarely associated with advanced AV blocks necessitating implantation of a permanent pacemaker [603]. Defecation syncope may also occur in patients in the context of alternation of intrinsic and pacemaker rhythms, requiring reprogramming of the device [604].

8.32 Aging

Aging attenuates the ECG potentials [481]; such changes in the precordial leads may be offset by the reduced thickness of the chest wall, bringing the heart closer to the recording electrodes. An increased incidence of atrial and ventricular ectopic beats, bundle branch blocks, pathological and non-pathological Q waves, T wave inversion and atrial fibrillation is seen, which is probably due to morphological and histological changes of the cardiac musculature, or associated ischemia and infarction. [605]; indeed differentiating such changes due to aging per se from those due to pathology is difficult [606]. Such changes in the atria with fibro-fatty regional replacement may be the substrate initiating and maintaining atrial fibrillation [607].

8.33 Gender

ECG is influenced by gender; accordingly left ventricular hypertrophy employs for its diagnosis different thresholds for amplitude criteria for the two sexes. Conversely, the performance of different ECG criteria differs between men and women [608]. The amplitude in some precordial leads is influenced by the positioning of electrodes in relation to the left breast [609]. The amplitude of ST segment and duration of QTc intervals varied among the three phases of the menstrual cycle [610]. P-R intervals are longer in men, while women have higher resting heart rates, longer QTc intervals and steeper slope of 24 h QT/RR dynamics, explaining their greater susceptibility to torsades de pointes during treatment with drugs that prolong QT interval [611, 612]. Further data relating to the influence of gender on the ECG can be found in ➋ Chap. 1.

8.34 Anthropometric Parameters

Anthropometric parameters influence the ECG. Thus the height, weight, configuration of different body parts, abdominal circumference, fat percentage, presence of obesity (see ➋ Sect. 8.26), and body habitus (see ➋ Sect. 8.25.2) need to be considered in research and practice. The magnitude of spatial atrial vectors has shown the greatest variability in reference to anthropometric parameters [613].

8.35 Race and Ethnicity

Race and ethnicity lead to differences in the ECG. The normal T wave amplitudes were greater in Chinese than in Americans, except for lead V_1, which was greater in Americans than in Chinese [614]. The prevalence of early transition in precordial leads, high R wave in lead V_1, and R and T wave amplitudes differed in various ethnic groups; also the incidence of left ventricular hypertrophy would be overestimated for some ethnic groups using fixed R wave amplitude criteria [615]. The prevalence of 1° AV block and ventricular extrasystoles is higher, and intraventricular blocks and atrial fibrillation lower, in African than Caucasian Americans [616–619]. The early repolarization pattern is more common in young black athletic males [620], and routine criteria for left ventricular hypertrophy do not apply to black Africans [621].

8.36 Normal Variants

It has long been recognized that inappropriate ECG interpretation has consequences often creating ECG-based cardiac invalidism [407]. Usually this is due to non-adherence to established ECG criteria of normalcy and/or lack of knowledge on normal variants on the part of the human interpreter. For professionals relying on automated ECG interpretations, problems arise with the occasional error in measurements, or employment of inappropriate diagnostic criteria by the automated algorithm. These problems could be easily corrected and are gradually being addressed.

8.36.1 P Waves

P wave abnormalities are often diagnosed inappropriately; the mere presence of a late negativity of the P wave in lead V_1 (area <1.0 mm^3) is a normal finding. "Left atrial enlargement" was ubiquitously present according to the interpretation of some of the earlier automated systems. Appearance of "transient P-pulmonale" is often seen in association with increased heart rate [120, 481, 482], and it is a normal response to exercise. Wandering atrial pacemaker, particularly in association with sinus bradycardia is a common finding in the young. Also "AV nodal" and "low atrial" activity with isorhythmic AV dissociation are commonly encountered. Many of the above are seen both in standard ECGs and Holter ECG recordings.

8.36.2 QRS Complexes

Notches, r′, rounding of peaks, W, or M-shaped QRS complexes, without increase in their duration, can be seen normally, although they are also encountered in patients with hypertension, septal fibrosis or as residuals from prior small myocardial infarctions. Elevated or depressed ST or PR segments due to atrial repolarization may hamper the measurement of the QRS duration. Some borderline QRS widening may disappear with exercise. The QRS duration in neonates is shorter than in adults [2]. Qs in QRS complexes in III may decrease or disappear with inspiration, or as a result of minor rightward shift of the frontal QRS axis during inspiration or exercise [482]. Deep but narrow Qs in inferior and lateral leads, often in association with large QRS complexes mimicking those encountered in left ventricular hypertrophy, are seen in normal adolescents and young adults, particularly male. Also Qs or QS, without associated ST segment and T changes in leads I and aVL may not be pathological in subjects with a vertical heart [481]. The pattern of "early transition" characterized by R/S > 1 in V_2–V_4 is frequently found in healthy subjects [615], often with a vertical QRS axis, while the "poor R-wave progression in V_1–V_2" ("pseudoinfarct" pattern), or with a QS in V_1 and V_2 (interpreted by some automated ECG interpretation algorithms as suggestive of anteroseptal myocardial infarction), are mostly not associated with such pathology [622]. Low voltage ECG in the limb leads or throughout all ECG leads, is occasionally a normal variant, while low voltage in leads V_3 and V_4 in women may be due to the underlying breast [609]. Transient augmentation in the QRS amplitude can be brought about by an increase in the heart rate in the setting of narrow QRS complex tachycardia [118]. Frontal QRS axes, −30° to 45° in the young, and more commonly 100° to 120° in the old, without identifiable cardiac pathology, are occasionally found.

8.36.3 ST Segment and T Waves

ST segment elevation, usually concave upwards starting from an r′ and an elevated J point with upright tall T waves involving particularly V_2–V_4, occasionally only II, III, and aVF, or rarely all ECG leads are seen in normal subjects and comprise the "early repolarization" normal variant (➋ Figs. 8.3 and ➋ 8.53). The ST segment elevation decreases in amplitude with mild exercise, as witnessed in the stress laboratory. The peaked T wave associated with early repolarization mimics the

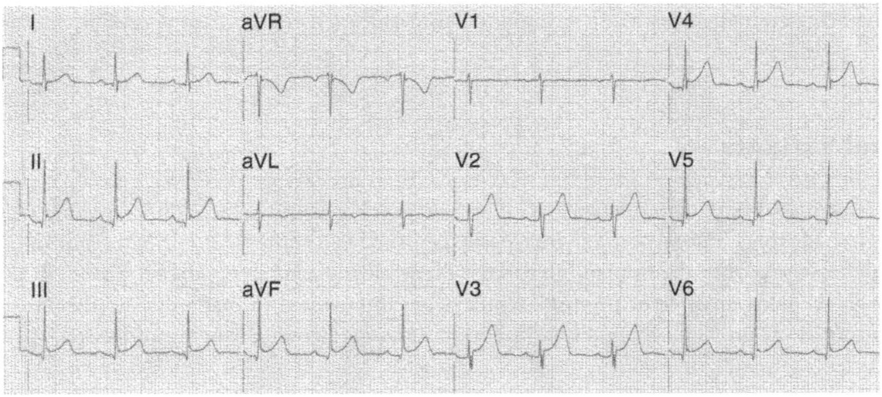

Fig. 8.53
ECG of a 37-year-old man with atypical for angina chest pain with a negative maximal exercise stress/thallium test, showing ST segment elevation of early repolarization type, involving all ECG leads, save for aVR, aVL, and V_1

one seen with hyperkalemia, but it is asymmetrical and not narrow-based; this T wave is often attributed to "metabolic abnormalities" by automated ECG interpretation systems. Although this ST segment elevation pattern is more common in the young, male, and particularly black individual [620, 623], it can be found in many other groups, and can be rarely associated with T wave inversion and notching of the downstroke of the R waves [624, 625]. The ST changes are stable, not accompanied by reciprocal ST depressions except in aVR, often diffuse as those noted in pericarditis, in contrast to those of ischemia or myocardial infarction. PR segment depression, thought to be due to atrial wall injury, and lower T wave amplitudes, changing over time, differentiate pericarditis from early repolarization. Although the characterization of early repolarization implies an overlapping of cardiac activation and recovery, this was not found with body surface isopotential mapping [626]. The similarities in the ECG of early repolarization, the "Osborn waves" of hypothermia, and the Brugada pattern have led to a reexamination of the mechanism of early repolarization. The cellular and ionic characteristics of Brugada pattern and early repolarization raise the possibility that the latter may not be benign after all, and that individuals with early repolarization may be at risk for life threatening arrhythmias under certain conditions [627]. The so-called post tachycardia syndrome is also characterized by ST depression [482], sometimes deeper than the ones of "nonspecific ST-T changes".

T-wave inversion, commonly seen in children, can be found mainly in leads V_1–V_3, in young or even middle age normal subjects, particularly women. The term "persistent juvenile pattern" is often used to describe such changes in adults [628], and has led to unnecessary coronary arteriography in normal individuals presenting with complaints of chest pain. Occasionally these T wave inversions are very deep [406], particularly in young black males. T wave inversion is noted in some leads, depending on the T wave axis. Shortened QTc mimicking hypercalcemia or digitalis effect is common in young healthy individuals (➋ Fig. 8.3), but occasionally seen in older adults. The congenital short QTc interval syndrome [40] is much shorter (<300 ms), than the one described herein.

8.36.4 Heart Rhythm and Conduction

Sinus arrhythmia is seen in all ages, and not necessarily in the presence of sinus bradycardia. Sinus tachycardia is frequent, and is occasionally unpleasant to some healthy subjects, who seek evaluation. Sinus bradycardia, rare PACs and PVCs, are found in normal subject. PR interval <120 ms suggestive of accelerated AV conduction is common, particularly in young subjects (➋ Fig. 8.54), with PR intervals even as low as 90 ms, especially in association with rapid heart rates; this is not due to Lown–Levine–Ganong syndrome, which should be diagnosed only in association with supraventricular

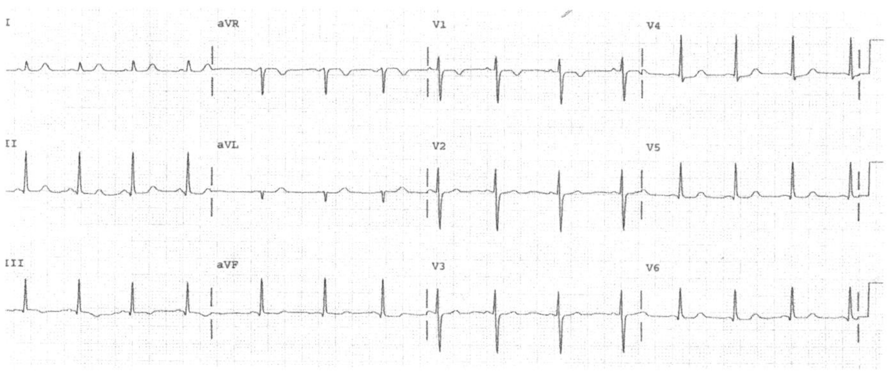

Fig. 8.54
ECG of a 29-year-old healthy lady showing a PR interval of 113 ms, with a sinus rhythm at a rate of 87 beats. min^{-1}, and with a frontal P wave axis of 58° and a QRS axis of 69°. T waves in V_1–V_3 suggest a "persistent juvenile" pattern

arrhythmias [629]. Mild to significant prolongation of PR interval, or Mobitz II AV block, particularly during sleep, are seen in normal young subjects [630].

8.37 Artifactual ECG Abnormalities

Artifactual ECG abnormalities are common, have many sources, and may result in confusion and difficulty in interpretation. When the ECG is in disagreement with the clinical state, an inquiry about ECG artifacts is in order.

8.37.1 Improper Electrode Positioning

Improper limb electrode positioning, particularly involving the reversal of the right and left arm electrodes, is frequent. The distortions of the ECG resulting from electrode misplacement are illustrated in ➋ Fig. 8.55 [631]. Reversal of the right arm and left leg electrodes creates the pattern of an inferior MI (➋ Fig. 8.56) [632]. The reversal of the leg electrodes does not change the ECG appearance, since the potential on the right and left ankles is similar while it does not matter on which leg the grounding electrode is placed. All types of artifactual ECG can be suspected by the marked difference in the morphology of the complexes in leads I and V_6 (➋ Fig. 8.57), save for the one shown in ➋ Fig. 8.55d. Although the changing polarity of leads I and aVR and the alteration of the other limb leads mimics dextrocardia (except in ➋ Fig. 8.55d), the unaltered V_1–V_6 leads can aid in the differentiation of artifactual ECGs from the ECG of dextrocardia (➋ Fig. 8.57).

With multi-channel ECG recorders, the inappropriate sequence in the positioning of V_1–V_6 electrodes leads to confusing ECG artifacts, with unaltered limb leads. The reversal(s) of electrodes at various points of the V_1–V_6 sequence result(s) in different patterns of R wave progression and/or regression (➋ Fig. 8.58). More frequent is the placement of all precordial electrodes higher (most common) or lower than their proper position. This has necessitated, when quantitative ECGs are employed serially, inclusion of a separate analysis of the limb leads [633]. Placing V_1–V_6 higher than appropriately on the thorax, results in poor R wave progression and mimics anterior myocardial infarction or RBBB or rSR pattern [632]. Problems with the recording of V_1–V_6 may arise in women when some of these leads are placed above or below the left breast [609], or when this is done with some variation in serial recordings. A device has been described to facilitate correct V_1–V_6 lead placement [634].

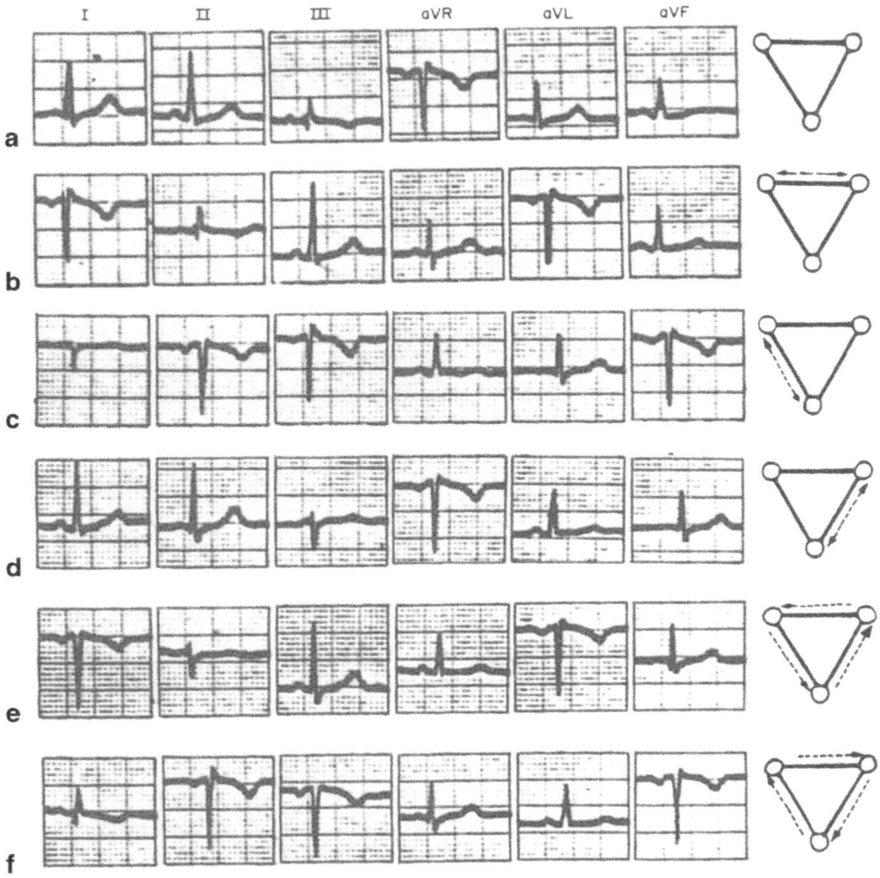

Fig. 8.55
Various patterns of ECG resulting from the incorrect positioning of limb electrodes: (a) normal; (b) reversed positioning of arm leads; (c) reversed positioning of the right arm and left leg leads; (d) reversed positioning of left-sided limb leads; (e) counterclockwise incorrect positioning of upper and lower limb leads; (f) clockwise incorrect placement of upper and lower limb leads (After Marriott [631]. © Williams and Wilkins, Baltimore, Maryland. Reproduced with permission)

8.37.2 Muscle Tremor and Other Movements During ECG Recording

Parkinsonism, the extrapyramidal syndrome, or shivering, result in muscle tremor distorting the isoelectric line, which by its coarse and fine undulations, may mimic atrial flutter (Figs. 8.59 and 8.60), or atrial fibrillation. The irregularity of the undulating baseline differentiates artifacts from atrial flutter. However, if the artifactual undulations of the baseline are regular, it may be problematic to differentiate artifacts superimposed on a regular atrial rhythm, from atrial flutter transmitted to the ventricles with a fixed AV block. Muscle tremor with sinus arrhythmia or other irregular rhythms may be mistaken for atrial fibrillation. Undulations from muscle tremor or insufficient relaxation of the peripheral musculature are of irregular frequency and amplitude, and may affect the limb leads more than the precordial leads. Applying the limb leads electrodes in the proximal part of the limbs may be necessary in patients with intense tremor. If the muscular tremor can be traced to cold environment, the ECG should be recorded in a room with an appropriate temperature. Sometimes AC interference or other electrical or mechanical artifacts, regular or quasi-regular, will have a similar effect on the ECG. Movements of the body or the attached electrodes cause coarse changes and shifts or wandering of the baseline. Body

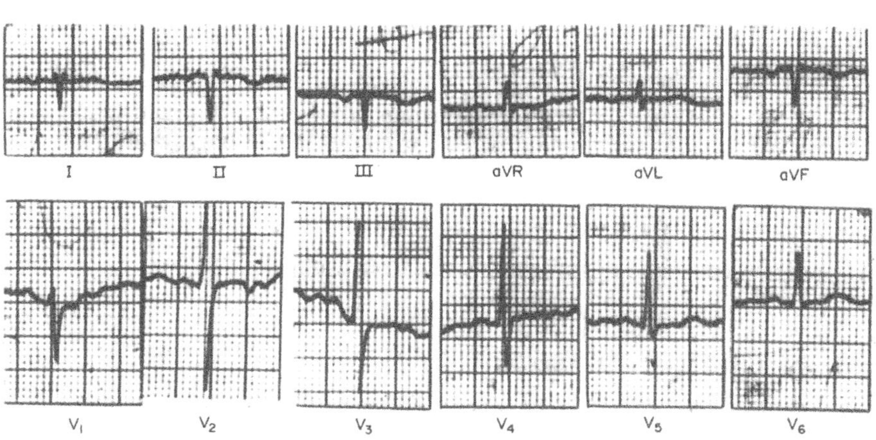

Fig. 8.56
Artifactual ECG resulting from the interchange of right arm and left leg lead connections

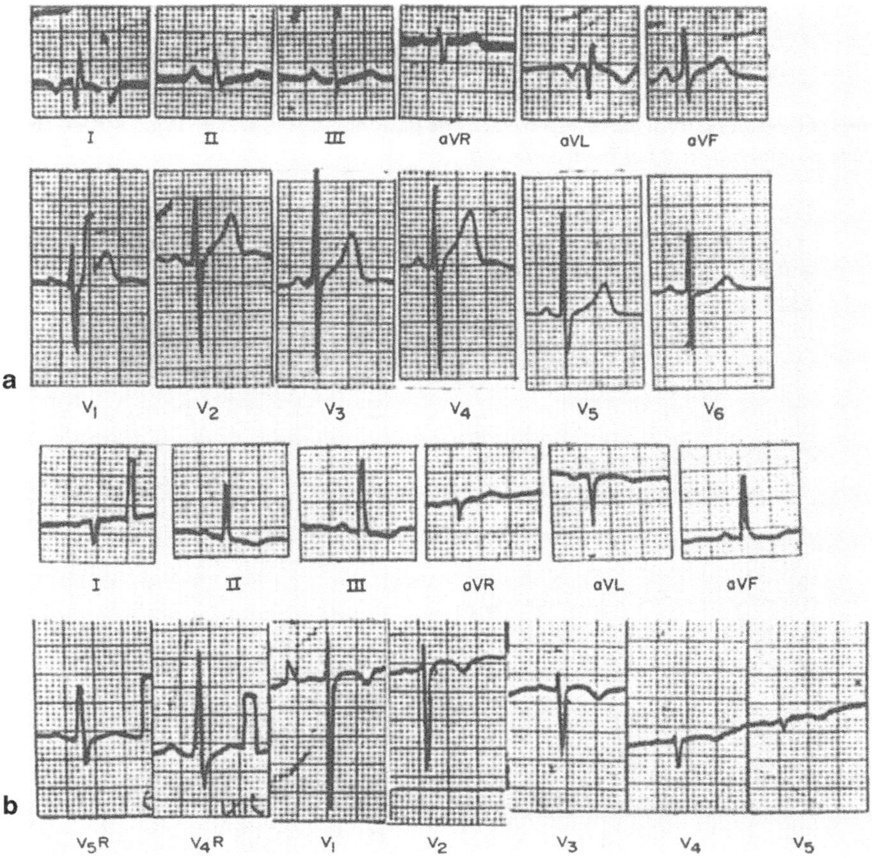

Fig. 8.57
(a) Artifactual ECG resulting from the reversal of right and left arm electrodes; (b) ECG correctly recorded in a young lady with dextrocardia, where there is a similarity between leads I and V_6. Leads from the right chest wall display larger QRS complexes than the ones from leads V_4 and V_5

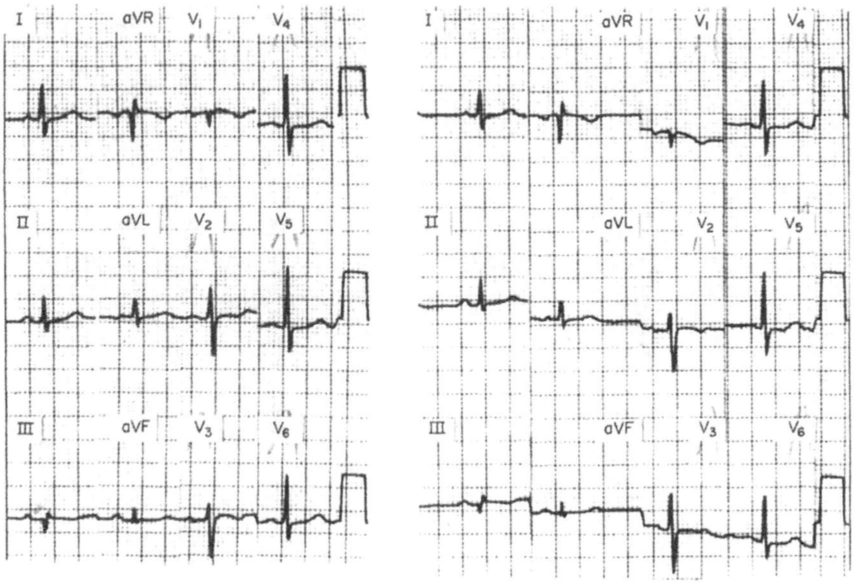

Fig. 8.58
Left **panel: artifactual ECG resulting from the reversed electrode positioning of V_2 and V_3, using a three-channel ECG recorder;** ***right*** **panel: electrode positioning error has been corrected**

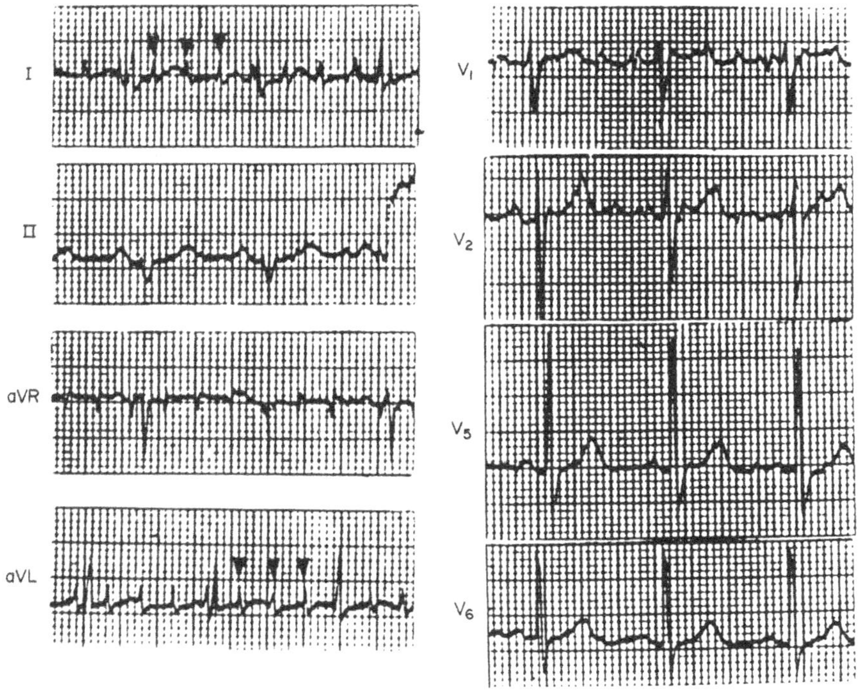

Fig. 8.59
Artifactual ECG, mimicking atrial flutter, resulting from tremor of limbs in a patient possibly suffering from the extrapyramidal syndrome

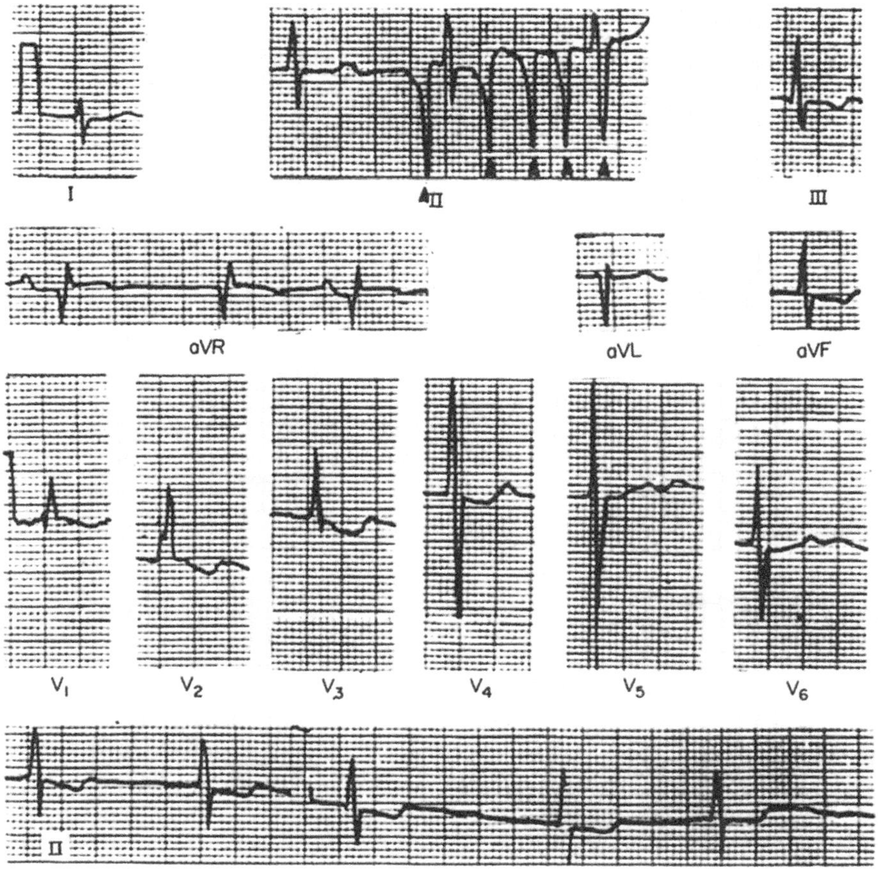

Fig. 8.60
Artifactual ECG (lead II) resulting from vigorous tremor of limbs

movements and poor skin-electrode contact may mimic arrhythmias, leading to improper therapies including implantation of devices [635]. Asymptomatic "pseudo-torsade de pointes" ventricular tachycardia has been recorded on telemetry in a patient with Parkinson's disease during urination [636]. Some of these artifacts can be traced to the respiratory movements, which if excessive in a particular patient, may necessitate recording the ECG with held respiration. Scrutinizing the ECG and the circumstances of its acquisition often resolve these mimicries, although repeating the ECG recording may occasionally be necessary. For ambulatory recordings, the multi-lead devices are preferred since occasionally 1 or 2 of the employed leads are uninterpretable due to artifacts.

8.37.3 Inappropriate Damping of the Stylus of the ECG Recorder

Inappropriate damping of the stylus of the ECG recorder will create distortion of signals. In an era of digital recorders, this applies only to equipment producing paper strip ECG recordings still in use. An underdamping causes an overshoot on the upswing and downswing of the signals (Fig. 8.61), and increase of the amplitude of all rapid deflections, i.e., the

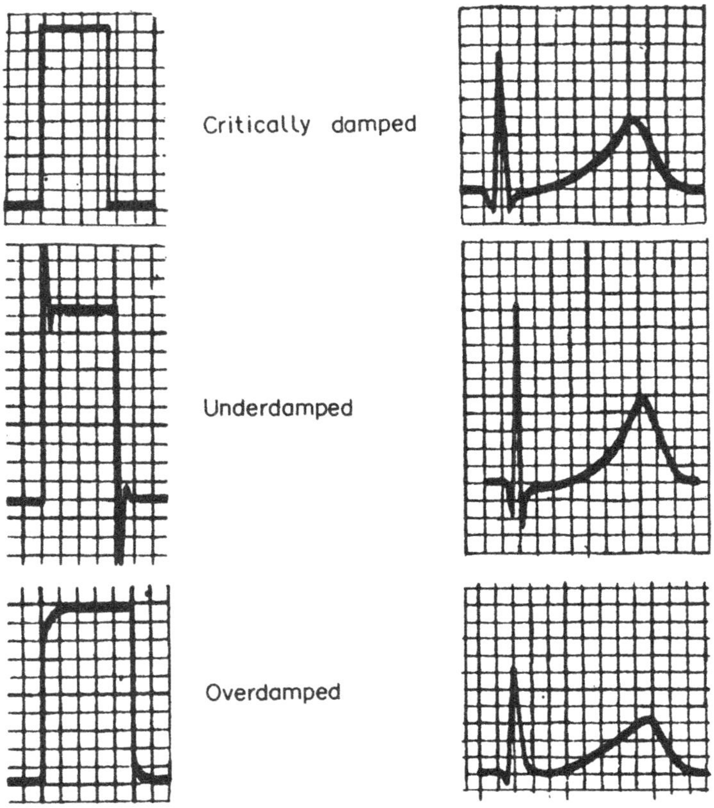

Fig. 8.61
The shape calibrations and corresponding different ECG morphologies resulting from critical damping, underdamping and overdamping of the stylus

Q, R, and S waves. In contrast, overdamping will record sharp angles or fast deflections with low fidelity (Fig. 8.61), all notches will become slurred, the QRS complexes may appear widened, and the ST segment falsely depressed (Fig. 8.62).

8.37.4 Wrong Speed or Wrong Switching During the ECG Recording

By recording at a faster chart paper speed, e.g., 50 mm/s, all components of the ECG appear widened (Fig. 8.63). This is occasionally intended for more accurate manual measurement of time intervals; however, if this is done by error it may confuse an inexperienced interpreter, unaware of the change. Diagnoses like prolonged P wave duration, 1° AV block, intraventricular conduction delay, prolonged QTc have been entertained prior to the reviewer noting the recording speed. Similar problems are encountered in continuous ambulatory ECG recorders due to mechanical malfunction. Another unusual artifactual ECG may occasionally be produced when a single-channel recorder is used and one fails to switch to the "V" lead position during precordial ECG recording, thus in turn generating a record with all V_1-V_6 leads being similar to lead aVF (Fig. 8.64). These artifacts, which may cause difficulty in interpretation, can be traced to an inexperienced operator of the ECG equipment, when an ECG technician is not available.

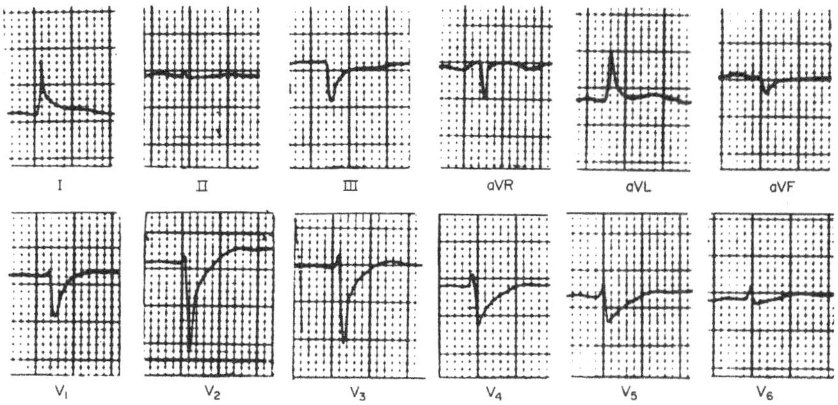

Fig. 8.62
Artifactual ECG resulting from an overdamped stylus

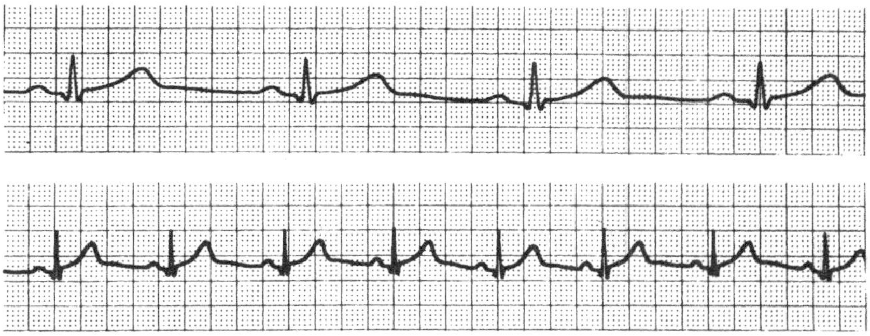

Fig. 8.63
"Artifactual" ECG caused by higher recording speed (50 mm s^{-1}) (*upper* panel), also shown at normal speed (25 mm s^{-1}) in the *lower* panel

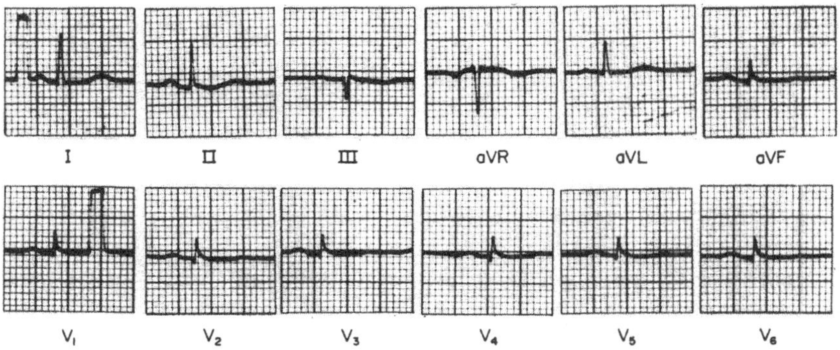

Fig. 8.64
***V_1–V_6* are similar to lead aVF, in an artifactual ECG caused by faulty switching during the recording of the precordial ECG leads**

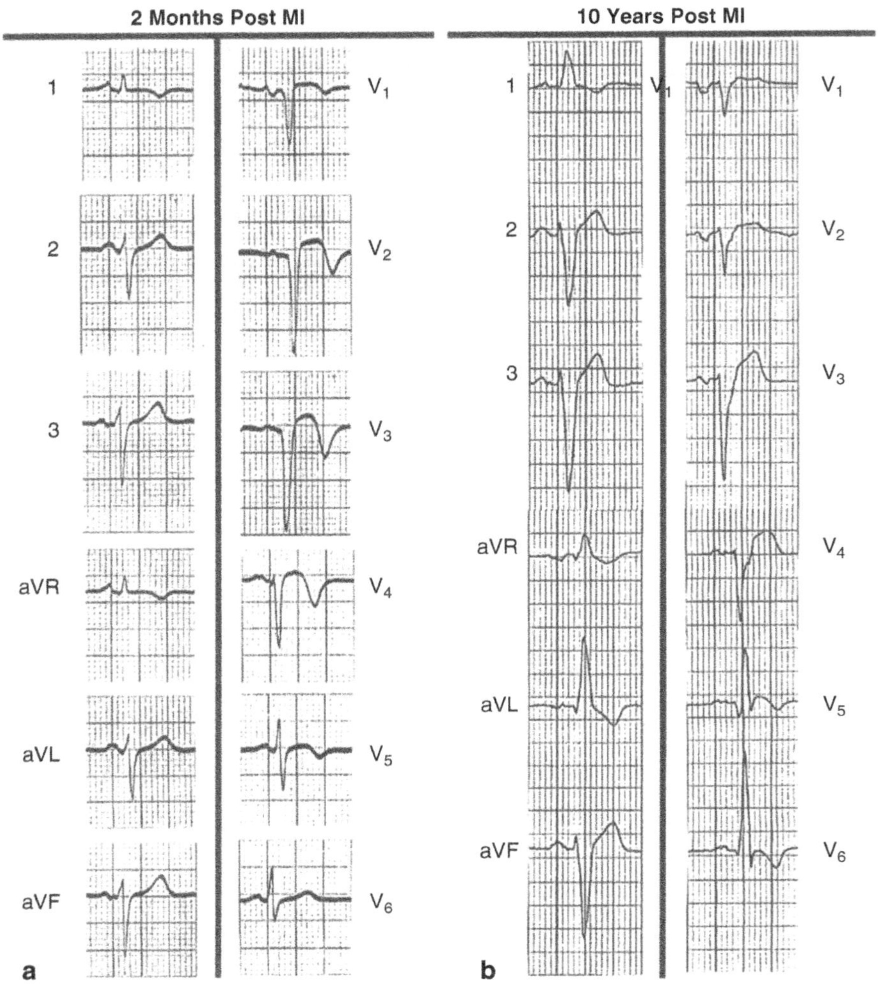

Fig. 8.65
ECG of a 55-year-old man who had suffered an extensive anterior myocardial infarction 10 years earlier (a) showing persistent ST segment elevation in lead V_5 (b) in the presence of left bundle branch block suggestive of a primary repolarization abnormality due to a ventricular aneurysm (consider this figure with Fig. 8.66) (Reproduced from Ref. [640]. With permission of the *Journal of Electrocardiology*)

8.37.5 Electric and Magnetic Fields

Sensing of the electromagnetic fields produces artifacts in the ECG. Proper grounding of the electrocardiograph and the patient prevents the characteristic fixed amplitude 50 or 60 Hz undulations of the electrical ac power lines, and higher frequencies from other electrical equipment in the environment. Magnetic fields are generated with the interaction of electrical power and the lead wires, and appear as a high frequency noise in the ECG; this distortion can be prevented by aligning all the lead wires with the patient's body in the head to foot axis. When feasible, unplugging some of the electrical devices (including the patient's bed), in the environment where the ECG is being recorded, contributes to an artifact-free record; similarly unplugging the electrocardiograph itself and operating it in "battery mode" is advisable.

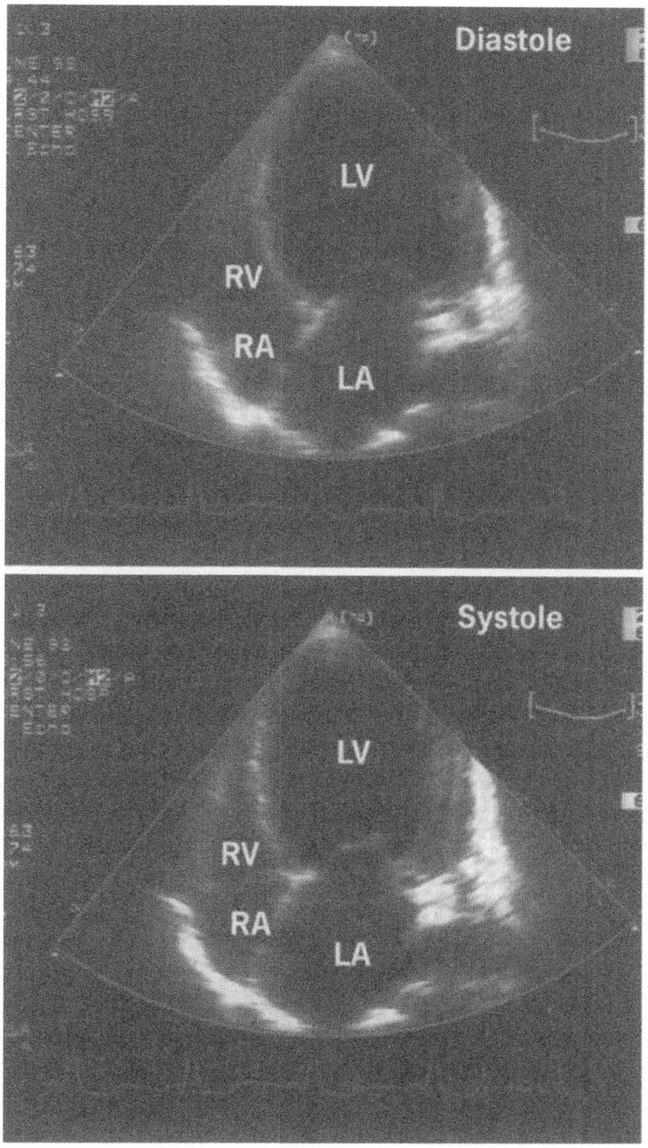

a

b

Fig. 8.66
An echocardiogram (four-chamber view) of the patient, whose ECG is shown in this figure, revealing an enormous ventricular aneurysm (VA). During systole (a) and diastole (b) the septum is thin and akinetic due to the VA, while the lateral wall displays thickening during systole. *LV* left ventricle, *RV* right ventricle, *LA* left atrium, *RA* right atrium (Reproduced from Ref. [640]. With permission of the *Journal of Electrocardiology*)

8.37.6 Other Sources of Artifactual ECGs

Unintentionally recording the ECG with an increased or decreased calibration for the entire ECG or only the precordial leads may create diagnostic problems in busy places, where scrutiny of the records is not routine. Unintentional under,

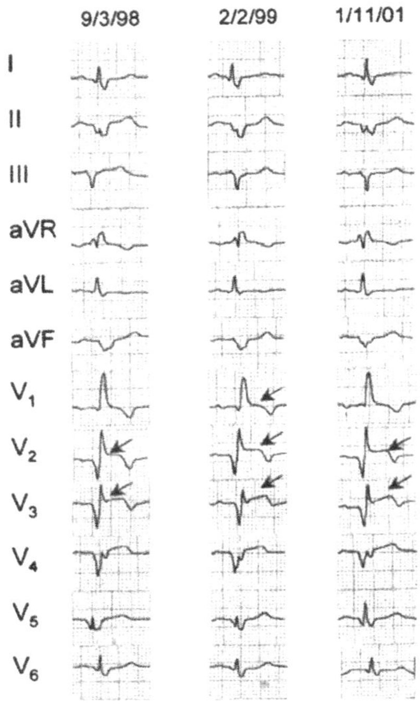

Fig. 8.67
ECG of a 67-year-old woman who had suffered an anterior myocardial infarction complicating by a ventricular aneurysm who had persistent ST segment elevation in leads V_1–V_3, suggestive of a primary repolarization change in the presence of right bundle branch block (Reproduced from Ref. [641]. With permission of the *Annals of Noninvasive Electrocardiology*)

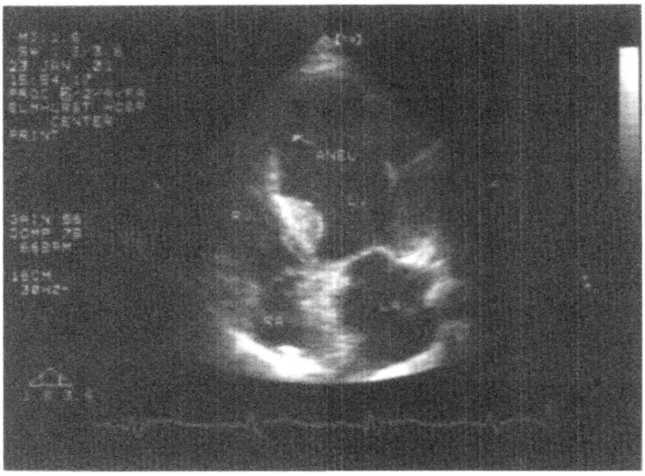

Fig. 8.68
An echocardiogram (four-chamber view) of the patient whose ECG is shown in Fig. 8.67, revealing a large ventricular aneurysm (Reproduced from Ref. [641]. With permission of the *Annals of Noninvasive Electrocardiology*)

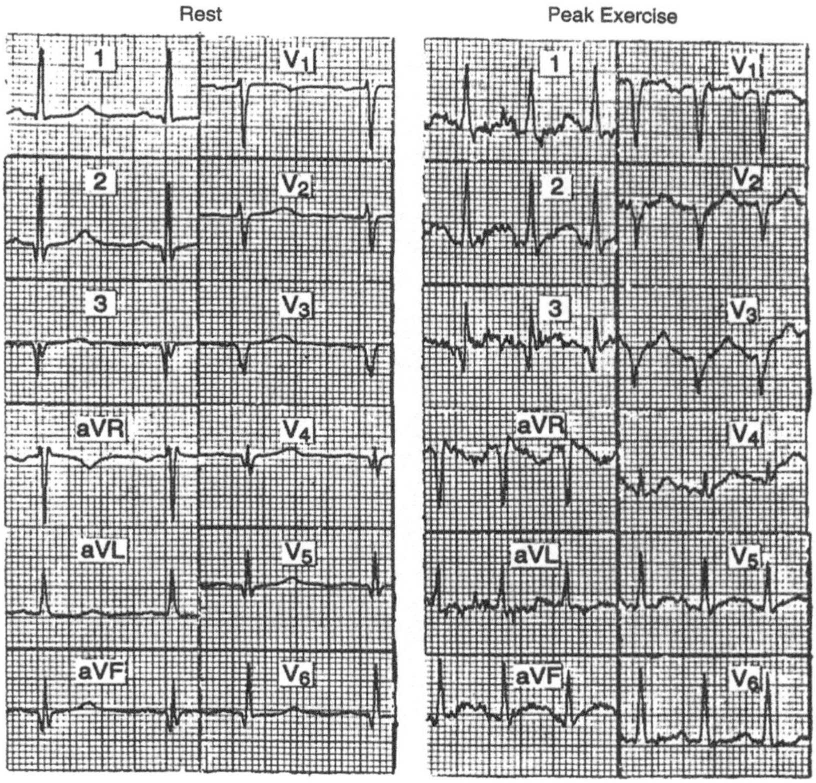

Fig. 8.69
Comparison of ECGs from rest, peak exercise stress test (94% of maximal predicted heart rate) and recovery phases of a 62-year-old woman did not disclose ischemic changes; note the enormous change in the P wave at peak exercise suggestive of left atrial abnormality. Compare with Fig. 8.70 (Reproduced from Ref. [642]. With permission of the *Journal of Electrocardiology*)

or over-calibration may be more of a problem when there is no automated interpretation provided by the ECG apparatus, since the latter's algorithm detects such alterations. Then "low voltage" ECG, left ventricular hypertrophy, P wave abnormalities, or major changes from previous tracings are diagnosed, before the recording mistake is detected.

8.38 Automated ECG Interpretation

Automated ECG interpretation is widely available in commercial electrocardiographs; both a routine and extended ECG interpretation can be generated instantly, with the hardcopy reports including different sets of ECG data measurements. Instant provision of measurements provides an advantage over manual assessment of the ECG when clinical decisions need to be implemented rapidly [637]. However, the presence of artifacts often complicates matters to the point that measurements become unreliable. Also, even with correct measurements, the final ECG diagnosis is often erroneous, but this is correctable by adopting appropriate criteria, or upgrading the algorithmic component dealing with the measurements-interpretation coupling. Thus, current experience shows that problems with automated ECG interpretation systems can be reduced to "inaccurate diagnoses" based on "accurate measurements". However, even today, automated ECG interpretation must be subject to human over-reading [638, 639]. Further discussion on this topic can be found in Chap. 5 of *Specialized Aspects of ECG*.

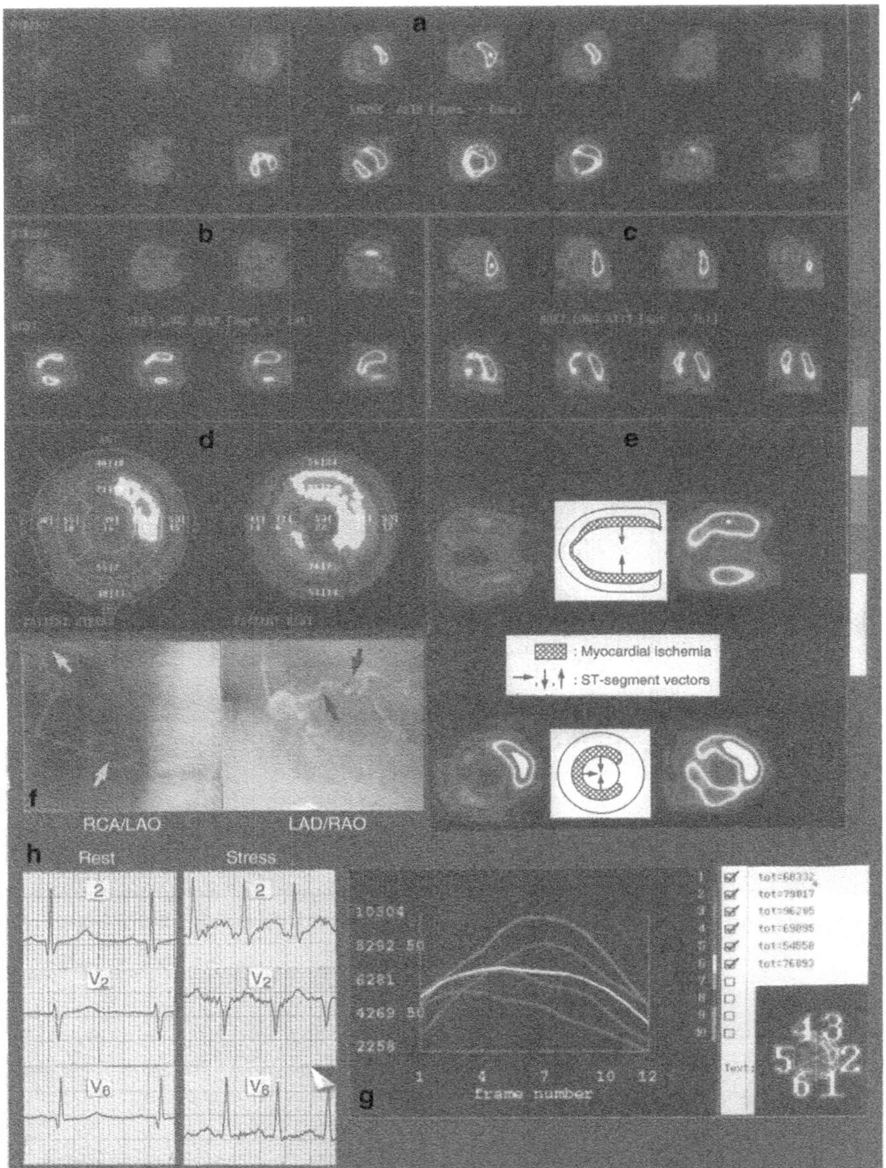

Fig. 8.70

Thallium myocardial imaging of the patient whose ECGs are shown in Fig. 8.69, revealing severe reversible perfusion defects involving many myocardial territories (A–D) selected ECG leads from the exercise stress test (H) severe stenosis of the right and left anterior descending coronary arteries on coronary arteriography (F) and the vectorial conceptualization explaining the association of ischemia in myocardial territories opposite each other with false negative exercise ECG due to electrical cancellation (Reproduced from Ref. [642]. With permission of the *Journal of Electrocardiology*)

8.39 New Ideas in Elecrocardiography

As the ever-expanding discovery of new ECG associations with various clinical entities goes on, new insights come to light. Some ECG "curiosities" start as such, and eventually find their way into the main stream of electrocardiography

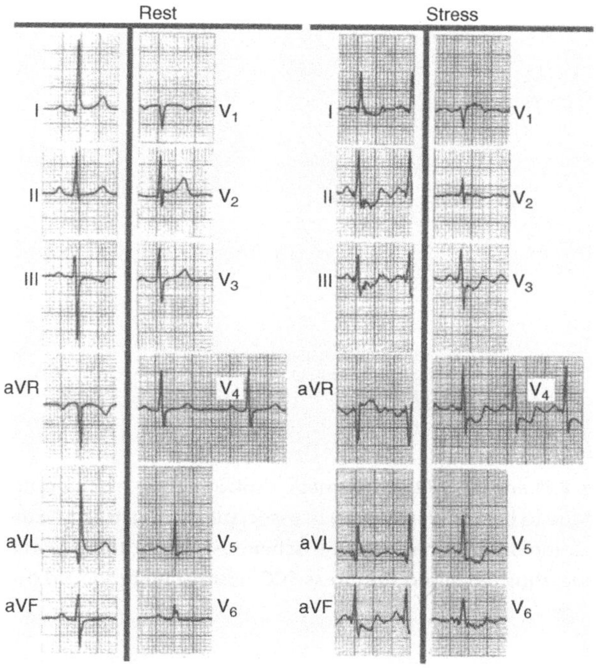

Fig. 8.71
Comparison of ECGs from rest, and peak exercise stress test of a 72-year-old man with severe three-vessel coronary artery disease showing ischemic changes. Compare with Fig. 8.72 (Reproduced from Ref. [643]. With permission of *Clinical Cardiology*)

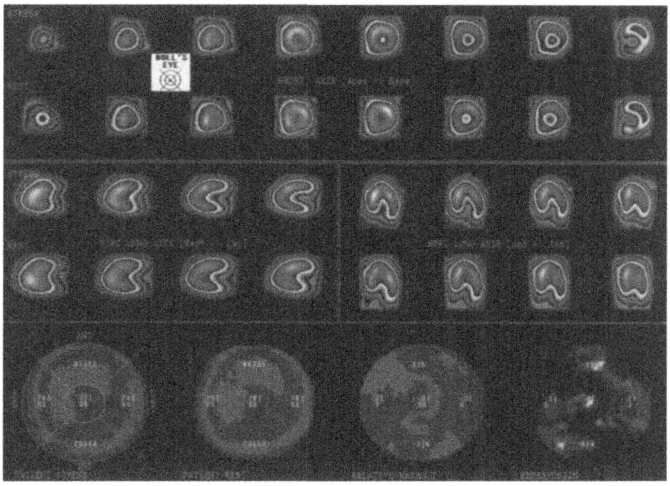

Fig. 8.72
Thallium myocardial imaging of the patient whose ECGs are shown in Fig. 8.70 revealing falsely negative appearances due to balanced severe myocardial ischemia (Reproduced from Ref. [643]. With permission of *Clinical Cardiology*)

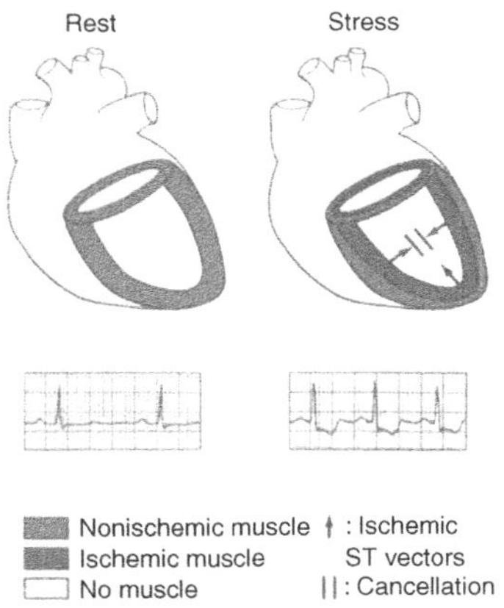

Fig. 8.73
Consider this figure with Figs. 8.71 and 8.72. A schematic explaining the mechanism of a false negative for ischemia thallium myocardial scintigram (due to balanced ischemia) in association with a true positive stress ECG; although electrical cancellation of ST segment depression occurs for most of the ischemic ventricle, the area of the ischemic apex remains unopposed by muscular ischemic tissue, thus rendering the stress ECG positive (Reproduced from Ref. [643]. With permission of *Clinical Cardiology*)

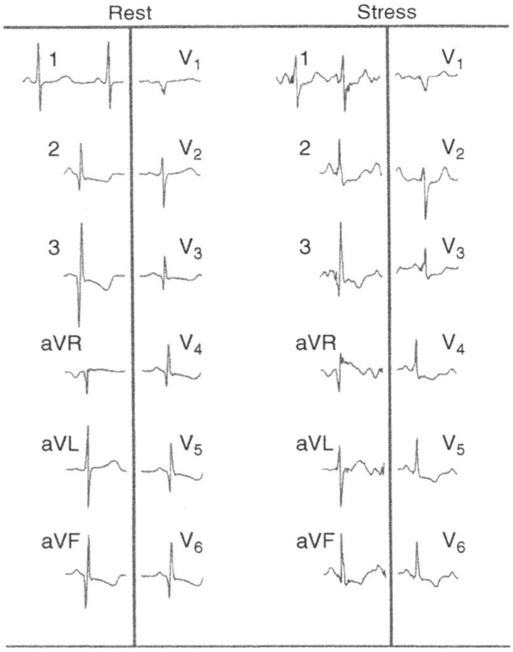

Fig. 8.74
Comparison of ECGs from rest, and peak exercise stress test of a 40-year-old woman with a previous inferior myocardial infarction revealed a transient reduction or disappearance of the infarctional Q waves in the stress ECG. Consider this figure with Fig. 8.75 (Reproduced from Ref. [644]. With permission of *Journal of Electrocardiology*)

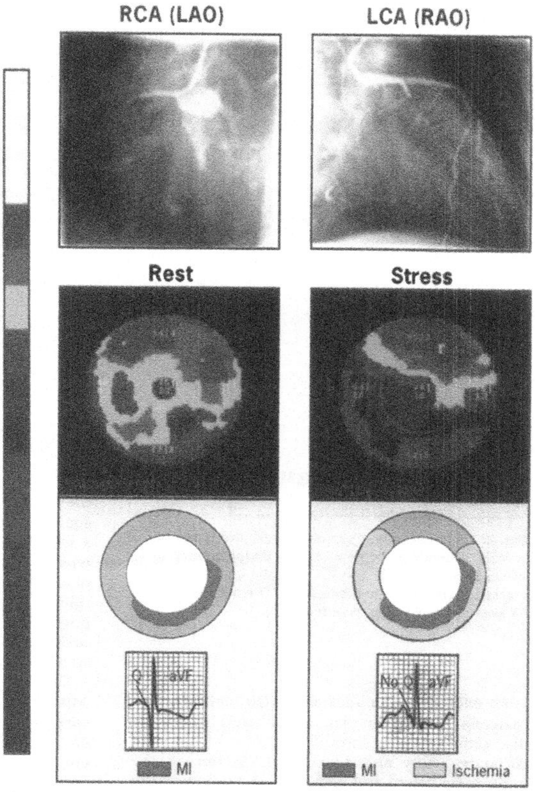

Fig. 8.75
Consider this figure with Fig. 8.74 Coronary arteriograms showed occluded right coronary artery (RCA) and left circumflex coronary artery, while the left anterior descending coronary artery had a 50% (LCA). Thallium myocardial scintigraphy disclosed severe reversible perfusion defects affecting among others the territory opposite the region of the old infarct (MI). The schematic explains the mechanism of transient disappearance of infarctional Q waves due to the transient incapacitation of the area opposite the MI, temporarily incapable to pull the early QRS vector away from the MI, and thus generate the Q wave (Reproduced from Ref. [644]. With permission of the *Journal of Electrocardiology*)

by being diagnostically useful. A few such examples include the diagnosis of left ventricular aneurysm in the presence of left bundle branch block from the ST segment elevation in the leads V_4–V_6 (Figs. 8.65 and 8.66) [640], left ventricular aneurysm in the presence of right bundle branch block from the ST segment elevation in the leads V_1–V_3 (Figs. 8.67 and 8.68) [641], an explanation for the false negative ECG diagnosis of exercise induced ischemia due to cancellation of the ST segment vectors from ischemic myocardial territories opposite each other ("ischemic ST segment counterpoise") (Figs. 8.69 and 8.70) [642], the false negative diagnosis of myocardial ischemia by myocardial scintigraphy in association with a positive exercise ECG (Figs. 8.71 and 8.72), and the role of the apical ischemia in producing such a discrepancy (Fig. 8.73) [643], and the transient reduction or disappearance of Q-waves from an old myocardial infarction due to exercise-induced ischemia in the territory opposite the infarct (Figs. 8.74 and 8.75) [644]. The employment of intracardiac electrograms obtained via a "saline ECG lead" from a central venous catheter for the detection of P waves (Fig. 8.76) [645] or the diagnosis of arrhythmias, is another example of an idea awaiting routine use.

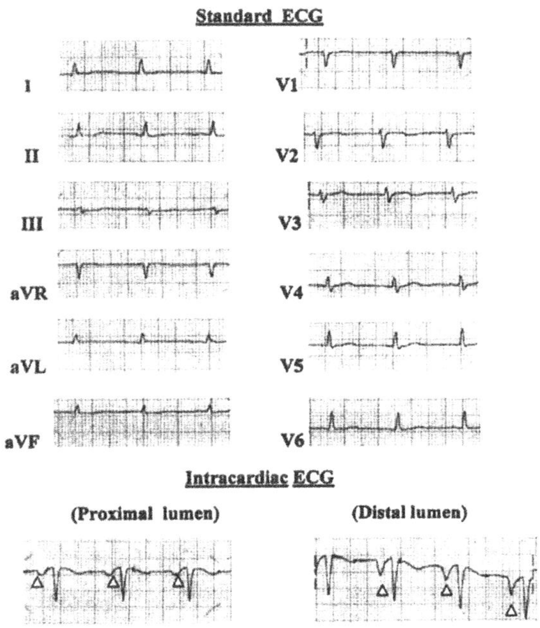

Fig. 8.76
Standard ECG of a 68-year-old woman with chronic renal failure and sepsis who suffered peripheral edema, showing attenuated ECG voltage and invisible P waves. Electrical connection of the one of the "V" leads with her saline-filled central venous (jugular) catheter enable recording of the P waves (Δ). Note the larger P waves recorded via the distal lumen versus the proximal lumen ("proximity effect") (Reproduced from Ref. [645]. With permission of *American Journal of Cardiology*)

References

1. Madias, J.E., R. Bazaz, H. Agarwal, M. Win, and L. Medepalli, Anasarca mediated attenuation of the amplitude of electrocardiogram complexes. A description of a heretofore unrecognized phenomenon. *J. Am. Coll. Cardiol.*, 2001;**38**: 756–764.
2. Surawicz, B., *Electrophysiologic Basis of ECG and Cardiac Arrhythmias.* Baltimore, MD: Williams & Wilkins, 1995.
3. Noble, D., *The Initiation of the Heart Beat*, 2nd edn. Oxford: Clarendon Press, 1979.
4. Fisch, C., S.B. Knoebel, H. Feigenbaum, K. Greenspan, Potassium and the monophasic action potential, electrocardiogram, conduction and arrhythmias. *Prog. Cardiovasc. Dis.*, 1966;**8**: 387–418.
5. Fisch, C., Relation of electrolyte disturbances to cardiac arrhythmias. *Circulation*, 1973;**47**: 408–419.
6. Ettinger, P.O., T.J. Regan, and H.A. Oldewurtel, Hyperkalemia, cardiac conduction, and the electrocardiogram. A review. *Am. Heart J.*, 1974;**88**: 360–371.
7. Watanabe, Y. and L.S. Dreifus, Interactions of quinidine and potassium on atrioventricular transmission. *Circ. Res.*, 1967;**20**: 434–446.
8. O'Neil, J.P. and E.K. Chung, Unusual electrocardiographic finding-Bifascicular block due to hyperkalemia. *Am. J. Med.*, 1976;**61**: 537–540.
9. Sekiya, S., S. Ichikawa, T. Tsutsumi, K. Harumi, Nonuniform action potential durations at different sites in canine left ventricle. *Jpn. Heart J.*, 1983;**24**: 935–945.
10. O'Reilly, M.V., D.P. Murnaghan, and M.B. Williams, Transvenous pacemaker failure induced by hyperkalemia. *J. Am. Med. Assoc.*, 1974;**228**: 336.
11. Barold, S.S., M.D. Falkoff, L.S. Ong, and R.A. Heinle, Hyperkalemia-induced failure of atrial capture during dual-chamber cardiac pacing. *J. Am. Coll. Cardiol.*, 1987;**10**: 467–469.
12. Dohrmann, M.L. and N.F. Goldschlager, Myocardial stimulation threshold in patients with cardiac pacemakers: Effect of physiologic variables, pharmacologic agents, and lead electrodes. *Cardiol. Clin.*, 1985;**3**: 527–537.
13. Surawicz, B., Relationship between electrocardiogram and electrolytes. *Am. Heart J.*, 1967;**73**: 814–834.
14. Levine, H.D., J.P. Vazifdar, B. Lown, J.P. Merrill, "Tent-shaped" T waves of normal amplitude in potassium intoxication. *Am. Heart J.*, 1952;**43**: 437–450.
15. Surawicz, B., H. Chlebus, and A. Mazzoleni, Hemodynamic and electrocardiographic effects of hyperpotassemia: Differences in response to slow and rapid increases in concentration of plasma K^+. *Am. Heart J.*, 1967;**73**: 647–664.

16. Van Mieghem, C., M. Sabbe, and D. Knockaert, The clinical value of the ECG in noncardiac conditions. *Chest*, 2004;**125**: 1561–1576.
17. Moulik, P.K., C. Nethaji, and A.A. Khaleeli, Misleading electrocardiographic results in patients with hyperkalemia and diabetic ketoacidosis. *BMJ*, 2002;**325**: 1346–1347.
18. Levine, H.D., S.H. Wanzer, and J.P. Merrill, Dialyzable currents of injury in potassium intoxication resembling acute myocardial infarction or pericarditis. *Circulation*, 1956;**13**: 29–36.
19. Madias, J.E. and N.E. Madias, Hyperkalemia-like ECG changes simulating acute myocardial infarction in a patient with hypokalemia undergoing potassium replacement. *J. Electrocardiol.*, 1989;**22**: 93–97.
20. Szerlip, H.M., J. Weiss, and I. Singer, Profound hyperkalemia without electrocardiographic manifestations. *Am. J. Kidney Dis.*, 1986;**7**: 461–465.
21. Surawicz, B., H.A. Braun, W.B. Crum, R.L. Kemp, S. Wagner, and S. Bellett, Quantitive analysis of the electrocardiographic patterns of hypopotassemia. *Circulation*, 1957;**16**: 750–763.
22. Gettes, L. and B. Surawicz, Effects of low and high concentrations of potassium on the simultaneously recorded Purkinje and ventricular action potentials of the perfused pig moderator band. *Circ. Res.*, 1968;**23**: 717–729.
23. Madias, J.E., N.E. Madias, and H.P. Gavras, Nonarrhythmogenicity of diuretic-induced hypokalemia. Its evidence in patients with uncomplicated hypertension. *Arch. Intern. Med.*, 1984;**144**: 2171–2176.
24. Cohn, J.N., P.R. Kowey, P.K. Whelton, and L.M. Prisant, New guidelines for potassium replacement in clinical practice: A contemporary review by the National Council on potassium in clinical practice. *Arch. Intern. Med.*, 2000;**160**: 2429–2436.
25. Krikler, D.M. and P.V.L. Curry, Torsade de pointes, an atypical ventricular tachycardia. *Br. Heart J.*, 1976;**38**: 117–120.
26. Leier, C.V., L. Dei Cas, and M. Metra, Clinical relevance and management of the major electrolyte abnormalities in congestive heart failure: Hyponatremia, hypokalemia, and hypomagnesemia. *Am. Heart J.*, 1994;**128**: 564–574.
27. Burton, D.R., Hypokalemia. *Clinical Physiology of Acid-Base and Electrolyte Disorders*, 4th edn. New York: McGraw-Hill, 1994, pp. 776–822.
28. Paes de Carvalho, A. and W.B. Langan, Influence of extracellular potassium levels on atrioventricular transmission. *Am. J. Physiol.*, 1963;**205**: 375–381.
29. Weidmann, S., Effects of calcium ions and local anaesthetics on electrical properties of Purkinje fibres. *J. Physiol. (Lond.)* 1955;**129**: 568–582.
30. Temte, J.V. and L.D. Davis, Effect of calcium concentration on the transmembrane potentials of Purkinje fibers. *Circ. Res.*, 1967;**20**: 32–44.
31. Lind, L. and S. Ljunghall, Serum calcium and the ECG in patients with primary hyperparathyroidism. *J. Electrocardiol.*, 1994;**27**: 99–103.
32. Shah, A.P., A. Lopez, R.Y. Wachsner, S.K. Meymandi, A.K. El-Bialy, and A.M. Ichiuji, Sinus node dysfunction secondary to hyperparathyroidism. *J. Cardiovasc. Pharmacol. Ther.*, 2004;**9**: 145–147.
33. Carpenter, C. and M.E. May, Case report: Cardiotoxic calcemia. *Am. J. Med. Sci.*, 1994;**307**: 43–44.
34. Reuter, H. and H. Scholz, The regulation of the calcium conductance of cardiac muscle by adrenaline. *J. Physiol. (Lond.)* 1977;**264**: 49–62.
35. Nierenberg, D.W. and B.J. Ransil, Q-aTc interval as a clinical indicator of hypercalcemia. *Am. J. Cardiol.*, 1979;**44**: 243–248.
36. Bronsky, D., A. Dubin, S.S. Waldstein, and D.S. Kushner, Calcium and the electrocardiogram. II. The electrocardiographic manifestations of hyperparathyroidism and of marked hypercalcemia from various other etiologies. *Am. J. Cardiol.*, 1961;**7**: 833–839.
37. Ellman, H., H. Dembin, and N. Seriff, The rarity of shortening of the QT interval in patients with hypercalcemia. *Crit. Care Med.*, 1982;**10**: 320–322.
38. Wagner, G.S., *Marriott's Practical Electrocardiography*, 10th edn. Philadelphia, PA: Lippincott Williams & Wilkins, 2001.
39. Sridharan, M.R. and L.G. Horan, Electrocardiographic J wave of hypercalcemia. *Am. J. Cardiol.*, 1984;**54**: 672–673.
40. Gussak, I., P. Brugada, J. Brugada, et al., Idiopathic short QT interval: A new clinical syndrome. *Cardiology*, 2000;**90**: 99–102.
41. Nekvasil, R., J. Stejskal, and A. Tuma, Detection of early onset neonatal hypocalcaemia in low birth weight infants by QTc and Q-oTc interval measurement. *Acta Paediatr. Acad. Sci. Hung.*, 1980;**21**: 203–210.
42. Lehmann, G., I. Deisenhofer, G. Ndrepepa, and C. Schmitt, ECG changes in a 25-year-old woman with hypocalcemia due to hypoparathyroidism. Hypocalcemia mimicking acute myocardial infarction. *Chest*, 2000;**118**: 260–262.
43. Johnson, J.D. and R. Jennings, Hypocalcemia and cardiac arrhythmias. *Am. J. Dis. Child* 1968;**115**: 373–376.
44. Griffin, J.H., Neonatal hypocalcemia and complete heart block. *Am. J. Dis. Child*, 1965;**110**: 672–675.
45. Kambara, H., B.J. Iteld, and J. Phillips, Hypocalcemia and intractable ventricular fibrillation. (Letter.) *Ann. Intern. Med.* 1977;**86**: 583–584.
46. Chang, C.J., S.A. Chen, C.T. Tai, et al., Ventricular tachycardia in a patient with primary hyperparathyroidism. *Pacing Clin. Electrophysiol.*, 2000;**23**: 534–537.
47. Kiewiet, R.M., H.H. Ponssen, E.N. Janssens, and P.W. Fels, Ventricular fibrillation in hypercalcaemic crisis due to primary hyperparathyroidism. *Neth. J. Med.*, 2004;**62**: 94–96.
48. Akiyama, T., J. Batchelder, J. Worsman, H.W. Moses, and M. Jedlinski, Hypocalcemic Torsades de Pointes. *J. Electrocardiol.*, 1989;**22**: 89–92.
49. Kearney, P., M. Reardon, and J. O'Hare, Primary hyperparathyroidism presenting as torsades de pointes. *Br. Heart J.*, 1993;**70**: 473.
50. Surawicz, B., M.G. MacDonald, V. Kaljot, and J.C. Bettinger, Treatment of cardiac arrhythmias with salts of ethylenediamine tetraacetic acid (EDTA). *Am. Heart J.*, 1959;**58**: 493–503.
51. Hoff, H.E., P.K. Smith, and A.W. Winkler, Electrocardiographic changes and concentration of calcium in serum following intravenous injection of calcium chloride. *Am. J. Physiol.*, 1939;**125**: 162–171.
52. Johnson, J.D. and R. Jennings, Hypocalcemia and cardiac arrhythmias. *Am. J. Dis. Child*, 1968;**115**: 373–376.
53. Voss, D.M. and E.H. Drake, Cardiac manifestations of hyperparathyroidism, with presentation of a previously unreported arrhythmia. *Am. Heart J.*, 1967;**72**: 235–239.
54. Seelig, M.S., Myocardial loss of functional magnesium. I. Effect on mitochondrial integrity and potassium retention. *Recent Adv. Stud. Cardiac Struct. Metab.*, 1972;**1**: 615–625.

55. Loeb, H.S., R.J. Pietras, R.M. Gunnar, and J.R. Tobin Jr., Paroxysmal ventricular fibrillation in two patients with hypomagnesemia. *Circulation*, 1968;**37**: 210–215.
56. Seelig, M.S., Electrocardiographic patterns of magnesium depletion appearing in alcoholic heart disease. *Ann. N. Y. Acad. Sci.*, 1969;**162**: 906–917.
57. Surawicz, B., Is hypomagnesemia or magnesium deficiency arrhythmogenic? *J. Am. Coll. Cardiol.*, 1989;**14**: 1093–1096.
58. Wellens, H.J., V.M. Cats, and D.R. Duren, Symptomatic sinus node abnormalities following lithium carbonate therapy. *Am. J. Med.*, 1975;**59**: 285–287.
59. Chih-Hsin, H., L. Ping-Yen, C. Jyh-Hong, Y. Tzung-Lieh, T. Hsiang-Yi, and L. Li-Jen, Electrocardiographic abnormalities as predictors for over-range lithium levels. *Cardiology*, 2005;**103**: 101–106.
60. Hermsmeyer, K., R. Rulon, and N. Sperelakis, Loss of the plateau of the cardiac action potential in hypertonic solutions. *J. Gen. Physiol.*, 1972;**59**: 779–793.
61. Bailey, J.C., Electrophysiological effects of hypertonic sucrose solutions on canine cardiac Purkinje fibers. *Circ. Res.*, 1981;**49**: 1112–1118.
62. Spitzer, K.W. and P.M. Hogan, The effects of acidosis and bicarbonate on action potential repolarization in canine cardiac Purkinje fibers. *J. Gen. Physiol.*, 1979;**73**: 199–218.
63. Barker, P.S., E.L. Schrader, and E. Ronzoni, The effects of alkalosis and of acidosis upon the human electrocardiogram. *Am. Heart J.*, 1939;**17**: 169–186.
64. Madias, J.E., K.M. Venkataraman, L.T. Synder, P.S. Vokonas, and W.B. Hood Jr., Experimental myocardial infarction. XI. Circulatory effects of hypoxia in intact conscious dogs with coronary occlusion. *Am. J. Cardiol.*, 1974;**23**: 796–802.
65. Broch, O.J., Calibrated hypoxemia test in normal subjects and coronary patients. II. The relation between ECG changes and oxygen saturation of blood. *Acta Med. Scand.*, 1972;**191**: 185–190.
66. Kiely, D.G., R.I. Cargill, and B.J. Lipworth, Effects of hypercapnia on hemodynamic, inotropic, lusitropic, and electrophysiologic indices in humans. *Chest*, 1996;**109**: 1215–1221.
67. Yasuma, F., M. Hirai, and J.I. Hayano, Differential effects of hypoxia and hypercapnia on respiratory sinus arrhythmia in conscious dogs. *Jpn. Circ. J.*, 2001;**65**: 738–742.
68. Rutherford, J.J., T.H. Clutton-Brock, and M.J. Parkes, Hypocapnia reduces the T wave of the electrocardiogram in normal human subjects. *Am. J. Physiol. Regul. Integr. Comp. Physiol.*, 2005;**289**: R148–R155.
69. Alexopoulos, D., J. Christodoulou, T. Toulgaridis, et al., Repolarization abnormalities with prolonged hyperventilation in apparently healthy subjects: Incidence, mechanisms and affecting factors. *Eur. Heart J.*, 1996;**17**: 1432–1437.
70. Rigatto, C., R. Foley, J. Jeffery, et al., Electrocardiographic left ventricular hypertrophy in renal transplant recipients: Prognostic value and impact of blood pressure and anemia. *J. Am. Soc. Nephrol.*, 2003;**14**: 462–468.
71. Gehi, A., J. Ix, M. Shlipak, S.S. Pipkin, and M.A. Whooley, Relation of anemia to low heart rate variability in patients with coronary heart disease (from the Heart and Soul Study). *Am. J. Cardiol.*, 2005;**95**: 1474–1477.
72. Nelson, C.V., P.W. Rand, E.T. Angelakos, and P.G. Hugenholtz, Effect of intracardiac blood on the special vectorcardiogram. 1. Results in the dog. *Circ. Res.*, 1972;**31**: 95–104.
73. Rosenthal, A., N.J. Restieaux, and S.A. Feig, Influence of acute variations in hematocrit on the QRS complex of the Frank electrocardiogram. *Circulation*, 1971;**44**: 456–465.
74. Lipsitz, L.A., F. Hashimoto, and L.P. Lubowsky, Heart rate and respiratory rhythm dynamics on ascent to high altitude. *Br. Heart J.*, 1995;**74**: 390–396.
75. Weilenmann, D., F. Duru, M. Schonbeck, et al., Influence of acute exposure to high altitude and hypoxemia on ventricular stimulation thresholds in pacemaker patients. *Pacing Clin. Electrophysiol.*, 2000;**23**: 512–515.
76. Kaufmann, P.A., C. Schirlo, V. Pavlicek, et al., Increased myocardial blood flow during acute exposure to simulated altitudes. *J. Nucl. Cardiol.*, 2001;**8**: 158–164.
77. Pan, A.W., J. He, Y. Kinouchi, H. Yamaguchi, and H. Miyamoto, Blood flow in the carotid artery during breath-holding in relation to diving bradycardia. *Eur. J. Appl. Physiol. Occup. Physiol.*, 1997;**75**: 388–395.
78. Mukerji, B., M.A. Alpert, and V. Mukerji, Right ventricular alterations in scuba divers: Findings on electrocardiography and echocardiography. *South Med. J.*, 2000;**93**: 673–676.
79. Ferrigno, M., B. Grassi, G. Ferretti, et al., Electrocardiogram during deep breath-hold dives by elite divers. *Undersea Biomed. Res.*, 1991;**18**: 81–91.
80. Rocha, I., E.I. de Oliveira, K.M. Spyer, and L.S. Carvalho, Interaction of the Bezold-Jarisch reflex with the urinary bladder function. *Rev. Port Cardiol.*, 2000;**19**: 977–988.
81. Hayashi, N., M. Ishihara, A. Tanaka, T. Osumi, and T. Yoshida, Face immersion increases vagal activity as assessed by heart rate variability. *Eur. J. Appl. Physiol. Occup. Physiol.*, 1997;**76**: 394–399.
82. Chu, C.S., T.H. Lin, Y.H. Lu, et al., Cold effect on qt dispersion in healthy subjects. *Kaohsiung J. Med. Sci.*, 2002;**18**: 236–240.
83. Saltykova, M., A. Capderou, O. Atkov, et al., Variations of intrathoracic amount of blood as a reason of ECG voltage changes. *Ann. Noninv. Electrocardiol.*, 2003;**8**: 321–332.
84. Whinnery, J.E., Acceleration induced voltage variations in the electrocardiogram during exhaustive simulated aerial combat maneuvering. *Aviat. Space Environ. Med.*, 1982;**53**: 147–152.
85. Osborn, J.J., Experimental hypothermia. Respiratory and blood pH changes in relation to cardiac function. *Am. J. Physiol.*, 1953;**175**: 389–398.
86. Surawitz, B. and T.K. Knilans,*Chou's Electrocardiography in Clinical Practice. Adult and Pediatric*, 5th edn. Philadelphia, PA: WB Saunders, 2001.
87. Okada, M., F. Nishimura, H. Yoshino, M. Kimura, and T. Ogino, The J wave in accidental hypothermia. *J. Electrocardiol.*, 1983;**16**: 23–28.
88. Gussak, I., P. Bjerregaard, T.M. Egan, and B.R. Chaitman, ECG phenomenon called the J wave. History, pathophysiology, and clinical significance. *J. Electrocardiol.*, 1995;**28**: 49–58.
89. Solomon, A., R.A. Barish, B. Browne, and E. Tso, The electrocardiographic features of hypothermia. *J. Emerg. Med.*, 1989;**7**: 169–173.
90. Strohmer, B. and M. Pichler, Atrial fibrillation and prominent J (Osborn) waves in critical hypothermia. *Int. J. Cardiol.*, 2004;**96**: 291–293.
91. Danzl, D.F. and R.S. Pozos, Accidental hypothermia. *N. Engl. J. Med.*, 1994;**331**: 1756–1760.
92. Trevino, A., B.M. Razi, B. Beller, and S. Antonio, The characteristic electrocardiogram of accidental hypothermia. *Arch. Intern. Med.*, 1971;**127**: 470–473.

93. Abbott, J.A. and M.D. Cheitlin, The non-specific camel-hump sign. *J. Am. Med. Assoc.*, 1976;**235**: 413–414.
94. Carrillo-Esper, R., L. Limon-Camacho, H.L. Vallejo-Mora, et al., Non-hypothermic J wave in subarachnoid hemorrhage. *Circulation*, 2004;**72**: 125–129.
95. Scherlag, B.J., C.G. Gunn, E.J. Berbari, and R. Lazzara, Peri-infarction block (1950)-Late potential (1980): Their relationship, significance and diagnostic implications. *Am. J. Cardiol.*, 1985;**55**: 839–841.
96. Nishida, K., A. Fujiki, K. Mizumaki, et al., Canine model of Brugada syndrome using regional epicardial cooling of the right ventricular outflow tract. *J. Cardiovasc. Electrophysiol.*, 2004;**15**: 936–941.
97. Fish, J.M. and C. Antzelevitch, Link between hypothermia and the Brugada syndrome. *J. Cardiovasc. Electrophysiol.*, 2004;**15**: 942–944.
98. Yan, G.X. and C. Antzelevitch, Cellular basis for the electrocardiographic J wave. *Circulation*, 1996;**93**: 372–379.
99. Wakita, R., I. Watanabe, Y. Okumura, et al., Brugada-like electrocardiographic pattern unmasked by fever. *Jpn. Heart J.*, 2004;**45**: 163–167.
100. Sanchez, J.M. and A.M. Kates, Brugada-type electrocardiographic pattern unmasked by fever. *Mayo. Clin. Proc.*, 2004;**79**: 273–274.
101. Morita, H., S. Nagase, K. Kusano, and T. Ohe, Spontaneous T wave alternans and premature ventricular contractions during febrile illness in a patient with Brugada syndrome. *J. Cardiovasc. Electrophysiol.*, 2002;**13**: 816–818.
102. Ryan, J.F. and L.G. Tedeschi, Sudden unexplained death in a patient with a family history of malignant hyperthermia. *J. Clin. Anesth.*, 1997;**9**: 66–68.
103. Jantzen, J.P., K. Erdmann, and P.P. Kleemann, Malignant hyperthermia susceptibility-successful management with a "stressfree" technique. *Acta Anaesthesiol. Belg.*, 1987;**38**: 107–113.
104. Zipes, D.P., P. Libby, R.O. Bonow, and E. Braunwald, *Braunwald's Heart Disease: A Textbook of Cardiovascular Medicine*, 7th edn. Philadelphia, PA: Elsevier Saunders, 2005.
105. Polikar, R., A.G. Burger, U. Scherrer, and P. Nicod, The thyroid and the heart. *Circulation*, 1993;**87**: 1435–1441.
106. Johnson, P.N., A.S. Freedberg, and J.M. Marshall, Action of thyroid hormone on the transmembrane potentials from sino atrial cells and atrial muscle cells in isolated atria of rabbits. *Cardiology*, 1973;**58**: 273–289.
107. Arnsdorf, M.F. and R.W. Childers, Atrial electrophysiology in experimental hyperthyroidism in rabbits. *Circ. Res.*, 1970;**26**: 575–581.
108. Jaeger, J.M., S.R. Houser, A.R. Freeman, J.F. Spann Jr., Effect of thyroid hormone on canine cardiac Purkinje fiber transmembrane potential. *Am. J. Physiol.*, 1981;**240**: H934–H940.
109. Binah, O., I. Rubinstein, and E. Gilat, Effects of thyroid hormone on the action potential and membrane currents of guinea pig ventricular myocytes. *Pflugers Arch.*, 1987;**409**: 214–216.
110. Sharp, N.A., D.S. Neel, and R.L. Parsons, Influence of thyroid hormone levels on the electrical and mechanical properties of rabbit papillary muscle. *J. Mol. Cell. Cardiol.*, 1985;**17**: 119–132.
111. Surawicz, B. and M.L. Mangiardi, Electrocardiogram in endocrine and metabolic disorders, in Clinical Electrocardiographic Correlations, J.C. Rios, Editor. Davis, Philadelphia, PA, 1977, pp. 243–266.
112. Hoffman, I. and R.D. Lowrey, The electrocardiogram in thyrotoxicosis. *Am. J. Cardiol.*, 1960;**6**: 893–904.
113. Benker, V.G., H. Preiss, H. Kreusen, et al., Ekg Veriinderungen bei Hyperthyreose. Untersuchungen an 542 patienten. *Z. Kardiol.*, 1974;**63**: 799–811.
114. Nakazawa, H., K. Sakurai, N. Hamada, N. Momotani, and K. Ito, Management of atrial fibrillation in the post-thyrotoxic state. *Am. J. Med.*, 1982;**72**: 903–906.
115. Sawin, C.T., Subclinical hyperthyroidism and atrial fibrillation. *Thyroid*, 2002;**12**: 501–503.
116. Pilapil, V.R. and D.G. Watson, Electrocardiogram in hyperthyroid children. *Am. J. Dis. Child*, 1970;**119**: 245–248.
117. Sanghvi, L.M. and K. Banerjee, Wolff-parkinson White syndrome associated with thyrotoxicosis. *Am. J. Cardiol.*, 1961;**8**: 431–437.
118. Wakimoto, H., N. Izumida, Y. Asano, et al., Augmentation of QRS wave amplitudes in the precordial leads during narrow QRS tachycardia. *J. Cardiovasc. Electrophysiol.*, 2000;**11**: 52–60.
119. Harumi, K. and T. Ouichi, Q-T prolongation syndrome (in Japanese). *Naika Mook* No.20. Tokyo. Kinbara, 1981: 210.
120. Lepeschkin, E., *Modern Electrocardiography*, vol. I. Baltimore, MD: Williams & Wilkins, 1951.
121. Fisher, J., Thyrotoxic periodic paralysis with ventricular fibrillation. *Arch. Intern. Med.*, 1982;**142**: 1362–1364.
122. Shih-Hua, L., Thyrotoxic periodic paralysis. *Mayo. Clin. Proc.*, 2005;**80**: 99–105.
123. Hsu, Y.J., Y.F. Line, T. Chau, J.T. Liou, S.W. Kuo, and S.H. Line, Electrocardiographic manifestations in patients with thyrotoxic periodic paralysis. *Am. J. Med.*, 2003;**326**: 128–132.
124. Boccalandro, C., L. Lopez, F. Boccalandro, and V. Lavis, Electrocardographic changes in thyrotoxic periodic paralysis. *Am. J. Cardiol.*, 2003;**91**: 775–777.
125. Kerber, R.E. and B. Sherman, Echocardiographic evaluation of pericardial effusion in myxedema. Incidence and biochemical and clinical correlations. *Circulation*, 1975;**52**: 823–827.
126. Vanhaelst, L., P. Neve, P. Chailly, and P.A. Bastenie, Coronary disease in hypothyroidism: Observations in clinical myxoedema. *Lancet*, 1967;**2**: 800–802.
127. Lee, J.K. and J.A. Lewis, Myxoedema with complete A-V block and Adams-Stokes disease abolished with thyroid education. *Br. Heart J.*, 1962;**24**: 253–256.
128. Hansen, J.E., Paroxysmal ventricular tachycardia associated with myxedema. A case report. *Am. Heart J.*, 1961;**61**: 692–697.
129. Macaulay, M.B. and R.J. Shepherd, Syncope in myxoedema due to transient ventricular fibrillation. *Postgrad. Med. J.*, 1971;**47**: 361–363.
130. Sun, Z.Q., W.A. Ojamaak-Coetzee, M. Artman, and I. Klein, Effects of thyroid hormone on action potential and repolarizing currents in rat ventricular myocytes. *Am. J. Physiol.*, 2000;**278**: E302–E307.
131. Surawicz, B., The pathogenesis and clinical significance of primary ST-T wave abnormalities, in Advances in electrocardiography, R.C. Schlant and J.W. Hurst, Editors. Grune and Stratton, New York, 1972.
132. Clayton, R.N., Cardiovascular function in acromegaly. *Endocr. Rev.*, 2003;**24**: 272–277.
133. Ciulla, M., M. Arosio, M.V. Barelli, et al., Blood pressure-independent cardiac hypertrophy in acromegalic patients. *J. Hypertens.*, 1999;**17**: 1965–1969.

134. Herrmann, B.L., C. Bruch, B. Saller, et al., Acromegaly: Evidence for a direct relation between disease activity and cardiac dysfunction in patients without ventricular hypertrophy. *Clin. Endocrinol. (Oxf.)*, 2002;**56**: 595–602.
135. Sugihara, N., M. Shimizu, Y. Kita, et al., Cardiac characteristics and postoperative courses in Cushing's syndrome. *Am. J. Cardiol.*, 1992;**69**: 1475–1480.
136. Bhattacharyya, A., S. Jagadeesan, R.J. Wolstenholme, and D.J. Tymms, Acute adrenocortical crisis and an abnormal electrocardiogram. *Hosp. Med.*, 1999;**60**: 908–909.
137. Rovetto, M.J. and A.M. Lefer, Electrophysiologic properties of cardiac muscle in adrenal insufficiency. *Am. J. Physiol.*, 1970;**218**: 1015–1019.
138. Bruch, C., N. Dagres, H. Wieneke, C. Herborn, K. Brandt-Mainz, and R. Erbel, Sinus node dysfunction with intermittent sinus arrest and AV-nodal escape rhythm as initial manifestation of pheochromocytoma. *Z. Kardiol.*, 2002;**91**: 81–87.
139. Dinckal, M.H., V. Davutoglu, S. Soydinc, and A. Kirilmaz, Phaeochromocytoma-induced myocarditis mimicking acute myocardial infarction. *Int. J. Clin. Pract.*, 2003;**57**: 842–843.
140. Takeno, Y., S. Eno, T. Hondo, K. Matsuda, and Z. Zushi, Pheochromocytoma with reversal of tako-tsubo-like transient left ventricular dysfunction: A case report. *J. Cardiol.*, 2004;**43**: 281–287.
141. Minami, J., M. Todoroki, T. Ishimitsu, and H. Matsuoka, Changes in heart rate variability before and after surgery in patients with pheochromocytoma. *Auton. Neurosci.*, 2004;**111**: 144–146.
142. Tzemos, N., G.P. McNeill, R.T. Jung, and T.M. MacDonald, Post exertional broad complex tachycardia in a normotensive patient: A rare presentation of phaeochromocytoma. *Scott. Med. J.*, 2001;**46**: 14–15.
143. Roshan, J., O.K. George, S. Vineet, P.V. George, and V.J. Jose, Torsade de pointes in a case of pheochromocytoma-an unusual presentation of an uncommon disease. *Indian Heart J.*, 2004;**56**: 248–249.
144. Viskin, S., R. Fish, A. Roth, P.J. Schwartz, and B. Belhassen, Clinical problem-solving. QT or not QT? *N. Engl. J. Med.*, 2000;**343**: 352–356.
145. Lopes, H.F., H.B. Silva, C. Frimm Cde, L.A. Bortolotto, G. Belotti, and F. Pileggi, A false diagnosis of hypertrophic myocardiopathy in pheochromocytoma. *Arq. Bras. Cardiol.*, 1995;**65**: 167–169.
146. Schuiki, E.R., R. Jenni, F.W. Amann, and W.H. Ziegler, A reversible form of apical left ventricular hypertrophy associated with pheochromocytoma. *J. Am. Soc. Echocardiogr.*, 1993;**6**: 327–331.
147. Salvador, M., F. Begasse, J. Guittard, and B. Chamontin, Value of the study of electrocardiographic P wave in pheochromocytoma. *Arch. Mal. Coeur. Vaiss.*, 1992;**85**: 39–43.
148. Senges, J., J. Brachmann, D. Pelzer, C. Hasslacher, E. Weihe, and W. Kubler, Altered cardiac automaticity and conduction in experimental diabetes mellitus. *J. Mol. Cell. Cardiol.*, 1980;**12**: 1341–1351.
149. Surawicz, B. and M.L. Mangiardi, Electrocardiogram in endocrine and metabolic disorders. *Cardiovasc. Clin. North Am.*, 1977;**77**: 243–246.
150. Huizar, J.F., L.A. Gonzalez, J. Alderman, and H.S. Smith, Sulfonylureas attenuate electrocardiographic ST-segment elevation during an acute myocardial infarction in diabetics. *J. Am. Coll. Cardiol.*, 2003;**42**: 1017–1021.
151. Ditchburn, C.J., J.A. Hall, M. de Belder, A. Davies, W. Kelly, and R. Bilous, Silent myocardial ischaemia in patients with proved coronary artery disease: A comparison of diabetic and non-diabetic patients. *Postgrad. Med. J.*, 2001;**77**: 395–398.
152. Coumel, P., N. Johnson, F. Extramiana, P. Maison-Blanche, and P. Valensi, Electrocardiographic changes and rhythm problems in the diabetic. *Arch. Mal. Coeur. Vaiss.*, 2000;**93**: 59–66.
153. Rodriguez-Moran, M. and F. Guerrero-Romero, Electrocardiographic changes and cardiovascular risk factors in patients with type-2 diabetes. *Salud. Publica. Mex.*, 1999;**41**: 12–17.
154. Pezzilli, R., P. Broccoli, P. Billi, and B. Barakat, Silent myocardial ischemia induced by hypoglycemia. *Panminerva. Med.*, 1998;**40**: 347–349.
155. Matsunaga, R., J. Miura, and T. Fujito, Ischemic change on electrocardiogram induced by hypoglycemia in a diabetic patient. *Jpn. Circ. J.*, 1998;**62**: 142–145.
156. Burch, G.E., R. Meyers, and J.A. Abildskov, A new electrocardiographic pattern observed in cerebrovascular accidents. *Circulation*, 1954;**9**: 719–723.
157. Makino, T. and R. Okada, A clinicopathological study of the T wave changes of the subarachnoidal hemorrhage (SAH). *Jpn. Heart J.*, 1982;**23** (Suppl I): 546–548.
158. Fentz, V. and J. Gormsen, Electrocardiographic patterns in patients with cerebrovascular accidents. *Circulation*, 1962;**25**: 22–28.
159. Shuster, S., The electrocardiogram in subarachnoid haemorrhage. *Br. Heart J.*, 1960;**22**: 316–320.
160. Di Pasquale, G., A. Andreoli, M. Lusa, et al., Cardiologic complications of subarachnoid hemorrhage. *J. Neurosurg. Sci.*, 1998;**42** (suppl 1): 33–36.
161. Di Pasquale, G., G. Pinelli, A. Andreoli, et al., Torsade de pointes and ventricular flutter-fibrillation following spontaneous cerebral subarachnoid hemorrhage. *Int. J. Cardiol.*, 1988;**18**: 163–172.
162. Cropp, G.J. and G.W. Manning, Electrocardiographic changes simulating myocardial ischemia and infarction associated with spontaneous intracranial hemorrhage. *Circulation*, 1960;**22**: 25–38.
163. Hersch, C., Electrocardiographic changes in subarachnoid haemorrhage, meningitis, and intracranial space-occupying lesions. *Br. Heart J.*, 1964;**26**: 785–793.
164. Hunt, D., C. McRae, and P. Zapf, Electrocardiographic and serum enzyme changes in subarachnoid hemorrhage. *Am. Heart J.*, 1969;**77**: 479–488.
165. Eisalo, A., J. Periisalo, and P.I. Halonen, Electrocardiographic abnormalities and some laboratory findings in patients with subarachnoid haemorrhage. *Br. Heart J.*, 1972;**34**: 217–226.
166. Harumi, K., Unpublished data. Yokohama: Showa University.
167. Surawicz, B., Electrocardiographic pattern of cerebrovascular accident. *J. Am. Med. Assoc.*, 1966;**197**: 913–914.
168. Valeriano, J. and J. Elson, Electrocardiographic changes in central nervous system disease. *Neurol. Clin.*, 1993;**11**: 257–272.
169. Brouwers, P.J., E.F. Wijdicks, D. Hasan, et al., Serial electrocardiographic recording in aneurysmal subarachnoid hemorrhage. *Stroke*, 1989;**20**: 1162–1167.

170. Dimant, J. and D. Grob, Electrocardiographic changes and myocardial damage in patients with acute cerebrovascular accidents. *Stroke*, 1977;**8**: 448–455.
171. Brit ton, M., U. de Faire, C. Helmers, K. Miah, and C. Ryding, Wester P0. Arrhythmias in patients with acute cerebrovascular-disease. *Acta Med. Scand.*, 1979;**205**: 425–428.
172. Norris, J.W. and V.C. Hachinski, Intensive care management of stroke patients. *Stroke*, 1976;**7**: 573–577.
173. Oppenheimer, S.M., D.F. Cechetto, and V.C. Hachinski, Cerebrogenic cardiac arrhythmias: Cerebral electrocardiographic influences and their role in sudden death. *Arch. Neurol.*, 1990;**47**: 513–519.
174. Jabaudon, D., J. Sztajzel, K. Sievert, T. Landis, and R. Sztajzel, Usefulness of ambulatory 7-day ECG monitoring for the detection of atrial fibrillation and flutter after acute stroke and transient ischemic attack. *Stroke*, 2004;**35**: 1647–1651.
175. Van der Ark, G., Cardiovascular changes with acute subdural hematoma. *Surg. Neurol.*, 1975;**3**: 305–308.
176. Lakusic, N., D. Mahovic, T. Babic, and D. Sporis, Changes in autonomic control of heart rate after ischemic cerebral stroke. *Acta Med. Croatica.*, 2003;**57**: 269–273.
177. Apak, I., K. Iltumur, Y. Tamam, and N. Kaya, Serum cardiac troponin T levels as an indicator of myocardial injury in ischemic and hemorrhagic stroke patients. *Tohoku. J. Exp. Med.*, 2005;**205**: 93–101.
178. Christensen, H., G. Boysen, A.F. Christensen, and H.H. Johannesen,. Insular lesions, ECG abnormalities, and outcome in acute stroke. *J. Neurol. Neurosurg. Psychiat.*, 2005;**76**: 269–271.
179. Greenhoot, J.H and D.D. Reichenbach, Cardiac injury and subarachnoid hemorrhage. A clinical, pathological, and physiological correlation. *J. Neurosurg.*, 1969;**30**: 521–531.
180. Connor, R.C.R., Heart damage associated with intracranial lesions. *Br. Med. J.*, 1968;**3**: 29–31.
181. Dixit, S., M. Castle, R.P. Velu, et al., Cardiac involvement in patients with acute neurologic disease. *Arch. Intern. Med.*, 2000;**160**: 3153–3158.
182. Connor, R.C.R., Heart damage associated with intracranial lesions. *BMJ*, 1968;**3**: 29–31.
183. Pollick, C., B. Cujec, S. Parker, and C. Tator, Left ventricular wall motion abnormalities in subarachnoid hemorrhage: An echocardiographic study. *J. Am. Coll. Cardiol.*, 1988;**12**: 600–605.
184. Kono, T., H. Morita, T. Kuroiwa, H. Onaka, H. Takatsuka, and A. Fujiwara, Left ventricular wall motion abnormalities in patients with subarachnoid hemorrhage: Neurogenic stunned myocardium. *J. Am. Coll. Cardiol.*, 1994;**24**: 636–640.
185. Pool, J.L., Vasocardiac effects of the circle of Willis. *AMA Arch. Neurol. Psychiat.*, 1957;**78**: 355–368.
186. Eisalo, A., J. Periisalo, and P.I. Halonen, Electrocardiographic abnormalities and some laboratory findings in patients with subarachnoid haemorrhage. *Br. Heart J.*, 1972;**34**: 217–226.
187. Pine, D.S., Tierney L Clinical problem-solving: A stressful interaction. *N. Engl. J. Med.*, 1996;**334**: 1530–1534.
188. Beard, E.F., J.W. Robertson, and R.C.L. Robertson, Spontaneous subarachnoid hemorrhage simulating acute myocardial infarction. *Am. Heart J.*, 1959;**58**: 755–759.
189. Doshi, R. and G. Neil-Dwyer, A clinicopathological study of patients following a subarachnoid hemorrhage. *J. Neurosurg.*, 1980;**52**: 295–301.
190. Tokgözoglu, S.L., M.K. Batur, M.A. Topçuoglu, O. Saribas, S. Kes, and A. Oto, Effects of stroke localization on cardiac autonomic balance and sudden death. *Stroke*, 1999;**30**: 1307–1311.
191. Jacob, W.A., A. van Bogaert, and M.H.A. De Groodt-Lasseel, Myocardial ultrastructure and haemodynamic reactions during experimental subarachnoid haemorrhage. *J. Mol. Cell. Cardiol.*, 1972;**4**: 287–298.
192. Shanlin, R.J., M.J. Sole, M. Rahimifar, C.H. Tator, and S.M. Factor, Increased intracranial pressure elicits hypertension, increased sympathetic activity, electrocardiographic abnormalities and myocardial damage in rats. *J. Am. Coll. Cardiol.*, 1988;**12**: 727–736.
193. McLeod, A.A., G. Neil-Dwyer, C.H.A. Meyer, P.L. Richardson, J. Cruickshank, and J. Bartlett, Cardiac sequelae of acute head injury. *Br. Heart J.*, 1982;**47**: 221–226.
194. Ackerman, M.J., Cardiac causes of sudden unexpected death in children and their relationship to seizures and syncope: Genetic testing for cardiac electropathies. *Semin. Pediatr. Neurol.*, 2005;**12**: 52–58.
195. Evrengul, H., H. Tanriverdi, D. Dursunoglu, et al., Time and frequency domain analyses of heart rate variability in patients with epilepsy. *Epilepsy Res.*, 2005;**63**: 131–139.
196. Griffith, T.W., On myotonia. *Q. J. Med.*, 1912;**5**: 229–247.
197. Evans, W., The heart in myotonia atrophica. *Br. Heart J.*, 1944;**6**: 41–47.
198. Church, S.C., The heart in myotonia atrophica. *Arch. Intern. Med.*, 1967;**119**: 176–181.
199. Olofsson, B.-O., H. Forsberg, S. Andersson, P. Bjerle, A. Henriksson, and I. Wedin, Electrocardiographic findings in myotonic dystrophy. *Br. Heart J.*, 1988;**59**: 47–52.
200. DeWind, L.T. and R.J. Jones, Cardiovascular observations in dystrophia myotonica. *J. Am. Med. Assoc.*, 1950;**144**: 299–303.
201. Petkovich, N.J., M. Dunn, and W. Reed, Myotonia dystrophica with A-V dissociation and Stokes-Adams attacks. A case report and review of the literature. *Am. Heart J.*, 1964;**68**: 391–396.
202. Finstere, J., C. Stollberger, and G. Meng, Cardiac involvement in facioscapulohumeral muscular dystrophy. *Cardiology*, 2005;**103**: 81–83.
203. Finsterer, J. and C. Stollberger, Cardiac involvement in primary myopathies. *Cardiology*, 2000;**94**: 1–11.
204. Berlit, P. and B. Stegaru-Hellring, The heart in muscular dystrophy: An electrocardiographic and ultrasound study of 20 patients. *Eur. Arch. Psychiat. Clin. Neurosci.*, 1991;**241**: 177–180.
205. De-Oliveira, J.M., M.P. Sambhi, and H.A. Zimmerman, The electrocardiogram in pectus excavatum. *Br. Heart J.*, 1958;**20**: 495–501.
206. Elisberg, E.I., Electrocardiographic changes associated with pectus excavatum. *Ann. Intern. Med.*, 1958;**49**: 130–141.
207. Wachtel, F.W., M.M. Ravitch, and A. Grishman, The relation of pectus excavatum to heart disease. *Am. Heart J.*, 1956;**52**: 21–37.
208. Dressier, W. and H. Roesler, Electrocardiographic changes in funnel chest. *Am. Heart J.*, 1950;**40**: 877–883.
209. Iakovlev, V.M., G.I. Nechaeva, and I.A. Viktorova, Clinical function of the myocardium and cardio- and hemodynamics in patients with pectus carinatum deformity. *Ter. Arkh.*, 1990;**62**: 69–72.
210. Kumar, U.K. and K.V. Sahasranam, Mitral valve prolapse syndrome and associated thoracic skeletal abnormalities. *J. Assoc. Physicians India*, 1991;**39**: 536–539.
211. Raggi, P., T.Q. Callister, N.J. Lippolis, and D.J. Russo, Is mitral valve prolapse due to cardiac entrapment in the chest cavity? A CT view. *Chest*, 2000;**117**: 636–642.

212. Chazan, R. and W. Droszcz, Electrocardiographic changes in patients with airway obstruction. *Pol. Arch. Med. Wewn.*, 1992;**87**: 237–241.
213. Efthimiou, J., A.B. Hassan, O. Ormerod, and M.K. Benson, Reversible T-wave abnormality in severe acute asthma: An electrocardiographic sign of severity. *Respir. Med.*, 1991;**85**: 195–202.
214. Gong, H. Jr., W.S. Linn, S.L. Terrell, et al., Altered heart-rate variability in asthmatic and healthy volunteers exposed to concentrated ambient coarse particles. *Inhal. Toxicol.*, 2004;**16**: 335–343.
215. Smith, R.P., M.K. Johnson, J. Ashley, S.T. Rudkin, and R.J. White, Effect of exercise induced hypoxaemia on myocardial repolarisation in severe chronic obstructive pulmonary disease. *Thorax*, 1998;**53**: 572–576.
216. Sarubbi, B., V. Esposito, V. Ducceschi, et al., Effect of blood gas derangement on QTc dispersion in severe chronic obstructive pulmonary disease: Evidence of an electropathy? *Int. J. Cardiol.*, 1997;**58**: 287–292.
217. Rudy, Y., The electrocardiogram and its relationship to excitation of the heart, in Physiology and Pathophysiology of the Heart, N. Sperelakis, Editor, 3rd edn. Kluwer, The Netherlands, 1995, p. 201.
218. McCord, J. and S. Borzak, Multifocal atrial tachycardia. *Chest*, 1998;**113**: 203–209.
219. Benditt, D.G., N. Samniah, S. Pham, et al., Effect of cough on heart rate and blood pressure in patients with "cough syncope". *Heart Rhythm*, 2005;**2**: 807–813.
220. Alonso-Fernandez, A., F. Garcia-Rio, M.A. Racionero, et al., Cardiac rhythm disturbances and ST-segment depression episodes in patients with obstructive sleep apnea-hypopnea syndrome and its mechanisms. *Chest*, 2005;**127**: 15–22.
221. Aydin, M., R. Altin, A. Ozeren, L. Kart, M. Bilge, and M. Unalacak, Cardiac autonomic activity in obstructive sleep apnea: Time-dependent and spectral analysis of heart rate variability using 24-hour Holter electrocardiograms. *Tex. Heart Inst. J.*, 2004;**31**: 132–136.
222. Nakamura, T., K. Chin, R. Hosokawa, et al., Corrected QT dispersion and cardiac sympathetic function in patients with obstructive sleep apnea-hypopnea syndrome. *Chest*, 2004;**125**: 2107–2114.
223. Valencia-Flores, M., A. Orea, M. Herrera, et al., Effect of bariatric surgery on obstructive sleep apnea and hypopnea syndrome, electrocardiogram, and pulmonary arterial pressure. *Obes. Surg.*, 2004;**14**: 755–762.
224. Stein, P.K., S.P. Duntley, P.P. Domitrovich, P. Nishith, and R.M. Carney, A simple method to identify sleep apnea using Holter recordings. *J. Cardiovasc. Electrophysiol.*, 2003;**14**: 467–473.
225. Madias, J.E., Amplitude of the electrocardiographic QRS complexes during and after severe pulmonary edema. *Ann. Noninvasive Electrocardiol.*, 2004;**9**: 192–197.
226. Rudy, Y., R. Wood, R. Plonsey, and J. Liebman, The effect of high lung conductivity on electrocardiographic potentials. Results from human subjects undergoing bronchopulmonary lavage. *Circulation*, 1982;**65**: 440–445.
227. Master, A.M., The electrocardiographic changes in pneumothorax in which the heart has been rotated: The similarity of some of these changes to those indicating myocardial involvement. *Am. Heart J.*, 1928;**3**: 472–483.
228. Littman, D., Electrocardiographic phenomena associated with spontaneous pneumothorax and mediastinal emphysema. *Am. J. Med. Sci.*, 1946;**212**: 682–690.
229. Armen, R.N. and T.V. Frank, Electrocardiogram patterns in pneumothorax. *Dis. Chest*, 1949;**15**: 709–719.
230. Copeland, R. and G. Omenn, Electrocardiographic changes suggestive of coronary artery disease in pneumothorax. Their reversibility with upright posture. *Arch. Intern. Med.*, 1970;**125**: 151–153.
231. Walston, A., D.L. Brewer, and C.S. Kitchens, The electrocardiographic manifestations of spontaneous left pneumothorax. *Ann. Intern. Med.*, 1974;**80**: 375–379.
232. Maheshwari, M. and S.R. Mittal, Right-sided pneumothorax simulating anterior wall myocardial infarction. *Indian Heart J.*, 2004;**56**: 73.
233. Sakabe, K., N. Fukuda, K. Wakayama, T. Nada, H. Shinohara, and Y. Tamura, Spontaneous pneumomediastium: A cause of T-wave inversion in electrocardiogram. *Int. J. Cardiol.*, 2004;**94**: 123–126.
234. Osswald, S., M. Roelke, S.S. O'Nunain, et al., Electrocardiographic pseudo-infarct patterns after implantation of cardioverter-defibrillators. *Am. Heart J.*, 1995;**129**: 265–272.
235. Madias, J.E., Comparison of P-waves recorded on the standard electrocardiogram, the "Lewis lead", and "saline-filled central venous catheter"-based intracardiac electrocardiogram. *Am. J. Cardiol.*, 2004;**94**: 474–478.
236. Eriksen, U.H., H. Molgaard, J. Ingerslev, and T.T. Nielsen, Fatal hemostatic complications following erroneous thrombolytic therapy in patients with suspected acute myocardial infarction. *Ugeskr. Laeger.*, 1993;**155**: 1392–1394.
237. Caruso, G., G.M. Trovato, A. Corsaro, and V. Sciuto, Correlative evaluation of electrocardiographic changes and spirometric parameters in pulmonary cardiopathy secondary to chronic obstructive bronchopneumopathy. *Recenti. Prog. Med.*, 1989;**80**: 468–470.
238. Lewczuk, J., Suggestive characteristics of inferior wall heart infarct in the EKG of patients with chronic cor pulmonale. *Pneumonol. Pol.*, 1989;**57**: 373–376.
239. Cutforth, R.H. and S. Oram, The electrocardiograms in pulmonary embolism. *Br. Heart J.*, 1958;**20**: 41–60.
240. Weber, D.M. and J.H. Phillips Jr., A re-evaluation of electrocardiographic changes accompanying acute pulmonary embolism. *Am. J. Med. Sci.*, 1966;**251**: 381–398.
241. Stein, P.D., J.E. Dalen, K.M. McIntyre, A.A. Sasahara, N.K. Wenger, and P.W. Willis III, The electrocardiograms in acute pulmonary embolism. *Prog. Cardiovasc. Dis.*, 1975;**17**: 2 47–57.
242. Hildner, F.J. and R.S. Ormond, Accuracy of the clinical diagnosis of pulmonary embolism. *J. Am. Med. Assoc.*, 1967;**202**: 567–570.
243. Ullman, E., W.J. Brady, A.D. Perron, et al., Electrocardiographic manifestations of pulmonary embolism. *Am. J. Emerg. Med.*, 2001;**19**: 514–519.
244. McGinn, S. and P.D. White, Acute cor pulmonale resulting from pulmonary embolism. Its clinical recognition. *J. Am. Med. Assoc.*, 1935;**104**: 1473–1480.
245. Sasahara, A., T.M. Hyers, C.M. Cole, et al. (eds.), The urokinase-pulmonary embolism trial. A national cooperative study. *Circulation*, 1973;**47** (Suppl. II): 1–12.
246. Chan, T.C., G.M. Vilke, M. Pollack, et al., Electrocardiographic manifestations: Pulmonary embolism. *J. Emerg. Med.*, 2001;**21**: 263–270.

247. Panos, R.J., R.A. Barish, W.W. Depriest, et al., The electrocardiographic manifestations of pulmonary embolism. *J. Emerg. Med.*, 1988;**6**: 301–307.
248. Lynch, R.E., P.D. Stein, and T.A. Bruce, Leftward shift of frontal plane QRS axis as a frequent manifestation of acute pulmonary embolism. *Chest*, 1972;**61**: 443–446.
249. Sreeram, N., E.C. Cheriex, J.L. Smeets, A.P. Gorgels, and H.J. Wellens, Value of the 12-lead electrocardiogram at hospital admission in the diagnosis of pulmonary embolism. *Am. J. Cardiol.*, 1994;**73**: 298–303.
250. Ferrari, E., A. Imbert, T. Chevalier, A. Mihoubi, P. Morand, and M. Baudouy, The ECG in pulmonary embolism: Predictive value of negative T waves in precordial leads-80 case reports. *Chest*, 1997;**111**: 537–543.
251. Daniel, K.R., D.M. Courtney, and J.A. Kline, Assessment of cardiac stress from massive pulmonary embolism with 12-lead ECG. *Chest*, 2001;**120**: 474–481.
252. Procacci, P.M., S.V. Savran, S.L. Schreiter, and A.L. Bryson, Prevalence of clinical mitral-valve prolapse in 1169 young women. *N. Engl. J. Med.*, 1976;**294**: 1086–1088.
253. Massie, B., E.H. Botvinick, D. Shames, M. Taradash, J. Werner, and N. Schiller, Myocardial perfusion scintigraphy in patients with mitral valve prolapse. *Circulation*, 1978;**57**: 19–26.
254. Digeos-Hasnier, S., X. Copie, O. Paziaud, et al., Abnormalities of ventricular repolarization in mitral valve prolapse. *Ann. Noninvasive Electrocardiol.*, 2005;**10**: 297–304.
255. Barlow, J.B. and W.A. Pocock, The problem of non ejection systolic clicks and associated mitral systolic murmurs: Emphasis on the billowing mitral leaflet syndrome. *Am. Heart J.*, 1975;**90**: 636–655.
256. DeMaria. A.N., E.A. Amsterdam, L.A. Vismara, A. Neumann, and D.T. Mason, Arrhythmias in the mitral valve prolapse syndrome. Prevalence, nature, and frequency. *Ann. Intern. Med.*, 1976;**84**: 656–660.
257. Devereux, R.B., J.K. Perloff, N. Reichek, and M.E. Josephson, Mitral valve prolapse. *Circulation*, 1976;**54**: 3–14.
258. Josephson, M.E., L.N. Horowitz, and J.A. Kastor, Paroxysmal supraventricular tachycardia in patients with mitral valve prolapse. *Circulation*, 1978;**57**: 111–115.
259. Winkle, R.A., M.G. Lopes, J.W. Fitzgerald, D.J. Goodwin, J.S. Schroeder, and D.C. Harrison, Arrhythmias in patients with mitral valve prolapse. *Circulation*, 1975;**52**: 73–81.
260. Shappell, S.D., C.E. Marshall, R.E. Brown, and T.A. Bruce, Sudden death and the familial occurrence of the mid-systolic click, late systolic murmur syndrome. *Circulation*, 1973;**48**: 1128–1134.
261. Kramer, H.M., P. Kligfield, R.B. Devereux, D.D. Savage, and R. Kramer-Fox, Arrhythmias in mitral valve prolapse. Effect of selection bias. *Arch. Intern. Med.*, 1984;**144**: 2360–2364.
262. Kligfield, P., C. Hochreiter, H. Kramer, et al., Complex arrhythmias in mitral regurgitation with and without mitral valve prolapse: Contrast to arrhythmias in mitral valve prolapse without mitral regurgitation. *Am. J. Cardiol.*, 1985;**55**: 1545–1549.
263. Lansdown, A.B.G., Viral infections and diseases of the heart. *Prog. Med. Virol.*, 1978;**24**: 70–113.
264. Morgera, T., A. Di Lenarda, L. Dreas, et al., Electrocardiography of myocarditis revisited: Clinical and prognostic significance of electrocardiographic changes. *Am. Heart J.*, 1992;**124**: 455–467.
265. Morgera, T., A. Salvi, E. Alberti, F. Silvestri, and F. Camerini, Morphological findings in apparently idiopathic ventricular tachycardia. An echocardiographic haemodynamic and histologic study. *Eur. Heart J.*, 1985;**6**: 323–334.
266. Feinstein, A.R., H.F. Wood, M. Spagnuolo, et al., Rheumatic fever in children and adolescents. A long-term epidemiologic study of subsequent prophylaxis, streptococcal infections, and clinical sequelae. VII. Cardiac changes and sequelae. *Ann. Intern. Med.*, 1964;**60** (Suppl. 5): 87–123.
267. Acquatella, H., F. Catalioti, J.R. Gomez-Mancebo, V. Davalos, and L. Villalobos, Long-term control of Chagas disease in Venezuela: Effects on serologic findings, electrocardiographic abnormalities and clinical outcome. *Circulation*, 1987;**76**: 556–562.
268. Maguire, J.H., K.E. Mott, J.S. Lehman, et al., Relationship of electrocardiographic abnormalities and seropositivity to Trypanosoma cruzi within a rural community in Northeast Brazil. *Am. Heart J.*, 1983;**105**: 287–294.
269. Villar, J.C., H. Leon, and C.A. Morillo, Cardiovascular autonomic function testing in asymptomatic T. cruzi carriers: A sensitive method to identify subclinical Chagas' disease. *Int. J. Cardiol.*, 2004;**93**: 189–1895.
270. Francis, J., M.A. Watanabe, and G. Schmidt, Heart rate turbulence: A new predictor for risk of sudden cardiac death. *Ann. Noninvasive Electrocardiol.*, 2005;**10**: 102–109.
271. Evrengul, H., D. Dursunoglu, V. Cobankara, et al., Heart rate variability in patients with rheumatoid arthritis. *Rheumatol. Int.*, 2004;**24**: 198–202.
272. Paradiso, M., M. Di Franco, A. Musca, et al., Ventricular late potentials in systemic sclerosis: Relationship with skin involvement. *J. Rheumatol.*, 2002;**29**: 1388–1392.
273. Algom, M., Z. Schlesinger, J. Madjar, S. Tal, D. Krakowsky, and K. Fried, Cardiovascular, skeletal and ophthalmologic manifestations in patients with Marfan's syndrome. *Isr. J. Med. Sci.*, 1989;**25**: 261–263.
274. Ansari, A., P.H. Larson, and H.D. Bates, Cardiovascular manifestations of systemic lupus erythematosus: Current perspective. *Prog. Cardiovasc. Dis.*, 1985;**27**: 421–434.
275. Laitinen, O., E. Kentala, and M. Leirisalo, Electrocardiographic findings in patients with connective tissue disease. *Scand. J. Rheumatol.*, 1978;**7**(4): 193–198.
276. Bagirova, V.V. and G.G. Bagirova, Cor pulmonale in various collagen diseases. *Kardiologiia*, 1978;**18**: 127–131.
277. Savage, D.D., S.F. Seides, C.E. Clark, et al., Electrocardiographic findings in patients with obstructive and nonobstructive hypertrophic cardiomyopathy. *Circulation*, 1978;**58**: 402–408.
278. Chen, C.Y. and W.G. Liang, Electrocardiographic patterns in patients with idiopathic hypertrophic cardiomyopathy. *Chin. Med. J.*, 1984;**33**: 393–402.
279. Braudo, M., E.D. Wigle, and J.D. Keith, A distinctive electrocardiogram in muscular subaortic stenosis due to ventricular septal hypertrophy. *Am. J. Cardiol.*, 1964;**14**: 599–607.
280. McKenna, W.J., S. Chetty, C.M. Oakley, and J.F. Goodwin, Arrhythmias in hypertrophic cardiomyopathy: Exercise and 48 hour ambulatory electrocardiographic assessment with and without beta adrenergic blocking therapy. *Am. J. Cardiol.*, 1980;**45**: 1–5.
281. Savage, D.D., S.F. Seides, B.J. Maron, D.J. Myers, and S.E. Epstein, Prevalence of arrhythmias during 24-hour electrocardiographic monitoring and exercise testing in patients with obstructive and nonobstructive hypertrophic cardiomyopathy. *Circulation*, 1979;**59**: 866–875.
282. Kon-No, Y., J. Watanabe, Y. Koseki, et al., Microvolt T wave alternans in human cardiac hypertrophy: Electrical instability and

abnormal myocardial arrangement. *J. Cardiovasc. Electrophysiol.*, 2001;**12**: 759–763.
283. Kuroda, N., Y. Ohnishi, A. Yoshida, A. Kimura, and M. Yokoyama, Clinical significance of T-wave alternans in hypertrophic cardiomyopathy. *Circ. J.*, 2002;**66**: 457–462.
284. Barletta, G., C. Lazzeri, F. Franchi, R. Del Bene, and A. Michelucci, Hypertrophic cardiomyopathy: Electrical abnormalities detected by the extended-length ECG and their relation to syncope. *Int. J. Cardiol.*, 2004;**97**: 43–48.
285. Frank, S. and E. Braunwald, Idiopathic hypertrophic subaortic stenosis. Clinical analysis of 126 patients with emphasis on the natural history. *Circulation*, 1968;**37**: 759–788.
286. Koga, Y., A. Yamaga, K. Hiyamuta, H. Ikeda, and H. Toshima, Mechanisms of abnormal Q waves in hypertrophic cardiomyopathy assessed by intracoronary electrocardiography. *J. Cardiovasc. Electrophysiol.*, 2004;**15**: 1402–1408.
287. Runquist, L.H., C.D. Nielsen, D. Killip, P. Gazes, and W.H. Spencer III, Electrocardiographic findings after alcohol septal ablation therapy for obstructive hypertrophic cardiomyopathy. *Am. J. Cardiol.*, 2002;**90**: 1020–1022.
288. Babuty, D., L. Fauchier, D. Nguyen, et al., Arrhythmias of primary hypertrophic cardiomyopathy *Arch. Mal. Coeur. Vaiss.*, 2003;**96**: 7–15.
289. Behr, E.R., P. Elliott, and W.J. McKenna, Role of invasive EP testing in the evaluation and management of hypertrophic cardiomyopathy. *Card. Electrophysiol. Rev.*, 2002;**6**: 482–486.
290. Kawai, S., H. Suzuki, H. Yamaguchi, et al., Ampulla cardiomyopathy ("Takotsubo" cardiomyopathy)-reversible left ventricular dysfunction: With ST segment elevation. *Jpn. Circ. J.*, 2000;**64**: 156–159.
291. Wittstein, I.S., D.R. Thiemann, J.A. Lima, et al., Neurohumoral features of myocardial stunning due to sudden emotional stress. *N. Engl. J. Med.*, 2005;**352**: 539–548.
292. Pavin, D., H. Le Breton, and C. Daubert, Human stress cardiomyopathy mimicking acute myocardial syndrome. *Heart*, 1997;**78**: 509–511.
293. Jonkaitiene, R. and V. Mizariene, Arrhythmogenic dilated cardiomyopathy. *Medicina (Kaunas)*, 2003;**39**: 673–676.
294. Matsuura, Y., W. Chin, T. Kurihara, et al., Tachycardia-induced cardiomyopathy: A case report. *J. Cardiol.*, 1990;**20**: 509–518.
295. Marcus, F.I. and G. Fontaine, Arrhythmogenic right ventricular dysplasia/cardiomyopathy: A review. *Pacing Clin. Electrophysiol.*, 1995;**18**: 1298–1314.
296. Mirvis, D.M., *Electrocardiography. A physiological Approach*. St. Louis, MO: Mosby, 1993.
297. Katz, L.N. and H. Wachtel, The diphasic QRS type of electrocardiogram in congenital heart disease. *Am. Heart J.*, 1937;**13**: 202–206.
298. Loperfido, F., A. Digaetano, P. Santarelli, et al., The evaluation of left and right ventricular hypertrophy in combined ventricular overload by electrocardiography: Relationship with the echocardiographic data. *J. Electrocardiol.*, 1982;**15**: 327–334.
299. Cabrera, E. and J.R. Monroy, Systolic and diastolic loading of the heart. II. Electrocardiographic data. *Am. Heart J.*, 1952;**43**: 669–686.
300. Hamby, R.I. and F. Raia, Electrocardiographic aspects of primary myocardial disease in 60 patients. *Am. Heart J.*, 1968;**76**: 316–328.
301. Goldberger, A., A specific ECG triad associated with congestive heart failure. *Pacing Clin. Electrophysiol.*, 1982;**5**: 593–599.
302. Trobec, R., B. Gersak, and R. Hren, Body surface mapping after partial left ventriculotomy. *Heart Surg. Forum*, 2002;**5**: 187–192.
303. Marriott, H.J.L., Electrocardiographic abnormalities, conduction disorders and arrhythmias in primary myocardial disease. *Prog. Cardiovasc. Dis.*, 1964;**7**: 99–114.
304. Tavel, M.E. and C. Fisch, Abnormal Q waves simulating myocardial infarction in diffuse myocardial diseases. *Am. Heart J.*, 1964;**68**: 534–537.
305. Flowers, N.C. and L.G. Horan, Electrocardiographic and vectorcardiographic features of myocardial disease, in Myocardial Disease, N.O. Fowler, Editor. Grune and Stratton, New York, 1973, pp. 181–211.
306. Stapleton, J.F., J.P. Segal, and W.P. Harvey, The electrocardiogram of myocardiopathy. *Prog. Cardiovasc. Dis.*, 1970;**13**: 217–239.
307. Childers, R., S. Lupovich, M. Sochanski, and H. Konarzewska, Left bundle branch block and right axis deviation: A report of 36 cases. *J. Electrocardiol.*, 2000;**33** Suppl: 93–102.
308. Zimetbaum, P.J., A.E. Buxton, W. Batsford, et al., Electrocardiographic predictors of arrhythmic death and total mortality in the multicenter unsustained tachycardia trial. *Circulation*, 2004;**110**: 766–769.
309. Shamim, W., M. Yousufuddin, M. Cicoria, D.G. Gibson, A.J. Coats, and M.Y. Henein, Incremental changes in QRS duration in serial ECGs over time identify high risk elderly patients with heart failure. *Heart*, 2002;**88**: 47–51.
310. Molhoek, S.G., L. VAN Erven, M. Bootsma, P. Steendijk, E.E. Van Der Wall, and M.J. Schalij, QRS duration and shortening to predict clinical response to cardiac resynchronization therapy in patients with end-stage heart failure. *Pacing Clin. Electrophysiol.*, 2004;**27**: 308–313.
311. Francis, J., M.A. Watanabe, and G. Schmidt, Heart rate turbulence: A new predictor for risk of sudden cardiac death. *Ann. Noninvasive Electrocardiol.*, 2005;**10**: 102–109.
312. Hohnloser, S.H., T. Klingenheben, D. Bloomfield, O. Dabbous, and R.J. Cohen, Usefulness of microvolt T-wave alternans for prediction of ventricular tachyarrhythmic events in patients with dilated cardiomyopathy: Results from a prospective observational study. *J. Am. Coll. Cardiol.*, 2003;**41**: 2220–2224.
313. Saksena, S. and A.J. Camm, *Electrophysiological Disorders of the Heart*. Philadelphia, PA: Elsevier Churchill Livingstone, 2005.
314. Rahman, J.E., E.F. Helou, R. Gelzer-Bell, et al., Noninvasive diagnosis of biopsy-proven cardiac amyloidosis. *J. Am. Coll. Cardiol.*, 2004;**43**: 410–415.
315. Kinoshita, O., M. Hongo, M. Takeda, and M. Sekiguchi, Body surface potential maps in patients with familial amyloid polyneuropathy. *J. Electrocardiol.*, 1993;**26**: 301–309.
316. Linhart, A., J.C. Lubanda, T. Palecek, et al., Cardiac manifestations in Fabry disease. *J. Inherit. Metab. Dis.*, 2001;**24** Suppl 2: 75–83.
317. Baudouy, P., P. Lombrail, I. Azancot, A. Piekarski, E. Martin, and R. Slama, Adiastole caused by a secondary cardiac hemochromatosis. Successful treatment with an iron chelating agent. *Arch. Mal. Coeur. Vaiss.*, 1983;**76**: 1240–1246.
318. Moiseev, S.V., E.N. Semenkova, and N.P. Shatkovskii, Heart involvement in hypereosinophilia: The restrictive or the dilated type? *Ter. Arkh.*, 1989;**61**: 79–81.
319. Bonnet, D., P. Rustin, A. Rotig, et al., Metabolic and genetic investigations in childhood cardiomyopathies. *Arch. Mal. Coeur. Vaiss.*, 1999;**92**: 1509–1514.

320. Hoskova, L., I. Malek, R. Krausova, M. Podzimkova, and J. Pirk, Electrocardiographic changes after heart transplantation. *Vnitr. Lek.*, 2002;**48** Suppl 1: 72–75.
321. Kolasa, M.W., J.C. Lee, J.E. Atwood, R.R. Marcus, and R.E. Eckart, Relation of QTc duration heterogeneity to morality following orthotopic heart transplantation. *Am. J. Cardiol.*, 2005;**95**: 431–432.
322. Stinson, E.B., E. Dong Jr, C.P. Hieber, J.S. Schroeder, and N.E. Shumway, Cardiac transplantation in man. I. Early rejection. *J. Am. Med. Assoc.*, 1969;**207**: 2233–2242.
323. Carzolari, V., A. Angelini, C. Basso, et al., Histologic findings in the conduction system after cardiac transplantation and correlation with electrocardiographic findings. *Am. J. Cardiol.*, 1999;**4**: 756–759.
324. Cooper, D.K., R.G. Charles, A.G. Rose, et al., Does the electrocardiogram detect early acute heart rejection. *Heart Transplant.*, 1985;**4**: 546–549.
325. Jamieson, S.W., B.A. Reitz, P.E. Oyer, C.P. Bieber, E.B. Stinson, and N.E. Shumway, Current management of cardiac transplant recipients. *Br. Heart J.*, 1979;**42**: 703–708.
326. Izrailtyan, I., J.Y. Kresh, R.J. Morris, et al., Early detection of acute allograft rejection by linear and nonlinear analysis of heart rate variability. *J. Thorac. Cadiovasc. Surg.*, 2000;**20**: 737–745.
327. Ali, A., M.R. Mehra, F.S. Malik, et al., Insights into ventricular repolarization abnormalities in cardiac allograft vasculopathy. *Am. J. Cardiol.*, 2001;**87**: 367–368.
328. Gao, S.Z., S.A. Hunt, V. Wiederhold, et al., Characteristics of serial electrocardiograms in heart transplant recipients. *Am. Heart J.*, 1991;**122**: 771–774.
329. Sandhu, J.S., E.I. Curtiss, W.P. Follansbee, et al., The scalar electrocardiogram of the orthotopic heart transplant recipient. *Am. Heart J.*, 1990;**119**: 917–923.
330. Eckart, R.E., M.W. Kolasa, N.A. Khan, M.D. Kwan, and M.E. Peele, Surface electrocardiography and histologic rejection following orthotopic heart transplantation. *Ann. Noninvas. Electrocardiol.*, 2005;**10**: 60–64.
331. Haberl, R., M. Weber, H. Reichenspurner, et al., Frequency analysis of the surface electrocardiogram for recognition of acute rejection after orthotopic cardiac transplantation in man. *Circulation*, 1987;**76**: 101–108.
332. Bernadic, M. and I. Sulkova, Classical electrocardiography and the Wigner distribution in the detection of rejection of heart transplants. *Bratisl. Lek. Listy.*, 2000;**101**: 223–225.
333. Zupan, I., B. Vrtovec, U.D. Breskvar, and T. Gabrijelcic, Noninvasive monitoring of rejection therapy based on intramyocardial electrograms after orthotopic heart transplantation. Initial experience with 14 cases. *Int. Immunopharmacol.*, 2005;**5**: 59–65.
334. Madias, C., B.J. Maron, J. Weinstock, N.A. Estes III, and M.S. Link, Commotio cordis-sudden cardiac death with chest wall impact. *J. Cardiovasc. Electrophysiol.*, 2007;**18**: 115–122.
335. Bianco, M., F. Colella, A. Pannozzo, et al., Boxing and "commotio cordis": ECG and humoral study. *Int. J. Sports Med.*, 2005;**26**: 151–157.
336. Franzius, C., H. Meyer-Hofmann, and A.E. Lison, Myocardial infarct and rhabdomyolysis after a high-voltage accident with successful resuscitation. *Dtsch. Med. Wochenschr.*, 1997;**122**: 400–406.
337. Lichtenberg, R., D. Dries, K. Ward, W. Marshall, and P. Scanlon, Cardiovascular effects of lightning strikes. *J. Am. Coll. Cardiol.*, 1993;**21**: 531–536.
338. Dec, W.G. Jr., T.A. Stern, and C. Welch, The effects of electroconvulsive therapy on serial electrocardiograms and serum cardiac enzyme values. *J. Am. Med. Assoc.*, 1985;**253**: 2525–2529.
339. Boriani, G., C. Valzania, M. Biffi, et al., Increase in QT/QTc dispersion after low energy cardioversion of chronic persistent atrial fibrillation. *Int. J. Cardiol.*, 2004;**95**: 245–250.
340. Chun, P.K., J.E. Davia, and D.J. Donohue, ST-segment elevation with elective DC cardioversion. *Circulation*, 1981;**63**: 220–224.
341. Eysmann, S.B., F.E. Marchlinski, A.E. Buxton, and M.E. Josephson, Electrocardiographic changes after cardioversion of ventricular arrhythmias. *Circulation*, 1986;**73**: 73–81.
342. Liaudet, L., R. Kehtari, and J.F. Enrico, Myocardial lesion secondary to defibrillation. Literature review and practical implications *Rev. Med. Suisse. Romande.*, 1993;**113**: 933–943.
343. Joglar, J.A., D.J. Kessler, P.J. Welch, et al., Effects of repeated electrical defibrillations on cardiac troponin I levels. *Am. J. Cardiol.*, 1999;**83**: 270–272.
344. Avitall, B., S. Port, R. Gal, et al., Automatic implantable cardioverter/defibrillator discharges and acute myocardial injury. *Circulation*, 1990;**81**: 1482–1487.
345. Spodick, D.H., Electrocardiogram in acute pericarditis. Distributions of morphologic and axial changes by stages. *Am. J. Cardiol.*, 1974;**33**: 470–474.
346. Shahar, A., H. Hod, G.M. Barabash, E. Kaplinsky, and M. Motro, Disappearance of a syndrome: Dressler's syndrome in the era of thrombolysis. *Cardiology*, 1994;**85**: 255–258.
347. Sapin, P.M., G. Koch, M.B. Blauwet, J.J. McCarthy, S.W. Hinds, and L.S. Gettes, Identification of false positive exercise tests with use of electrocardiographic criteria: A possible role for atrial repolarization waves. *J. Am. Coll. Cardiol.*, 1991;**18**: 127–135.
348. Kudo, Y., F. Yamasaki, Y. Doi, and T. Sugiura, Clinical correlates of PR-segment depression in asymptomatic patients with pericardial effusion. *J. Am. Coll. Cardiol.*, 2002;**39**: 2000–2004.
349. Hull, E., The electrocardiogram in pericarditis. *Am. J. Cardiol.*, 1961;**7**: 21–32.
350. Ginzton, L.E. and M.M. Laks, The differential diagnosis of acute pericarditis from the normal variant: New electrocardiographic criteria. *Circulation*, 1982;**65**: 1004–1009.
351. Spodick, D.H., "Low voltage ECG" and pericardial effusion; practical and conceptual problems. *Chest*, 1979;**75**: 113–114.
352. Spodick, D.H., Low voltage with pericardial effusion: Complexity of mechanisms. *Chest*, 2003;**124**: 2044–2045.
353. Surawicz, B. and C. Fisch, Cardiac alternans: Diverse mechanisms and clinical manifestations. *J. Am. Coll. Cardiol.*, 1992;**20**: 483–499.
354. Bruch, C., A. Schmermund, N. Dagres, et al., Changes in QRS voltage in cardiac tamponade and pericardial effusion: Reversibility after pericardiocentesis and after anti-inflammatory drug treatment. *J. Am. Coll. Cardiol.*, 2001;**38**: 219–226.
355. Dalton, J.C., R.J. Pearson, and P.D. White, Constrictive pericarditis: A review and long term follow-up of 78 cases. *Ann. Intern. Med.*, 1956;**45**: 445–458.
356. Evans, W. and F. Jackson, Constrictive pericarditis. *Br. Heart J.*, 1952;**14**: 53–59.
357. Abe, S., N. Watanabe, S. Ogura, et al., Myocardial metastasis from primary lung cancer: Myocardial infarction-like ECG changes and pathologic findings. *Jpn. J. Med.*, 1991;**30**: 213–218.
358. Tremel, F., O. Orliaguet, J.E. Lanney, O. Guenot, and E. Arnaud Crozat, Metastasis stimulating a myocardial infarction. *Arch. Mal. Coeur. Vaiss.*, 2003;**96**: 59–61.

359. Hammerschmidt, S., C. Pohlink, H. Wirtz, and T. Rother, Alternating electric heart axis in a patient with small cell lung cancer. *Dtsch. Med. Wochenschr.*, 2004;**129**: 19–22.
360. Shiono, J., H. Horigome, S. Yasui, T. Miyamoto, et al., Electrocardiographic changes in patients with cardiac rhabdomyomas associated with tuberous sclerosis. *Cardiol. Young*, 2003;**13**: 258–263.
361. Komiya, N., S. Isomoto, M. Hayano, T. Kugimiya, and K. Yano, The influence of tumor size on the electrocardiographic changes in patients with left atrial myxoma. *J. Electrocardiol.*, 2002;**35**: 53–57.
362. Rozanski, J.J. and M. Kleinfeld, Alternans of the ST segment of T wave. A sign of electrical instability in Prinzmetal's angina. *Pacing Clin. Electrophysiol.*, 1982;**5**: 359–365.
363. Puletti, M., C. Borgia, S.M. Erba, G. Jacobellis, and M. Curione, ST segment alternams in myocardial infarct: Apropos of a case. *G Ital. Cardiol.*, 1983;**13**: 208–211.
364. Rozanski, J.J. and M. Kleinfeld, Occurrence of ST segmental electrical alternans during exercise test. *Pacing Clin. Electrophysiol.*, 1981;**4**: 339–340.
365. Sochanski, M., T. Feldman, K.G. Chua, A. Benn, and R. Childers, ST segment alternans during coronary angioplasty. *Cathet. Cardiovasc. Diagn.*, 1992;**27**: 45–48.
366. Usher, B.W. and R.L. Popp, Electrical alternans: Mechanism in pericardial effusion. *Am. Heart J.*, 1972;**83**: 459–463.
367. Hamburger, W.W., L.N. Katz, and O. Saphir, Electrical alternans: A clinical study with a report of two necropsies. *J. Am. Med. Assoc.*, 1936;**106**: 902–905.
368. Gehi, A.K., R.H. Stein, L.D. Metz, and J.A. Gomes, Microvolt T-wave alternans for the risk stratification of ventricular tachyarrhythmic events: A meta-analysis. *J. Am. Coll. Cardiol.*, 2005;**46**: 75–82.
369. Bloomfield, D.M., R.C. Steinman, P.B. Namerow, et al., Microvolt T-wave alternans distinguishes between patients likely and patients not likely to benefit from implanted cardiac defibrillator therapy: A solution to the Multicenter Automatic Defibrillator Implantation Trial (MADIT) II conundrum. *Circulation*, 2004;**110**: 1885–1889.
370. Burgess, M.J., L.S. Green, K. Millar, and J.A. Abildskov, The sequence of normal ventricular recovery. *Am. Heart J.*, 1972;**84**: 660–669.
371. Autenreith, G., B. Surawicz, and C.S. Kuo, Sequence of repolarization on the ventricular surface in the dog. *Am. Heart J.*, 1975;**89**: 463–469.
372. Abildskov, J.A., Effects of activation sequence on the local recovery of ventricular excitability in the dog. *Circ. Res.*, 1976;**38**: 240–243.
373. Toyoshima, H. and M.J. Burgess, Electrotonic interaction during canine ventricular repolarization. *Circ. Res.*, 1978;**43**: 348–356.
374. Rosenbaum, M.B., H.H. Blanco, M.V. Elizari, J.O. Lizzari, and J.M. Davidenko, Electrotonic modulation of the T wave and cardiac inemory. *Am. J. Cardiol.*, 1982;**50**: 213–222.
375. Rosenbaum, M.B., H.H. Blanco, M.V. Elizari, J.O. Lizzari, and H.M. Vetulli, Electrotonic modulation of ventricular repolarization and cardiac memory, in Frontiers of Cardiac Electrophysiology, M.B. Rosenbaum and M.V. Elizari, Editors. Nijhoff, Boston, MA, 1983, pp. 67–99.
376. Hoffman, B.F., Electrotonic modulation of the T wave. *Am. J. Cardiol.*, 1982;**50**: 361–362.
377. Surawicz, B., Transient T wave abnormalities in intermittent bundle branch block. *Am. J. Cardiol.*, 1982;**50**: 363–364.
378. Rosen, M.R., What is cardiac memory? *J. Cardiovasc. Electrophysiol.*, 2000;**11**: 1289–1293.
379. Surawicz, B., What is cardiac memory? *J. Cardiovasc. Electrophysiol.*, 2001;**12**: 390–391.
380. Chung, E.K., *Principles of Cardiac Arrhythmias*, 3rd edn. Philadelphia,PA: Williams & Wilkins, 1983, pp. 348–349.
381. Ranganathan, N., V. Sivaciyan, and R.C. Chisholm, Effects of post-extrasystolic potentiation on systolic time intervals. *Am. J. Cardiol.*, 1978;**42**: 14–22.
382. Shvilkin, A., K.K.L. Ho, M.R. Rosen, and M.E. Josephson, T-vector direction differentiates postpacing from ischemic T-wave inversion in precordial leads. *Circulation*, 2005;**111**: 969–974.
383. Colleran, J.A., V. Papademetriou, P. Narayan, et al., Electrocardiographic abnormalities suggestive of myocardial ischemia during upper gastrointestinal bleeding. *Am. J. Cardiol.*, 1995;**75**: 312–314.
384. Khairy, P. and P. Marsolais, Pancreatitis with electrocardiographic changes mimicking acute myocardial infarction. *Can. J. Gastroenterol.*, 2001;**15**: 522–526.
385. Wani, M. and S. Hishon, ECG record during changes in oesophageal pH. *Gut*, 1990;**31**: 127–128.
386. Christensen, M., H.W. Hendel, V. Rasmussen, et al., Endoscopic retrograde cholangiopancreatography causes reduced myocardial blood flow. *Endoscopy*, 2002;**34**: 797–800.
387. Rosenberg, J., K. Stausholm, I.B. Andersen, et al., No effect of oxygen therapy on myocardial ischaemia during gastroscopy. *Scand. J. Gastroenterol.*, 1996;**31**: 200–205.
388. Patterson, K.W., N. Noonan, N.W. Keeling, et al., Hypoxemia during outpatient gastrointestinal endoscopy: The effects of sedation and supplemental oxygen. *J. Clin. Anesth.*, 1995;**7**: 136–140.
389. Holm, C., M. Christensen, V. Rasmussen, et al., Hypoxaemia and myocardial ischaemia during colonoscopy. *Scand. J. Gastroenterol.*, 1998;**33**: 769–772.
390. Jones, R. and S. Lydeard, Irritable bowel syndrome in the general population. *BMJ*, 1992;**304**: 87–90.
391. Frais, M.A. and K. Rodgers, Dramatic electrocardiographic T-wave changes associated with gastric dilatation. *Chest*, 1990;**98**: 489–490.
392. Ishikawa, K., T. Nagasawa, and H. Shimadu, Influence of hemodialysis on electrocardiographic wave forms. *Am. Heart J.*, 1979;**97**: 5–11.
393. Madias, J.E. and V. Narayan, Augmentation of the amplitude of electrocardiographic QRS complexes immediately after hemodialysis: A study of 26 hemodialysis sessions of a single patient, aided by measurements of resistance, reactance, and impedance. *J. Electrocardiol.*, 2003;**36**: 263–271.
394. Madias, J.E., P waves in patients with changing edematous states: Implications on interpreting repeat P wave measurements in patients developing anasarca or undergoing hemodialysis. *Pacing Clin. Electrophysiol.*, 2004;**27**: 749–756.
395. Urso, S., M. Garozzo, F. Milone, and G. Battaglia, Cardiovascular risk markers in hemodialysis patients. *Int. J. Artif. Organs*, 2004;**27**: 1083–1090.
396. Morales, M.A., C. Gremigni, P. Dattolo, et al., Signal-averaged ECG abnormalities in haemodialysis patients. Role of dialysis. *Nephrol. Dial. Transplant.*, 1998;**13**: 668–673.
397. Fukuta, H., J. Hayano, S. Ishihara, et al., Prognostic value of heart rate variability in patients with end-stage renal disease on chronic haemodialysis. *Nephrol. Dial. Transplant.*, 2003;**18**: 318–325.

398. Tezcan, U.K., B. Amasyali, I. Can, et al., Increased P wave dispersion and maximum P wave duration after hemodialysis. *Ann. Noninvasive Electrocardiol.*, 2004;**9**: 34–38.
399. Suzuki, R., K. Tsumura, T. Inoue, H. Kishimoto, and H. Morii, QT interval prolongation in the patients receiving maintenance hemodialysis. *Clin. Nephrol.*, 1998;**49**: 240–244.
400. Madias, J.E., Increases in P-wave duration and dispersion after hemodialysis are totally (or partially) due to the procedure-induced alleviation of the body fluid overload: A hypothesis with strong experimental support. *Ann. Noninvasive Electrocardiol.*, 2005;**10**: 129–133.
401. Birkhofer, A., G. Schmidt, and H. Forstl, Heart and brain – the influence of psychiatric disorders and their therapy on the heart rate variability. *Fortschr. Neurol. Psychiatr.*, 2005;**73**: 192–205.
402. Mont, L., J. Castro, B. Herreros, et al., Reversibility of cardiac abnormalities in adolescents with anorexia nervosa after weight recovery. *J. Am. Acad. Child Adolesc. Psychiat.*, 2003;**42**: 808–813.
403. Vanderdonckt, O., M. Lambert, M.C. Montero, B. Boland, and C. Brohet, The 12-lead electrocardiogram in anorexia nervosa: A report of 2 cases followed by a retrospective study. *J. Electrocardiol.*, 2001;**34**: 233–242.
404. Reilly, J.G., S.A. Ayis, I.N. Ferrier, S.J. Jones, and S.H. Thomas, QTc-interval abnormalities and psychotropic drug therapy in psychiatric patients. *Lancet*, 2000;**355**: 1048–1052.
405. Hollister, L.E., Electrocardiographic screening in psychiatric patients. *J. Clin. Psychiat.*, 1995;**56**: 26–29.
406. Goldberger, A.L., *Myocardial Infarction. Electrocardiographic Differential Diagnosis*, 4th edn. St. Louis, MO: Mosby Year Book, 1991.
407. Goldman, M.J., Normal variants in the electrocardiogram leading to cardiac invalidism. *Am. Heart J.*, 1960;**59**: 71–77.
408. Brady, W.J. and D. Roberts, and F. Morris, The nondiagnostic ECG in the chest pain patient: Normal and nonspecific initial ECG presentations of acute MI. *Am. J. Emerg. Med.*, 1999;**17**: 394–397.
409. Quyyumi, A.A., Current concepts of pathophysiology, circadian patterns, and vasoreactive factors associated with myocardial ischemia detected by ambulatory electrocardiography. *Cardiol. Clin.*, 1992;**10**: 403–415.
410. Bertolet, B.D., A.F. Boyette, C.A. Hofmann, et al., Prevalence of pseudoischemic ST-segment changes during ambulatory electrocardiographic monitoring. *Am. J. Cardiol.*, 1992;**70**: 818–820.
411. Madias, J.E., The earliest electrocardiographic sign of acute transmural myocardial infarction. *J. Electrocardiol.*, 1977;**10**: 193–196.
412. Prinzmetal, M., A. Ekmekci, R. Kennamer, J.K. Kwoczynski, H. Shubin, and H. Toyoshima, Variant form of angina pectoris, previously undelineated syndrome. *J. Am. Med. Assoc.*, 1960;**174**: 1794–1800.
413. Madias, J.E. and M. Attari, Exercise-triggered transient R-wave enhancement and ST-segment elevation in II, III, and aVF ECG leads: A testament to the “plasticity” of the QRS complex during ischemia. *J. Electrocardiol.*, 2004;**37**: 121–126.
414. Madias, J.E., Ventricular tachycardia-like complexes in acute myocardial infarction. *Chest*, 1985;**88**: 644.
415. Barnhill, J.E., J.P. Wikswo Jr, A.K. Dawson, et al., The QRS complex during transient myocardial ischemia: Studies in patients with variant angina pectoris and in a canine preparation. *Circulation*, 1985;**71**: 901–911.
416. Jacobson, D. and V. Schrire, Giant T wave inversion. *Br. Heart J.*, 1966;**28**:768–775, 417.
417. Wyss, S., M. Holzmann, F. Schaub, G. Forster, and E. Hohnloser, Abnorme Repolarisationsbilder nach Adams-Stokes’schen Anfällen. *Cardiologia*, 1962;**40**: 169–190.
418. Yamour, B.J., M.R. Sridharan, J.F. Rice, and N.C. Flowers, Electrocardiographic changes in cerebrovascular hemorrhage. *Am. Heart J.*, 1980;**99**: 294–300.
419. Surawicz, B. and E. Lepeschkin, The electrocardiographic pattern of hypopotassemia with and without hypocalcemia. *Circulation*, 1953;**8**: 801–823.
420. Vincent, G.M., J.A. Abildskov, and M.J. Burgess, QT interval syndromes. *Prog. Cardiovasc. Dis.*, 1974;**16**: 523–530.
421. Fowler, N.O., D. McCall, T.-C. Chou, J.C. Holmes, and I.B. Nanenson, Electrocardiographic changes and cardiac arrhythmias in patients receiving psychotropic drugs. *Am. J. Cardiol.*, 1976;**37**: 223–230.
422. Pruitt, R.D., E.W. Dennis, and S.A. Kinard, The difficult electrocardiographic diagnosis of myocardial infarction. *Prog. Cardiovasc. Dis.*, 1963;**6**: 85–106.
423. Cook, R.W., J.E. Edwards, and R.D. Pruitt, Electrocardiographic changes in acute subendocardial infarction, I and II. *Circulation*, 1958;**18**: 603–622.
424. Ogawa, H., K. Hiramori, K. Haze, et al., Classification of non-Q-wave myocardial infarction according to electrocardiographic changes. *Br. Heart J.*, 1985;;**4**: 473–478.
425. Miwa, K., H. Kambara, C. Kawai, and T. Murakami, Two electrocardiographic patterns with or without transient T-wave inversion during recovery periods of variant anginal attacks. *Jpn. Circ. J.*, 1983;**47**: 1415–1422.
426. Taylor, G.J., R.S. Crampton, R.S. Gibson, P.T. Stebbins, M.T.G. Waldman, and G.A. Beller, Prolonged QT interval at onset of acute myocardial infarction in predicting early phase ventricular tachycardia. *Am. Heart J.*, 1981;**102**: 16–24.
427. Ahnve, S., E. Gilpin, E.B. Madsen, V. Froelicher, H. Henning, and J. Ross Jr., Prognostic importance of QTc interval at discharge after acute myocardial infarction: A multicenter study of 865 patients. *Am. Heart J.*, 1984;**108**: 395–400,
428. Wheelan, K., J. Mukharji, R.E. Rude, et al., Sudden death and its relation to QT interval prolongation after acute myocardial infarction: Two-year follow-up. *Am. J. Cardiol.*, 1986;**57**: 745–750.
429. Sakamoto, T., C. Tei, M. Murayama, et al., Giant T wave inversion as a manifestation of asymmetrical apical hypertrophy (AAH) of the left ventricle. Echocardiographic and ultrasono-cardiotomographic study. *Jpn. Hearl J.*, 1976;**17**: 611–629.
430. Yamaguchi, H., T. Ishimura, S. Nishiyama, et al., Hypertrophic nonobstructive cardiomyopathy with giant negative T waves (apical hypertrophy). Ventriculographic and echocardiographic features in 30 patients. *Am. J. Cardiol.*, 1979;**44**: 401–412.
431. Kereiakes, D., D.J. Anderson, L. Crouse, and K. Chatterjee, Apical hypertrophic cardiomyopathy. *Am. Heart J.*, 1983;**105**: 855–856.
432. Ino, T., M. Iwahara, K. Nishimoto, et al., Infantile hypertrophic cardiomyopathy with QT prolongation. *Jpn. Heart J.*, 1986;**27**: 893–899.
433. Abildskov, J.A., K. Millar, M.J. Burgess, and W. Vincent, The electrocardiogram and the central nervous system. *Prog. Cardiovasc. Dis.*, 1970;**13**: 210–216.

434. Hammer, W.J., A.J. Luessenhop, and A.M. Weintraub, Observations on the electrocardiographic changes associated with subarachnoidal hemorrhage with special reference to their genesis. *Am. J. Med.*, 1975;**59**: 427–433.
435. Levine, H.D., Non-specificity of the electrocardiogram associated with coronary artery disease. *Am. J. Med.*, 1953;**15**: 344–355.
436. Hurch, G.E., R. Meyers, and J.A. Abildskov, A new electrocardiographic pattern observed in cerebrovascular accidents. *Circulation*, 1954;**9**: 719–723.
437. Cropp, G.J. and G.W. Manning, Electrocardiographic changes simulating myocardial ischemia and infarction associated with spontaneous intracranial hemorrhage. *Circulation*, 1960;**22**: 25–38.
438. Hersch, C., Electrocardiographic changes in subarachnoidal haemorrhage, meningitis, and intracranial space occupying lesions. *Br. Heart J.*, 1965;**26**: 785–793.
439. Miura, T., K. Tsuchihashi, E. Yoshida, K. Kobayashi, K. Shimamoto, and O. Iimura, Electrocardiographic abnormalities in cerebrovascular accidents. *Jpn. J. Med.*, 1984;**23**: 22–26.
440. Jachuck, S.J., P.S. Ramani, F. Clark, and R.M. Kalbag, Electrocardiographic abnormalities associated with raised intracranial pressure. *Br. Med. J.*, 1975;**1**: 242–244.
441. Goldstein, D.S., The electrocardiogram in stroke: Relationship to pathophysiological type and comparison with prior tracings. *Stroke*, 1979;**10**: 253–259.
442. Hayashi, S., J. Watanabe, S. Miyagawa, S. Tamakuma, and H. Nagaki, Studies of electrocardiographic patterns in cases with neurosurgical lesions. *Jpn. Heart J.*, 1961;**2**: 92–111.
443. Hrunninkhuis, L.G.H., Electrocardiographic abnormalities suggesting myocardial infarction in a patient with severe cranial trauma. *Pacing Clin. Electrophysiol.*, 1983;**6**: 1336–1340.
444. Tamura, K., T. Tamura, S. Yoshida, M. Inui, and N. Fukuhara, Transient recurrent ventricular fibrillation due to hypopotassemia with special note on the U wave. *Jpn. Heart J.*, 1967;**8**: 652–660.
445. Lepeschkin, E., H. Marchet, G. Schroeder, et al., Effect of epinephrine and norepinephrine on the electrocardiogram of 100 normal subjects.*Am. J. Cardiol.*, 1960;**5**: 594–603.
446. Mashima, S., Effects of insulin on the electrocardiogram. *Jpn. Heart J.*, 1960;**1**: 56–71.
447. Struthers, A.D., J.L. Reid, R. Whitesmith, and J.C. Rodger, Effect of intravenous adrenaline on electrocardiogram, blood pressure, and serum potassium. *Br. Heart J.*, 1983;**49**: 90–93.
448. Prinzmetal, M., Y. Hashimoto, A. Hayashi, et al., Effects of propranolol and epinephrine on the electrophysiology of the heart. *Jpn. Heart J.*, 1970;**11**: 478–488.
449. Giotti, A., F. Ledda, and P.F. Mannaioni, Effects of noradrenaline and isoprenaline, in combination with IX and p receptor blocking substances, on the action potential of cardiac Purkinje fibres. *J. Physiol. (Lond.)*, 1973;**229**: 99–113.
450. Nathan, D. and G.W. Heeler Jr., Electrophysiologic correlates of the inotropic effects of isoproterenol in canine myocardium. *J. Mol. Cell. Cardiol.*, 1975;**7**: 1–15.
451. Ueda, H., Y. Yanai, S. Murao, et al., Electrocardiographic and vectorcardiographic changes produced by electrical stimulation of the cardiac nerves. *Jpn. Heart J.*, 1964;**5**: 359–372.
452. Yanowitz, F., J.H. Preston, and J.A. Abildskov, Functional distribution of right and left stellate innervation to the ventricles. Production of neurogenic electrocardiographic changes by unilateral alteration of sympathetic tone. *Circ. Res.*, 1966;**18**: 416–428.
453. Murayama, M., K. Harumi, S. Mashima, K. Shimomura, and S. Murao, Prolongation of ventricular action potential due to sympathetic stimulation. *Jpn. Heart J.*, 1977;**18**: 259–265.
454. Autenrieth, G., H. Surawicz, C.S. Kuo, and M. Arita, Primary T wave abnormalities caused by uniform and regional shortening of ventricular monophasic action potential in dog. *Circulation*, 1975;**51**: 668–676.
455. Randall, W.C., M. Szentivanyi, J.H. Pace, J.S. Wechsler, and M.P. Kaye, Patterns of sympathetic nerve projections onto the canine heart. *Circ. Res.*, 1968;**22**: 315–323.
456. Piscatelli, R.L. and L.M. Fox, Myocardial injury from epinephrine overdosage. *Am. J. Cardiol.*, 1968;**21**: 735–737.
457. Wexler, H., J. Kuaity, and E. Simonson, Electrocardiographic effects of isoprenaline in normal subjects and patients with coronary atherosclerosis. *Br. Heart J.*, 1971;**33**: 759–764.
458. Murayama, M., S. Mashima, K. Shimomura, K. Takayanagi, Y.Z. Tseng, and S. Murao, An experimental model of giant negative T wave associated with QT prolongation produced by combined effect of calcium and isoproterenol. *Jpn. Heart J.*, 1981;**22**: 257–265.
459. Sayer, W.J., M. Moser, and T.W. Mattingly, Pheochromocytoma and the abnormal electrocardiogram. *Am. Heart J.*, 1954;**48**: 42–53.
460. Cheng, T.O. and T.T. Bashour, Striking electrocardiographic changes associated with pheochromocytoma. *Chest*, 1976;**70**: 397–399.
461. Van Vliet, P.D., H.B. Hurchell, and J.L. Titus, Focal myocarditis associated with pheochromocytoma. *N. Engl. J. Med.*, 1966;**274**: 102–108.
462. Rona, G., Catecholamine cardiotoxicity. *J. Mol. Cell Cardiol.*, 1985;**17**: 291–306.
463. Dessertenne, F., La tachycardie ventriculaire a deux foyers opposes variables. *Arch. Mal. Coeur. Vaiss.*, 1966;**59**: 263–272.
464. Soffer, J., L.S. Dreifus, and E.L. Michelson, Polymorphous ventricular tachycardia associated with normal and long QT intervals. *Am. J. Cardiol.*, 1982;**49**: 2021–2029.
465. Kernohan, R.J., Post-paroxysmal tachycardia syndrome. *Br. Heart J.*, 1969;**31**: 803–806.
466. Myerson, R.M. and A.H. Clagett Jr., Transient inversion of T waves after paroxysmal tachycardia. *J. Am. Med. Assoc.*, 1952;**148**: 193–196.
467. Tsutsumi, T., K. Izumo, S. Sekiya, and K. Harumi, Post-pacing T loop abnormalities. *Jpn. Heart J.*, 1985;**26**: 897–908.
468. Richter von Arnauld, H.P., H. Kirsch, C. Gauwerky, and K.W. Westermann, Schrittmacherarrhythmie durch ungewohnliche T-Welleninhibierung bei einem externen Demand-Schrittmacher. *Z. Kreilaufforsch.*, 1974;**63**: 637–642.
469. Denes, P., A. Pick, R.H. Miller, R.J. Pietras, and K.M. Rosen, A characteristic precordial repolarization abnormality with intermittent left bundle-branch block. *Ann. Intern. Med.*, 1978;**89**: 55–57.
470. Wood, M.A., J.P. DiMarco, and D.E. Haines, Electrocardiographic abnormalities after radiofrequency catheter ablation of accessory bypass tracts in the Wolff-Parkinson-White syndrome. *Am. J. Cardiol.*, 1992;**70**: 200–204.
471. Surawicz, B., Transient T wave abnormalities after cessation of ventricular preexcitation: Memory of what? *J. Cardiovasc. Electrophysiol.*, 1996;**7**: 51–59.

472. MacAlpin, R.N., W.A. Weidner, A.A. Kattus Jr., and W.N. Hanafee, Electrocardiographic changes during selective coronary cineangiography. *Circulation*, 1966;**34**: 627–637.
473. Klein, H.O., H. Gross, and I.L. Rubin, Transient electrocardiographic changes simulating myocardial infarction during open-heart surgery. *Am. Heart J.*, 1970;**79**: 463–470.
474. Martin, G.R. and P. Stanger, Transient prolongation of the QTc interval after balloon valvuloplasty and angioplasty in children. *Am. J. Cardiol.*, 1986;**58**: 1233–1235.
475. Hultgren, H.N., M. Miyagawa, W. Buch, and W.W. Angell, Ischemic myocardial injury during cardiopulmonary bypass surgery. *Am. Heart J.*, 1973;**85**: 167–176.
476. Benchimol, A., K.B. Desser, and J.A. Schumacher, Electrocardiographic changes during selective aortocoronary saphenous vein bypass graft angiography in man. *Am. J. Cardiol.*, 1973;**31**: 23–29.
477. Toshima, H., Y. Ohkita, and M. Shingu, Clinical features of acute coxsackie B viral myocarditis. *Jpn. Circ. J.*, 1979;**43**: 441–444.
478. Brody, D.A., A theoretical analysis of intracavitary blood mass influence on the heart-lead relationship. *Circ. Res.*, 1956;**4**: 731–738.
479. Feldman, T., K.M. Borow, A. Neumann, R.M. Lang, and R.W. Childers, Relation of electrocardiographic R-wave amplitude to changes in left ventricular chamber size and position in normal subjects. *Am. J. Cardiol.*, 1985;**55**: 1168–1174.
480. Wilson, F.N., F.D. Johnston, F. Rosenbaum, et al., The precordial electrocardiogram. *Am. Heart J.*, 1944;**27**: 19–85.
481. Holzmann, M., *Clinical Electrocardiography. A Textbook for Practitioners and Students.* Translated by Douglas Robertson, London: Staples Press, 1952.
482. Sodi-Pallares and R.M. Calder, *New Bases of Electrocardiography*. St. Louis, MO: The CV Mosby, 1956.
483. Mason, R.E. and I. Likar, A new system of multiplelead exercise electrocardiography. *Am. Heart J.*, 1966;**71**: 196–205.
484. Madias, J.E., Comparability of the standing and supine standard electrocardiograms, and standing, sitting, and supine stress electrocardiograms. *J. Electrocardiol.*, 2006;**39**(2): 142–149.
485. Jones, A.Y., C. Kam, K.W. Lai, et al., Changes in heart rate and R-wave amplitude with posture. *Chin. J. Physiol.*, 2003;**46**: 63–69.
486. Yeragani, V.K., R. Pohl, V.C. Jampala, R. Balon, J. Kay, and G. Igel, Effect of posture and isoproterenol on beat-to-beat heart rate and QT variability. *Neuropsychobiology*, 2000;**41**: 113–123.
487. Pharand, C., J.B. Nasmith, J.C. Rajaonah, B. Dube, and A.R. LeBlanc, Distinction between myocardial ischemia and postural changes in continuous ECG monitoring based on ST-segment amplitude and vector orientation-preliminary results. *Can. J. Cardiol.*, 2003;**19**: 1023–1029.
488. Dieuaide, F.R.,The ECG as an aid in the diagnosis of adhesive pericardial mediastinitis. *Arch. Int. Med.*, 1925;**35**: 362–370.
489. Ruttkay-Nedecky, I., Effects of respiration and heart position on the cardiac electric field, in The Theoretical Basis of Electrocardiology, C.V. Nelson and D.B. Geselowitz, Editors. Clarendon Press, Oxford, 1976, p. 120.
490. Madias, J.E., The Impact of changing edematous states on the QRS duration: Implications for cardiac resynchronization therapy and implantable cardioverter/defibrillator implantation *Europace*, 2005;**7**: 158–164.
491. Ishikawa, K., A.S. Berson, and H.W. Pipberger, Electrocardiographic changes due to cardiac enlargement. *Am. Heart J.*, 1971;**81**: 635–643.
492. Madias, J.E., Standard electrocardiographic and signal-averaged electrocardiographic changes in congestive heart failure. *Congest. Heart Fail.*, 2005;**11**: 266–271.
493. Fuenmayor, A.J., C.J. Vasquez, A.M. Fuenmayor, et al., Hemodialysis changes the QRS amplitude in the electrocardiogram. *Int. J. Cardiol.*, 1993;**41**: 141–145.
494. Madias, J.E. and V. Narayan, Augmentation of the amplitude of electrocardiographic QRS complexes immediately following hemodialysis: A study of 26 hemodialysis sessions of a single patient, aided by measurements of resistance/reactance/impedance. *J. Electrocardiol.*, 2003;**36**: 263–271.
495. Madias, J.E., Concealment of electrocardiographically based diagnosis of left ventricular hypertrophy by anasarca. *Am. J. Hypertens.*, 2004;**17**: 897–903.
496. Madias, J.E., Masking of the diagnoses of P-pulmonale, P-mitrale, and biatrial abnormality by anasarca peripheral edema. *Congest. Heart Fail.*, 2006;**12**(1): 20–24.
497. Madias, J.E., Significance of shortening of the mean QRS duration of the standard electrocardiogram in patients developing peripheral edema. *Am. J. Cardiol.*, 2002;**89**: 1444–1446.
498. Madias, J.E., QTc Interval in patients with changing edematous states: Implications on interpreting repeat QTc interval measurements in patients with anasarca of varying etiology, and those undergoing hemodialysis. *Pacing Clin. Electrophysiol.*, 2005;**28**: 54–61.
499. Belalcazar, A. and R. Patterson, Monitoring lung edema using the pacemaker pulse and skin electrodes. *Physiol. Meas.*, 2005;**26**: S153–S163.
500. Srar, G.W., G.W. Wagner, S.V. Behar, et al., Vectocardiographic criteria for the diagnosis of inferior myocardial infarction. *Circulation*, 1974;**49**: 829–836.
501. Frank, S., J.A. Colliver, and A. Frank, The electrocardiogram in obesity: Statistical analysis of1,029 patients. *J. Am. Coll. Cardiol.*, 1986;**7**: 295–299.
502. Valencia-Flores, M., A. Orea, and M. Herrera, Effect of bariatric surgery on obstructive sleep apnea and hypopnea syndrome, electrocardiogram, and pulmonary arterial pressure. *Obes. Surg.*, 2004;**14**: 755–762.
503. Singh, B.N., T.D. Gaarder, T. Kanegae, M. Goldstein, J.Z. Montgomerie, and H. Mills, Liquid protein diets and torsade de pointes. *J. Am. Med. Assoc.*, 1978;**240**: 115–119.
504. Brown, J.M., J.F. Yetter, M.J. Spicer, and J.D. Jones, Cardiac complications of protein-sparing modified fasting. *J. Am. Med. Assoc.*, 1978;**240**: 120–122.
505. Bhagwat, A.R. and P.J. Engel, Heart disease and pregnancy. *Cardiol. Clin.*, 1995;**13**: 163–168.
506. Lee, S.H., S.A. Chen, T.J. Wu, et al., Effects of pregnancy on first onset and symptoms of paroxysmal supraventricular tachycardia. *Am. J. Cardiol.*, 1995;**76**: 675–678.
507. Copeland, G.D. and T.N. Stern, Wenckebach periods in pregnancy and puerperium. *Am. Heart J.*, 1958;**56**: 291–298.
508. Veille, J.C., D.W. Kitzman, and A.E. Bacevice, Effects of pregnancy on the electrocardiogram in healthy subjects during strenuous exercise. *Am. J. Obstet. Gynecol.*, 1996;**175**: 1360–1364.
509. Oram, S., *Clinical Heart Disease*, 2nd edn. London: Heinemann, 1981, p. 703.
510. Cremer, M., Ueber die direkte Ableitung der Aktionsstrome des mensch lichen Herzens vom Oesophagus und iiber das Elektrokardiogramm des Fotus. *Munchener. Med. Woch. MMW Muench. Med. Wochenschr.*, 1906;**53**: 811–813.

511. de Smoler, P.E., H.C. Smith, and S. Karchmer, Correlation of fetal heart rate, maternal heart rate, and age of pregnancy. *Am. J. Obstet. Gynecol.*, 1975;**121**: 62–65.
512. Maekawa, M. and J. Toyoshima, The foetal electrocardiogram on the human subject. *Acta Sch. Med. Univ. Kioto*, 1930;**12**: 519–520.
513. Advances in fetal electrocardiography. *J. Perinat. Med.*, 1986;**14**: 345–452.
514. Van Oosterom, A., Spatial filtering of the fetal electrocardiogram. *J. Perinat. Med.*, 1986;**14**: 411–419.
515. Jenkins, H.M.L., Technical progress in fetal electrocardiography-A review. *J. Perinat. Med.*, 1986;**14**: 365–370.
516. Murray, H.G., The fetal electrocardiogram: Current clinical developments in Nottingham. *J. Perinat. Med.*, 1986;**14**: 399–404.
517. Cerrutti, S., G. Baselli, S. Civardi, et al., Variability analysis of the fetal heart rate signals as obtained from abdominal electrocardiographic readings. *J. Perinat. Med.*, 1986;**14**: 445–452.
518. Luzietti, R., R. Erkkola, U. Hasbargen, et al., European Community Multicentre Trial "Fetal ECG Analysis During Labour": The P-R interval. *J. Perinat. Med.*, 1997;**25**: 27–34.
519. Rosen, K.G., Fetal electrocardiogram waveform analysis in labour. *Curr. Opin. Obstet. Gynecol.*, 2005;**17**: 147–150.
520. Assaleh, K. and H. Al-Nashash, A novel technique for the extraction of fetal ECG using polynomial networks. *IEEE Trans. Biomed. Eng.*, 2005;**52**: 1148–1152.
521. Mochimaru, F., Y. Fujimoto, and Y. Ishikawa, The fetal electrocardiogram by independent component analysis and wavelets. *Jpn. J. Physiol.*, 2004;**54**: 457–463.
522. Tongsong, T., A. Iamthongin, C. Wanapirak, et al., Accuracy of fetal heart-rate variability interpretation by obstetricians using the criteria of the National Institute of Child Health and Human Development compared with computer-aided interpretation. *J. Obstet. Gynaecol. Res.*, 2005;**31**: 68–71.
523. Becker, A. and H.K. Hellerstein, Effects of drinking iced water on the T loop of the spatial vectorcardiogram and on the spatial ventricular gradient. *J. Electrocardiol.*, 1969;**2**: 145–157.
524. Scardi, S. and C. Pandullo, Supraventricular tachyarrhythmia of a variable degree of atrial synchronization caused by drinking cold water. *G. Ital. Cardiol.*, 1985;**15**: 454–455.
525. Gillinov, A.M. and T.W. Rice, Prandial atrial fibrillation: Off-pump pulmonary vein isolation with hiatal hernia repair. *Ann. Thorac. Surg.*, 2004;**78**: 1836–1838.
526. Ng, G.A., E.W. Lau, and M.J. Griffith, Temperature-sensitive focal atrial tachycardia in the left atrium. *J. Cardiovasc. Electrophysiol.*, 2000;**11**: 324–327.
527. Tanabe, T. and Y. Goto, Unstable angina pectoris-changes in the ST-T segment during daily activities such as bathing, eating, defecating and urinating. *Jpn. Circ. J.*, 1983;**47**: 451–458.
528. Routledge, H.C., S. Chowdhary, J.H. Coote, and J.N. Townend, Cardiac vagal response to water ingestion in normal human subjects. *Clin. Sci. (Lond.)*, 2002;**103**: 157–162.
529. Farb, A. and S.A. Valenti, Swallow syncope. *Md. Med. J.*, 1999;**48**: 151–154.
530. Wilmshurst, P.T., Tachyarrhythmias triggered by swallowing and belching. *Heart*, 1999;**81**: 313–315.
531. Shea, M.J., J.E. Deanfield, R.A. Wilson, C.M. Delandsheere, and A.P. Selwyn, Silent myocardial ischemia during mastication. *Am. J. Med.*, 1987;**82**: 357–360.
532. Figueras, J., B.N. Singh, W. Ganz, and H.J. Swan, Haemodynamic and electrocardiographic accompaniments of resting postprandial angina. *Br. Heart J.*, 1979;**42**: 402–409.
533. Lu, C.L., X. Zou, W.C. Orr, and J.D. Chen, Postprandial changes of sympathovagal balance measured by heart rate variability. *Dig. Dis. Sci.*, 1999;**44**: 857–861.
534. Corovic, N., Z. Durakovic, and M. Misigoj-Durakovic, Dispersion of the corrected QT interval in the electrocardiogram of the ex-prisoners of war. *Int. J. Cardiol.*, 2003;**88**: 279–283.
535. Galetta, F., F. Franzoni, F. Prattichizzo, M. Rolla, G. Santoro, and F. Pentimone, Heart rate variability and left ventricular diastolic function in anorexia nervosa. *Adolesc. Health*, 2003;**32**: 416–421.
536. Franzoni, F., E. Mataloni, R. Femia, and F. Galetta, Effect of oral potassium supplementation on QT dispersion in anorexia nervosa. *Acta Paediatr.*, 2002;**91**: 653–656.
537. Swenne, I., Heart risk associated with weight loss in anorexia nervosa and eating disorders: Electrocardiographic changes during the early phase of refeeding. *Acta Paediatr.*, 2000;**89**: 447–452.
538. Lorsheyd, A., D.W. de Lange, M.L. Hijmering, et al., PR and OTc interval prolongation on the electrocardiogram after binge drinking in healthy individuals. *Neth. J. Med.*, 2005;**63**: 59–63.
539. Gowda, R.M., I.A. Khan, B.C. Vasavada, and T.J. Sacchi, Alcohol-triggered acute myocardial infarction. *Am. J. Ther.*, 2003;**10**: 71–72.
540. Nishimura, F.T., T. Fukunaga, H. Kajiura, et al., Effects of aldehyde dehydrogenase-2 genotype on cardiovascular and endocrine responses to alcohol in young Japanese subjects. *Auton. Neurosci.*, 2002;**102**: 60–70.
541. Papaioannou, G.I. and J. Kluger, Ineffective ICD therapy due to excessive alcohol and exercise. *Pacing Clin. Electrophysiol.*, 2002;**25**: 1144–1145.
542. Steinbigler, P., R. Haberl, B. Konig, and G. Steinbeck, P-wave signal averaging identifies patients prone to alcohol-induced paroxysmal atrial fibrillation. *Am. J. Cardiol.*, 2003;**91**: 491–494.
543. Denison, H., S. Jern, R. Jagenburg, C. Wendestam, and S. Wallerstedt, ST-segment changes and catecholamine-related myocardial enzyme release during alcohol withdrawal. *Alcohol.* 1997;**32**: 185–194.
544. Gould, L., C.V. Reddy, K.C. Oh, et al., Electrophysiologic properties of coffee in man. *J. Clin. Pharmacol.*, 1979;**19**: 46–55.
545. Newcombe, P.F., K.W. Renton, P.M. Rautaharju, C.A. Spencer, and T.J. Montague, High-dose caffeine and cardiac rate and rhythm in normal subjects. *Chest*, 1988;**94**: 90–94.
546. Myers, M.G. and L. Harris, High dose caffeine and ventricular arrhythmias. *Can. J. Cardiol.*, 1990;**6**: 95–98.
547. Graboys, T.B., C.M. Blatt, and B. Lown, The effect of caffeine on ventricular ectopic activity in patients with malignant ventricular arrhythmia. *Arch. Intern. Med.*, 1989;**149**: 637–639.
548. Frost, L. and P. Vestergaard, Caffeine and risk of atrial fibrillation or flutter: The Danish Diet, Cancer, and Health Study. *Am. J. Clin. Nutr.*, 2005;**81**: 578–582.
549. Newby, D.E., J.M. Neilson, D.R. Jarvie, and N.A. Boon, Caffeine restriction has no role in the management of patients with symptomatic idiopathic ventricular premature beats. *Heart*, 1996;**76**: 355–357.
550. Hirsch, J.A., B. Bishop, and J.L. York, Role of parasympathetic (vagal) cardiac control in elevated heart rates of smokers. *Addict. Biol.*, 1996;**1**: 405–413.

551. Pope, C.A. 3rd, D.J. Eatough, D.R. Gold, et al., Acute exposure to environmental tobacco smoke and heart rate variability. *Environ. Health Perspect.*, 2001;**109**: 711–716.
552. Aparici, M., A.L. Fernandez Gonzalez, and J. Peteiro, 24-hour ambulatory electrocardiographic registry: Differences between smokers and non-smokers and habit breaking effects. *Med. Clin. (Barc.)*, 1993;**100**: 125–127.
553. Peters, R.W., N.L. Benowitz, S. Valenti, G. Modin, and M.L. Fisher, Electrophysiologic effects of cigarette smoking in patients with and without chronic beta-blocker therapy. *Am. J. Cardiol.*, 1987;**60**: 1078–1082.
554. Sperry, R.E., J.L. Vacek, and G.S. Smith, The effects of smoking on the signal-averaged electrocardiogram in normal subjects. *Chest*, 1991;**99**: 121–122.
555. Harrigan, R.A. and W.J. Brady, ECG abnormalities in tricyclic antidepressant ingestion. *Am. J. Emerg. Med.*, 1999;**17**: 387–393.
556. Groleau, G., R. Jotte, and R. Barish, The electrocardiographic manifestations of cyclic antidepressant therapy and overdose: A review. *J. Emerg. Med.*, 1990;**8**: 597–605.
557. Frishman, W.H., H.M. Sung, H.C. Yee, et al., Cardiovascular toxicity with cancer chemotherapy. *Curr. Probl. Cardiol.*, 1996;**21**: 225–286.
558. Hanley, P.C., D.R. Holmes Jr, P.R. Julsrud, et al., Use of conventional and newer radiographic contrast agents in cardiac angiography. *Prog. Cardiovasc. Dis.*, 1986;**28**: 435–448.
559. Zukerman, L.S., T.D. Friehling, N.M. Wolf, et al., Effect of calcium-binding additives on ventricular fibrillation and repolarization changes during coronary angiography. *J. Am. Coll. Cardiol.*, 1987;**10**: 1249–1253.
560. Brennan, E., P.R. Mahrer, and V.J. Aharonian, Incidence and presumed etiology of ventricular fibrillation during coronary angioplasty. *Am. J. Cardiol.*, 1991;**67**: 769–770.
561. Missri, J. and R.M. Jeresaty, Ventricular fibrillation during coronary angiography: Reduced incidence with nonionic contrast media. *Cathet. Cardiovasc. Diagn.*, 1990;**19**: 4–7.
562. Lange, R.A. and L.D. Hillis, Cardiovascular complications of cocaine use. *N. Engl. J. Med.*, 2001;**345**: 351–8.
563. Satran, D., C.R. Henry, C. Adkinson, C.I. Nicholson, Y. Bracha, and T.D. Henry, Cardiovascular manifestations of moderate to severe carbon monoxide poisoning. *J. Am. Coll. Cardiol.*, 2005;**45**: 1513–1516.
564. Lee, D., T.L. Hsu, C.H. Chen, S.P. Wang, and M.S Chang, Myocardial infarction with normal coronary artery after carbon monoxide exposure: A case report. *Zhonghua Yi Xue Za Zhi (Taipei)*, 1996;**57**: 355–359.
565. Weaver, L.K., R.O. Hopkins, K.J. Chan, et al., Hyperbaric oxygen for acute carbon monoxide poisoning. *N. Engl. J. Med.*, 2002;**347**: 1057–1067.
566. Katzman, G.M. and D.G. Penney, Electrocardiographic responses to carbon monoxide and cyanide in the conscious rat. *Toxicol. Lett.*, 1993;**69**: 139–153.
567. Saadeh, A.M., N.A. Farsakh, and M.K. Al-Ali, Cardiac manifestations of acute carbamate and organophosphate poisoning. *Heart*, 1997;**77**: 461–464.
568. Karki, P., J.A. Ansari, S. Bhandary, and S. Koirala, Cardiac and electrocardiographical manifestations of acute organophosphate poisoning. *Singapore Med. J.*, 2004;**45**: 385–389.
569. Vahter, M. and G. Concha, Role of metabolism in arsenic toxicity. *Pharmacol. Toxicol.*, 2001;**89**: 1–5.
570. Pain, A. and A. Wingfield, Electrocardiographic changes due to emetine therapy. *Trans. R. Soc. Trop. Med. Hyg.*, 1968;**62**: 221–226.
571. Chulay, J.D., H.C. Spencer, and M. Mugambi, Electrocardiographic changes during treatment of leishmaniasis with pentavalent antimony (sodium stibogluconate). *Am. J. Trop. Med. Hyg.*, 1985;**34**: 702–709.
572. Mashour, N.H., G.I. Lin, and W.H. Frishman, Herbal medicine for the treatment of cardiovascular disease, clinical considerations. *Arch. Intern. Med.*, 1998;**158**: 2225–2234.
573. Gonzalez-Romero, S., J.A. Gonzalez-Hermosillo, A. Gonzalez, M.E. Flores, and G. Mijangos Vargas, The electrocardiographic changes in patients stung by scorpions. *Arch. Inst. Cardiol. Mex.*, 1991;**61**: 15–20.
574. Hannukainen, J.C., U.M. Kujala, J. Toikka, et al., Cardiac structure and function in monozygotic twin pairs discordant for physical fitness. *J. Appl. Physiol.*, 2005;**99**: 535–541.
575. Shetler, K., R. Marcus, V.F. Froelicher, et al., Heart rate recovery: Validation and methodologic issues. *J. Am. Coll. Cardiol.*, 2001;**38**: 1980–1987.
576. Raczak, G., G.D. Pinna, M.T. La Rovere, et al., Cardiovagal response to acute mild exercise in young healthy subjects. *Circ. J.*, 2005;**69**: 976–980.
577. Turitto, G., E.B. Caref, G. El-Attar, et al., Optimal target heart rate for exercise-induced T-wave alternans. *Ann. Noninvasive Electrocardiol.*, 2001;**6**: 123–128.
578. Chiba, T., M. Yamauchi, N. Nishida, T. Kaneko, K. Yoshizaki, and N. Yoshioka, Risk factors of sudden death in the Japanese hot bath in the senior population. *Forensic Sci. Int.*, 2005;**149**: 151–158.
579. Ishikawa, K., C. Shirato, and A. Yanagisawa, Electrocardiographic changes due to sauna bathing. Influence of acute reduction in circulating blood volume on body surface potentials with special reference to the Brody effect. *Br. Heart J.*, 1983;**50**: 469–475.
580. Tanabe, T. and Y. Goto, Unstable angina pectoris-changes in the ST-T segment during daily activities such as bathing, eating, defecating and urinating. *Jpn. Circ. J.*, 1983;**47**: 451–458.
581. Pokan, R., M. Huonker, M. Schumacher, et al., ECG of the athlete's heart. *Acta Med. Austriaca*, 1994;**21**: 76–82.
582. Langdeau, J.B., L. Blier, H. Turcotte, G. O'Hara, and L.P. Boulet, Electrocardiographic findings in athletes: The prevalence of left ventricular hypertrophy and conduction defects. *Can. J. Cardiol.*, 2001;**17**: 655–659.
583. Pelliccia, A., F.M. Di Paolo, and B.J. Maron, The athlete's heart: Remodeling, electrocardiogram and preparticipation screening. *Cardiol. Rev.*, 2002;**10**: 85–90.
584. Biffi, A., B.J. Maron, L.Verdile, et al., Impact of physical deconditioning on ventricular tachyarrhythmias in trained athletes. *J. Am. Coll. Cardiol.*, 2004;**44**: 1053–1058.
585. Turkmen, M., I. Barutcu, A.M. Esen, et al., Assessment of QT interval duration and dispersion in athlete's heart. *J. Int. Med. Res.*, 2004;**32**: 626–632.
586. Lonati, L.M., G. Magnaghi, C. Bizzi, and G. Leonetti, Patterns of QT dispersion in athletic and hypertensive left ventricular hypertrophy. *Ann. Noninvasive Electrocardiol.*, 2004;**9**: 252–256.
587. Masini, V., M. Rocchi, and M. Santini, Dynamic ECG in normal subjects. *G Ital. Cardiol.*, 1980;**10**: 1267–1279.
588. Zhuang, Z., X. Gao, and S. Gao, The relationship of HRV to sleep EEG and sleep rhythm. *Int. J. Neurosci.*, 2005;**115**: 315–327.

589. Molnar, J., F. Zhang, J. Weiss, F.A. Ehlert, and J.E. Rosenthal, Diurnal pattern of QTc interval: How long is prolonged? Possible relation to circadian triggers of cardiovascular events. *J. Am. Coll. Cardiol.*, 1996;**27**: 76–83.
590. Zhong, X., H.J. Hilton, G.J. Gates, et al., Increased sympathetic and decreased parasympathetic cardiovascular modulation in normal humans with acute sleep deprivation. *J. Appl. Physiol.*, 2005;**98**: 2024–2032.
591. Guo, Y.F. and P.K. Stein, Circadian rhythm in the cardiovascular system: Considerations in non-invasive electrophysiology. *Card. Electrophysiol. Rev.*, 2002;**6**: 267–272.
592. Schuchert, A., G. Behrens, and T. Meinertz, Diurnal variations of the ventricular pacing threshold in patients with cardiac pacemakers are not related to changes in autonomic tone. *Am. J. Cardiol.*, 2000;**86**: 226–229.
593. Dilaveris, P.E., P. Farbom, V. Batchvarov, A. Ghuran, and M. Malik, Circadian behavior of P-wave duration, P-wave area, and PR interval in healthy subjects. *Ann. Noninvasive Electrocardiol.*, 2001;**6**: 92–97.
594. Yeragani, V.K., R. Berger, R. Pohl, and R. Balon, Effect of age on diurnal changes of 24-hour QT interval variability. *Pediatr. Cardiol.*, 2005;**26**: 39–44.
595. Drory, Y., I. Shapira, E.Z. Fisman, and A. Pines, Myocardial ischemia during sexual activity in patients with coronary artery disease. *Am. J. Cardiol.*, 1995;**75**: 835–837.
596. Drory, Y., E.Z. Fisman, Y. Shapira, and A. Pines, Ventricular arrhythmias during sexual activity in patients with coronary artery disease. *Chest*, 1996;**109**: 922–924.
597. Masini, V., E. Romei, and A.T. Fiorella, Dynamic electrocardiogram in normal subjects during sexual activity. *G. Ital. Cardiol.*, 1980;**10**: 1442–1448.
598. Sztajzel, J., M. Periat, V. Marti, P. Krall, and W. Rutishauser, Effect of sexual activity on cycle ergometer stress test parameters, on plasmatic testosterone levels and on concentration capacity. A study in high-level male athletes performed in the laboratory. *J. Sports Med. Phys. Fitness*, 2000;**40**: 233–239.
599. Wilmshurst, P.T., Tachyarrhythmias triggered by swallowing and belching. *Heart*, 1999;**81**: 313–315.
600. Lowenstein, L. and A. Hussein, Transient ischemic ECG changes in a patient with acute cholecystitis without a history of ischemic heart disease. *Harefuah*, 2000;**138**: 449–450.
601. Contaldo, F., M.R. Di Paolo, C. Mazzacano, G. Di Biase, and D. Giumetti, Hypopotassemia and prolongation of the Q-T interval in a patient with severe malnutrition caused by bulimia and post-prandial vomiting. *Recenti. Prog. Med.*, 1990;**81**: 266–268.
602. Brignole, M., Neurally-mediated syncope. *Ital. Heart J.*, 2005;**6**: 249–255.
603. Mikhail, M.S., D. Thangathurai, J.F. Viljoen, and P.A. Chandraratna, Atrioventricular block secondary to straining. *Crit. Care Med.*,1987;**15**: 705–706.
604. Rudas, L., A. Kardos, L. Halmai, T. Torok, I. Pap, and Z. Hegedus, Defecation syncope following pacemaker implantation. *Orv. Hetil.*, 1997;**138**: 81–82.
605. Molander, U., D.K. Dey, V. Sundh, and B. Steen, ECG abnormalities in the elderly: Prevalence, time and generation trends and association with mortality. *Aging Clin. Exp. Res.*, 2003;**15**: 488–493.
606. Roffe, C., Ageing of the heart. *Br. J. Biomed. Sci.*, 1998;**55**: 136–148.
607. Becker, A.E., How structurally normal are human atria in patients with atrial fibrillation? *Heart Rhythm*, 2004;**1**: 627–631.
608. Alfakih, K., K. Walters, T. Jones, J. Ridgway, A.S. Hall, and M. Sivananthan, New gender-specific partition values for ECG criteria of left ventricular hypertrophy: Recalibration against cardiac MRI. *Hypertension*, 2004;**44**: 175–179.
609. Colaco, R., P. Reay, C. Beckett, T.C. Aitchison, and P.W. Mcfarlane, False positive ECG reports of anterior myocardial infarction in women. *J. Electrocardiol.*, 2000;**33** Suppl: 239–244.
610. Endres, S., K.A. Mayuga, A. Cristofaro, T. Taneja, J.J. Goldberger, and A.H. Kadish, Menstrual cycle and ST height. *Ann. Noninvasive Electrocardiol.*, 2004;**9**: 121–126.
611. James, A.F., S.C. Choisy, and J.C. Hancox, Recent advances in understanding sex differences in cardiac repolarization. *Prog. Biophys. Mol. Biol.*, 2007;**94**(3): 265–319.
612. Sredniawa, B., A. Musialik-Lydka, P. Jarski, Z. Kalarus, and L. Polonski, Circadian and sex-dependent QT dynamics. *Pacing Clin. Electrophysiol.*, 2005;**28** Suppl 1:S211–S216.
613. Regecova, V. and D. Andrasyova, Relation between anthropometric indicators and electrocardiogram variability. *Vnitr. Lek.*, 2002;**48**: Suppl 1: 120–129.
614. Xie, Z., C. Wang, and M. Li, Electrocardiographic T-wave amplitude of normal population and its correlation with age, sex and race. *Hunan Yi Ke Da Xue Xue Bao*, 1999;**24**: 335–340.
615. Mansi, I.A. and I.S. Nash, Ethnic differences in electrocardiographic amplitude measurements. *Ann. Saudi. Med.*, 2004;**24**: 459–464.
616. Upshaw, C.B. Jr., Comparison of the prevalence of first-degree atrioventricular block in African-American and in Caucasian patients: An electrocardiographic study III. *J. Natl. Med. Assoc.*, 2004;**96**: 756–760.
617. Simpson, R.J. Jr, W.E. Cascio, P.J. Schreiner, R.S. Crow, P.M. Rautaharju, and G. Heiss, Prevalence of premature ventricular contractions in a population of African American and white men and women: The Atherosclerosis Risk in Communities (ARIC) study. *Am. Heart J.*, 2002;**143**: 535–540.
618. Upshaw, C.B. Jr., Lower prevalence of intraventricular block in African-American patients compared with Caucasian patients: An electrocardiographic study II. *J. Natl. Med. Assoc.*, 2003;**95**: 818–824.
619. Upshaw, C.B. Jr., Reduced prevalence of atrial fibrillation in black patients compared with white patients attending an urban hospital: An electrocardiographic study. *J. Natl. Med. Assoc.*, 2002;**94**: 204–208.
620. Klatsky, A.L., R. Oehm, R.A. Cooper, N. Udaltsova, and M.A. Armstrong, The early repolarization normal variant electrocardiogram: Correlates and consequences. *Am. J. Med.*, 2003;**115**: 171–177.
621. Niakara, A., N. Ouedraogo, L.V. Nebie, N.J. Kabore, and C.A. Megnigbeto, Routine electrocardiographic criteria for the diagnosis of left ventricular hypertrophy: Performance in Black Africans. *Ann. Cardiol. Angeiol. (Paris)*, 2002;**51**: 193–198.
622. MacAlpin, R.N., Clinical significance of QS complexes in V_1 and V_2 without other electrocardiographic abnormality. *Ann. Noninvasive Electrocardiol.*, 2004;**9**: 39–47.
623. Kambara, H. and J. Phillips, Long-term evaluation of early repolarization syndrome (normal variant RS-T segment elevation). *Am. J. Cardiol.*, 1976;**38**: 157–156.
624. Mirvis, D.M., Evaluation of normal variation in S-T segment patterns by body surface isopotential mapping: S-T segment elevation in absence of heart disease. *Am. J. Cardiol.*, 1982;**50**: 122–128.

625. Mirvis, D.M., The electrogenesis of terminal QRS notches in normal subjects. *J. Electrocardiol.*, 1983;**16**: 113–121.
626. Mirvis, D.M., Evaluation of normal variation in S-T segment patterns by body surface isopotential mapping: S-T segment elevation in absence of heart disease. *Am. J. Cardiol.*, 1982;**50**: 122–128.
627. Gussak, I. and C. Antzelevitch, Early repolarization syndrome: Clinical characteristics and possible cellular and ionic mechanisms. *J. Electrocardiol.*, 2000;**33**: 299–309.
628. Page, H.L. Jr and W.B. Campbell, Electrocardiography: Persistent juvenile T wave pattern. *J. Tenn. Med. Assoc.*, 1974;**67**: 306.
629. Lown, B., W.F. Ganong, and S.A. Levine, The syndrome of short P-R interval, normal QRS complex and paroxysmal rapid heart action. *Circulation*, 1952;**5**: 693–706.
630. Brodsky, M., D. Wu, P. Denes, C. Kanakis, and K.M. Rosen, Arrhythmias documented by 24 hour continuous electrocardiographic monitoring in 50 male medical students without apparent heart disease. *Am. J. Cardiol.*, 1977;**39**: 390–395.
631. Marriott, H.J.L., *Practical Electrocardiography*. Baltimore, MD: Williams & Wilkins, 1983, pp. 33–35.
632. Peberdy, M.A. and J.P. Ornato, Recognition of electrocardiographic lead misplacements. *Am. J. Emerg. Med.*, 1993;**11**: 403–405.
633. Madias, J.E., A comparison of 2-lead, 6-lead, and 12-lead ECGs in patients with changing edematous states: Implications for the employment of quantitative electrocardiography in research and clinical applications. *Chest*, 2003;**124**: 2057–2063.
634. Herman, M.V., D.A. Ingram, J.A. Levy, J.R. Cook, and R.J. Athans, Variability of electrocardiographic precordial lead placement: A method to improve accuracy and reliability. *Clin. Cardiol.*, 1991;**14**: 469–476.
635. Knight, B.P., F. Pelosi, G.F. Michaud, et al., Clinical consequences of electrocardiographic artifact mimicking ventricular tachycardia. *N. Engl. J. Med.*, 1999;**341**: 1270–1274, 278.
636. Krantz, M.J. and J.A. Garcia, Pseudo-torsade de pointes with underlying wandering pacemaker. *Clin. Cardiol.*, 2005;**28**: 355.
637. Ripa, R.S., E. Persson, B. Heden, et al., Comparison between human andautomated electrocardiographic waveform measurements for calculating the Anderson-Wilkins acuteness score in patients with acute myocardial infarction. *J. Electrocardiol.*, 2005;**38**: 96–99.
638. Poon, K., P.M. Okin, and P. Kligfield, Diagnostic performance of a computer-based ECG rhythm algorithm. *J. Electrocardiol.*, 2005;**38**: 235–238.
639. Hamilton, R.M., A.B. Houston, K. McLeod, and P.W. Macfarlane, Evaluation of pediatric electrocardiogram diagnosis of ventricular hypertrophy by computer program compared with cardiologists. *Pediatr. Cardiol.*, 2005;**26**: 373–378.
640. Madias, J.E., A. Kaminetsky, and N. Sonlanki, Myocardial infarction-induced ventricular aneurysm in the presence of complete left bundle branch block. *J. Electrocardiol.*, 1999;**32**: 179–183.
641. Madias, J.E., R. Ashtiani, H. Agarwal, V.K. Narayan, M. Win, and A. Sinha, Diagnosis of ventricular aneurysm and other severe segmental left ventricular dysfunction consequent to a myocardial infarction in the presence of right bundle branch block: ECG correlates of a positive diagnosis made via echocardiography and/or contrast ventriculography. *Ann. Noninvasive Electrocardiol.*, 2005;**10**: 53–59.
642. Madias, J.E., M. Mahjoub, and J. Valance, The paradox of negative exercise stress ECG/positive thallium scintigram. Ischemic ST-segment counterpoise as the underlying mechanism. *J. Electrocardiol.*, 1996;**29**: 243–248.
643. Madias, J.E., P. Knez, and M.T. Win, True-positive exercise electrocardiogram/false-negative thallium-201 scintigram: A proposal of a mechanism for the paradox. *Clin. Cardiol.*, 2000;**23**: 625–629.
644. Madias, J.E., B. Manyam, M. Khan, V. Singh, and C. Tziros, Transient disappearance of Q waves of previous myocardial infarction due to exercise-induced ischemia of the contralateral noninfarcted myocardium. *J. Electrocardiol.*, 1997;**30**: 97–103.
645. Madias, J.E., V. Narayan, and M. Attari, Detection of P waves via a "saline-filled central venous catheter electrocardiographic lead" in patients with low electrocardiographic voltage due to anasarca. *Am. J. Cardiol.*, 2003;**91**: 910–914.

9 The Electrocardiogram in Congenital Heart Disease

Jerome Liebman

P. W. Macfarlane et al. (eds.), *Electrocardiology*, DOI 10.1007/978-0-85729-874-4_9,

9.1 Introduction

The electrocardiogram in congenital heart disease has often been discussed in terms of specific types of electrocardiograms for specific types of lesions. Indeed, in the pages, which follow, certain such relationships do occur. However, the relationships are usually based upon specific mechanisms, some of which are well understood (including cardiovascular hemodynamics) and some of which are not. Close analysis reveals that most of the time the electrocardiogram is not specific for a specific lesion, but that the hemodynamics determine the changes from normal. An exception is the abnormal superior vector associated with endocardial cushion defect. Therefore, an understanding of the electrocardiogram of infants, children and young adults with congenital heart diseases necessitates an understanding of the hemodynamics of the various lesions. Consequently, accompanying the discussion of each lesion will be a brief delineation of pertinent hemodynamics. Since these hemodynamics are usually not contaminated by effects of coronary artery disease, the related atrial and ventricular hypertrophy tends to be relatively "pure" as compared to hypertrophy in the older adult. On the other hand, there are specific problems which complicate matters in infants and children, particularly the problem of the heart being so large in relation to the chest – the proximity effect. [1–6] This proximity effect not only accentuates anterior over posterior sources in terms of magnitude but may significantly distort the orientation of the various sources differently in different parts of the chest [1–6]. These effects plus lung effects and various inhomogeneities appear to be particularly important in children [7–12]. Another problem relates to the often considerable differences in normal values from one age-group to another, particularly in early infancy [8, 9, 11–13]. Appropriate statistics for electrocardiography must also be utilized [14, 15].

Despite the obvious differences between infants and, children on the one hand and the older adult on the other, the basic principles of the electrocardiographic interpretations are not different per se [10]. Furthermore, there are no differences in basic principles when interpreting the electrocardiogram of people with congenital heart disease. The interpretation must be based upon known physics, physiology and pathology [3, 4, 8, 10].

The term electrocardiography is used for

(a) The two lead systems of standard electrocardiography with scalar display, namely the standard limb leads and the precordial leads [8, 9]
(b) Orthogonal electrocardiography with scalar and/or vector display [16–20]
(c) Electrocardiographic body surface potential mapping (BSPM) [21, 22]

In this chapter, standard electrocardiography, and Frank system [16] and McFee–Parungao system [17] orthogonal electrocardiography, will be utilized, often contiguously. In all figures showing simultaneous X, Y and Z scalars, the paper speed is 50 div s^{-1}. It seems probable that some form of BSPM is part of the future of electrocardiography, but its inclusion in this chapter will be minimal; it is discussed in detail in ➋ Chaps. 9 and ➋ 10 of *Cardiac Arrhythmias and Mapping Technique*.

The approach to interpretation of the electrocardiogram must also reflect improvements in the understanding of anatomical, physical and electrophysiological phenomena. Terminology, as much as possible, must be based upon appropriate principles, the past not being revered simply because of usage. The term "axis deviation," for example, is not appropriate since "axis" as utilized, refers to the mean QRS vector in the frontal plane. There are many areas of the heart being depolarized early, other areas late and other areas later yet. These areas cannot be averaged.

The only axes of use are the X, Y and Z axes, representing left-right, inferior-superior, and anterior-posterior directions. Although, there are many areas of interpretation where understanding is deficient, pattern reading is not generally reliable. Perhaps, the major element necessary for appropriate interpretation of hypertrophy is the knowledge of the sequence of activation "what is being depolarized and when" [8–10, 21–26].

A most useful way to appreciate "what is being depolarized and when" (while interpreting the standard electrocardiogram), is to utilize vector analysis, despite the known inaccuracies. Each lead on the chest, for example, is best viewed as a projection of the cardiac vector (see ➋ Chaps. 10, ➋ 11 of *Basic Electrocardiology: Cardiac Electrophysiology, ECG Systems and Mathematical Modeling*, and ➋ 1), despite the fact that this projection is distorted by many things, including proximity effects and various inhomogeneities. The vector loop in the frontal plane of standard electrocardiography is only minimally useful even though proximity distortion is not a factor, particularly because of the very poor X axis as represented in lead I. This poor X axis is the major distorting factor in Burger's scalene triangle [27]. The vector loop in the horizontal plane of standard electrocardiography is extremely useful, however, despite the distortion of the cardiac vector. For an explicit description of the simple methodology for construction of the vector loop from standard limb or precordial leads, see previous publications [8–10]. Considerable reference will be made in this chapter to such vector loops – hence the use of terms such as "terminal vector" in the standard ECG.

The electrocardiographer must also have available all normal values for the various types of useful parameters, including the quantitative limits for specific leads. These values must be utilized within the guidelines of appropriate statistics [13, 14]. The normal limits of the ECG in infants and children are discussed in ➋ Chap. 1 and a comprehensive list of tables is presented in the Appendices. Many of these tables were produced as a result of the work of the author [8, 9]. A separate paper dealing with statistical treatment of data has also been prepared by the author and is presented in the Appendices. For convenience a small summary table of principal limits of normality is presented in the ➋ Table 9.1.

In the following pages, common and otherwise important congenital cardiac diseases will be discussed and representative electrocardiograms will be illustrated. Whenever pertinent, the hemodynamics will be illustrated utilizing the box diagram, as shown for a normal child [28, 29] in ➋ Fig. 9.1.

9.2 Atrial Septal Defect (Ostium Secundum Type)

Atrial septal defect (ASD) is not a disease usually recognized in early infancy [28]. Since compliance of the right ventricle in the newborn period is diminished as compared to that of the left ventricle, there is no left-to-right shunt at that time. At the same time, there is no stimulus to prevent the newborn's pulmonary arterioles and small muscular arteries (resistance vessels) from maturing normally (rapidly) into thin-walled, very compliant vessels. Such "adult-type" vessels can allow up to three to four times normal flow without increasing pulmonary artery pressure. In the first weeks to months after birth, as compliance of the right ventricle slowly increases compared to that of the left ventricle, a left-to-right shunt develops, albeit very slowly. As the left-to-right shunt slowly increases, selective hypertrophy gradually develops so that the ventricle is conditioned to prevent congestive heart failure. The hypertrophy causes a decrease in compliance of the right ventricle resulting in the slow development of the left-to-right shunt because of "feed back" mechanisms. By the time a large left-to-right shunt is present through the ASD, the resistance vessels are thin-walled and the pulmonary artery pressure is rarely more than 35–40 mm Hg systolic. The consequence is a right ventricle, which is complaint, is a little thicker than normal, but is dilated. Very few children with atrial septal defect are diagnosed as such between 1 and 2 years of age. Most then remain very stable throughout childhood. The box diagrams ➋ Fig. 9.2 for atrial septal defect include the volume of work in each chamber. There is increased volume of work of both the right atrium and right ventricle (although there is increased volume entering the left atrium, it immediately goes through the nonrestrictive ASD so that there is no increased work for the left atrium).

Table 9.1

Approximate upper limits of normal subjects used as a pediatric ECG "ready-reckoner" (ECG standards 95%)

Age	Heart rate (beats min^{-1})	PR (s)	QRS (s)	QT (s)	V_5 R	V_5 S	aVF R	aVF S	V_2 R	V_2 S
0–24 h	145	0.12	0.08	0.32	18.0	24.0				
1–7 days	175	0.12	0.08	0.31	19.3	16.2	10.5	3.1	31.1	34.1
8–30 days	190	0.11	0.07	0.30	27.0	12.3	12.4	3.8	29.0	25.7
1–3 months	190	0.13	0.08	0.28	20.7	12.7	13.8	3.1	27.4	34.1
3–6 months	179	0.13	0.08	0.30	25.5	15.4	18.5	3.4	28.6	26.5
6–12 months	177	0.13	0.08	0.30	24.7	8.0	16.4	3.7	24.4	30.1
1–3 years	163	0.15	0.08	0.31	27.7	7.0	16.6	3.8	22.5	32.1
3–5 years	132	0.15	0.08	0.38	30.0	5.8	16.7	3.0	22.8	28.8
5–8 years	115	0.16	0.08	0.37	31.2	6.6	14.8	3.4	22.0	35.3
8–12 years	107	0.17	0.08	0.42	30.0	4.4	17.8	3.7	16.9	35.6
12–16 years	102	0.16	0.08	0.42	26.7	5.0	19.7	3.8	18.4	41.0

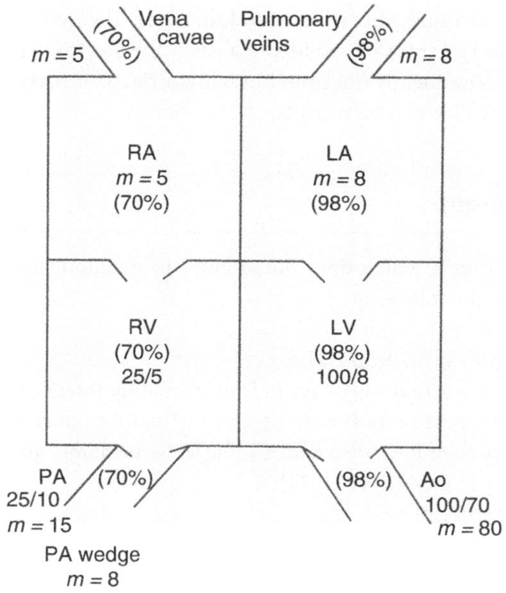

Fig. 9.1

Hemodynamics of a normal child, utilizing the box diagram: RA, right atrium; RV, right ventricle; PA, pulmonary artery; PA wedge, pulmonary artery wedge (an estimate of pulmonary venous pressure); LA, left atrium; LV, left ventricle; Ao, aorta; *m*, mean pressure. Numbers indicate pressures in mm Hg. Numbers in parentheses are percentage oxygen saturations

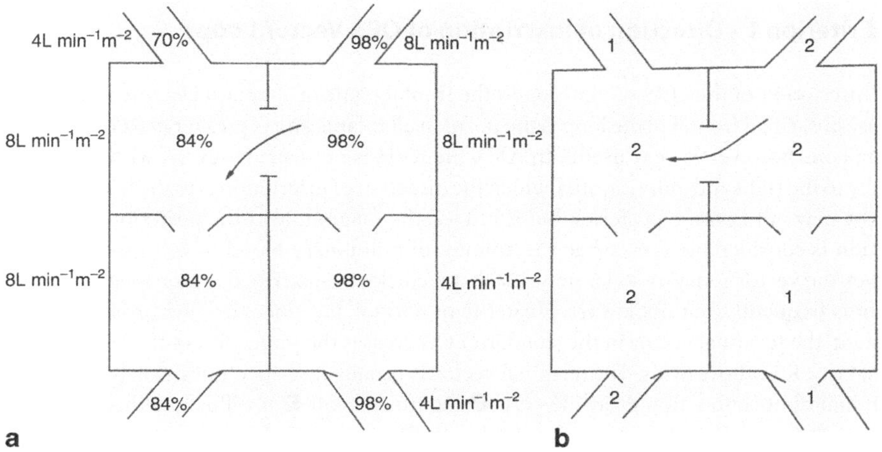

Fig. 9.2

Box diagrams of atrial septal defect (ASD). In (a), the volume in each blood vessel and chamber is in 1 min^{-1} m^{-2}. It is assumed that 41 min^{-1} m^{-2} is the normal cardiac output. Note the increase in oxygen saturation (expressed as percentages) at the atrial level. The calculated pulmonary:systemic (P:S) flow ratio is 2:1. In (b), ASD is shown, utilizing the normal cardiac output as 1 unit of cardiac output. Therefore, 1 unit returns to the venae cavae and 1 unit goes across the ASD, resulting in 2 units of volume in the RA, 2 units in the RV, 2 units in the PA, 2 units in the pulmonary veins (PV), 2 units in the LA, 1 unit in the LV, and 1 unit in the Ao. Therefore, this box diagram delineates an ASD with a 2:1 P:S flow ratio as in (a)

All of the above is for the most common ASD (the secundum type). The dynamics of partial anomalous pulmonary venous return and the sinus venosus type of ASD are identical, as is the electrocardiogram. The exception is that in the sinus venosus lesion the pacemaker is frequently not sinus but is low atrial or atrioventricular (AV) junctional. The ostium primum type of ASD will be discussed later in this chapter.

9.2.1 Right Atrial Enlargement

Right atrial enlargement (RAE) is a term which does not attempt to distinguish between hypertrophy and dilatation. The most useful criteria for RAE are the following.

(a) Standard electrocardiography (ECG) [8, 9, 30–32]:
  (i) Increased magnitude of first portion of P wave in lead II (mainly inferior)
  (ii) Increased magnitude of first portion of P wave in lead V_1.(mainly anterior) and
  (iii) Increased negative magnitude of P wave in lead V_1 if lead V_2 is mainly anterior
(b) Orthogonal electrocardiography (VCG) [8, 9, 33, 34]:
  (i) Increased magnitude of P anterior
  (ii) Increased spatial vector magnitude (SVA) at the time of maximum P anterior
  (iii) Increased P magnitude inferior

9.2.2 Right Ventricular Hypertrophy with Terminal Right Conduction Delay

Criteria for right ventricular hypertrophy (RVH) are many [8, 9, 35], with the most sensitive being an increased magnitude of the terminal QRS vector to the right, and analysis of the direction of inscription of the vector loop in the horizontal plane. It is appropriate at this time to delineate all the criteria for RVH, while being more specific about ASD. Then, for other defects where pure RVH is present, reference can be made to these criteria.

9.2.2.1 RVH Criterion 1 – Direction of Inscription of QRS Vector Loops

The direction of inscription of the QRS vector loop in the frontal plane of standard electrocardiography is not generally useful. A clockwise-inscribed frontal plane loop is the norm in all infants and is present in 62% of teenagers [35]. Analysis of the horizontal plane, however, is very useful. In ASD, the RVH is not usually severe, with the initial QRS loop being inscribed normally to the right and anterior, after which the direction of inscription is to the left and anterior. The terminal vector then may or may not become posterior, but if it does, the magnitude of the posterior QRS vector is usually very small. The variation is considerable even when the amount of pulmonary blood flow is essentially the same from case to case. Sometimes the vector remains so far anterior that a clockwise-inscribed vector loop results. The terminal QRS vector to the right is frequently, but not always, greater than normal, but since the QRS projection posteriorly is usually small or nonexistent, the terminal vector in the standard ECG crosses the projection of the V_4R and V_1 lead vectors. The result is a terminal r or R in those leads. The terminal vector is usually inscribed quite slowly, so that the ECG diagnosis is RVH with terminal right conduction delay [36–39]. ➋ Figures 9.3 and ➋ 9.4 illustrate this.

➋ Plates 9.1 and ➋ 9.2 are BSPMs of the same child as in ➋ Fig. 9.4. These maps were recorded with 180 electrodes. ➋ Plate 9.1 is from 36 to 46 ms of the QRS; while ➋ Plate 9.2 is from 48 to 58 ms. On the side is the color scale, from 0 to $-2,550\ \mu$ V, and from 0 to $+2,640\ \mu$ V. At the bottom is a magnitude factor, which represents the total of the instantaneous value from each of the 180 electrodes. The frontal and horizontal plane vectorcardiograms, derived from appropriate leads from among the 180, are also simultaneously drawn. The red dots each indicate the six maps of the QRS BSPM 2 ms apart. As with the scale factor, the yellow to orange to red are negative values, while the increasing intensity green to red are positive values. Each map (from clavicle to waist) is divided into four sections. The left border is the right axillary line and the right border is also the right axillary line. Therefore, the viewer should consider the maps as the chest unrolled. Therefore, the four sections are the right anterior chest, left anterior chest, left posterior chest and right posterior chest.

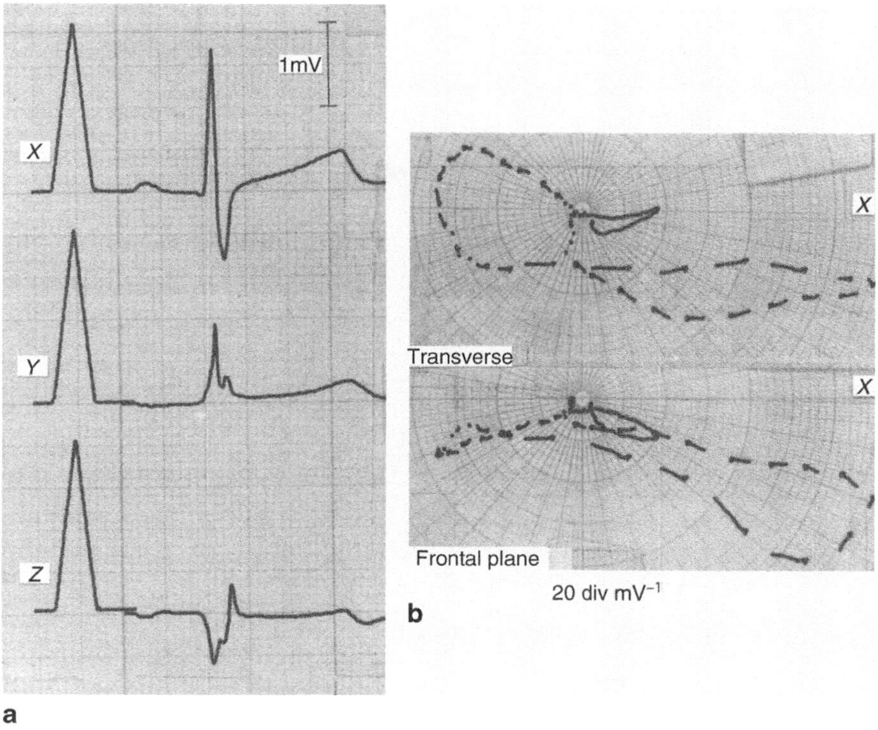

Fig. 9.3
Frank-system orthogonal electrocardiogram with (a), simultaneous *X*, *Y* and *Z* orthogonal scalars plus (b), horizontal and frontal plane vectorcardiograms. In this and all similar figures of this article, the scalar ECG traces are at 50 div s^{-1}. The large regular peaks preceding the traces in (a) are the standardizations. The direction of inscription in (b) is away from the "hook" on each mark; e.g., mainly clockwise in the frontal plane. The patient is a 15-year-old male with a sinus venosus type of ASD, including partial anomalous pulmonary venous return to the superior vena cava. The diagnosis of RVH with terminal right conduction delay was straightforward and typical, just as in ASD secundum. Note, however, that the P vector (lead *Y*) is superior, a low atrial pacemaker being common in sinus venosus ASD (After Liebman et al. [8]. © Williams and Wilkins, Baltimore, MD. Reproduced with permission)

Note in ➋ Plate 9.1 at 38 ms that there is a notch (just to the left of the sternum) in the positive zone. This notch gradually expands, becoming less and less positive, so that it eventually loses positivity. At 48 ms, an extension of the negative has fitted into the notch (➋ Plate 9.2), which continues to expand in area and magnitude. This entire process depicts epicardial right ventricular breakthrough. It has begun very late and is very prolonged, typical of atrial septal defect. The average normal time for epicardial right ventricular breakthrough is 25 ms, with the negative extension being from the right superior area rather than the central superior zone. In addition, after the onset of breakthrough there is considerable positivity to the right and anteriorly, arising from the right ventricle. This is not seen in the normal subject. We have documented previously [37–39] that in right bundle branch block there is no epicardial right ventricular breakthrough. In the past, it has been stated that in atrial septal defect, there is incomplete right bundle branch block. Our BSPM data clearly documents that the diagnosis in ASD is RVH with terminal right conduction delay, and that there is no right bundle branch block.

Obviously, in RVH in general there is a spectrum based upon the severity of the hemodynamics. Therefore, it is not considered useful to describe types of RVH. (With ASD, there is a spectrum even with very little variation in hemodynamics.) It is also not considered useful to diagnose volume overload versus pressure overload on the basis of the type of activation sequence. Any diagnostic criteria that have been developed to do so most likely indicate differences in severity.

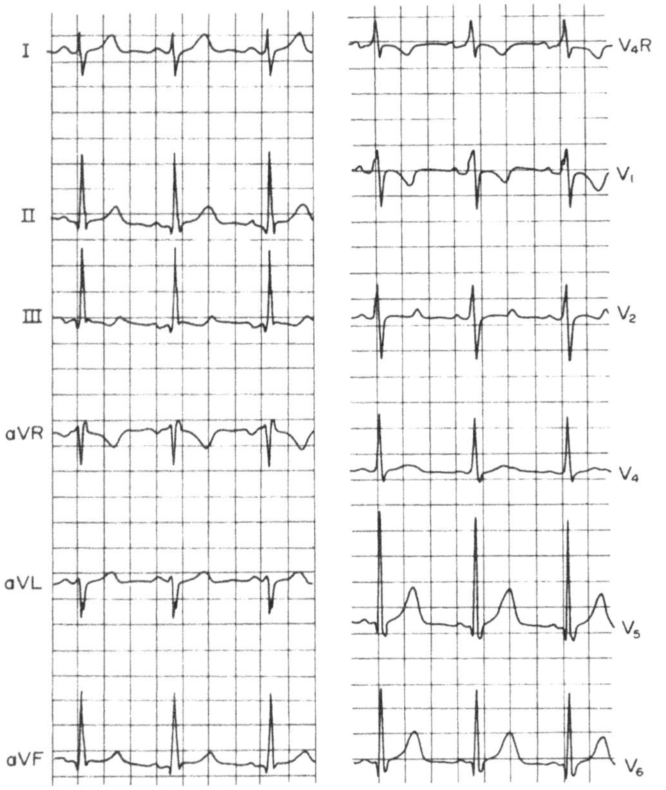

Fig. 9.4
Standard ECG (with six simultaneous leads in limb and chest leads) of a 9½-year-old boy with a large secundum ASD. This type of ECG is unusual for an ASD. Note that the R waves in V_4R, V_1, V_2 are prolonged in duration (in V_2 above 0.03 s). In this child's VCG, the diagnosis of RVH with terminal right conduction delay was straightforward although the terminal vector was posterior (and well to the right). Why there was not a prominent terminal vector the right in the standard ECG is not clear, but the reason why there is no terminal R in the right chest leads is because the rightward posterior or terminal projection was too far posterior to cross the projections of the V_4R and V_1 lead vectors (see Fig. 9.5) (After Liebman et al. [8]. © Williams and Wilkins, Baltimore, MD. Reproduced with permission)

A terminal right conduction delay from right ventricular volume overload, is likely in ASD, although mild to moderate pulmonic stenosis may result in an almost identical ECG [40].

9.2.2.2 RVH Criterion 2 – Initial QRS Vector Loop to the Left and Anterior

This is uncommon except in severe RVH. This criterion is unlikely to be met in ASD, where the RVH is not marked.

9.2.2.3 RVH Criterion 3 – Main or Mean QRS Horizontal Plane Vector to the Right

This is only found when RVH is severe enough, and therefore is not usually seen in ASD.

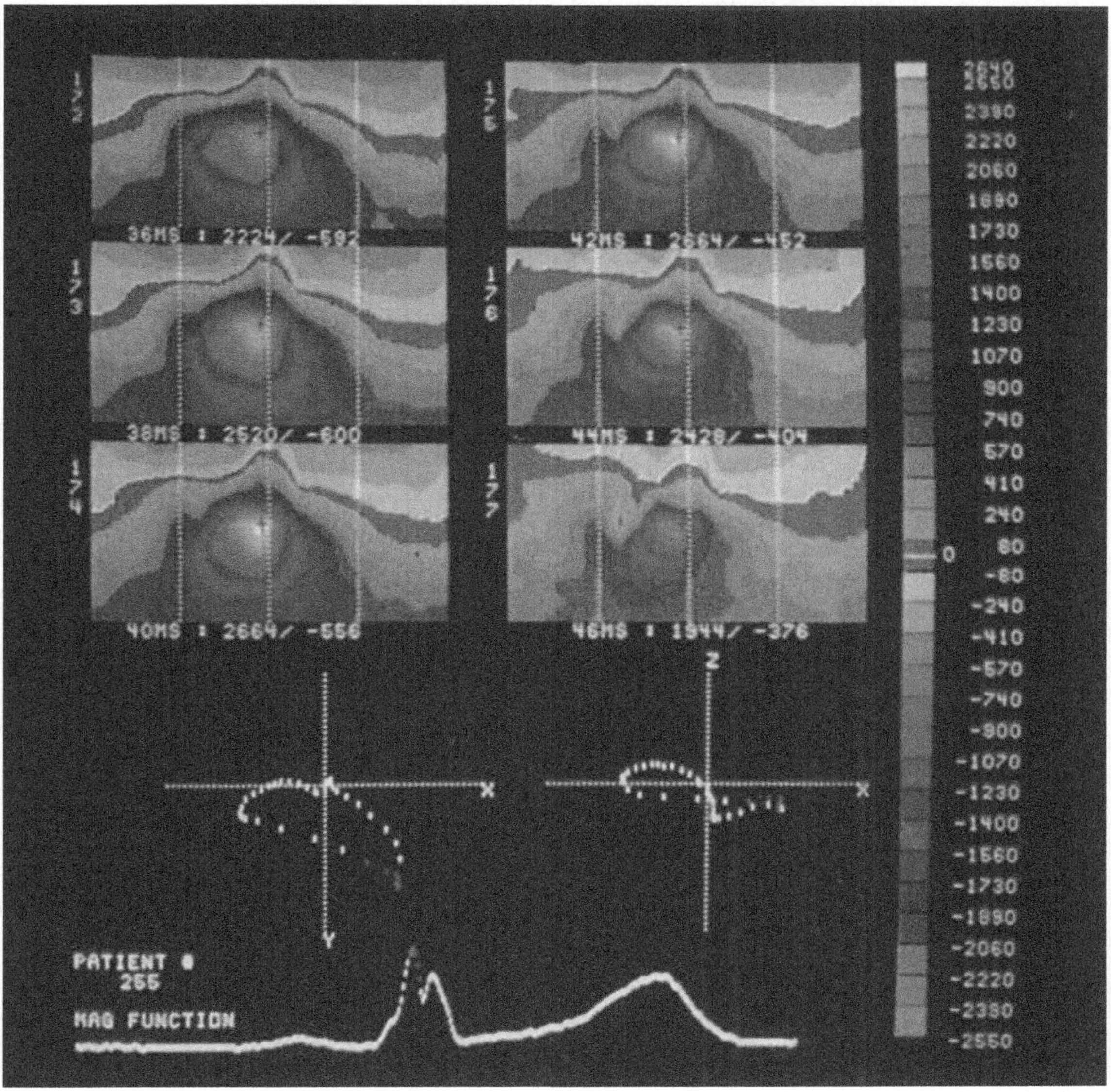

Plate 9.1

Body-surface potentia map of the subject of Fig. 9.4 from 36 to 45 ms of the QRS (See Sect. 9.2.2.1 for detail)

9.2.2.4 RVH Criterion 4 – Main or Mean QRS Vector Abnormally Anterior

This is common, but by itself is an unreliable sign of RVH. Proximity effect, particularly in preschool children, or in the presence of chest deformities such as pectus excavatum, may cause overreading of RVH. This is so, on occasion, even in older children.

As an important aside, note that main QRS vectors are much more meaningful than are mean vectors. In utilizing main vectors, the electrocardiographer is considering activation sequences. In RVH, there may be two main vectors: the first vector to the left and anterior, the second (terminal) vector to the right and posterior (or anterior). The result is that after 1 month, and certainly after 2 months of age, the presence of two main vectors provides a criterion for RVH. If the first vector is abnormally to the left, then additional left ventricular hypertrophy (LVH) must be diagnosed. However,

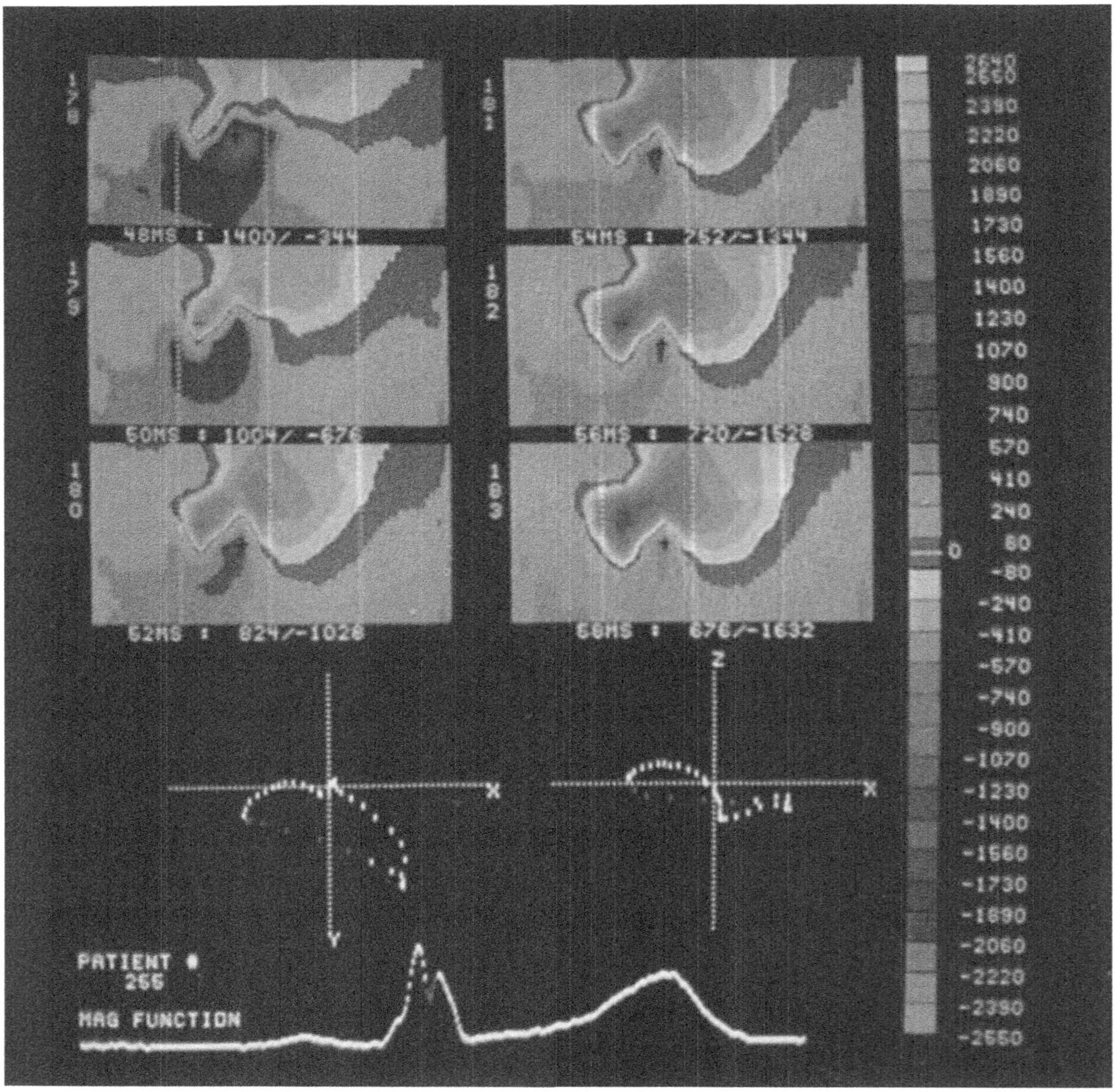

Plate 9.2

Body-surface potentia map of the subject of Fig. 9.4 from 45 to 58 ms of the QRS (See Sect. 9.2.2.1 for details)

it must be appreciated that this LVH may be diagnosed inappropriately in ASD, since the anterior right ventricle, because of its increased volume, may cause a proximity effect artifact in leads V_5 and V_6.

9.2.2.5 RVH Criterion 5 – Mean QRS Vector in the Frontal Plane to the Right

This has been called right axis deviation (RAD), a standard ECG term which is not appropriate. The use of axis deviation as a parameter for diagnosis is not recommended since the only true orthogonal axes are the X, Y and Z axes.

If RAD is present in the standard 12-lead ECG with nothing else to suggest RVH, a mean QRS to the right should be ignored. As with Burger's scalene triangle [27], the X axis of lead I is poor. The prominent S in lead I may be owing to distortion of the right-left lead by superior-inferior forces, often present without a prominent S in lead V_5. In orthogonal electrocardiography, a mean vector to the right is a reliable indicator of RVH.

9.2.2.6 RVH Criterion 6 – Increased Magnitude of Terminal Rightward QRS Vector Loop

This is manifested by an increased terminal X to the right, or a deep S in V_5, and is the most sensitive measurement criterion for RVH [35]. To be certain of its reliability, a deep S in V_6 as well is helpful.

9.2.2.7 RVH Criterion 7 – A Terminal r or R′ in V_4R and V_1

This has been the most misunderstood criterion for RVH (particularly in ASD), and points out a major reason why pattern reading, or the identification of a particular criterion in one lead, may be fraught with error. ➋ Figure 9.5 is explanatory. A terminal r or R in V_4R or V_1 indicates only that the terminal projection crosses the perpendicular to the V_4R or V_1 lead vector. When the terminal QRS vector is markedly posterior, a large terminal vector to the right is necessary in order to cross the perpendicular to the V_4R or V_1 lead vector, whereas when the terminal vector is minimally posterior, or is anterior, only a small magnitude terminal QRS vector to the right is necessary to cross the perpendicular to the V_4R or V_1 lead vector. In ASD, where the terminal vector is of decreased magnitude posteriorly, the characteristic terminal r or R is expected. In normal people, because of large variation in how far posterior the main body of the vector "loop" projects, as well as how much to the anterior the most rightward portion of the terminal QRS vector extends, it is difficult to correlate the magnitude of the terminal r or R′. This helps explain the normal variant rsŕ in the right chest leads, particularly when

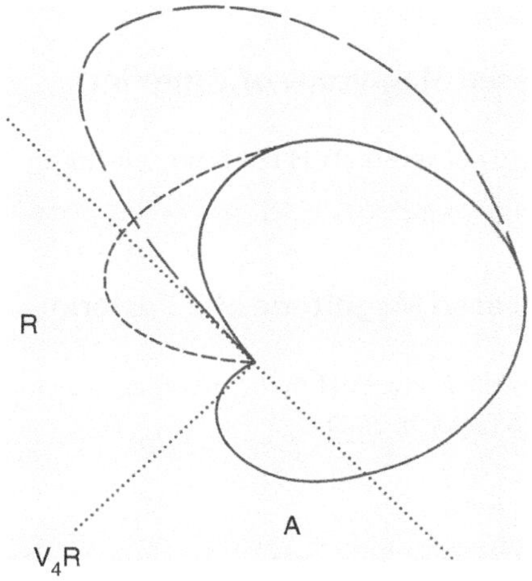

Fig. 9.5
A diagrammatic representation of a transverse vector loop with two different terminal vectors: A, anterior; R, right. The V_4R lead axis is depicted as well as the perpendicular to the projection of the V_4R lead (*dotted line*). Both terminal vectors extend about equally to the right, with the more posterior projection (*dashes*) slightly further to the right. The more anterior terminal vector (*bold dashes*) crosses the perpendicular to the V_4R lead axis, as well as the perpendicular to the V_1 lead axis (not depicted). Therefore, for the more anterior terminal rightward vector, V_4R (and V_1) would project on those chest leads as rSr′ complexes, whereas for the more posterior terminal rightward vector, V_4R (and V_1) would project on those chest leads as rS complexes (After Liebman et al. [8]. © Williams and Wilkins, Baltimore, MD. Reproduced with permission)

there is not a deep S in V_5 and V_6, and when the S (Z axis posterior) is relatively small. The deeper the S in V_2, the more significant is the r′ in V_4R and V_1 as an indicator of RVH.

There are times when, in the right chest leads, there is a small voltage terminal r in V_4R and/or V_1 without a deep S in V_5. This is likely to represent a proximity effect and is usually a normal variant. (Despite the fact that is represents a proximity effect, it may also be the only clue, in a particular tracing, to the diagnosis of mild RVH.) An orthogonal electrocardiogram with vector display will usually help determine whether RVH is present.

The rsŕ or rsŔ has, of course, been called "incomplete right bundle branch block" by the majority of electrocardiographers. Clearly this is incorrect, for the reasons described above. Furthermore, even though in ASD there is right ventricular dilatation and terminal right conduction delay on the ECG of almost all patients, there is no right bundle branch block. This has been documented in the body-surface potential map in that there is definite epicardial right ventricular breakthrough [37–39] (➋ Plate 9.1). (In order to make sure that there is no confusion with the terminology of the past, the author has discarded the term "incomplete right bundle branch block," even when it is truly present, in favor of the term partial right bundle branch block (partial RBBB). Partial RBBB, in congenital heart diseases, is usually seen as a consequence of certain types of cardiac surgery and is only infrequently seen in the nonoperative state [37–39]. It is very rare for children with ASD who have not undergone operation to have partial RBBB.)

9.2.2.8 RVH Criterion 8 – Increased Magnitude of Z Anterior

This is only relatively reliable. It is necessary to be cautious about the tall initial r or R. It is easy to overread RVH where there is a tall spiking R wave of brief duration as part of an RS complex. Most of the time, particularly in the preschool child, the cause is a proximity effect because the heart is so close to the chest wall at those ages. It is preferred that the duration of the initial QRS (e.g., R in V_1) be at least 30 ms in order to suggest the diagnosis of RVH. Although an increased R/S ratio in V_1 is commonly used to diagnose RVH, it is a very soft unreliable sign. (Z anterior corresponds to an R wave in V_1, V_2, in the orthogonal ECG, e.g., ➋ Fig. 9.3.)

9.2.2.9 RVH Criterion 9 – Increased Magnitude of Y Inferior

This involves a tall R in aVF. It may be part of severe RVH but is not a factor in ASD.

9.2.2.10 RVH Criterion 10 – Increased Magnitude of Z Posterior

This is a deep S in V_1, V_2. It may be part of severe RVH in the presence of a clockwise-inscribed horizontal plane "loop" terminating well posterior, but it is not a factor in ASD.

9.2.2.11 RVH Criterion 11 – Abnormal Ratios of Specific Magnitudes

An example of this is an increased ratio of the magnitude of Z anterior to Z posterior (a weak criterion) and/or an increased ratio of the magnitude of X terminal right to X left (an excellent criterion). Normal standards for orthogonal electrocardiography are present for many, although not all, age groups and very few standards are available for the standard 12-lead ECG. The concept, however, must always be considered. It is particularly useful in the presence of abnormally low voltage from various causes, including lung disease. However, overreading of RVH in the standard ECG is very common when the R/S ratio in lead V_1 is utilized, as mentioned above. The error appears especially when the tall initial R is of brief duration, presumably part of a proximity effect. Proximity effect is most common in the preschool child, but can be recognized at all ages.

9.2.2.12 RVH Criterion 12 – Increased Magnitude of the Terminal R in AVR

This is a reliable criterion, but when present the diagnosis is usually obvious from other criteria.

9.2.2.13 RVH Criterion 13 – Increased Magnitude of the Maximal Spatial Vector to the Right

This is known as MSVR. In general it is an excellent criterion, but it is not useful in ASD (see ➋ Sect. 9.5).

9.2.2.14 RVH Criterion 14 – Abnormally Prolonged QRS Duration

On average, the QRS is prolonged, but the variation is so great that the criterion is only of limited value. Most often, a clearly prolonged QRS duration is part of RBBB, but, occasionally, it is seen as part of ASD, with considerable terminal right conduction delay.

9.2.2.15 RVH Criterion 15 – T-Wave Abnormality

This is not useful in ASD (see ➋ Sect. 9.5).

9.2.2.16 RVH Criterion 16 – ST Segment Abnormality

With severe RVH, ST-segment abnormality may occur, although it is not as common or extensive as in severe LVH. The abnormal ST-segment vector is directed posterior and to the left, so that it is recognized in the standard ECG as ST depression in the right chest leads. It is not expected in ASD.

9.2.2.17 RVH Criterion 17 – T Vector Anterior Leftward

An upright T wave in leads V_4R and V_1 after age 72 h is abnormal, and is indicative of RVH. It does not appear to occur in ASD.

9.3 Atrial Septal Defect (Ostium Primum Type)

This condition is considered here without mitral valve abnormality. The horizontal plane electrocardiogram of the ostium primum defect without mitral regurgitation is identical to that of the ostium secundum type [41]. All else being equal, the amount of RVH is dependent upon the amount of left-to-right shunt. However, because this is an endocardial cushion defect, an abnormally superior vector loop is present (➋ Fig. 9.6). (The term "abnormally superior vector" is utilized instead of the inaccurate and inappropriate term, "left axis deviation.") It is specifically defined, in the frontal plane, as initial inferior, usually rotating counterclockwise, and terminally superior. In addition to the premise that axis deviation is a term that is inaccurate and not useful (mean vector is preferred), a normal mean vector is usually further to the left than is the abnormally superior vector. Another term commonly used is left anterior hemiblock, since the electrocardiogram is identical. However, here the term left anterior hemiblock is reserved for that of an abnormally superior vector loop which develops after a disease or surgical injury, in situations where the ECG was previously known to demonstrate a normal inferior vector.

The genesis of the congenital abnormally superior vector almost always implies an endocardial cushion defect, even when it is part of other congenital lesions such as tricuspid atresia or double outlet right ventricle. It can also be part of the Noonan syndrome, for reasons not completely clear, although there may be some left ventricular cardiomyopathy in patients with Noonan's syndrome.

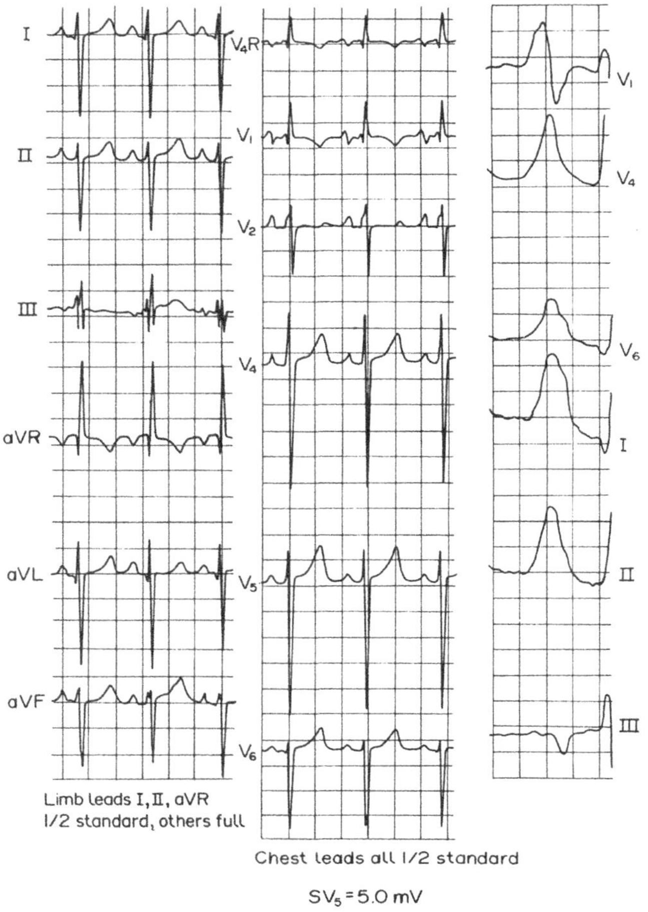

Fig. 9.6
Standard ECG in a 2½-year-old child with a large ASD of the ostium primum type. On the right is a simultaneous recording of the P wave in leads V_1, V_4, V_6, I, II, III at 4 x standard and 100 mms^{-1} for purposes of atrial analysis. The first portion of the P wave is of increased magnitude inferiorly and anteriorly, so that there is right atrial enlargement. No left atrial enlargement is present. There is the classical abnormally superior maximum QRS vector of endocardial cushion defects (with initial QRS inferior, as it must be to make the diagnosis). There is more marked RVH than is usual, yet right ventricular pressure is only minimally above normal (After Liebman et al. [8])

Whether the left anterior branch has been surgically injured or whether the abnormally superior vector is congenital as in patients with endocardial cushion defect, BSPMs have shown late and prolonged superior activation [42]. The genesis of the initial inferior activation is related to the fact that whereas the left side of the septum is activated by the posterior branch of the left bundle, the initial superior vector in the normal person is the result of activation of the left anterior branch of the left bundle. Therefore, when there is a true "abnormally superior vector loop" or left anterior hemiblock, the normal initial superior activation does not occur. The consequence is an initial inferior vector [43, 44].

9.4 Single Atrium

The true single atrium is rare, but since it includes the area of the ostium primum, an endocardial cushion defect is part of the lesion. Therefore, an abnormally superior vector is present.

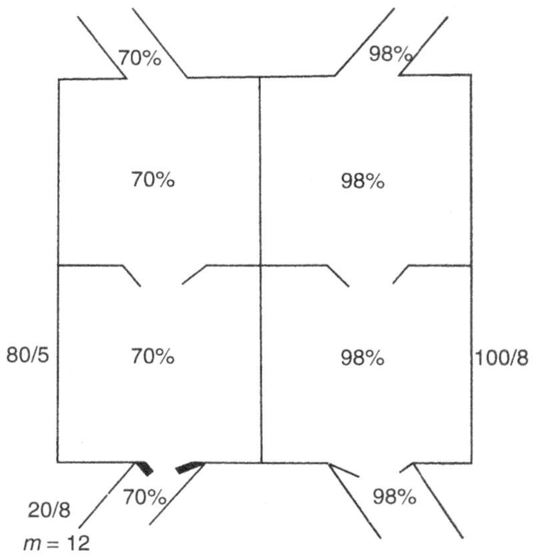

Fig. 9.7
Box diagram of pulmonic stenosis with intact ventricular septum. The oxygen saturations are normal. The right ventricular pressure is elevated, in this case to near systemic level

9.5 Pulmonic Stenosis with Intact Ventricular Septum

Pulmonic stenosis (PS) is, almost invariably, purely valvular. Infundibular pulmonic stenosis, when present as the only lesion, is believed to have been associated with a ventricular septal defect (VSD), which had previously closed. Occasionally, an anomalous right ventricular muscle bundle could have been the cause of the PS, although here too, a VSD has often been present. The spectrum of severity in valvular PS is from a trivial narrowing with minimal or no increase in right ventricular pressure (RV pressure), to that of extremely severe narrowing resulting in suprasystemic pressure in the right ventricle. The hemodynamics, therefore, is that of pure pressure overloading of the right ventricle (➊ Fig. 9.7). Occasionally with suprasystemic RV pressure there is a right-to-left shunt at the atrial level through a foramen ovale. The hemodynamic consequence is cyanosis and less than normal volume in the right ventricle. The pressure and volume in the left ventricle remain normal.

RAE is expected with increased pressure overload of the right ventricle, since compliance of the right ventricle is diminished. RVH is common in PS and the various criteria for RVH from ➊ Sect. 9.2.2 in the presence of PS are discussed here.

9.5.1 RVH Criterion 1 in Pulmonic Stenosis

In the mildest PS, the ECG may be normal. With slightly increased RV pressure, the activation sequence remains normal, with an increased QRS terminal vector to the right, often associated with a decreased posterior projection. Therefore, there will be a terminal r or R in V_4R and/or V_1, since the terminal vector crosses the V_4R and/or V_1 lead vectors (➊ Fig. 9.8). This can occur, of course, without terminal right conduction delay, but the latter is sometimes present in the RVH of the pure pressure load hypertrophy of PS. As expected, since there is a spectrum of severity of valvular PS, the RVH severity varies. As the PS increases, the maximum QRS vector is less posterior and the terminal vector is more to the right so that the horizontal plane may show a crossed loop with two main vectors. With increased severity, the vector loop is almost entirely anterior, with a clockwise direction of inscription (➊ Fig. 9.9). Rarely, in severe PS, the terminal QRS vector is markedly posterior with a clockwise direction of QRS loop inscription. With increased severity, the initial QRS is to the

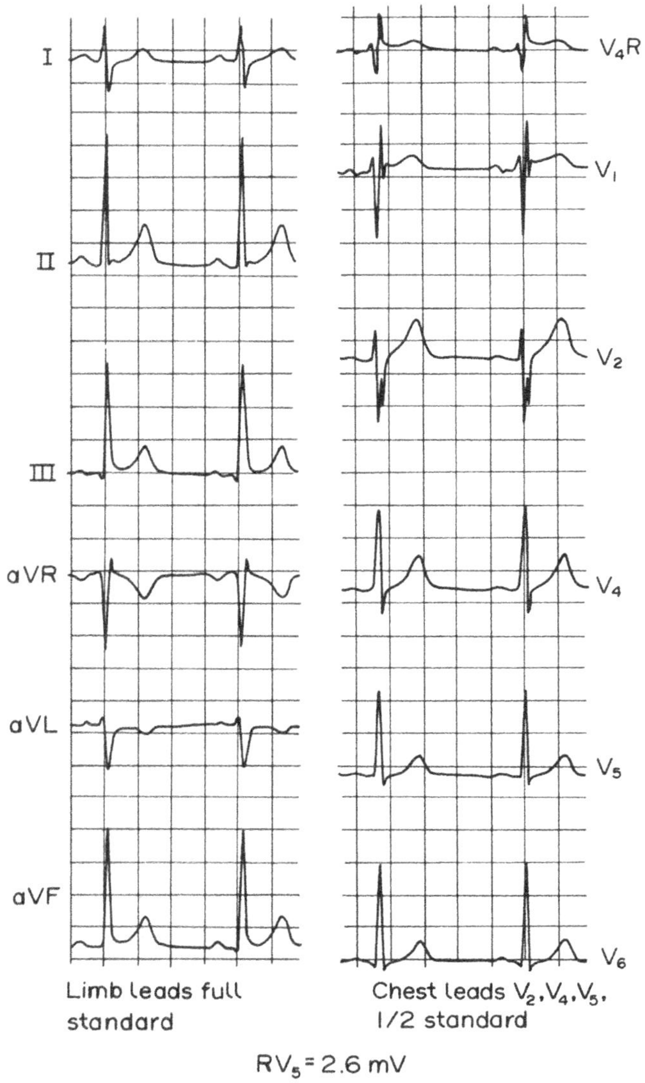

Fig. 9.8
Standard 12-lead ECG of a 17-year-old male who had surgery for moderately severe valvular pulmonic stenosis (PS), via the pulmonary artery. The right ventricle was not entered and RBBB did not develop. The RVH gradually decreased until it stabilized with this ECG. Mild residual PS remains. There is trivial RVH on the basis of the anterior T vector and terminal R′ in V_4R and V_1 (After Liebman et al. (1982). © Williams and Wilkins, Baltimore, MD. Reproduced with permission)

left and anterior, suggesting suprasystemic right ventricular pressure [40] (➜ Fig. 9.10). The mechanism for the initial QRS to the left in severe pulmonic stenosis has been hypothesized utilizing body surface potential maps [24, 45, 46].

9.5.2 RVH Criterion 2 in Pulmonic Stenosis

When the PS is very severe, the initial QRS is frequently to the left and anterior. Suprasystemic pressure must then be considered, although the mechanism can only be hypothesized. The ECG of initial QRS activation is due mainly to four

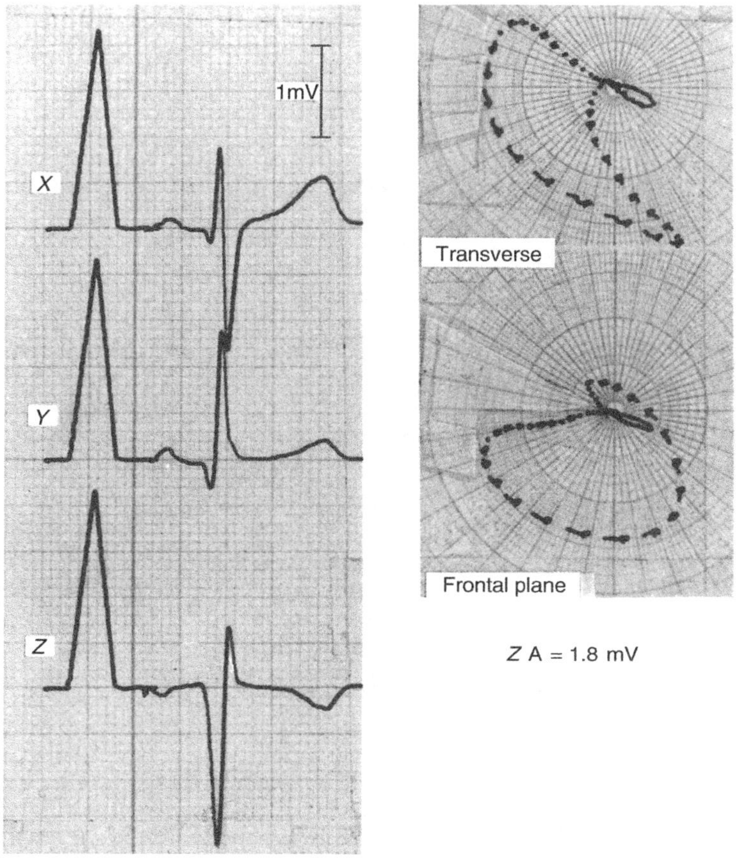

Fig. 9.9
Frank-system orthogonal ECG of a 20-month-old female with valvular PS and RV pressure just under systemic level. The initial QRS is to the right, consistent with the RV pressure being less than suprasystemic. The wide open clockwise vector indicates considerable RVH. There are two main vectors, the first to the left and anterior, the second to the right and posterior. The magnitude left is within normal limits so that additional LVH is not present. (In the standard ECG, the initial vector to the left may be *above* the 95th percentile and additional LVH diagnosed, yet the cause in this case is only a proximity effect because the right ventricle is so large that the V_5 lead is too close to it. This artifact is *less* likely in the Frank or axial (McFee–Parungao) orthogonal ECG systems) (After Liebman et al. [8]. © Williams and Wilkins, Baltimore, MD. Reproduced with permission)

components, namely the left septum 1/2 to 2/3 down the septum, the free posterior wall adjacent to the left septum, the right septum (somewhat more inferior than the left septum), and the right ventricular endocardium. (A fifth area responsible for initial superior activation has been discussed above.) Immediately following is activation of the free anterior wall including the portion near the septum. Rotation of the septum owing to the high RV pressure appears to be an insignificant factor in the presence of pressure overloading, so that aspects of initial activation as described above appear most important. Right septal hypertrophy could also be a factor, but this cannot be anatomically documented. The most likely hypothesis is that the marked hypertrophy of the anterior wall inferior to the position of normal initial activation extends to the left of the position of normal initial activation. It is also possible that the sequence of initial activation has changed so that different components become more important. The answers may not be easily available, but perhaps they will be found through detailed studies involving endocardial and epicardial mapping in humans. Body surface mapping appears to have confirmed the above hypothesis [45, 46].

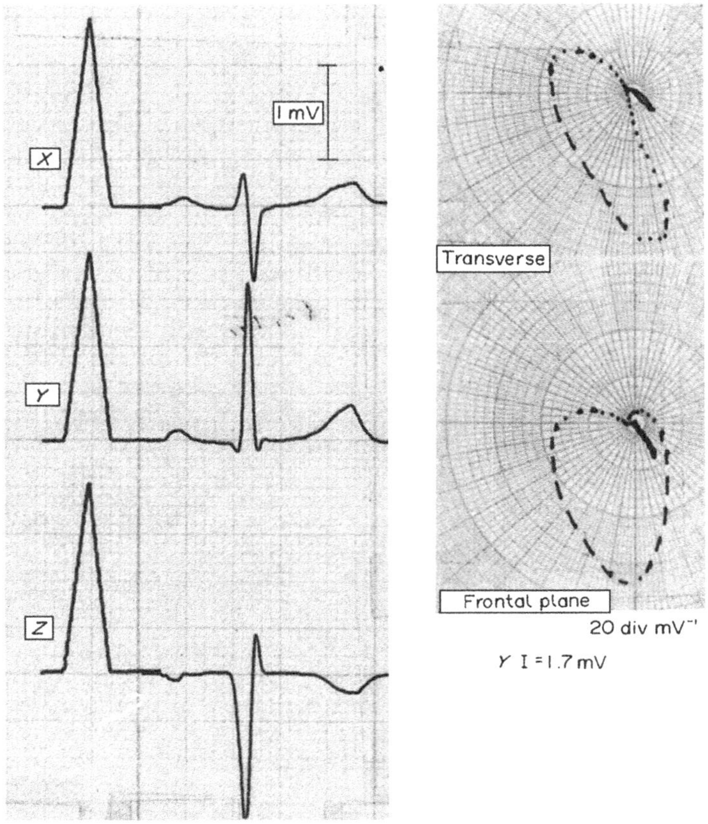

Fig. 9.10
Frank-system orthogonal ECG of a 3-year-old female with valvular PS and RV pressure above systemic level. The initial QRS to the left is consistent with suprasystemic RV pressure, although not all patients with PS and intact ventricular septum and initial QRS to the left have suprasystemic pressure. However, when initial QRS is *not* to the left, the suprasystemic RV pressure is not likely to be present

Occasionally the initial leftward QRS vector is far enough to the left so that the V_4R and/or V_1 lead vectors are not crossed. The result is a qR complex in those leads. The qR in V_4R and V_1, therefore, provides another indication of severity. A qR in V_2, because the initial QRS vector is to the left and posterior, is also very occasionally seen and is an indication of even greater severity. Usually in such patients, however, the VCG does not demonstrate this vector to be to the left and posterior (because V_2 is not reliably comparable to lead Z).

9.5.3 RVH Criterion 6 in Pulmonic Stenosis

This criterion is the single most reliable criterion of RVH and in known PS has been shown to provide at least as good an index for estimation of RV pressure as the more tediously calculated MSVR [35].

9.5.4 RVH Criterion 7 in Pulmonic Stenosis

As described above, an rsŕ or rsŔ pattern is very common in the ECG associated with pure valvular PS even though there is pressure overload. With increased severity of the PS, the right chest leads demonstrate a pure R (because the vector is mostly anterior) or a qR when the initial QRS is well to the left.

9.5.5 RVH Criterion 13 in Pulmonic Stenosis

In PS this criterion has been used as a specific predictor of the RV pressure in valvular PS with intact ventricular septum. Present data indicates a correlation coefficient of 0.65 – 0.70 for the Frank system (lower with McFee–Parungao) [35], although the originally published data claimed much higher correlation. In any case, the confidence interval for specific patients is so wide that the criterion is best used considering the individual patient as his or her own control, just as for magnitude of the terminal QRS vector to the right; e.g., when looking for change over a period of time.

9.5.6 RVH Criteria 16 and 17 in Pulmonic Stenosis

With very severe PS, ST-T abnormality may be present. There may be ST depression in the right chest leads and/or the T vector may be abnormally posterior and, usually, to the left. Very occasionally, the T vector may even be to the right so that the T is inverted from V_4R to V_5 (➋ Fig. 9.11). The deviation of T from QRS is less in the frontal than horizontal planes. A special T abnormality must be mentioned which is not related to severity and is not well understood. An anterior leftward T vector is abnormal after age 72 h (T upright V_4R, V_1, V_2, as well as V_5, V_6) (➋ Fig. 9.12). This empiric indication of RVH may be present in mild PS even in the presence of a normal QRS.

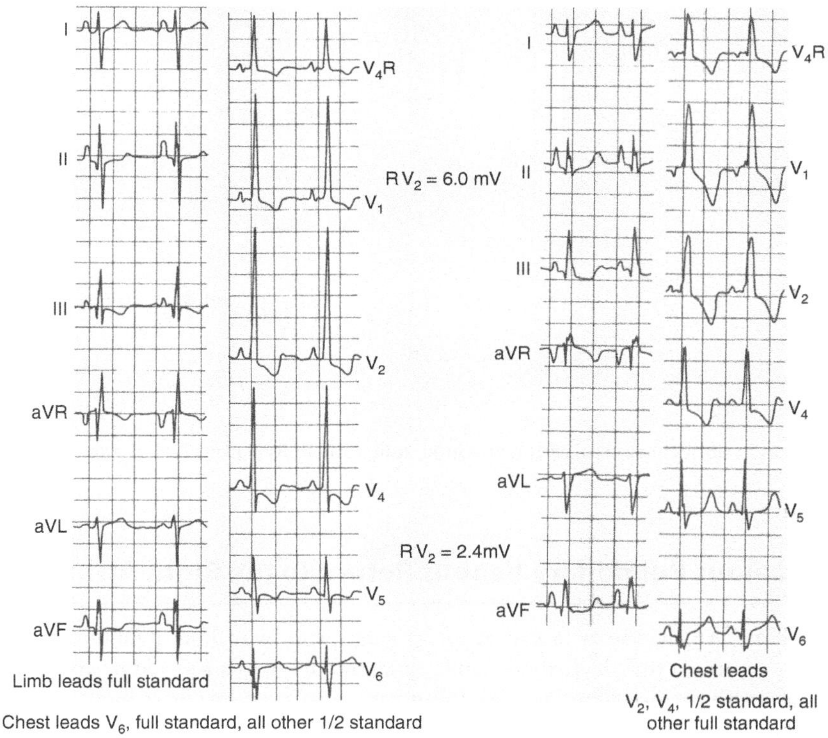

Fig. 9.11
Standard ECG before (*left*) and after (*right*) surgery in a 22-month-old male with severe PS and suprasystemic RV pressure. Note that initial QRS is *not* to the left (a rare exception) but there is marked ST and T abnormality so that the T vector is to the right and posterior. Right atrial hypertrophy is also present. Following surgery (the surgeon had to enter the right ventricular outflow tract via the pulmonary artery) advanced RBBB developed. (A few years later, the RBBB resolved.) (After Liebman et al. [8]. © Williams and Wilkins, Baltimore, Maryland. Reproduced with permission)

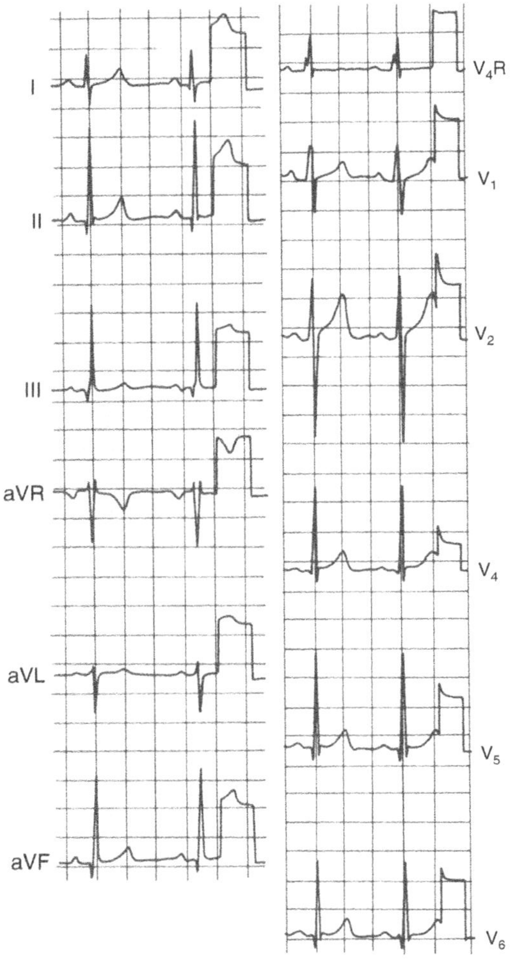

Fig. 9.12
Note the anterior T waves in right chest lead, an unexplained indication of RVH after 72 h of age

9.6 Total Anomalous Pulmonary Venous Return to the Right Atrium

This condition, known as TAPVR, comes in two major varieties, with or without pulmonary venous obstruction. In either case, the RVH is severe, so that the hemodynamic variations are not considered pertinent to this section. In the majority of patients after early infancy, there is no significant pulmonary venous obstruction. Almost invariably, the four pulmonary veins drain into a common pulmonary venous trunk, which has not been normally incorporated into the left atrium. Drainage is then via a systemic vein, frequently primitive, to the right superior vena cava, left superior vena cava or coronary sinus, and thereafter, to the right atrium. The result (see Fig. 9.13) is a tremendous volume overload of the right side of the heart. As with atrial septal defect, and for similar reasons, there is only moderate elevation of RV pressure, although since the increase in pulmonary blood flow is obligatory and early, there may be a significant RV pressure elevation in some cases. Another significant aspect is that, because there has been decreased volume into the left atrium and left ventricle in utero, as well as after birth, the left atrium and left ventricle may be small. In addition embryologically, since the common trunk has not been incorporated into the primitive left atrium, the resulting left

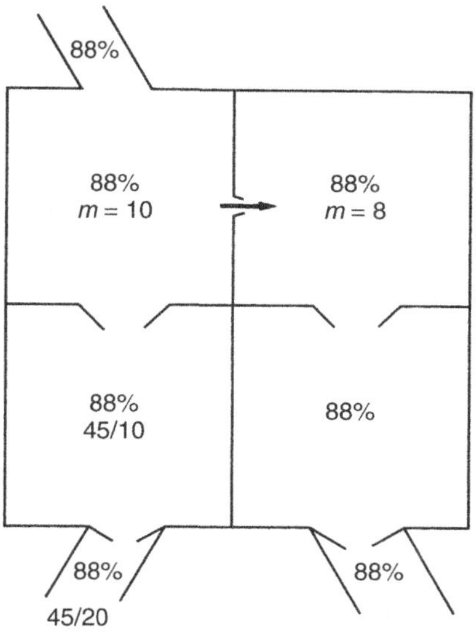

Fig. 9.13
Box diagram in total anomalous pulmonary venous return (TAPVR) with low pulmonary vascular resistance, so that the pulmonary artery pressure is only minimally elevated. The common pulmonary venous trunk (posterior to left atrium) drains into a systemic vein and then into the superior vena cava. Therefore there is a very large volume overload into the right atrium and ventricle estimated as at least four times normal. The left atrium is embryologically small and the left ventricle may also be small, contributing to the marked RVH. The ventricular septum usually bows into the left ventricle

atrium may be very small. In patients with pulmonary venous obstruction, the usual anatomy is that the systemic vein from the common trunk drains below the diaphragm to the portal vein or even hepatic vein. The pulmonary venous obstruction is in the liver and is intense. The increase in volume work of the right ventricle may be minimal, but because of the severe elevation of pulmonary venous pressure in utero, the pulmonary vascular resistance is greatly elevated. Usually, the pulmonary artery pressure is suprasystemic. In both the unobstructed and obstructed types of TAPVR, the former mainly because of volume overload, the latter mainly because of pressure overload, the RVH is severe (➋ Fig. 9.14). The small left ventricle adds to the RVH. The two types of TAPVR cannot be separated on the basis of the ECG. With increased volume and pressure in the right atrium, as well as decreased compliance of the right ventricle, RAE is usually considerable.

9.6.1 RVH Criterion 1 in TAPVR

The initial QRS is usually to the left and may be posterior. At the time of activation of the free walls of each ventricle, the right ventricle usually dominates. More often than not, the maximum QRS vector does not ever go posterior, so that after reaching a brief maximal deflection to the left, the vectors are anterior and to the right. A clockwise horizontal plane vector usually results, with the main vector well to the right and anterior.

9.6.2 RVH Criterion 2 in TAPVR

For the reasons described for severe PS in ➋ Sect. 9.5.2, the initial QRS is usually to the left and anterior. In addition, the large volume right ventricle together with the small left ventricle results in the lower septum bowing into the left ventricle. Consequently, the initial QRS is often even posterior as well as to the left (➋ Fig. 9.15).

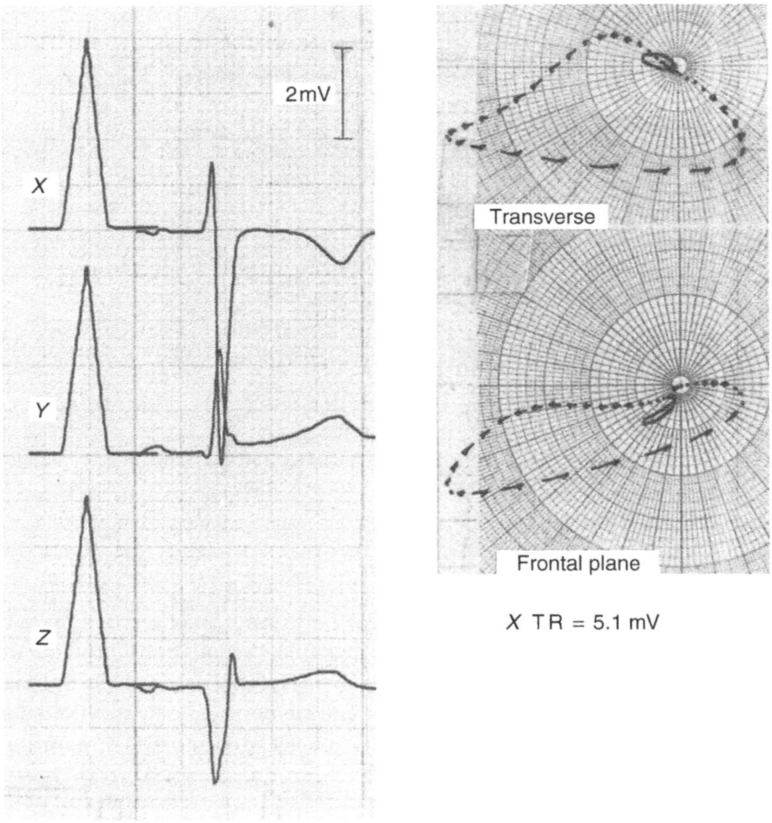

Fig. 9.14
McFee-Parungao system orthogonal ECG and vector loops of a 7 year old male with TAPVR and low pulmonary vascular resistance. The magnitude of the terminal vector of the right (XTR) is remarkably large, even for the McFee-Parungao system, where voltages are greater than in the Frank system. The T vector to the right and posterior, is very abnormal although there was only volume overload. In the standard ECG, the T wave was inverted from V_4r through V_6 (After Liebman et al. [8]. © Williams and Wilkins, Baltimore, MD (1982). Reproduced with permission)

9.7 Hypoplastic Left Ventricle Syndrome

In the most severe form of the hypoplastic left ventricle syndrome, there is little or no left ventricular cavity, with no blood in it. There is a hypoplastic ascending aorta, aortic atresia and mitral atresia. Therefore, all pulmonary venous flow must go through a usually restrictive atrial opening into the right atrium, right ventricle and pulmonary artery. There is a high pulmonary vascular resistance, so that there is a right-to-left shunt through a patent ductus arteriosus into the descending aorta. Therefore, even in cases where the hypoplastic left ventricle syndrome is less severe, for example, with aortic stenosis and/or mitral stenosis instead of atresia, the RVH is severe (➔ Fig. 9.16). There is marked volume and pressure overload, to which is added the small left ventricle.

In addition to RAE, there is marked left atrial enlargement (LAE) as well. The left atrial pressure is very high and there is volume overload, with the only egress being the restrictive atrial opening.

The direction of inscription of the QRS vector loop and the initial portion are similar to those of the marked RVH of total anomalous pulmonary venous return. In approximately half of the children with hypoplastic left ventricle syndrome, the initial QRS is posterior as well as to the left (➔ Fig. 9.17). Very infrequently the initial QRS is to the right. Rarely, the

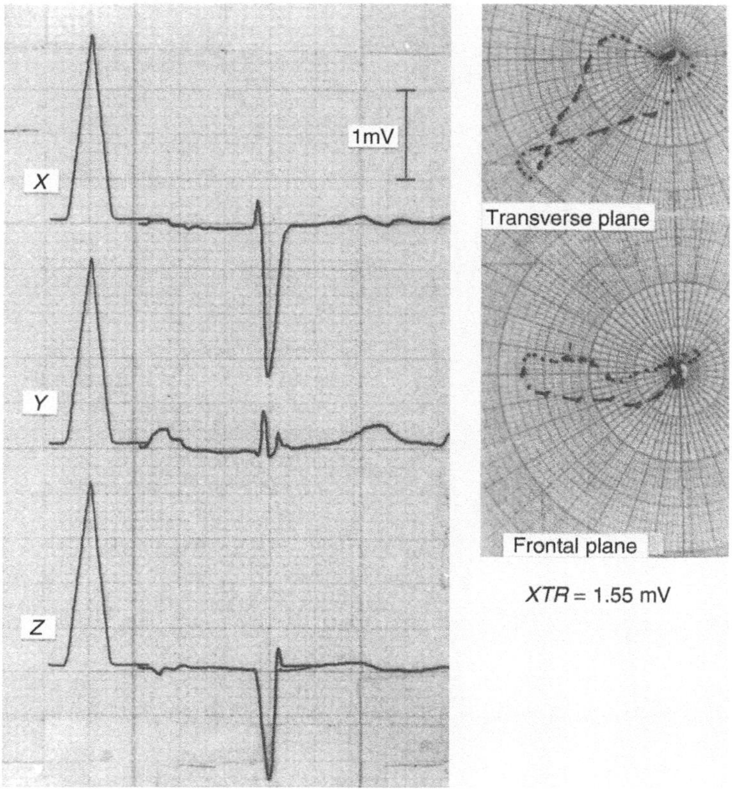

Fig. 9.15
Frank system orthogonal ECG and vector loops of a 16 month old male with TAPVR to the superior vena cava and low pulmonary vascular resistance. There was marked right ventricular volume overload as in Fig. 9.14. The initial QRS is to the left, indicating the severity of the RVH, but it is also posterior, consistent with even more severe RVH. The fact that the septum is bowed into the left ventricle contributes to this unusual QRS (After Liebman et al. [8]. © Williams and Wilkins, Baltimore, MD (1982). Reproduced with permission)

ECG may show good left chest potentials [47], most likely because of the large volume right ventricle extending well to the left, providing a proximity effect.

9.8 Complicated Coarctation of the Aorta

The most common combination of lesions making up this syndrome is that of severe coarctation of the aorta (in the normal position near the left subclavian artery) together with a ventricular septal defect and/or patent ductus arteriosus. Although the pulmonary vascular resistance after birth remains high, the resistance to flow through the coarctation is even greater, so that there is an early left-to-right shunt. Consequently, the left ventricle is hypertrophied and dilated owing to great pressure and volume work. Nonetheless, the ECG often demonstrates pure RVH (Fig. 9.18). It is believed that the effects in utero are responsible. Prior to birth, the right ventricle, working against the newborn's very high pulmonary vascular resistance, sends blood through the ductus arteriosus and then, presumably, through the coarctation. It is hypothesized that prior to birth this extra work of the right ventricular myocardium results in cellular hyperplasia, which persists after birth. Thus, there is hypertrophy of more cells. In addition, because of left ventricular failure after birth, there is a high pulmonary venous pressure, resulting in pulmonary hypertension. Although simple coarctation is

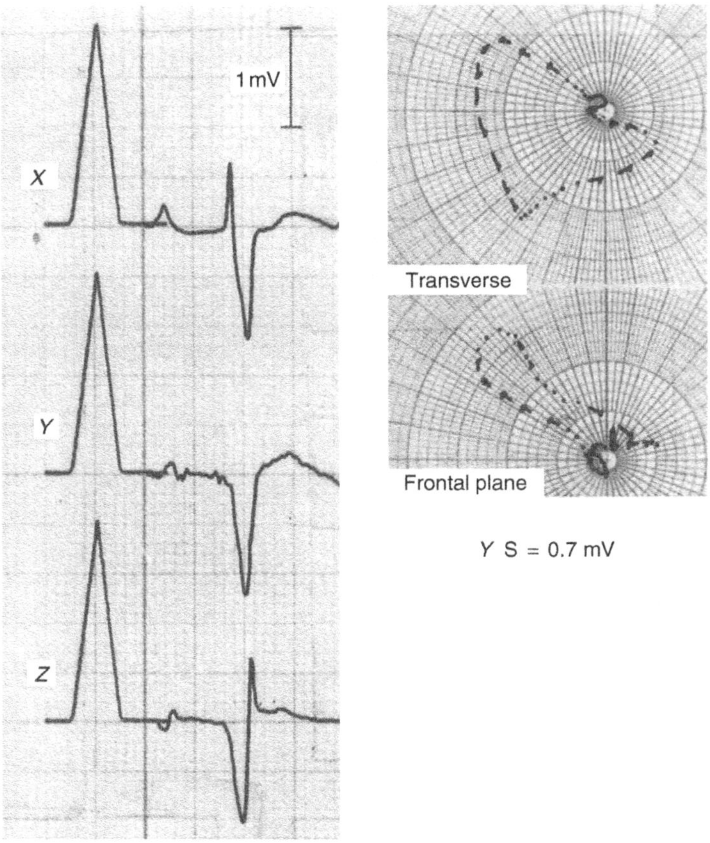

Fig. 9.16
Frank system orthogonal ECG with vector loops of a 5 day old male with the hypoplastic LV syndrome. The initial QRS is to the left, is part of the severe RVH. There is also ST abnormality as manifested in the unclosed ST segment directed posterior in the transverse plane. The elevation of ST in the Z lead is derived from the same observation. The frontal plane is unusual being entirely superior. It is not related to an "abnormally superior QRS vector" since the initial QRS is not inferior. Explanations can only be hypothesized (After Liebman et al. [8]. © Williams and Wilkins, Baltimore, MD (1982). Reproduced with permission)

expected to have pure LVH, the infant with severe narrowing occasionally has pure RVH. Although this usually changes to LVH in a few months, occasionally it may persist (➋ Fig. 9.19). Many years after successful surgery for simple coarctation of the aorta BSPM has shown mild RVH in many [48]. The mechanism is believed to be cellular hyperplasia with hypertrophy shortly after birth.

9.9 Transposition of the Great Arteries with Intact Ventricular Septum

The hemodynamics of transposition of the great arteries is one of constant change after birth. In most cases, the anatomy demonstrates in addition only a foramen ovale, no atrial septal defect, with minimal left-to-right shunt and right -to-left shunt at that level. The ductus arteriosus, because of low systemic PO_2, remains open for a variable, but brief, period of days, allowing some low-oxygen blood to go from the aorta to the pulmonary artery. Pulmonary vascular resistance does not decrease as rapidly as in normal babies, so that pulmonary blood flow (and thus left ventricular flow) is only a little above normal. Left ventricular pressure (LV pressure) gradually decreases over the first few days. On balance, the work of the left ventricle is a little above normal and this, together with the right ventricle working against systemic pressure,

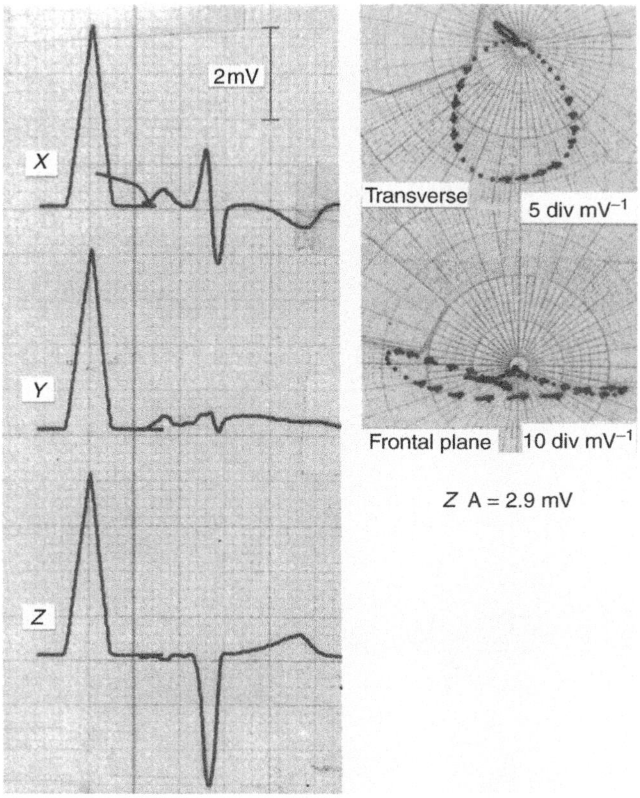

Fig. 9.17
Frank system orthogonal ECG with vector loops in a 6 year old female with the hypoplastic left ventricle syndrome (unusually old for this condition). The RVH is severe with the initial QRS vector directed left and posterior (as in half such babies) and the T vector to the right posterior (After Liebman et al. [8]. © Williams and Wilkins, Baltimore, MD (1982). Reproduced with permission)

usually results in a normal vectorcardiogram (➋ Fig. 9.20). Occasionally, there is some right ventricular hypertrophy. After successful balloon atrial septostomy, the pulmonary vascular resistance usually decreases and the ductus arteriosus closes. There is then significant bi-directional shunting at the atrial level. The volume of work of the systemic right ventricle is above normal and that of the left ventricle is very much increased. However, because of the low pulmonary vascular resistance, LV pressure is quite low; for example, 40 mmHg. Therefore, pure, often considerable, RVH can be expected (➋ Fig. 9.21). Then, if an "atrial switching" operation, such as the Mustard or Senning procedure, is successfully accomplished, the result is that left ventricular volume is normal with low left ventricular pressures. Consequently, the RVH is now severe (➋ Fig. 9.22). In many such patients, there is significant pulmonic stenosis, but the expected additional LVH is often not recognized. After successful arterial switching surgery (now a standard of care), the electrocardiogram usually gradually normalizes.

9.10 Tetralogy of Fallot

In tetralogy of Fallot (TOF), by definition, there is a nonrestrictive ventricular septal defect (so that the RV and LV pressures are equal), with pulmonic stenosis being severe enough so that resistance to flow into the pulmonary artery is greater than resistance to flow into the aorta. The result is a right-to-left shunt. Although an overriding aorta is not necessary to create the hemodynamics, it is usually present in the embryological TOF. In the maximally severe TOF,

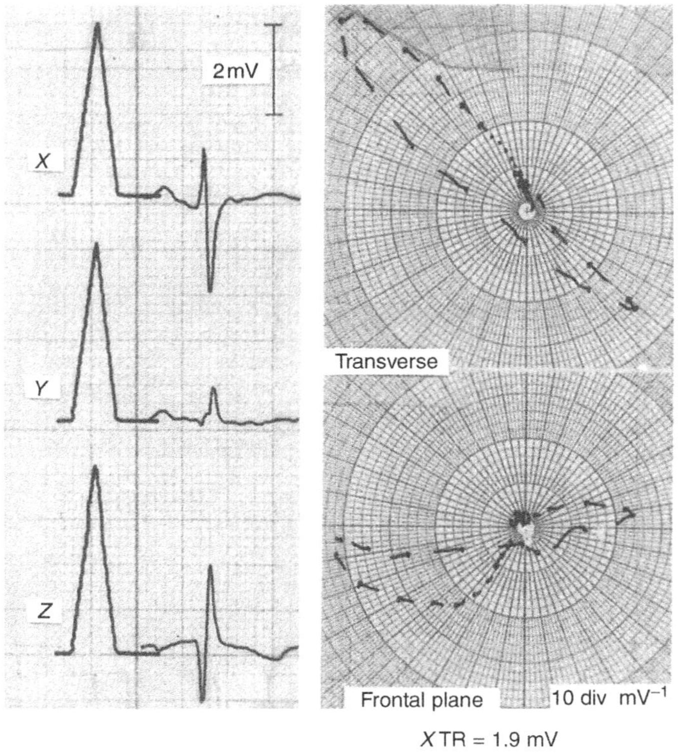

Fig. 9.18
Frank system orthogonal ECG with vector loops in a 3 month old male with coarctation of the aorta, ventricular septal defect and mitral stenosis. The RVH is considerable. The horizontal plane vector loop is clockwise with the large terminal right vector (XTR) markedly posterior. (The large terminal right posterior projection is part of the RVH. The diagnosis of additional LVH would be an error) (After Liebman et al. [8]. © Williams and Wilkins, Baltimore, MD (1982). Reproduced with permission)

there is pulmonary atresia, so that 100% of right ventricular blood goes from right to left through the VSD. The pulmonary blood flow is then by way of a ductus arteriosus or bronchial arteries. A typical moderately severe TOF, with 50% of right ventricular blood going from right to left through the VSD, is depicted in Fig. 9.23.

Right ventricular volume work is normal, at systemic pressure, while left ventricular volume work is less than normal, at normal pressure. Pure RVH, therefore, is expected. (Note that if a systemic-pulmonary artery shunt is created, there is increased left ventricular volume work to accompany the RV pressure work) so that LVH may also develop.

With regard to the effect on atria, RAE is usually found in TOF. The effect on ventricles is discussed according to the criteria laid down in Sect. 9.2.2.

9.10.1 RVH Criterion 1 in TOF

Because the hypertrophy is usually severe, the RVH is much as described for severe valvular PS with intact ventricular septum. An exception is that in the most severe form, often associated with the lowest arterial oxygen saturation, the clockwise-inscribed vector loop turns quickly to the right (after beginning to the left) before terminating markedly posterior. The result in the standard ECG is often that the only QRS complexes where R > S are V_4R and V_1 (Figs. 9.24 and 9.25). Occasionally, the only complex with R > S is V_4R, so that unless there is an orthogonal VCG, the diagnosis of RVH may be difficult to make. Careful vector analysis of the chest leads, however, should reveal that the horizontal plane is rotated clockwise (Fig. 9.26).

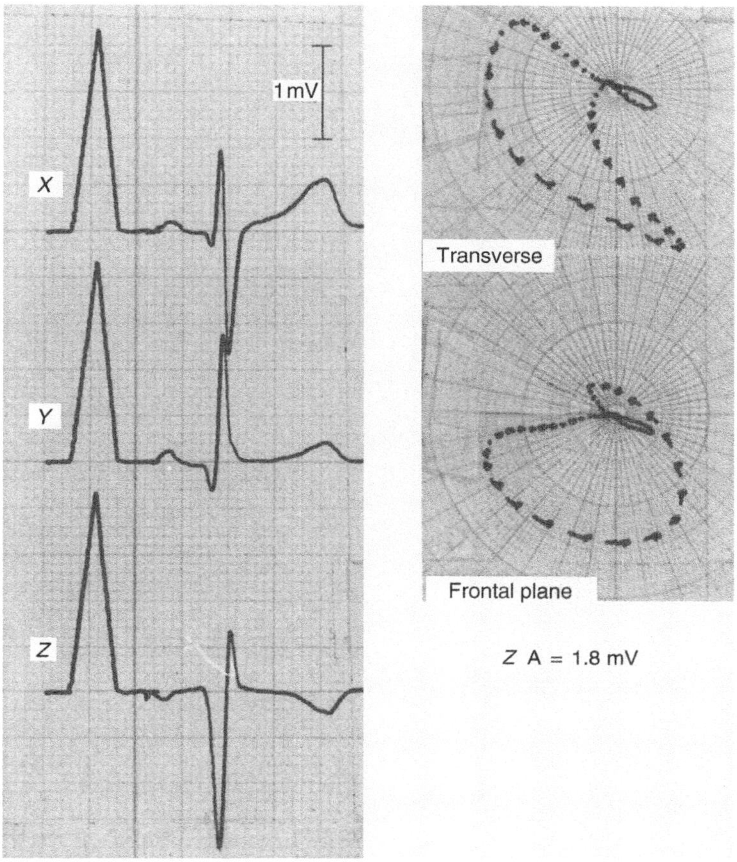

Fig. 9.19
Frank system orthogonal ECG with vector loops in a 21 year old female with severe simple coarctation of the aorta. The diagnosis is RVH with no evidence for additional LVH

9.10.2 RVH Criterion 2 in TOF

The initial QRS vectors are usually to the left and anterior (➋ Figs. 9.27 and ➋ 9.28) since the RVH is severe.

9.10.3 RVH Criterion 9 in TOF (R in AVF)

The abnormally tall R in aVF by itself, in the presence of prominent left chest potentials, suggests the diagnosis of left ventricular hypertrophy since the more inferior ventricle is the left ventricle. However, it is an error, in the presence of significant RVH, to diagnose additional LVH when an abnormally tall R in aVF is present. In this case, the prominent inferior vector is part of RVH, presumably from hypertrophy of the inferior right ventricle. This criterion is extremely common in the presence of TOF (➋ Fig. 9.24).

9.10.4 RVH Criterion 16 and 17 in TOF

ST-T abnormally (with the T vector well to the right and posterior) is very unusual in TOF, even when very severe, but can occur (➋ Fig. 9.25).

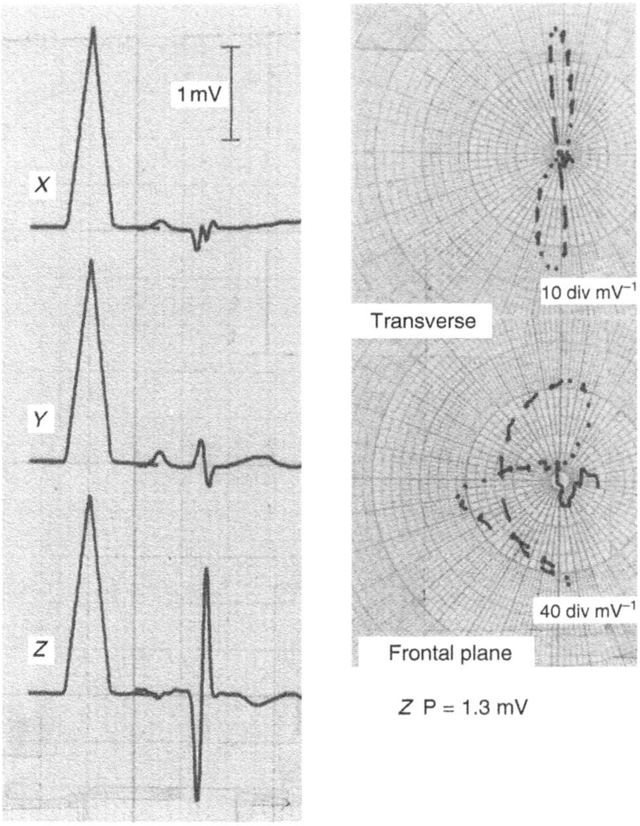

Fig. 9.20
Frank system orthogonal ECG with vector loops in a 5 day old with simple transposition of the great arteries with intact ventricular septum (the frontal plane vector loop is at 40 div(mv^{-1}) (so that voltage is quite low). The ECG is normal (very unusual)

9.11 Obstruction of Outflow From the Left Atrium

This includes congenital mitral stenosis (multiple varieties), supravalvular stenosing ring, and cor triatriatum. All of these have the same pathophysiology, unrelated to the varying embryology. The cause of the RVH is elevation of pulmonary venous pressure. Should the obstruction be significant in the newborn period, when the fetal thick-walled pulmonary arterioles remain, the RVH may be severe. Should the obstruction become significant later in life, it may take time, as the pulmonary arterioles become more muscular once again, before significant RVH develops. Both left and right atrial hypertrophy (LAE and RAE, respectively) will be present [8, 33, 49–53]. The reliability of the reading of LAE is only fair although reliability of reading RAE is very good.

9.12 Nonrestrictive LV-RV Communication with Pulmonary Vascular Disease

An example of this is ventricular septal defect. The degree of RAE or RVH depends upon the severity of the pulmonary vascular disease, just as in tetralogy of Fallot, where the degree of RAH or RVH depends upon the severity of the pulmonic stenosis. The box diagram in ➋ Fig. 9.29 is explanatory.

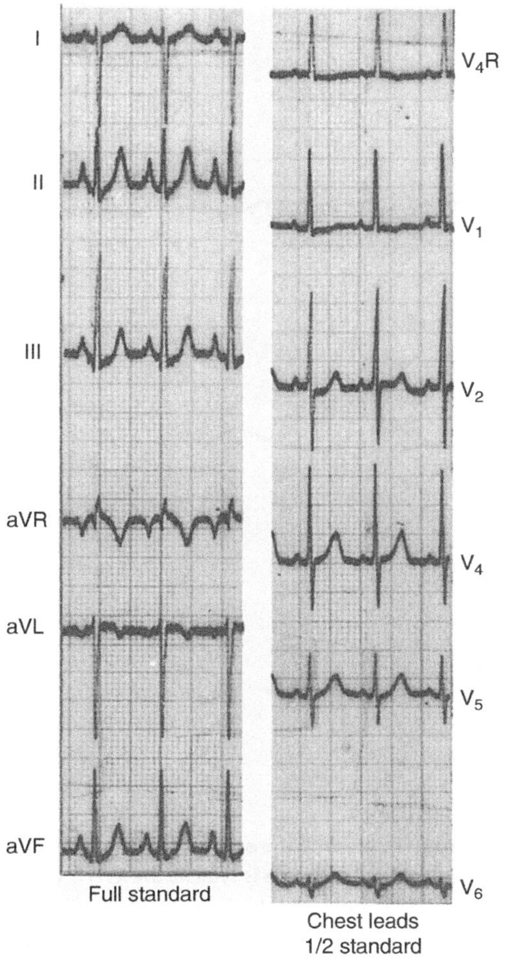

Fig. 9.21
Standard ECG in a 3 month old male with simple transposition of the great arteries and intact ventricular septum. A balloon atrial septostomy had been done in the newborn period. The RVH is moderate. Note that the initial QRS is to the left. Right atrial hypertrophy is present on the basis of the first part of the P wave inferior and anterior having a large magnitude

However, in patients with large ventricular septal defect, there is likely to have been a period before the pulmonary vascular disease developed when there was significant left-to-right shunt. Therefore, there may be less RVH than in TOF, owing to previous hemodynamics.

9.13 Patent Ductus Arteriosus

In pediatrics, the isolated patent ductus arteriosus (PDA) must be discussed in two contexts. First, there is the PDA associated with the newborn, usually prematurely born, often with respiratory distress syndrome; and second, there is PDA that is congenitally open, and manifest after the newborn period. The ductus in the former is presumed to be kept open mainly because of the hypoxia associated with the pulmonary disease. The flow through it is from left-to-right, so that the left atrium and left ventricle are enlarged. However, because of the high pulmonary venous pressure

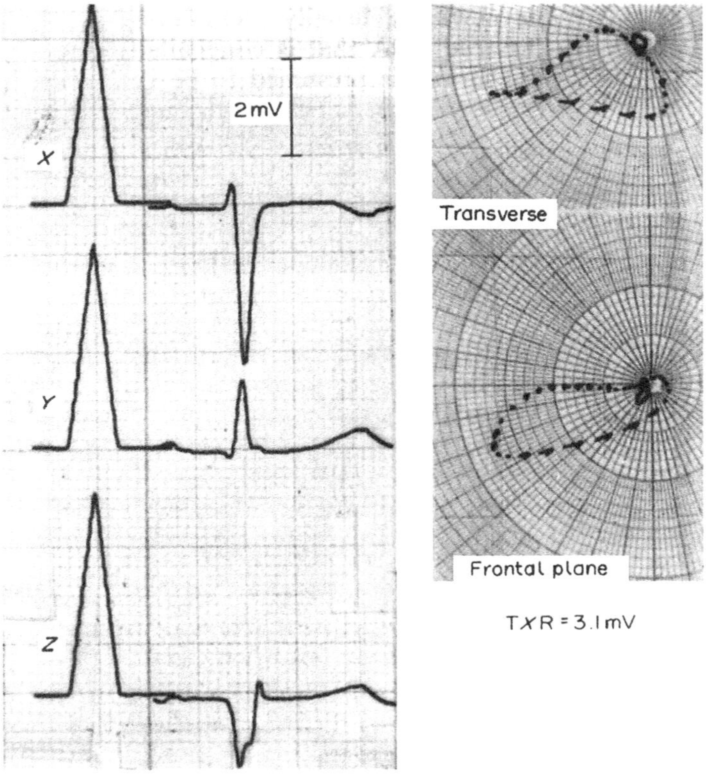

Fig. 9.22
Frank-system orthogonal ECG in a 6-year-old female with transposition of the great arteries who had undergone a successful atrial switching procedure (Mustard) in the first year of life. As is typical, the RVH is very severe with initial QRS to the left, most of the clockwise-inscribed QRS vector loop to the right and the T vector posterior right. After successful Mustard operations, the right ventricle is at systemic level, and the left ventricle is usually at less than half systemic level (After Liebman et al. [8]. © Williams and Wilkins, Baltimore, MD. Reproduced with permission)

as well as the lung disease per se, there is likely to be significant pulmonary hypertension. Therefore, the right ventricle is involved as well. In addition, the prematurely born baby has a very low voltage and has less of the newborn's right ventricular dominance [54]. Finally, the ductus tends to open and close, the hemodynamics changing rapidly. Consequently, the ECG is not reliably useful in evaluation. The ECG is very useful, however, in the evaluation of the "true" congenital PDA.

The left-to-right shunt through the "true" PDA is not usually significant until a number of weeks after birth, related to a more gradual decrease in pulmonary vascular resistance than in normal babies. The ductus itself, because of its length, has considerable resistance, so that the majority of PDAs are associated with no more than moderate pulmonary hypertension and usually less. The work of the heart is, therefore, volume work of the left ventricle (➊ Fig. 9.30).

There is left atrial enlargement (LAE), a term which does not attempt to distinguish between hypertrophy and dilatation. The most useful criteria for LAE are the following [8, 33, 49–53]:

(a) Standard electrocardiography [3, 16, 17, 29–31]:
   (i) Increased duration of second portion of P wave (i.e., when P is m-shaped)
   (ii) Increased P terminal force in V_1 (>0.003 mVs)
   (iii) Increased time between first and second peak of P

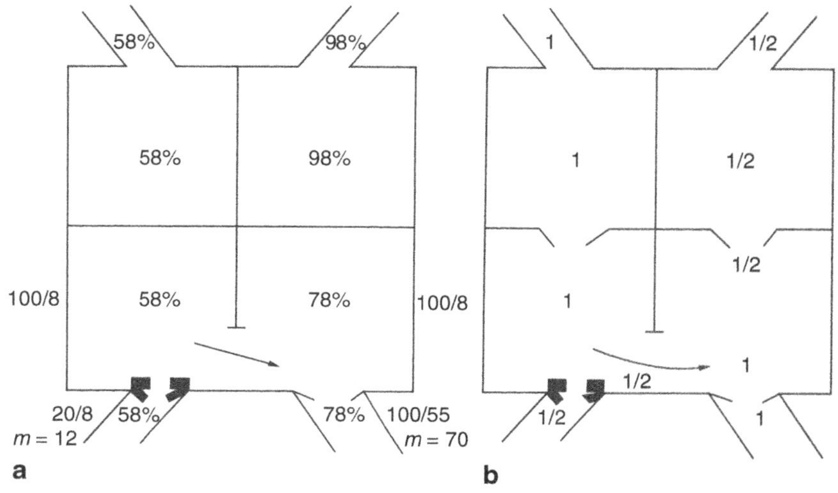

Fig. 9.23
Box diagram typical of tetralogy of Fallot. In (a), the right and left ventricular pressures are equal. Resistance to flow past the severe pulmonary stenosis is much greater than is systemic artery vascular resistance. Therefore, there is considerable right-to-left shunt and no left-to-right shunt. The systemic arterial oxygen saturation is only 78%. In (b), the outputs into the pulmonary artery and aorta, and volumes in each entering great vein and each chamber are delineated. The right ventricle at systemic pressure sends blood through the severely stenotic right ventricular outflow tract and into the aorta as well. Only one-half normal volume enters the left ventricle, which sends less than the normal volume into the aorta at normal pressure. Therefore, the ECG is that of pure RVH

(b) Orthogonal electrocardiography [3, 32–34]:
- (i) Increased P terminal force
- (ii) Increased duration second portion of P
- (iii) Increased magnitude posterior of second portion of P
- (iv) Increased time between first and second peak of P
- (v) Increased spatial magnitude at the time of maximum posterior (SVP)

9.13.1 Left Ventricular Hypertrophy

Criteria for left ventricular hypertrophy are many [35], with the most sensitive being an increased magnitude posterior in the presence of a normally inscribed horizontal plane vector loop. It is appropriate at this time to delineate all the criteria for LVH while being more specific about PDA. Then, for other defects where pure LVH is present, reference can be made to these criteria.

9.13.1.1 LVH Criterion 1 – Direction of Inscription of QRS Vector Loops

The QRS vector loops may have exactly the same configuration as in the normal, so that after infancy there is a normal initial QRS vector to the right and anterior, followed by the vector being increasingly to the left, first anterior, then clearly posterior, ending slightly to the right and posterior. However, the spatial voltage will be larger than normal. (Occasionally, particularly in severe hypertrophy, the most distal portion of the loop is to the left, but inscribed clockwise. The genesis of this is presumed to be an intraventricular conduction abnormality involving the left bundle, associated with fibrosis.) A newborn with a wide-open counterclockwise-inscribed vector loop indicates LVH no matter what the voltage.

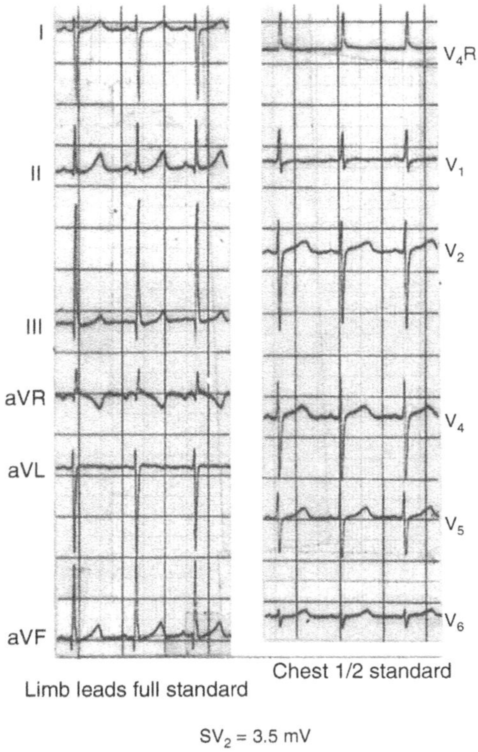

Fig. 9.24
Standard ECG of a 4½-year-old male with TOF and marked RVH. There is a wide open clockwise horizontal plane vector loop which extends quickly to the right and posterior. The loop is not shown but can be derived from the standard ECG as discussed in Chap. 11 of *Basic Electrocardiology: Cardiac Electrophysiology, ECG Systems and Mathematical Modeling*. The posterior projection is very large (3.5 mV) (not part of LVH) and there is also a prominent inferior vector, seen frequently in TOF

The direction of inscription in the frontal plane usually remains clockwise. Only occasionally does LVH cause counterclockwise inscription in the frontal plane, usually in older children with very severe LVH, but the maximum QRS vector will still be mainly inferior.

In PDA, the initial QRS vector is usually normally rightward and anterior, with normal horizontal plane direction of inscription and increased voltage both to the left and posterior.

9.13.1.2 LVH Criterion 2 – Initial QRS vector

An initial QRS vector to the left and anterior [45, 46, 55, 56] (a manifestation of severe LVH) is not usually seen in PDA. However, a large initial QRS to the right and anterior, and frequently superior, is very common. This is left septal hypertrophy, not LVH per se. (Proximity effect, particularly in the preschool child, may cause a prominent initial anterior vector, sometimes also rightward, contributing to an erroneous diagnosis of left septal hypertrophy.)

9.13.1.3 LVH Criterion 3 – Abnormally Posterior Angle of the Main or Mean QRS Vector

This is only a fair sign of LVH because of so much normal variability.

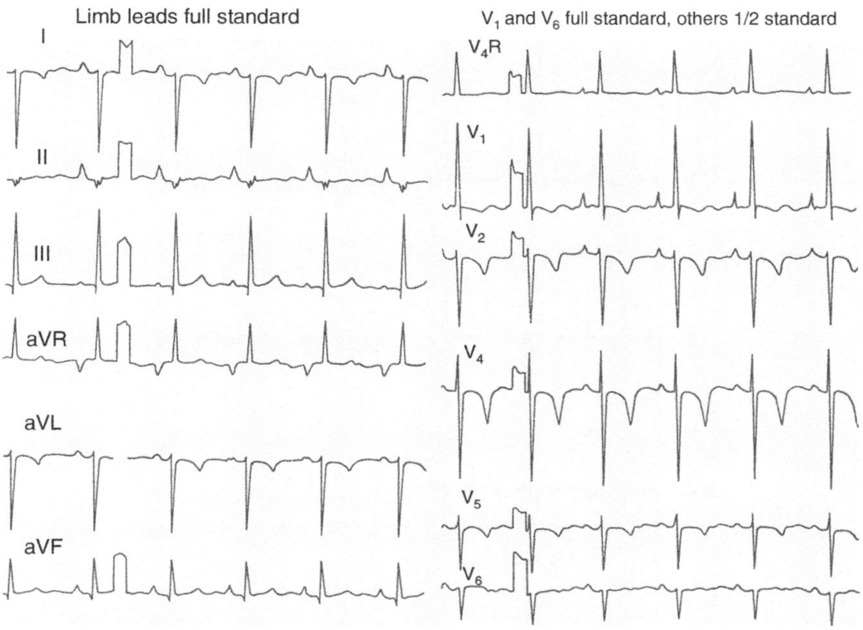

Fig. 9.25
Standard ECG of a 10-year-old with severe TOF and very severe RVH (as well as right atrial hypertrophy). What is unusual for TOF is the marked T abnormality, the T being to the right and posterior. The maximum QRS vector is also posteriorly directed (and to the right) as in Fig. 9.24

9.13.1.4 LVH criterion 4 – Horizontal Plane Vector Loop Progressing Rapidly from Anterior to Posterior

This causes the loop to be posterior by about 20 ms. The differential diagnosis is anterior myocardial infarction, rare in children, so that the criterion is excellent.

9.13.1.5 LVH Criterion 5 – Increased Magnitude of Leftward QRS Vector

This gives increased X to the left and tall R in V_5, V_6. This is an excellent sign of LVH. If V_6 is greater than V_5, even though neither is above 97.5 percentile, LVH should be considered. In the latter, a very wide, broad leftward loop has been projected, which remains to the left for a long time.

9.13.1.6 LVH Criterion 6 – Increased Magnitude of Inferior QRS Vector

This leads to increased Y inferior and a tall R in aVF. In the presence of a normal horizontal plane vector loop with good left chest potential (which need not be abnormally high), a clearly large inferior vector suggests LVH. The left ventricle is the more inferior ventricle. However, pure marked RVH is frequently associated with a large inferior vector, but, as noted above, even mild RVH or LVH can be associated with a high magnitude inferior vector.

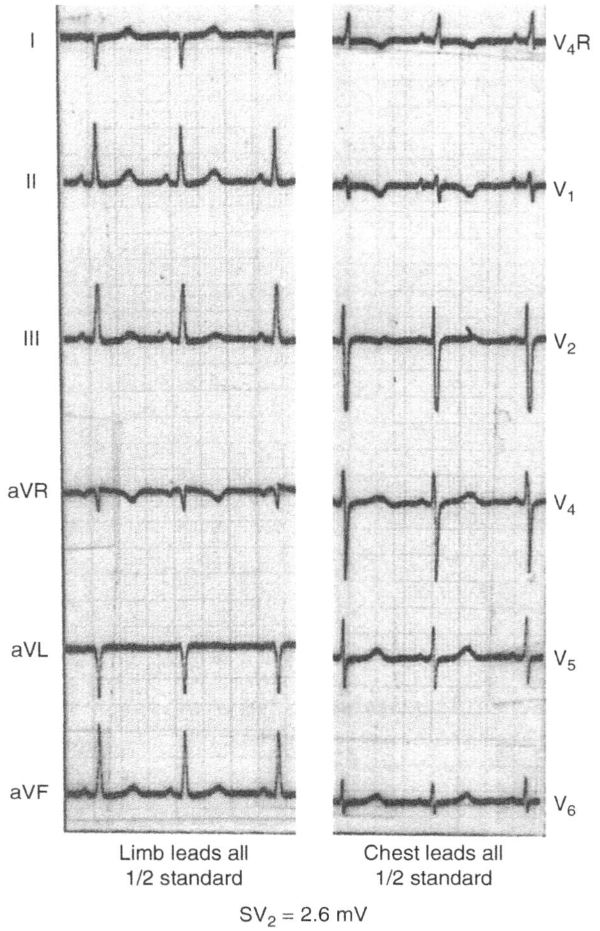

Fig. 9.26
Standard ECG of a 5-year-old female with TOF and moderately severe RVH. As in Figs. 9.24 and 9.25, the initial QRS is to the left and the QRS transverses quickly to the right and posterior. The difference here is that not only does V_2 demonstrate rS, but so does V_1. Therefore, without V_4R (and/or the orthogonal ECG) RVH would be difficult to diagnose. Note that all leads are half standard size (After Liebman et al. [8]. © Williams and Wilkins, Baltimore, MD. Reproduced with permission)

9.13.1.7 LVH Criterion 7 – Increased Magnitude of Posterior QRS Vector

This means increased Z posterior, with a deep S in V_1, V_2. The abnormally posterior maximum QRS vector is probably the single best criterion for LVH (although lung disease, with high residual volume, may cause decreased anterior forces, and therefore, an abnormally posterior vector) [57]. In severe RVH, a clockwise-inscribed horizontal plane vector loop may terminally swing far posterior, so that additional LVH is sometimes diagnosed. This would be in error for in such a case the genesis of the posterior forces is presumed to be late posterior right ventricular potentials occurring after the left ventricle has completed activation. If, with a counterclockwise horizontal plane vector loop, the X left and Z posterior are at the upper limit of normal in magnitude, LVH is likely. A Z posterior at the upper limit of normal together with a quite small X left may be part of an abnormally posterior horizontal plane QRS vector angle and is a weak sign of LVH.

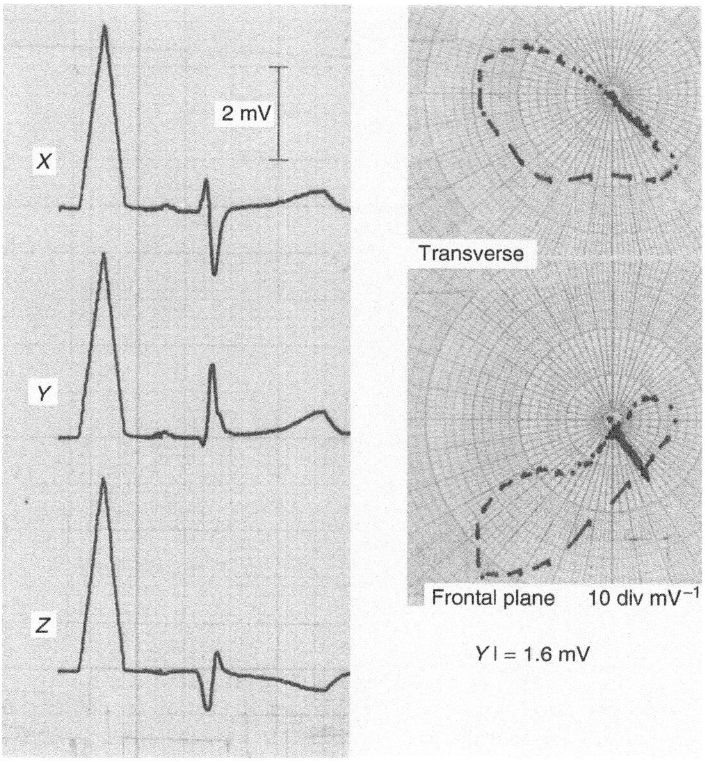

Fig. 9.27
Frank-system orthogonal ECG of a 4-year-old with TOF. As is typical, the direction of inscription is wide open clockwise with the initial QRS to the left. The T in the horizontal plane overlays the initial QRS (After Liebman et al. [8]. © Williams and Wilkins, Baltimore, MD. Reproduced with permission)

9.13.1.8 LVH Criterion 8 – Increased Magnitude of Terminal Rightward QRS Vector in the Presence of an Abnormally Posterior Maximum QRS Vector

This is frequently a manifestation of posterobasal LVH rather than combined ventricular hypertrophy. However, it is often not possible to distinguish the difference.

9.13.1.9 LVH Criterion 9 – Abnormal Ratios of Specific Magnitudes

An example of this is a decreased magnitude of the ratio of Z anterior to Z posterior. Other ratios are less reliable. It is particularly useful in the presence of low voltage from various causes. The major differential is that of lung disease with a high residual volume. A good clue is that, in lung disease, the X left is also decreased in magnitude, more than merely by the low voltage per se, since there is frequently air in the lateral left chest wall in cystic fibrosis [57] as well as in the anterior chest.

9.13.1.10 LVH Criterion 10 – Increased Magnitude of R in aVL

This is a reliable criterion, but, when met, the diagnosis is usually obvious from other criteria. An important note of caution is that in the presence of an abnormally superior maximum QRS vector, the magnitude of R in aVL will be

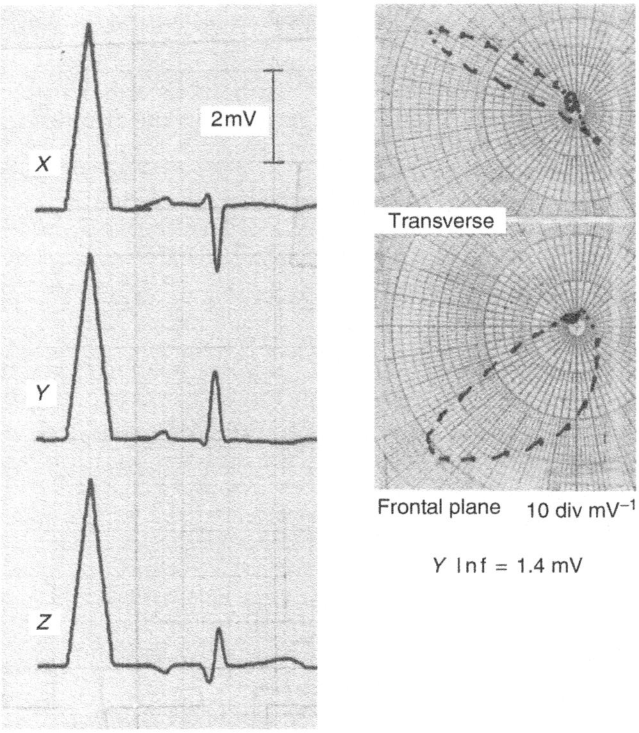

Fig. 9.28
Frank-system orthogonal ECG of a 1-day-old baby boy with a maximal TOF, which indicates non-restrictive VSD, pulmonary atresia and 100% right-to-left shunt. The pulmonary blood flow in the 1-day-old child was via a small ductus arteriosus. The RVH is severe with a wide open clockwise vector loop (normal for this age), but with most of the terminal vector to the right and posterior. The T vector is to the right and posterior, but that could be normal for this age

increased because the direction of the vector is similar to that of the lead vector for aVL; in such cases, therefore, the criterion cannot be utilized.

9.13.1.11 LVH Criterion 11 – Increased Magnitude of the Maximal Spatial Vector to the Left (MSVL)

This is, in general, an excellent criterion, but the measurement of Z posterior by itself is probably just as good, and simpler. (See Sect. 9.14 for specific use.)

9.13.1.12 LVH Criterion 12 – Abnormally Prolonged QRS Duration

On average, the QRS is prolonged, but the criterion is only fair because the variation is so great.

9.13.1.13 LVH Criterion 13 – T-Wave Abnormality

There are two types of T-wave abnormality. The first, very common in PDA, is a large magnitude T vector in the normal direction (increased left and/or inferior). By itself the criterion is not useful, for tall T waves can be present in many

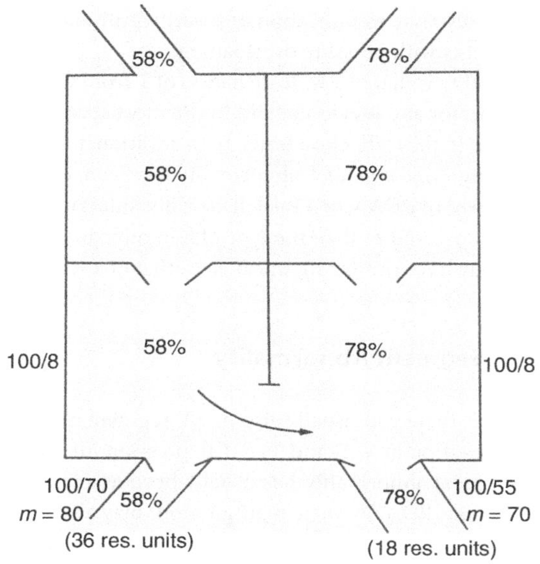

Fig. 9.29
Box diagram of a patient with non-restrictive VSD and pulmonary vascular disease, so that resistance to flow into the pulmonary artery is higher than resistance to flow into the aorta. The amount of right-to-left shunt is exactly the same as in the patient with TOF depicted in ➋ Fig. 9.23. Oxygen saturations are given as percentage values

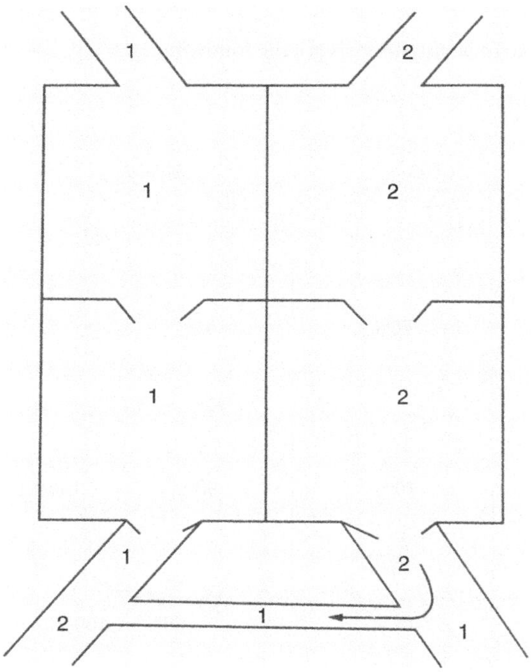

Fig. 9.30
Box diagram of a patient with a patent ductus arteriosus and moderate left-to-right shunt (2/1 pulmonary/systemic flow ratio). On the basis of the volume work alone, there is pure LVH. However, the larger the ductus, the greater the pulmonary artery (and thus right ventricular) pressure

situations including hyperkalemia. It is also not an indication of severity. Although often present in volume overloading, tall T waves can also be present in patients with pressure overloading.

The second type of T-wave abnormality is that of a wide deviation of T from QRS (i.e., increased QRS-T angle). When LVH is severe, the T vector is more anterior and less to the left. In the most severe cases, the T vector will be so much to the anterior that the T waves are upright in the right chest leads. If, in addition, the T vector is to the right, the T in the left chest leads will also be negative. Although this type of T abnormality has been associated with severe pressure overload, it is also seen in the pure volume overload of PDA when the left-to-right shunt is very large. Severity of the hypertrophy, perhaps with fibrosis, seems to be the cause, rather than the type of hemodynamics, for example, pressure versus volume overloading. A low-voltage T vector may have similar significance to that of a wide QRS-T angle.

9.13.1.14 LVH criterion 14 – ST-Segment Abnormality

When the T-wave abnormality is severe, there will usually also be ST-segment abnormality, manifested by depression in the X leads (V_5, V_6) and sometimes elevation in V_4R and V_1. ST depression inferiorly, in Y or aVF, may also be present. As in the T-wave abnormality, ST-segment abnormality has usually been associated with severe pressure overload, but severe volume overload, as in a large shunt PDA or aortic regurgitation, may also be responsible.

9.14 Aortic Stenosis (Valvular)

Whereas PDA provides the prototype for left ventricular volume overload, aortic stenosis (AS) provides the example usually given for pure pressure overload. However, valvular stenosis, because of the frequent narrow pulse pressure causing less coronary perfusion when severe and the need for perfusion of very thick muscle, has the additional problem of that poor perfusion (➋ Fig. 9.31).

The ECG criteria of importance in aortic stenosis are the following.

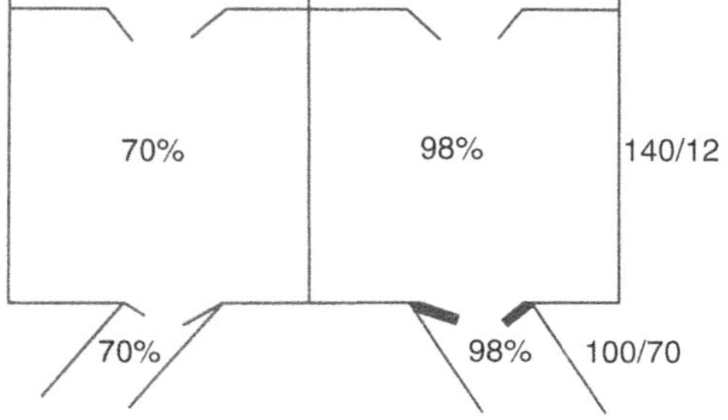

Fig. 9.31
Box diagram of a patient with pure valvular aortic stenosis. The oxygen saturations are normal. The amount of stenosis is moderate in this case, with a 40 mm systolic gradient. Note that the end-diastolic pressure in the left ventricle is, as is typical, only somewhat elevated. Although there is consequent elevation of the left atrial pressure, there is usually, no dilatation

9.14.1 LVH Criterion 1 in Aortic Stenosis

The direction of inscription of the vector loop is typical of that in LVH, but there are a number of important specifics for this lesion. First, the more severe the stenosis, the more likely is the initial QRS to be oriented to the left and anterior [45, 46, 55, 56] (➋ Fig. 9.32). Second, in the more severe cases, the QRS forces are often directed posterior so early that anterior myocardial infarction may not be able to be differentiated (➋ Fig. 9.33). Third, posterobasal LVH is common, although there seems to be little or no relationship to severity (➋ Fig. 9.32). Fourth, in severe cases, the vector turns posterior very early, then turns laterally so that there is a crossed (figure-of-eight) loop. It may be that the posterobasal area is being activated early, as in left bundle branch block (LBBB). Under any circumstance it is likely that considerable

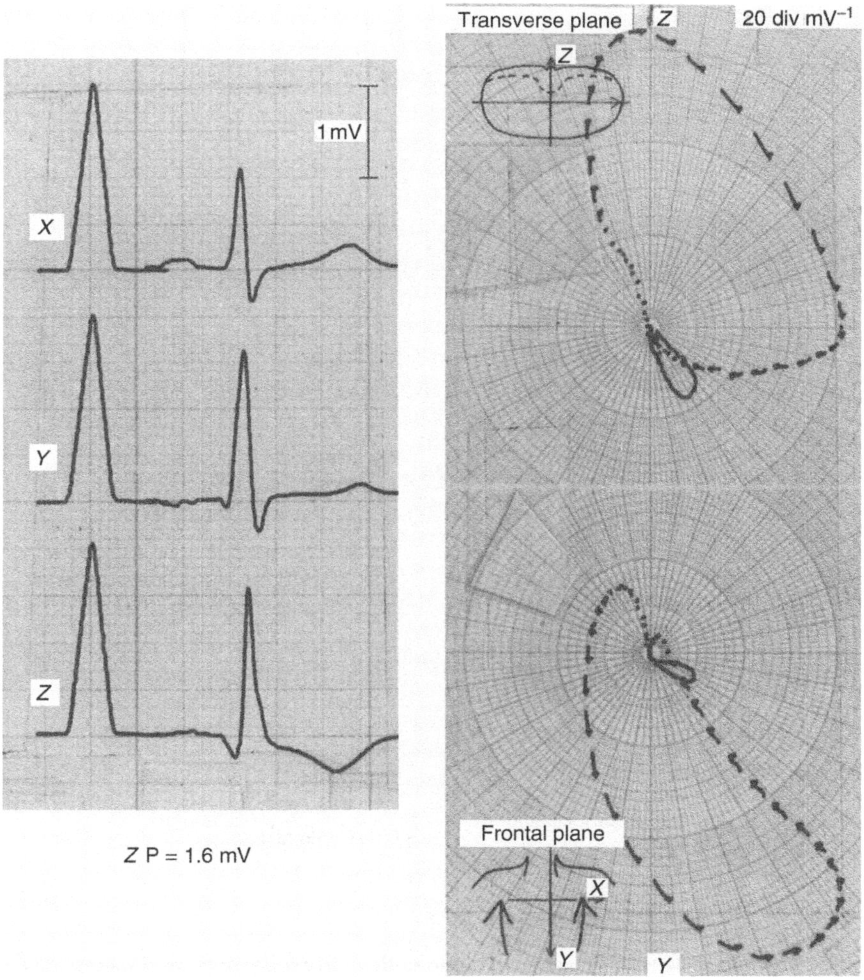

Fig. 9.32
Frank-system orthogonal ECG of an 18-year-old male operated upon 1 year previously for severe valvular aortic stenosis. The QRS had not significantly changed, although the T-vector had been further to the right. (Note that, as is usual, the frontal plane vector loop is wide open and clockwise inscribed, despite the severe LVH) (After Liebman et al [8]. © Williams and Wilkins, Baltimore, MD. Reproduced with permission)

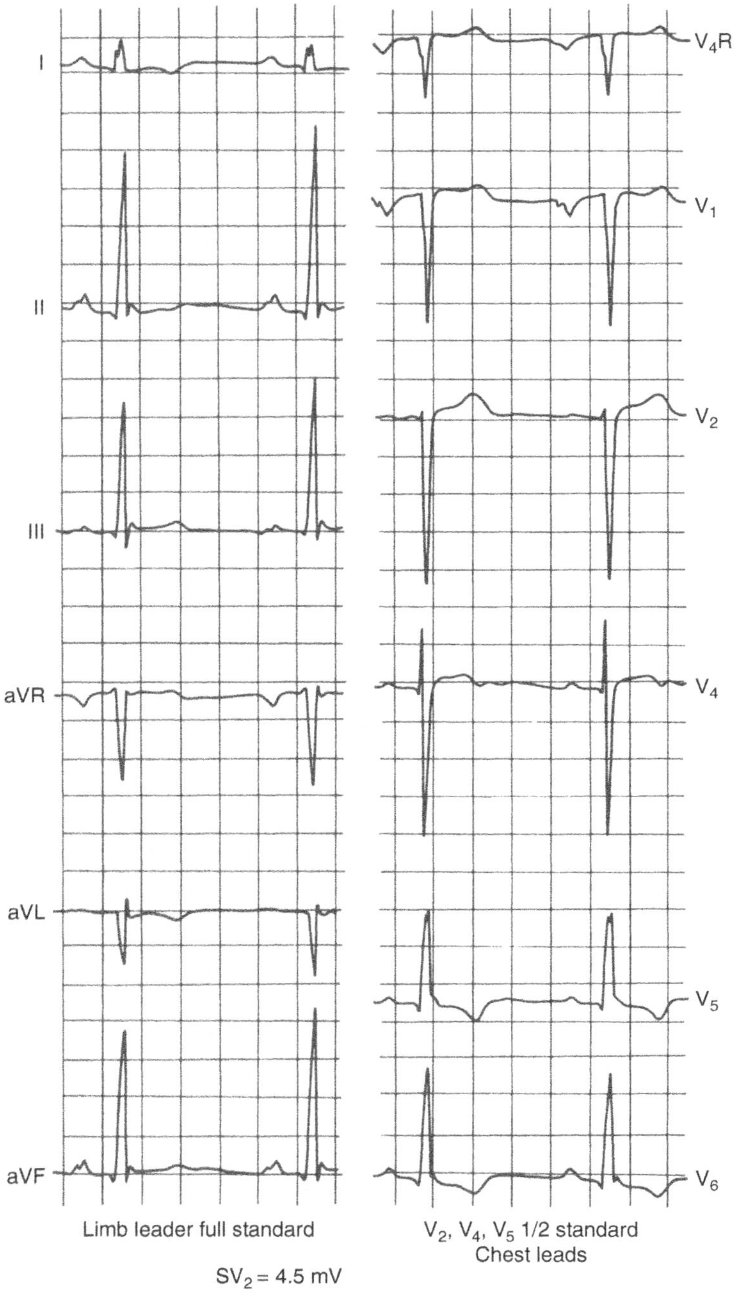

Fig. 9.33
Standard ECG of an 18-year-old male with severe coarctation of the aorta (operated upon successfully at age 2 years) and two further operations for severe valvular aortic stenosis. The first operation was a valvotomy and the second for aortic valve replacement. The initial QRS is to the right, anterior, superior (normal). The horizontal plane direction of inscription in the ECG appears to be counterclockwise with considerable midportion slowing, but with the VCG the vector goes well posterior before going to the left as in many patients with left bundle branch block (LBBB). Nonetheless, the diagnosis is intraventricular conduction abnormality as part of marked LVH since the initial QRS is normal. (The T vector is well to the right and posterior, very abnormal, and could be part of either severe LVH or LBBB) (After Liebman et al. [8]. © Williams and Wilkins, Baltimore, MD. Reproduced with permission)

fibrosis is present. If the initial QRS is to the right, then intraventricular conduction abnormality (perhaps due to fibrosis) is suggested, as part of severe LVH (➋ Fig. 9.33). If the initial QRS is to the left, then differentiation from LBBB may not be possible.

9.14.2 LVH Criterion 2 in Aortic Stenosis

The initial QRS activation includes at least five major components:

(a) The left septum, 1/2 to 2/3 down the septum
(b) The posterior free wall of the left ventricle near the left septum where activation begins, stimulated by the posterior branch of the left bundle
(c) The right septum, stimulated by a branch of the right bundle from the base of the anterior papillary muscle
(d) The right ventricular endocardium, stimulated by branches from the right bundle via the moderator band
(e) Up the septum from stimulation by the left anterior branch of the left bundle, which causes the normal QRS to be initially superior left or right and anterior or posterior.

As stated above, in severe valvular AS, the initial QRS is frequently to the left. Data [56] shows that in a series of 70 patients severe enough to need surgery, the initial QRS was to the left in half, and when it was to the right, the magnitude was small. In another series of 63 catheterized patients, 41 had systolic gradients less than 50 mmHg, of which, in 37 the initial QRS was to the right. Of 22 who had systolic gradients greater than 50 mmHg and/or need surgery, the initial QRS was to the right in only three. The etiology of the initial QRS vector to the left in the more severe cases is not known, but it could be hypothesized that hypertrophy of the free posterior wall near the left septum may provide the answer. Studies in BSPM [45, 46] have confirmed this hypothesis. Fibrosis of the left septum, which could surely cause the initial QRS to be to the left, has not been confirmed in pathologic studies. Left septal hypertrophy is not usually seen in valvular aortic stenosis, but is frequently recognized in fixed subvalvular stenosis, where the initial QRS to the left is very unusual.

9.14.3 LVH Criterion 4 in Aortic Stenosis

This criterion, which involves the QRS vector turning posterior very rapidly (so that anterior myocardial infarction is in the differential diagnosis) is common in significant aortic stenosis (➋ Fig. 9.33).

9.14.4 LVH Criterion 7 in Aortic Stenosis

An increased magnitude of the Z posterior is an excellent parameter. Correlations of peak LV pressure with the magnitude of the Z posterior in the Frank system gives an estimated R value of 0.65 for prediction of the pressure. The confidence interval is wide, however, so that it is beneficial using only the patient himself or herself as his or her own control. As severity increases, the magnitude of Z posterior increases (➋ Fig. 9.34).

9.14.5 LVH Criterion 8 in Aortic Stenosis

This is common in significant aortic stenosis, where the prominent terminal vector to the right and posterior occurs without pulmonary hypertension or other evidence of a hypertrophied right ventricle (➋ Fig. 9.32), and suggests posterobasal LVH.

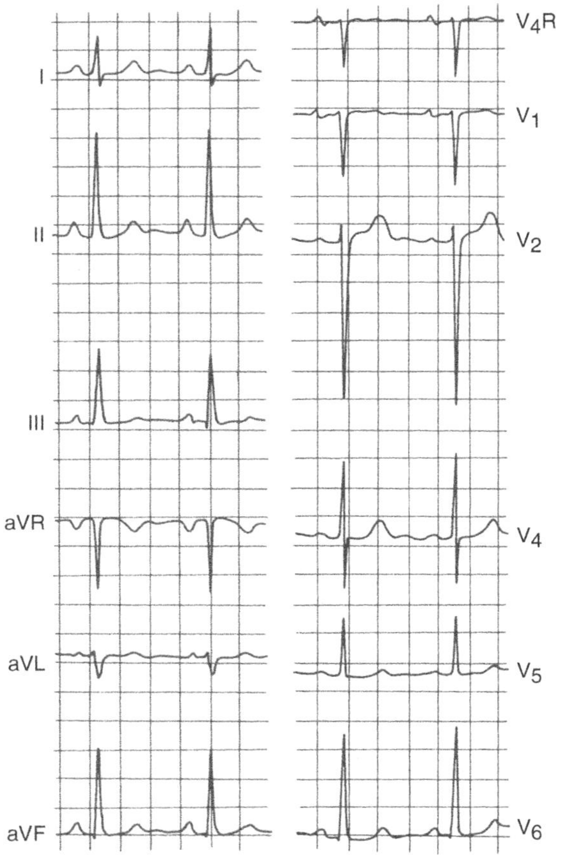

Fig. 9.34
Standard ECG of a 16-year-old male with severe aortic stenosis. There is minimal if any ST-segment abnormality, and the T-wave abnormality is minimal, with the maximum T vector being well anterior, but not to the left. The initial QRS is minimally to the right. The posterior projection is of extremely large magnitude. Another sign of LVH in this ECG is that the magnitude of the *X* left in V_6 is at least as great as in V_5 (After Liebman et al. [8]. © Williams and Wilkins, Baltimore, MD. Reproduced with permission)

9.14.6 LVH Criterion 11 in Aortic Stenosis

This measure, at one time, was considered to have a very strong correlation with LV pressure, but data indicates that its usefulness is essentially the same as for the magnitude of the Z posterior (Frank system). However, as a parameter for LVH per se, it is an excellent parameter.

9.14.7 LVH Criterion 13 in Aortic Stenosis

There may be a T-wave abnormality in significant valvular aortic stenosis without ST-segment abnormality. The T vector may be markedly anterior, although still to the left (Fig. 9.32), and on occasion the T vector magnitude may be increased.

Neither abnormality is worrisome, but if the T vector is to the right as well as anterior, and if the T vector magnitude is decreased, then there is great concern indicating the need for immediate intervention. This can be compared to the presence of secondary T-wave abnormalities in LVH in the adult (see ➋ Chap. 3).

9.14.8 LVH Criterion 14 in Aortic Stenosis

Depressed ST segment in the left chest or X leads and/or aVF (Y leads) indicate that perfusion may not be adequate for the great mass of left ventricular muscle. (ST-segment abnormalities, particularly with a low-magnitude T vector and/or T vector to the right, usually indicates the need for immediate surgery or balloon valvuloplasty). This finding, it should be made clear, is not because of severe pressure overload, but because of "severity" per se. It can occur in association with a large PDA or severe aortic regurgitation, as an example.

9.15 Aortic Stenosis (Fixed, Subvalvular)

Everything stated above for valvular aortic stenosis holds for fixed subvalvular aortic stenosis except for one difference, for which no explanation is available. This relates to the initial QRS vector, which, in severe cases, is only rarely to the left. In fact, it may be abnormally to the right, as in left septal hypertrophy (➋ Fig. 9.35). As part of the same studies cited above [55, 56], seven of eight patients with fixed subvalvular aortic stenosis, a systolic gradient greater than 50 mm Hg and needing surgery, had initial QRS vectors directed to the right and anterior of greater magnitude than normal.

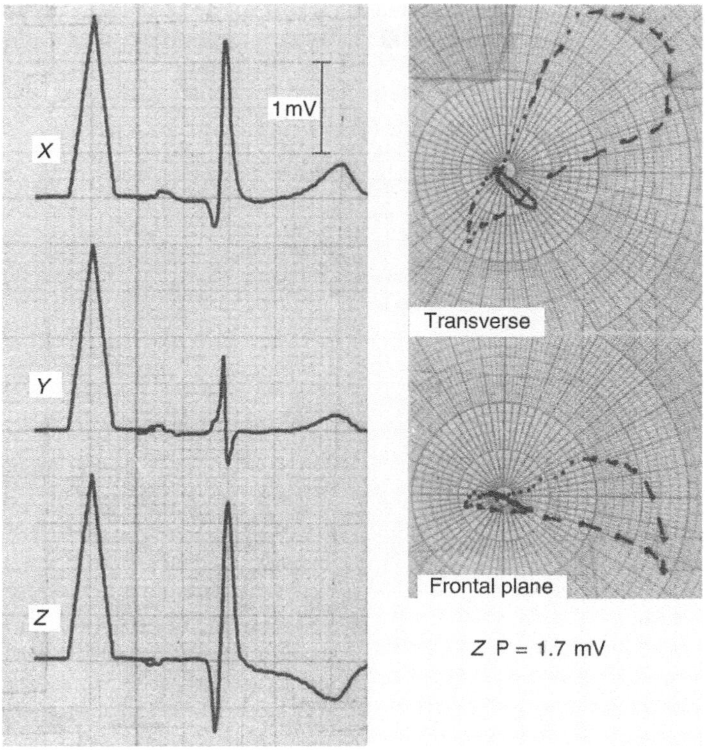

Fig. 9.35
Frank-system orthogonal ECG of a 14-year-old male with subvalvular aortic stenosis. Note the typical large magnitude initial QRS to the right and anterior

9.16 Cardiomyopathy

Primary cardiomyopathies (congestive or restrictive) are part of this discussion, whereas hypertrophic cardiomyopathies (with or without obstruction) are not. Cardiomyopathies per se are usually not considered congenital. However, an increasing number of infants are being recognized, often with primary cardiomyopathy, without systemic disease. Many are familial. Of the familial cardiomyopathies (including what used to be termed endocardial fibroelastosis), an increasing number of affected infants are being documented as having specific abnormalities of mitochondrial energy metabolism. It is not the purview of this section to delineate these diseases; just two things will be pointed out. First, the majority, when severe, have LVH with ST and T abnormalities as previously described, although LBBB may be present. Second (a critical piece of information) is, that the patient and the electrocardiogram are almost invariably categorized as normal in the newborn period. One reported family where all five children had severe cardiomyopathy [58] provides information of particular interest. The electrocardiogram, followed from the newborn period in three of the five, became abnormal at 2 months of age, before the patients' disease became clinically evident shortly thereafter. Another sibling had been evaluated on many occasions, with normal electrocardiograms, only to become ill as a teenager, with severe LVH and ST-segment and T-wave abnormality along with severe congestive heart failure.

9.17 Coarctation of the Aorta After Infancy

Isolated coarctation of the aorta is almost always located in the same place, near the origin of the original ductus arterious, and near the left subclavian artery. Although some patients with this anatomy can be very ill in early infancy, with heart failure and pulmonary hypertension, the majority of patients with simple coarctation after infancy are not associated with congestive heart failure. There will also usually not be very much elevation of left ventricular end-diastolic, and thus pulmonary venous, pressure. Therefore, pulmonary hypertension is not expected. Consequently, the ECG demonstrates pure LVH. In addition, because there is high aortic pressure (➋ Fig. 9.36), coronary flow and perfusion are adequate. Therefore,

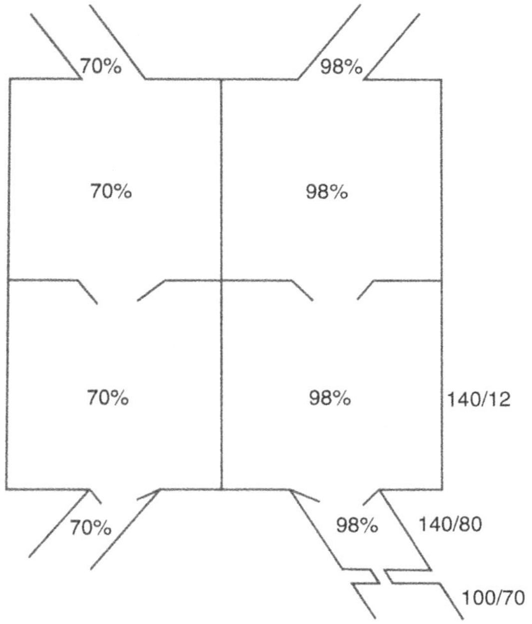

Fig. 9.36
Box diagram of a patient with simple coarction of the aorta, of moderate severity, with 40 mm systolic gradient and moderate increase in left ventricular end-diastolic pressure. Unlike the situation in valvular of subvalvular aortic stenosis (see ➋ Fig. 9.31), the driving force for coronary blood flow is high, so that myocardial perfusion is usually adequate

ST-segment and T-wave abnormalities are usually not present. Although the type of LVH is usually not distinctive, it is very common to have posterobasal LVH. As part of the posterobasal LVH the terminal vector to the right may be so great that there is often a terminal r or R in V_4R and V_1. Such standard ECG's have often erroneously been diagnosed as "incomplete right bundle branch block." In many teenagers and young adults, many years after successful coarctation surgery, rsr' is often recognized. This has been shown using BSPM to reflect RVH, as described above [48]. The mechanism is believed to be hypertrophy of more cells (hyperplasia) shortly after birth.

9.18 Anomalous Origin of the Left Coronary Artery in the Older Child

When the left coronary artery originates from the pulmonary artery and the right coronary artery originates from the aorta normally, the coronary flow depends upon the development of adequate intercoronary collaterals and the extent of lowering of pulmonary vascular resistance. There are children with this anomaly who progress through infancy without transmural myocardial infarction [59], presumably because intercoronary collaterals are adequate, resulting in considerable flow from the right coronary system into the left coronary artery system. Since pulmonary vascular resistance is normal, flow is through the left coronary artery into the pulmonary artery, resulting in left-to-right shunt. The latter per se results in volume work in the left ventricle so that there may be LVH. In addition, there is some "steal" from the left ventricle into the pulmonary artery causing some left ventricular disease, though usually not enough to result in ST-segment and T-wave abnormality. Finally, because of the steal from the myocardium there may be papillary muscle dysfunction and significant mitral regurgitation. The result is even more severe LVH, with no special aspects that specifically point to the diagnosis of anomalous left coronary artery from the pulmonary artery. (On the other hand, if there are not enough intercoronary collaterals and/or the left coronary artery is very small, there is little flow into the left coronary artery system. The result is very poor perfusion of the left ventricular myocardium so that there is LVH with ST-T abnormality. However, this latter ECG is not pure, since there will usually also be anterolateral wall myocardial infarction as manifested by a deep broad Q in lead aVL.)

9.19 Congenital Mitral Regurgitation

There are many causes of isolated congenital mitral regurgitation, with no other cardiac abnormalities, although it is always necessary to rule out an anomalous left coronary artery. Among these, the diagnosis of endocardial cushion defect with pure mitral regurgitation is not common. Therefore, the frontal plane vector is inferior and the severity of the LVH (due to a pure volume overload) (➋ Figs. 9.37 and ➋ 9.38), depends upon the magnitude of the regurgitation.

Of particular interest for discussion is the magnitude of the regurgitation of the abiotrophy of the mitral valve associated with Marfan's syndrome, which may result in extremely severe mitral regurgitation in infancy. The LVH is extremely severe, often with ST-T abnormalities, even though the hypertrophy is caused by a pure volume overload. After infancy, the mitral regurgitation in Marfan's syndrome is usually mild and is associated with prolapsed mitral valve.

A second lesion for discussion is the pure mitral regurgitation associated with prolapsed mitral valve [60] (➋ Fig. 9.39). This is also a congenital lesion, often familial (mother and daughter), even though the diagnosis is rarely made before the immediate preschool period. In childhood, the mitral regurgitation is rarely enough to cause LVH on the ECG. Nonetheless, T-wave abnormality is very common, the T vector being markedly anterior and sometimes superior as well [60] (➋ Fig. 9.40). Strikingly, an electrocardiogram taken a few hours later may be normal, the variation with time being remarkable. Prominent U waves are often present. There are hypotheses for the etiology of the T-wave abnormality, but there is no knowledge. LVH is not responsible.

9.20 Congenital Aortic Regurgitation

Congenital aortic regurgitation is a lesion which varies in severity from the trivial to the moderately severe. The LVH on the ECG depends upon the severity of the leak. The most severe cases are often not caused by valve problems per se but

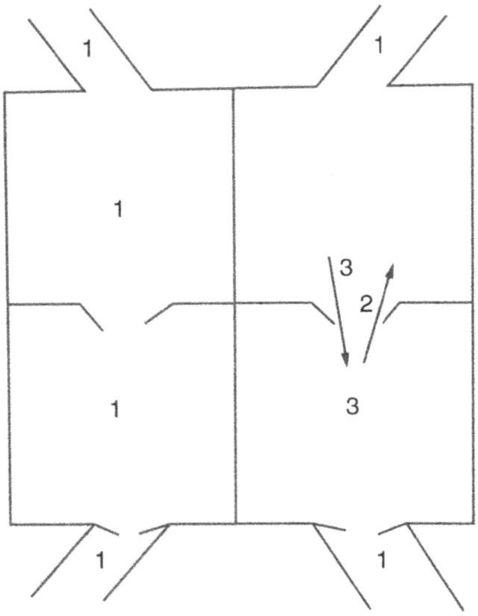

Fig. 9.37
Box diagram of a patient with moderate mitral valve regurgitation so that for each unit of blood ejected into the aorta, two units regurgitate into the left atrium. The result is three times normal volume of the left atrium (so that there is left atrial dilatation) and three times normal volume work of the left ventricle. LAH and LVH are expected

by a "tunnel" – a fistula between the root of the aorta and the left ventricular outflow tract. The sinuses of valsalva are not involved, with aneurysm caused by ruptured sinus of valsalva being mainly a disease of adulthood. One type of T-wave abnormality, common in congenital aortic regurgitation, is a large magnitude T vector in the normal direction. This T-wave abnormality is of little concern. On occasion, in severe cases, there may be the more common ST-T abnormality of great concern, similar to that seen in severe aortic stenosis, even though aortic regurgitation causes volume overload (Fig. 9.41). Commonly present in aortic regurgitation is a large initial QRS vector to the right and anterior, providing evidence of left septal hypertrophy.

9.21 Systemic Arterial Fistula

Cerebral arterial fistula is included in this discussion. The hemodynamics are similar to that of patent ductus arterious without pulmonary hypertension. There is pure volume overload of the left ventricle, although there may be enough increased systemic venous flow to the superior venacava to cause additional RVH.

9.22 Coronary Arterial Fistula

Coronary arterial fistula is a special type of systemic arterial fistula. Pure LVH occurs only when the fistula is into the left ventricle or left atrium, and such cases are rare [61]. In addition to the LVH, there may be ST-T abnormality, which is not related to hypertrophy per se, but to inadequate perfusion. When the fistula is into the right side of the heart there may be RVH owing to the right heart volume overload.

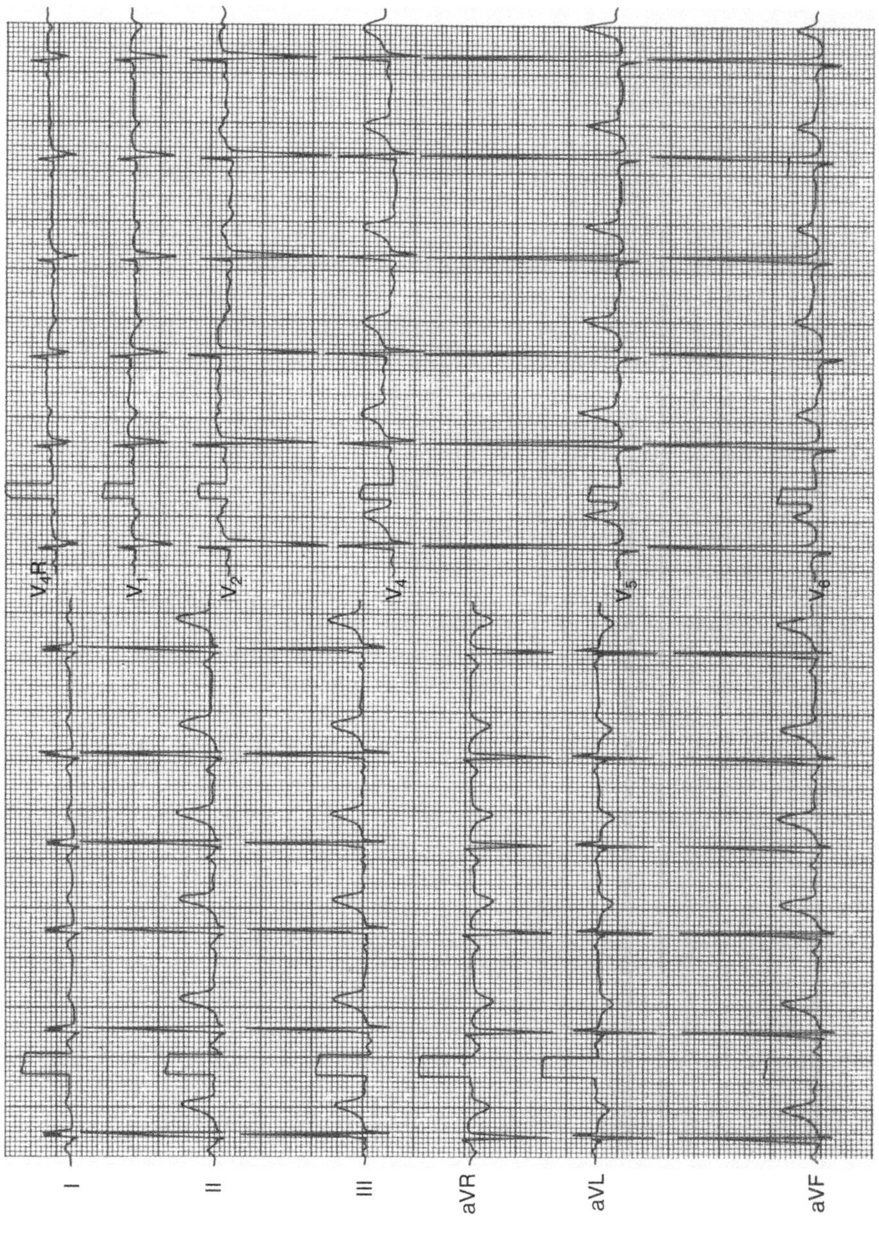

■ Fig. 9.38
Standard ECG of a 9-year-old female with severe congenital mitral regurgitation. Angiography demonstrated considerable dilatation of the left atrium and left ventricle. The left atrial enlargement is diagnosed because of the very prolonged second part of the P wave (see ➲ Fig. 9.50. for enlargement). There is a left septal hypertrophy (increased magnitude of initial QRS forces to the right and anterior) while the QRS loop is wide open and inscribed counterclockwise with increased magnitude posteriorly to left (QRS loop is not shown here)

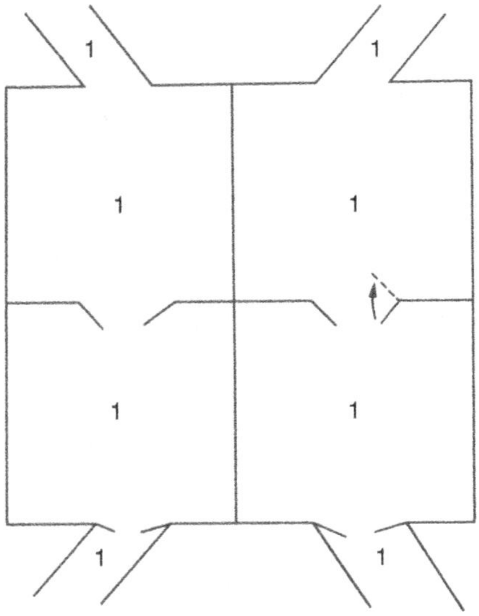

Fig. 9.39
Box diagram of a patient with prolapsed mitral valve (almost always the posterior leaflet). This diagram depicts no significant regurgitation. The actual leak may be nonexistent and, in children, rarely more than minimal. An important exception is the rare infant with severe mitral regurgitation associated with Marfan's syndrome.

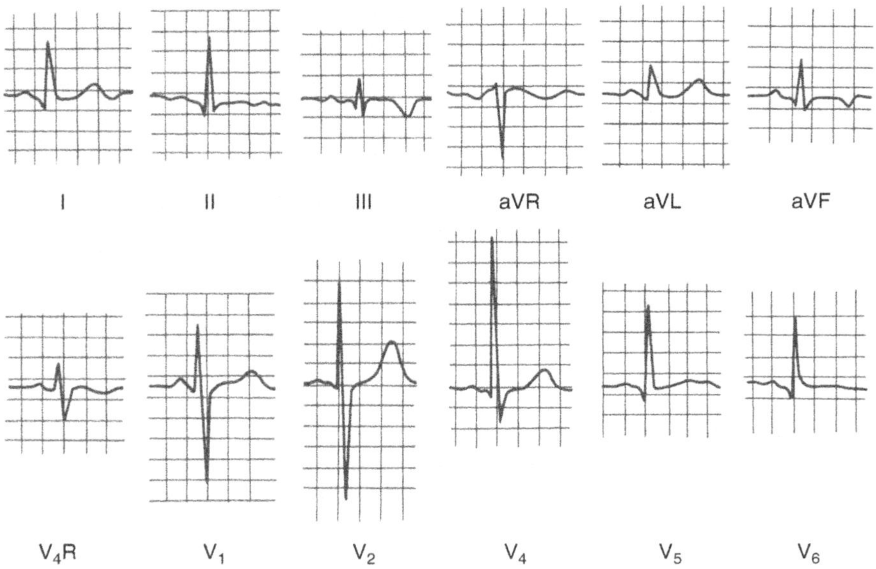

Fig. 9.40
Standard ECG of an 11-year-old female with prolapsed mitral valve and trivial mitral regurgitation. The T vector is abnormally anterior and superior. There is no LVH (After Liebman et al. [8]. © Williams and Wilkins, Baltimore, MD. Reproduced with permission)

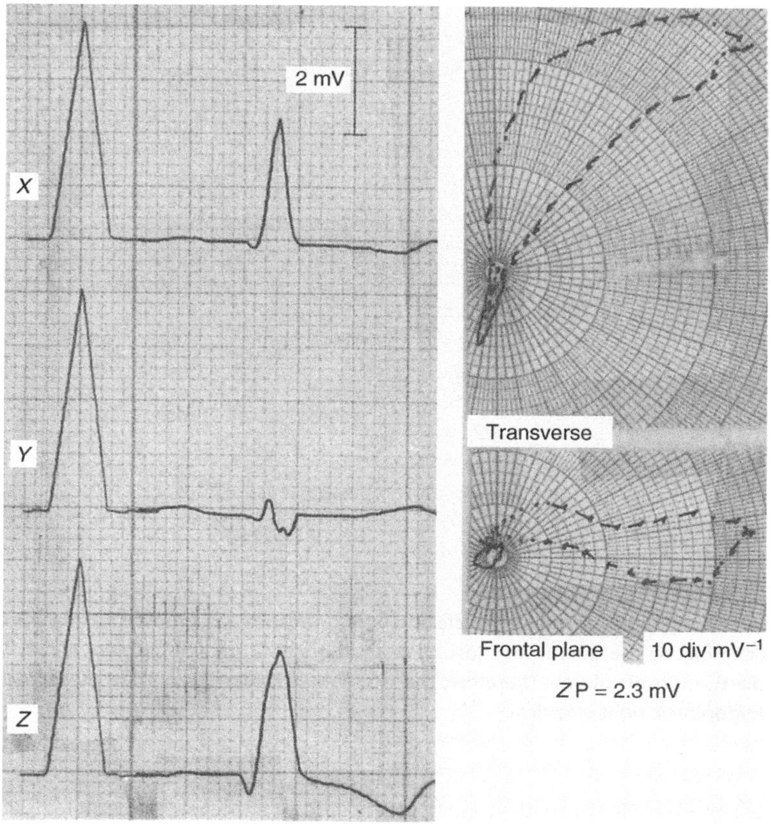

Fig. 9.41
Frank-system orthogonal ECG in a 23-year-old male who had been operated upon at age 18 years for severe aortic regurgitation. The operation was a plication and aortic stenosis was created. The left ventricle was not entered. The T direction, opposite to the direction of the QRS vector, was present *before* surgery and is part of the severe LVH. The QRS vector turns posteriorly so quickly that anterior myocardial infarction had to be considered. The reason for the mainly superior QRS vector is not known (After Liebman et al. [8]. © Williams and Wilkins, Baltimore, MD. Reproduced with permission)

9.23 Hypoplastic Right Ventricle with Pulmonary Atresia

The box diagram in ➋ Fig. 9.42 describes the hemodynamics of hypoplastic RV with pulmonary atresia. Note that a ventricular septal defect is not part of the lesion. Since no blood can leave the right ventricle, the entire systemic cardiac output goes right to left through an atrial opening. Babies with this lesion are "patent ductus dependent," with the only pulmonary artery blood flow coming from the aorta via the ductus. The flow then drains from the lungs, via the pulmonary veins, to the left atrium. Therefore, if as in ➋ Fig. 9.42, the pulmonary artery blood flow is half of the normal systemic blood flow, then the left atrium and left ventricle handle 3/2 times the normal volume. The volume overload of the left ventricle, as well as the hypoplastic right ventricle, results in an ECG that demonstrates considerable LVH (➋ Fig. 9.43). Since, prior to surgery, the patients are newborns, the LVH is often diagnosed mainly on the basis of the direction of inscription of the vector loop, which is wide open as seen in the frontal plane and counterclockwise inscribed in the transverse view. Specific magnitude increases may also be present, but conduction abnormalities and ST-T abnormalities are usually not. As a result of the hypoplastic right ventricle, the septum and left ventricle are differently positioned from normal, which must be considered in making ECG interpretations.

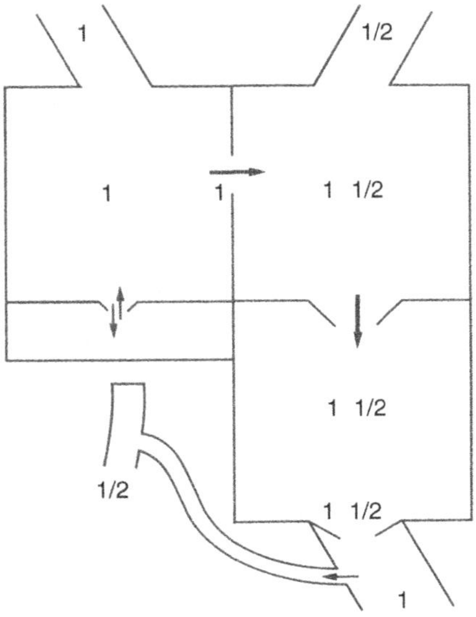

Fig. 9.42
Box diagram of a patient with hypoplastic right ventricle and pulmonary atresia. This is a ductal-dependent lesion, the entire pulmonary blood flow coming via the ductus arteriosus. Presuming half normal pulmonary blood flow, the left atrium and left ventricle each handle 1½ units of volume. Therefore, there is marked LVH on account of the increased volume work of the left ventricle, plus the hypoplastic right ventricle

Surgery is absolutely necessary for the patient's survival, including relief of right ventricular outflow obstruction and, more important, a systemic pulmonary artery connection. The latter causes even more volume load on the left ventricle. Should the surgery result in an increased volume of the right ventricle, the ECG only rarely reflects it. The surgical systemic-pulmonary connection accentuates the LVH.

9.24 Hypoplastic Right Ventricle with Tricuspid Atresia

The box diagram in Fig. 9.44 describes the hemodynamics of hypoplastic RV with tricuspid atresia. In this case, a ventricular septal defect is present (although spontaneous closure is common). Since no blood can enter the right ventricle through the atretic tricuspid valve, the entire systemic cardiac output goes through an atrial opening into the left atrium and left ventricle. Flow then goes left to right through the VSD to enter the right ventricle and pulmonary artery. As in the hypoplastic right ventricle with pulmonary atresia, if there is one-half normal pulmonary blood flow, left ventricular volume work is 3/2 times normal. Consequently, with the hypoplastic right ventricle and the left ventricular volume overload, there is considerable LVH on the ECG. LVH in the newborn period is often diagnosed on the basis of the direction of inscription of the vector loop – wide open with counterclockwise inscription in the transverse plane. With aging, specific magnitude increases become more important, and with the need for a systemic to pulmonary artery shunt procedure, the LVH becomes more severe.

Two aspects of the ECG are of great interest. The first is that usually the frontal plane will demonstrate an abnormally superior QRS vector typical of that in endocardial cushion defects (Figs. 9.45 and 9.46). Studies have shown that the ventricular septal defect is almost always posterior [62] and is believed to be an endocardial cushion defect. (On the other hand, in the presence of tricuspid atresia with transposition, the frontal plane QRS vector is inferiorly directed and associated with an anterior VSD [62].) The second aspect of the ECG of great interest is the occasional unusual ECG suggesting left lateral well fibrosis with initial QRS to the right and extending posterior before going left [8] (Fig. 9.46). The latter has not been seen in newborns in the author's experience, so it is presumed that it is acquired,

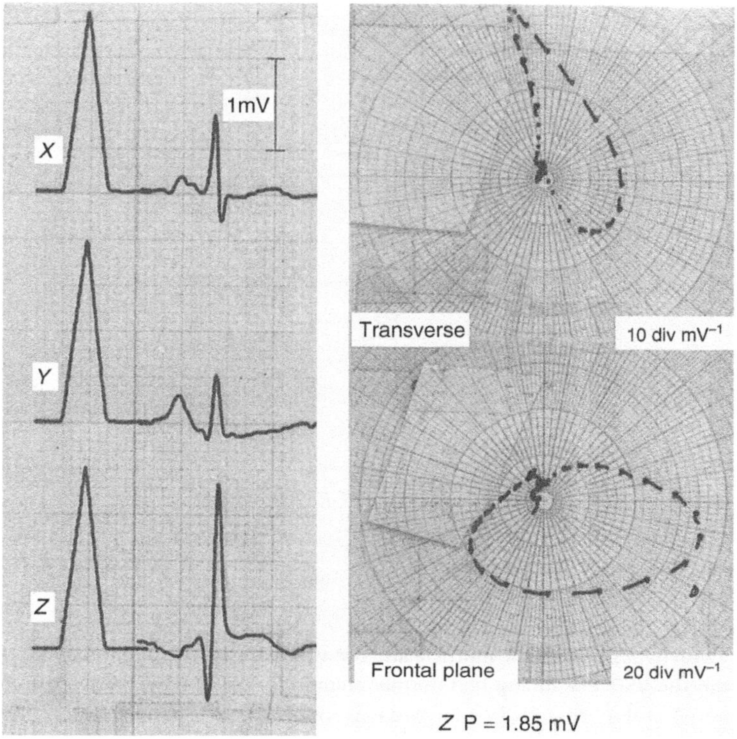

Fig. 9.43
Frank-system orthogonal ECG of a 1-day-old male baby with hypoplastic right ventricle and pulmonary atresia. Note the wide open counterclockwise direction of inscription in the horizontal plane, indicative of LVH in a newborn. Note also the large magnitude of the first portion of the P wave (lead *Y*, inferior; lead Z, anterior) indicative of RAH (After Liebman et al. [8]. © Williams and Wilkins, Baltimore, MD. Reproduced with permission)

in association with the longstanding volume overload. Left ventricular cardiomyopathy is relatively common, part of the same etiology.

As with the hypoplastic right ventricle with pulmonary atresia, the proper ECG interpretation may be impeded by the different position of the septum and left ventricle, although the LVH per se is easily diagnosed in both.

9.25 Biventricular (Combined Ventricular) Hypertrophy

For further information see Liebman et al. [8].

9.25.1 Left Ventricular Disease with Pulmonary Venous Hypertension

Any of the lesions described above with pure LVH may be associated with elevated pulmonary venous pressure, and thus pulmonary hypertension (➋ Fig. 9.47). Therefore, RVH can be present in addition to LVH. When the left ventricular dysfunction occurs in the newborn period, at which time the pulmonary arterioles are still thick walled, pulmonary venous hypertension causes pulmonary artery hypertension more quickly and more severely. Should the left ventricular disease be treated, medically or surgically, so that dysfunction becomes less, then the RVH may resolve even though there is enough left ventricular abnormality to continue to cause LVH.

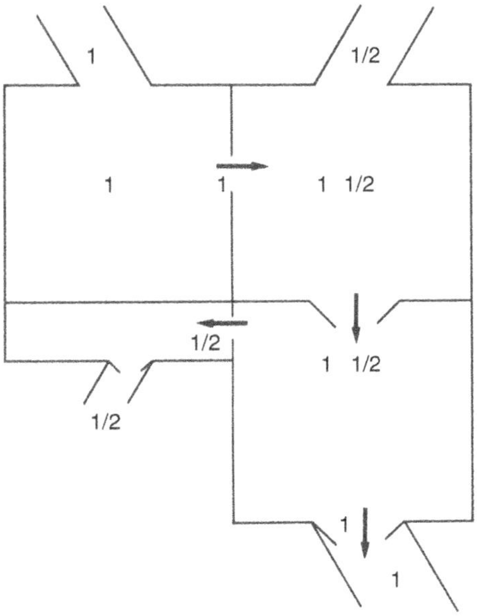

Fig. 9.44
Box diagram of a patient with hypoplastic right ventricle and tricuspid atresia. The pulmonary blood is dependent upon the left-to-right shunt through the VSD. Presuming half normal pulmonary blood flow, the left atrium and left ventricle each handle $1\frac{1}{2}$ units of volume. Therefore there is LVH for two reasons (The VSD is almost always posterior in the endocardial cushion position)

9.25.2 Two Separate Lesions with Dynamics for LVH and RVH

There are numerous cardiac lesions, which predispose to the presence of biventricular (combined ventricular) hypertrophy. These are now discussed.

9.25.2.1 Ventricular Septal Defect

The prototype of biventricular hypertrophy (BVH) is the ventricular septal defect. Before discussing the electrocardiogram in ventricular septal defect (VSD), some aspects of the physiology and pathophysiology must be discussed. By definition, in the largest defects (nonrestrictive), the RV pressure is the same as that of the left ventricle. Therefore, in the absence of pulmonary stenosis, systemic level pulmonary hypertension is present. The determination of shunting depends, in such cases, on the difference in vascular resistance in the pulmonary and systemic circulations. As a result of transmission of systemic pressure into the pulmonary resistance vessels, the newborn's arterioles mature slowly. It is usually only after some weeks that a left-to-right shunt becomes significant. A baby of 6 weeks may have a nonrestrictive VSD with a pulmonary to systemic flow ratio of 3/1. The left ventricle and left atrium have three times normal blood flow, so that there is LAE and LVH. The right ventricle shares in some of the volume overload, although much of the increased pulmonary artery blood flow reaches the pulmonary artery via a left ventricular thrust almost directly into the pulmonary artery. RVH is certainly present, however, because of the high pressure. With increasingly smaller sized defects, the right ventricular and pulmonary artery pressures are, perhaps, 3/4, 2/3, or even 1/2, systemic level, irrespective of the amount of left-right shunt. In fact, despite the restrictive nature of the defects, the pulmonary to systemic flow ratio can still be large, for example, 3/1 or more, because of low pulmonary vascular resistance. When the defects are so restrictive that

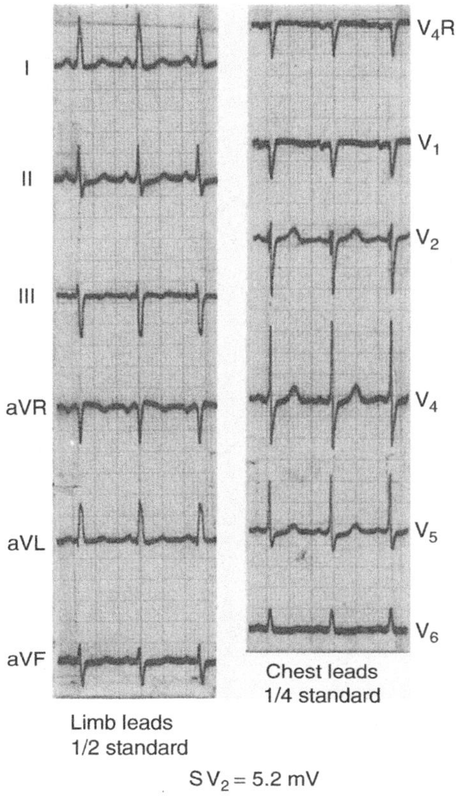

Fig. 9.45
Standard ECG of a 19-month-old male with hypoplastic right ventricle and tricuspid atresia, who had had a systemic to pulmonary artery shunt because the VSD had spontaneously closed. The horizontal plane is wide open with counterclockwise inscription in the transverse plane and the voltages to the left and posterior are of very great magnitude. LVH is considerable although there is no ST-T abnormality. There is also an abnormally superior maximum QRS vector, since the VSD had been in the endocardial cushion defect position (After Liebman et al. [8]. © Williams and Wilkins, Baltimore, MD. Reproduced with permission)

the pressure is less than half systemic, including normal, it is unusual after infancy for the pulmonary to systemic flow ratio to be more than 2/1. This is because the small size of the defect itself provides too much resistance to blood flow to allow a large left-to-right shunt. Finally, to add to the complexity of the ECG interpretation, there is the problem of the lesion being dynamic. First, the defect tends to become smaller with age, and second, in large defects, where surgery is not undertaken till after early infancy, pulmonary vascular disease may occasionally develop.

In summary, VSD is a lesion which is expected to cause BVH. The volume overload is mainly left ventricular, although the right ventricle shares in it, albeit less so (Figs. 9.48 and 9.49). There is also right ventricular pressure overload, dependent upon the size of the defect, since the larger the defect the greater the magnitude of the right ventricular and pulmonary artery hypertension. Therefore, prediction of the amount of left-to-right shunt through the VSD is based mainly on the amount of LVH, whereas prediction of the size of the defect and thus the amount of pulmonary hypertension is based mainly on the amount of RVH. This predictability is reasonable in the first year of life, but because of the problem of the dynamic nature of the lesion, becomes less reliable after that. In general, when only LVH is present, the defect is quite restrictive, so that there is little or no pulmonary hypertension present. When there is only RVH, there should be concern that the defect is large, perhaps with an increased pulmonary vascular resistance, so that there is little left-to-right shunt.

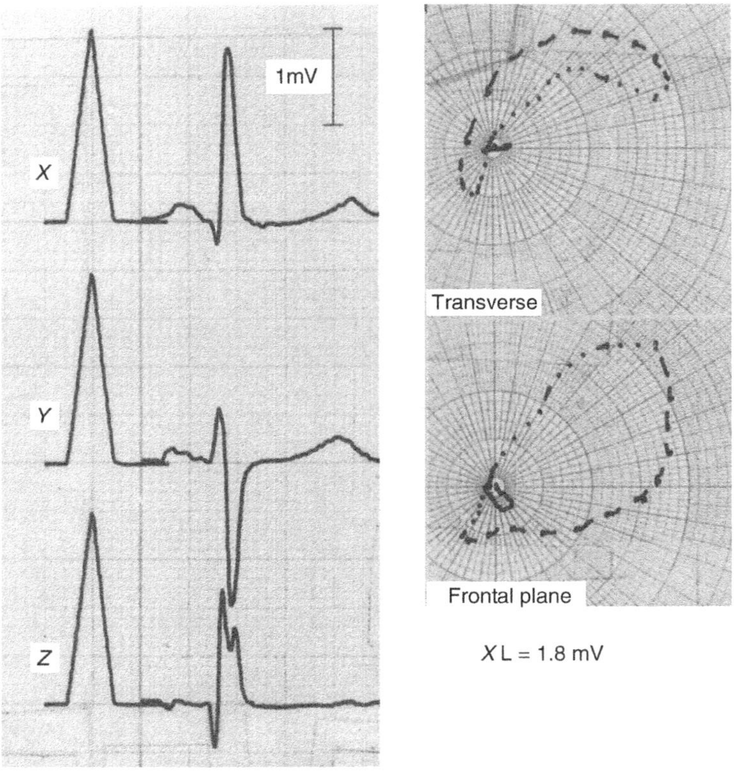

Fig. 9.46
Frank-system orthogonal ECG of a 9-year-old female with hypoplastic right ventricle and tricuspid atresia, who had had no surgery. The frontal plane QRS vector loop is typical, beginning inferior, and rotating counterclockwise, mainly superior. The transverse plane demonstrates considerable conduction abnormality. The initial QRS portion is to the right and anterior, then swings posterior while still well to the right, so that the QRS is inscribed clockwise. A left lateral wall myocardial infarction must be considered (but autopsy 4 years later, death following the Fontan procedure, demonstrated no infarction). The left ventricle was myopathic, however, with considerable hypertrophy and replacement fibrosis (After Liebman et al. [8]. © Williams and Wilkins, Baltimore, MD. Reproduced with permission)

The degree of BVH should reflect the amount of left-to-right shunt and the size of the defect, but accuracy can only be approximate.

A VSD may also cause combined atrial enlargement. The larger the left-to-right shunt, the larger the volume overload of the left atrium. Meanwhile, the higher the RV pressure, the less is the compliance of the right ventricle, so that RAE may be present. The most commonly recognized, however, is pure LAE because the volume overload of the left atrium is dominant.

9.25.3 Biatrial Enlargement

For further discussion see Liebman et al. [8] and Ishikawa et al. [34]. Simultaneous registration of various leads is particularly useful in diagnosing biatrial enlargement (BAE) (Fig. 9.50), particularly when the magnitude is increased (e.g., four times normal standard) and the speed of the paper is 100 mm s $^{-1}$. The author has usually utilized simultaneous

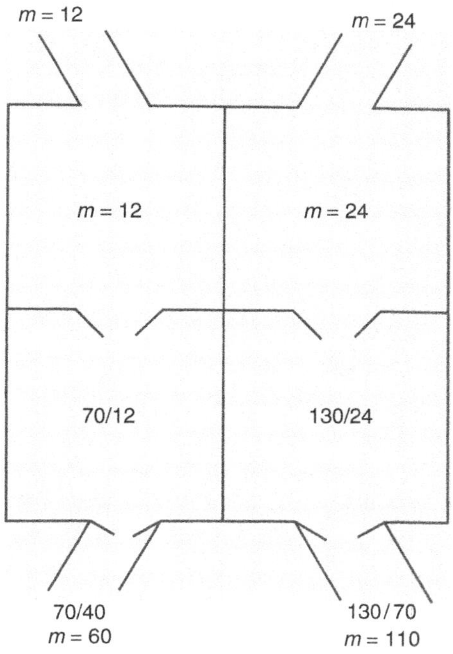

Fig. 9.47
Box diagram of a patient with left ventricular cardiomyopathy and secondary pulmonary hypertension. The left ventricular end-diastolic pressure is 24 mmHg, so that there is elevated pulmonary venous pressure (*m* = mean pressure in mmHg). Reflex pulmonary hypertension may result

leads V_1, V_4, V_6, I, II and III, but other combinations can be useful. It is important to be able to delineate the first portion of the P wave (especially along its inferior and anterior lead axes) from the terminal portion (to the left). If only three simultaneous leads are available, leads II, V_1 and V_5 or V_6 would usually be most useful.

The most useful criteria for BAE are the following.

(a) Standard ECG:
- (I) Increased P magnitude inferior and/or anterior (first part) plus an increased duration of P (the latter owing to increased duration of second part of P)
- (II) Increased P magnitude inferior and/or anterior (first part) plus increased magnitude posterior (second part)
- (III) Increased P magnitude inferior and/or anterior (first part) plus increased P terminal force
- (IV) Increased P magnitude inferior and/or anterior (first part) plus increased time between first and second peaks (the latter in normal infants is usually not more than 0.02 s apart, and in adolescents, rarely exceeds 0.04 s [3])

(b) Orthogonal ECG:
- (I) Increased P magnitude inferior and/or anterior (first part) plus increased duration of P (owing to increased duration second part)
- (II) Increased spatial vector magnitude of P anterior (SVA) plus increased duration of P
- (III) Increased P magnitude inferior and/or anterior (first part) and/or SVA plus increased magnitude posterior (second part)
- (IV) Increased P magnitude inferior and/or anterior (first part) and/or SVA plus increased magnitude of P spatial vector posterior
- (V) Increased P magnitude inferior and/or anterior (first part) and/or SVA plus increased time between peaks
- (VI) Increased P magnitude inferior and/or anterior (first part) and/or SVA plus increased P terminal force

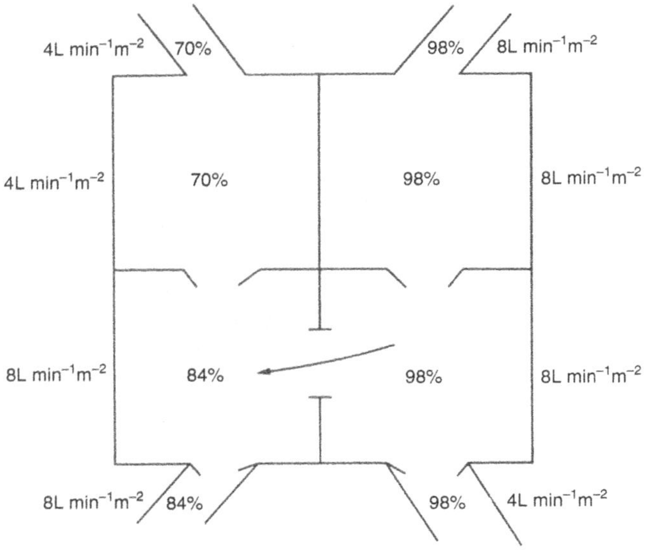

Fig. 9.48
Box diagram of a child with a VSD with left-to-right shunt so that the P/S flow ratio is 2/1 (*P* pulmonary flow, *S* systemic flow). The systemic cardiac output is normal. There is an increase in oxygen saturation in the right ventricle

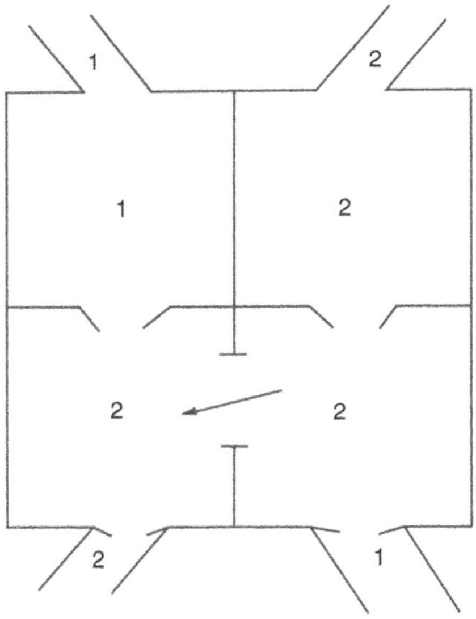

Fig. 9.49
Box diagram of same child as in Fig. 9.48, with a 2/1 P/S flow ratio. The left atrium and left ventricle each has twice normal volume, while the left ventricle must eject blood into the right ventricle, although some is ejected directly into the pulmonary artery. There is LVH and there *may* be some additional mild RVH based on the passive volume work of the right ventricle. However, the larger the VSD, the higher the RV pressure, so that RVH is expected

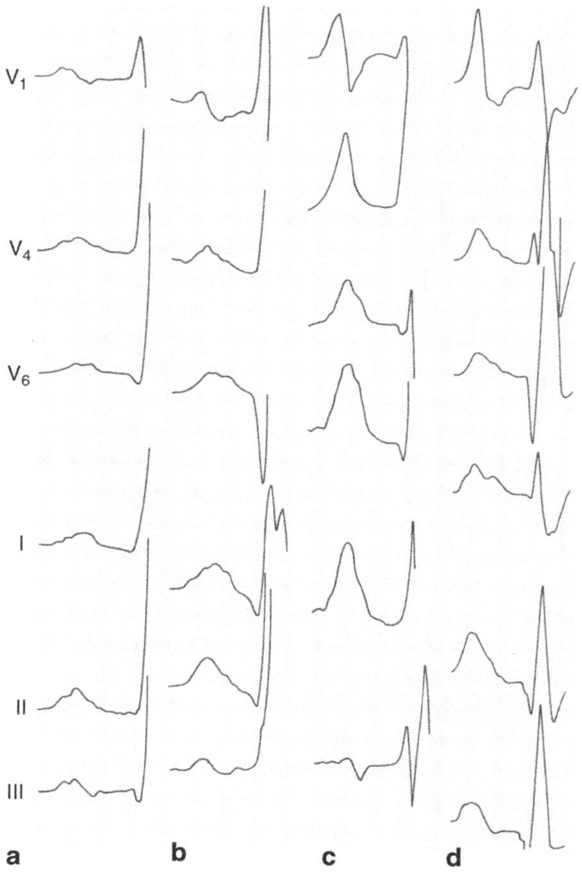

Fig. 9.50
Four representative ECGs for P-wave analysis. The simultaneous tracings of leads V_1, V_4, V_6, I, II and III are recorded at 100 mm s^{-1} and at four times standard calibration. The first ECG (a) is normal, (b) shows LAH, (c) shows RAH and (d) shows BAH (After Liebman et al. [8]. © Williams and Wilkins, Baltimore, MD. Reproduced with permission)

The fact that there is a dynamic reason to have BVH does not necessarily mean that there should be combined atrial hypertrophy (BAH). Neither or only one atrium may be enlarged or hypertrophied. Volume overload, of course, causes atrial enlargement, whereas decreased ventricular compliance, as with ventricular pressure overload or cardiomyopathy, causes mainly atrial hypertrophy. In general, RAH is much better recognized with the ECG than is LAH. Obviously, also, RAH or LAH may be present without hypertrophy of the ventricle on the same side. The prime examples are the expected RAH in the presence of the hypoplastic right ventricle syndrome and the expected LAH in the presence of the hypoplastic left ventricle syndrome.

9.25.4 Criteria for Biventricular Hypertrophy

Biventricular hypertrophy and relevant criteria are discussed further in Liebman et al. [8].

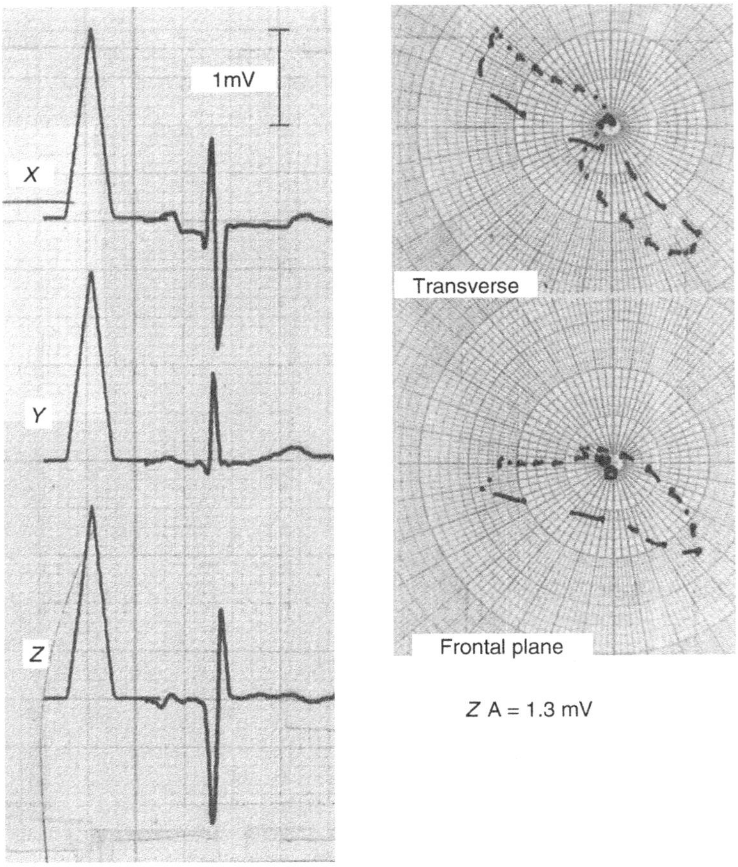

Fig. 9.51
Frank-system orthogonal ECG of a 5½-week-old baby boy with TOF. There are two main vectors, the first being to the left and anterior, the second to the right and posterior. From the activation sequence, RVH is clear. There is no additional LVH, since the first main vector is not abnormally to the left (After Liebman et al. [8]. © Williams and Wilkins, Baltimore, MD. Reproduced with permission)

9.25.4.1 BVH Criterion 1 – Direction of Inscription of QRS Vector Loops

(a) There are many variations of BVH where the direction of inscription is particularly useful. The presence of two main vectors in the transverse plane often provides excellent evidence. The most common situation is that of the first vector being abnormally to the left as well as anterior and the second vector being abnormally to the right as well as posterior. After 1 month of life, RVH is definite (➋ Fig. 9.51), and LVH is additionally diagnosed if the leftward vector is of increased magnitude. (An increased magnitude posterior QRS vector in this situation is not enough.) Most commonly, the first limb of the QRS vector loop is inscribed counterclockwise and the second limb clockwise.

(b) The activation sequence may be exactly as normal, with a wholly counterclockwise transverse QRS loop and large magnitude leftward and/or posterior projections. (In the newborn period, such a loop indicates LVH without abnormal magnitudes.) However, if the anterior projection is also very large and prolonged, then additional RVH is diagnosed. In the same situation, if the terminal right QRS magnitude is increased, RVH should also be suggested; but if the corresponding vector is abnormally posterior, then the large rightward vector may indicate posterobasal LVH rather than additional RVH (➋ Fig. 9.52).

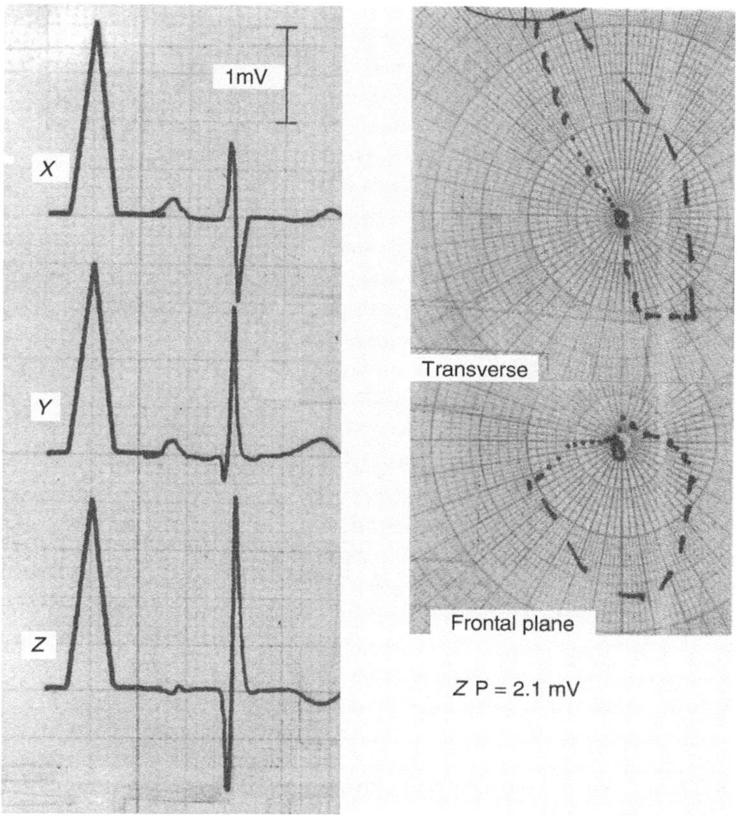

Fig. 9.52
Frank-system orthogonal ECG of a 3-week-old baby boy with a large VSD and large left-to-right shunt at an unusually early age. Both the posterior and inferior projections are of increased magnitude. LVH is clear, and the terminal projection to the right is also of increased magnitude, so that additional RVH is likely. It is possible, however, that the terminal projection to the right may be due to posterobasal LVH (After Liebman et al. [8]. © Williams and Wilkins, Baltimore, MD. Reproduced with permission)

(c) If the transverse plane is inscribed wholly clockwise, pure RVH is the usual diagnosis; but if it is also abnormally to the left, additional LVH should be considered (➲ Fig. 9.53). However, this latter diagnosis can be an error, since a large dilated right ventricle can cause considerable proximity effect upon the lead projections on the left chest. A definite error is to diagnose additional LVH if, with the presence of a wholly clockwise transverse plane loop, there is a large terminal rightward posterior projection. This terminal posterior projection is probably derived from the right ventricle after the left ventricle has completed activation, and is a manifestation of severe RVH.

9.25.4.2 BVH Criterion 2 – Decreased QRS Magnitude Posteriorly and/or to the Left, with a Large Terminal QRS Vector to the Right

These provide excellent criteria with the caution that a terminal right posterior QRS vector may be a possible manifestation of posterobasal LVH instead of additional RVH. In the standard ECG, the BVH may be missed, even though it is clearly

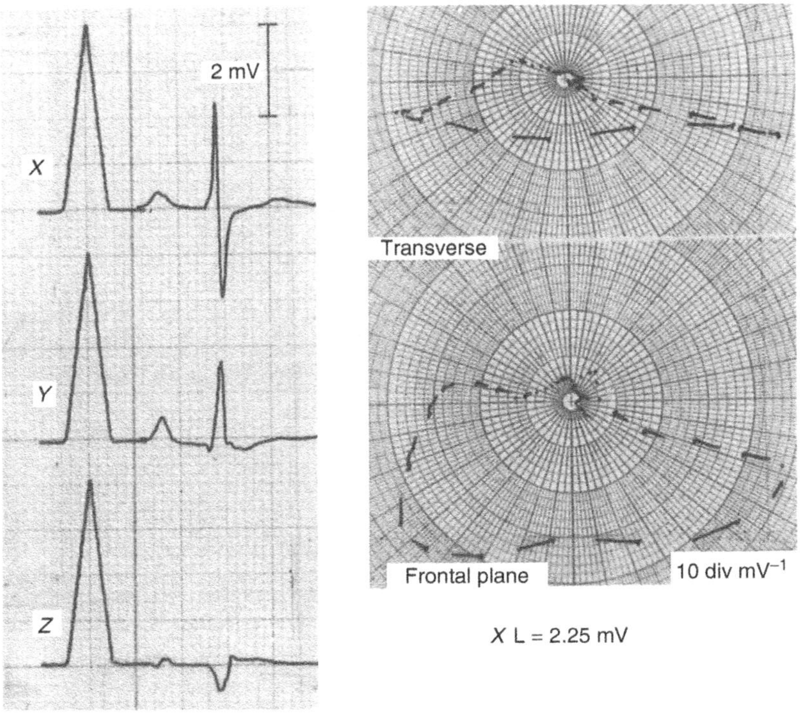

Fig. 9.53
Frank-system orthogonal ECG in a 4-month-old baby boy with a large VSD and large left-to-right shunt. There are two main vectors in the transverse plane, although the inscription is wholly clockwise, indicative of RVH. The magnitude to the left is increased indicative of additional LVH. It is unlikely that the latter is caused by the proximity effect, although the very large heart in the small chest of a baby makes it possible (After Liebman et al. [8]. © Williams and Wilkins, Baltimore, MD. Reproduced with permission)

present in the Frank- or McFee-system orthogonal VCG. The abnormally posterior QRS vector may cause the projection of the large terminal rightward vector not to cross the perpendiculars to leads V_4R and V_1. If, on the standard ECG, there is a deep S wave in V_5 or V_6, then the lack of a terminal r or R in V_4R or V_1 is not missed, except that, for reasons unknown, the large terminal QRS vector to the right may be present in the VCG, without a deep S in V_5 or V_6 in the standard ECG.

9.25.4.3 BVH Criterion 3 – Increased Magnitude Anterior Along with Definite Evidence for LVH

The anterior portion provides only a soft sign for additional RVH. The initial anterior limb should be broad and of at least 0.03 s duration (after infancy). A large initial rightward anterior QRS vector could be caused by left septal hypertrophy, whereas a tall spiking initial anterior vector reflected in the right chest leads is commonly caused by proximity effect – particularly in preschool children.

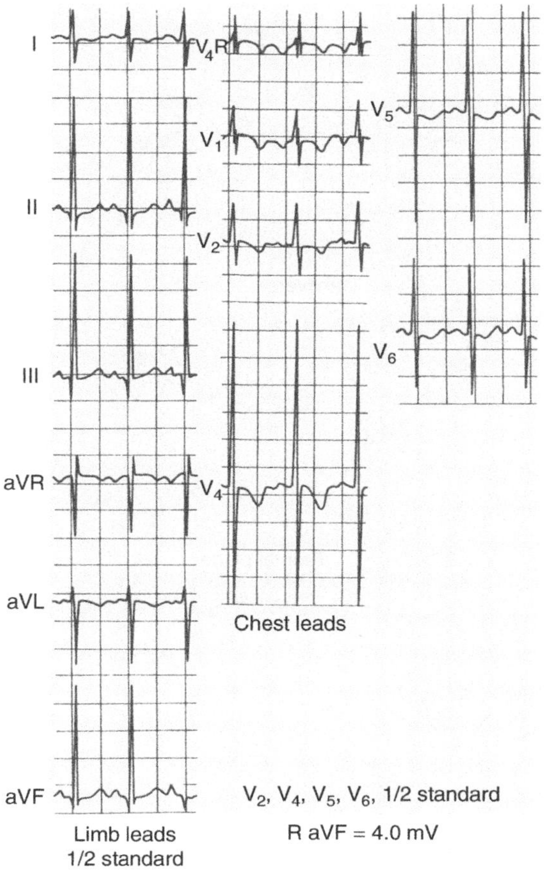

Fig. 9.54
Standard ECG of a 2-month-old baby boy with a large VSD and large left-to-right shunt. The voltages are exceptionally high. In lead V_4, the combined QRS magnitude is greater than 10.0 mV. The QRS appearances in V_4, V_5 demonstrate the Kaltz-Wachtel phenomenon

9.25.4.4 BVH Criterion 4 – Increased Magnitude Inferior Vector (Increased Y Inferior, Tall R in aVF) in the Presence of RVH as Diagnosed in the Transverse Plane

In the presence of good left ventricular potential and the absence of very severe RVH, additional LVH can be considered. However, if the RVH is severe, the increased magnitude inferior is part of the RVH. Such an ECG is common, for example, in tetralogy of Fallot.

9.25.4.5 BVH Criterion 5 – Katz-Wachtel phenomenon

This is a "pattern" and is not generally useful, although it is commonly discussed, particularly in relation to ventricular septal defect. It was originally described as "tall R and S waves in the mid-chest leads, together with tall R and S waves in two of the three 'bipolar' standard limb leads [63]." The biphasic nature of the QRS was believed to be caused by the

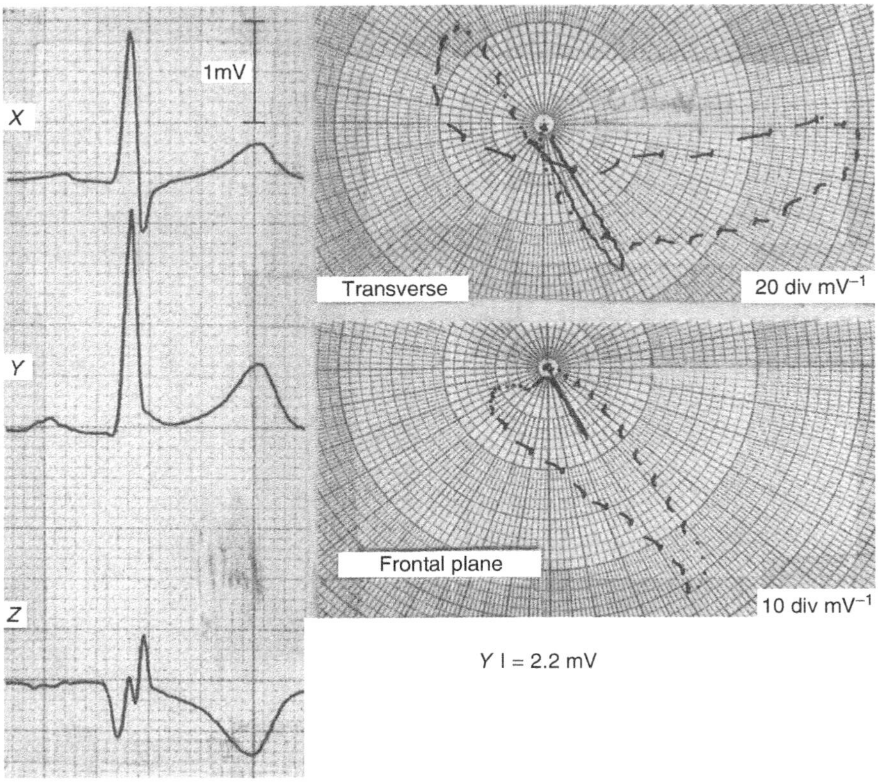

Fig. 9.55
Frank-system orthogonal ECG of a 17-year-old with a small VSD (once significantly larger). LVH is present on the basis of the increased magnitude inferior vector. The activation sequence, where the QRS vector moves to the right without going posterior, indicates RVH. There is also some terminal right conduction delay. The mild BVH reflects previous dynamics (After Liebman et al. [8]. © Williams and Wilkins, Baltimore, MD. Reproduced with permission)

opening in the septum, but of course that is not true. The manifestation of BVH is that of a wide-open counterclockwise transverse plane vector loop with the first limb markedly anterior and the second decidedly posterior (➋ Fig. 9.54).

9.25.4.6 BVH Criterion 6 – Definite ECG Evidence of Hypertrophy of One Ventricle, with Suggested ECG Evidence of Hypertrophy for the Other

This is a nonspecific but valid criterion, and an overlap of much that has been said above.

9.25.4.7 BVH Criterion 7 – ST and T Abnormality

With the present level of knowledge, ST and T abnormality in the presence of hypertrophy indicates severity, but cannot be used to diagnose hypertrophy per se.

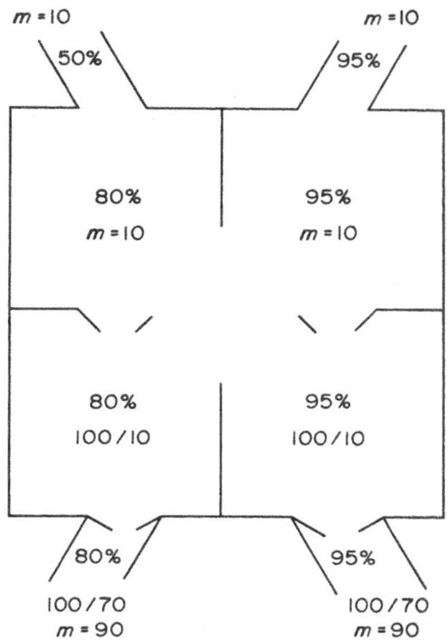

Fig. 9.56
Box diagram of a patient with complete AV canal. Note the communication among all four chambers. Left and right atrial pressures are equal, and LV and RV pressures are equal. There must be systemic level pulmonary hypertension. In this case, there is a large left-to-right shunt at the atrial level, although severe mitral and/or tricuspid regurgitation is possible

9.25.4.8 Addendum

As a result of the dynamic nature of the lesion, BVH may be recognized although the lesion has become very small. The ECG thus reflects previous dynamics (Fig. 9.55).

9.25.5 False-Positive Criteria for BVH

9.25.5.1 BVH Criterion 8 – Mean QRS Vector to the Right in the Frontal Plane of Standard ECG in the Presence of Definite LVH

The LVH is best diagnosed in the chest leads, the transverse plane, but the mean QRS vector to the right may help in diagnosing additional RVH. However, it is often an artifact of the poor lead I, so it is not reliable. However, if present in Frank or McFee vectorcardiograms, the horizontal plane would show the large terminal vector to the right, as well, and BVH would be the correct diagnosis.

9.25.5.2 BVH Criterion 9 – Clockwise Inscription of the Frontal Plane in the Presence of Definite LVH

This is similar to criterion 8 and is not an indicator of BVH since the clockwise frontal plane in the standard ECG is normal in most children.

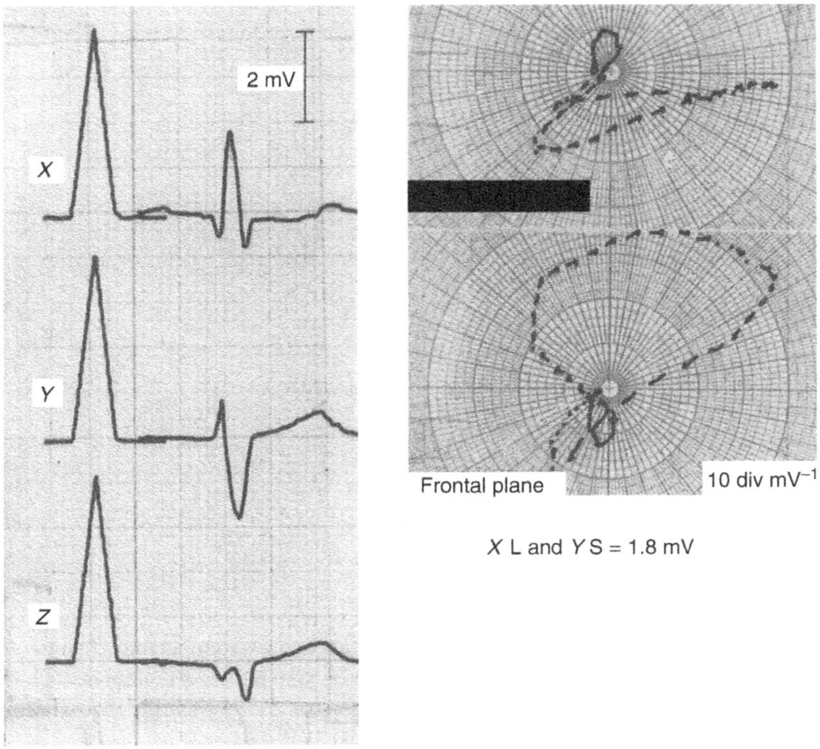

Fig. 9.57
Frank-system orthogonal ECG of a 15-month-old female with a partial AV canal. There is a large left-to-right shunt at both the atrial and ventricular levels with the RV pressure at 2/3 systemic level. There is a typical "abnormally superior vector" and BVH. The RVH is diagnosed on the basis of the mainly clockwise-inscribed anterior loop, as seen in the transverse plane, with the increased QRS magnitude projection to the left

9.25.5.3 BVH Criterion 10 – Mean QRS Vector to the Left in the Frontal Plane in the Presence of Definite RVH

Frequently, the inscription in the frontal plane will be counterclockwise. This is only a fair sign unless there is increased magnitude to the left (R in lead I or aVL). But this, too, is unreliable since a leftward frontal vector causes the projection on lead aVL to increase in magnitude.

9.25.5.4 BVH Criterion 11 – Abnormally Superior Maximum QRS Vector in the Presence of Definite RVH

This is not a sign of BVH, for the abnormally superior vector indicates a conduction defect involving the left anterior branch of the left bundle. The abnormally superior vector may also cause the R wave in lead I and/or aVL to be of increased magnitude.

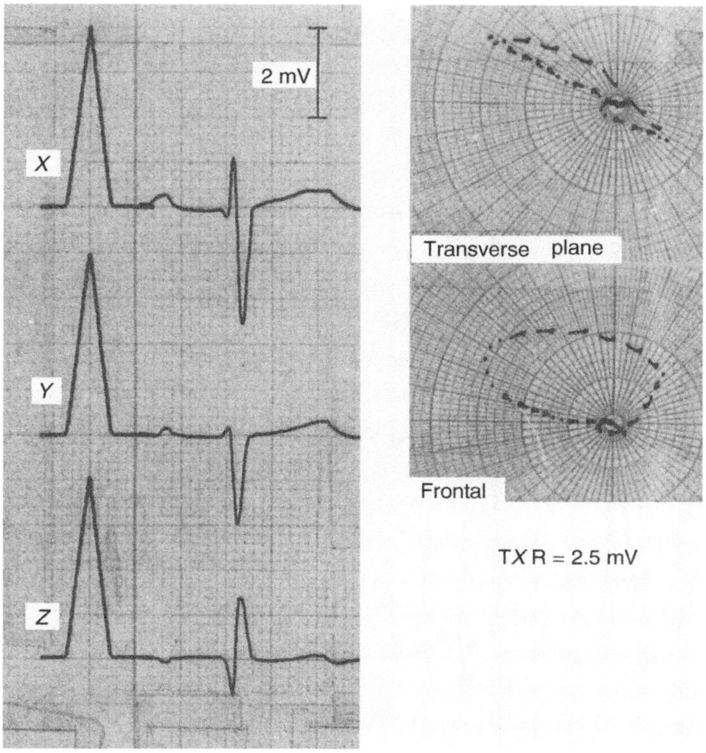

Fig. 9.58
Frank-system orthogonal ECG of a 5-year-old male with complete AV canal and increased pulmonary vascular resistance. There is a small left-to-right and right-to-left shunt plus significant mitral regurgitation. There is a typical "abnormally superior QRS vector." Although RVH is marked, with the very large terminal QRS vector to the right, additional LVH is suggested because the transverse plane loop is inscribed counterclockwise (After Liebman et al. [8]. © Williams and Wilkins, Baltimore, MD. Reproduced with permission)

9.26 Atrioventricular Canal

No matter how extensive the endocardial cushion defect, whether a simple ostium primum defect without mitral regurgitation, or a simple VSD in the endocardial cushion position, a complete atrioventricular (AV) canal, or any intermediate form, an abnormally superior maximum QRS vector is expected. Only very occasionally is such a vector not present (the uncommon exception being especially seen in Down syndrome).

In the Complete AV canal, the shunting is complex and may be in diastole as well as systole. Diastolic flow can be right to left, from right atrium to left ventricle, or left to right, from left atrium to right ventricle. Systolic flow is from left atrium to right atrium as well as left ventricle to right ventricle. Left-to-right atrial flow may also occur in diastole. Since a nonrestrictive ventricular septal communication is usually part of the lesion, by definition, there is left-to-right shunt at the ventricular level as long as pulmonary vascular resistance is less than systemic vascular resistance. Mitral regurgitation and, less often, tricuspid regurgitation may also be part of the lesion. The left-to-right shunt at the ventricular level as well as mitral regurgitation cause left ventricular volume overload, whereas left ventricle to right atrial communication and left-to-right shunting at the atrial level cause right ventricular volume overload. Tricuspid regurgitation also causes right ventricular volume overload. Since there is systemic pressure in the right ventricle and pulmonary artery, there is also

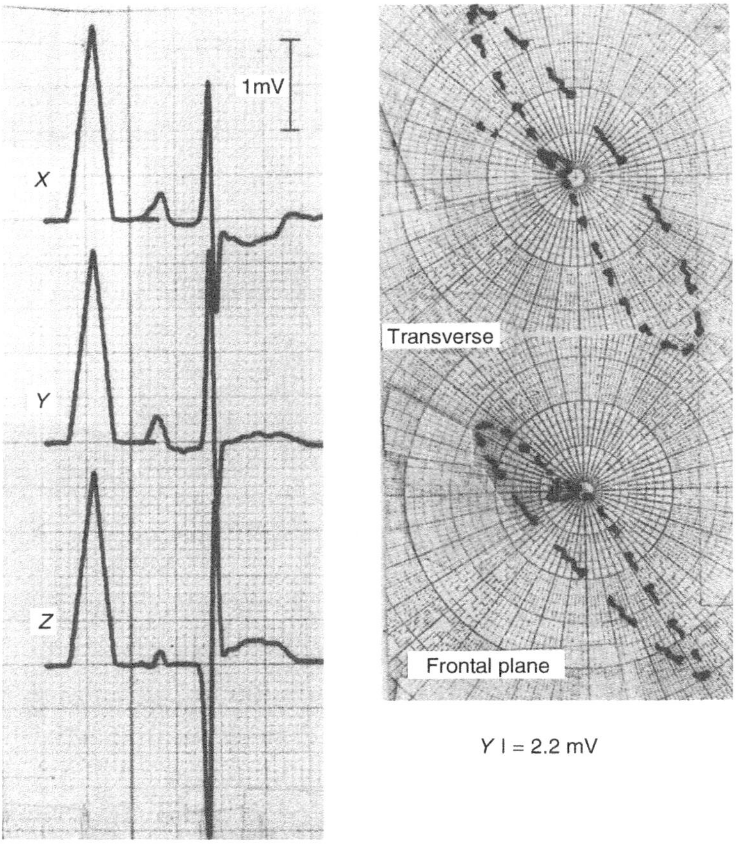

Fig. 9.59
Frank-system VCG of a 6-week-old baby girl with a true truncus arteriosus and elevated pulmonary vascular resistance. The left-to-right shunt was small. The VCG loop exhibits counterclockwise inscription in the transverse plane. There is also a large inferior vector as well as prominent anterior and posterior forces. BVH is present, although the LVH is dominant. The hemodynamics have not been well predicted (After Liebman et al. [8]. © Williams and Wilkins, Baltimore, MD. Reproduced with permission)

RV pressure overload (➋ Fig. 9.56). It should be evident that it would be very difficult on the basis of the ECG per se to predict the hemodynamics (➋ Figs. 9.57 and ➋ 9.58). The information must be complementary to other aspects of the clinical picture. Even patients with little or no left-to-right shunt because of pulmonary vascular disease may have LVH in addition to the marked RVH if there is mitral regurgitation, or if the left ventricle is reflecting previous hemodynamics. BVH can, of course, occur in a variety of lesions besides the above.

9.27 Large PDA (and the Common A-P Window)

The PDA with left-to-right shunt, as described previously, is associated with LVH. However, in the presence of larger PDA (and the connection is shorter), the resistance to flow through it decreases and the pressure in the pulmonary artery increases. The nonrestrictive PDA is quite uncommon and is associated, by definition, with systemic pressure pulmonary

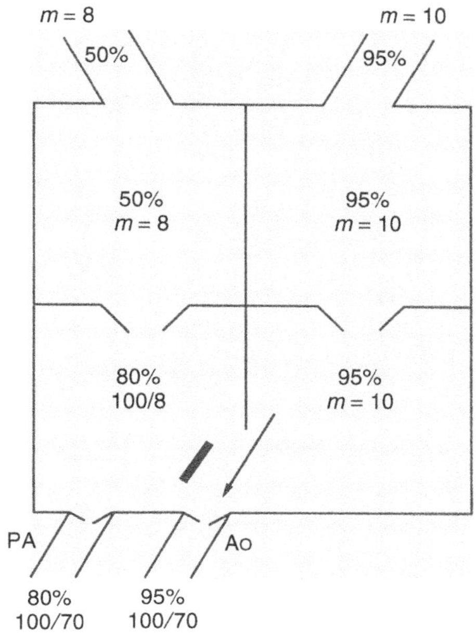

Fig. 9.60
Box diagram of a patient with double outlet right ventricle (DORV) where the VSD is subaortic. As a result of the double conus, there is usually considerable muscle separating the origin of the aorta and pulmonary artery. Therefore, very little of the right ventricle blood goes into the aorta and the patient is usually quite pink, acting like one with a simple large VSD

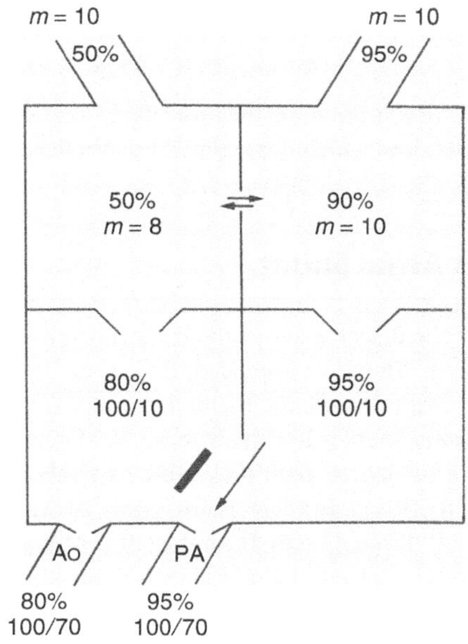

Fig. 9.61
Box diagram of a patient with DORV where the VSD is subpulmonic (Taussig-Bing complex). As a result of the double conus, there is considerable muscle separating the origin of the aorta and pulmonary artery. Therefore, very little of the right ventricle blood goes out through the pulmonary artery. The physiology is that of transposition of the great arteries with RV and pulmonary artery pressures at systemic level

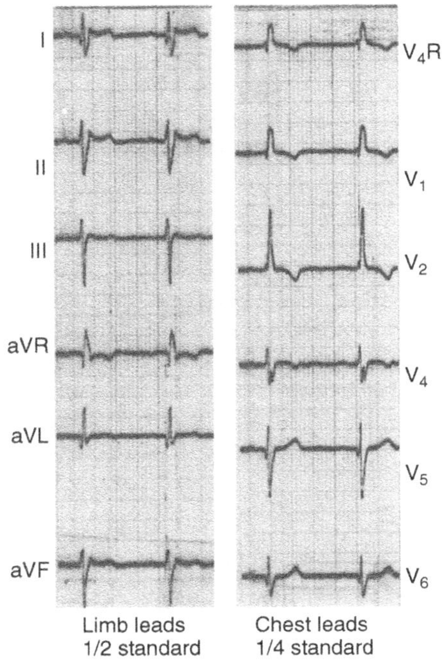

Fig. 9.62
Standard ECG recorded postoperatively from a 6½-year-old male with DORV. There is RBBB. The abnormally superior maximum QRS vector was present preoperatively as well, as in some patients with DORV where the VSD is subaortic and in the endocardial cushion position

hypertension. The higher the pulmonary artery pressure, the more likely it is that there will be additional RVH. The same principles, of course, hold for the A-P window, which is usually nonrestrictive.

9.28 Left Ventricle to Right Atrial Shunt

This is an unusual form of VSD where the defect is above the tricuspid valve ring. Consequently, left ventricular flow through the defect is into the right atrium. There are important differences from that of the more common VSD (from left ventricle to right ventricle), for no matter how large the defect, there is no transmission of systemic pressure into the right ventricle. Therefore, on that basis, there is less likely to be RVH. On the other hand, since all the left-to-right flow is into the right atrium, then all of the left-to-right flow must passively flow from the right atrium into the right ventricle. Therefore, on this latter basis, RVH is *more* likely. There is none of the aspect encountered in the more common VSD where some of the left-to-right shunt flows directly from the left ventricle to the pulmonary artery. Obviously, the presence or absence of RVH in this lesion is not very helpful in estimating pulmonary hypertension. RAE, on the other hand, is definitely more likely than in the common VSD.

9.29 Ostium Primum ASD with Mitral Regurgitation

The hemodynamics of this lesion are quite straightforward. With a larger left-to-right shunt, the RVH with terminal right conduction delay is greater, as in the secundum ASD. With considerable mitral regurgitation, the LVH is great.

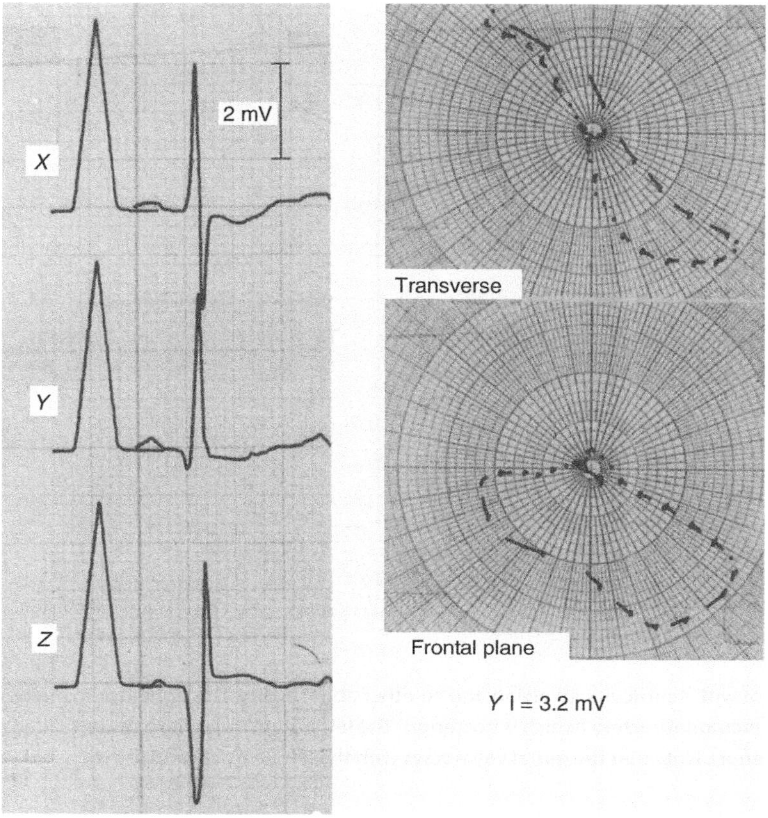

Fig. 9.63
Frank-system orthogonal ECG in a 9-week-old male with simple severe coarction of the aorta, and who is not in congestive heart failure. There is considerable LVH with large magnitude inferior and leftward vectors in the presence of a counterclockwise-inscribed transverse plain "loop." However, there is also considerable RVH since the terminal QRS vector to the right (2.0 mV) is abnormally large

However, if the ostium primum opening is large, the regurgitant flow acts as though it is going directly into the right atrium, and some actually does. Therefore, unlike pure mitral regurgitation, LAH is not present. It is present only when the ostium primum opening is small, while the mitral regurgitation is considerable.

9.30 True Truncus Arteriosus

Since the VSD is very large, RV pressure is at systemic level and since, in infancy, in the most common type I truncus, pulmonary vascular resistance is low, the left ventricle provides most of the work of the increase in pulmonary blood flow. BVH is, therefore, part of the lesion. In general, just as in large VSD, with low pulmonary vascular resistance, the left ventricle dominates, and if pulmonary vascular resistance is increased, the right ventricle dominates. Pulmonary vascular disease frequently develops very rapidly, so that the progression to pure RVH on the ECG is ominous. However, particularly because of varying streaming patterns from left ventricle to right ventricle and left ventricle to aorta or pulmonary artery, predictability is not reliable (Fig. 9.59).

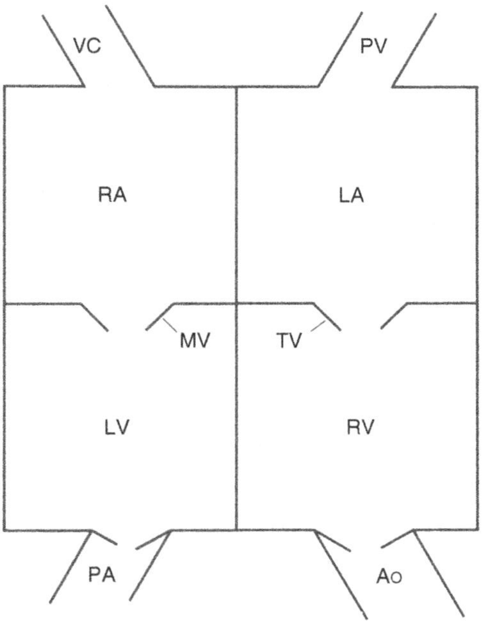

Fig. 9.64
Box diagram of a patient with ventricular inversion and no other abnormality. The right atrium drains into the right-sided left ventricle and then the pulmonary artery (which is posterior). The left atrium drains into the left-sided right ventricle and then the aorta (which is anterior). Note that the mitral valve stays with the left ventricle and the tricuspid valve stays with the right ventricle

9.31 Double Outlet Right Ventricle

The dynamics of this lesion are of great interest and very variable, because of variable anatomy. The VSD may be subaortic (➋ Fig. 9.60) so that the patient acts like that of a simple nonrestrictive VSD, with LVH dominant on the ECG. There may be severe pulmonic stenosis in addition to the non-restrictive VSD so that the patient may be cyanotic, acting like that of TOF. Pure RVH may be present, but if so, usually with much more left chest potential than in TOF. There may even be BVH despite the severe PS. The VSD may be subpulmonic so that the pathophysiology is like that of transposition with large VSD (➋ Fig. 9.61). (Additional pulmonic stenosis in the presence of the subpulmonic VSD is not common.) The VSD can also be not preferentially committed to either great artery, in which case, LVH is likely to be dominant; the VSD can be restrictive so that in addition to RVH, the additional LVH may be very severe, even with ST-T abnormality. Finally, particularly when in the subaortic position, the VSD is commonly an endocardial cushion type, resulting in an abnormally superior maximum QRS vector on the ECG (➋ Fig. 9.62).

9.32 Coarctation of the Aorta Late in Infancy

The electrocardiogram in simple severe coarctation of the aorta in infancy is of great interest. It is known that in early infancy pure RVH is common because of the dynamics in utero plus, in those with congestive heart failures, there is pulmonary hypertension secondary to pulmonary venous hypertension. However, even after increased pulmonary venous pressure is no longer present and after the expected LVH has finally developed, additional RVH may persist for a long time. The explanation is again, presumed to be related to, the dynamics in utero and attendant cellular hyperplasia [48] (➋ Fig. 9.63).

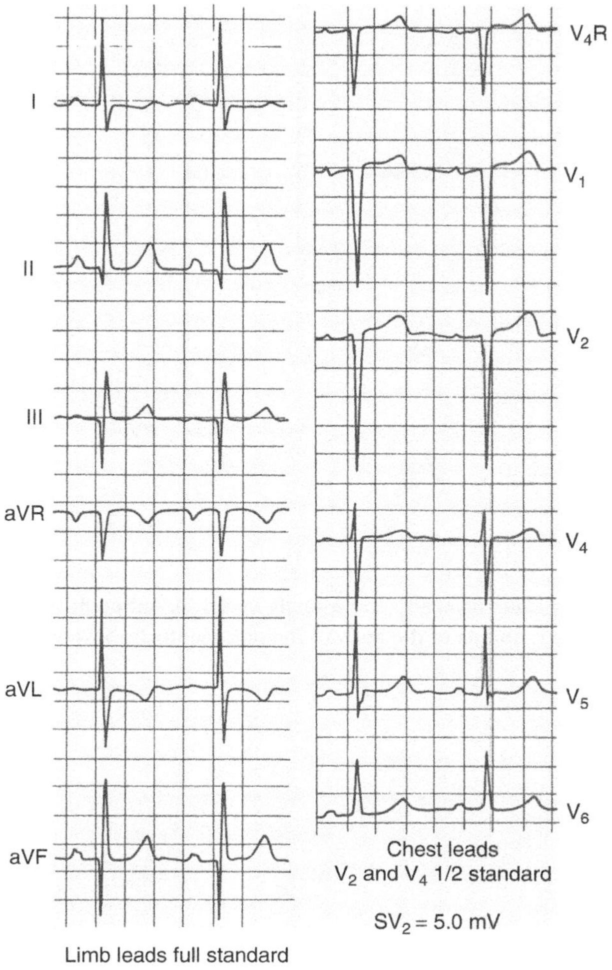

Fig. 9.65
Standard ECG of an 11½-year-old male with ventricular inversion (L transposition) and, as the only other abnormality, left AV valve (tricuspid) regurgitation. The initial QRS activation is straight to the left and only slightly anterior. There is a very large magnitude initial superior vector. There is a wide open counterclockwise direction of inscription, with the magnitude posterior very large. LVH is diagnosed, although this is a right ventricle on the left side (After Liebman et al. [8]. © Williams and Wilkins, Baltimore, MD. Reproduced with permission)

9.33 Special Lesions

There are a number of lesions where the ECG is of particular interest.

9.33.1 Ventricular Inversion

In this lesion, the right atrial blood goes into the right-sided left ventricle, from which the pulmonary artery arises. The left atrial blood enters the left-sided right ventricle from which the aorta arises (Fig. 9.64). Although ventricular

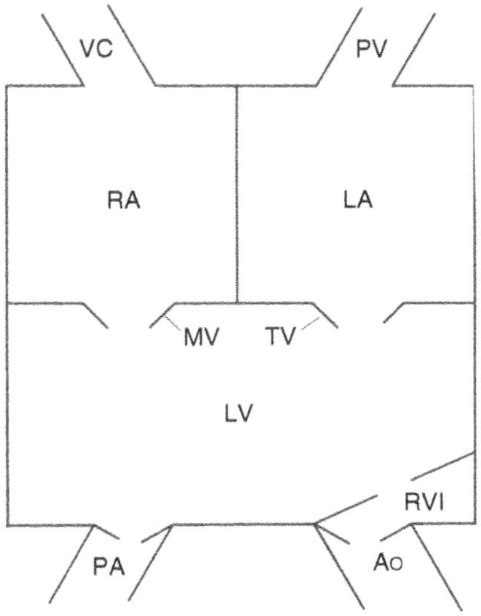

Fig. 9.66
Box diagram of a patient with ventricular inversion and a single ventricle. Although seeimingly complex, it is really quite similar to that of Fig. 9.64. There is aplasia of the body of the right ventricle, however, so that only the right ventricular infundibulum (RVI) remains

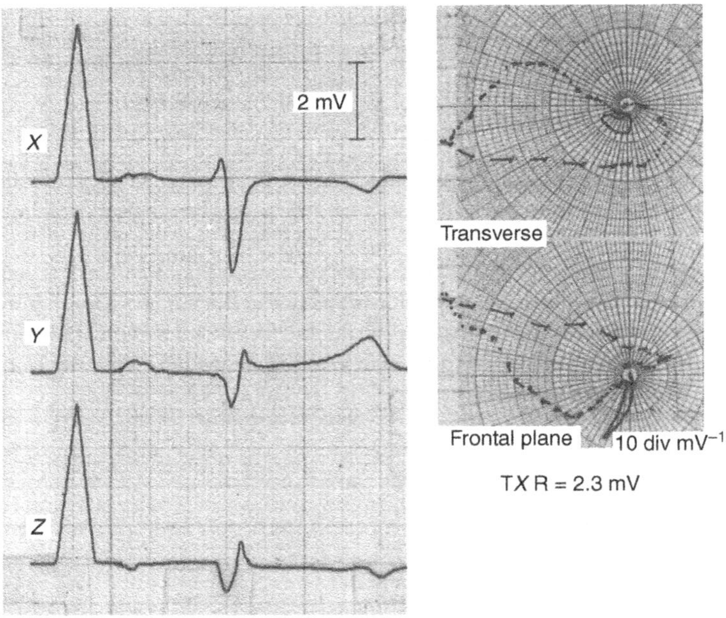

Fig. 9.67
Frank-system orthogonal ECG of a 24-year-old male with single ventricle (SV), who had pulmonary artery banding procedure at the age of 4 years. The SV is of the most common type with ventricular inversion and L transposition. There is no AV valve regurgitation. Note that the initial superior vector is very large and that the initial QRS forces are to the left and very slightly posterior. There is marked "RVH" associated with the pulmonary artery band

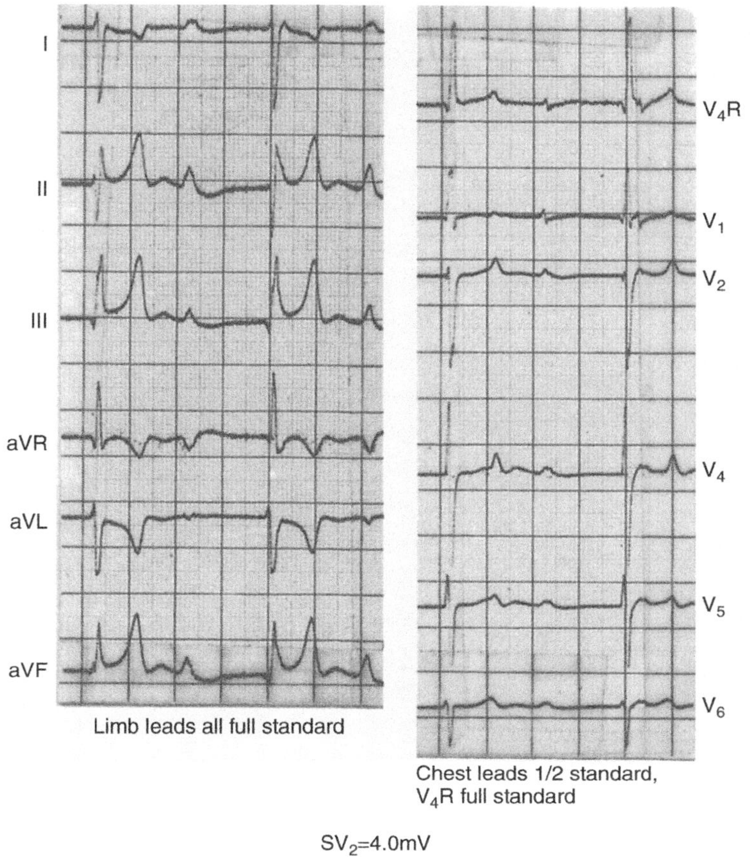

Fig. 9.68
Standard ECG of same patient as in Fig. 9.67 4 years previously (there was no significant difference). Although the initial QRS is to the left and slightly posterior, the large magnitude initial QRS superior force seen in the VCG is not reflected in the ECG. Note that the patient has complete AV block, a finding which is very common in ventricular inversion

inversion can be associated with no other anomalies, usually something else is present, such as ventricular septal defect, left-sided atrioventricular valve insufficiency or pulmonic stenosis. However, the most common abnormality is actually a variety of single ventricle (see Sect. 9.33.2). Obviously, the ECG must reflect the hemodynamics of the particular abnormalities, but of special interest is initial QRS activation. The left bundle branches are on the right side, since the left ventricle is on the right side, and, of course, the right bundle branch is on the left side. Therefore, the vector of initial QRS activation may be from right to left depending upon other aspects of initial activation. The anatomy of the ventricles is such that the septum is almost vertical rather than at an angle. Therefore, the expected right-to-left activation is usually *not* to the left and posterior, although this can occur. It is usually straight left. This usually produces q waves in V_4R and V_1, but not V_2 (although this can occur), but, of course, no small q wave in V_5 and V_6. Meanwhile, because of the vertical septum, initial activation is straight up the septum, so that in the superior inferior leads (for example, aVF) there is often a large initial Q wave (Fig. 9.65). This may even be the larger magnitude wave in lead aVF; or be entirely superior. This is of course not an abnormally superior vector for, to make that diagnosis, the initial QRS vector must be inferior.

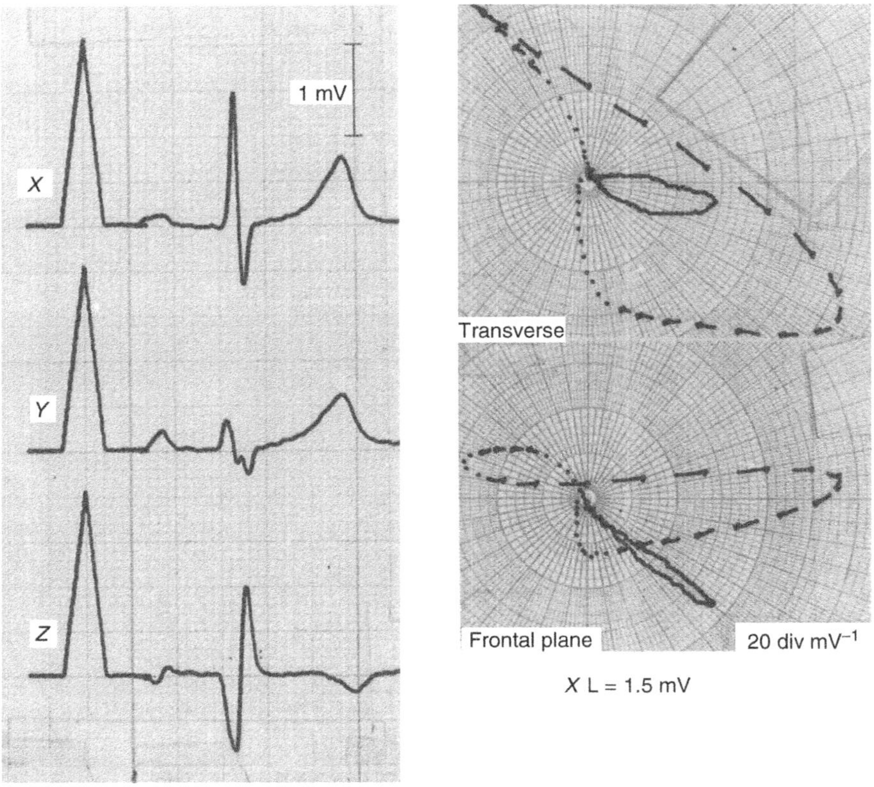

Fig. 9.69
Frank-system orthogonal ECG of a 6½-year-old male with single ventricle, no ventricular inversion and D loop transposition of the great arteries. The initial QRS loop is normal and the standard ECG, as well as the Frank-system ECG, gave no clue to single ventricle. There was a large left-to-right shunt. The ECG shows enough terminal right conduction delay to suggest partial RBBB. Complete repair (septation) had been successfully accomplished (After Liebman et al. [8]. © Williams and Wilkins, Baltimore, MD. Reproduced with permission)

9.33.2 Single Ventricle

By definition, in single ventricle, both AV valves enter one ventricle even if one of the AV valves is atretic. By far the most common single ventricle is, in actual fact, a form of ventricular inversion with an unusual abnormality; that of hypoplasia of the body of the right ventricle. As a result of the ventricular inversion, the single left ventricle is on the right and a right ventricular infundibulum (connected by the bulboventricular foramen) is on the left. The pulmonary artery arises on the right from the single left ventricle, whereas the aorta arises on the left from the right ventricular infundibulum (➋ Fig. 9.66). The classical initial QRS of ventricular inversion may be present (➋ Figs. 9.67 and ➋ 9.68), but other than that there are no other reliable electrocardiographic clues to single ventricle. The conduction system is, however, very specifically known [64].

There used to be a dictum that single ventricle is associated electrocardiographically with deep S waves in all the precordial leads. This presupposed that single ventricle was caused by an absent septum, with all else normal. That type of

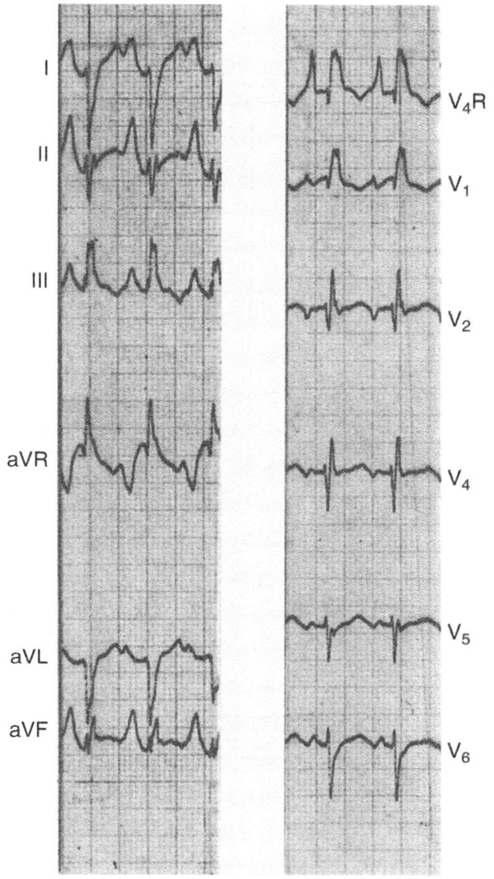

Fig. 9.70
Standard ECG of an 18-month-old female with Ebstein's anomaly. There is marked RAH (note tall P in leads II and V_4R). The QRS complex demonstrates a prominent terminal vector to the right and anterior which is inscribed very slowly (advanced RBBB)

single ventricle is quite rare, and even when present, such an ECG is not usually found (Fig. 9.69). In general, however, for most varieties of single ventricle, severe PS is associated with pure RVH, and BVH is likely to indicate that severe PS is not present.

9.33.3 Ebstein's Anomaly

Ebstein's anomaly is very variable in its anatomy and severity. The tricuspid valve is very abnormal and there is displacement of the valve into the right ventricle. The result is a small ineffective functioning right ventricle. Intracavitary electrocardiography reveals a right ventricular electrocardiogram at a varying distance on the right atrial side of the valve. The degree of tricuspid regurgitation varies from none to considerable, and the amount of right-to-left shunt at the atrial level varies from none to considerable.

The electrocardiogram usually demonstrates right atrial hypertrophy, which is often marked. In addition, there is advanced RBBB because of the abnormal development and position of the bundle (Lev, M., personal communication) (Fig. 9.70), with the generalized voltage often less than usual for advanced RBBB. (There may be great variation in the

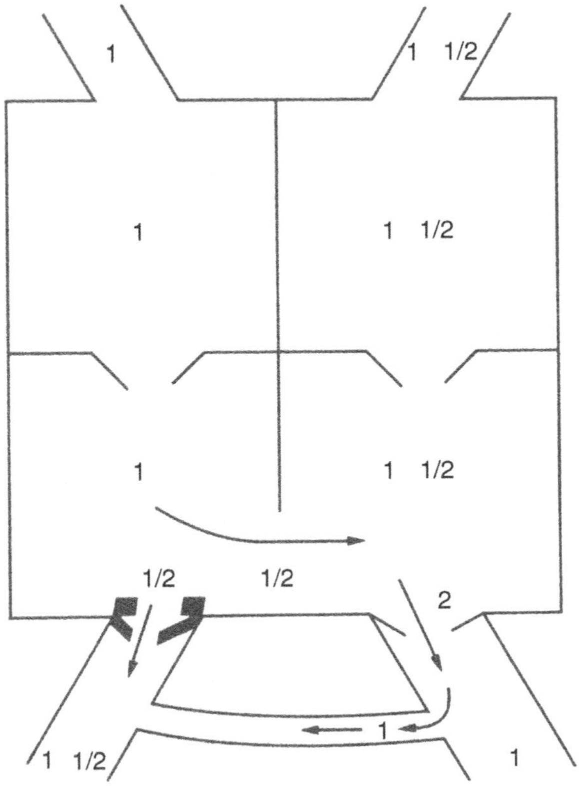

Fig. 9.71
Box diagram of a patient with TOF who has had a systemic-pulmonary shunt surgically placed. In the unoperated patient with TOF (Fig. 9.23) where the pulmonary blood flow is one-half normal, the left ventricle handles between one-half normal and normal volume, depending upon how much right ventricular blood flows into the aorta directly. For a shunt where one unit of cardiac output flows from aorta to pulmonary artery, the entire volume must be handled by the left ventricle. Therefore, the left ventricle handles between $1\frac{1}{2}$ and 2 times normal volume, depending upon how much right ventricular blood flows into the aorta directly

degree and variety of RBBB in Ebstein's anomaly.) Finally, in a large number of cases, there is evidence for an accessory connection usually entering the anterior high lateral portion of the right ventricle. The resulting electrocardiogram is that of the classical pre excitation and simulation of LBBB. Even without the Wolff-Parkinson-White (WPW) syndrome, atrial arrhythmias are very common.

9.33.4 Dextrocardia

Interpretation of the electrocardiogram is very difficult, not so much because the heart is in the right chest, but because of the complex anatomic relationship of the chambers often present. In the presence of abdominal situs inversus, there is atrial situs inversus and usually there is no pathology. In that situation, when there is a cardiac abnormality, interpretation

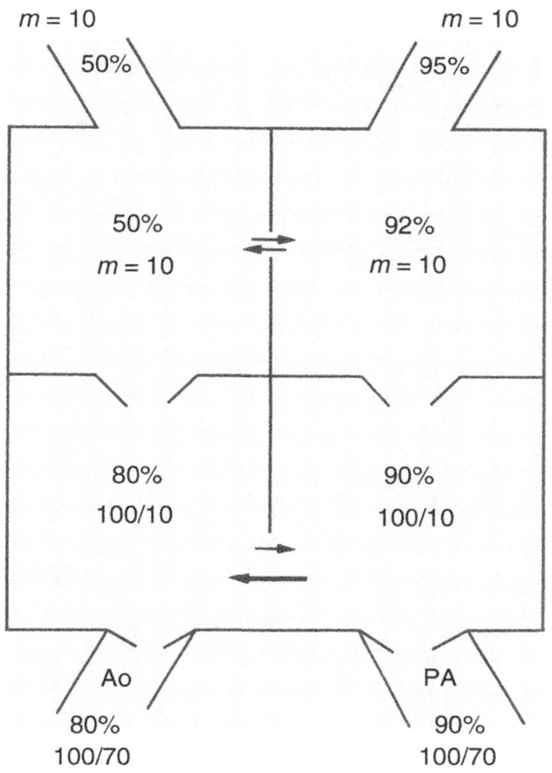

Fig. 9.72
Box diagram of a patient with transposition of the great arteries (TGA) with a nonrestrictive VSD. The right and left ventricular and, of course, aorta and pulmonary artery systolic pressures are equal. (Should pulmonary stenosis be present, the ventricular pressures would be unaffected, but pulmonary artery pressures would be less. Should the VSD be smaller, then LV pressure would be less). The flow patterns through the atrial and ventricular openings are complex. The amount of left-to-right and right-to-left shunt theoretically should be equal, but the difficult calculations rarely come out that way. With low pulmonary vascular resistance, the expected is a larger left atrial to right atrial shunt at the atrial level, and a larger right-to-left shunt at the ventricular level. In the above box diagram, there is a small right-to-left shunt and trivial left-to-right shunt at the atrial level, plus a small right-to-left shunt and a large left-to-right shunt at the ventricular level. In this case pulmonary vascular resistance is high

of the electrocardiogram is not difficult. On the other hand, normal abdominal situs together with normal atrial situs are usually associated with complex disease. A particular use of the electrocardiogram has been to determine the relationship of the atria to each other. However, there may be many errors for many reasons, including the frequent left atrial pacemaker. Since the left atrium is on the same side as that of the stomach bubble, the chest x-ray provides a far more reliable method than does the ECG. If there is a transverse liver, however, the ECG is extremely helpful.

On the other hand, by utilizing the initial QRS forces, ventricular relationships are often readily determined with the electrocardiogram [65]. For example, in situs inversus, if the initial QRS vector is directed to the left, anterior and superior, then it is surmised that the morphologic left ventricle is to the right of the morphologic right ventricle, and that this morphologic ventricle is also posterior to the morphologic right ventricle. Thus, this information can be utilized in deciding which ventricle is hypertrophied and can also be used in a complementary way in interpreting

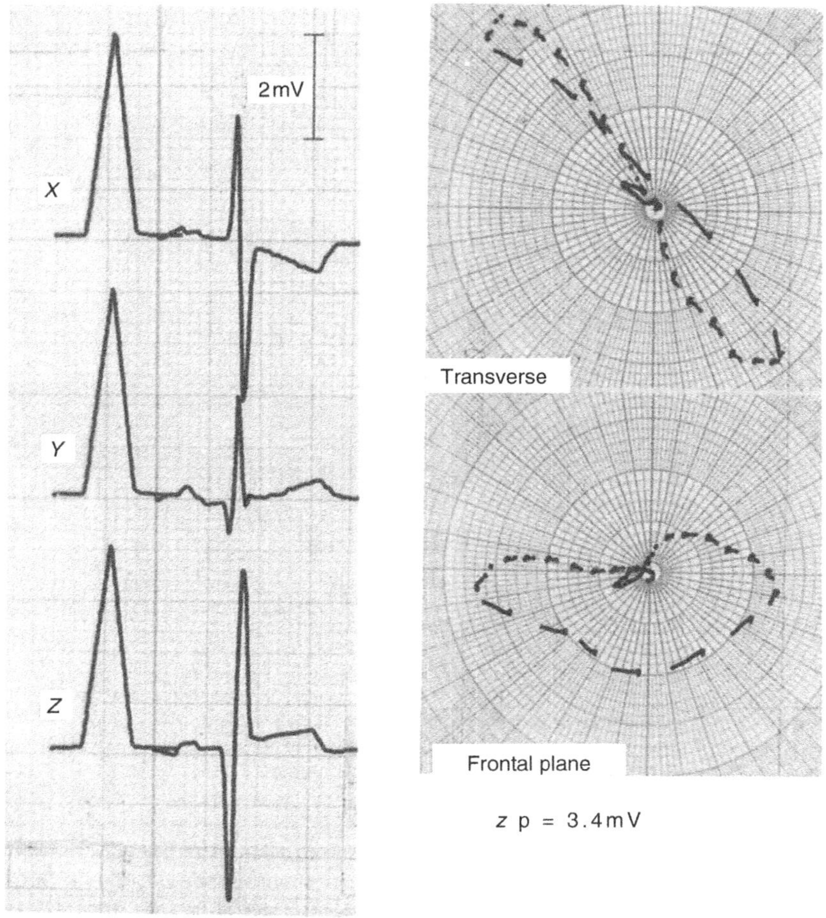

Fig. 9.73
McFee–Parungao (axial) system orthogonal ECG in a 3½-month-old baby girl with TGA and a large VSD. There are two main vectors, the first to the left and anterior (with the QRS magnitude left above normal) and the second to the right and posterior. BVH is clear (After Liebman et al. [8]. © Williams and Wilkins, Baltimore, MD. Reproduced with permission)

echocardiographic, cardiac catheterization, and angiographic data. Although the above type of analysis can be very useful, it must be remembered that unpredictable rotations as well as hypertrophy may cause many errors.

9.33.5 Tetralogy of Fallot with Systemic-Pulmonary Shunt

As described in Sect. 9.10, TOF is a lesion associated with pure RVH. The addition of a systemic-pulmonary shunt provides left ventricular volume work and increased left-sided potential (Fig. 9.71). The ECG is very sensitive in this regard. If a child is born with an embryologic TOF but less severe pulmonic stenosis, there may be left-to-right shunt. Such a patient may show BVH. It is then common as the child grows older for the pulmonic stenosis to become more severe, the child to become cyanotic from the right-to-left shunt, the left-to-right shunt to disappear and the ECG to show pure RVH. Then such a patient may need a systemic-pulmonary shunt, and once again develop BVH. In terms of the major parameter of the LVH in this situation, an increased posterior QRS projection is not useful for reasons described previously. An increased magnitude to the left, particularly as part of a vector loop with two main vectors, is very reliable.

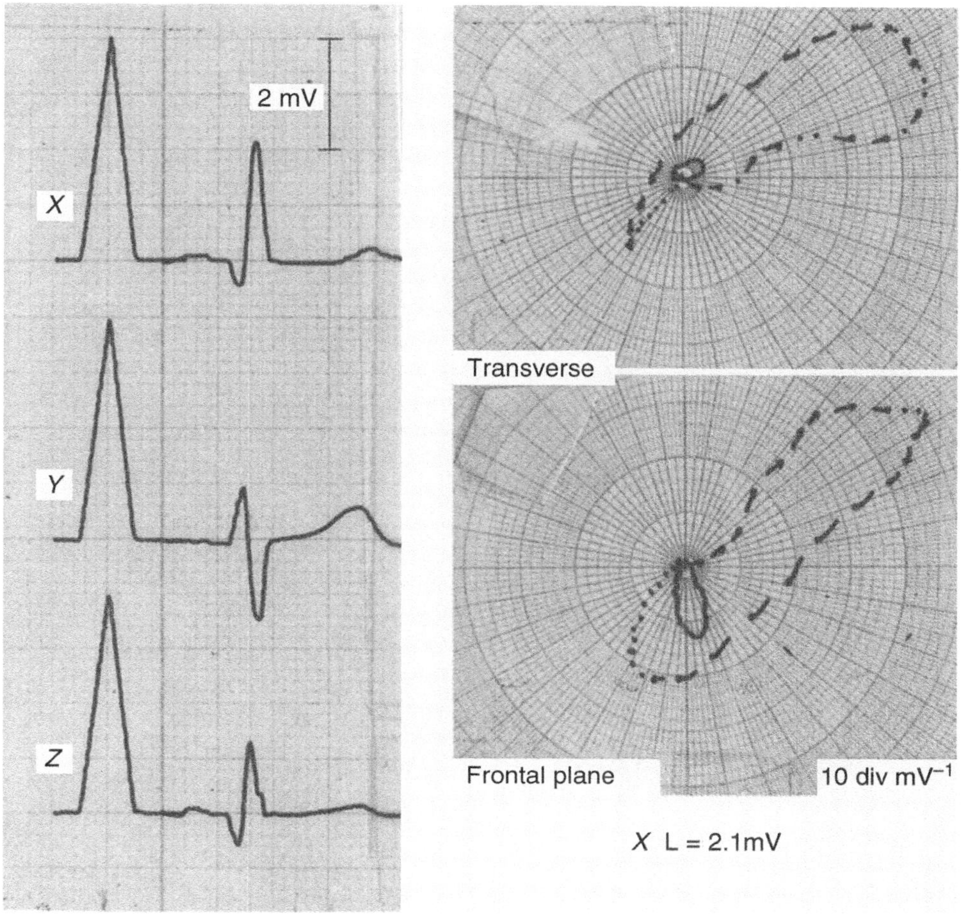

Fig. 9.74
Frank-system orthogonal ECG in a 3-year-old asymptomatic female referred to a heart murmur (caused by considerable mitral regurgitation). There was a significant left-to-right atrial shunt at the pulmonary artery level owing to retrograde flow from the large right coronary artery into the left coronary artery by way of intercoronary collaterals. The left coronary artery drained into the left pulmonary artery. An area of the left lateral left ventricular wall did not contract. The initial QRS is to the right, anterior, superior, but then extends to the right and posterior before extending left. (It would appear that the posterobasal left ventricle is depolarizing before any left lateral wall). In the *X* lead, the initial QRS right is prolonged. Left lateral and myocardial infarction is the diagnosis, owing to anomalous left coronary artery (ALCA). (ALCA with manifest infarction in the older child is not common. Usually, the infarctions occur in infants with fewer intercoronary collaterals) (After Liebman et al. [8]. © Williams and Wilkins, Baltimore, MD. Reproduced with permission)

9.33.6 Transposition of the Great Arteries with Large VSD

Since the right ventricle is the systemic ventricle, it is at systemic pressure; RVH is, therefore, expected. If a VSD is present and is nonrestrictive, the left ventricle is also at systemic pressure. Should pulmonary vascular resistance be low, then there will be considerably increased pulmonary blood flow and increased volume work of the left ventricle (➋ Fig. 9.72) so that BVH may be present on the ECG (➋ Fig. 9.73). Should there be a high pulmonary vascular resistance, there is less pulmonary blood flow and pure RVH is more likely. It is said that significant pulmonic stenosis lends itself to additional LVH, presumably because of high LV pressure as well as continued increased volume. Experience shows, however, that

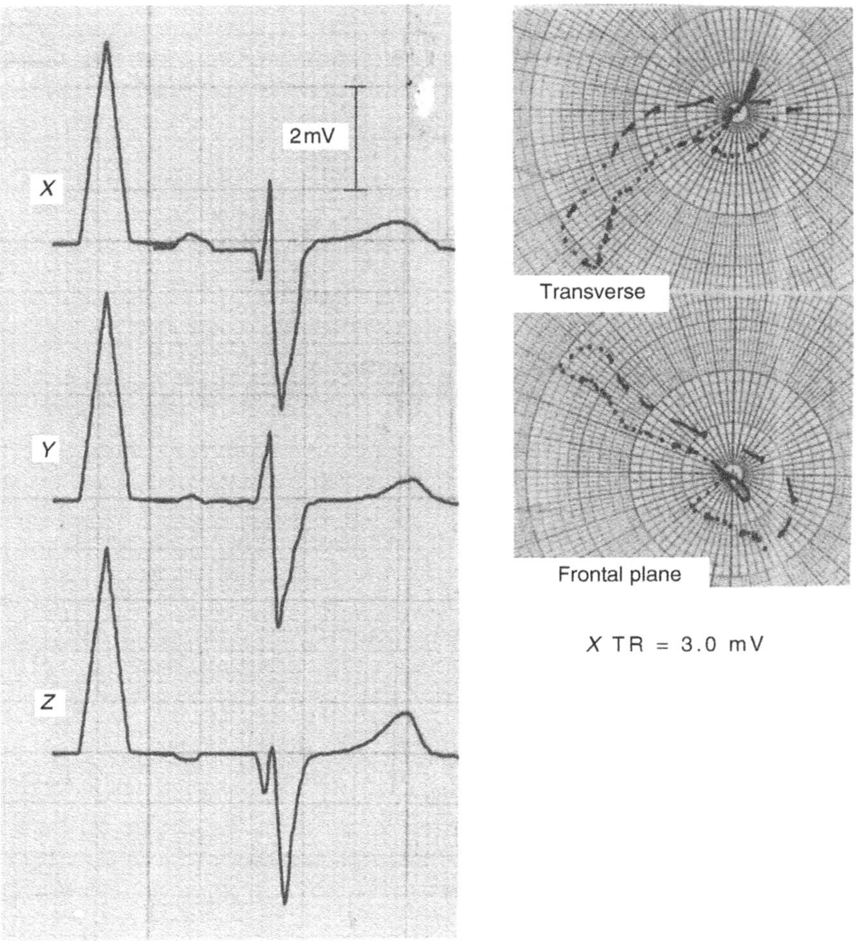

Fig. 9.75
McFee–Parungao system orthogonal ECG of a 5-year-old male who had had complete repair for TOF 1 year previously. There is a large terminal vector loop to the right and anterior, which is very slowly inscribed. There is advanced RBBB. In the frontal plane, the initial QRS force is inferior, and most of the vector loop is superior, so that there is an "abnormally superior maximum QRS vector." Since this patient, prior to surgery, had a normal inferior maximum QRS vector with initial superior QRS forces, it is preferable to term this left anterior division block (left anterior hemiblock)

the finding is unreliable because with the increasing pulmonic stenosis, left ventricular volume decreases, resulting in less LVH. On the other hand, in the presence of an intact ventricular septum, PS results in increased LV pressure, so there is hemodynamic reason for *more* LVH.

9.33.7 Anomalous Left Coronary Artery in the Infant

Babies born with anomalous left coronary artery are recognized almost invariably by 3 months of age. The hearts are large, congestive heart failure is considerable and the ECG documents a left lateral wall myocardial infarction (Fig. 9.74). As a result of lack of opposition from lateral wall potentials, the initial QRS stays to the right for a long time as the QRS vector turns posterior. The ECG differential is that of left septal hypertrophy, but in the latter, the duration is not great and the QRS vector turns to the left before traversing posterior. The latter is readily recognized with the vector loop display but

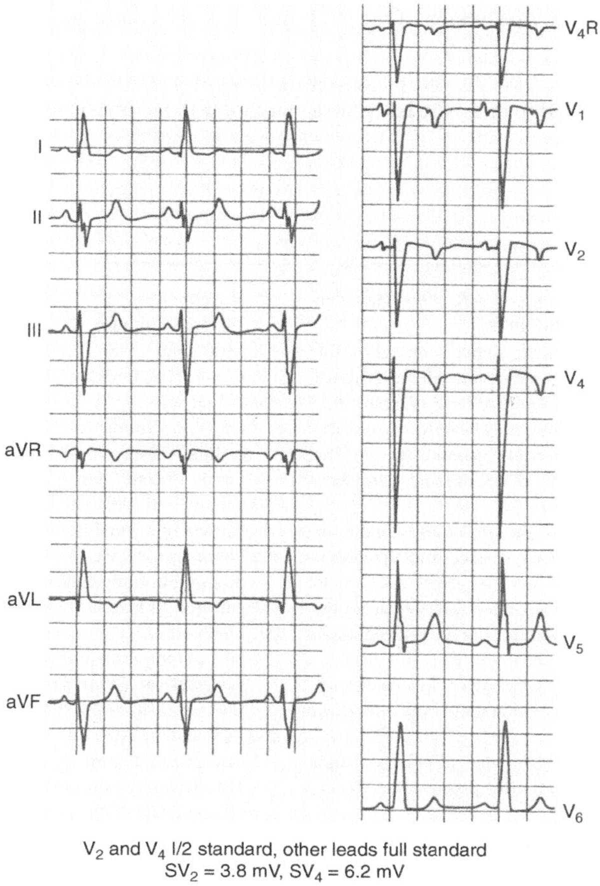

Fig. 9.76
Standard ECG of a 2-year-old female with TGA, a large VSD in the endocardial cushion area and pulmonic stenosis (the typical abnormally superior maximum QRS vector had been present prior to surgery). A Mustard procedure had been done, and attempts had been made to relieve some of the pulmonic stenosis via the pulmonary artery, so that some of the left ventricular outlow area was excised. The ECG result included partial LBBB. The initial QRS is to the left and anterior and there is midventricular slowing. There is no T-wave abnormality (A VCG would be needed, however, for better delineation)

is difficult to be sure of with a standard ECG. The lesion where a similar ECG may be seen is that of the hypoplastic right ventricle with tricuspid atresia, but the abnormally superior maximum QRS vector in the latter is distinctive (see Fig. 9.46).

9.33.8 Postoperative RBBB, Left Anterior Hemiblock and LBBB

Postoperative RBBB is very common, is usually advanced, but can be partial. Only infrequently is the advanced RBBB caused by damage to the proximal right bundle. Most often it is because of damage to the right bundle after ventriculotomy with incision into the moderator band. Although traditional definitions would allow the ECG interpretation of "complete" RBBB for all such patients, we have recently documented, utilizing body-surface potential mapping, that there is a great spectrum of "complete" RBBB [66]. Therefore, the term advanced RBBB appears to be more appropriate. Occasionally, the advanced RBBB is associated with an abnormally superior maximum QRS vector not present prior to surgery, in which case it is presumed that the left anterior branch of the left bundle has been damaged (➋ Fig. 9.75). Postoperative partial RBBB is also often recognized.

Postoperative advanced LBBB is becoming increasingly common, particularly as more complex lesions are being surgically corrected and as the need to enter the left ventricle in order to facilitate such surgery increases (➋ Fig. 9.76).

References

1. Rush, S., *An Atlas of Heart-Lead Transfer Coefficients*. Hanover, NH: University Press of New England, 1975.
2. Rudy, Y. and R. Plonsey, The eccentric spheres model as the basis for the study of the role of geometry and inhemogeneites in electrocardiography. *IEEE Trans. Biomed. Eng.*, 1979;**26**: 392.
3. Rudy, Y., R. Plonseyi, and J. Liebman, The effects of variations in conductivity and geometrical parameters on the electrocardiogram using an eccentric spheres model. *Circ. Res.*, 1979;**44**: 104–111.
4. Rudy, Y. and R. Plonsey, A comparison of volume conductor and source geometry effects on body surface and epicardial potentials. *Circ. Res.*, 1980;**46**: 283.
5. Rudy, Y. and R. Plonsey, Comments on the effects of variations in the size of the heart on the magnitude of ECG potentials. *J. Electrocardiol.*, 1980;**13**: 79.
6. Ishikawa, K., A.S. Berson, and H.W. Pipberger, Electrocardiographic changes due to cardiac enlargement. *Am. Heart J.*, 1971;**81**: 635.
7. Rudy, Y., R.Wood, R. Plonsey, and J. Liebman, The effects of high lung conductivity on electrocardiographic potentials. *Circulation*, 1982;**65**: 440–445.
8. Liebman, J., R. Plonsey, and P.C.Gillette, Editors, *Pediatric Electrocardiography*. Baltimore, MD: Williams and Wilkins, 1982.
9. Liebman, J. and R. Plonsey, Electrocardiolography in heart disease, in *Infants, Children and Adolescents*, 2nd edn., Chapter 3, A.J. Moss, F.H. Adams, and G.C. Emmanouilides, Editors. Baltimore, MD: Williams and Wilkins, 1983, pp. 18–61.
10. Liebman, J. and R. Plonsey, Basic principles for understanding electrocardiography. *Paediatrican*, 1973;**2**: 251–268.
11. Davignon, A., P. Rautaharju, E. Boiselle E, et al., Normal electrocardiogrophic standards for infants and children. *Pediatr. Cardiol.*, 1979;**I**: 133–152.
12. Macfarlane, P.W. and T.D.V. Lawrie, Tables of normal limits, in *Comprehensive Electrocardiology*, Vol. 3. New York: Pergamon Press, 1989, pp. 1442–1526.
13. Liebman, J., Tables of normal limits for standard and orthogonal pediatric ECG, in *Comprehensive Electrocardiology*, Vol. 3. New York: Pergamon Press, 1989, pp. 1475–1494, 1509–1517.
14. Downs, T.D. and J. Liebman, Statistical methods for vectorcardiographic directions. *IEEE Trans. Biomed. Eng.*, 1969;**16**: 87–94.
15. Liebman, J., Linear and directional statistics, in *Comprehensive Electrocardiology*, Vol. 3. New York: Pergamon Press, 1989, pp. 1522–1526.
16. Frank, E., An accurate, clinically practical system for spatial vectorcardiography. *Circulation*, 1956;**13**: 737–749.
17. McFee. R. and A. Parungoa,. An orthogonal lead system for clinical electrocardiography. *Am. Heart J.*, 1961;**62**: 93–100.
18. Young, E., J. Liebman, and A.S. Nadas, The normal vectorcardiogram in children. *Am. J Cardiol.*, 1960;**5**: 457–463.
19. Hugenholtz, P.G. and J.Liebman, The orthogonal vectorcardiogram in 100 normal children (Frank system) with some comparative data recorded by the cube system. *Circulation*, 1962;**26**: 891–901.
20. Rautaharju, P.M., A. Davignon, F. Soumis, et al., Evolution of QRS-T relationships from birth to adolescence in Frank lead orthogonal electrocardiograms of 1492 normal children. *Circulation*, 1979;**60**: 196–204.
21. Taccardi, B., Distribution of heart potentials on the thoracic surface of normal human subjects. *Circ. Res.*, 1963;**12**: 341–352.
22. Liebman, J., C.W. Thomas, Y. Rudy, and R. Plonsey, Electrocardiographic body surface potential maps of the QRS of normal children. *J. Electrocardiol.*, 1981;**12**: 249–260.
23. Liebman, J., The electrocardiogram of the future, body surface potential mapping (Keynote Lecture), in *21st International Congress on Electrocardiography*, Yokohama, Japan, July 4–7, 1994; *Jpn. Heart J.*, 1994;**35**(Suppl. 1): 69–73.
24. Liebman, J., The body surface potential map in congenital heart disease, in *Einthoven 2002: 100 years of Electrocardiography*, M.J. Schalij, et al., Editors. Leiden: The Einthoven Foundation, 2002, pp. 215–220.
25. Durrer, D., R.Th. van Dam, G.E. Freud, M.J. Janse, F.L. Meijler, and R.C. Arzbaecher, Total excitation of the isolated human heart. *Circulation*, 1970;**41**: 899–912.
26. Scher, A.M. and M.S. Spach, Cardiac depolarization and repolarization and the electrocardiogram, in *Handbook of Physiology, Section 2: The Cardiovascular System, Vol. I: The Heart*, R.M. Berne, N. Speralakis, and S.R. Geiger, Editors. Bethesda, MD: American Physiological Society, 1979, pp. 357–392.
27. Burger, H.C. and J.L. van Milaan, Heart vector and leads, Part II. *Br. Heart J.*, 1947;**9**: 154–160.
28. Liebman, J., G. Borka, and S. Hirschfeld, The heart, in *Care of the High Risk Neonate*, M.H. Klaus and A.A. Fanaroff, Editors. Philadelphia, PA: Saunders, 1979, pp. 294–323.
29. Nadas, A.S. and D.C. Fyler, *Pediatric Cardiology*, 3rd edn. Philadelphia, PA: Saunders, 1972.
30. Spach, M.S., T.D. King, R.C. Barr, D.E. Boaz, M.N. Morrow, and S. Herman-Giddens, Electrical potential distribution surrounding the atria during depolarization and repolarization of the dog. *Circ. Res.*, 1969;**24**: 857–873.
31. Puech, P., The P wave: correlations of surface and intra-atrial electrograms, in *Complex Electrocardiography 2*, C. Fisch, Editor. Philadelphia, PA: Davis, 1974; *Cardivasc. Clin.*, 1974;**6**(1).
32. Reynolds, J.L., The electrocardiographic recognition of right atrial abnormality in children. *Am. Heart J.*, 1971;**81**: 748–759.
33. Ferrer, P.L. and R.C. Ellison. The Frank scalar atrial vectorcardiogram in normal children. *Am. Heart J.*, 1974;**88**: 467–475.
34. Ishikawa, K., P.M. Kini, and H.V.P. Pipberger, Wave analysis in 2464 orthogonal electrocardiograms from normal subjects and patients with atrial overload. *Circulation*, 1973;**48**: 565–574.

35. Lee, M H., J. Liebman, and W.Mackay. Orthogonal electrocardiograph correlation study of 100 children with pure cardiac defects, in *Vectorcardiography 3*, I. Hoffman and R.I. Hamby, Editors. Amsterdam: North-Holland, 1976, pp. 181–198.
36. Zhou, S. H., J. Liebman, A.M. Dubin, et al., Using 12-lead ECG and synthesized VCG in detection of right ventricular hypertrophy with terminal right conduction delay versus partial RBBB in the pediatric population. *J. Electrocardiol.*, 2001;**34**(Suppl.): 249–257.
37. Liebman, J., Y. Rudy, P.J. Diaz, et al., Body surface potential mapping: partial right bundle branch block vs right ventricular hypertrophy with terminal right conduction delay. *J.Am. Coll. Cardiol.*, 1984;**3**: 496.
38. Liebman, J., C.W. Thomas, Y. Rudy, et al., Partial right bundle-branch block vs right ventricular hypertrophy with terminal conduction delay. Differentiation using a color-displayed body-surface potential mapping system, in *Electrocardiology 83*, I. Ruttkáy-Nedecky and P.MacFarlane, Editors. Amsterdam: Excerpta Medica, 1984, pp. 218–225.
39. Liebman, J., Y. Rudy, and C.W. Thomas. RVH with terminal right conduction delay versus partial right bundle branch block (utilizing body surface potential maps), in *Fundamental and Pediatric Electrocardiography*, J. Liebman, R. Plonsey, and Y. Rudy, Editors. Boston, MA: Nijhoff, 1986, pp. 389–398.
40. Mehran-Pour, M., A.Whitney, J. Liebman, et al., Quantification of the Frank and McFee-Parungao orthogonal electrocardiogram in valvular pulmonic stenosis. Correlations with hemodynamic measurement. *J. Electrocardiol.*, 1979;**12**: 69–76.
41. Liebman, J. and A.S. Nadas, The vectorcardiogram on the differential diagnosis of atrial septal defect in children. *Circulation*, 1960;**72**: 956–975.
42. Spach, M.S., J.P. Boineau, E.C. Long, et al., Genesis of the vectorcardiogram (electrocardiogram) in endocardial cushion defects, in *Vectorcardiography – 1965*, I. Hoffman and R.C. Taymor, Editors. Amsterdam: North-Holland, 1966, pp. 307–326.
43. Liebman, J., R. Plonsey, and Y. Rudy, *Pediatric and Fundamental Electrocardiography*. Boston, MA: Martinus Nijhoff, 1987.
44. Liebman. J., C.W. Thomas, and Y. Rudy, Conduction abnormalities and ventricular hypertrophy, in *Body Surface Electrocardiographic Mapping*, D. Mirvis, Editor. Boston, MA: Kluwer Academic, 1988, pp. 153–166.
45. Liebman, J., The initial QRS left as part of severe obstructive hypertrophy. Body surface potential mapping in children with severe aortic stenosis and pulmonic stenosis, in *Proceedings of the 24th International Congress on Electrocardiology*, Bratislava, June 24–28, 1997, p. 53.
46. Liebman, J., What's old, what's new in non-arrhythmia electrocardiology. Annual Harumi Lecture of the International Society of Computerization, in *Electrocardiology (ISCE)*, April 30, 2004; *J Electrocardiol.*, 2004;**37**(Suppl.): 152–165.
47. Strong, W B., J. Liebman, and E. Perrin, Hypoplastic left ventricle syndrome. Electrocardiographic evidence of left ventricular hypertrophy. *Am. J. Dis. Child.*, 1970;**120**: 511–514.
48. Liebman, J., C.W.Thomas, and Y. Rudy, ECG body surface potential mapping many years after successful surgery for coarctation of the aorta. *J. Electrocardiol.*, 1993;**26**: 25–41.
49. Macruz, R., J.K. Perloff, and R.B. Case, A method for the electrocardiographic recognition of atrial enlargement. *Circulation*, 1958;**17**: 882–889.
50. Morris J.J. Jr., E.H. Estes Jr., R.E. Whalen, et al., P wave analysis in valvular heart disease. *Circulation*, 1964;**29**: 242–252.
51. Banerjea, J.C. and S.K. Mukherjee, Some observations in left atrial enlargement in the electrocardiogram. *Indian Heart J.*, 1978;**20**: 264.
52. Ishikawa, K. and H.V. Pipberger, Critical evaluation of the twin peaked P wave (pseudo-P mitrale) in orthogonal electrocardiograms. *J. Electrocardiol.*, 1980;**13**: 181–184.
53. Ferrer, P.L. and R.C. Ellison, Detection of atrial overload in congenital heart disease by the Frank scalar atrial vectorcardiogram. *Circulation*, 1973;**48**(Suppl. IV): 82. [Abstract.]
54. Liebman, J., H.C. Romberg, and T.D. Downs, The Frank QRS vectorcardiogram in the premature infant, in *Vectorcardiography 1965*, I. Hoffman and R.C. Taymor, Editors. Amsterdam: North-Holland, 1966.
55. Liebman, J., R. Plonsey, and J.L. Ankeney, The initial QRS vector in ventricular hypertrophy, in *Proceedings of the IXth International Congress on Electrocardiology*, Tokyo, 1982; *Jpn. Heart J.*, 1982;**23**(Suppl. 1): 480–482.
56. Ankeney, J.L., T.S. Tzeng, and J. Liebman, Surgical therapy for congenital aortic valvular stenosis: a 23 year experience. *J. Thorac. Cardiovasc. Surg.*, 1983;**85**: 41–48.
57. Liebman, J., C.F. Doershuk, C. Rapp, et al., The vectorcardiogram in cystic fibrosis. Diagnostic significance and correlation with pulmonary function tests. *Circulation*, 1967;**35**: 552–567.
58. Lee, M.H., J. Liebman, A.G. Steinberg, E.V. Perrin, and V.Whitman, Familial occurrence of endocardial fibroelastosis in three siblings, including identical twins. *Pediatrics*, 1973;**52**: 402–411.
59. Liebman, J., H.K. Hellerstein, J.L. Ankeney, et al., The problem of the anomalous left coronary artery arising from the pulmonary artery in older children. *N. Engl. J. Med.*, 1963;**269**: 486–494.
60. Sreenivasan, V.V., J. Liebman, D.S. Linton, et al., Posterior mitral regurgitation in girls possibly due to posterior papillary muscle dysfunction. *Pediatrics*, 1968;**42**: 276–290.
61. Agusti, R., J. Liebman, J.Ankeney, et al., Congenital right coronary artery to left atrium fistula. *Am J. Cardiol.*, 1967;**19**: 428–433.
62. Bharati, S. and M. Lev, The conduction system in tricuspid atresia with and without regular (d-) transposition. *Circulation*, 1977;**56**: 423–439.
63. Katz, L.N. and H. Wachtel, The diphasic QRS type of electrocardiogram in congenital heart disease. *Am. Heart J.*, 1937;**13**: 202–206.
64. Bharati, S. and M. Lev, The course of the conduction system in single ventricle with inverted (L-) loop and inverted (L-) transposition. *Circulation*, 1975;**51**: 723–730.
65. Liebman, J., S.L. Miller, and I.H. Gessner. The initial QRS vector in children, in *Vectorcardiography*, 2 edn., I. Hoffman, Editor. Amsterdam: North-Holland, 1971, pp. 645–648.
66. Liebman, J., Y. Rudy, P. Diaz, et al., The spectrum of right bundle branch block as manifested in electrocardiographic body surface potential maps. *J. Electrocardiol.*, 1984;**17**: 329–346.

10 Electrocardiography in Adult Congenital Heart Disease

Paul Khairy · Ariane J. Marelli

P. W. Macfarlane et al. (eds.), *Electrocardiology*, DOI 10.1007/978-0-85729-874-4_10,

10.1 Introduction

Adult congenital heart disease (ACHD) is a growing subspecialty of cardiology with a rapidly expanding patient population [1–4]. In an earlier era, more than half of all children born with congenital defects died before reaching adulthood [5]. With current care, nearly 90% of such infants are expected to thrive into their adult years [1, 3, 6]. In North America, outpatient visits in ACHD tertiary care centers increased by 400% in 1999 and continue to rise [3].

Despite these successes, it is now appreciated that early surgical interventions were "reparative" and not "curative." Symptoms and complications may surface many years after quiescent courses in childhood. As such, meticulous clinical assessment and follow-up is warranted. As the growing population of survivors with ACHD ages and health needs rise, an increasing number of caregivers will be exposed to such patients at some point in their careers. The 12-lead electrocardiogram (ECG) remains an invaluable cornerstone in the clinical appraisal of adults with congenital heart disease that, in certain circumstances, provides diagnostic and/or prognostic information. It is, therefore, timely and appropriate that a chapter be dedicated to this topic.

In ➋ Chap. 9, detailed ECG criteria associated with congenital heart defects in children and their hemodynamic consequences were extensively reviewed. Isolated lesions of the left and right ventricular outflow tracts have also been addressed elsewhere. This chapter provides a clinical perspective to ECG interpretation in ACHD, emphasizing practical and pathognomonic ECG findings in the more frequent congenital defects encountered in adults, stressing the particularities associated with adults as opposed to children. As a result of hemodynamic or hypoxic stress imposed by the original cardiac malformation and/or postoperative sequelae from reparative surgery [7], arrhythmias figure prominently among the issues encountered in ACHD [8]. Thus, when discussing ECG findings for the varied pathologies, examples of associated common arrhythmias will be presented. First, an overview of the conduction system and its variations in congenital heart disease will be provided to facilitate an understanding of ECG patterns in ACHD.

10.2 Anatomy of the Conduction System in Congenital Heart Disease

10.2.1 Sinus Node

In the morphologically normal heart, a spindle-shaped sinus node is usually located epicardially in the sulcus terminalis, at the junction between the venous portion of the right atrium and the base of the right atrial appendage. Normal sinus activation, therefore, results in a typical P-wave axis between 15° and 75°. Most patients with congenitally malformed hearts have normally positioned atrial chambers, or "atrial situs solitus." This arrangement is usually associated with normal sinus node location. The position of the sinus node may, however, vary with the atrial chambers and their appendages.

10.2.2 Juxtaposition of the Atrial Appendages

Juxtaposition of the atrial appendages refers to a condition whereby both atrial appendages are located on the same side of the arterial pedicle rather than each being ipsilateral to its respective atrium. Right juxtaposition, with the left atrial appendage on the right side, adjacent to the right atrial appendage, is exceedingly rare and not associated with a malpositioned sinus node. However, left juxtaposition is more common and is accompanied by a displaced sinus node. While the sulcus terminalis remains an important landmark, the sinus node is more anteriorly positioned and may be located inferior to the crista terminalis [9]. Left juxtaposition may herald an abnormal ventriculoarterial connection, such as discordant or double outlet right ventricle, and is frequently found in tricuspid atresia [10].

10.2.3 Situs Inversus and Heterotaxy Syndromes

In "atrial situs inversus," the atria are positioned in mirror-image fashion, with the right atrium and its sinus node on the individual's left side. Consequently, the P-wave axis shifts to between 105° and 165°, with a P-wave that is often negative in lead I and most positive in lead III.

Heterotaxy syndromes refer to disorders of lateralization whereby the arrangement of abdominal and thoracic viscera differ from situs solitus and situs inversus. These syndromes are often associated with severe congenital cardiac malformations, and although there is much variability, are generally characterized as either right atrial isomerism (asplenia syndrome) or left atrial isomerism (polysplenia syndrome). Patients with right atrial isomerism often have two separate sinus nodes, at the junctions of right- and left-sided superior vena cavae with atrial chambers [11, 12]. On the ECG, this is often reflected by a P-wave axis that fluctuates as the prevailing pacemaker shifts from one sinus node to the other (➲ Fig. 10.1) [13]. In contrast, the majority of hearts with left atrial isomerism do not have a histologically recognizable sinus node. When present, it is hypoplastic and located posteroinferiorly, far from the orifice of the superior vena cava [12, 14]. As a result, slow atrial rates and junctional escape rhythms are common (➲ Fig. 10.2) [14].

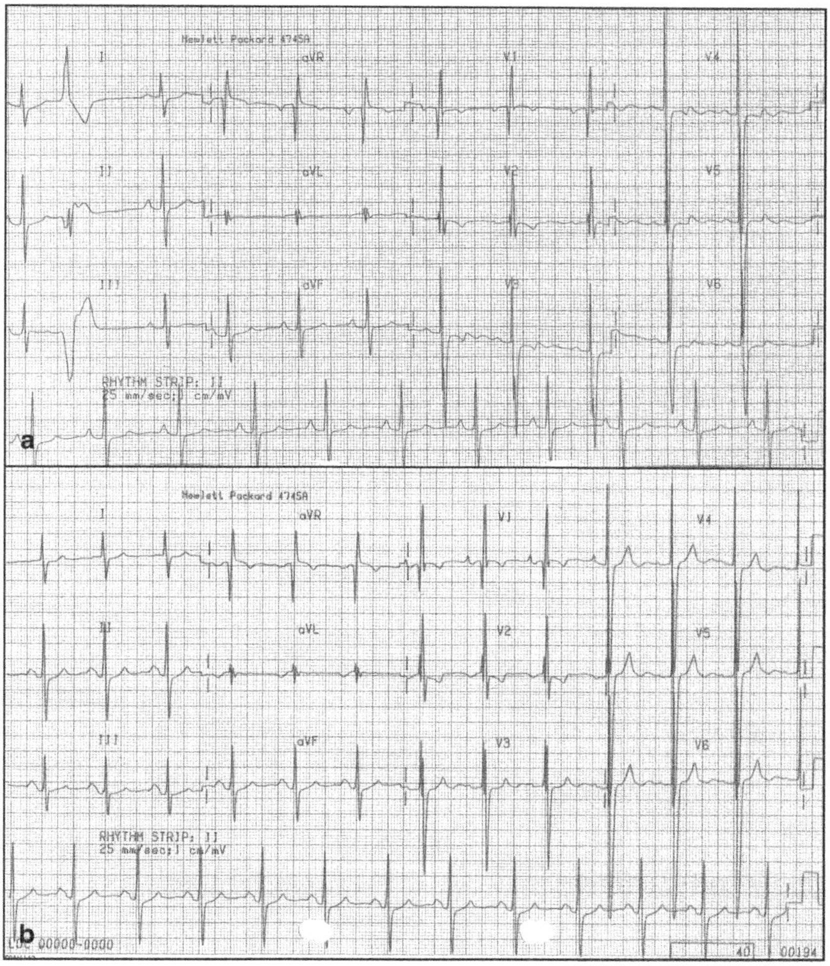

Fig. 10.1
12-lead electrocardiogram (ECGs) of a 37-year-old man with heterotaxy syndrome of the asplenia type. Note the difference in P-wave axis and morphology between panels a and b, indicating a shift in the governing pacemaker. In panel a, the P-wave axis is 65° and is positive in lead I, monophasic in the inferior leads, and predominantly negative in lead V1. In panel b, the P-wave axis is 90°, notched in the inferior leads, and predominantly positive in lead V1

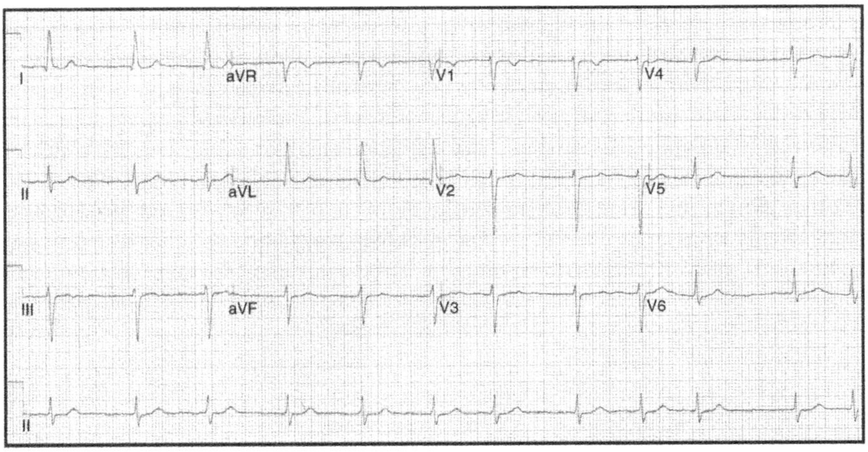

Fig. 10.2
A 12-lead ECG of a 42-year-old woman with heterotaxy syndrome of the polysplenia type. Note the absence of clearly identifiable P-waves. The irregular rate suggests underlying atrial fibrillation. However, multiple cardioversion attempts failed to interrupt this rhythm, even briefly. A junctional rhythm was present at birth and sinus node function was never confirmed

10.2.4 AV Node and His-Purkinje System

In normal hearts, the atrioventricular (AV) node is located at the apex of Koch's triangle, delimited on one side by the septal leaflet of the tricuspid valve and on another side by the tendon of Todaro that extends from the Eustachian valve (guarding the opening of the inferior vena cava) to the central fibrous body. The mouth of the coronary sinus forms the base of this triangle. The common bundle, or bundle of His, extends from the AV node and is the only pathway of myocardial continuity between the atria and the ventricles. In simple septal defects and/or valvar stenosis, the AV conduction system generally assumes its normal pattern. However, displacement of the AV conduction system occurs in congenital defects associated with malaligned atrial and ventricular septae, discordant AV arrangements, and single ventricles.

10.2.5 AV Canal Defect

Atrioventricular canal defects (AVCD) are associated with a displaced AV conduction system, as the compact AV node occupies an inferior position outside of Koch's triangle, anterior to the mouth of the coronary sinus and adjacent to where posterior rims of atrial and ventricular septae unite [15–17]. The common bundle extends along the lower rim of the ventricular septum. This inferior course and the relative hypoplasia of the left anterior hemifascicle gives rise to the superior QRS axis typical of AVCD [18, 19].

10.2.6 Congenitally Corrected Transposition of the Great Arteries

In "congenitally corrected" transposition of the great arteries, or L-TGA, atrioventricular and ventriculo-arterial discordance coexist such that the atrial situs is normal but the right ventricle is sub-aortic and leftward and the left ventricle is sub-pulmonary and rightward. L-TGA is associated with marked displacement of the AV conduction system. The AV node is located outside of Koch's triangle, displaced anteriorly and slightly more laterally [20, 21]. An elongated common bundle of His runs medially toward the septum to the site of fibrous continuity between the right-sided mitral valve and the pulmonary artery. The common bundle then courses along the anterior rim of the pulmonary valve and, if a ventricular septal defect (VSD) is present, continues along its upper rim [20, 21].

10.2.7 Tricuspid Atresia

Patients with tricuspid atresia have an imperforated fibrous AV connection. The septal leaflet of the tricuspid valve that normally forms one border of Koch's triangle is absent. Therefore, the usual anatomic landmarks demarcating the location of the AV node cannot be applied. Pathologic studies in tricuspid atresia have suggested that the compact AV node is typically situated on the floor of the right atrium, adjacent to an abnormally formed central fibrous body [22, 23]. A small "dimple" lined with endocardium is found just anterior to the mouth of the coronary sinus and has been considered to indicate the theoretical site of the absent tricuspid valve [22]. The AV node is found within the confines of the coronary sinus, tendon of Todaro, and right atrial "dimple." It pierces the central fibrous body to become the penetrating bundle of His, along the left side of the septum. The remaining course of the His-Purkinje system is related to some extent on the presence and location of associated VSDs. In general, the His-bundle is further leftward and away from more anterior septal defects [23].

10.2.8 Other Forms of Single Ventricle Physiology

In considering the course of the conduction system and potential for AV block in other types of single ventricle physiology, it is important to note the type of ventricular looping and whether the dominant ventricle is right or left. The most conspicuous abnormalities in the location of the AV conduction system occur in single ventricles with AV discordance and AVCD. In the case of an L-looped single left ventricle, two AV nodes may be present, with a posterior node that does not usually make contact with the ventricular septum [17]. The elongated course of the common bundle renders it susceptible to fibrous degeneration and complete AV block [24]. With ventricular D-looping and a dominant right ventricle, the AV node is positioned within its usual landmarks and the common bundle enters the ventricular septum directly [25].

10.3 Electrocardiography in Adult Congenital Heart Disease (ACHD)

10.3.1 Ostium Secundum Atrial Septal Defect

Defects of the atrial septum constitute at least 30% of all congenital heart disease seen in adults and ostium secundum atrial septal defect (ASD) is twice more prevalent in females than males (4). Adults with a secundum-type ASD most commonly have underlying sinus rhythm. However, the incidence of atrial fibrillation and/or flutter with unrepaired ASDs is approximately 20% and increases with age [26, 27]. Surgical closure may decrease the occurrence of atrial arrhythmias, but appears less effective in older individuals [26–29]. Gatzoulis et al. [26] retrospectively reviewed 218 adults with surgical closure of an isolated ASD. Over a mean postoperative follow-up of 3.8 years, 60% of patients with preoperative atrial flutter or fibrillation continued to have arrhythmias and 2.3% developed new-onset arrhythmias. All patients with persistent and new arrhythmias were over 40 years of age at surgery. Attie et al. [27] randomized 521 adults 40 years and older to surgical ASD closure versus medical therapy. Over a median of 7.3 years, new-onset atrial flutter or fibrillation occurred in 7.4% and 8.7% of patients with surgical and medical therapy, a nonsignificant difference.

The impact of transcatheter ASD device closure remains to be determined. One retrospective study of 132 patients found that all persistent arrhythmias remained after closure [29]. Of those with prior paroxysmal atrial tachyarrhythmias, two-thirds were free of symptomatic recurrence at a mean of 17 months. The incidence of symptomatic paroxysmal and persistent atrial fibrillation or flutter was 17 and 11%/year, respectively. Age $\geqslant$ 55 years was a risk factor for atrial tachyarrhythmias after transcatheter device closure.

A typical ECG in the adult with an ASD has a QRS complex with an rSr′ or rsR′ configuration over the right precordial leads [30–39]. This is likely a manifestation of right ventricular overload rather than a true conduction delay in the right bundle branch [40]. In contrast to a sharp and narrow r′ not exceeding 5 mm in the rSr′ pattern found in 2.4% of normal hearts, the r′ associated with an ASD is broader and somewhat slurred [32, 34]. As a result of prolonged terminal forces, QRS duration is lengthened but often remains within the upper limit of normal. However, a complete right bundle branch block pattern is not infrequent with increasing age. Also, q-waves in the inferior leads are occasionally observed although poorly defined.

While PR prolongation is seen in 6–19% of patients, progression toward higher degree AV block is uncommon [39, 41, 42], with complete AV block rarely reported [43]. The QRS axis is usually between 0° and 180° and is often vertical. Right axis deviation is commonly seen in adults with associated pulmonary vascular disease [44, 45]. In contrast, left axis deviation is rare but has been described in some hereditary forms such as Holt–Oram syndrome [43, 46]. In older individuals, it may represent an acquired left anterior fascicular block. ECG criteria for right atrial enlargement are met in approximately 35% of patients [30, 32–34, 36–39].

A notch near the apex of the R-wave in the inferior leads, termed "crochetage," has been correlated with ASD [35]. In a study of 1,560 adults and adolescents including 459 normal subjects and 1,101 patients with various forms of congenital heart disease, this pattern was identified in 73.1% of those with ASDs [47]. Among patients with ASDs, its incidence increased with larger anatomic defects or greater left-to-right shunts, even in the presence of pulmonary hypertension. The specificity of this sign in diagnosing ASD was 92% when present in all three inferior limb leads. Early disappearance of this pattern was observed in 35.1% of surgically repaired patients, although the right bundle branch block pattern persisted. In a second study, the "crochetage" pattern was observed in at least one inferior limb lead in 31.7% of preoperative patients with a secundum ASD [48]. The specificity of the "crochetage pattern" for detecting a secundum ASD was 86.1% and > 92% when present in at least one and in all three inferior limb leads, respectively. Typical ECG features are depicted in ➋ Figs. 10.3 and ➋ 10.4.

10.3.2 Ventricular Septal Defect

Ventricular septal defects (VSD) are the most common congenital heart malformation in the pediatric population, but often close spontaneously or cause symptoms of congestive heart failure that prompt surgical intervention prior to adulthood [49]. Although a VSD can occur anywhere along the interventricular septum, effects on the conduction system and arrhythmias in unoperated patients are most likely related to hemodynamic consequences, not specific location [50]. Adults most commonly present with small restrictive VSDs or large unrestrictive VSDs with Eisenmenger's complex.

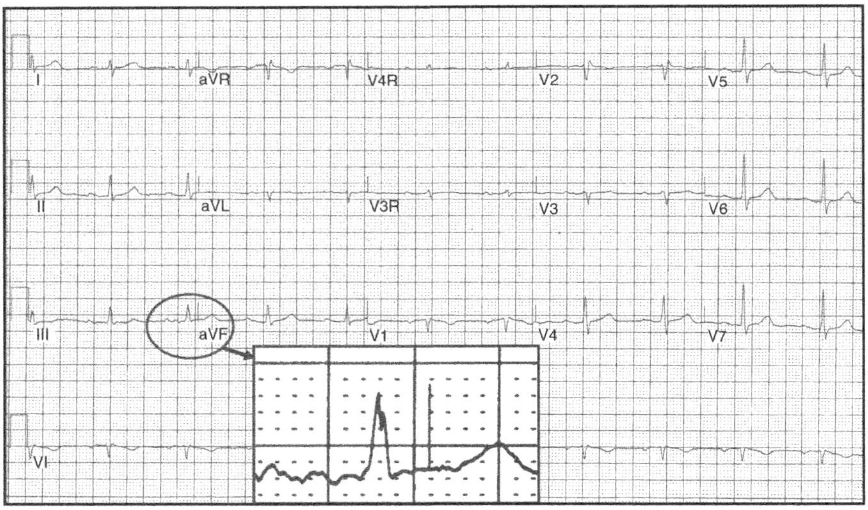

Fig. 10.3
15-lead ECG in a 53-year-old woman with a secundum atrial septal defect (ASD). Note the rSr′ QRS pattern over the right precordial leads, with a broad and slurred r′. The QRS axis is vertical and the PR interval measures 200 ms. Encircled and magnified in the insert is the "crochetage" pattern over the inferior leads, characterized by a notch near the R-wave apex

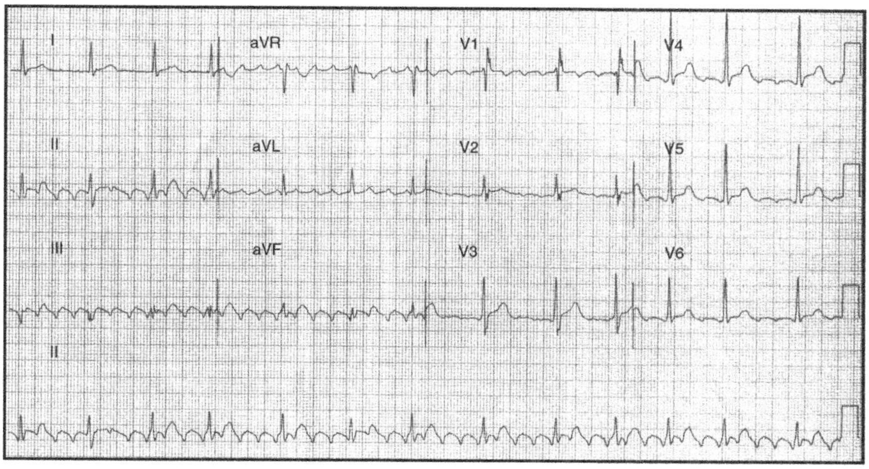

Fig. 10.4
12-lead ECG in a 58-year-old man with a secundum ASD. Intra-atrial reentrant tachycardia developed 21 years after surgical repair. Note the classic "saw tooth" pattern of flutter waves with a cycle length of 230 ms and variable AV conduction, compatible with typical counterclockwise atrial flutter. The patient underwent successful transcatheter ablation of the cavotricuspid isthmus

Either way, defects of the membranous septum, or "perimembranous" VSDs, are located in the left ventricular outflow beneath the aortic valve and account for the majority of VSDs [4].

In a review comparing 439 patients with unoperated VSDs to a control population, a higher prevalence of isolated premature ventricular contractions (PVC), couplets, and multiform PVCs was noted [50]. Non-sustained or sustained ventricular tachycardia occurred in 5.7% of patients. The most powerful independent predictor for high-grade ectopy was higher mean pulmonary artery pressure. Despite these ventricular arrhythmias, sudden cardiac death is reportedly uncommon but has been described in patients with cardiac hypertrophy and progressive fibrosis of the conduction system [51–54]. In patients with surgically repaired VSDs, late sudden death occurs in about 4% [55, 56]. Risk factors for mortality include age greater than 5 years at time of surgery, pulmonary vascular resistance greater than 7 Woods units, and complete heart block [56]. Transcatheter VSD closure is an alternative to surgery in selected patients. Although long-term follow-up is not yet available, complete heart block is a recognized complication [57–59].

Electrocardiographic findings in isolated VSDs are highly dependent on the hemodynamic effects of the left-to-right shunt, i.e., degree of left ventricular volume overload and right ventricular pressure overload. Small defects often produce normal tracings, with the exception of increased ventricular ectopy and the occasional rsr′ pattern over the right precordial leads [60, 61]. Large VSDs are associated with right and sometimes left atrial enlargement, with broad notched P-waves in leads I and II and negative terminal forces in lead V1. The PR interval is normal or mildly prolonged [60, 61]. The QRS axis usually shifts moderately rightward and evidence for biventricular hypertrophy is found in 23–61% of cases [62]. As shown in ➋ Fig. 10.5, the Katz–Wachtel phenomenon may be seen, with large equiphasic RS complexes over the midprecordial leads [63]. The R-wave amplitude in V1 may meet right ventricular hypertrophy criteria and deep Q-waves may be present over the lateral precordial leads. A right bundle branch block has been reported in 30–60% of patients and appears independent of whether the VSD was repaired through an atrial or ventricular incision [56, 64, 65]. Right bundle branch block with left-axis deviation is seen in 3–15% of patients [56, 65]. First-degree AV block occurs in about 10% of patients and the incidence of complete heart block on long-term follow-up is 1–3% [56, 65].

Eisenmenger's complex refers to flow reversal across a VSD when pulmonary vascular resistance exceeds systemic levels. Evidence for biventricular hypertrophy is often lacking, as right ventricular hypertrophy and pulmonary hypertension predominate. In adults, rightward QRS axis deviation is often present, as are peaked P-waves in lead II and tall monophasic R-waves in V1 [66, 67].

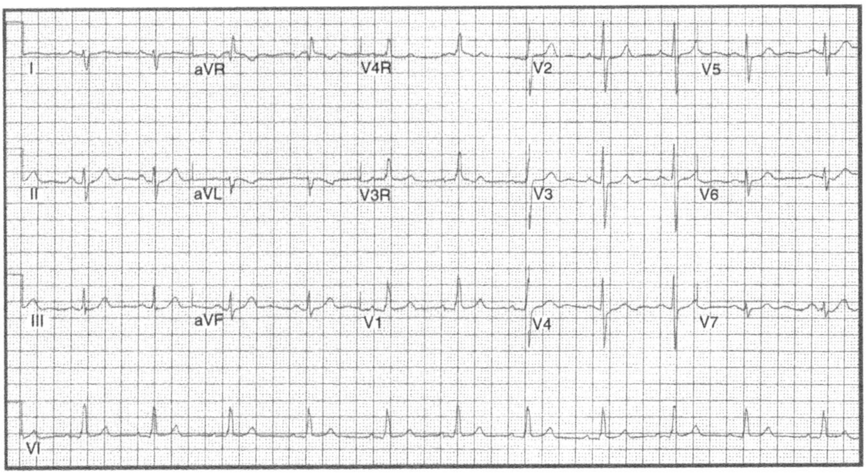

Fig. 10.5
15-lead ECG in a 45-year-old woman with a moderate ventricular septal (VSD). Note the broad notched P-wave in lead II, normal PR interval, and right axis deviation. The R-wave amplitude in V1 meets right ventricular hypertrophy criteria. "Katz–Wachtel" phenomenon is present, with large equiphasic RS complexes over the mid-precordial leads that reflect biventricular hypertrophy

10.3.3 Atrioventricular Canal Defect

The most common presentations of AVCD in adulthood are either a partial defect, consisting of a primum ASD and cleft mitral valve, or surgically repaired complete AVCD. Less commonly, an unoperated patient with a complete AVCD that includes a large primum ASD, inlet VSD, and cleft mitral valve presents with Eisenmenger's physiology or with spontaneous closure of the inlet VSD by way of aneurysm formation. In addition to ECG findings associated with the displaced AV conduction system, electrocardiographic findings reflect the dominant physiology of the defect, e.g., large left-to-right atrial shunt and mitral regurgitation in partial AVCD and Eisenmenger's physiology in an unrepaired complete AVCD [4].

Following surgical repair of AVCD, atrial fibrillation or flutter may develop in 5% of patients [68, 69]. Persistent complete AV block occurs in 1–7% in the immediate postoperative period and approximately 2% thereafter [69–72]. Prolonged infra-Hisian conduction time may be a marker for increased risk of late AV block, even in the presence of a normal PR interval [73]. Although increased ventricular ectopy has been described in up to 30% of patients, complex ventricular arrhythmias occur most commonly in the setting of left ventricular dysfunction [69].

Distinctive ECG features in the adult with AVCD, displayed in ➋ Fig. 10.6, involve the PR interval, right ventricular activation pattern, and QRS axis. First-degree AV block is present in over 50% of patients and is most commonly due to intraatrial conduction delay, although acquired postoperative AV block may occur [73–78]. In 18 patients with AVCD, electrophysiologic studies revealed supra-Hisian first-degree AV block in five patients, and intraatrial conduction delay in the majority [55]. The QRS pattern in right precordial leads may be similar to ostium secundum ASD, with delay in right ventricular activation. Interestingly, this is thought to result from conduction along a longer than normal right bundle branch that emanates from the inferiorly displaced common bundle; not from delayed parietal conduction [74].

As previously mentioned, a superior QRS axis is a hallmark of AVCD with left axis deviation that may be moderate or extreme. Q-waves are present in leads I and aVL and S waves in II, III, and aVF that characteristically have a notched upstroke [74–77]. Nonetheless, an intermediate QRS axis and right axis deviation have been described. One study assessed the QRS axis in 135 patients with typical AVCD and 9 patients with atypical forms of AVCD characterized by a well-formed atrial septum, milder downward displacement of the AV valves, and shorter length of the ostium primum defect [79]. All nine patients with atypical AVCD had an unusual mean frontal QRS axis compared with 6 of 135 patients (4%) with typical

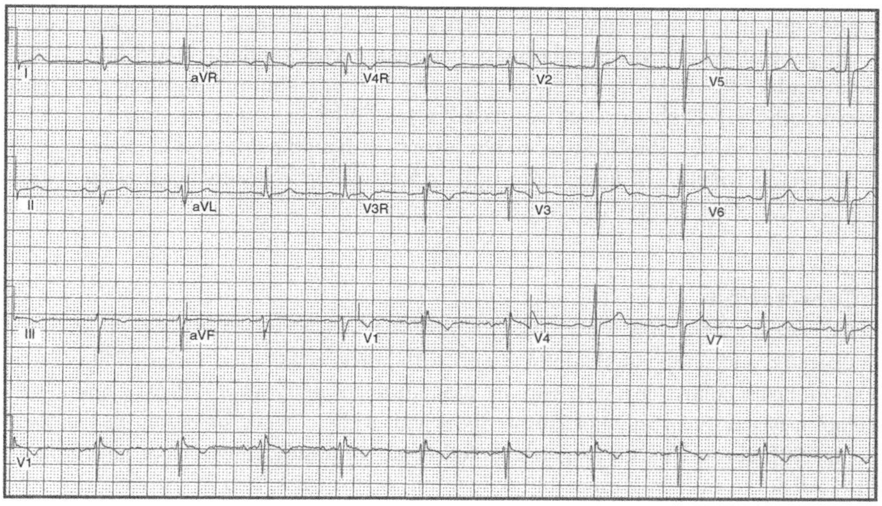

Fig. 10.6
15-lead ECG in a 42-year-old man with a surgically repaired Atrioventricular canal defects (AVCD). Note the rSr′ QRS pattern over the right precordial leads, similar to secundum ASD. The PR interval is prolonged and the typical superior QRS axis is present. S-waves in leads II, III, and aVF have a characteristically notched upstroke

AVCD. It was, therefore, speculated that this atypical morphology, supposedly related to the degree of posteroinferior displacement of the conduction system, explained in part the observed differences in QRS axis.

10.3.4 Patent Ductus Arteriosus

Most patients with moderate or large patent ductus arteriosus (PDA) will have undergone ductal ligation in infancy. The majority of adults with PDA fall into one of two categories: a fortuitously discovered PDA on echocardiography or Eisenmenger's physiology with irreversible pulmonary vascular obstructive disease [4]. In the former case, the ECG is expected to be normal, whereas in the latter case, ECG findings are dominated by Eisenmenger's physiology. In patients with a moderate size PDA, sinus rhythm is usually present although atrial fibrillation may occur in older individuals [80, 81]. Evidence for left atrial enlargement may be present and PR prolongation is found in 10–20% [82]. The QRS axis is generally normal. Left ventricular volume overload may be characterized by deep S-waves in V1 and tall R-waves in leads V5 and V6 that are accompanied by nonspecific repolarization changes [81, 82].

10.3.5 Pulmonary Stenosis

The obstruction of the right ventricular outflow tract can occur at the level of the pulmonary valve, below, or above it, either in the main pulmonary artery trunk or at one or both of its branches. As a group, these lesions represent a spectrum of unoperated and postoperative anomalies that are among the most commonly encountered in the adult with congenital disease. Isolated congenital valvar pulmonary stenosis is reported to occur in 10% of all patients with congenital heart disease. In adults, pulmonary atresia, supravalvar, and branch pulmonary artery stenosis are commonly encountered in the setting of tetralogy of Fallot (TOF). Congenital branch pulmonary artery stenosis can occur in isolation but is not usually associated with substantial right ventricular pressure overload. ECG features of primary infundibular stenosis or double-chambered right ventricle vary depending on the presence or absence of an associated VSD and/or concomitant valvar pulmonary stenosis [4].

Criteria for right ventricular hypertrophy in the presence of valvar pulmonary stenosis were extensively reviewed in a previous chapter. In general, the severity of pulmonary stenosis correlates with the R to S ratio in leads V1 and V6, and R-wave amplitude in lead V1 [83, 84]. The PR interval is typically normal but prolongation may reflect increased right atrial size and pressure [85, 86]. High amplitude peaked P-waves in lead II are commonly found in severe pulmonary stenosis, but not consistently so [87]. The QRS axis may be normal with mild pulmonary stenosis but is deviated rightward with moderate or severe obstruction. The degree of right axis deviation is positively correlated with right ventricular pressure [83].

10.3.6 Aortic Coarctation

Complications of operated and unoperated adult patients with aortic coarctation include left ventricular hypertrophy, systemic hypertension, heart failure, aortic dissection, premature coronary artery disease, and cerebrovascular events [88, 89]. In a population-based study, only 1 of 536 survivors with aortic coarctation repair died suddenly during the first 20 years of follow-up [90]. However, with longer-term follow-up, nine sudden deaths occurred, two of which resulted from aortic rupture. All seven sudden presumably arrhythmic deaths transpired in patients with advanced ventricular dysfunction [90].

In adults with uncomplicated aortic coarctation, the ECG usually exhibits normal sinus rhythm. Unlike children with concomitant left-to-right interatrial shunts, left but not right atrial enlargement is often seen [91]. The PR interval is usually normal and the QRS axis is normal or displaced leftward. Persistent right ventricular hypertrophy beyond infancy is rare. Left ventricular hypertrophy commonly occurs, with the most sensitive ECG criterion being increased QRS voltage [92], as demonstrated in ➋ Fig. 10.7.

10.3.7 Ebstein's Anomaly

In Ebstein's anomaly, the tricuspid valve is displaced apically, creating an "atrialized" portion of the right ventricle that is morphologically and electrically right ventricle but functionally right atrium [93]. Differences in clinical presentation

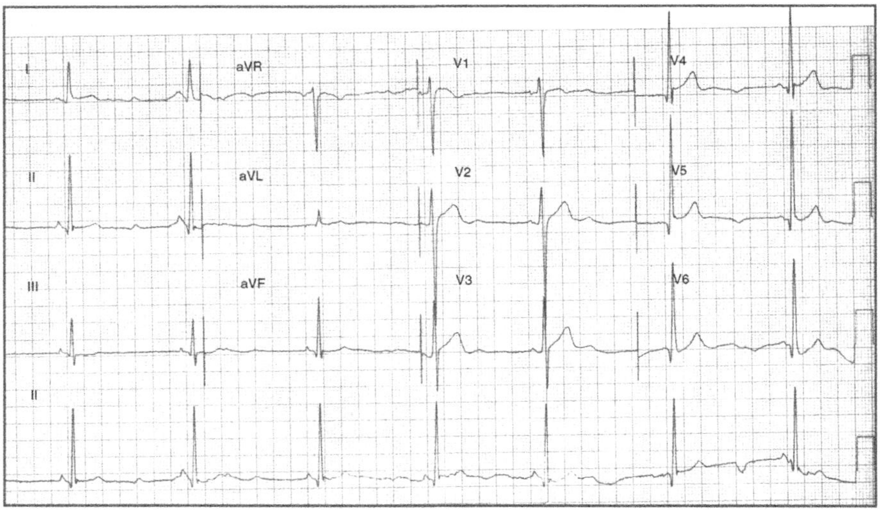

Fig. 10.7
12-lead ECG in a 26-year-old man with aortic coarctation surgically repaired at 6 years of age, with recoarctation repair at 17 years. Note the voltage criteria for left ventricular hypertrophy with an R-wave in lead II > 2.0 mV, R-wave in lead V5 > 3.0 mV, and sum of S-wave in lead V1 and R-wave in lead V5 or V6 > 3.5 mV. The QRS duration exceeds 90 ms

result from a wide spectrum of lesion severity as determined by degree of tricuspid leaflet tethering, relative proportion of atrialized and true right ventricle, and presence or absence of right ventricular outflow tract obstruction. A patent foramen ovale or secundum ASD is a common associated feature. The presence of tricuspid regurgitation with an enlarged right atrium, left-to-right shunting, and accessory pathways provide the substrate for most atrial arrhythmias. Mechanical stimulation of the "atrialized" ventricle may provoke ventricular arrhythmias, but spontaneous ventricular tachycardia is otherwise uncommon in the absence of associated malformations [94].

The ECG is invaluable in the adult with Ebstein's anomaly for clinical diagnosis, detection of accessory pathways, and characterization of arrhythmias, as exemplified in ➋ Figs. 10.8 and ➋ 10.9. Indeed, accessory AV and atriofascicular pathways are found in 25% and are more often right-sided and multiple than accessory pathways in structurally normal hearts [93, 95, 96] ventricular tachyarrhythmias including AV reciprocating tachycardia, ectopic atrial tachycardia, and atrial fibrillation or flutter occur in 30–40% of patients, constituting the most common presentation in adolescents and adults [97, 98]. Tolerance to tachyarrhythmia is dependent on the severity of Ebstein's malformation that can range from mild and asymptomatic to severe, with associated tricuspid regurgitation, cyanosis, and hemodynamic compromise. The role of arrhythmias in the etiology of sudden death, reported in 3–4% of patients [97], remains poorly defined. Sudden death may occur from severe cyanosis or from rapid conduction of atrial fibrillation or flutter to the ventricles via high risk or multiple pathways [96].

In Ebstein's anomaly, P-waves are characteristically tall and broad due to prolonged conduction in the enlarged right atrium and have been coined "Himalayan" [99, 100]. First-degree AV block is often present as a result of intraatrial conduction delay, with a PR interval than can be markedly prolonged [101]. Naturally, the PR interval may be shortened in the presence of an accessory AV or atriofascicular pathway. As the right ventricle is diminutive, low amplitude QRS complexes are characteristically seen over the right precordial leads [102, 103]. Due to the "atrialized" portion of the right ventricle, the QRS complex typically exhibits right ventricular conduction delay of the right bundle branch

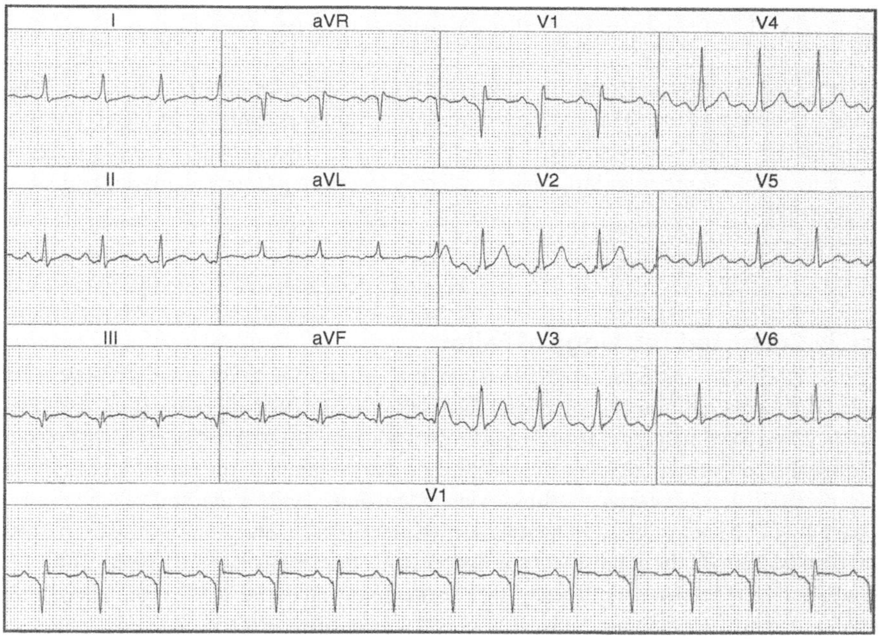

◘ Fig. 10.8
12-lead ECG in a 39-year-old man with Ebstein's anomaly and palpitations. Note the short PR interval, delta wave, and wide QRS complex consistent with ventricular preexcitation. The delta wave axis (i.e., negative in leads V1, III, and aVF and positive in leads I and aVL) suggests a right-sided posteroseptal accessory pathway. This pathway was deemed "high risk" as preexcited atrial fibrillation up to 245 bpm occurred. It was successfully ablated

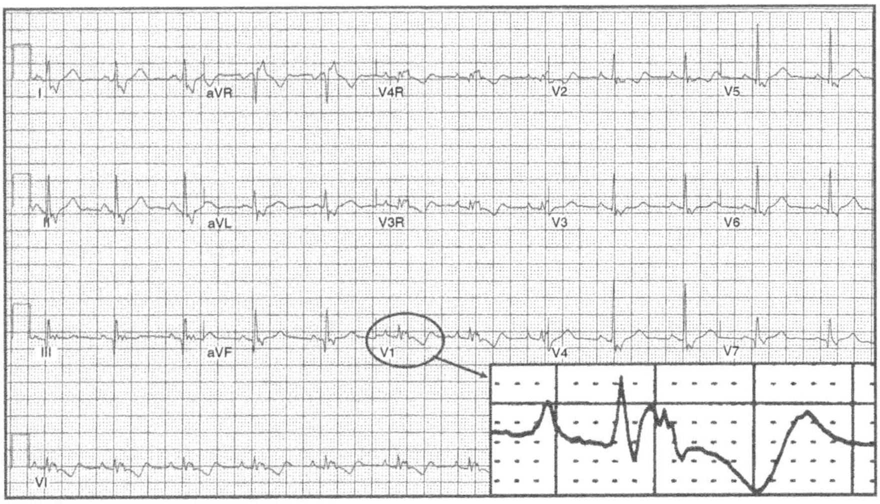

Fig. 10.9
15-lead ECG in a 33-year-old woman with Ebstein's anomaly. *Encircled* and magnified in the insert, a low-amplitude multiphasic "bizarre" QRS complex is seen over the right precordial leads with a right bundle branch block pattern. P-waves are broad and somewhat tall. The QRS axis is normal and Q-waves are notable in leads V1, II, III, and aVF

type that is often atypical and multiphasic [99–101]. In unoperated patients with Ebstein's anomaly, signal-averaged ECGs almost universally identify late potentials that correspond to delayed conduction across the "atrialized" right ventricle [104].

In the absence of ventricular preexcitation, the QRS axis is generally normal but occasionally leftward [105, 106]. In about 50% of patients, Q-waves are noted in lead V1 and may extend as far as lead V4 [107, 108]. T-wave inversion in leads V1–V4 is also common [107, 108]. Q-waves may be present in leads II, III, and aVF [105, 107]. It has been hypothesized that these Q-waves reflect right ventricular intracavitary potentials resulting from the inferior and leftward displacement of the tricuspid valve [107].

10.3.8 Surgically Corrected Tetralogy of Fallot

Tetralogy of Fallot is the most common cyanotic heart disease, accounting for approximately 10% of all congenital heart malformations [109]. Corrective surgery has been performed for over 40 years with excellent results [110]. However, atriotomies are commonly performed, predisposing to the late development of intraatrial reentrant tachycardia (IART) [111, 112]. Patients with IART may have typical isthmus-dependent flutter and/or incision-related macroreentrant circuits [113–116]. Development of IART may herald worsening ventricular function and tricuspid regurgitation [111, 112, 117, 118]. Moreover, sudden cardiac death is the single most common cause of mortality late after repair [119]. In a cohort study of 793 patients with repaired TOF followed for 35 years, 10% developed atrial flutter, 11.9% experienced sustained ventricular tachycardia (➋ Fig. 10.10), and 8.3% died suddenly [112]. Very few arrhythmic events occurred the first 5–10 years following corrective surgery. Thereafter, a slow but steady decline in freedom from atrial and ventricular arrhythmias and sudden cardiac death was observed [112, 120–122].

In adults with surgically corrected TOF, baseline sinus rhythm is commonly seen, with P-waves of normal axis, duration, and amplitude, although somewhat peaked [123–128]. The QRS axis is typically normal or rightwardly displaced with underlying right ventricular hypertrophy. In the presence of a right bundle branch block, criteria for right ventricular hypertrophy include an R′ in V1 $\geqslant$ 15 mm and right axis deviation of the initial vector that represents unblocked

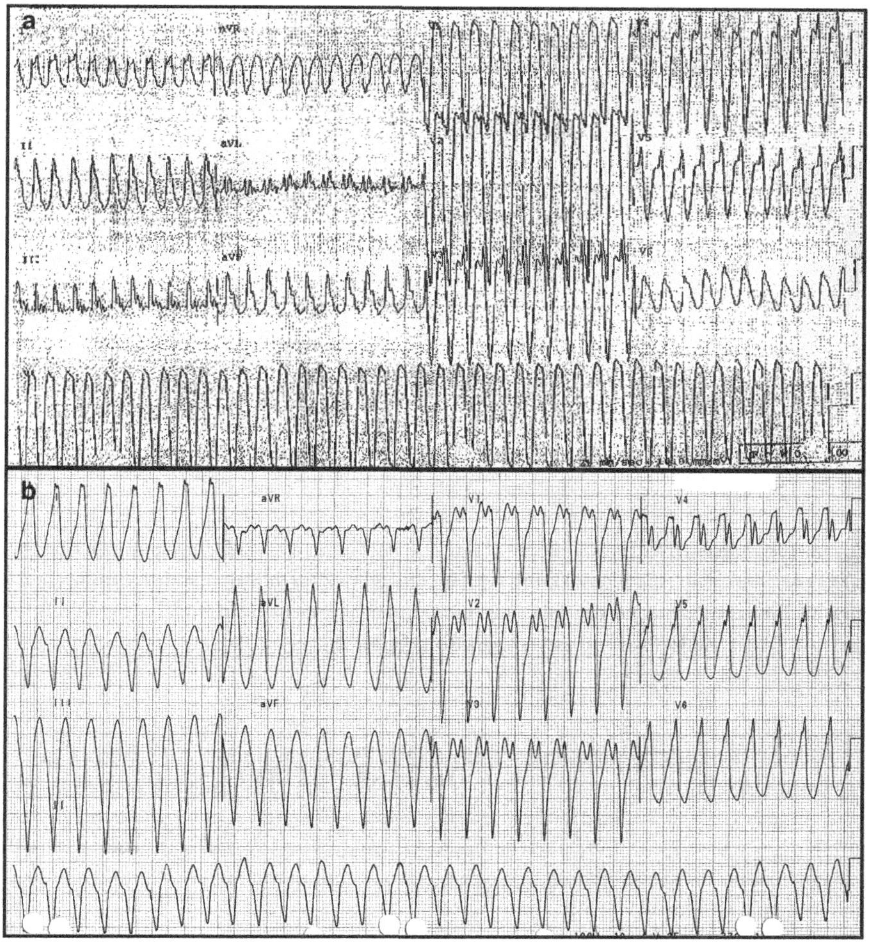

Fig. 10.10
ECG examples of clinical monomorphic ventricular tachycardia in adults with corrected tetralogy of Fallot. In Panel a, a 34-year-old man with surgically repaired tetralogy of Fallot presented with a wide-complex tachycardia at 240 bpm. Left bundle branch block morphology and inferior axis reflect the typical right ventricular outflow tract origin. Panel b depicts ventricular tachycardia at 195 bpm in a 46-year-old man with surgically repaired tetralogy of Fallot. While the QRS complex is of left bundle branch morphology, consonant with a right ventricular source, the superior QRS axis suggests an origin remote from the outflow tract

forces [129, 130]. Left axis deviation should raise the suspicion of an associated AVCD, although left anterior hemiblock may be present in 5–10% of adults [124, 131]. Right bundle branch block is the rule following repair, even in the absence of a ventriculotomy incision [123–126]. Early lengthening of the QRS interval post TOF repair results from surgical injury to the right bundle branch and myocardium [132], whereas later broadening reflects right ventricular dilation [133, 134].

Given the small but undeniable risk of ventricular arrhythmias and sudden cardiac death post TOF repair, considerable efforts have been directed toward identifying predictors allowing stratification of patients into high- and low-risk categories. In the largest cohort study to date [112], a QRS interval $\geqslant$ 180 ms (RR 8.8), as shown in ❷ Fig. 10.11, and an annual increase in QRS duration (RR 1.1 for each 1 ms increase/year) were independent risk factors for sustained ventricular tachycardia. Patients with ventricular tachycardia or sudden cardiac death were more likely to have increased

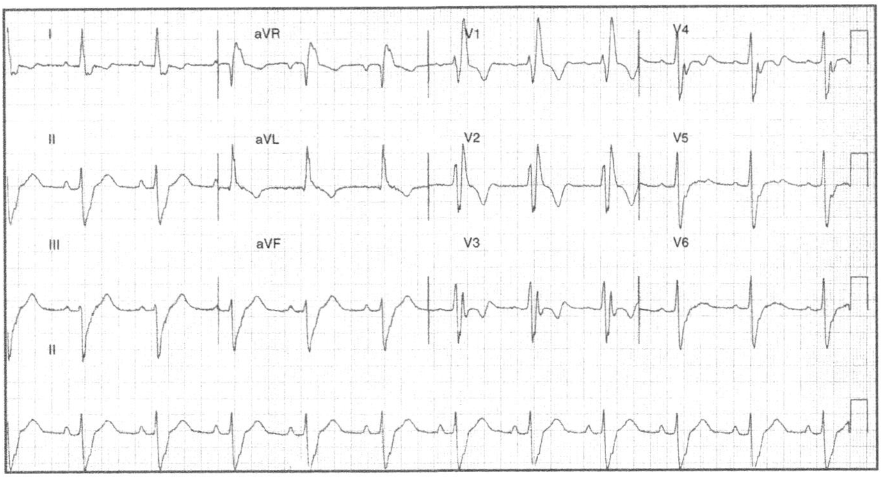

Fig. 10.11
12-lead ECG of a 50-year-old man with surgically repaired tetralogy of Fallot. Note the characteristic right bundle branch block morphology. The QRS duration of 192 ms is associated with increased risk for ventricular arrhythmias and sudden death. The tall R′ in V1 and deep S-waves in V5 and V6 suggest right ventricular hypertrophy in the context of mild residual pulmonary stenosis. First-degree AV block and left axis deviation are also present

cardiothoracic ratios, at least moderate pulmonary and tricuspid regurgitation, and peripheral pulmonary stenosis. A greater degree of QT dispersion was also noted, believed to reflect increased heterogeneity in myocardial repolarization. Other reported risk factors have included frequent ectopic beats [135], increased right ventricular systolic pressures [121, 136, 137], complete heart block [121, 138], and increased JT dispersion [139, 140]. The induction of sustained ventricular tachycardia on electrophysiologic study is a powerful independent predictor of susceptibility to clinical ventricular tachycardia or sudden death [141].

10.3.9 Congenitally Corrected Transposition of the Great Arteries

Patients with isolated L-TGA may remain asymptomatic and undiagnosed well into their adult years. As depicted in Fig. 10.12, the 12-lead ECG can provide critically important diagnostic information. The anatomy of the conduction system in L-TGA was previously reviewed, explaining the vulnerable AV conduction system with its fragile common bundle. In a study of 107 patients with L-TGA, complete AV block occurred in 22% [142]. Risk of AV block was estimated to be 2% per year, irrespective of associated anomalies. On electrophysiologic testing, the site of AV block was found to be above or within the area that generated His-like electrograms [143–145]. This finding is consistent with clinical and pathological observations: a stable narrow QRS escape rhythm often accompanies complete AV block [142] and fibrosis of the common bundle is noted histologically [144, 146, 147]. As the AV node and elongated bundle appear particularly susceptible to catheter or surgical trauma, caution should be exercised with manipulation to these areas. Complete AV block follows surgical repair of an associated VSD in over 25% of patients [142, 148–150].

L-TGA has also been referred to as "ventricular inversion," as the ventricles and associated bundle branches are reversed. The sinus node is positioned in its usual location such that the P-wave axis and morphology are typically normal. However, the ventricular septum that is normally activated from left-to-right is depolarized in the opposite direction, producing the ECG pattern characteristic of L-TGA [151–154]. The usual "septal" q-waves over left precordial leads and small initial R-waves over the right precordial leads are absent. Instead, Q-waves are present over the right precordial leads, consonant with right-to-left septal activation. Moreover, as the septum is activated in a superior direction, Q-waves, which

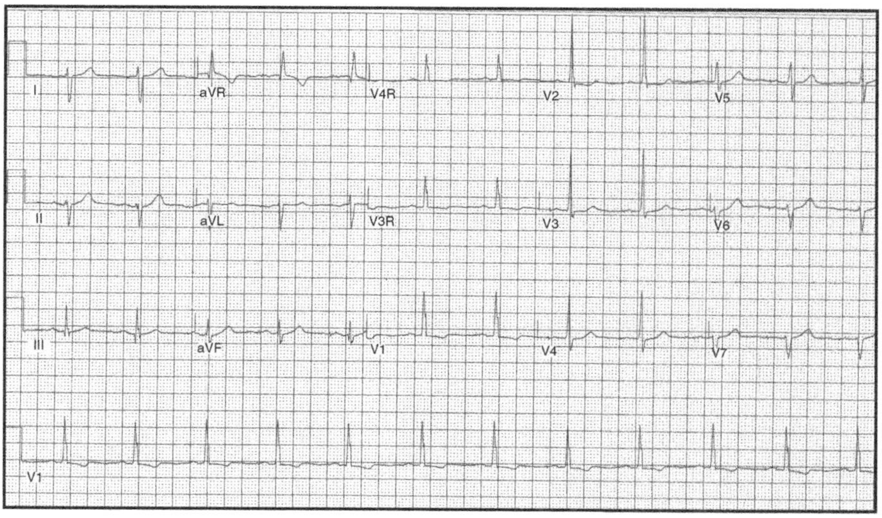

Fig. 10.12
15-lead ECG of a 25-year-old man with L-TGA. Note the first-degree AV block, normal P-wave axis, left QRS axis deviation, and absent septal q-waves. Broad Q-waves are seen over the right precordial leads. In inferior leads, Q-waves are deepest in lead III. T-waves are positive in all precordial leads

are not uncommonly broad, are seen in leads III and aVF, typically most pronounced in lead III. Thus, left axis deviation is the rule. Interestingly, in > 80% of patients, positive T-waves are present over all precordial leads, attributed to the side-by-side nature of the inverted ventricles [151–154]. In patients with associated Ebstein's malformation of the tricuspid valve, left-sided accessory pathways may be present [155–158].

10.3.10 Complete Transposition of the Great Arteries and Intraatrial Baffle

In "complete" transposition of the great arteries, or D-TGA, the atrioventricular relationship is preserved but ventriculo-arterial discordance is present. D-TGA accounts for 5–7% of all congenital cardiac malformations [109]. In the absence of a shunt allowing for mixing between parallel systemic and pulmonary circulations, D-TGA is incompatible with life. In 1959, Senning introduced an intraatrial baffle repair redirecting systemic and pulmonary venous return without grafts or prostheses [159]. In 1964, Mustard described an alternate technique for intraatrial baffle repair using a pericardial patch [160]. Although arterial switch surgery [161] has supplanted atrial correction as the procedure of choice, the majority of adults with D-TGA have had intraatrial baffle repairs. Late arrhythmic complications include sinus node dysfunction, atrial tachyarrhythmias, and sudden cardiac death [90, 162–169].

Of 478 patients with Mustard repairs, the actuarial rate of loss of sinus rhythm was 39% at 10 years and 60% at 20 years [165]. By 20 years after repair, atrial flutter had occurred in 24%. Loss of coordinated atrial activity and rapid ventricular rates can result in severe symptoms and hemodynamic compromise. Atrial arrhythmias are associated with impaired ventricular function [170, 171] and increased risk of sudden death in some, but not all, studies [172]. In a retrospective multicenter case-control study that identified 47 patients with D-TGA and Mustard or Senning surgery who experienced sudden death, risk factors included the presence of symptoms of arrhythmia or heart failure and history of documented atrial fibrillation or flutter [173]. ECG criteria, chest X-ray, and Holter findings were not predictive of sudden death and medical therapy and pacemakers were not found to be protective.

Characteristic ECG findings, exemplified by ➋ Figs. 10.13 and ➋ 10.14, are found in adults with D-TGA and intraatrial baffle repair [174, 175]. As sinus node dysfunction is highly prevalent, atrial and junctional rhythms may be seen. In simple D-TGA, AV node function is preserved. However, intraatrial conduction delay may result in a prolonged PR interval.

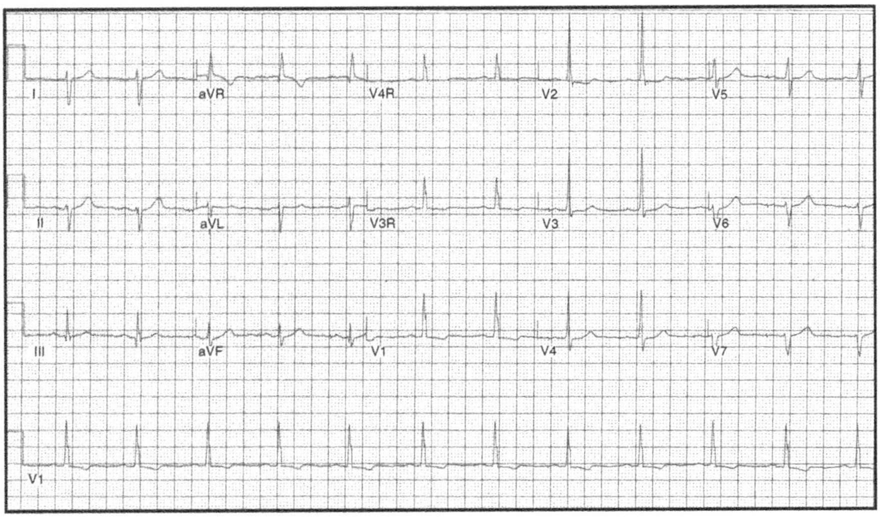

Fig. 10.13
15-lead ECG of a 29-year-old woman with D-TGA and Mustard procedure. Note the normal PR interval, right axis deviation, and right ventricular hypertrophy. Absent q-waves, small r-waves, and deep S-waves over leads V5–V7 reflect the diminutive left ventricle. A pacemaker was implanted for sinus node dysfunction; bipolar atrial pacing spikes precede the eighth and 11th P-wave

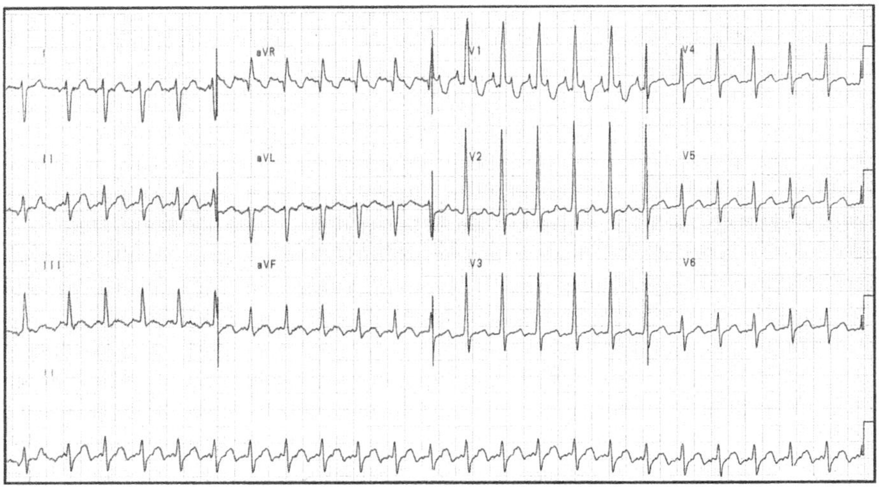

Fig. 10.14
12-lead ECG in a 38-year-old woman with D-TGA and Mustard procedure. Note the intraatrial reentrant tachycardia (IART) cycle length of 215 ms with 2:1 AV conduction. Right axis deviation, right ventricular hypertrophy, and a diminutive left ventricle are also present

AV block is more common in the presence of surgical repair of an associated VSD and/or tricuspid regurgitation [176]. Despite corrected physiology, the right ventricle remains systemically positioned. Thus, ECG criteria for right ventricular hypertrophy are usually present, with right axis deviation [174, 175]. Right atrial enlargement may likewise be present [174]. Conversely, the subpulmonary left ventricle is diminutive with decreased terminal forces reflected in the absence of q-waves, small r-waves, and deep S-waves over the left precordial leads.

10.3.11 Single Ventricle Physiology with Fontan Surgery

Developed in 1971 as surgical palliation for tricuspid atresia, the Fontan procedure has undergone multiple modifications to become the procedure of choice for various forms of single ventricle physiology [177]. Atrial arrhythmias after the Fontan procedure are among the more challenging problems in the field of adult congenital electrophysiology. These arrhythmias occur in the context of single functional ventricles and may be associated with substantial morbidity and mortality. Rapid hemodynamic deterioration and heart failure can ensue. Depending on the particular type of repair, IART or atrial fibrillation may occur in up to 57% of patients [178]. Tachycardia circuits can be complex and/or multiple [113, 116, 179, 180]. Patients with failing Fontans and refractory atrial arrhythmias should be considered for surgical conversion to a lateral tunnel or extracardiac conduit with concomitant arrhythmia surgery [181–185]. On short- to medium-term follow-up, advantages of the extracardiac in comparison to the intracardiac lateral tunnel Fontan include a decreased incidence of sinus node dysfunction [186], although not consistently so [187].

Given the heterogeneity of the multiple morphologic types of single ventricles, the ECG appearance is highly variable. At mid-term follow-up, sinus node dysfunction occurs in 13–16% of patients with classic Fontans (i.e., right atrium to pulmonary artery anastamosis) and increases with duration of follow-up [188–190]. In patients with tricuspid atresia, the PR interval is usually normal with tall and broad P-waves. Left axis deviation is characteristic [191–194], as shown in ❯ Fig. 10.15. In the absence of a functional right ventricle, left ventricular forces are unopposed, as manifested by small r-waves and deep S-waves over the right precordial leads and tall R-waves over the left precordial leads.

In the most common subtype of double-inlet left ventricle, i.e., with ventriculo-arterial discordance, AV conduction is often abnormal, with PR prolongation and increased risk of complete heart block [195, 196]. As in L-TGA, Q-waves are absent over the left precordial leads and may be present over the right precordial leads. Q-waves may also be seen in leads II, III, and aVF [195, 197]. In a series of 18 patients with univentricular hearts of right ventricular morphology, 12 had double inlet, four absent right, and two absent left AV connections [198]. ECG revealed right ventricular hypertrophy in all and 11 had a superior frontal QRS axis. An example of an ECG in an adult with a hypoplastic left ventricle is provided in ❯ Fig. 10.16.

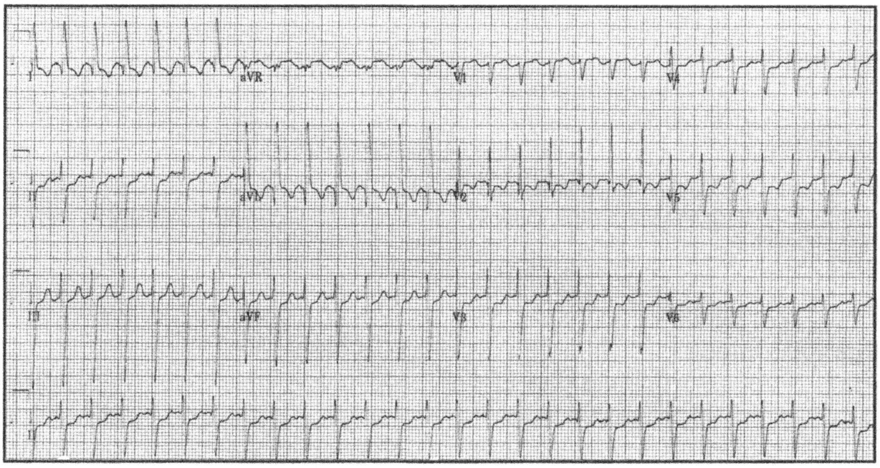

Fig. 10.15
12-lead ECG in a 31-year-old woman with tricuspid atresia, ASD, and VSD, status post old-style Fontan later revised to an extracardiac conduit with a right atrial Maze procedure. An IART with a ventricular response rate of 167 bpm was electrically cardioverted. Note the characteristic left axis deviation

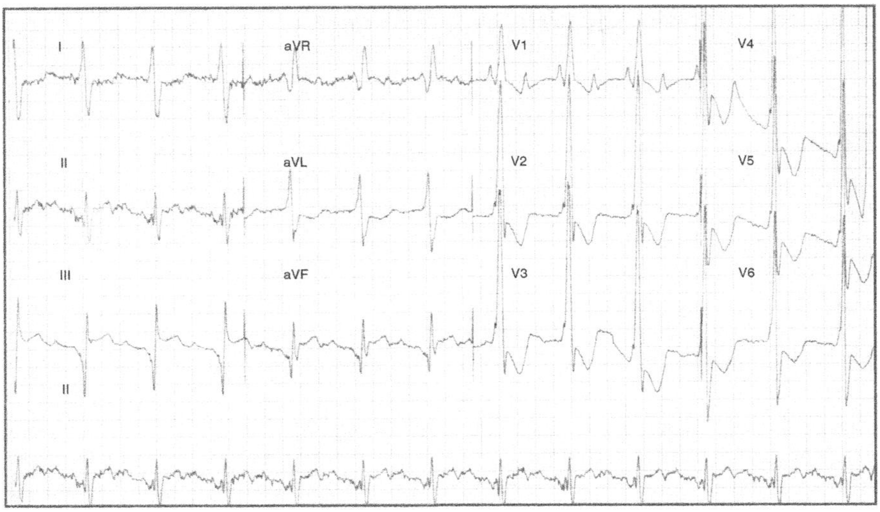

Fig. 10.16
12-lead ECG in a 24-year-old man with mitral atresia and hypoplastic left ventricle status post old-style Fontan. Note the IART at a cycle length of 370 ms with 2:1 AV conduction. Right ventricular hypertrophy criteria are met and the frontal QRS axis is superior, typical of univentricular hearts of right ventricular morphology

10.3.12 Cardiac Malpositions

In dextrocardia with situs inversus, also called mirror-image dextrocardia, the ventricles are inverted, as are the viscera and the atria. The heart usually functions normally and the diagnosis is often fortuitous. In mesocardia, the heart is centrally located in the chest with normal atrial and visceral anatomy. The apex is central or rightwardly displaced on chest radiography. Typically, no associated cardiac malformations are present. When dextrocardia with situs solitus occurs, as illustrated in Fig. 10.17, the ventricles are inverted, but not the viscera or atria. Associated severe cardiac malformations are typical [4].

The ECG is of considerable diagnostic importance in dextrocardia with situs inversus. As previously discussed, the right atrium and sinus node are positioned on the patient's left side, yielding a P-wave axis that remains inferiorly oriented but rightwardly displaced. In the absence of an ectopic focus, P-waves are upright in aVR and inverted in I and aVL [199–202]. Ventricular depolarization and repolarization occur in an inverse fashion. In lead I, the QRS is predominantly negative with T-wave inversion. Right precordial leads resemble the left precordial leads of normal hearts, aVL resembles aVR, and vice versa. Thus, left ventricular hypertrophy is manifested by tall R-waves in V1 and V2. Right ventricular hypertrophy is reflected by deeper Q-waves and small R-waves in lead I and taller R-waves over right lateral chest leads (e.g., V5R and V6R) [199, 200].

10.3.13 Coronary Anomalies

Isolated ectopic or anomalous origins of the coronary arteries are seen in 0.6–1.5% of patients undergoing coronary angiography [203]. The prognosis is favorable if the anomalous coronary artery does not course between the pulmonary artery and aorta. The most common anomalies are not associated with myocardial ischemia and include ectopic origin of the left circumflex artery from the right sinus of Valsalva; anomalous origin of the right coronary artery from the left sinus, and anomalous origin of the left main coronary artery from the right sinus. In coronary-cameral fistulas, the ECG is typically normal until volume overload of the receiving chamber occurs with or without ischemic changes related to coronary steal [204–206].

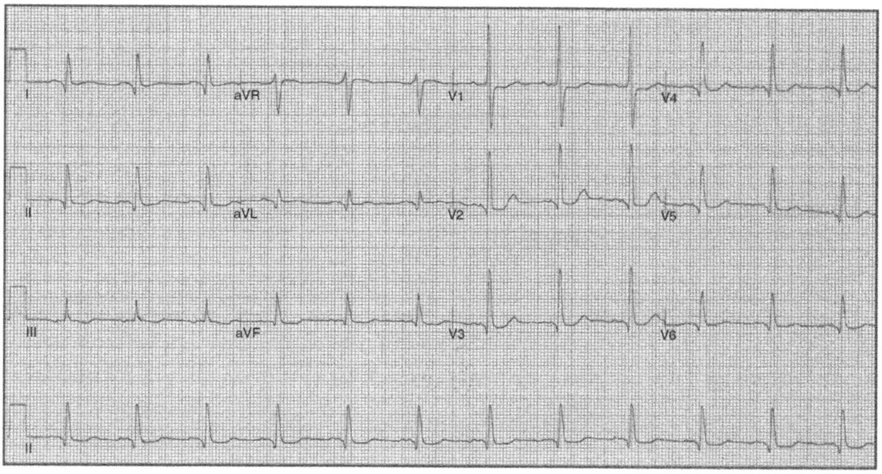

Fig. 10.17
12-lead ECG in a 45-year-old man with situs solitus, dextrocardia, anomalous pulmonary venous return, single atrium, and pulmonary stenosis. The P-wave vector is directed leftward and somewhat inferiorly, with an axis of 30° that is consistent with atrial situs solitus and normal position of the sinus node. Note the reverse R-wave progression pattern, with decreasing amplitude from leads V1 to V6. The pathologic Q-wave in lead I may reflect right ventricular hypertrophy in the setting of pulmonary stenosis

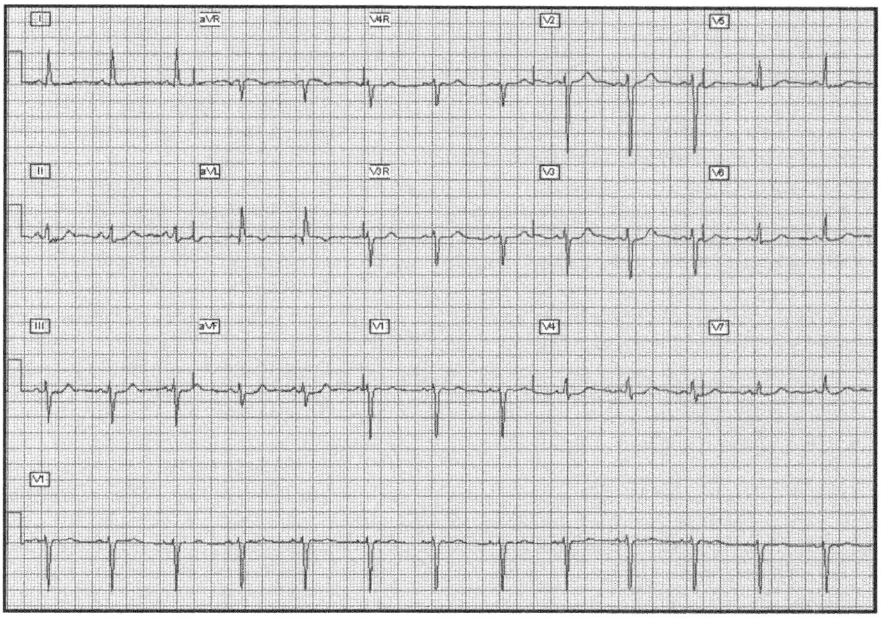

Fig. 10.18
15-lead ECG in a 35-year-old woman with anomalous origin of the left coronary artery from the pulmonary artery. She presented with chest pain at 13 years of age and underwent a Takeuchi repair. Note the loss of R-wave amplitude with no R-wave progression over precordial leads V1–V3, consistent with an old anteroseptal myocardial infarction

The ECG is useful in the diagnosis of anomalous origin of the left coronary artery from the pulmonary trunk. This is the most common anomaly associated with myocardial ischemia, with 25% of cases surviving to adolescence or adulthood [207]. As a result of decreased perfusion pressure and hypoxemic blood flow through the left coronary artery, anterolateral myocardial infarction usually occurs prior to the clinical recognition of this entity. The 12-lead ECG, therefore, displays pathologic Q-waves in leads I, aVL, and V4–V6 that are typically deep [208–214]. In addition, the posterobasal portion of the left ventricle appears to selectively hypertrophy [211]. This may result in left axis deviation, a pattern consistent with left ventricular hypertrophy, and nonspecific repolarization changes [208–211, 214]. Anteroseptal myocardial infarction patterns have also been described, as depicted in ➋ Fig. 10.18.

References

1. Perloff, J.K. and C.A. Warnes, Challenges posed by adults with repaired congenital heart disease. *Circulation*, 2001;**103**(21): 2637–2643.
2. Warnes, C.A., R. Liberthson, G.K. Danielson, et al., Task force 1: the changing profile of congenital heart disease in adult life. *J. Am. Coll. Cardiol.*, 2001;**37**(5): 1170–1175.
3. Gatzoulis, M.A., S. Hechter, S.C. Siu, and G.D. Webb, Outpatient clinics for adults with congenital heart disease: increasing workload and evolving patterns of referral. *Heart*, 1999;**81**(1):57–61.
4. Marelli, A. and Moodie D. Adult congenital heart disease, in *Textbook of Cardiovascular Medicine*, 2nd edn., E. Topol, Editor. Philadelphia, PA: Lippincott Williams & Wilkins, 2002, pp. 709–731.
5. Moller, J.H., K.A. Taubert, H.D. Allen, E.B. Clark, and R.M. Laurer, Cardiovascular health and disease in children: current status. *Circulation*, 1994;**89**: 923–930.
6. Gatzoulis, M.A. and G.D. Webb, Adults with congenital heart disease: a growing population, in *Diagnosis and Management of Adult Congenital Heart Disease*, M.A. Gatzoulis and G.D. Webb, From chapter P.E.F. Daubeney, Editors. London: Churchill Livingston, 2003, pp. 3–6.
7. Kanter, R.J. and A. Garson, Jr., Atrial arrhythmias during chronic follow-up of surgery for complex congenital heart disease. *Pacing Clin. Electrophysiol.*, 1997;**20**(2 Pt 2): 502–511.
8. Engelfriet, P., E. Boersma, E. Oechslin, et al., The spectrum of adult congenital heart disease in Europe: morbidity and mortality in a 5 year follow-up period. *Eur. Heart J.*, 2005; **26**(21): 2325–2333.
9. Ho, S.Y., J.L. Monro, and R.H. Anderson, Disposition of the sinus node in left-sided juxtaposition of the atrial appendages. *Br. Heart J.*, 1979;**41**(2): 129–132.
10. Anjos, R.T., S.Y. Ho, and R.H. Anderson, Surgical implications of juxtaposition of the atrial appendages. A review of forty-nine autopsied hearts. *J. Thorac. Cardiovasc. Surg.*, 1990;**99**(5): 897–904.
11. Rossi, L., S. Montella, C. Frescura, and G. Thiene, Congenital atrioventricular block in right atrial isomerism (asplenia). A case due to atrionodal discontinuity. *Chest*, 1984;**85**(4):578–580.
12. Dickinson, D.F., J.L. Wilkinson, K.R. Anderson, A. Smith, S.Y. Ho, and R.H. Anderson, The cardiac conduction system in situs ambiguus. *Circulation*, 1979;**59**(5): 879–885.
13. Wren, C., F.J. Macartney, and J.E. Deanfield, Cardiac rhythm in atrial isomerism. *Am. J. Cardiol.*, 1987;**59**(12): 1156–1158.
14. Momma, K., A. Takao, and T. Shibata, Characteristics and natural history of abnormal atrial rhythms in left isomerism. *Am. J. Cardiol.*, 1990;**65**(3): 231–236.
15. Moorman, A.F.M., F. de Jong, M.M.F.J. Denyn, and W.H. Lamers. Development of the cardiac conduction system. *Circ. Res.*, 1998;**82**: 629–644.
16. Anderson, R.H. and S.Y. Ho, The morphology of the specialized atrioventricular junctional area: the evolution of understanding. *Pacing Clin. Electrophysiol.*, 2002;**25**(6): 957.
17. Anderson, R.H. and S.Y. Ho, The morphology of the cardiac conduction system. *Novartis Found. Symp.*, 2003;**250**: 6–17.
18. Campbell, R.M., M. Dick, P. Hees, and D.M. Behrendt, Epicardial and endocardial activation in patients with endocardial cushion defect. *Am. J. Cardiol.*, 1983;**51**(2): 277–281.
19. Borkon, A.M., D.R. Pieroni, P.J. Varghese, C.S. Ho, and R.D. Rowe. The superior QRS axis in ostium primum ASD: a proposed mechanism. *Am. Heart J.*, 1975;**90**(2): 215–221.
20. Anderson, R.H., R. Arnold, and J.L. Wilkinson, The conducting system in congenitally corrected transposition. *Lancet*, 1973;**1**(7815): 1286–1288.
21. Anderson, R.H., A.E. Becker, R. Arnold, and J.L. Wilkinson, The conducting tissues in congenitally corrected transposition. *Circulation*, 1974;**50**(5): 911–923.
22. Guller, B., J.W. DuShane, and J.L. Titus. The atrioventricular conduction system in two cases of tricuspid atresia. *Circulation*, 1969;**40**(2): 217–226.
23. Bharati, S. and M. Lev, The conduction system in tricuspid atresia with and without regular (d-) transposition. *Circulation*, 1977;**56**(3): 423–429.
24. Bharati, S. and M. Lev, The course of the conduction system in single ventricle with inverted (L-) loop and inverted (L-) transposition. *Circulation*, 1975;**51**(4): 723–730.
25. Wilkinson, J.L., D. Dickinson, A. Smith, and R.H. Anderson, Conducting tissues in univentricular heart of right ventricular type with double or common inlet. *J. Thorac. Cardiovasc. Surg.*, 1979;**77**(5): 691–698.
26. Gatzoulis, M.A., M.A. Freeman, S.C. Siu, G.D. Webb, and L. Harris, Atrial arrhythmia after surgical closure of atrial septal defects in adults. *N. Engl. J. Med.*, 1999;**340**(11): 839–846.
27. Attie, F., M. Rosas, N. Granados, C. Zabal, A. Buendia, and J. Calderon, Surgical treatment for secundum atrial septal defects in patients > 40 years old. A randomized clinical trial. *J. Am. Coll. Cardiol.*, 2001;**38**(7): 2035–2042.
28. Donti, A., M. Bonvicini, and A. Placci, et al., Surgical treatment of secundum atrial septal defect in patients older than 50 years. *Ital. Heart J.*, 2001;**2**(6): 428–432.
29. Silversides, C.K., S.C. Siu, P.R. McLaughlin, et al., Symptomatic atrial arrhythmias and transcatheter closure of atrial septal defects in adult patients. *Heart*, 2004;**90**(10): 1194–1198.

30. Zufelt, K., H.C. Rosenberg, M.D. Li, and G.I. Joubert, The electrocardiogram and the secundum atrial septal defect: a reexamination in the era of echocardiography. *Can. J. Cardiol.*, 1998;**14**(2): 227–232.
31. Tan, K.T., A. Takao, A. Hashimoto, and T. Sato, Electrocardiogram of secumdum type atrial septal defect simulating endocardial cushion defect. *Br. Heart. J.*, 1975;**37**(2): 209–215.
32. Mori, H., K. Mikawa, T. Niki, T. Nagao, and S. Matsumo, QRS waves of the spatial velocity electrocardiogram in atrial septal defect. *Jpn. Heart J.*, 1972;**13**(5): 407–417.
33. Boineau, J.P., M.S. Spach, and C.R. Ayers, Genesis of the electrocardiogram in atrial septal defect. *Am. Heart J.*, 1964;**68**: 637–651.
34. Dreifus, L.S., S. Bender, H. Goldberg, and D.F. Downing, The electrocardiogram in atrial septal defect. *Dis. Chest*, 1959;**36**: 521–527.
35. Rodriguez-Alvarez, A., G. Martinez De Rodriguez, A.M. Goggans, et al., The vectorcardiographic equivalent of the "crochetage" of the QRS of the electrocardiogram in atrial septal defect of the ostium secundum type. Preliminary report. *Am. Heart J.*, 1959;**58**: 388–394.
36. Burch, G.E. and N. Depasquale, The electrocardiogram and ventricular gradient in atrial septal defect. *Am. Heart J.*, 1959;**58**(2): 190–203.
37. Toscano Barboza, E., R.O. Brandenburg, and H.J. Swan, Atrial septal defect; the electrocardiogram and its hemodynamic correlation in 100 proved cases. *Am. J. Cardiol.*, 1958;**2**(6): 698–713.
38. Milnor, W.R. and C.A. Bertrand, The electrocardiogram in atrial septal defect; a study of twenty-four cases, with observations on the RSR'-V1 pattern. *Am. J. Med.*, 1957;**22**(2): 223–233.
39. Barber, J.M. and O. Magidson, Atrial septal defect with special reference to the electrocardiogram. *Br. Heart J.*, 1950;**12**(2): 203–204.
40. Sung, R.J., D.M. Tamer, A.S. Agha, A. Castellanos, R.J. Myerburg, and H. Gelband, Etiology of the electrocardiographic pattern of "incomplete right bundle branch block" in atrial septal defect: an electrophysiologic study. *J. Pediatr.*, 1975;**87**(6 Pt 2): 1182–1186.
41. Anderson, P.A., M.C. Rogers, R.V. Canent Jr., and M.S. Spach, Atrioventricular conduction in secundum atrial septal defects. *Circulation*, 1973;**48**(1): 27–31.
42. Clark, E.B. and J.D. Kugler, Preoperative secundum atrial septal defect with coexisting sinus node and atrioventricular node dysfunction. *Circulation*, 1982;**65**(5): 976–980.
43. Emanuel, R., K. O'Brien, J. Somerville, K. Jefferson, and M. Hegde, Proceedings: association of secundum atrial septal defect with abnormalities of atrioventricular conduction or left axis deviation: a new syndrome. *Br. Heart J.*, 1976;**38**(5): 536.
44. Yamaki, S., T. Horiuchi, M. Miura, Y. Suzuki, E. Ishizawa, and T. Takahashi, Pulmonary vascular disease in secundum atrial septal defect with pulmonary hypertension. *Chest*, 1986; **89**(5): 694–698.
45. Heath, D., H.F. Helmholz Jr., H.B. Burchell, J.W. Dushane, and J.E. Edwards, Graded pulmonary vascular changes and hemodynamic findings in cases of atrial and ventricular septal defect and patent ductus arteriosus. *Circulation*, 1958; **18**(6): 1155–1166.
46. Emanuel, R., K. O'Brien, J. Somerville, K. Jefferson, and M. Hegde, Association of secundum atrial septal defect with abnormalities of atrioventricular conduction or left axis deviation. Genetic study of 10 families. *Br. Heart J.*, 1975;**37**(10): 1085–1092.
47. Heller, J., A.A. Hagege, B. Besse, M. Desnos, F.N. Marie, and C. Guerot, "Crochetage" (notch) on R wave in inferior limb leads: a new independent electrocardiographic sign of atrial septal defect. *J. Am. Coll. Cardiol.*, 1996;**27**(4): 877–882.
48. Cohen, J.S., D.J. Patton, and R.M. Giuffre, The crochetage pattern in electrocardiograms of pediatric atrial septal defect patients. *Can. J. Cardiol.*, 2000;**16**(10): 1241–1247.
49. Therrien, J., A. Dore, W. Gersony, et al., CCS Consensus Conference 2001 update: recommendations for the management of adults with congenital heart disease. Part I. *Can. J. Cardiol.* 2001;**17**(9): 940–959.
50. Liberman, L., S. Kaufman, M. Alfayyadh, A.J. Hordof, and H.D. Apfel, Noninvasive prediction of pulmonary artery pressure in patients with isolated ventricular septal defect. *Pediatr. Cardiol.*, 2000;**21**(3): 197–201.
51. Cohle, S.D., E. Balraj, and M. Bell, Sudden death due to ventricular septal defect. *Pediatr. Dev. Pathol.*, 1999;**2**(4): 327–332.
52. Sarubbi, B., L.M. Gerlis, S.Y. Ho, and J. Somerville, Sudden death in an adult with a small ventricular septal defect and an aneurysmal membranous septum. *Cardiol. Young*, 1999;**9**(1): 99–103.
53. Byard, R.W., Ventricular septal defect and sudden death in early childhood. *J. Paediatr. Child Health*, 1994;**30**(5): 439–440.
54. Smith, N.M. and S.Y. Ho, Heart block and sudden death associated with fibrosis of the conduction system at the margin of a ventricular septal defect. *Pediatr. Cardiol.*, 1994;**15**(3): 139–142.
55. Fournier, A., M.L. Young, O.L. Garcia, D.F. Tamer, and G.S. Wolff, Electrophysiologic cardiac function before and after surgery in children with atrioventricular canal. *Am. J. Cardiol.*, 1986;**57**(13): 1137–1141.
56. Moller, J.H., C. Patton, R.L. Varco, and C.W. Lillehei, Late results (30 to 35 years) after operative closure of isolated ventricular septal defect from 1954 to 1960. *Am. J. Cardiol.*, 1991;**68**(15): 1491–1497.
57. Knauth, A.L., J.E. Lock, S.B. Perry, et al., Transcatheter device closure of congenital and postoperative residual ventricular septal defects. *Circulation*, 2004;**110**(5): 501–507.
58. Thanopoulos, B.D. and M.L. Rigby, Outcome of transcatheter closure of muscular ventricular septal defects with the Amplatzer ventricular septal defect occluder. *Heart*, 2005;**91**(4): 513–516.
59. Pedra, C.A., S.R. Pedra, C.A. Esteves, F. Chamie, L.A. Christiani, and V.F. Fontes, Transcatheter closure of perimembranous ventricular septal defects. *Expert Rev. Cardiovasc. Ther.*, 2004;**2**(2): 253–264.
60. Papadopoulos, C., Y.C. Lee, and L. Scherlis, Isolated ventricular septal defect. Electrocardiographic, vectorcardiographic and catheterization data. *Am. J. Cardiol.* 1965;**16**(3): 359–368.
61. Toscano-Barboza, E., and J.W. Dushane, Ventricular septal defect: correlation of electrocardiographic and hemodynamic findings in 60 proved cases. *Am. J. Cardiol.*, 1959;**3**(6): 721–732.
62. Riggs, T., S. Mehta, S. Hirschfeld, G. Borkat, and J. Liebman, Ventricular septal defect in infancy: a combined vectorgraphic and echocardiographic study. *Circulation*, 1979;**59**(2): 385–394.
63. Katz, L.N. and H. Wachtel, The diphasic QRS type of electrocardiogram in congenital heart disease. *Am. Heart J.*, 1937;**13**: 22.
64. Kidd, L., D.J. Driscoll, W.M. Gersony, et al., Second natural history study of congenital heart defects: results of treatment of patients with ventricular septal defects. *Circulation*, 1993;**87**(Suppl. 1): I-38–I-59.
65. Blake, S., E. Chung, H. Wesley, and K. Hallidie-Smith, Conduction defects, ventricular arrhythmias, and late death after

surgical closure of ventricular septal defect. *Br. Heart J.*, 1982;**47**: 305–315.
66. Cantor, W.J., D.A. Harrison, J.S. Moussadji, et al., Determinants of survival and length of survival in adults with Eisenmenger syndrome. *Am. J. Cardiol.*, 1999;**84**(6): 677–681.
67. Saha, A., K.G. Balakrishnan, P.K. Jaiswal, et al., Prognosis for patients with Eisenmenger syndrome of various aetiology. *Int. J. Cardiol.*, 1994;**45**(3): 199–207.
68. Vetter, V.L. and L.N. Horowitz, Electrophysiologic residua and sequelae of surgery for congenital heart defects. *Am. J. Cardiol.*, 1982;**50**(3): 588–604.
69. Daliento, L., G. Rizzoli, M.C. Marchiori, et al., Electrical instability in patients undergoing surgery for atrioventricular septal defect. *Int. J. Cardiol.*, 1991;**30**(1): 15–21.
70. McGrath, L.B. and L. Gonzalez-Lavin, Actuarial survival, freedom from reoperation, and other events after repair of atrioventricular septal defects. *J. Thorac. Cardiovasc. Surg.*, 1987;**94**(4): 582–590.
71. Culpepper, W., J. Kolff, C.Y. Lin, et al., Complete common atrioventricular canal in infancy – surgical repair and postoperative hemodynamics. *Circulation*, 1978;**58**(3): 550–558.
72. Rastelli, G.C., P.A. Ongley, J.W. Kirklin, and D.C. McGoon, Surgical repair of the complete form of persistent common atrioventricular canal. *J. Thorac. Cardiovasc. Surg.*, 1968;**55**(3): 299–308.
73. Jacobsen, J.R., P.C. Gillette, B.N. Corbett, M. Rabinovitch, and D.G. McNamara, Intracardiac electrography in endocardial cushion defects. *Circulation*, 1976;**54**(4): 599–603.
74. Boineau, J.P., E.N. Moore, and D.F. Patterson, Relationship between the ECG, ventricular activation, and the ventricular conduction system in ostium primum ASD. *Circulation*, 1973;**48**(3): 556–564.
75. Feldt, R.H., J.W. DuShane, and J.L. Titus, The atrioventricular conduction system in persistent common atrioventricular canal defect: correlations with electrocardiogram. *Circulation*, 1970;**42**(3): 437–444.
76. Durrer, D., J.P. Roos, and R.T. van Dam, The genesis of the electrocardiogram of patients with ostium primum defects (ventral atrial septal defects). *Am. Heart J.*, 1966;**71**(5): 642–650.
77. Coelho, E., S. Sequerra Amran, and E.S.A. Bordalo, Electrocardiogram and vectorcardiogram of ostium secundum and ostium primum. *Cardiologia*, 1960;**37**: 319–330.
78. Waldo, A.L., G.A. Kaiser, F.O. Bowman Jr., and J.R. Malm, Etiology of prolongation of the P-R interval in patients with an endocardial cushion defect. Further observations on internodal conduction and the polarity of the retrograde P wave. *Circulation*, 1973;**48**(1): 19–26.
79. Suzuki, K., Y. Murakami, K. Tatsuno, et al., Atypical form of atrioventricular septal defect without left axis deviation: relation between morphology and unusual QRS axis. *Br. Heart J.*, 1993;**70**(2): 180–184.
80. Cosh, J.A., Patent ductus arteriosus; a follow-up study of 73 cases. *Br. Heart J.*, 1957;**19**(1): 13–22.
81. Marquis, R.M., H.C. Miller, R.J. McCormack, M.B. Matthews, and A.H. Kitchin, Persistence of ductus arteriosus with left to right shunt in the older patient. *Br. Heart J.*, 1982;**48**(5): 469–484.
82. Mirowski, M., F. Arevalo, G.A. Medrano, and F.A. Cisneros, Conduction disturbances in patent ductus arteriosus. A study of 20 cases before and after surgery with determination of the P-R index. *Circulation*, 1962;**25**: 807–813.
83. Danilowicz, D., J.I. Hoffman, and A.M. Rudolph, Serial studies of pulmonary stenosis in infancy and childhood. *Br. Heart J.*, 1975;**37**(8): 808–818.
84. Rasmussen, K. and S.J. Sorland, Prediction of right ventricular systolic pressure in pulmonary stenosis from combined vectorcardiographic data. *Am. Heart J.*, 1973;**86**(3): 318–328.
85. Yahini, J.H., M.J. Dulfano, and M. Toor, Pulmonic stenosis. A clinical assessment of severity. *Am. J. Cardiol.*, 1960;**5**: 744–757.
86. Macruz, R., J.K. Perloff, and R.B. Case, A method for the electrocardiographic recognition of atrial enlargement. *Circulation*, 1958;**17**(5): 882–889.
87. Abrahams, D.G. and P. Wood, Pulmonary stenosis with normal aortic root. *Br. Heart J.*, 1951;**13**(4): 419–448.
88. Vriend, J.W. and B.J. Mulder, Late complications in patients after repair of aortic coarctation: implications for management. *Int. J. Cardiol.*, 2005;**101**(3): 399–406.
89. Toro-Salazar, O.H., J. Steinberger, W. Thomas, A.P. Rocchini, B. Carpenter, and J.H. Moller, Long-term follow-up of patients after coarctation of the aorta repair. *Am. J. Cardiol.*, 2002;**89**(5): 541–547.
90. Silka, M.J., B.G. Hardy, V.D. Menashe, and C.D. Morris. A population-based prospective evaluation of risk of sudden cardiac death after operation for common congenital heart defects. *J. Am. Coll. Cardiol.*, 1998;**32**(1): 245–251.
91. Gaum, W.E., T.C. Chou, and S. Kaplan, The vectorcardiogram and electrocardiogram in supravalvular aortic stenosis and coarctation of the aorta. *Am. Heart J.*, 1972;**84**(5): 620–628.
92. Glancy, D.L., A.G. Morrow, A.L. Simon, and W.C. Roberts, Juxtaductal aortic coarctation. Analysis of 84 patients studied hemodynamically, angiographically, and morphologically after age 1 year. *Am. J. Cardiol.*, 1983;**51**(3): 537–551.
93. Ho, S.Y., D. Goltz, K. McCarthy, et al., The atrioventricular junctions in Ebstein malformation. *Heart*, 2000;**83**(4): 444–449.
94. Smith, W.M., J.J. Gallagher, C.R. Kerr, et al., The electrophysiologic basis and management of symptomatic recurrent tachycardia in patients with Ebstein's anomaly of the tricuspid valve. *Am. J. Cardiol.*, 1982;**49**(5): 1223–1234.
95. Hebe, J., Ebstein's anomaly in adults. Arrhythmias: diagnosis and therapeutic approach. *Thorac. Cardiovasc. Surg.*, 2000;**48**(4): 214–219.
96. Attie, F., M. Rosas, M. Rijlaarsdam, et al., The adult patient with Ebstein anomaly. Outcome in 72 unoperated patients. *Medicine* (Baltimore), 2000;**79**(1): 27–36.
97. Celemajer, D., C. Bull, J. Till, et al., Ebstein's anomaly: presentation and outcome from fetus to adult. *J. Am. Coll. Cardiol.*, 1994;**23**: 170–176.
98. Gentles, T., A. Calder, P. Clarkson, and J. Neutze, Predictors of long-term survival with Ebstein's anomaly of the tricuspid valve. *Am. J. Cardiol.*, 1992;**69**: 377–381.
99. Hernandez, F.A., R. Rochkind, and H.R. Cooper, The intracavitary electrocardiogram in the diagnosis of Ebstein's anomaly. *Am. J. Cardiol.*, 1958;**1**(2): 181–190.
100. Van Lingen, B. and S.R. Bauersfeld, The electrocardiogram in Ebstein's anomaly of the tricuspid valve. *Am. Heart J.*, 1955;**50**(1): 13–23.
101. Macruz, R., J. Tranchesi, M. Ebaid, F. Pileggi, A. Romero, and L.V. Decourt, Ebstein's disease. Electrovectorcardiographic and radiologic correlations. *Am. J. Cardiol.*, 1968;**21**(5): 653–660.
102. Kastor, J.A., B.N. Goldreyer, M.E. Josephson, et al., Electrophysiologic characteristics of Ebstein's anomaly of the tricuspid valve. *Circulation*, 1975;**52**(6): 987–995.

103. Genton, E. and S.G. Blount Jr., The spectrum of Ebstein's anomaly. *Am. Heart. J.*, 1967;**73**(3): 395–425.
104. Tede, N.H., K. Shivkumar, J.K. Perloff, et al., Signal-averaged electrocardiogram in Ebstein's anomaly. *Am. J. Cardiol.*, 2004; **93**(4): 432–436.
105. Follath, F. and K.A. Hallidie-Smith, Unusual electrocardiographic changes in Ebstein's anomaly. *Br. Heart J.*, 1972;**34**(5): 513–519.
106. Schiebler, G.L., P. Adams Jr., R.C. Anderson, K. Amplatz, and R.G. Lester, Clinical study of twenty-three cases of Ebstein's anomaly of the tricuspid valve. *Circulation*, 1959;**19**(2): 165–187.
107. Bialostozky, D., G.A. Medrano, L. Munoz, and R. Contreras, Vectorcardiographic study and anatomic observations in 21 cases of Ebstein's malformation of the tricuspid valve. *Am. J. Cardiol.*, 1972;**30**(4): 354–361.
108. Kumar, A.E., D.C. Fyler, O.S. Miettinen, and A.S. Nadas, Ebstein's anomaly. Clinical profile and natural history. *Am. J. Cardiol.*, 1971;**28**(1): 84–95.
109. Brickner, M.E., L.D. Hillis, and R.A. Lange, Congenital heart disease in adults. Second of two parts. *N. Engl. J. Med.* 2000;**342**(5): 334–342.
110. Lillehei, C.W., M. Cohen, and H.E. Warden, Direct vision intracardiac surgical correction of the tetralogy of Fallot, pentalogy of Fallot, and pulmonary atresia defects: report of the first ten cases. *Ann. Surg.*, 1955;**142**: 418–445.
111. Li, W. and J. Somerville, Atrial flutter in grown-up congenital heart (GUCH) patients. Clinical characteristics of affected population. *Int. J. Cardiol.*, 2000;**75**(2–3): 129–137.
112. Gatzoulis, M.A., S. Balaji, S.A. Webber, et al., Risk factors for arrhythmia and sudden cardiac death late after repair of tetralogy of Fallot: a multicentre study. *Lancet*, 2000;**356**(9234): 975–981.
113. Delacretaz, E., L.I. Ganz, K. Soejima, et al., Multi atrial macro-re-entry circuits in adults with repaired congenital heart disease: entrainment mapping combined with three-dimensional electroanatomic mapping. *J. Am. Coll. Cardiol.*, 2001;**37**(6): 1665–1676.
114. Nakagawa, H., N. Shah, K. Matsudaira, et al., Characterization of reentrant circuit in macroreentrant right atrial tachycardia after surgical repair of congenital heart disease: isolated channels between scars allow "focal" ablation. *Circulation*, 2001;**103**(5): 699–709.
115. Triedman, J.K., M.E. Alexander, B.A. Love, et al., Influence of patient factors and ablative technologies on outcomes of radiofrequency ablation of intra-atrial re-entrant tachycardia in patients with congenital heart disease. *J. Am. Coll. Cardiol.*, 2002;**39**(11): 1827–1835.
116. Triedman, J.K., K.J. Jenkins, S.D. Colan, J.P. Saul, and E.P. Walsh, Intra-atrial reentrant tachycardia after palliation of congenital heart disease: characterization of multiple macroreentrant circuits using fluoroscopically based three-dimensional endocardial mapping. *J. Cardiovasc. Electrophysiol.*, 1997;**8**(3): 259–270.
117. Harrison, D.A., S.C. Siu, F. Hussain, C.J. MacLoghlin, G.D. Webb, and L. Harris, Sustained atrial arrhythmias in adults late after repair of tetralogy of fallot. *Am. J. Cardiol.*, 2001;**87**(5): 584–588.
118. Therrien, J., S.C. Siu, L. Harris, et al., Impact of pulmonary valve replacement on arrhythmia propensity late after repair of tetralogy of Fallot. *Circulation*, 2001;**103**(20): 2489–2494.
119. Gillette, P.C. and A. Garson Jr., Sudden cardiac death in the pediatric population. *Circulation*, 1992;**85**(Suppl. 1): 164–169.
120. Nollert, G., T. Fischlein, S. Bouterwek, C. Bohmer, W. Klinner, and B. Reichart, Long-term survival in patients with repair of tetralogy of Fallot: 36-year follow-up of 490 survivors of the first year after surgical repair. *J. Am. Coll. Cardiol.*, 1997;**30**(5): 1374–1383.
121. Jonsson, H., T. Ivert, L.A. Brodin, and R. Jonasson, Late sudden deaths after repair of tetralogy of Fallot. Electrocardiographic findings associated with survival. *Scand. J. Thorac. Cardiovasc. Surg.*, 1995;**29**(3): 131–139.
122. Bricker, J.T., Sudden death and tetralogy of Fallot. Risks, markers, and causes. *Circulation*, 1995;**92**(2): 158–159.
123. Roberts, D.L., H.R. Wagner, and E.C. Lambert, The electrocardiogram in tetralogy of Fallot. *J. Electrocardiol.*, 1972;**5**(2): 155–161.
124. Feldt, R.H., J.W. DuShane, and J.L. Titus, The anatomy of the atrioventricular conduction system in ventricular septal defect and tetralogy of fallot: correlations with the electrocardiogram and vectorcardiogram. *Circulation*, 1966;**34**(5): 774–782.
125. Landtman, B. and M.D. Wolf, Total correction of tetralogy of Fallot: II. Changes in the electrocardiogram following surgery. *Circulation*, 1965;**31**: 394–402.
126. Mirowski, M., A. Mehrizi, and H.B. Taussig, The electrocardiogram in patients with both great vessels arising from the right ventricle combined with pulmonary stenosis. An analysis of 22 cases with special reference to the differential diagnosis from the tetralogy of Fallot. *Circulation*, 1963;**28**: 1116–1127.
127. Depasquale, N.P. and G.E. Burch, The electrocardiogram, vectorcardiogram, and ventricular gradient in the tetralogy of Fallot. *Circulation*, 1961;**24**: 94–109.
128. Pileggi, F., J. Bocanegra, J. Tranchesi, et al., The electrocardiogram in tetralogy of Fallot: a study of 142 cases. *Am. Heart J.*, 1960;**59**: 667–680.
129. Gardberg, M. and I.L. Rosen, The electrocardiogram and vectorcardiogram in right ventricular hypertrophy and right bundle branch block. *Dis. Chest.*, 1959;**36**: 407–422.
130. Milnor, W.R. Electrocardiogram and vectorcardiogram in right ventricular hypertrophy and right bundle-branch block. *Circulation*, 1957;**16**(3): 348–367.
131. DiSciascio, G. and L.M. Bargeron Jr., The electrocardiogram in tetralogy of Fallot with complete atrioventricular canal. *Tex. Heart Inst. J.*, 1982;**9**(2): 163–167.
132. Norgard, G., M.A. Gatzoulis, F. Moraes, et al., Relationship between type of outflow tract repair and postoperative right ventricular diastolic physiology in tetralogy of Fallot: implications for long-term outcome. *Circulation*, 1996;**94**(12): 3276–3280.
133. Gatzoulis, M.A., J.A. Till, J. Somerville, and A.N. Redington, Mechanoelectrical interaction in tetralogy of Fallot. QRS prolongation relates to right ventricular size and predicts malignant ventricular arrhythmias and sudden death. *Circulation*, 1995;**92**(2): 231–237.
134. Till, J.A., M.A. Gatzoulis, J.E. Deanfield, J. Somerville, W. Gregory, and A.N. Redington, Evolution of QRS prolongation following repair of tetralogy of Fallot: implications for symptomatic arrhythmia and sudden death. *Circulation*, 1995;**92** (Suppl.): 1707.
135. Harrison, D.A., L. Harris, S.C. Siu, et al., Sustained ventricular tachycardia in adult patients late after repair of tetralogy of Fallot. *J. Am. Coll. Cardiol.*, 1997;**30**(5): 1368–1373.
136. Garson, A. Jr., M.R. Nihill, D.G. McNamara, and D.A. Cooley, Status of the adult and adolescent after repair of tetralogy of Fallot. *Circulation*, 1979;**59**: 1232–1240.

137. Katz, N.M., E.H. Blackstone, J.W. Kirklin, and A.D. Pacifico, Late survival and symptoms after repair of tetralogy of Fallot. *Circulation*, 1982;**65**: 403–410.
138. Hokanson, J.S. and J.H. Moller, Significance of early transient complete heart block as a predictor of sudden death late after operative correction of tetralogy of Fallot. *Am. J. Cardiol.*, 2001;**87**(11): 1271–1277.
139. Berul, C.I., S.L. Hill, R.L. Geggel, et al., Electrocardiographic markers of late sudden death risk in postoperative tetralogy of Fallot children. *J. Cardiovasc. Electrophysiol.*, 1997;**8**(12): 1349–1356.
140. Vogel, M., J. Sponring, S. Cullen, J.E. Deanfield, and A.N. Redington, Regional wall motion and abnormalities of electrical depolarization and repolarization in patients after surgical repair of tetralogy of Fallot. *Circulation*, 2001;**103**(12): 1669–1673.
141. Khairy, P., M.J. Landzberg, M.A. Gatzoulis, et al., Value of programmed ventricular stimulation after tetralogy of Fallot repair: a multicenter study. *Circulation*, 2004;**109**(16): 1994–2000.
142. Huhta, J.C., J.D. Maloney, D.G. Ritter, D.M. Ilstrup, and R.H. Feldt, Complete atrioventricular block in patients with atrioventricular discordance. *Circulation*, 1983;**67**(6): 1374–1377.
143. Daliento, L., D. Corrado, G. Buja, N. John, A. Nava, and G. Thiene, Rhythm and conduction disturbances in isolated, congenitally corrected transposition of the great arteries. *Am. J. Cardiol.*, 1986;**58**(3): 314–318.
144. Gillette, P.C., U. Busch, C.E. Mullins, and D.G. McNamara, Electrophysiologic studies in patients with ventricular inversion and "corrected transposition". *Circulation*, 1979;**60**(4): 939–945.
145. Amikam, S., J. Lemer, Y. Kishon, E. Riss, and H.N. Neufeld, Complete heart block in an adult with corrected transposition of the great arteries treated with permanent pacemaker. *Thorax*, 1979;**34**(4): 547–549.
146. Foster, J.R., A.N. Damato, L.E. Kline, M. Akhtar, and J.N. Ruskin, Congenitally corrected transposition of the great vessels: localization of the site of complete atrioventricular block using his bundle electrograms. *Am. J. Cardiol.*, 1976;**38**(3): 383–387.
147. Rosen, K.M., H.S. Loeb, R.M. Gunnar, and S.H. Rahimtoola, Mobitz type II block without bundle-branch block. *Circulation*, 1971;**44**(6): 1111–1119.
148. de Leval, M.R., P. Bastos, J. Stark, J.F. Taylor, F.J. Macartney, and R.H. Anderson, Surgical technique to reduce the risks of heart block following closure of ventricular septal defect in atrioventricular discordance. *J. Thorac. Cardiovasc. Surg.*, 1979;**78**(4): 515–526.
149. McGrath, L.B., J.W. Kirklin, E.H. Blackstone, A.D. Pacifico, J.K. Kirklin, and L.M. Bargeron, Jr., Death and other events after cardiac repair in discordant atrioventricular connection. *J. Thorac. Cardiovasc. Surg.*, 1985;**90**(5): 711–728.
150. Hwang, B., F. Bowman, J. Malm, and E. Krongrad, Surgical repair of congenitally corrected transposition of the great arteries: results and follow-up. *Am. J. Cardiol.*, 1982;**50**(4): 781–785.
151. Victorica, B.E., B.L. Miller, and I.H. Gessner, Electrocardiogram and vectorcardiogram in ventricular inversion (corrected transposition). *Am. Heart J.*, 1973;**86**(6): 733–744.
152. Okamura, K., A. Takao, A. Hashimoto, S. Hosoda, and K. Mimori, Electrocardiogram in corrected transposition of the great arteries with and without associated cardiac anomalies. *J. Electrocardiol.*, 1973;**6**(1): 3–10.
153. Fernandez, F., J. Laurichesse, L. Scebat, and L. Lenegre, Electrocardiogram in corrected transposition of the great vessels of the bulbo-ventricular inversion type. *Br. Heart J.*, 1970;**32**(2): 165–171.
154. Namin, E.P., R.A. Arcilla, and B.M. Gasul, The vectorcardiogram and electrocardiogram in corrected transposition of the great vessels. *Dis. Chest.*, 1963;**44**: 313–314.
155. Bokeriia, L.A., A. Revishvili, and M.M. Makhmudov, Syndrome of ventricular preexcitation and corrected transposition of the great vessels with insufficiency of the arterial atrioventricular valve of the Ebstein anomaly type. *Kardiologiia*, 1984;**24**(12): 94–95.
156. Rogers, J.H. Jr. and P.S. Rao, Ebstein's anomaly of the left atrioventricular valve with congenital corrected transposition of the great arteries. Diagnosis by intracavitary electrocardiography. *Chest*, 1977;**72**(2): 253–256.
157. Brugada, J., V. Valls, R. Freixa, et al., Radiofrequency ablation of a posteroseptal atrioventricular accessory pathway in a left-sided tricuspid ring with Ebsteinlike anomaly in a patient with congenitally corrected transposition of the great arteries. *Pacing Clin. Electrophysiol.*, 2000;**23**(1): 133–136.
158. Keller, N. and M.R. Soorensen, Corrected transposition of the great arteries with a left-sided Ebstein-like anomaly and WPW-syndrome. A case diagnosed by two-dimensional echocardiography. *Ugeskr Laeger*, 1981;**143**(31): 1971–1972.
159. Senning, A., Surgical correction of transposition of the great vessels. *Surgery*, 1959;**45**: 966–980.
160. Mustard, W.T., Successful two stage correction of transposition of the great vessels. *Surgery*, 1964;**55**: 469–472.
161. Jatene, A.D., V.F. Fontes, P.P. Paulista, et al., Anatomic correction of transposition of the great vessels. *J. Thorac. Cardiovasc. Surg.*, 1976;**72**(3): 364–370.
162. Wilson, N.J., P.M. Clarkson, B.G. Barratt-Boyes, et al., Long-term outcome after the mustard repair for simple transposition of the great arteries. 28-year follow-up. *J. Am. Coll. Cardiol.*, 1998;**32**(3): 758–765.
163. Janousek, J., T. Paul, I. Luhmer, M. Wilken, J. Hruda, H.C. Kallfelz, Atrial baffle procedures for complete transposition of the great arteries: natural course of sinus node dysfunction and risk factors for dysrhythmias and sudden death. *Z. Kardiol.*, 1994;**83**(12): 933–938.
164. Gatzoulis, M.A., J. Walters, P.R. McLaughlin, N. Merchant, G.D. Webb, and P. Liu, Late arrhythmia in adults with the mustard procedure for transposition of great arteries: a surrogate marker for right ventricular dysfunction? *Heart*, 2000;**84**(4): 409–415.
165. Gelatt, M., R.M. Hamilton, B.W. McCrindle, et al., Arrhythmia and mortality after the Mustard procedure: a 30-year single-center experience. *J. Am. Coll. Cardiol.*, 1997;**29**(1): 194–201.
166. Stark, J., M.J. Tynan, K.W. Ashcraft, E. Aberdeen, and D.J. Waterston, Obstruction of pulmonary veins and superior vena cava after the Mustard operation for transposition of the great arteries. *Circulation*, 1972;**45**(Suppl. 1): 1116–1120.
167. Benatar, A., R. Tanke, M. Roef, E.J. Meyboom, and H.J. Van de Wal, Mid-term results of the modified Senning operation for cavopulmonary connection with autologous tissue. *Eur. J. Cardiothorac. Surg.*, 1995;**9**(6): 320–324.
168. Kirjavainen, M., J.M. Happonen, and I. Louhimo, Late results of Senning operation. *J. Thorac. Cardiovasc. Surg.*, 1999;**117**(3): 488–495.

169. Khairy, P., M.J. Landzberg, J. Lambert, and C.P. O'Donnell, Long-term outcomes after the atrial switch for surgical correction of transposition: a meta-analysis comparing the Mustard and Senning procedures. *Cardiol. Young.*, 2004;**14**(3): 284–292.
170. Puley, G., S. Siu, M. Connelly, et al., Arrhythmia and survival in patients > 18 years of age after the mustard procedure for complete transposition of the great arteries. *Am. J. Cardiol.*, 1999;**83**(7): 1080–1084.
171. Li, W., J. Somerville, D.G. Gibson, and M.Y. Henein, Disturbed atrioventricular electromechanical function long after Mustard operation for transposition of great arteries: a potential contributing factor to atrial flutter. *J. Am. Soc. Echocardiogr.*, 2001;**14**(11): 1088–1093.
172. Sarkar, D., C. Bull, R. Yates, et al., Comparison of long-term outcomes of atrial repair of simple transposition with implications for a late arterial switch strategy. *Circulation*, 1999;**100**(Suppl. 19): II176–II181.
173. Kammeraad, J.A., C.H. van Deurzen, N. Sreeram, et al., Predictors of sudden cardiac death after Mustard or Senning repair for transposition of the great arteries. *J. Am. Coll. Cardiol.*, 2004;**44**(5): 1095.
174. Khoury, G.H., R.M. Shaher, R.S. Fowler, and J.D. Keith, Preoperative and postoperative electrocardiogram in complete transposition of the great vessels. *Am. Heart J.*, 1966;**72**(2): 199–205.
175. Shaher, R.M. and D.C. Deuchar, The electrocardiogram in complete transposition of the great vessels. *Br. Heart J.*, 1966;**28**(2): 265–275.
176. Bharati, S. and M. Lev, The conduction system in simple, regular (D-), complete transposition with ventricular septal defect. *J. Thorac. Cardiovasc. Surg.*, 1976;**72**(2): 194–201.
177. Fontan, F. and E. Baudet, Surgical repair of tricuspid atresia. *Thorax*, 1971;**26**(3): 240–258.
178. Gatzoulis, M.A., M.D. Munk, W.G. Williams, and G.D. Webb, Definitive palliation with cavopulmonary or aortopulmonary shunts for adults with single ventricle physiology. *Heart*, 2000;**83**(1): 51–57.
179. Love, B.A., K.K. Collins, E.P. Walsh, and J.K. Triedman, Electroanatomic characterization of conduction barriers in sinus/atrially paced rhythm and association with intra-atrial reentrant tachycardia circuits following congenital heart disease surgery. *J. Cardiovasc. Electrophysiol.*, 2001;**12**(1): 17–25.
180. Triedman, J.K., M.E. Alexander, C.I. Berul, L.M. Bevilacqua, and E.P. Walsh, Electroanatomic mapping of entrained and exit zones in patients with repaired congenital heart disease and intra-atrial reentrant tachycardia. *Circulation*, 2001;**103**(16): 2060–2065.
181. Setty, S.P., K. Finucane, J.R. Skinner, and A.R. Kerr, Extracardiac conduit with a limited maze procedure for the failing Fontan with atrial tachycardias. *Ann. Thorac. Surg.*, 2002;**74**(6): 1992–1997.
182. Petko, M., R.J. Myung, G. Wernovsky, et al., Surgical reinterventions following the Fontan procedure. *Eur. J. Cardiothorac. Surg.*, 2003;**24**(2): 255–259.
183. Agnoletti, G., A. Borghi, G. Vignati, and G.C. Crupi, Fontan conversion to total cavopulmonary connection and arrhythmia ablation: clinical and functional results. *Heart*, 2003;**89**(2): 193–198.
184. Mavroudis, C., C.L. Backer, B.J. Deal, C. Johnsrude, and J. Strasburger, Total cavopulmonary conversion and maze procedure for patients with failure of the Fontan operation, *J. Thorac. Cardiovasc. Surg.*, 2001;**122**(5): 863–871.
185. Mavroudis, C., B.J. Deal, and C.L. Backer, The beneficial effects of total cavopulmonary conversion and arrhythmia surgery for the failed Fontan. *Semin. Thorac. Cardiovasc. Surg. Pediatr. Card. Surg. Annu.*, 2002;**5**: 12–24.
186. Nurnberg, J.H., S. Ovroutski, V. Alexi-Meskishvili, P. Ewert, R. Hetzer, and P.E. Lange, New onset arrhythmias after the extracardiac conduit Fontan operation compared with the intraatrial lateral tunnel procedure: early and midterm results. *Ann. Thorac. Surg.*, 2004;**78**(6): 1979–1988.
187. Kumar, S.P., C.S. Rubinstein, J.M. Simsic, A.B. Taylor, J.P. Saul, and S.M. Bradley, Lateral tunnel versus extracardiac conduit Fontan procedure: a concurrent comparison. *Ann. Thorac. Surg.*, 2003;**76**(5): 1389–1396.
188. Cohen, M.I., G. Wernovsky, V.L. Vetter, et al., Sinus node function after a systematically staged Fontan procedure. *Circulation*, 1998;**98**(Suppl. 19): II352–II358.
189. Manning, P.B., J.E. Mayer Jr., G. Wernovsky, S.B. Fishberger, and E.P. Walsh, Staged operation to Fontan increases the incidence of sinoatrial node dysfunction. *J. Thorac. Cardiovasc. Surg.*, 1996;**111**(4): 833–839.
190. Chan, D.P., D.A. Bartmus, W.D. Edwards, and C.B. Porter, Histopathologic abnormalities of the sinus node compared with electrocardiographic evidence of sinus node dysfunction after the modified Fontan operation: an autopsy study of 14 cases. *Tex. Heart Inst. J.*, 1992;**19**(4): 278–283.
191. Davachi, F., R.V. Lucas Jr., and J.H. Moller, The electrocardiogram and vectorcardiogram in tricuspid atresia. Correlation with pathologic anatomy. *Am. J. Cardiol.*, 1970;**25**(1): 18–27.
192. Gamboa, R., W.M. Gersony, and A.S. Nadas, The electrocardiogram in tricuspid atresia and pulmonary atresia with intact ventricular septum. *Circulation*, 1966;**34**(1): 24–37.
193. Neill, C.A. and A.J. Brink, Left axis deviation in tricuspid atresia and single ventricle; the electrocardiogram in 36 autopsied cases. *Circulation*, 1955;**12**(4): 612–619.
194. Kroop, I.G. and A. Grishman, The variability of the electrocardiogram in congenital tricuspid atresia. *J. Pediatr.*, 1950;**37**(2): 231–237.
195. Davachi, F. and J.H. Moller, The electrocardiogram and vectorcardiogram in single ventricle. Anatomic correlations. *Am. J. Cardiol.*, 1969;**23**(1): 19–31.
196. Shaher, R.M., The electrocardiogram in single ventricle. *Br. Heart J.*, 1963;**25**: 465–473.
197. Elliott, L.P., H.D. Ruttenberg, R.S. Eliot, and R.C. Anderson, Vectorial analysis of the electrocardiogram in common ventricle. *Br. Heart J.*, 1964;**26**: 302–311.
198. Shinebourne, E.A., K.C. Lau, G. Calcaterra, and R.H. Anderson, Univentricular heart of right ventricular type: clinical, angiographic and electocardiographic features. *Am. J. Cardiol.*, 1980;**46**(3): 439–445.
199. Momma, K. and L.M. Linde, Cardiac rhythms in dextrocardia. *Am. J. Cardiol.*, 1970;**25**(4): 420–427.
200. Campbell, M. and D.C. Deuchar, Dextrocardia and isolated laevocardia. II. Situs inversus and isolated dextrocardia. *Br. Heart J.*, 1966;**28**(4): 472–487.
201. Mirowski, M., C.A. Neill, H.T. Bahnson, and H.B. Taussig, Negative P waves in lead I in dextroversion: differential diagnosis from mirror-image dextrocardia, with a report of a successful

closure of a ventricular septal defect in a patient with dextroversion associated with agenesis of the right lung. *Circulation*, 1962;**26**: 413–420.
202. Campbell, M. and G. Reynolds, The significance of the direction of the P wave in dextrocardia and isolated laevocardia. *Br. Heart J.*, 1952;**14**(4): 481–488.
203. Click, R., D. Holmes, R. Vlietstra, A. Kosinski, and R. Kronmal, Anomalous coronary arteries: location, degree of atherosclerosis and effect on survival-a report from the Coranary Artery Surgery Study. *J. Am. Coll. Cardiol.*, 1989;**13**(3): 531–537.
204. Haravon, A., M. Franklin, and M.J. Krauthamer, Congenital coronary artery to left ventricle fistula with angina pectoris. Coronary steal syndrome? *N. Y. State. J. Med.*, 1972;**72**(17): 2196–2200.
205. Moro-Serrano, C., J. Martinez, A.H. Madrid, et al., Ventricular tachycardia in a patient with congenital coronary arteriovenous fistula. *Am. Heart J.*, 1992;**124**(2): 503–505.
206. McNamara, J.J. and R.E. Gross, Congenital coronary artery fistula. *Surgery*, 1969;**65**(1): 59–69.
207. Wilson, C., P. Dlabal, R. Holeyfield, C. Akins, and D. Knauf, Anomalous origin of left coronary artery from pulmonary artery: case reports and review of literature concerning teenagers and adults. *J. Thorac. Cardiovasc. Surg.*, 1977;**73**(6): 887–893.
208. Perry, L.W. and L.P. Scott, Anomalous left coronary artery from pulmonary artery: report of 11 cases; review of indications for and results of surgery. *Circulation*, 1970;**41**(6): 1043–1052.
209. Flaherty, J.T., M.S. Spach, J.P. Boineau, R.V. Canent, Jr., R.C. Barr, and D.C. Sabiston Jr., Cardiac potentials on body surface of infants with anomalous left coronary artery (myocardial infarction). *Circulation*, 1967;**36**(3): 345–358.
210. Vanderhauwaert, L.G., G.L. Stalpaert, and L. Verhaeghe, Anomalous origin of the left coronary artery from the pulmonary artery; a therapeutic problem. *Am. Heart. J.*, 1965;**69**: 538–543.
211. Burch, G.E. and Depasquale N.P., The anomalous left coronary artery: an experiment of nature. *Am. J. Med.*, 1964;**37**: 159–161.
212. Rudolph, A.M., N.L. Gootman, N. Kaplan, and M. Rohman, Anomalous left coronary artery arising from the pulmonary artery with large left-to-right shunt in infancy. *J. Pediatr.*, 1963;**63**: 543–549.
213. Cumming, G.R. and C.C. Ferguson, Anomalous origin of the left coronary artery from the pulmonary artery, functioning as a coronary arteriovenous fistula. *Am. Heart J.*, 1962;**64**: 690–695.
214. Keith, J.D., The anomalous origin of the left coronary artery from the pulmonary artery. *Br. Heart J.*, 1959;**21**(2): 149–161.

Index

Note: The page numbers that appear in bold type indicates a substantive discussion of the topic.

C

D

I

J

K

L

M

Q

R

S

U

V

W

The manufacturer's authorised representative in the EU is Springer Nature Customer Service Centre GmbH, Europaplatz 3, 69115 Heidelberg, Germany. If you have any concerns regarding our products, please contact ProductSafety@springernature.com

Printed and bound by CPI Group (UK) Ltd, Croydon, CR0 4YY
13/10/2026
02232694-0003